DENDRITIC CELLS
Biology and Clinical Applications

Cover illustration: *In vitro*-derived chimpanzee dendritic cells localize in the lymph node paracortex after subcutaneous injection. Endogenous interdigitating dendritic cells fluoresce green with an antibody to MHC class II; injected dendritic cells appear orange due to double-labelling with antibody and a red plasma membrane dye added prior to injection. For further details see Chapter 31. Courtesy of the Center for Biologic Imaging, University of Pittsburgh, USA.

DENDRITIC CELLS
Biology and Clinical Applications

Edited by

Michael T. Lotze
Departments of Surgery and Molecular Genetics and Biochemistry
University of Pittsburgh Cancer Institute
USA

Angus W. Thomson
Departments of Surgery and Molecular Genetics and Biochemistry
Thomas E. Starzl Transplantation Institute
University of Pittsburgh
USA

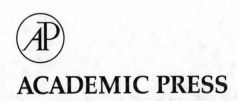

A Harcourt Science and Technology Company

San Diego San Francisco New York Boston London Sydney Tokyo

This book is printed on acid-free paper.

Academic Press
A Harcourt Science and Technology Company
32 Jamestown Road, London NW1 7BY, UK
http://www.academicpress.com

Academic Press
A Harcourt Science and Technology Company
525 B Street, Suite 1900, San Diego, California 92101-4495, USA
http://www.academicpress.com

ISBN 0-12-455860-7

Library of Congress Card Number: 98-86759

A catalogue record for this book is available from the British Library

Printed in Great Britain by Bookcraft (Bath) Ltd, Midsomer Norton, Somerset. UK

00 01 02 03 04 RB 8 7 6 5 4 3 2

Contents

Contributors

Sebastian Amigorena CJF 95-01 INSERM, Institut Curie, 12 rue Lhomond, 75006 Paris, France

Jonathan M. Austyn Nuffield Department of Surgery, University of Oxford, John Radcliffe Hospital, Headington, Oxford OX3 9DC, UK

David Avigan Department of Medicine, Beth Israel-Deaconess Medical Center, Harvard Medical School, Boston, MA 02115, USA

Jacques Banchereau Department of Immunology, Baylor Research Institute, 2nd Floor Hobitzelle, 3500 Gaston Avenue, Dallas, TX 75246, USA

Simon M. Barratt-Boyes Department of Infectious Diseases and Microbiology, University of Pittsburgh, Pittsburgh, PA 15261, USA

Armin Bender Department of Dermatology, University of Erlangen, Hartmannstrasse 14, D-91054 Erlangen, Germany

Francine Brière Schering-Plough, Laboratory for Immunological Research, 27 Chemin des Peupliers, BP 11, 69571 Dardilly, France

Christophe Caux Schering-Plough, Laboratory for Immunological Research, 27 Chemin des Peupliers, BP 11, 69571 Dardilly, France

Marina Cella Basel Institute for Immunology, Grenzacherstrasse 487, CH-4005 Basel, Switzerland

Benedict J. Chambers Microbiology and Tumor Biology Center, Karolinska Institute, S-171 77 Stockholm, Sweden

S. Citterio CNR, Centre of Cellular and Molecular Pharmacology, Via Vanvitelli 32, I-20129 Milan, Italy

Georgina J. Clark Mater Medical Research Institute, Mater Misericordiae Hospitals, South Brisbane, Queensland 4101, Australia

Mary T. Crowley Department of Immunology IMM-25, The Scripps Research Institute, 10550 North Torrey Pines Road, La Jolla, CA 92037, USA

Marie Cumberbatch Zeneca Central Toxicology Laboratory, Alderley Park, Macclesfield, Cheshire SK10 4TJ, UK

Rebecca J. Dearman Zeneca Central Toxicology Laboratory, Alderley Park, Macclesfield, Cheshire SK10 4TJ, UK

F.G.A. Delemarre Department of Immunology, Faculty of Medicine, Erasmus University of Rotterdam, PO Box 1738, Rotterdam, The Netherlands

Elena Delgado Laboratory of Cellular Physiology and Immunology, The Rockefeller University, 1230 York Avenue, New York, NY 10021-6399, USA

A.J. Demetris Department of Pathology, Division of Transplantation, University of Pittsburgh Medical Center, 15th Floor, Biomedical Science Tower, 200 Lothrop Street, Pittsburgh, PA 15213, USA

H.A. Drexhage Department of Immunology, Faculty of Medicine, Erasmus University of Rotterdam, PO Box 1738, Rotterdam, The Netherlands

Bertrand Dubois Schering-Plough, Laboratory for Immunological Research, 27 Chemin des Peupliers, BP 11, 69571 Dardilly, France

Anneke Engering Basel Institute for Immunology, Grenzacherstrasse 487, CH-4005 Basel, Switzerland

Clemens Esche Biological Therapeutics Program, University of Pittsburgh Cancer Institute, Pittsburgh, PA 15213, USA

Louis D. Falo, Jr. Department of Dermatology, University of Pittsburgh, Pittsburgh, PA 15261, USA

Hassan Farhood Biological Therapeutics Program, University of Pittsburgh Cancer Institute, 15th Floor, Biomedical Science Tower, 200 Lothrop Street, Pittsburgh, PA 15213, USA

U. Fascio Department of Biology, University of Milan, Milan, Italy

Jérôme Fayette Schering-Plough, Laboratory for Immunological Research, 27 Chemin des Peupliers, BP 11, 69571 Dardilly, France

J.V. Forrester Department of Ophthalmology, University of Aberdeen Medical School, Foresterhill, Aberdeen AB25 2ZD, UK

M. Foti CNR, Centre of Cellular and Molecular Pharmacology, Via Vanvitelli 32, I-20129 Milan, Italy

Sarah Frankel Division of Retrovirology, and Division of AIDS and Emerging Infectious Disease Pathology, Walter Reed Army Institute of Research, Rockville, MD, USA

J.J. Fung Division of Transplantation, Department of Surgery, University of Pittsburgh Medical Center, 15th Floor, Biomedical Science Tower, 200 Lothrop Street, Pittsburgh, PA 15213, USA

Anne Galy Karmanos Cancer Institute, Wayne State University, 110 East Warren Avenue, Detroit, MI 48201, USA

Wendy S. Garrett Department of Cell Biology and Section of Immunobiology, Yale University School of Medicine, New Haven, CT 06520, USA

Katia Georgopoulos Cutaneous Biology Research Center, Harvard Medical School, Massachusetts General Hospital, Charlestown, MA, USA

Giampiero Girolomoni Laboratory of Immunology, Istituto Dermopatico dell'Immacolata, IRCCS, Via Monti di Creta 104, I-00167 Rome, Italy

Jianlin Gong Division of Cancer Pharmacology, Dana-Farber Cancer Institute, Harvard Medical School, 44 Binney Street, Cambridge, MA 02115, USA

Angela Granelli-Piperno Laboratory of Cellular Physiology and Immunology, The Rockefeller University, 1230 York Avenue, New York, NY 10021-6399, USA

F. Granucci CNR, Centre of Cellular and Molecular Pharmacology, Via Vanvitelli 32, I-20129 Milan, Italy

Stephen T. Haley Department of Anatomy, Division of Immunobiology, Medical College of Virginia, Virginia Commonwealth University, Richmond, VA 23298-0678, USA

Derek N.J. Hart Mater Medical Research Institute, Mater Misericordiae Hospitals, South Brisbane, Queensland 4101, Australia

J.A. Hartley University Medicine, Southampton General Hospital, Tremona Road, Southampton SO16 6YD, UK

Christine Heufler Department of Dermatology, University of Innsbruck, Anichstrasse 35, A-6020 Innsbruck, Austria

S.T. Holgate University Medicine, Southampton General Hospital, Tremona Road, Southampton SO16 6YD, UK

P.G. Holt Division of Cell Biology, TVW Telethon Institute for Child Health Research, PO Box 855, West Perth, WA 6872, Australia

Giandomenica Iezzi Basel Institute for Immunology, Grenzacherstrasse 487, CH-4005 Basel, Switzerland

Ralf Ignatius Laboratory of Cellular Physiology and Immunology, The Rockefeller University, 1230 York Avenue, New York, NY 10021-6399, USA

Kayo Inaba Laboratory of Immunology, Department of Zoology, Kyoto University, Kitashirakawa-Oiwake-cho, Sakyo-ku, Kyoto 606-01, Japan

Ronald Jaffe Department of Pathology, University of Pittsburgh Children's Hospital, 15th Floor, Biomedical Science Tower, 200 Lothrop Street, Pittsburgh, PA 15213, USA

Eckhart Kämpgen Department of Dermatology, University of Würzburg, Würzburg, Germany.

Zoher Kapasi Department of Rehabilitative Medicine, Division of Physical Therapy, Emory University School of Medicine, Atlanta, GA 30322, USA

Samia J. Khoury Center for Neurologic Diseases, Brigham and Women's Hospital, Harvard Medical School, Boston, MA, USA

Ian Kimber Zeneca Central Toxicology Laboratory, Alderley Park, Macclesfield, Cheshire SK10 4TJ, UK

Stella C. Knight Antigen Presentation Research Group, Imperial College School of Medicine at Northwick Park Institute for Medical Research, Harrow, Middlesex HA1 3UJ, UK

Franz Koch Department of Dermatology, University of Innsbruck, Anichstrasse 35, A-6020 Innsbruck, Austria

Donald Kufe Division of Cancer Pharmacology, Dana-Farber Cancer Institute, Harvard Medical School, 44 Binney Street, Boston, MA 02115, USA

Antonio Lanzavecchia Basel Institute for Immunology, Grenzacherstrasse 487, CH-4005 Basel, Switzerland

Adriana Larregina Molecular Medicine Unit, Department of Medicine, Stopford Building, University of Manchester, Oxford Road, Manchester M13 9PT, UK

Serge Lebecque Schering-Plough, Laboratory for Immunological Research, 27 Chemin des Peupliers, BP 11, 69571 Dardilly, France

P.J.M. Leenen Department of Immunology, Faculty of Medicine, Erasmus University of Rotterdam, PO Box 1738, Rotterdam, The Netherlands

LiMing Liu Center for Neurologic Diseases, Brigham and Women's Hospital, Harvard Medical School, 221 Longwood Avenue, Boston, MA 02115, USA

Yong-Jun Liu DNA Research Institute, Palo Alto, CA 94304, USA

Hans-Gustaf Ljunggren Microbiology and Tumor Biology Center, Karolinska Institute, S-171 77 Stockholm, Sweden

David Lo Department of Immunology IMM-25, The Scripps Research Institute, 10550 North Torrey Pines Road, La Jolla, CA 92037, USA

Anna Lokshin Biological Therapeutics Program, University of Pittsburgh Cancer Institute, Pittsburgh, PA 15213, USA

Michael T. Lotze Division of Surgical Oncology and Biological Therapeutics, Department of Surgery, University of Pittsburgh Cancer Institute, 15th Floor, Biomedical Science Tower, 200 Lothrop Street, Pittsburgh, PA 15213, USA

Anne Lozier Unit of Transdepartmental Immunotherapy, Institut Gustave-Roussy, 39 rue Camille Desmouline, 94805 Villejuif Cedex, France

Lina Lu Division of Transplant Surgery, Department of Surgery, University of Pittsburgh Medical Center, 15th Floor, Biomedical Science Tower, 200 Lothrop Street, Pittsburgh, PA 15213, USA

Manfred Lutz Department of Dermatology, University of Erlangen, Hartmannstrasse 14, D-91054 Erlangen, Germany

P.G. McMenamin Department of Anatomy and Human Biology, University of Western Australia, Nedlands, WA 6907, Australia

G. Gordon MacPherson Sir William Dunn School of Pathology, University of Oxford, South Parks Road, Oxford OX1 3RE, UK

A.S. McWilliam Division of Cell Biology, TVW Telethon Institute for Child Health Research, PO Box 855, West Perth, WA 6872, Australia

Eugene Maraskovsky Department of Immunobiology, Immunex Corporation, 51 University Street, Seattle, WA 98101, USA

M. Martino CNR, Centre of Cellular and Molecular Pharmacology, Via Vanvitelli 32, I-20129 Milan, Italy

M.K. Matyszak CNR, Centre of Cellular and Molecular Pharmacology, Via Vanvitelli 32, I-20129 Milan, Italy

Dieter Maurer Department of Dermatology, University of Vienna Medical School, Waehringer Guertel 18–20, A-1090 Vienna, Austria

Ira Mellman Department of Cell Biology and Section of Immunobiology, Yale University School of Medicine, New Haven, CT 06520, USA

Adrian Morelli Molecular Medicine Unit, Department of Medicine, Stopford Building, University of Manchester, Oxford Road, Manchester M13 9PT, UK

N. Murase Division of Transplantation, Department of Surgery, University of Pittsburgh Medical Center, 15th Floor, Biomedical Science Tower, 200 Lothrop Street, Pittsburgh, PA 15213, USA

Yasuhiko Nishioka Department of Surgery, University of Pittsburgh Medical Center, 15th Floor, Biomedical Science Tower, 200 Lothrop Street, Pittsburgh, PA 15213, USA

Michio Ogawa Department of Surgery II, Kumamoto University Medical School, 1-1 Honjo, Kumamoto 860, Japan

Jean Pieters Basel Institute for Immunology, Grenzacherstrasse 487, CH-4005 Basel, Switzerland

Melissa Pope Laboratory of Cellular Physiology and Immunology, The Rockefeller University, 1230 York Avenue, New York, NY 10021-6399, USA

Bali Pulendran Department of Immunobiology, Immunex Corporation, 51 University Street, Seattle, WA 98101, USA

Dahui Qin Departments of Microbiology and Immunology, Division of Immunobiology, Medical College of Virginia, Virginia Commonwealth University, Richmond, VA 23298-0678, USA

Paul Racz Department of Pathology and Körber Laboratory for AIDS Research, Bernhard-Nocht-Institute for Tropical Medicine, Hamburg, Germany

K. Radosevic Department of Immunology, Faculty of Medicine, Erasmus University of Rotterdam, PO Box 1738, Rotterdam, The Netherlands

Graça Raposo UMR144 CNRS, Institut Curie, 12 rue Lhomond, 75006 Paris, France

Armelle Regnault CJF 95-01 INSERM, Institut Curie, 12 rue Lhomond, 75006 Paris, France

I.G. Reischl University Medicine, Southampton General Hospital, Tremona Road, Southampton SO16 6YD, UK

Maria Rescigno CNR, Centre of Cellular and Molecular Pharmacology, Via Vanvitelli 32, I-20129 Milan, Italy

Paola Ricciardi-Castagnoli CNR, Centre of Cellular and Molecular Pharmacology, Via Vanvitelli 32, I-20129 Milan, Italy

M. Rittig Department of Anatomy, University of Erlangen, Krankenhausstrasse 9, D-91054 Erlangen, Germany

Claudia Röder Department of Dermatology, University of Erlangen, Hartmannstrasse 14, D-91054 Erlangen, Germany

Nikolaus Romani Department of Dermatology, University of Innsbruck, Anichstrasse 35, A-6020 Innsbruck, Austria

P. Rovere HSR, Department of Internal Medicine, University of Milan, Italy

Mariolina Salio Basel Institute for Immunology, Grenzacherstrasse 487, CH-4005 Basel, Switzerland

Federica Sallusto Basel Institute for Immunology, Grenzacherstrasse 487, CH-4005 Basel, Switzerland

Mohamed H. Sayegh Laboratory of Immunogenetics and Transplantation, Brigham and Women's Hospital, Harvard Medical School, Boston, MA, USA

Doris Scheidegger Basel Institute for Immunology, Grenzacherstrasse 487, CH-4005 Basel, Switzerland

Gerold Schuler Department of Dermatology, University of Erlangen, Hartmannstrasse 14, D-91054 Erlangen, Germany

A.E. Semper University Medicine, Southampton General Hospital, Tremona Road, Southampton SO16 6YD, UK

Ken Shortman PO Royal Melbourne Hospital, The Walter and Eliza Hall Institute of Medical Research, Melbourne, Victoria 3050, Australia

Michael R. Shurin University of Pittsburgh Cancer Institute, Division of Surgical Oncology and Biological Therapeutics, 3471 Fifth Avenue, 300 Kaufmann Building, Pittsburgh, PA 15213, USA

T.E. Starzl Department of Surgery, Division of Transplantation, University of Pittsburgh Medical Center, 15th Floor, Biomedical Science Tower, 200 Lothrop Street, Pittsburgh, PA 15213, USA

Ralph M. Steinman Laboratory of Cellular Physiology and Immunology, The Rockefeller University, 1230 York Avenue, New York, NY 10021-6399, USA

Raymond J. Steptoe Thomas E. Starzl Transplantation Institute, University of Pittsburgh Medical Center, 15th Floor, Biomedical Science Tower, 200 Lothrop Street, Pittsburgh, PA 15213, USA

Georg Stingl Department of Dermatology, University of Vienna Medical School, Waehringer Guertel 18–20, A-1090 Vienna, Austria

Walter J. Storkus University of Pittsburgh Medical Center, 15th Floor, Biomedical Science Tower, 200 Lothrop Street, Pittsburgh, PA 15213, USA

P.A. Stumbles Division of Cell Biology, TVW Telethon Institute for Child Health Research, PO Box 855, West Perth, WA 6872, Australia

Andras K. Szakal Department of Anatomy, Division of Immunobiology, Medical College of Virginia, Virginia Commonwealth University, Richmond, VA 23298-0678, USA

Klara Tenner-Racz Department of Pathology and Körber Laboratory for AIDS Research, Bernhard-Nocht-Institute for Tropical Medicine, Hamburg, Germany

John G. Tew Departments of Microbiology and Immunology, Division of Immunobiology, Medical College of Virginia, Virginia Commonwealth University, Richmond, VA 23298-0678, USA

Angus W. Thomson Department of Surgery and Thomas E. Starzl Transplantation Institute, University of Pittsburgh Medical Center, 15th Floor, Biomedical Science Tower, 200 Lothrop Street, Pittsburgh, PA 15213, USA

Beatrice Thurner Department of Dermatology, University of Erlangen, Hartmannstrasse 14, D-91054 Erlangen, Germany

Shannon J. Turley Department of Cell Biology, Yale University School of Medicine, New Haven, CT 06520, USA

Thomas Tüting Department of Dermatology, J. Gutenberg-University, Langenbeckstrasse 1, D-55131 Mainz, Germany

Stéphane Vandenabeele Schering-Plough, Laboratory for Immunological Research, 27 Chemin des Peupliers, BP 11, 69571 Dardilly, France

Antonella Viola Basel Institute for Immunology, Grenzacherstrasse 487, CH-4005 Basel, Switzerland

Cara C. Wilson University of Pittsburgh Medical Center, 15th Floor, Biomedical Science Tower, 200 Lothrop Street, Pittsburgh, PA 15213, USA

Jiuhua Wu Departments of Microbiology and Immunology, Division of Immunobiology, Medical College of Virginia, Virginia Commonwealth University, Richmond, VA 23298-0678, USA

Li Wu PO Royal Melbourne Hospital, The Walter and Eliza Hall Institute of Medical Research, Melbourne, Victoria 3050, Australia

Yasuo Yamaguchi Department of Surgery II, Kumamoto University Medical School, 1-1 Honjo, Kumamoto 860, Japan

James W. Young Division of Hematologic Oncology, Department of Medicine, Memorial Sloan-Kettering Cancer Center, 1275 York Avenue, New York, NY 10021, USA

Laurence Zitvogel Unit of Transdepartmental Immunotherapy, Institut Gustave-Roussy, 39 rue Camille Desmouline, 94805 Villejuif Cedex, France

Preface

> Fighting in the forefront of the Greeks, the Athenians crushed at Marathon the might of the gold bearing Medes.
>
> Simonides, c. 556–468 B.C.

This volume represents a special effort to bring together in one place the information that would allow a scientifically oriented clinician, or even nonimmunologically oriented scientist, to appreciate the important role of this previously obscure cell. The notion of having an entire book dedicated to a single cell, albeit one as important as the dendritic cell (DC), is one which could be met with disapprobation in some quarters. It does, however, reflect the importance which the authors (who completed their task admirably) and the editors have placed on the extraordinarily important role this cell has in dictating the initiation and persistence of the adaptive immune response. Indeed, all aspects of the 'fight' during the acute natural immune response but in particular the chronic inflammatory immune response associated with cancer, chronic infectious diseases, autoimmunity, and transplantation are importantly related to DC biology. While the first report of DC by Ralph Steinman and Zanvil Cohn, 25 years ago, posited an important role for this cell in immune regulation, this volume's role is not solely celebratory (but it does have those elements!).

It has thus been appreciated for the last 25 years that DC are specialized antigen-presenting cells (APC) with a unique ability to prime effective immune responses. This may give them a special importance in several human disease states known to have an immunological basis. While great strides were made in the understanding of the role of specific T cells and antibodies in mediating allergy, autoimmunity, graft rejection, infectious disease, and tumor immunity over this period, it was also clear that these effector cells and molecules represented the end stage of an immune response, the outcome of which was probably determined at its very initiation by the type of APC, the nature and state of the antigen, and the cytokine conditions under which the antigen was first presented. As is usually the case in science, testing of ideas must await development of new techniques and reagents. Several opportunities presented themselves in the 1970s with the discovery and cloning of the first few cytokines, especially interferon-α and IL-2. This allowed for the first time use of immunologically important molecules themselves as means to manipulate immune responses or to support the growth and expansion of T cells and NK cells *in vitro*. This in turn led to the identification and characterization of the T cell receptor for antigen and examination of disease-specific T cell responses. T cells that mediate graft rejection, T cells specific for tumor antigens, and T cells specific for autoantigens were studied for their biology and function, as well as being used as reagents to fully define disease-specific antigens and the genes that encode them. The important role of cytokines, as well as the number of identifiable cytokines, continued to rise throughout that same period, now with possibly as many as 20–21 so-called 'interleukins' in addition to the colony-stimulating factors and interferons. Their pivotal role in directing the immune response was unveiled. An important outcome from this work has been the understanding of the polarity of the immune response at the T cell level, T_H1 vs T_H2 and Tc1 vs Tc2. The helper T cell response that develops as predominately T_H1 type (in the presence of and producing T_H1-type cytokines, IL-2, IFN-γ, GM-CSF) supports the development of cytotoxic T cells (CTL), often of the Tc1 type. Alternatively, the T_H2-type response (developed in the presence of and producing the T_H2-type cytokines, IL-4, IL-10) supports the development of humoral immunity and Tc2-type CTL. In systems where this can be tested *in vivo*, this dichotomy translates into a life or death, or disease or no disease situation. During this same period, understanding of immunoglobulin gene rearrangements and the advent of monoclonal antibody technology truly revolutionized all of the biological sciences, perhaps one of the greatest gifts that immunologists have yet bestowed on their nonimmunological colleagues.

So how is this complex adaptive system initiated and maintained? We now believe that the DC plays an important role in initiating and maintaining immune reactivity. The sequential steps in the choreography from its birth in the bone marrow, maturation there or in the thymus or secondary lymphatic tissues, traversion of the initial endothelial barriers into virtually all tissues, sensitivity to inflammatory initiators and tissue damage, injury or 'danger', and transformation into a 'mature cell' capable of migrating across the lymphatic or postcapillary venules to enter secondary lymphoid sites, interacting with the resident T cells and B cells to rapidly screen and select immunological suitors make it one of the most versatile of dance partners. Not only does it have the potential to come into contact with all cells in all tissues, its athletic potential as the 'track star of immunology' makes it a marathon contender of the first order. And, just like the marathon runner who crossed the Plains of Marathon, after delivering its message in the lymph node or spleen, this cell dies, to be born again, Athena-like, in the bone marrow every day.

The last five years have been particularly dizzying with application of cytokines now to the culture and maintenance of DC. Just as the advances in T cell and B cell biology required means to grow and maintain these cells, the use of GM-CSF and IL-4 or TNF has made their study and application in preclinical and clinical disease models feasible. Prior studies, restricted by the relatively limiting numbers of these cells from any one site in tissue or blood, have now been extended by extraordinary new knowledge available from advances in these relatively simple and straightforward culture techniques. This new knowledge has emphasized the importance of the very early events in the priming of the immune response and turned full attention to the DC. As we prepare these comments, some of the important issues in DC migration and recruitment via specialized chemokines including MIP-3 and and their receptors CCR6 and CCR7, as well as the preferred source of antigenic material for DC (apoptotic cells and bodies) are just coming to light. These and other recent insights will require some time to become integrated into the growing corpus of information and raise important additional questions about these centrally important cells. This volume celebrates them and, when it enters the second edition, hopefully many of the issues raised here will have been successfully addressed and new ones raised.

We appreciate the careful assistance of our publishers from Academic Press, Tessa Picknett, Duncan Fatz, Lilian Leung and Emma White for their belief in the importance of this project, their patience, and persistence. To our families and in particular to

Joan and Robyn, our spouses, acknowledgment for their gifts of time and support. To our students and colleagues who make the intellectual challenges and the great social role of science a pleasure and vocation, our gratitude and hopes for the future.

Michael T. Lotze
Angus W. Thomson

REFERENCE

Steinman, R.M. and Cohn, Z.A. (1973). Identification of a novel cell type in peripheral lymphoid organs of mice. I. Morphology, quantitation, tissue distribution. *J. Exp. Med.* **137** (5), 1142–1162.

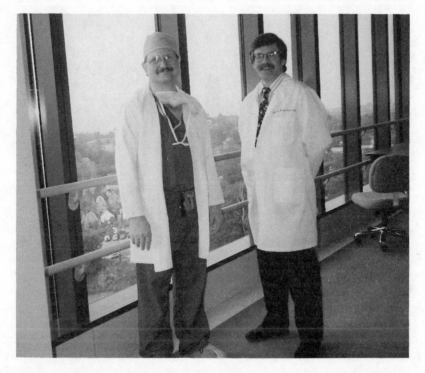

Drs Lotze (left) and Thomson (right) pictured in the Biomedical Science Tower of the University of Pittsburgh Medical Center.

Introduction

Ralph M. Steinman

Laboratory of Cellular Physiology and Immunology, Rockefeller University, New York, USA

Jacques Banchereau

Baylor Institute for Immunology Research, Dallas, Texas, USA

Congratulations to Drs Lotze and Thomson for pulling together an extensive series of articles on dendritic cell biology, as of 1999. It seems to be more difficult for scientists to find time to write these chapters. We are all too busy contributing to and keeping up with our fields, and with biomedicine on a broader scale. Everything moves so quickly, so we worry that our writing will soon be outdated. Yet books still have their place. They provide an historical record, as nothing else can, that quickly relates the state of thinking at a particular time. For the reader, either newcomer or oldtimer, books remain an effective way to keep in touch with a broad array of topics. Here we introduce some of the established and emerging themes that are considered in this volume.

ESTABLISHED THEMES

Dendritic Cells as Nature's Adjuvant

Some of the common themes of the book have motivated scientists for a long time to study dendritic cells (DC). These themes relate to their capacity to stimulate T cell-dependent immunity. One is the potency of DC. This is manifest in the small numbers of DC and low levels of antigen that are used to stimulate immunity, and the strength of the ensuing lymphocyte response. Other recurring themes are the abilities of DC to stimulate primary or quiescent lymphocytes, and to do so *in vivo*, in animals and patients. However, the chapters also deal with newer targets for the adjuvant effects of DC, such as their stimulatory effects on B cells and possible roles in T cell tolerance rather than immunity.

Improved Methods for Dendritic Cell Isolation and Identification

The wave of advances and activity in DC biology in large part reflects the easier access to these cells. This is the result of methods that generate large numbers of DC from either proliferating progenitors or, in the case of human blood monocytes, nonproliferating

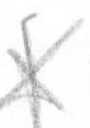

Table 1. Developmental stages of dendritic cells

- Precursor DC (DC_{pre}), patrolling through blood and lymphoid organs
- Immature DC (DC_{imm}) residing within virtually every tissue in ambush to capture any pathogen that passes by
- Mature DC (DC_{mat}) usually residing within lymphoid organs and responsible for T cell stimulation and perhaps tolerance.

precursors. The criteria for identifying the mature immunostimulatory form of DC, both in cytokine-driven culture and from primary tissues, are proving to be consistent in many laboratories and many settings. The cells are large, dendritic or very irregular in shape, motile, nonadherent, poorly phagocytic or nonphagocytic for many particulates, rich in MHC products and costimulators (like CD40, CD54, CD86), lacking in key differentiation markers of other lineages (like CD3, 14, 16, 19/20), and, when tested as inducers of T cell immunity, unusually potent. New markers are becoming available, particularly in the human system: e.g., the CD83 immunoglobulin superfamily member.

Defining Dendritic Cells

As just mentioned, mature DC have common and distinctive features regardless of the species or tissue or method that is used. However, there is complexity at several other levels. DC can take up, process and, following maturation, present antigen. Yet the DC that take up antigen characteristically lack cardinal features of mature DC, such as the very irregular cell shape and very high levels of surface MHC products, the CD86 costimulator, and the CD83 marker. DC select and eventually stimulate antigen-specific naive T cells, but there are also situations where DC can stimulate B cells and can delete or anergize T cells. These differences currently are thought to reflect the function of distinct subsets of DC, but the origin of these subsets and the molecular basis for these new functions need to be unraveled. DC are of hematopoietic origin, but there are some different phenotypes and developmental pathways that may reflect separate lineages (distinct progenitors) or the effects of distinct cytokines and stromal cells. Currently there is evidence for three pathways: one that gives rise to typical Langerhans cells with Birbeck granules and E-cadherin; a second that shares more features with monocytes like CD14 during development; and a third lymphoid subset that lacks the myeloid marker CD11b and, during development, CD11c, but can express (in mice only) the T cell marker CD8. Nonetheless, it is still evident that DC encompass three stages of development, for which we suggest the terms precursors, immature, and mature (Table 1).

EMERGING THEMES

The current text, instead of emphasizing the past, reports on a number of newer areas that certainly will be rapidly outdated because the topics are attracting a lot of attention.

Molecular Genetic Approaches to Dendritic Cells

Laboratories are screening ESTs and cDNAs from DC, looking for genes that are expressed either uniquely or relatively selectively. The products are starting to come in: chemokines and chemokine receptors, proteases and antiproteases, new members of the killer inhibitory receptor family with ITIM motifs, new members of the TNF-receptor family, and lectin-like receptors for antigen uptake. More new molecules will come, hopefully to include molecules that will approach several gaps: to selectively identify immature and mature DC, especially in tissues *in vivo*, to help explain DC development at the signaling and transcriptional levels, and to account for known DC migratory patterns, tissue localization and specific functions.

Cell Biology of Antigen Uptake and Processing

The availability of more abundant populations of DC, particularly the immature stage that is specialized for antigen capture, is finally making it possible to exploit DC to study mechanisms of antigen presentation. Another methodological breakthrough is looming, i.e., monoclonal antibodies that allow one to directly visualize MHC–peptide complexes. Together these advances are revealing that no cell has such abundant MIIC (MHC class II-rich compartments) as DC, and no cell can express such high levels of MHC–peptide complexes. MHC class I-mediated presentation has not been as intensively studied to date. This will not be for long, given the identification of several new pathways for charging DC MHC class I products including nonreplicating forms of viruses, apoptotic cells, and the products of genes that have been transfected into DC using many different vectors.

Infectious Disease and Vaccines

There are many examples—HIV-1, SIV, measles, and perhaps CMV and KSHV—where DC are not simply antigen-presenting cells for infectious agents but, in addition, represent safe havens for pathogens and conspirators in pathogenesis. The flip side of the coin—targeting the biology of DC to design better vaccines—is underexploited. DC are the cell to target, given their physiological role as controllers of immunity and their known capacities to elicit strong B and T (CD4 and CD8; T_H1/T_H2 and Tc1/Tc2) cell responses, including IL-12 production and protective cytolytic T lymphocytes. Can DC be used in the demanding settings of tumors (see below) or even for new types of vaccines that would induce tolerance towards allergy and autoimmunity? These seem like fantasies right now, but a rationale is being put into place.

Dendritic Cells as Adjuvants for Immunotherapy

Trials are being undertaken in many centers to use DC to induce human immune responses to viral and other tumor antigens. Our feeling is that this field will need time to ripen, i.e., to identify the best sources of DC, to learn to charge them with relevant antigens, to determine doses and routes of administration, to measure the immune responses well, to target the immune T cells to the tumor, and finally to identify settings that result in clinical efficacy. Immunotherapy is challenging at so many biological levels. No one should be content with the lovely data that have already emerged from mice, since there is so much to do in the realm of DC-mediated, clinical immunotherapy as just mentioned.

Two other aspects of tumor immunology are emerging as well. One is learning how DC behave *in situ* in the context of human tumors—are DC in the tumor, are DC functions blocked, can one mobilize DC to present tumor antigens *in vivo* and not simply charge them *ex vivo* with antigens? A second is the realization that DC can exert a killing activity against selected tumors, and that DC express recognition receptors that are shared with natural killer (NK) cells.

Dendritic Cells and B Cell Responses

The prior emphasis on antigen presentation to T cells was well deserved, but now comes the new evidence that B cells may be controlled directly by DC. The first tissue culture experiments record large effects at the levels of cell proliferation, immunoglobulin secretion and immunoglobulin switching with a particular effect on IgA. *In vivo* experiments are likewise being energized, given the need to understand the contributions of DC to the plasma cell reaction (antibody response) and germinal center formation and function.

Multiple Dendritic Cell Developmental Pathways, Possibly Lineages

The evidence for different pathways of DC development will surely help in understanding DC function *in vivo*. First, there is the Langerhans cell pathway that yields, in the presence of GM-CSF and TNF and very quickly from marrow progenitors, DC that express E-cadherin and Birbeck granules including the ill-defined LAG antigen. Is this pathway reserved for the skin and other stratified squamous epithelia, or do other epithelia, as in the airway, have comparable cells? Second, there is the monocyte-related pathway that does not yield typical Langerhans cells in the presence of GM-CSF and TNF, but instead expresses monocyte related markers like high levels of CD68 and CD14 and for relatively long periods in development. This pathway may give rise to the DC that are found in the interstitial spaces of many tissues such as heart, kidney, and lung. Third, there is the enigmatic lymphoid pathway, DC that are thought to be related in lineage to T cells rather than phagocytes. This pathway likely provides DC for the thymic medulla and the T cell areas of lymphoid tissues. So far, these three pathways are delineated more by markers than by functional distinctions, with the exceptions being that the monocyte-related pathway has B cell stimulating properties and the lymphoid pathway is proposed to function in tolerance and regulating immunity.

The cytokines for generating these DC are at the moment complex, perhaps confusing. In marrow cultures, especially mouse marrow, some use IL-4 together with GM-CSF, while some omit IL-4. With human $CD34^+$ cells, TNF is used together with GM-CSF, but some emphasize TGF in addition. With blood monocytes, IL-4 is important for generating immature DC, while TNF and other factors induce maturation. IL-3 is held to be special for the lymphoid pathway, yet recently a progenitor that is responsive to IL-3 and expresses 'myeloid' M-CSF receptors has been reported. Then there are the impressive effects of Flt-3 ligand *in vivo* on DC numbers. In a reciprocal vein, cytokines that inhibit DC development are of new interest, the best candidate now being IL-10.

Another important puzzle relates to the stimuli for DC maturation to the final T cell stimulatory stage of differentiation. DC respond to many TNF family members like TNF, CD40, TRANCE/RANK. Yet why are there so many TNF-like stimuli? Is each TNF receptor on DC associated with a distinct set of biological functions? Is the TNF-receptor pathway the key to understanding DC maturation?

Dendritic Cells in Immunogenicity and Tolerance

Immunogenicity has been the focus of DC research for so long that their potential importance in tolerance surprises many. However, this dual role, as controllers of immunity and tolerance, makes a lot of sense. New information is leading to the conclusion that DC may tolerize the repertoire to self, both centrally in the thymus and peripherally in lymphoid organs. So when antigen enters the immune system, the DC more selectively elicit immune responses to foreign epitopes, since the repertoire has already been tolerized to many self-antigens that the cell could present. Perhaps immunity vs tolerance reflects the key distinction for separate lymphoid vs myeloid pathways for development, although there may be other mechanisms whereby DC function in both T cell stimulation (immunity) and T cell death and anergy (self-tolerance).

Thanks to all the contributors to this volume. In keeping with the new emphasis on both immunity and tolerance, you have portrayed a stimulating period in DC research, and the waiting time for resolving many of the topics in this volume will hopefully be tolerable.

I ORIGIN OF DENDRITIC CELLS

CHAPTER 1
Hematopoietic Cell Fate and the Development of Dendritic Cells

Anne Galy[1], Katia Georgopoulos[2] and Li Wu[3]
[1]Karmanos Cancer Institute, Wayne State University, Detroit, Michigan, USA; [2]Cutaneous Biology Research Center, Harvard Medical School, Massachusetts General Hospital, Charlestown, Massachusetts, USA; [3]The Walter and Eliza Hall Institute of Medical Research, Melbourne, Victoria, Australia

INTRODUCTION

Charles de Gaulle once said about France: 'How can anyone govern a nation that has two hundred and forty-six different kinds of cheese?' Similarly, it is perplexing to define what governs the production of blood cells, which provide functions as diverse as tissue oxygenation, tissue repair, blood clotting and the capacity to sustain immune responses. It is our interest to understand how cells of the immune system are produced and more precisely how the mutually interactive lymphocytes and antigen-presenting dendritic cells (DC) are born. Blood cell diversity is created by genetic and molecular changes that control the differentiation, survival and proliferation of multipotential hematopoietic progenitors and of hematopoietic stem cells (HSC). It is generally thought that the development of HSC into mature cells is a gradual process rather than an abrupt event because discrete steps can be recognized, and different cells can be isolated along that process. In that respect there is a lot of information available on the stages of production of T cells (Godfrey and Zlotnik, 1993) and B cells (Hardy *et al.*, 1991). In these two lineages of cells, the events occurring between the stage of recognizable commitment and the stage of mature effector have been exquisitely defined. Understandably, the definition of specification and recognizable commitment may evolve as we better understand what determines these two putative steps in the cell fate decision determination process. Hematopoietic progenitors exist at precommitment stages with potential to differentiate into more than one lineage. In such cells, genes common to the development of subsequent lineages may be found. We will discuss in this chapter evidence that lymphocytes and DC share common hematopoietic progenitors and utilize similar sets of genes for their development.

Dendritic Cells: Biology and Clinical Applications
ISBN 0-12-455860-7

CELL TYPES UNDERGOING DEVELOPMENTAL DECISION CHECKPOINTS

A large body of work has led to the isolation to relative homogeneity of rare and highly primitive populations of HSC. As a corollary of such studies, nonprimitive hematopoietic progenitors have often been identified and distinguished from HSC or from mature cells based on differences in durability of multilineage engraftment, radioprotective ability, physical properties, membrane markers, metabolic activity, or cell-cycle status. To this effect, variable combinations of the murine markers Sca-1, Sca-2, c-kit, Lin (a cocktail of markers of mature committed granulocytes, erythrocytes, T cells, B cells, monocytes), Thy-1, CD34, and retention of the mitochondrial dye Rhodamine 123 have been useful (Spangrude *et al.*, 1988; Antica *et al.*, 1994; Morrison *et al.*, 1995; Morel *et al.*, 1996; Morel *et al.*, 1998). Cells that can give rise to several lineages but not to all hematopoietic lineages represent possible developmental checkpoints of hematopoietic differentiation.

Human Studies

The expression of the high molecular weight isoform of CD45 on $CD34^+$ bone marrow (BM) cells has been useful in identifying progenitor cells with lineage-restricted potential. Indeed, $CD34^+$ $CD45RA^+$ BM cells are distinct from primitive HSC based on phenotype and function. Unlike HSC, $CD34^+$ $CD45RA^+$ BM cells lack Thy-1, express CD38 and HLA-DR, cannot repopulate the marrow cavity of bone fragments implanted into SCID mice, and cannot sustain the long-term production of the primitive cobblestone-forming cells in cultures on BM stroma *in vitro* (Baum *et al.*, 1992; Craig *et al.*, 1993, 1994; Gunji *et al.*, 1993; Huang and Terstappen, 1994; Murray *et al.*, 1995, Galy *et al.*, 1995a). The differentiation potential of $CD34^+$ $CD45RA^+$ cells is restricted to lymphocytes and to myeloid cells (granulocytes and monocytes) lacking erythroid potential in conventional assays using cytokines such as erythropoietin and c-kit ligand (Craig *et al.*, 1994; Galy *et al.*, 1995a). In contrast, there is an increased level of commitment for T cells and NK cells in $CD34^+$ $CD45RA^+$ cells (Galy *et al.*, 1995a). In particular, it is possible to recognize within BM $CD34^+$ $CD45RA^+$ cells a small subset of cells expressing CD10 but no lineage-associated markers (Lin) such as CD19, CD2, CD14, CD15, CD56, and glycophorin A. Such $CD34^+$ Lin^- $CD10^+$ cells represent approximately 5% of $CD34^+$ Lin^- cells in adult BM. As predicted from their inclusion within $CD45RA^+$ cells, the $CD34^+$ Lin^- $CD10^+$ cells do not display HSC activity such as marrow repopulation or self-renewal. Their differentiation potential is restricted to the production of lymphocytes and DC and they cannot produce myeloid cells (granulocytes or monocytes), erythrocytes, mast cells or platelets in spite of stimulation with multiple growth factors (Galy *et al.*, 1995b). Within $CD34^+$ Lin^- $CD10^+$ cells there are progenitor cell clones with multiple potential for B lymphoid, NK lymphoid, and DC differentiation. Kinetics studies and precursor frequency calculations indicate that $CD34^+$ Lin^- $CD10^+$ BM cells are readily committed into the lymphocytic lineages. Such was confirmed by an independent study of $CD34^+$ $CD19^-$ B cell precursors expressing the IL-7Rα chain, a population that is largely superimposable with the $CD34^+$ $CD19^-$ (Lin^-) $CD10^+$ cell population. Such $CD34^+$ IL-7Rα^+ $CD19^-$ cells express TdT, RAG-1, the transcription factor Pax5, and are pre-pro-B cells enriched in

B lymphoid clonogenic precursors, thus confirming that there is an increased lymphoid 'fitness' in this population (Ryan *et al.*, 1997).

Cells with the $CD34^+$ Lin^- $CD10^+$ phenotype represent the elusive BM lymphoid 'stem cell' proposed by Gore *et al.* (1991) that has the unexpected ability to produce DC as well. Because of their ability to produce T cells rapidly (although not durably) and because of their overall differentiation potential, it is tempting to speculate that $CD34^+$ Lin^- $CD10^+$ cells could leave the BM to colonize the thymus (Ardavin *et al.*, 1993; Marquez *et al.*, 1995; Res *et al.*, 1996).

Murine Studies

Multipotent yet lineage-restricted progenitor cells have been well characterized in the murine thymus. Immature thymocytes with the phenotype Thy-1^{lo}, $CD4^{lo}$, Sca-2^+, c-kit^+, $CD25^-$ are not yet irreversibly committed to the T cell lineage and produce NK cells, B cells and DC. However, they have no myeloid or erythroid differentiation potential (reviewed in Shortman and Wu, 1996). In murine BM, cells with a restricted differentiation potential have been isolated recently. Approximately 25% of $CD34^+$ murine BM cells express CD45RA. Like their human counterparts, murine $CD34^+$ $CD45RA^+$ BM cells are depleted of erythroid precursors but enriched in lymphoid progenitor cells (Galy *et al.*, 1997). A recent report describes clonogenic common lymphoid progenitors in murine BM expressing the IL-7Rα chain but no lineage markers (Kondo *et al.*, 1997). Such cells do not have detectable myeloid (granulocyte and monocyte) or erythroid differentiation potential, and thus appear to be very similar to the human $CD34^+$ $CD10^+$ IL-7Rα^+ population (Galy *et al.*, 1995b; Ryan *et al.*, 1997).

Overall, the study of hematopoietic cell fate is much facilitated by the identification of cell surface markers on progenitor cells having various levels of differentiation potential. Such markers are useful in isolating cells. Table 1 lists some of the markers that can be useful in human BM.

HETEROGENEITY WITHIN THE DC LINEAGE

DC constitute a seemingly coherent group of hematopoietic cells characterized by their unusual dendritic morphology, by their potent antigen-presenting capability and by their lack of lineage-specific markers such as CD3, CD19, CD16, CD14, which distinguishes them respectively from T cells, B cells, NK cells, and monocytes. In spite of their importance in the immune system, DC have been called ontogenetic orphans (Peters, 1996) because their hematopoietic lineage affiliation is unclear.

Phenotypic and Functional Heterogeneity

DC are rare but ubiquitous cells. Various denominations of DC include veiled cells in lymphatic ducts, DC in peripheral blood or interstitial spaces of organs, interdigitating cells in lymphoid organs, and Langerhans cells (LC) in the epidermis. Considerable phenotypic and functional heterogeneity has now been documented within the DC system (O'Doherty *et al.*, 1993; Austyn, 1996; Takamizawa *et al.*, 1997; Kronin *et al.*, 1996; Süss and Shortman, 1996). Clearly, it is important to understand the reasons for this diversity.

Table 1. Markers of human BM progenitor and HSC

Cell type	Combined markers	Biological properties	Lineage differentiation potential	References
HSC pool	$CD34^+$ $Thy\text{-}1^+$ $CD38^{lo}$ $HLADR^{lo/-}$ $CD45RA^-$ $CD10^-$ $CD19^-$ $CD2^-$ $CD71^{lo}$ $c\text{-}kit^{+lo}$	Marrow repopulation Thymus repopulation Long-term culture-initiating cells, multilineage Clonogenic activity	E, G, M, L, DC	Baum *et al.* (1992) Craig *et al.* (1993) Gunji *et al.* (1993) Craig *et al.* (1994) Huang and Terstappen (1994) Murray *et al.* (1995) Galy *et al.* (1995a)
Multipotent progenitor pool	$CD34^+$ $Thy\text{-}1^-$ $CD38^+$ $HLADR^+$ $CD45RA^-$ $CD10^-$ $CD19^-$ $CD2^-$	Thymus repopulation Clonogenic activity	E, G, M, L, DC	Murray *et al.* (1995) Galy *et al.* (1995a)
Lineage-restricted pool	$CD34^+$ $Thy\text{-}1^-$ $CD38^+$ $HLADR^+$ $CD45RA^+$ $CD10^-$ $CD19^-$ $CD2^-$	Thymus repopulation CFU-GM Committed lymphoid progenitor	G, M, L, DC	Craig *et al.* (1994) Galy *et al.* (1995a)
Lymphoid-related progenitor	$CD34^+$ $Thy\text{-}1^-$ $CD38^+$ $HLADR^+$ $CD45RA^+$ $CD10^+$ $CD19^-$ $CD2^-$ $IL\text{-}7R\alpha^+$ $c\text{-}kit^{lo/-}$ Tdt^+	Thymus repopulation Committed lymphoid progenitor Lymphoid-related DC progenitor	L, DC	Galy *et al.* (1995b) Ryan (1997)

Markers not indicated for a given population may be absent or may not have been tested yet. E = erythroid, G = granulocytes, M = monocytes, L = lymphocytes (T, B, NK).

Evidence for Distinct Hematopoeitic Lineages of DC

Functional differences between several types of DC may merely reflect differences in the maturation or activation status of the same cells. For instance, cultured LC can acquire the phenotypic, morphological and functional characteristics of lymphoid DC *in vitro* (Romani *et al.*, 1989). On the other hand, and not in a mutually exclusive fashion, there is strong evidence that separate hematopoietic lineages of DC exist.

Lymphoid-Related DC

The development of some DC appears to be tightly related to that of lymphocytes. As detailed above, human DC can arise from a clonogenic common lymphoid progenitor $CD34^+$ Lin^- $CD10^+$ BM progenitor cell that is not capable of differentiating into monocytes upon exposure to multiple cytokines (Galy *et al.*, 1995b).

A number of cell surface markers are shared by lymphocytes and DC, including in humans and mice the markers CD1, CD4, CD8, CD2, and BP-1 (Wu *et al.*, 1991a; Vremec *et al.*, 1992; Sotzik *et al.*, 1994; Takamizawa *et al.*, 1997). It may attest to the existence of common precursors. Indeed, precursors for DC are found along T cell precursors within the thymus. In mice, the early intrathymic precursor population, the '$CD4^{lo}$ precursor' ($CD3^-$, $CD8^-$, $CD4^{low}$, $CD44^+$ $CD25^-$, c-kit^+) can also produce T, B, and NK cells but not cells of the myeloid or erythroid lineages (Wu *et al.*, 1991b; Ardavin *et al.*, 1993; Matsuzaki *et al.*, 1993; Wu *et al.*, 1995; Wu *et al.*, 1996). It was further demonstrated that cells that lie a step downstream of the $CD4^{lo}$ precursor are no longer able to generate B cells and NK cells but can still produce T cells and DC, thus indicating a strong lineage relationship between DC and T cells. The splenic and thymic DC progeny of the $CD4^{lo}$ precursor express homogeneously the $CD8\alpha\alpha$ homodimer in contrast with normal splenic DC and the splenic progeny of BM cells which consist of $CD8^+$ and $CD8^-$ DC (Wu *et al.*, 1996). It suggests that, in mice, a subclass of DC ($CD8^+$) and T cells shares a common precursor stage. In man, immature thymocytes expressing CD34 with low levels of CD38 are precursors to T cells, NK cells, and DC. Limiting dilution analysis has shown that there are common clones for NK lymphocytes and DC in the human thymus (Marquez *et al.*, 1995; Res *et al.*, 1996). These results imply that some DC may be more closely related to lymphocytes than to myeloid cells and thus may share similar genetic control of their development.

Monocyte-Derived DC

Monocytes can generate immunostimulatory DC. The change occurs without proliferation and is induced by GM-CSF and IL-4 (Zhou and Tedder, 1996, and our own observations). There are many similarities between monocytes/macrophages and resident DC as they share some morphological traits, and functional or phenotypic resemblance (reviewed in Peters, 1996). For instance, resident DC in the liver can efficiently phagocytose particles (Matsuno *et al.*, 1996), and skin LC express a number of markers common to macrophages such as Fc receptors, ATPase, and nonspecific esterase. GM-CSF or related cytokines such as IL-3 appear to be essential for the growth of monocytes as well as DC (Inaba *et al.*, 1993; Caux *et al.*, 1996). Monocyte-derived DC may not represent a stable population of cells because the phenotype is transient.

Myeloid DC

In spite of their relationship, DC and monocytes can also develop independently in 'myeloid' cell growth conditions.

It is possible to grow, from BM, pure colonies of DC (DC-CFU) that are distinct from mixed DC-myeloid CFU, therefore indicating that myeloid cells and DC can have distinct clonogenic precursors at some point in their development (Young *et al.*, 1995). Two distinct pathways have been described for the production of DC from $CD34^+$ cord blood progenitor cells in response to GM-CSF and TNF-α. CD34$^+$ cord blood cells may differentiate into the CD14$^-$ CD1$^+$ pathway to produce DC with strong T cell stimulatory characteristics and markers of LC. Alternatively, CD34$^+$ cells also differentiate along a CD14$^+$ CD1$^-$ intermediate stage that is bipotential for DC and monocytes and generates DC with preferential capacity to process antigen and the unique ability to activate naive B cells (Caux *et al.*, 1996).

The nature of the progenitor cells that respond to GM-CSF and TNF-α is not yet clear but may include blood CD34$^+$ CLA$^+$ cells that are enriched in LC precursors (Strunk *et al.*, 1997). In fetal BM, CD34$^+$ cells expressing low to negative levels of the IL-3Rα chain respond to GM-CSF and TNF-α by producing LC with Birbeck granules (Olweus *et al.*, 1997). In contrast, fetal BM cells expressing CD34 and high levels of the IL-3Rα chain respond to GM-CSF and TNF-α by producing DC without evidence of Birbeck granules (Olweus *et al.*, 1997). Such DC express themselves high levels of the IL-3Rα chain and are found in secondary peripheral lymphoid organs. This suggests that, possibly, a DC lineage distinct from that of LC could exist. Indeed, TGF-β mutant mice are found to lack LC but not lymph node DC (Borkowski *et al.*, 1996).

It is not yet clear how so-called 'myeloid' and lymphoid progenitors relate to each other. Further studies aimed at clarifying the relationship between the myeloid DC progenitors and the lymphoid-related progenitors are necessary. Different effects of cytokines such as GM-CSF or Flt3-ligand may be useful to understand the differentiation/growth requirements of various DC lineages (Saunders *et al.*, 1996; Maraskovsky *et al.*, 1996; Vremec *et al.*, 1997).

TARGETED MUTATIONS WITH HEMATOPOIETIC LINEAGE-SPECIFIC EFFECTS

Like other developmental biology systems, hematopoiesis provides a fertile ground for studying the transcriptional control of cell fate. Master regulators of hematopoiesis include DNA binding proteins such as GATA-2, tal-1/scl, AML-1, and PEBP2/CBF (Tsai *et al.*, 1994; Porcher *et al.*, 1996; Niki *et al.*, 1997). Targeted mutations in mice to abrogate the function of such genes profoundly disrupt blood cell formation and are usually lethal to the embryo. Presumably, such proteins are required for the development of HSC or of multipotential progenitors. In a more specific fashion, some transcription factors appear to be critical only for the production of one lineage and therefore may control commitment into this lineage of cells. Those include GATA-1 and Rbtn2, which are critical for erythroid development, c/EBPα, which is indispensable for granulocyte formation, and PU.1 for myeloid and lymphoid formation (reviewed in Orkin, 1996; Tenen *et al.*, 1997). Within the immune system, B cell production is singly dependent upon having the functional transcription factor genes *sox4*, *E2A*, *EBF*, or *Pax5* (Bain *et al.*, 1994; Urbanek *et al.*, 1994; Zhuang *et al.*, 1994; Lin and Grosschedl, 1995; Schilham *et al.*, 1996). An *Id1* transgene acting as a dominant negative regulator of basic helix–loop–helix (bH-L-H) transcription factors such as E2A specifically blocks B cell development (Sun, 1994). For T cell formation, GATA-3 is required and the HMG-box protein TCF-1 is necessary for the transition of immature single positive to double positive T cells (Verbeek *et al.*, 1995; Ting *et al.*, 1996). Possibly bH-L-H proteins determine the fate of common T and NK progenitors, since overexpression of the H-L-H dominant negative regulator Id3 blocks T cell differentiation but spares NK production in the thymus (Heemskerk *et al.*, 1997). Critical regulators in the formation and maintenance of lymphoid lineages are zinc finger proteins encoded by the *Ikaros* gene family.

Ikaros Regulates the Development of Lymphocytes and DC

Ikaros is a member of the Kruppel family of zinc finger DNA-binding proteins. Alternatively spliced transcripts of *Ikaros* encode a family of proteins with potential DNA binding sites in many T cell and B cell-associated genes such as the promoter and enhancer regions of CD3γ, δ and ε, the TCR α and β genes, the CD4 silencer, in the NF-κB sites of the IL-2Rα, β-interferon and class II MHC genes, in the HIV-LTR, in the LYF element of the TdT promoter, the EBF sites of the Igα promoter, and in the promoters of granzyme B, B29, TNF R p75 and BP-1 (Wargnier *et al.*, 1995; Babichuk *et al.*, 1996; Molnar *et al.*, 1996; Santee and Owen-Schaub, 1996; Thompson *et al.*, 1996). The *Ikaros* gene family which is abundantly expressed in lymphoid tissues is required for the development of all classes of lymphocytes (Georgopoulos *et al.*, 1994). *Ikaros* itself is a tumor suppressor gene in T cells and differentially controls the development of fetal and adult lymphocytes (Wang *et al.*, 1996). Interestingly, and further evidence for a developmental relationship between lymphocytes and DC, it was found that *Ikaros* controls the production of DC.

A mutation in the N-terminal DNA binding domain of Ikaros eliminates the protein products of exons 3 and 4 which encode the three N-terminal zinc fingers thus impairing sequence-specific DNA binding of the isoforms Ik1, Ik2, Ik3, and Ik4. As a result of this mutation, a truncated protein with two remaining C-terminal zinc fingers is produced that is transcriptionally inert but capable of dimerization with wild-type Ikaros or its partners and therefore acts in a dominant negative fashion (DN$-/-$). Germline transmission of this mutation (DN$-/-$) in mice is not lethal but confers a severely immunodeficient phenotype and mice often succumb to infections within a month. Mice altogether lack T cells, B cells, NK cells, and their earliest recognizable precursors. T cells are absent and thymuses are rudimentary, lacking their T cell compartment. Epidermal $\gamma\delta$ T cells are also absent. B cells expressing CD45R, CD43, or sIgM are undetectable in bone marrow and in the spleen. Cytolytic NK cell activity is absent. Contrasting with these severe immune deficiencies, DN $-/-$ animals have only minor alterations in the production of erythrocytes and myeloid cells. Platelets, monocytes and macrophages are produced abundantly. Spleens are enlarged but with no sign of extramedullary lymphoid activity. Interestingly, DN $-/-$ animals are partially deficient in cells of the DC lineage. Thymic DC expressing MHC class II, CD11c, and CD8α cannot be found in the Ikaros DN $-/-$ mice (Wu *et al.*, 1997). In the enlarged spleens of DN $-/-$ animals, both MHC class II^{++} CD8α^+ and MHC class II^{++} CD8α^- DC types are absent. However, contrasting with the lack of 'lymphoid DC', DN $-/-$ mice have skin Langerhans cells expressing high levels of MHC class II antigens. Bone marrow transplantation chimeras were created between mutant and wild-type congenic mice to exclude the possibility of environmental control on DC development. Results showed that chimeras lack mutant-derived lymphocytes and mutant-derived DC. This demonstrates that the defect in lymphoid cell production and in DC production in DN $-/-$ mice are both autonomous and result from alterations in hematopoietic cells but are not due to environmental factors (Wu *et al.*, 1997).

A different type of *Ikaros* null mutation was prepared to further investigate the role of Ikaros protein interactions in the development of the hemo-lymphoid system. A deletion in the last translated exon removes the C-terminal zinc fingers which are involved in dimerization and other protein interactions that contribute to transcriptional regulation. The resulting protein is very unstable and not detectable at the cellular level. Homozygotic mice with the null C –/– mutation show profound alterations of the lymphoid and DC systems, but the effects are selectively different between fetal and adult hematopoiesis. Throughout gestation and in the neonatal period, mice lack thymocytes and their identifiable precursors. A small number of thymocyte precursors (10-fold fewer than wild type) appear 3–5 days after birth and originally expand in a polyclonal fashion. T cells differentiate preferentially into the TCR $\alpha\beta$ lineage and numbers of $\gamma\delta$ T cells are severely reduced. Consistent with altered fetal T cell development, the subset of Vγ3 T cells is absent in these mice. NK cells are absent, as well as fetal and adult B cells of the conventional or of the B-1a lineages. In the thymus of C–/– mutants, which have on average a 2-fold to 5-fold lower cellularity than wild-type mice, it is possible to find cells with the characteristics of thymic DC (large size, high levels of MHC class II antigens, expression of CD11c and of CD8α and DEC-205). However, thymic DC in C–/– animals are in much reduced numbers (15-fold reduction) compared to wild-type animals. In the spleen, only one of the two types of splenic DC is found, the CD8α^+ DEC 205$^+$ cells, that is similar to the thymic subset. BM transplantation experiments determined that wild-type cells contributed to engraftment of myeloid cells, erythroid cells, CD8$^+$ and CD8$^-$ DC, T cells, B cells, and NK cells. In contrast, C–/– derived hematopoietic progenitors contributed to myeloid cells, some T cells, some CD8α^+ DEC 205$^+$ DC but not to B cell and not to CD8$^-$ DEC 205$^-$ DC. Thus the selective defect in the development of Ikaros C–/– cells is also autonomous and not environmentally determined.

In addition to the severe effects on immune cells, there are some effects on the hematopoietic progenitor and stem cell compartment in C–/– and DN–/– Ikaros mutant mice (Nichogiannopoulou, in preparation). These findings support a role of Ikaros at the level of a primitive multipotent progenitor, possibly HSC. Findings of Ikaros mRNA in Sca-1$^+$ c-kit$^+$ murine BM cells (Morgan *et al.*, 1997) and in CD34$^+$ Lin$^-$ CD45RA$^-$ Thy-1$^+$ human BM cells (A. Galy, in preparation) support a possible role of Ikaros at an early stage of hematopoietic differentiation. The differential effects between the N-terminal and C-terminal mutations of Ikaros suggest that heterodimerization partners of Ikaros in HSC and lymphoid progenitors may play an important role to further drive T-lymphoid cell fate (Morgan *et al.*, 1997; Morgan, unpublished results).

While Ikaros could control the development of separate progenitors of DC and of lymphocytes, it seems more likely, in the view of existing common progenitors of lymphocytes and DC, that a common precursor could be the target of action of Ikaros to determine cell fate specification, proliferation, or survival. In support of this, Ikaros mRNA is found in the bipotential lymphoid-DC CD34$^+$ Lin$^-$ CD10$^+$ BM progenitor (Galy *et al.*, 1997). Ikaros mRNA is also detected in human thymocytes and in human mature DC and therefore is likely to play a role in the development of the human lymphoid and DC systems as well (A. Galy, in preparation). Overall, *Ikaros* gene family members are essential for the development not only of lymphocytes but also of DC. It is surprising that the *Ikaros* DN–/– mutation has such a profound effect on the pool of peripheral DC, sparing the development of LC. This provides further evidence that separate subtypes of DC utilize different genes for their development. A provocative possibility supported by these data and by the phenotype of Ikaros mutant mice is that lymphoid DC and LC may constitute different hematopoietic lineages.

CONCLUSION

We speculate that differentiation of HSC into lymphocytes in BM occurs incrementally and involves precommitment (i.e. loss of erythroid and of myeloid potential) prior to final specification of any one of the lymphoid or DC lineages. We hypothesize that the differentiation of HSC into lymphocytes and DC proceeds sequentially along the intermediary steps that are depicted in Plate 1.1. Markers indicated in Table 1 are useful in identifying various stages of progenitor cells and provide a scaffold that can be used to link functional and phenotypic studies. Presumably, multiple genes must be activated ahead of time to control such predifferentiation programs. Perhaps *Ikaros* is one such gene as it is already expressed prior to final commitment. Interestingly, the development of some (but not all) DC appears to be strongly correlated with that of lymphocytes. Much work remains to be done to establish lineal relationships between the different types of DC such as the monocyte-derived DC, LC, and CD34-derived DC. It will be important to determine the relative contribution of each hematopoietic pathway to the pool of peripheral DC and it will be important to define whether different hematopoietic lineages of DC produce cells with distinct functions.

REFERENCES

Antica, M., Wu, L. Shortman, K. and Scollay, R. (1994). Thymic stem cells in the mouse bone marrow. *Blood* **84**, 111–117.

Ardavin, C., Wu, L. Li, C.-L. and Shortman, K. (1993). Thymic dendritic cells and T cells develop simultaneously in the thymus from a common precursor population. *Nature* **362**, 761–763.

Austyn, J.M. (1996). New insights into the mobilization and phagocytic activity of dendritic cells. *J. Exp. Med.* **183**, 1287–1292.

Babichuk, C.K., Duggan, B.L. and Bleakley, R.C. (1996). In vivo regulation of murine granzyme B gene transcription in activated primary T cells. *J. Biol. Chem.* **271**, 16485–16493.

Bain, G., Robanus Maandag, E., Izon, D., Amsen, D., Kruisbeek, A., Weintraub, B., Krop, I., Schlissel, M., Feeney, A., van Roon, M., van der Valk, M., te Riele, H., Berns, H. and Murre, C. (1994). E2A proteins are required for proper B cell development and initiation of immunoglobulin gene rearrangements. *Cell* **79**, 885–892.

Baum, C.M., Weissman, I.L., Tsukamoto, A.S., Buckle A.M. and Peault, B. (1992). Isolation of a candidate human hematopoietic stem cell population. *Proc. Natl Acad. Sci. USA* **89**, 2804–2808.

Borkowski, T.A., Letterio, J., Farr, A.G. and Udey, M. (1996). A role for endogenous transforming growth factor β1 in Langerhans cell biology: The skin of transforming growth factor β1 null mice is devoid of epidermal Langerhans cells. *J. Exp. Med.* **184**, 2417–2422.

Caux, C., Vanbervliet, B., Massacrier, C., Dezutter-Dambuyant, C., de Saint-Vis, B., Jacquet, C., Yoneda, K., Imamura, S., Schmitt, D. and Banchereau, J. (1996). $CD34^+$ hematopoietic progenitors from human cord blood differentiate along two independent dendritic cell pathways in response to GM-CSF + TNFα. *J. Exp. Med.* **184**, 695–706.

Craig, W., Kay, R., Cutler, R.L. and Lansdorp, P.M. (1993). Expression of Thy-1 on human hematopoietic progenitor cells. *J. Exp. Med.* **177**, 1331–1342.

Craig, W., Poppema, S., Dragowska, L.M.T. and Lansdorp, P.M. (1994). CD45 isoform expression on human haemopoietic cells at different stages of development. *Br. J. Haematol.* **88**, 24–30.

Galy, A.H.M., Cen, D., Travis, M., Chen, S. and Chen, B.P. (1995a). Delineation of T-progenitor cell activity within the CD34$^+$ compartment of adult bone marrow. *Blood* **85**, 2770–2778.
Galy, A., Travis, M., Cen, D. and Chen, B.P. (1995b). Human T, B, natural killer and dendritic cells arise from a common bone marrow progenitor cell subset. *Immunity* **3**, 459–473.
Galy, A., Morel, F., Hill, B. and Chen, B.P. (1997). Hematopoietic progenitor cells of lymphocytes and dendritic cells. *J. Immunother.* **21**, 132–141.
Georgopoulos, K., Bigby, M., Wang, J.H., Molnar, A., Wu, P., Winandy, S. and Sharpe, A. (1994). The Ikaros gene is required for the development of all lymphoid lineages. *Cell* **79**, 143–156.
Godfrey, D. and Zlotnik, A. (1993). Control points in early T-cell development. *Immunol. Today* **14**, 547–553.
Gore, S.D., Kastan, M.B. and Civin, C.I. (1991). Normal human bone marrow precursors that express terminal deoxynucleotidyl transferase include T-cell precursors and possible lymphoid stem cells. *Blood* **77**, 1681–1690.
Gunji, Y., Nakamura, M., Osawa, H., Nagayoshi, K., Nakauchi, H., Miura, Y., Yanagisawa, M. and Suda, T. (1993). Human primitive hematopoietic progenitor cells are more enriched in KITlow cells than in KIThigh cells. *Blood* **82**, 3283–3289.
Hardy, R.R., Carmack, C.E., Shinton, S.A., Kemp, J.D. and Hayakawa, K. (1991). Resolution and characterization of pro-B and pre-pro-B cell stages in normal mouse bone marrow. *J. Exp. Med.* **173**, 1213–1225.
Heemskerk, M., Blom, B., Nolan, G., Stegmann, A., Bakker, A., Weijer, K., Res, P. and Spits, H. (1997). Inhibition of T cell and promotion of natural killer cell development by the dominant negative helix loop helix factor Id3. *J. Exp. Med.* **186**, 1597–1602.
Huang, S. and Terstappen, L.W. (1994). Lymphoid and myeloid differentiation of single human CD34$^+$, HLA$^-$DR$^+$, CD38$^-$ hematopoietic stem cells. *Blood* **83**, 1515–1526.
Inaba, K., Inaba, M., Deguchi, M., Hagi, K., Yasumizu, R., Ikehara, S., Muramatsu, S. and Steinman, R.M. (1993). Granulocytes, macrophages, and dendritic cells arise from a common major histocompatibility complex class II-negative progenitor in mouse bone marrow. *Proc. Natl. Acad. Sci. USA* **90**, 3038–3042.
Kondo, M., Weissman, I.L. and Akashi, K. (1997). Identification of clonogenic common lymphoid progenitors in mouse bone marrow. *Cell* **91**, 661–672.
Kronin, V., Winkel, K., Suss, G., Kelso, A., Heath, W., Kirberg, J., von Boehmer, H. and Shortman, K. (1996). A subclass of dendritic cells regulates the response of naive CD8 T cells by limiting their IL-2 production. *J. Immunol.* **157**, 3819–3827.
Lin, H. and Grosschedl, R. (1995). Failure of B-cell differentiation in mice lacking the transcription factor EBF. *Nature* **376**, 263–267.
Maraskovsky, E., Brasel, K., Teepe, M., Roux, E., Lyman, S.D., Shortman, K. and McKenna, H.J. (1996). Dramatic increase in the numbers of functionally mature dendritic cells in Flt3 ligand-treated mice: multiple dendritic cell subpopulations identified. *J. Exp. Med.* **184**, 1953–1962.
Marquez, C., Trigueros, C., Fernandez, E. and Toribio, M.L. (1995). The development of T and non-T-cell lineages from CD34$^+$ human thymic precursors can be traced by differential expression of CD44. *J. Exp. Med.* **181**, 475–483.
Matsuno, K., Ezaki, T., Kudo, S. and Uehara, Y. (1996). A life stage of particle-laden rat dendritic cells in vivo: their terminal division, active phagocytosis, and translocation from the liver to the draining lymph. *J. Exp. Med.* **183**, 1865–1878.
Matsuzaki, Y., Gyotoku, J., Ogawa, M., Nishikawa, S., Katsura, Y., Gachelin, G. and Nakauchi, H. (1993). Characterization of c-kit positive intrathymic stem cells that are restricted to lymphoid diferentiation. *J. Exp. Med.* **178**, 1283–1292.
Molnar, A., Wu, P., Largespada, D.A., Scherer, V.A., Copeland, N.G., Jenkins, N.A., Bruns, G. and Georgopoulos, K. (1996). The Ikaros gene encodes a family of lymphocyte restricted zinc finger DNA binding proteins, highly conserved in human and mouse. *J. Immunol.* **156**, 585–592.
Morel, F., Szilvassy, S.J., Travis, M., Chen, B. and Galy, A. (1996). Primitive hematopoietic cells in murine bone marrow express the CD34 antigen. *Blood* **88**, 3774–3784.
Morel, F., Galy, A., Chen, B. and Szilvassy, S. (1998). Equal distribution of competitive long-term repopulating stem cells in the CD34$^+$ and CD34$^-$ fractions of Thy-1^{low} Lin$^{-/low}$ Sca-1$^+$ bone marrow cells. *Exp. Hematol.* **26**, 440–448.
Morgan, B., Sun, L., Avithal, N., Andrikopoulos, K., Ikeda, T., Gonzales, E., Wu, P., Neben, S. and Georgopoulos, K. (1997). Aiolos, a lymphoid restricted transcription factor that interacts with Ikaros to regulate lymphocyte differentiation. *EMBO J.* **16**, 2004–2013.

Morrison, S., Uchida, N. and Weissman, I.L. (1995). The biology of hematopoietic stem cells. *Annu. Rev. Cell Dev. Biol.* **11**, 35–71.

Murray, L., Chen, B., Galy, A., Chen, S., Tushinski, R., Uchida, N., Negrin, R., Tricot, G., Jagannath, S., Vesole, D., Barlogie, B., Hoffman, R. and Tsukamoto, A. (1995). Enrichment of human hematopoietic stem cell activity in the $CD34^+$ $Thy\text{-}1^+$ Lin^- subpopulation from mobilized peripheral blood. *Blood* **85**, 368–378.

Niki, M., Okada, H., Takano, H., Kuno, J., Tani, K., Hibino, H., Asano, S., Ito, Y., Satake, M. and Noda, T. (1997). Hematopoiesis in the fetal liver is impaired by targeted mutagenesis of a gene encoding a non-DNA binding subunit of the transcription factor, polyomavirus enhancer binding 2/core binding factor. *Proc. Natl Acad. Sci. USA* **94**, 5697–5702.

O'Doherty, U., Steinman, R.M., Peng, M., Cameron, P.U., Gezelter, S., Kopeloff, I., Swiggard, W.J., Pope, M. and Bhardwaj, N. (1993). Dendritic cells freshly isolated from human blood express CD4 and mature into typical immunostimulatory dendritic cells after culture in monocyte-conditioned medium. *J. Exp. Med.* **178**, 1067–1078.

Olweus, J.A.B., Warnke, R., Thompson, P., Carballido, J., Picker, L.J. and Lund-Johansen, F. (1997). Dendritic cell ontogeny: a human dendritic cell lineage of myeloid origin. *Proc. Natl Acad. Sci. USA* **94**, 12551–12556.

Orkin, S. (1996). Development of the hematopoietic system. *Curr. Opin. Genet. Dev.* **6**, 597–602.

Peters, J.H., Gieseler, R., Thiele, B. and Steinbach, F. (1996). Dendritic cells: from ontogenetic orphans to myelomonocytic descendants. *Immunol. Today* **17**, 273–278.

Porcher, C., Swat, W., Rockwell, K., Fujiwara, Y., Alt, F.W. and Orkin, S. (1996). The T cell leukemia oncoprotein SCL/tal-1 is essential for development of all hematopoietic lineages. *Cell* **86**, 47–57.

Res, P., Martínez-Cáceres, E., Jaleco, A. C., Staal, F., Noteboom, E., Weijer, K. and Spits, H. (1996). $CD34^+$ $CD38^{dim}$ cells in the human thymus can differentiate into T, natural killer, and dendritic cells but are distinct from pluripotent stem cells. *Blood* **87**, 5196–5206.

Romani, N., Lenz, A., Glassel, H., Stossel, H., Stanzl, U., Majdic, O., Fritsch, P. and Schuler G. (1989). Cultured human Langerhans cells resemble lymphoid dendritic cells in phenotype and function. *J. Invest. Dermatol.* **93**, 600–609.

Ryan, D.H., Nuccie, B.L., Ritterman, I., Liesveld, J., Abboud, C. and Insel, R. (1997). Expression of interleukin-7 receptor by lineage-negative human bone marrow progenitors with enhanced lymphoid proliferative potential and B-lineage differentiation capacity. *Blood* **89**, 929–940.

Santee, S.M. and Owen-Schaub, L.B. (1996). Human tumor necrosis factor receptor p75/80 (CD120b) gene structure and promoter characterization. *J. Biol. Chem.* **271**, 21151–21159.

Saunders, D., Lucas, K., Ismaili, J., Wu, L., Maraskovsky, E., Dunn, A. and Shortman, K. (1996). Dendritic cell development in culture from thymic precursor cells in the absence of granulocyte/macrophage colony stimulating factor. *J. Exp. Med.* **184**, 2185–2196.

Schilham, M.W., Oosterwegel, M.A., Moerer, P., Ya, J., de Boer, P.A., van de Wetering, M., Verbeek, S., Lamers, W.H., Kruisbeek, A., Cumano, A. and Clevers, H. (1996). Defects in cardiac outflow tract formation and pro-B lymphocyte expansion in mice lacking sox-4. *Nature* **380**, 711–714.

Shortman, K. and Wu, L. (1996). Early T lymphocyte progenitors. *Annu. Rev. Immunol.* **14**, 29–47.

Sotzik, F., Rosenberg, Y., Boyd, A.W., Honeyman, M., Metcalf, D., Scollay, R., Wu, L. and Shortman, K. (1994). Assessment of CD4 expression by early T precursor cells and by dendritic cells in the human thymus. *J. Immunol.* **152**, 3370–3377.

Spangrude, G.J., Muller-Sieburg, C.E., Heinfeld, S. and Weissman, I.L. (1988). Two rare populations of mouse $Thy\text{-}1^{lo}$ bone marrow cells repopulate the thymus. *J. Exp. Med.* **167**, 1671–1683.

Strunk, D., Egger, C., Leitner, G., Hanau, D. and Stingl, G. (1997). A skin homing molecule defines the Langerhans cell progenitor in human peripheral blood. *J. Exp. Med.* **185**, 1131–1136.

Sun, X. (1994). Constitutive expression of the Id1 gene impairs mouse B cell development. *Cell* **79**, 893–900.

Suss, G. and Shortman, K. (1996). A subclass of dendritic cells kills CD4T cells via Fas/Fas-ligand-induced apoptosis. *J. Exp. Med.* **183**, 1789–1796.

Takamizawa, M., Rivas, A., Fagnoni, F., Benike, C., Kosek, J., Hyakawa, H. and Engleman, E. (1997). Dendritic cells that process and present nominal antigens to naive T lymphocytes are derived from $CD2^+$ precursors. *J. Immunol.* **158**, 2134–2142.

Tenen, D., Hromas, R., Licht, J. and Zhang, D. (1997). Transcription factors, normal myeloid development, and leukemia. *Blood* **90**, 489–519.

Thompson, A., Wood, W., Gilly, M., Damore, M., Omori, S. and Wall, R. (1996). The promoter and 5′ flanking sequences controlling human B29 gene expression. *Blood* **87**, 666–673.

Ting, C.N., Olson, M.C., Barton, K.P. and Leiden, J.M. (1996). Transcription factor GATA-3 is required for development of the T-cell lineage. *Nature* **384**, 474–478.

Tsai, F.Y., Keller, G., Kuo, F., Weiss, M., Chen, J., Rosenblatt, M., Alt, F.W. and Orkin, S. (1994). An early haematopoietic defect in mice lacking the transcription factor GATA-2. *Nature* **371**, 221–226.

Urbanek, P., Wang, Z.Q., Fetka, I., Wagner, E.F. and Busslinger, M. (1994). Complete block of early B cell differentiation and altered patterning of the posterior midbrain in mice lacking Pax5/BSAP. *Cell* **79**, 901–912.

Verbeek, S., Izon, D., Hofhuis, F., Robanus-Maandag, E., te Riele, H., van de Wetering, M., Osterwegel, M., Wilson, A., MacDonald, H.R. and Clevers, H. (1995). An HMG-box containing T-cell factor required for thymocyte differentiation. *Nature* **374**, 70–74.

Vremec, D., Zorbas, M., Scollay, R., Saunders, D.J., Ardavin, C.F., Wu, L. and Shortman, K. (1992). The surface phenotype of dendritic cells purified from mouse thymus and spleen: Investigation of the CD8 expression by a subpopulation of dendritic cells. *J. Exp. Med.* **176**, 47–58.

Vremec, D., Lieschke, G., Dunn, A., Robb, L., Metcalf, D. and Shortman, K. (1997). The influence of granulocyte/macrophage colony-stimulating factor on dendritic cell levels in mouse lymphoid organs. *Eur. J. Immunol.* **27**, 40–44.

Wang, J.H., Nichogiannopoulou, A., Wu, L., Sun, L., Sharpe, A., Bigby, M. and Georgopoulos K. (1996). Selective defects in the development of the fetal and adult lymphoid system in mice with an Ikaros null mutation. *Immunity* **5**, 537–549.

Wargnier, A., Legros-Maida, S., Bosselut, R., Bourge, J.G., Lafaurie, C., Ghysdael, C.J., Sasportes, M. and Paul, P. (1995). Identification of human granzyme B promoter regulatory elements interacting with activated T cell specific proteins: implications of Ikaros and CBF binding sites in promoter activation. *Proc. Natl Acad. Sci. USA* **92**, 6930–6934.

Wu, L., Scollay, R., Egerton, M., Pearse, M., Spangrude, G.J. and Shortman, K. (1991a). CD4 expressed on earliest T-lineage precursor cells in the adult murine thymus. *Nature* **349**, 71–74.

Wu, L., Antica, M., Johnson, G.R., Scollay, R. and Shortman, K. (1991b). Developmental potential of the earliest precursor cells from the adult mouse thymus. *J. Exp. Med.* **174**, 1617–1627.

Wu, L., Vremec, D., Ardavin, C., Winkel, K., Gabriele, S., Georgiou, H., Maraskovsky, E., Cook, W. and Shortman, K. (1995). Mouse thymus dendritic cells: kinetics of development and changes in surface markers during maturation. *Eur. J. Immunol.* **25**, 418–425.

Wu, L., Li, C. and Shortman, K. (1996). Thymic dendritic cell precursors: relationship to the T lymphocyte lineage and phenotype of the dendritic cell progeny. *J. Exp. Med.* **184**, 903–911.

Wu, L., Nichogiannopoulou, A., Shortman, K. and Georgopoulos, K. (1997). Cell autonomous defect in dendritic cell populations of Ikaros mutant mice points to a developmental relationship with the lymphoid lineage. *Immunity* **7**, 483–492.

Young, J.W., Szabolcs, P. and Moore, M.A.S. (1995). Identification of dendritic cell colony-forming units among normal human CD34$^+$ bone marrow progenitors that are expanded by c-*kit*-ligand and yield pure dendritic cell colonies in the presence of granulocyte/macrophage colony-stimulating factor and tumor, necrosis factor α. *J. Exp. Med.* **182**, 1111–1120.

Zhou, L.J. and Tedder, T.F. (1996). CD14$^+$ monocytes can differentiate into functionally mature CD83$^+$ dendritic cells. *Proc. Natl Acad. Sci. USA* **93**, 2588–2592.

Zhuang, Y., Soriano, P. and Weintraub, H. (1994). The helix–loop–helix gene E2A is required for B cell formation. *Cell* **79**, 875–884.

CHAPTER 2
Thymic Dendritic Cells

Ken Shortman and Li Wu
The Walter and Eliza Hall Institute of Medical Research, Melbourne, Victoria, Australia

> ... thymocytes and thymic accessory cells were a concordant pair ... (they) could arise from a bipotential precursor that diverges into these separate lineages after colonization of the epithelial thymic rudiment.
>
> J. B. Turpen and P. B. Smith
> on the developing thymus of *Xenopus laevis*

INTRODUCTION

Dendritic cells (DC) of the thymus (Ardavin, 1997) are considered to have a biological role which differs from that of the DC in other tissues. The overall function of the peripheral DC system is to collect and present foreign antigens to mature T cells and initiate immune responses, whereas the function of thymic DC is to present self-antigens to developing T cells and initiate apoptosis, in other words to mediate negative selection and so induce self-tolerance. This oversimplified view ignores the extensive apoptotic T cell death associated with peripheral immune responses and ignores the phenomenon of peripheral T cell tolerance. Nevertheless, it serves to pose the question of whether thymic DC are fundamentally different from those of other tissues. The question was first posed experimentally by Matzinger and Guerder (1989), who showed that splenic DC, if introduced into fetal thymus organ cultures, were also able to produce negative selection. Subsequent work has demonstrated that other antigen-presenting cells, including thymic cortical epithelial cells, are able to initiate the death of immature $CD4^+8^+$ thymocytes, if the affinity for the peptide–MHC complex or the amount of peptide presented is high enough (Tanaka *et al*., 1993; Sprent and Webb, 1995). These studies suggest that it is the developmental state of the T cell, rather than the type of antigen-presenting cell, that determines the outcome of the T cell–DC interaction. However, it remains possible that thymic DC do have additional undiscovered mechanisms to promote negative selection, especially the negative selection that occurs after positive selection, among the semimature thymocytes found in the medulla (Kishimoto and Sprent, 1997).

Even if thymic DC prove to be equipped with the same mechanisms for signaling T cells as the DC found elsewhere, their different overall role and particular location may imply a different developmental history. The paradigm of DC life history is that of the

Dendritic Cells: Biology and Clinical Applications
ISBN 0-12-455860-7

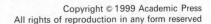

Langerhans cell, a migratory cell whose function changes with location, as presented elsewhere in this volume. The essential features are a sentinel phase in peripheral non-lymphoid tissue where antigens are ingested and processed, a phase of maturation and migration when antigen uptake declines but costimulatory function increases, and finally in lymph nodes a phase of antigen presentation and T cell activation. An important issue is whether this model applies at all to the DC within the thymus, where the entry of migratory antigen-presenting cells from the bloodstream would be expected to delete from the T cell repertoire the possibility of responding to the foreign antigens collected in the peripheral environment.

The origin, development and nature of thymic DC will be considered with these issues in mind.

MOUSE THYMIC DENDRITIC CELLS

Localization and Isolation

The majority of DC in the mouse thymus are localized in the medulla and at the cortico-medullary junction (reviewed by Sprent and Webb, 1995; Ardavin, 1997). A similar medullary localization of DC is seen in the rat thymus (Duijvestijn and Barclay, 1984). Although the proportion of DC in thymus suspensions is lower than for spleen or lymph nodes, the incidence in the medullary zone where the DC are concentrated is comparable with that in the T cell areas of other lymphoid tissues.

Thymic DC are in close contact with T lineage cells, as are the interdigitating DC of spleen or lymph nodes (Steinman *et al.*, 1997). Gentle dissociation of thymic tissue by digestion with collagenase (rather than trypsin) will release pre-existing DC–thymocyte complexes or 'rosettes', held together by adhesion molecules; these rosettes can then be separated by unit-gravity sedimentation or elutriation (Kyewski *et al.*, 1982; Shortman *et al.*, 1989; Shortman and Vremec, 1991).

DC may be purified from such rosettes, or directly from suspensions of dissociated and digested thymus tissue, where mature DC represent only about 0.1% of all cells (Vremec *et al.*, 1992; Winkel *et al.*, 1994). An important first step for good yield is to dissociate the DC–thymocyte complexes by adding EDTA and/or using calcium- and magnesium-free media. Selection of the 3–5% lowest density cells by density centrifugation provides a substantial enrichment of the mature DC. Further enrichment can be obtained by immunodepletion of T-lineage cells and other non-DC thymus components, although care is needed to avoid loss of the DC, which express Fc receptors, express certain T cell markers (CD8, CD2), and pick up low levels of certain T cell surface molecules (e.g. Thy-1). Fluorescence-activated sorting for cells expressing one or more characteristic DC markers (CD11c; high levels of class II MHC) is needed to obtain a completely pure DC preparation.

Phenotype

The features of thymic DC have been reviewed recently by Ardavin (1997). The DC freshly isolated from the thymus may need to be incubated for several hours in culture medium to recover a dendritic morphology (Fig. 1a); even then, the appearance of

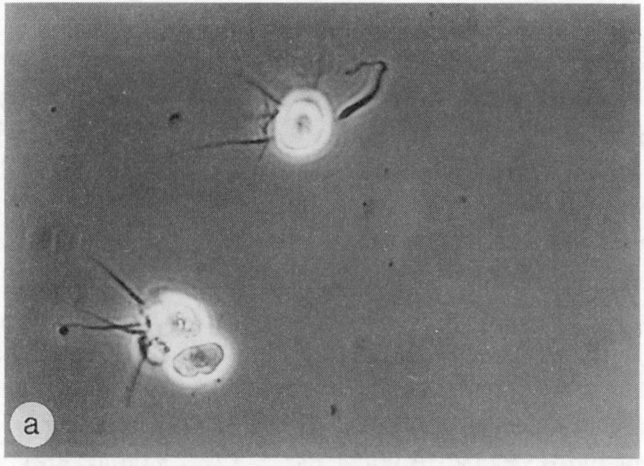

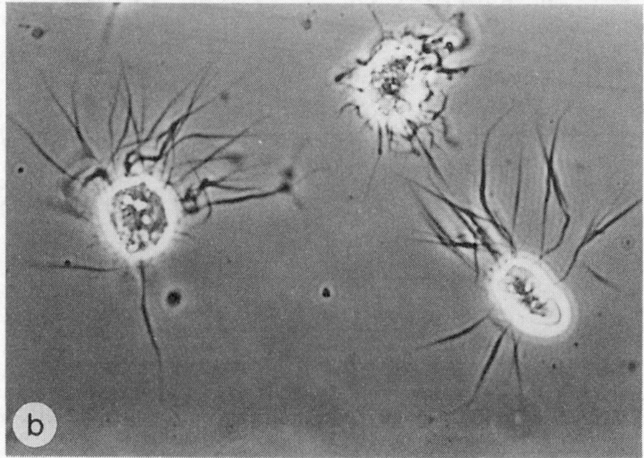

Fig. 1. The appearance under phase-contrast microscopy of DC purified from the mouse (a) or the human (b) thymus. The DC were isolated by a procedure involving collagenase digestion, EDTA treatment, low-density separation, immunomagnetic bead depletion and finally sorting for cells expressing high levels of class II MHC (Vremec et al., 1992; Winkel et al., 1994). They were then incubated in culture medium for several hours to regenerate a dendritic form. (Magnification ×1500.) Reproduced from Winkel et al. (1994) with kind permission of Elsevier Science-NL, Sara Burgerhartstraat 25, 1055 KV, Amsterdam, The Netherlands.

dendrites and other DC characteristics is less florid than on DC grown in culture using GM-CSF or on DC derived from the Langerhans cells of skin explants. The mature thymic DC, like the mature DC from other lymphoid organs, die rapidly in basic culture media, most having lost viability within 24 h (Winkel *et al*., 1997); this suggests they are end-cells with an inherently limited life span. However, certain factors can extend the culture survival time of a proportion of the DC by about one day; these include the T cell products GM-CSF and CD40 ligand, suggesting that interaction with T cells *in vivo* may extend the DC life span.

Thymic DC express the characteristic pan-DC markers, such as high levels of class I and especially class II MHC, and relatively high levels of the β_2 integrin CD11c (Crowley *et al*., 1989; Vremec *et al*., 1992; Vremec and Shortman, 1997). A subpopulation expressing lower surface levels of class II MHC but higher levels of CD45 has been delineated and interpreted as being a less mature form of thymic DC (Ardavin, 1997). Freshly isolated mouse thymic DC express CD80 and CD86 (B7/1 and B7/2), as well as CD40, suggesting they are already mature in their capacity to interact with T cells (Vremec and Shortman, 1997). They also express adhesion molecules, including VCAM-1 and ICAM-1 (L. Wu, unpublished).

Some of the surface markers on mouse thymic DC indicate that they represent a particular DC subtype. Thymic DC express the interdigitating DC marker NLDC-145, now known as the multi-lectin domain molecule DEC-205 (Crowley *et al.*, 1989; Witmer-Pack *et al.*, 1995; Vremec and Shortman, 1997). They express several molecules found on early thymus precursor cells, including Sca-2 and c-kit (Vremec and Shortman, 1997). They show only very low surface levels of the macrophage marker Mac-1 (CD11b). However, they express a number of surface molecules normally characteristic of lymphoid cells, including CD8α (Vremec *et al.*, 1992; Vremec and Shortman, 1997). As illustrated in Fig. 2, the pattern of surface markers on the thymic DC resembles closely that seen on one of the two DC populations of mouse spleen. The DC phenotype common to thymus and spleen is CD8α^+ DEC-205$^+$ HSA$^+$ CD11b$^-$, whereas the DC phenotype found in spleen but not to a significant level in thymus is CD8α^- DEC-205$^-$ HSA$^-$ CD11b$^+$ (Crowley *et al.*, 1989; Vremec and Shortman, 1997). Section studies indicate that thymic DC express Fas-ligand (French *et al.*, 1997), as do the CD8α^+ DC of spleen (Süss and Shortman, 1996).

The apparent presence of 'lymphoid' markers on mouse thymic DC is of particular interest but the significance of these needs to be viewed with caution. Because of the

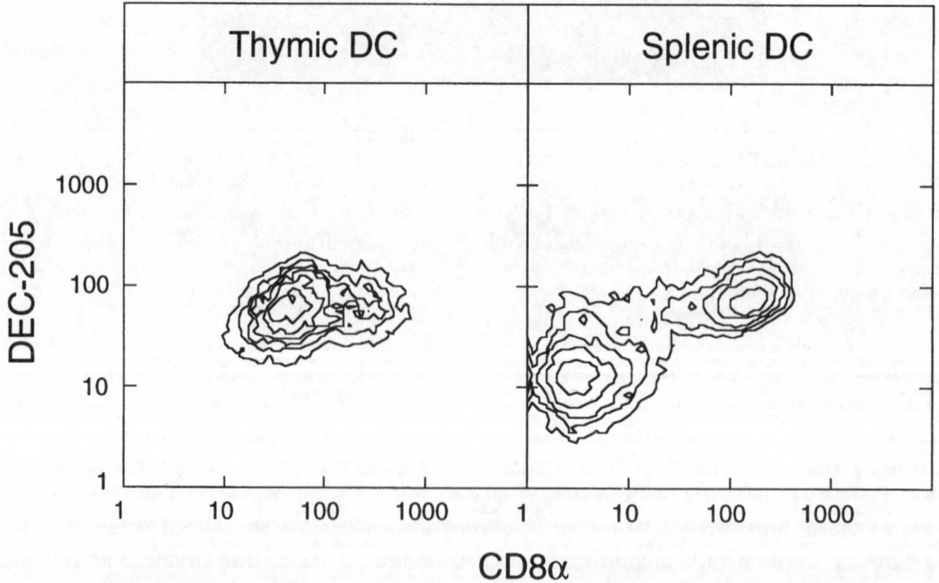

Fig. 2. Comparison of the surface phenotype of the DC populations of mouse thymus and mouse spleen. DC were isolated as in Fig. 1, and stained for class II MHC, CD8α and DEC-205. The DC were then gated during flow cytometric analysis as high class II MHC cells with typical DC light scatter characteristics, and the gated cells were analyzed for CD8α and DEC-205 expression. Full details are in Vremec and Shortman (1997). The data were generated by L. Wu and D. Vremec.

tight association of DC with thymocytes, T cell surface components can readily be picked up by the DC, probably when the T cell–DC complexes are being dissociated during isolation. Thus much if not all of the Thy-1 on the surface of thymic DC was shown to originate from T lineage cells, since in bone marrow chimeras made using Thy 1.1 and Thy 1.2 congenic precursor cells, where the thymocytes expressed only one or the other Thy-1 allotype, the thymic DC were found to have on their surface both allotypes (Shortman *et al.*, 1995). Such absorbed components are generally lost on overnight culture of DC (Wu *et al.*, 1995); earlier isolation procedures involving overnight culture avoided these problems by providing an inbuilt washing stage (Crowley *et al.*, 1989). However, isolation involving culture at 37°C has its own problems, since certain surface molecules are then induced or upregulated. One example is CD25, the IL-2Rα chain, which is only expressed on a small proportion of freshly isolated thymic DC, but which is expressed at high levels on most thymic DC after overnight culture, especially with GM-CSF (Vremec and Shortman, 1997). Only the IL-2Rα chain, not the IL-2Rβ chain, is so induced (D. Vremec, unpublished data). However, such induction of CD25, although it is a 'lymphoid' marker, appears to be a characteristic of most DC from most species (MacPherson *et al.*, 1989).

CD8 is one of the lymphoid markers found on thymic DC that appears to be a normal surface component produced by the DC themselves. The CD8 is neither eliminated nor induced by culture (Wu *et al.*, 1995). The CD8 is present largely as an $\alpha\alpha$ homodimer (such as is found on $\gamma\delta$ T cells) rather than as the $\alpha\beta$ heterodimer found on most T cells. Thymic DC, and the corresponding population of splenic DC, express mRNA for CD8α but not for CD8β (Vremec *et al.*, 1992). The level of CD8α can be as high as on T cells. In some strains such as C57BL/6 (Fig. 2), thymic DC show a spread of CD8α expression from medium to high; there is evidence of an increase in CD8α with maturation (Wu *et al.*, 1995). In other strains such as Balb/c, the level of expression on thymic DC is more uniformly high (Wu *et al.*, 1995). Some particular inductive factor in the lymphoid tissue environment must switch on CD8α during DC development, since the DC generated in culture from intrathymic DC precursors lack CD8α expression (Saunders *et al.*, 1996). However, such an inductive factor is not unique to the thymus since certain DC populations found in the spleen, and even found in the spleens of athymic mice, also express CD8α (Fig. 2). In addition, when the intrathymic precursor is transferred intravenously into irradiated recipients, it produces CD8α^+ DC in the spleen as well as the thymus (Wu *et al.*, 1996). Although CD8α serves as a useful marker for one type of DC, at least *in vivo*, there is no evidence so far for a functional role for this surface component. Mice with the CD8α gene disrupted have normal DC levels in thymus and spleen and have all DC populations present as assessed by markers other than CD8α; in addition, no differences are apparent in their functional interaction with T cells (Kronin *et al.*, 1997).

Another lymphoid marker found on most mouse thymus DC is the early B cell marker BP-1, a glutamyl aminopeptidase. BP-1 is not expressed at all by spleen or lymph node DC and to date it is the only surface marker which distinguishes thymic DC from all other DC, including the otherwise similar CD8α^+ DC of spleen (Wu *et al.*, 1995; Vremec and Shortman, 1997). BP-1 appears to be produced by the DC themselves, since it is not washed off the DC surface on culture and BP-1 mRNA is found in the DC (Wu *et al.*, 1995). However, BP-1 is not a constitutive product of thymic DC and appears to be induced during DC development by some factor in the thymic environment. The DC which develop in the thymus following transfer of the thymic

DC precursor express BP-1, but the DC which develop in the spleen following intravenous transfer of the same precursor, or which develop in culture from the same precursor, all lack BP-1 (Saunders *et al.*, 1996; Wu *et al.*, 1996).

Function

Thymic DC form part of the thymic stroma, which induces and directs T cell development (Boyd *et al.*, 1993). Kyewski (1987) found, by isolating thymic rosettes, that DC interact with developing T cells at a relatively late stage after the initial entry of T precursors into the thymus; this fits with the location of most DC in the medullary area where the more mature T cells are found. As reviewed by Sprent and Webb (1995), the evidence that DC mediate negative selection of thymocytes is strong. The negative selection occurring post positive selection in the medullary zone, as the T lineage cells are developing mature T cell characteristics, may be exclusively mediated by DC (Kishimoto and Sprent, 1997). The role of thymic DC in negative selection has recently been confirmed by Brocker and colleagues (1997), who targeted expression of a class II MHC to DC by using a CD11c promoter, and showed that such restricted expression produced negative but not positive selection in the thymus.

Based on negative selection and antigen presentation studies, thymic DC are able to process and present not just endogenous thymic self-antigens but also blood-borne protein antigens such as the C5 complement component (Kyewski *et al.*, 1986; Stockinger and Hausmann, 1994). Blood-borne proteins appear to have greater access to the thymic medulla, where the DC are concentrated, than to the thymic cortex. However, the limits of access of antigens to the medulla, and of the antigen uptake and processing capacity of thymic DC compared to other DC, have not yet been established. It is clear, however, that isolated thymic DC are capable not only of inducing apoptosis in immature thymocytes (Tanaka *et al.*, 1993), but also of stimulating proliferation in mature T cells (Kyewski *et al.*, 1986; Guéry and Adorini, 1995; Saunders *et al.*, 1996). Thymic DC seem, by this basic test, fully capable of presenting antigens so as to activate mature T cells into cycle, which fits with their surface expression of the costimulatory molecules CD80 and CD86 at levels comparable with those of spleen or lymph node DC (Vremec and Shortman, 1997). This strongly supports the concept that it is the developmental state of the T lineage cell which determines whether the interaction with a DC leads to clonal deletion or to an immune response.

Despite their evident capacity to present antigens and activate T cells, some aspects of the thymic DC–T cell interaction may differ from that of at least some immunostimulatory peripheral DC. In culture studies the CD8α^+ DEC-205$^+$ CD11b$^-$ splenic DC (Fig. 2) have been found to display distinct 'regulatory' effects on the T cells they activate, leading to reduced responses compared to that given by the CD8α^- DEC-205$^-$ CD11b$^+$ DC. The CD8α^+ splenic DC are poor inducers of interleukin-2 production by CD8 T cells, compared to the CD8α^- DC (Kronin *et al.*, 1996). In addition the CD8α^+ splenic DC express a surface Fas-ligand and induce apoptotic death in a proportion of the activated CD4 T cells (Süss and Shortman, 1996). Thus it is possible that thymic DC, which are also CD8α^+ DEC-205$^+$ CD11b$^-$, are members of a group of DC with regulatory function, a group having representatives in the peripheral lymphoid tissue as well as being the major DC type in the thymus. The interaction of thymic DC with T cells has not as yet been examined with these issues in mind.

Development

Thymic DC of mice and rats have been shown in many studies (e.g. Barclay and Mayrhofer, 1981) to be bone marrow derived, and so to differ in origin from thymic stromal epithelial cells. It has been formally demonstrated, by reconstitution of the irradiated thymus with purified Ly-5 congenic multipotent hematopoietic stem cells, that thymic DC are derived originally from the same multipotent precursor that produces erythroid, myeloid and lymphoid cells (Ardavin *et al*., 1993). The lineage relationships and developmental control mechanisms downstream of this multipotent progenitor are of more current interest.

It had been assumed that the DC of the thymus have a common origin with other DC and that they arrive in the thymus preformed as migratory DC from the bloodstream. It is now clear that the thymus contains early DC precursors lacking the morphological features or surface markers of either mature or immature DC (Ardavin *et al*., 1993; Wu *et al*., 1995). This has led to the opposite view that all thymic DC are endogenously generated and do not follow the migratory Langerhans cell model. This endogenous generation model overcomes the paradox that importation of foreign antigens, as presented by migratory DC, would cause deletion of the potentially responsive developing T cells. However, it should be emphasized that the entry of some migratory DC into the thymus has not as yet been excluded. It remains possible that some part of the thymic medulla is accessible to migratory DC and that they could initiate an immune response by the most mature medullary thymocytes, those that have matured beyond the window of tolerance (Kishimoto and Sprent, 1997). Experimental testing of this possibility is required.

The DC of the mouse and rat thymus have a short life span and rapid turnover, substantially faster than thymic macrophages, at least as judged by irradiated reconstitution models (Kyewski *et al*., 1986; Kampinga *et al*., 1990; Wu *et al*., 1995). Transfer of an intrathymic DC precursor into an irradiated recipient thymus (Fig. 3) demonstrates that 7 days are required to generate thymic DC with mature phenotype (high class II MHC and CD11c), and that these DC then last for 14 days before disappearing from the thymus. This loss probably represents death rather than exit from the organ, since few if any DC can be detected among recent thymic emigrants (L. Wu, unpublished data). In addition, the DC of similar phenotype in the periphery are at normal levels in athymic 'nude' mice, indicating that they were not of thymic origin (D. Vremec and K. Shortman, unpublished data). The life span of DC within the thymus is therefore about as short as that of a T-lineage cell from the time of its acquisition of a functioning T cell receptor to the time of intrathymic death or maturation and exit. This implies that each cohort of developing T cells in the thymus is accompanied by a parallel cohort of freshly generated DC, a system that would help ensure that negative selection is largely restricted to newly synthesized or recently processed self-antigens.

The nature of the intrathymic DC precursor in the adult mouse thymus provided some surprises and new insights into the origin of thymic DC. The earliest precursor of the T-lineage cells in the thymus had been identified by Wu *et al*. (1991a,b) as a rare population (1 per 3000 thymocytes) with a phenotype differing from most early thymocytes ($CD4^{lo}$ $CD8^-$ $CD3^-$ $CD25^-$ $CD44^+$ Thy 1^{lo} c-kit^+ Sca-1^+ Sca-2^+ class II MHC^-) and with T cell antigen receptor genes still in germline state. This 'low CD4' precursor appeared to be lymphoid-restricted, able on intravenous transfer to form T

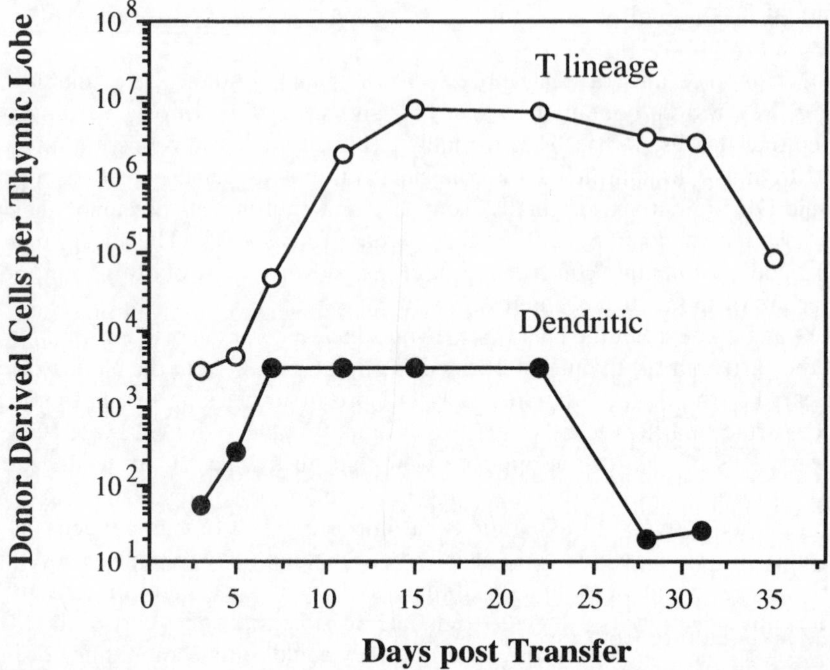

Fig. 3. The generation of both DC and T-lineage thymocytes in an irradiated recipient thymus following intrathymic transfer of purified thymic low CD4 precursors. Full details are in Wu *et al.* (1995). The precursor cells were isolated from Ly 5.2 mice and transferred into Ly 5.1 congenic mice. The T-lineage progeny were analyzed directly on thymus suspensions as Ly 5.2^+ Thy 1^+ cells. The DC progeny were analyzed as Ly 5.2^+ class II MHC^{hi} $CD11c^+$ cells after preliminary enrichment by the DC isolation procedure of Fig. 1.

cells and B cells (Wu *et al.*, 1991a) as well as NK cells (Matsuzaki *et al.*, 1993), but not able to produce a detectable level of erythroid or myeloid cells. A limited ability to form macrophage colonies in culture was the only myeloid potential noted; this low (~1%) colony-forming cell incidence suggested either a contaminant or a multipotent potential by a very minor subset of these precursors. This apparently lymphoid-restricted low CD4 precursor population was then shown by Ardavin *et al.* (1993) to produce DC, as well as T cells, in the thymus of irradiated recipient mice. Although the ratio of DC to T-lineage cell produced was low (1:1000) (Fig. 3; Wu *et al.*, 1995), this is close to the normal thymic DC to T-lineage cell ratio, suggesting that this precursor has the capacity to form all thymic DC. Further studies (Wu *et al.*, 1996) have shown that the capacity to produce DC extends down the T-lineage precursor pathway to the $CD4^-$ 8^- 44^+ 25^+ progenitor, which has already lost the potential to form B cells and NK cells and is devoid of myeloid potential; the capacity to form DC is only lost at the $CD4^-$ 8^- 44^- 25^+ stage, the point where rearrangement of the T cell antigen-receptor β-gene commences. Furthermore, these early thymus precursors, if transferred intravenously, produced only the $CD8\alpha^+$ DC type in recipient spleens, in contrast to multipotent bone marrow precursors which produced both $CD8\alpha^-$ and $CD8\alpha^+$ DC (Wu *et al.*, 1996). Thus it is unlikely that the DC production was due to a trace contamination of the precursors by multipotent stem cells or by myeloid precursor cells. This evidence pointed to a lymphoid rather than myeloid origin for thymic DC.

The adoptive transfer approach has now been extended by studies of DC development in culture (Saunders *et al.*, 1996; Lucas *et al.*, 1998). The early T-precursor populations purified from the adult mouse thymus have produced pure populations of DC after 3–5 days of culture, with very high cloning efficiency; 70% of all precursors formed DC, the remaining 30% dying rapidly in culture. This excludes the possibility that DC were derived from a trace contaminant in the precursor preparations, but does not prove that DC and T cells can be produced from the one cell; it is possible that all the T cells obtained by adoptive transfer from this T-precursor population were derived from the 30% of cells which died in these cultures. The DC produced were functional in ability to activate T cells and they expressed markers typical of mature interdigitating DC (class II MHC; CD11c; DEC-205; CD80; CD86). However, they lacked expression of both CD8α and BP-1, markers found on thymic DC *in vivo*. In view of the high cloning efficiency, it is unlikely that a potential to generate a different or minor DC type has been revealed in culture; it is more likely that the factors required to induce these particular markers have not been reproduced in the culture system.

The cytokines required for generating DC from the purified intrathymic precursors (Saunders *et al.*, 1996; Lucas *et al.*, 1998) differed from the cytokines required to produce DC in culture from myeloid precursors or from blood monocytes (discussed elsewhere in this volume). In particular, no DC were produced from the thymic precursors using the usual combination of GM-CSF and TNF-α, and the myeloid hormone GM-CSF was not required at all in the final effective cytokine mix. The optimal mix was complex and included TNFα, IL-1, IL-3, IL-7, SCF, Flt3 ligand and CD40 ligand; TNF-α and IL-1 were essential, not only for DC maturation but also for initiation of division in the precursors. These distinct cytokine requirements point to a different lineage origin for thymic DC.

Some aspects of these cytokine requirements have now been checked in intact mice. By using GM-CSF transgenic mice, or GM-CSF null or GM-CSF receptor null mice, the level of DC in the thymus was found to show only marginal changes with GM-CSF levels or GM-CSF-dependent signals (Vremec *et al.*, 1997). Even the spleen of these mice showed only relatively minor changes in DC levels and a clear dependence on GM-CSF was only apparent amongst the lymph node DC. This contrasts with the striking elevation in DC levels in spleen and thymus when Flt3 ligand is administered to mice (Maraskovsky *et al.*, 1996), as discussed elsewhere in this volume.

Overall, these results suggest that in mice thymic DC are of lymphoid rather than myeloid origin. Arguing by analogy, they also suggest that the related CD8α^+ DEC-205$^+$ CD11c$^-$ DC population found in spleen and at lower levels in lymph nodes is likewise lymphoid derived. The DC precursor studies thus provide a rationale for the incidence of lymphoid markers on thymic DC. However, in view of the lack of direct clonal evidence for a single precursor with both DC and T cell developmental capabilities, the term 'lymphoid-related' is preferable to 'lymphoid-derived'. It remains possible that the intrathymic DC and T lineages are parallel rather than identical pathways at the early precursor level, with the precursors sharing identical surface phenotype. What is clear is that the thymic DC developmental pathway in the mouse differs in many respects from that of myeloid-derived DC.

Some caveats are now in order. As discussed previously, the entry of some migratory DC of different origin from the bloodstream into the thymus has not been ruled out. In addition, many of the above conclusions are based on the reconstitution of the irradiated thymus by precursors selected for T-lineage potential; this may give a strong bias to one type of DC precursor. Other DC precursors and DC developmental pathways not linked to T cell development are not excluded by this data. In particular, E. Donsky and I. Goldschneider (personal communication), studying nonirradiated parabiotic mice, have evidence for thymic DC development from blood-borne precursors that continuously enter the thymus throughout adult life, a development not linked to the intermittent entry of T-lineage precursors. Nevertheless, the predominance of the single CD8α^+ DC type within the thymus (Fig. 2) argues that a single type of DC precursor dominates thymic DC development.

HUMAN THYMIC DENDRITIC CELLS

General

This chapter is based primarily on studies of the rodent thymus, where cell transfer and other experimental procedures are more readily available. Human thymic DC appear similar to those of the mouse in histological sections and their immunological role is believed to be the same. Yet some features of the DC of the human thymus clearly differ from those of the mouse thymus. Studies on DC development and lineage origin in the human thymus are approaching the point where direct comparison can be made with the data from the mouse thymus, but issues such as a lymphoid versus myeloid origin are not yet settled. However, evidence for linkage of T cell and DC development via some form of common intrathymic precursor is emerging; the question is the nature of that precursor. It is of interest that even in the frog, thymic lymphoid cells and thymic accessory DC appear to form a concordant pair, developing from a common precursor (Turpen and Smith, 1986).

Localization, Isolation, Phenotype, Function

In the human thymus, DC are localized in the medulla and cortico-medullary junction, where they are in close contact with T-lineage cells (Pelletier *et al.*, 1986). DC may be isolated from the human thymus in good yield using a procedure basically similar to that used for mouse DC (Winkel *et al.*, 1994). An important difference in technical detail is the antibodies used for immunodepletion. In contrast to the isolation of mouse DC, anti-CD8 and anti-CD2 may be used to remove T lymphoid cells, but anti-CD4 cannot be employed since it is expressed on human thymic DC (Sotzik *et al.*, 1994; Winkel *et al.*, 1994). The isolated DC, if incubated in culture medium for a short period to recover morphological form, have a typical dendritic appearance with numerous cytoplasmic extensions (Fig. 1). In this respect they have a more extreme dendritic form than the corresponding population isolated from the mouse thymus. Like the DC from the mouse thymus, the isolated human thymus DC are efficient at presenting antigen and initiating proliferation of T cells in culture (Sotzik *et al.*, 1994; Winkel *et al.*, 1994; Guéry and Adorini, 1995). Human thymic DC express high levels of class II

MHC and are $CD45RA^+$, ICAM-1^+, LFA-1^+, $B7^+$. They are negative for many macrophage and lymphoid markers, being $CD1^- 2^- 3^- 7^- 14^- 16^- 19^- 56^- 34^-$ and $CD11b^-$ (Sotzik *et al.*, 1994; Winkel *et al.*, 1994; Guéry and Adorini, 1995). These surface markers are in line with the properties of mouse thymic DC. Some discrepancies in the reported surface antigen phenotype of human thymus DC may result from incubation at 37°C, which can upregulate certain markers (such as CD1) and downregulate others (such as CD4); in addition, protease action can strip markers from the DC surface, and selective extraction of particular DC types could bias the analyses. Although earlier reports suggested otherwise, freshly isolated human thymic DC have been shown to express $CD11c^+$ (Winkel *et al.*, 1994), although a proportion of $CD11c^-$ DC are present (Mavaddat, unpublished data); mouse thymic DC are virtually all $CD11c^+$. Likewise, in contrast to earlier reports most freshly isolated human thymus DC are very strongly positive for CD4 (Sotzik *et al.*, 1994; Winkel *et al.*, 1994). Human thymic DC differ most obviously from mouse thymus DC in being mainly $CD4^+ 8^-$ rather than $CD4^- 8^+$ (Winkel *et al.*, 1994); the significance of this difference is not clear. The presence of CD4 on human thymus DC does, however, render these DC susceptible to infection with HIV-1 (Cameron *et al.*, 1996).

Development

The search for committed or partially committed precursors of DC or T cells in the embryonic and infant human thymus is complicated by the likely presence of a form of multipotent stem cell capable of generating all hematopoietic lineages (Shortman and Wu, 1996). A similar situation exists in the embryonic mouse thymus, but not in the adult mouse thymus where multipotent progenitors are at extremely low levels if present at all (Shortman and Wu, 1996). A lymphoid-restricted precursor, able to form DC but not myeloid cells, has been identified in human bone marrow (Galy *et al.*, 1995), but not so far in the human thymus.

It has been possible to generate DC in culture from early precursor populations isolated from the human thymus. Márquez and colleagues (1995) found that culture of $CD34^+$ $CD44^{int}$ thymocytes from post-natal human thymus with IL-7 led to the parallel development of two lineages, one of T-lymphoid cells, the other monocytes plus DC. Both progressed via $CD1^+$ $CD4^+$ intermediate stages, which were separable based on CD44 expression; CD44 expression increased along the monocyte/DC pathway but decreased along the T lymphocyte pathway. Although this suggests an early common T/DC precursor, these may have been separate progenitors from the first. The results differ from those with the mouse in pointing to a linked monocyte–DC myeloid pathway.

Res and colleagues (1996) have isolated a $CD34^+$ $CD38^{lo}$ precursor population from fetal human thymus and demonstrated that these cells differ in surface phenotype from the multipotent stem cells of fetal liver or bone marrow; however, there was no formal test of whether these thymic precursors had lost myeloid developmental potential. This $CD34^+$ $CD38^{lo}$ population showed T precursor activity on transfer into fetal mouse thymus cultures. It also produced either NK cells or DC in culture, depending on the cytokines used. The cloning frequency for each indicated that at least some of these $CD34^+$ 38^{lo} precursors had the capacity to form both cell types. This fits with a linked DC and T cell precursor and a DC origin from a lymphoid precursor, as in the mouse.

However, the possibility that these precursors were multipotent, with the capacity to form all hematopoietic cells including monocytes and granulocytes, has not been excluded; it is significant that the cytokines used to generate the DC were TNF-α, SCF and GM-CSF, a mixture usually used to generate myeloid-related DC and one that does not generate DC from the mouse lymphoid-committed precursor.

In summary, the current evidence indicates that there is a link between T-lineage and DC development in the human as in the mouse thymus, with a common early precursor for both occurring within the thymus. However, this precursor in the human thymus might be multipotent, or at least still able to generate monocytes and macrophages as well as T cells and DC. To date there is no clear evidence that human thymic DC are distinct from the myeloid-related DC generated in culture or found in human peripheral lymphoid organs. Further studies are required to establish whether the lineage origin and developmental pathway of human thymic DC are similar to or differ from that of the mouse. However, much the same can be said at present of human and murine DC in general.

REFERENCES

Ardavin, C. (1997). Thymic dendritic cells. *Immunol. Today* **18**, 350–361.

Ardavin, C., Wu, L., Li, C. and Shortman, K. (1993). Thymic dendritic cells and T cells develop simultaneously within the thymus from a common precursor population. *Nature* **362**, 761–763.

Barclay, A.N. and Mayrhofer, G. (1981). Bone marrow origin of Ia-positive cells in the medulla of rat thymus. *J. Exp. Med.* **153**, 1666–1671.

Boyd, R.L., Tucek, C.L., Godfrey, D.I., Izon, D.J., Wilson, T.J., Davidson, N.J., Bean, A.G., Ladyman, H.M., Ritter, M.A. and Hugo, P. (1993). The thymic microenvironment. *Immunol. Today* **14**, 445–459.

Brocker, T., Riedinger, M. and Karjalainen, K. (1997). Targeted expression of major histocompatibility complex (MHC) class II molecules demonstrates that dendritic cells can induce negative but not positive selection of thymocytes in vivo. *J. Exp. Med.* **185**, 541–550.

Cameron, P.U., Lowe, M.G., Sotzik, F., Coughlan, A.F., Crowe, S.M. and Shortman, K. (1996). The interaction of macrophage and non-macrophage tropic isolates of HIV-1 with thymic and tonsillar dendritic cells in vitro. *J. Exp. Med.* **183**, 1851–1856.

Crowley, M., Inaba, K., Witmer-Pack, M. and Steinman, R.M. (1989). The cell surface of mouse dendritic cells: FACS analysis of dendritic cells from different tissues including thymus. *Cell. Immunol.* **118**, 108–125.

Duijvestijn, A.M. and Barclay, A.N. (1984). Identification of the bone marrow derived Ia positive cells in the rat thymus: a morphological and cytochemical study. *J. Leukocyte Biol.* **36**, 561–568.

French, L.E., Wilson, A., Hahne, M., Viard, I., Tschopp, J. and MacDonald, H.R. (1997). Fas ligand expression is restricted to nonlymphoid thymic components in situ. *J. Immunol.* **159**, 2196–2202.

Galy, A., Travis, M., Cen, D. and Chen, B. (1995). Human T, B, natural killer and dendritic cells arise from a common bone marrow progenitor subset. *Immunity* **3**, 459–473.

Guéry, J.-C. and Adorini, L. (1995). Dendritic cells are the most efficient in presenting endogenous naturally processed self-epitopes to class II-restricted T cells. *J. Immunol.* **154**, 536–544.

Kampinga, J., Nieuwenhuis, P., Roser, B. and Aspinall, R. (1990). Differences in turnover between thymic medullary dendritic cells and a subset of cortical macrophages. *J. Immunol.* **145**, 1659–1663.

Kishimoto, H. and Sprent, J. (1997). Negative selection in the thymus includes semimature T cells. *J. Exp. Med.* **185**, 263–271.

Kronin, V., Winkel, K., Süss, G., Kelso, A., Heath, W., Kirberg, J., von Boehmer, H. and Shortman, K. (1996). A subclass of dendritic cells regulates the response of naive CD8 T cells by limiting their IL-2 production. *J. Immunol.* **157**, 3819–3827.

Kronin, V., Vremec, D., Winkel, K., Classon, B.J., Miller, R.G., Mak, T.W., Shortman, K. and Süss, G. (1997). Are $CD8^+$ dendritic cells veto cells? The role of CD8 on dendritic cells in the regulation of CD4 and CD8 T cell responses. *International Immunol.* **9**, 1061–1064.

Kyewski, B.A. (1987). Seeding of thymic microenvironments defined by distinct thymocyte–stromal cell interactions is developmentally controlled. *J. Exp. Med.* **166**, 520–538.

Kyewski, B.A., Rouse, R.V. and Kaplan, H.S. (1982). Thymocyte rosettes: multicellular complexes of lymphocytes and bone marrow-derived stromal cells in the mouse thymus. *Proc. Natl Acad. Sci. USA* **79**, 5646–5650.

Kyewski, B.A., Fathman, C.G. and Rouse, R.V. (1986). Intrathymic presentation of circulating non-MHC antigens by medullary dendritic cells. An antigen-dependent microenvironment for T cell differentiation. *J. Exp. Med.* **163**, 231–246.

Lucas, K., Vremec, D., Wu, L. and Shortman, K. (1998). A linkage between dendritic cell and T-cell development in the mouse thymus: the capacity of sequential T-cell precursors to form dendritic cells in culture. *Dev. Comp. Immunol.*, in press.

MacPherson, G.G., Fossum, S. and Harrison, B. (1989). Properties of lymph-borne (veiled) dendritic cells in culture. II. Expression of the IL-2 receptor: role of GM-CSF. *Immunology* **68**, 108–113.

Maraskovsky, E., Brasel, K., Teepe, M., Roux, E.R., Lyman, S.D., Shortman, K., and McKenna, H.J. (1996). Dramatic increase in the numbers of functionally mature dendritic cells in mice treated with Flt3 ligand: multiple dendritic cell subpopulations identified. *J. Exp. Med.* **184**, 1953–1962.

Márquez, C., Trigueros, C., Fernández, E. and Toribio, M.L. (1995). The development of T and non-T cell lineages from $CD34^+$ human thymic precursors can be traced by the differential expression of CD44. *J. Exp. Med.* **181**, 475–483.

Matsuzaki, Y., Gyotoku, J., Ogawa, M., Nishikawa, S., Katsura, Y., Gachelin, G., and Nakauchi, H. (1993). Characterization of c-kit positive intrathymic stem cells that are restricted to lymphoid differentiation. *J. Exp. Med.* **178**, 1283–1291.

Matzinger, P. and Guerder, S. (1989). Does T-cell tolerance require a dedicated antigen-presenting cell? *Nature* **338**, 74–76.

Pelletier, M., Tautu, C., Landry, D., Montplaisir, S., Chardrand, C. and Perreault, C. (1986). Characterization of human thymic dendritic cells in culture. *Immunology* **58**, 263–270.

Res, P., Martinez-Cáceras, E., Jaleco, A.C., Staal, F., Noteboom, E., Weijer, K., and Spits, H. (1996). $CD34^+$ $CD38^{dim}$ cells in the human thymus can differentiate into T, natural killer, and dendritic cells but are distinct from pluripotent stem cells. *Blood* **87**, 5196–5206.

Saunders, D., Lucas, K., Ismaili, J., Wu, L., Maraskovsky, E., Dunn, A., Metcalf, D., and Shortman, K. (1996). Dendritic cell development in culture from thymic precursor cells in the absence of granulocyte-macrophage colony-stimulating factor. *J. Exp. Med.* **184**, 2185–2196.

Shortman, K. and Vremec, D. (1991). Different subpopulations of developing thymocytes are associated with adherent (macrophage) or non-adherent (dendritic) thymic rosettes. *Dev. Immunol.* **1**, 225–235.

Shortman, K. and Wu, L. (1996). Early T lymphocyte progenitors. *Annu. Rev. Immunol.* **14**, 29–47.

Shortman, K., Vremec, D., D'Amico, A., Battye, F. and Boyd, R. (1989). Nature of the thymocytes associated with dendritic cells and macrophages in thymic rosettes. *Cell. Immunol.* **119**, 85–100.

Shortman, K., Wu, L., Ardavin, C., Vremec, D., Sotzik, S., Winkel, K. and Süss, G. (1995). Thymic dendritic cells: surface phenotype, developmental origin and function. In *Dendritic Cells in Fundamental & Cinical Immunology* (eds J. Banchereau and D. Schmitt), Plenum, New York, pp. 21–29.

Sotzik, F., Rosenberg, Y., Boyd, A.W., Honeyman, M., Metcalf, D., Scollay, R., Wu, L. and Shortman, K. (1994). Assessment of CD4 expression by early T-precursor cells and by dendritic cells in the human thymus. *J. Immunol.* **152**, 3370–3377.

Sprent, J. and Webb, S.R. (1995). Intrathymic and extrathymic clonal deletion of T cells. *Curr. Opin. Immunol.* **7**, 196–205.

Steinman, R.M., Pack, M. and Inaba, K. (1997). Dendritic cells in the T-cell areas of lymphoid organs. *Immunol. Rev.* **156**, 25–37.

Stockinger, B. and Hausmann, B. (1994). Functional recognition of in vivo processed self antigen. *Int. Immunol.* **6**, 247–254.

Süss, G. and Shortman, K. (1996). A subclass of dendritic cells kills CD4 T cells via Fas/Fas-ligand-induced apoptosis. *J. Exp. Med.* **183**, 1789–1796.

Tanaka, Y., Mamalaki, C., Stockinger, B. and Kioussis, D. (1993). In vitro negative selection of $\alpha\beta$ T cell receptor transgenic thymocytes by conditionally immortalized thymic cortical epithelial cell lines and dendritic cells. *Eur. J. Immunol.* **23**, 2614–2621.

Turpen, J.B. and Smith, P.B. (1986). Analysis of hemopoietic lineage of accessory cells in the developing thymus of *Xenopus laevis. J. Immunol.* **136**, 412–421.

Vremec, D. and Shortman, K. (1997). Dendritic cell subtypes in mouse lymphoid organs: cross-correlation of surface markers, changes on incubation and differences between thymus, spleen and lymph nodes. *J. Immunol.* **159**, 565–573.

Vremec, D., Lieschke, G.J., Dunn, A.R., Robb, L., Metcalf, D. and Shortman, K. (1997). The influence of granulocyte/macrophage colony-stimulating factor on dendritic cell levels in mouse lymphoid organs. *Eur. J. Immunol.* **27**, 40–44.

Vremec, D., Zorbas, M., Scollay, R., Saunders, D.J., Ardavin, C.F., Wu, L. and Shortman, K. (1992). The surface phenotype of dendritic cells purified from mouse thymus and spleen: investigation of the CD8 expression by a subpopulation of dendritic cells. *J. Exp. Med.* **176**, 47–58.

Winkel, K., Sotzik, F., Vremec, D., Cameron, P.U. and Shortman, K. (1994). CD4 and CD8 expression by human and mouse thymic dendritic cells. *Immunol. Lett.* **40**, 93–99.

Winkel, K.D., Kronin, V., Krummel, M.F. and Shortman, K. (1997). The nature of the signals regulating CD8 T cell proliferative responses to CD8α^{+} or CD8α^{-} dendritic cells. *Eur. J. Immunol.* **27**, 3350–3359.

Witmer-Pack, M.D., Swiggard, W.J., Mirza, A., Inaba, K. and Steinman, R.M. (1995). Tissue distribution of the DEC-205 protein that is detected by the monoclonal antibody NLDC-145. II. Expression *in situ* in lymphoid and nonlymphoid tissues. *Cell. Immunol.* **163**, 157–162.

Wu, L., Antica, M., Johnson, G.R., Scollay, R. and Shortman, K. (1991a). Developmental potential of the earliest precursor cells from the adult thymus. *J. Exp. Med.* **174**, 1617–1627.

Wu, L., Scollay, R., Egerton, M., Pearse, M., Spangrude, G.J. and Shortman, K. (1991b). CD4 expressed on earliest T-lineage precursor cells in the adult murine thymus. *Nature* **349**, 71–74.

Wu, L., Vremec, D., Ardavin, C., Winkel, K., Suss, G., Georgiou, H., Maraskovsky, E., Cook, W. and Shortman, K. (1995). Mouse thymus dendritic cells: kinetics of development and changes in surface markers during maturation. *Eur. J. Immunol.* **25**, 418–425.

Wu, L., Li, C.-L. and Shortman, K. (1996). Thymic dendritic cell precursors: relationship to the T-lymphocyte lineage and phenotype of the dendritic cell progeny. *J. Exp. Med.* **184**, 903–911.

CHAPTER 3
Cell Fate Development in the Myeloid System

James W. Young
Division of Hematologic Oncology, Department of Medicine, Memorial Sloan-Kettering Cancer Center, New York, New York, USA

INTRODUCTION

Hematopoiesis is the regulated development of leukocytes, erythrocytes, and platelets from both primitive stem cells and downstream progenitors. Stem cells are operationally defined as those most primitive, uncommitted progenitors with a unique capacity for long-term self-renewal and an ability to reconstitute hematopoiesis in a lethally irradiated host. Stem cells, as well as the earliest clonogenic progenitors, are pluripotent insofar as lineage commitment is not yet determined and differentiation can still occur along multiple alternative pathways. Self-renewal vs differentiation of stem cells and early progenitors is a stochastic, or random process (Moore, 1991; Ogawa, 1995). As cell division proceeds, clonogenic capacity, or the ability to form hematopoietic colonies, declines, and lineage restriction becomes increasingly specific. This process of survival, proliferation, lineage specificity, and terminal differentiation is regulated by many different cytokines, both stimulatory and/or inhibitory, acting at many different stages of hematopoiesis (Moore, 1991).

Bone marrow is the principal repository of hematopoiesis in the normal adult, where bulk progenitors are readily identified by the expression of CD34. Within the CD34$^+$ compartment the earliest progenitors (long-term culture-initiating cells, LTC-IC) lack CD38 and class II MHC (Sutherland *et al.*, 1989; Terstappen *et al.*, 1991; Civin, 1990), as well as the CD33 epitope which characterizes commitment toward myeloid differentiation (Civin, 1990). Other accessible sources of sizable populations of CD34 cells include placental and umbilical cord blood, as well as cytokine-stimulated or cytokine-elicited peripheral blood (commonly termed peripheral blood stem cells, or PBSC).

Dendritic cells represent a distinct pathway of myeloid differentiation in all human and animal models studied, although human dendritic cells are the focus of this chapter. Within the myeloid system, there is emerging evidence that dendritic cells which terminally differentiate along different pathways perform distinct functions. There is also evidence of a dendritic cell precursor shared with lymphocytes (Galy *et al.*, 1995; Saunders *et al.*, 1996; Grouard *et al.*, 1997; Vremec and Shortman, 1997), the dendritic cell progeny of which may be important in central and peripheral tolerance; the reader is referred to the respective chapters for further information.

Dendritic Cells: Biology and Clinical Applications
ISBN 0-12-455860-7

DENDRITIC CELLS CONSTITUTE A DISTINCT PATHWAY FOR MYELOID DIFFERENTIATION

The bone marrow origin of dendritic cells was first demonstrated in transplant chimeras soon after their original discovery by Steinman in the mouse (Steinman *et al.*, 1974; Katz *et al.*, 1979; Pugh *et al.*, 1983; Volc-Platzer *et al.*, 1984). These dendritic cells proved to be myeloid rather than lymphoid, notwithstanding recent evidence for the latter (Galy *et al.*, 1995; Saunders *et al.*, 1996; Grouard *et al.*, 1997; Vremec and Shortman, 1997). Myeloid dendritic cells lack lymphocyte antigen receptors and rearrange neither Ig nor T cell receptor genes (Kampgen *et al.*, 1994). As do macrophages and granulocytes, dendritic cells also maintain expression of CD33 (Thomas *et al.*, 1993), an epitope that characterizes the earliest myeloid commitment of CD34 precursors. Like all other myeloid cells, dendritic cells are responsive to GM-CSF. However, dendritic cells do not respond to the more lineage-restricted macrophage and granulocyte colony-stimulating factors, M-CSF and G-CSF; and a dendritic cell-specific cytokine per se has not yet been identified.

The distinction of mature dendritic cells from mononuclear and polymorphonuclear phagocytes is made on the basis of their unusual morphology and motility *in vitro* and *in vivo*; the abundance of costimulatory, adhesive, and MHC molecules; and their extreme potency in initiating T cell proliferative and cytolytic responses (Flechner *et al.*, 1988; Young and Steinman, 1988; Freudenthal and Steinman, 1990; Young and Steinman, 1990; Inaba *et al.*, 1987; O'Doherty *et al.*, 1993; Steinman, 1991; Hart, 1997; Steinman, 1997; Banchereau and Steinman, 1998). Mature dendritic cells also lack CD14, a receptor that is more abundant on macrophages and some granulocytes and which mediates the response of phagocytes to complexes of lipopolysaccharide (LPS) and LPS binding protein (Wright *et al.*, 1990). Dendritic cells have few receptors for immune complexes or C3 and its fragments, although low levels of CD32 and CD11b can be found on immature forms. Lastly, mature dendritic cells have usually not been reported to have myeloperoxidase and lysozyme, enzymes that support the phagocytic activity of other myeloid populations. Therefore, in general, the pathway of myeloid dendritic cell differentiation relinquishes the phagocytic properties shared to some extent with macrophages in particular, in exchange for the very high levels of MHC and accessory molecules that support dendritic cells' efficient antigen presentation and costimulation of quiescent T cells (Reis e Sousa *et al.*, 1993; Romani *et al.*, 1989; Koch *et al.*, 1995; Witmer-Pack *et al.*, 1987; Heufler *et al.*, 1988).

PROLIFERATING DENDRITIC CELL PRECURSORS IN SUSPENSION CULTURES

The first reports of dendritic cell development in the early 1990s used GM-CSF with or without additional cytokines, notably TNF-α, and demonstrated that dendritic cells developed alongside macrophages and granulocytes (Reid *et al.*, 1990; Caux *et al.*, 1992; Reid *et al.*, 1992; Santiago-Schwarz *et al.*, 1992). This was true in both murine and human systems, although exogenous TNF-α has never proved to be as critical in murine as in human cultures, presumably because of sufficient endogenous production. TNF-α has pleotropic effects on hematopoiesis and was of interest in dendritic cell development for several reasons. TNF-α has been shown to recruit primitive, transferrin receptor (TfR)-negative progenitors to become TfR positive and responsive to other growth factors like IL-3 and GM-CSF (Caux *et al.*, 1993). TNF-α mediates the latter effect directly, at least in part, because it downmodulates receptors for some of the more lineage-restricted cytokines, while increasing receptors for GM-CSF (Jacobsen *et al.*, 1992; Moore, 1991; Shieh *et al.*, 1989; Shieh *et al.*, 1991; Caux *et al.*, 1990; Caux *et al.*, 1991), to which myeloid dendritic cells are universally responsive.

Murine studies pioneered by Inaba and colleagues identified class II MHC-negative precursors in both blood (Inaba *et al.*, 1992b) and marrow (Inaba *et al.*, 1992a) that proliferated and differentiated into dendritic cells, granulocytes, and macrophages in the presence of GM-CSF. After nonadherent granulocytes were washed away early in these cultures, proliferating clusters that released large numbers of nonadherent dendritic cells could be enriched away from macrophages, which remained adherent to tissue culture plastic. These Ia-negative precursors were far more abundant in marrow than blood. Approximately five million dendritic cells could be generated from the marrow of two murine femurs over 7–8 days' culture (Inaba *et al.*, 1992a).

The murine dendritic cell progeny that developed under these *in vitro* conditions displayed typical motile, sheet-like cytoplasmic veils or processes, with abundant class II MHC molecules and the usual complement of other surface markers. The dendritic cells were also notably potent stimulators of resting T cells, and even more compelling was their capacity to migrate and home to T cell regions in draining lymph nodes. The growth of these dendritic cells was not supported by other lineage-specific factors like G-CSF and M-CSF, nor could the commitment to terminal dendritic cell differentiation be reversed.

Although the first indication that a human progenitor for dendritic cells could be expanded *in vitro* was based on clonogenic assays (Reid *et al.*, 1990; see below), most of the early human work used suspension cultures of $CD34^+$ cells in the presence of defined cytokines (Reid *et al.*, 1992; Caux *et al.*, 1992; Santiago-Schwarz *et al.*, 1992). Starting with bulk or $CD34^+$ enriched populations of cord blood cells, investigators showed that mixtures of macrophages and dendritic cells were generated after 2–3 weeks' culture in GM-CSF and TNF-α (Santiago-Schwarz *et al.*, 1992). Although as many as 40% of these cells displayed some characteristics of dendritic cells, they were not potent stimulators of T cell responses. Caux and colleagues further detailed the generation of dendritic cells from $CD34^+$ precursors, also in cord blood and under the aegis of GM-CSF and TNF-α (Caux *et al.*, 1992). Candidate dendritic cells, which numbered between 20% and 50% of the progeny, were identified by their characteristic stellate morphology, array of typical surface epitopes (e.g., CD80/86, CD11a, CD18, CD54, class II MHC), and potent stimulatory capacity for quiescent allogeneic $CD4^+$ T cells. At least 20% of the progeny also had identifiable Birbeck granules which characterize Langerhans cells.

Large numbers of dendritic cells have also been generated in liquid cultures of $CD34^+$ cells from normal human bone marrow (Szabolcs *et al.*, 1995), which is the principal repository of hematopoietic function in adults. Dendritic cells, macrophages, and granulocytes (principally eosinophilic precursors owing to the effects of GM-CSF), developed in the same cultures with GM-CSF and TNF-α. The addition of c-*kit* ligand, or stem cell factor, increased expansion 10- to 15-fold over that achieved by GM-CSF and TNF-α alone, but did not directly influence dendritic cell differentiation per se. It did permit more detailed phenotypic and functional assessments of dendritic cell progeny than had previously been feasible. Approximately 50% of the $CD34^+$ progeny were class II MHC positive under these conditions, including both adherent $CD14^+$ macrophages and nonadherent $CD14^-$ dendritic cells in a ratio of approximately 4:1. This nevertheless represented a substantial expansion of dendritic cells, with absolute yields from 5 to 10 ml of cellular bone marrow, approximating the usual steady-state yield of $\sim 10^6$ dendritic cells from a 450–500 ml unit of peripheral blood.

Dendritic cells that terminally differentiated during 2 weeks' culture could therefore be sorted cytofluorographically with respect to the presence or absence of CD14 among the class II MHC-positive progeny. Only the cells in the $CD14^-$ HLA-$DR^{++/+++}$ fraction were nonadherent, motile, and had the cytologic and phenotypic features of dendritic cells (Szabolcs *et al.*, 1995). In the critical test of potent immunostimulatory function, dendritic cells exceeded the stimulatory capacity of the sorted $CD14^+$/HLA-DR^+ macrophages by at least 1.5 to 2 logs.

A DISTINCT CLONOGENIC CD34⁺ PROGENITOR OF HUMAN DENDRITIC CELLS

Bulk Cultures of Murine Ia Negative Progenitors

The development of murine dendritic cells was followed in clonogenic assays using class II MHC-negative precursors in bone marrow (Inaba *et al.*, 1993a). GM-CSF-supported colonies were individually plucked, disrupted, and enriched for each of the respective myeloid cell types found in the colonies, i.e., granulocytes, macrophages, and dendritic cells. Neither exogenous TNF nor IL-4 was added to these cultures. Dendritic cell progeny displayed the usual veiled cytoplasmic morphology, expressed abundant class II MHC, lacked macrophage and granulocyte-specific markers, and potently stimulated resting allogeneic T cells in the mixed leukocyte reaction. Although dendritic cells constituted only 0.5–1.5% of the myeloid progeny, this was proportional to dendritic cell representation in most sites where myeloid cells are found *in vivo*, just as it was for the macrophage and granulocyte progeny.

Clonogenic Cultures of Bulk Human CD34⁺ Progenitors

Evidence that a human progenitor for dendritic cells could be expanded *in vitro* was first reported by Reid *et al.* in 1990, using unselected precursors from bone marrow and the peripheral blood of patients recovering from chemotherapy (Reid *et al.*, 1990). Mixed colonies of macrophages and dendritic cells grew in the presence of lectin-conditioned medium which likely contained GM-CSF and other active cytokines. These investigators subsequently demonstrated that the human dendritic cell precursor in bone marrow was in fact $CD34^+$ and responsive to GM-CSF and TNF-α under serum-free conditions (Reid *et al.*, 1992). Unselected bulk bone marrow mononuclear cells generated rare candidate colonies of dendritic cells only. However, their identification was based only on morphology and CD1a expression, and the cloning efficiency was $<0.05\%$. To the extent that cytokines like GM-CSF can induce CD1 expression on monocytes (Kasinrerk *et al.*, 1993), CD1 is not always specific for dendritic or Langerhans cells. Limited cell yields did not permit further phenotyping or functional assays in these earliest studies.

Capitalizing on the contribution of an early-acting cytokine like c-*kit* ligand (stem cell factor) in synergy with GM-CSF and TNF-α, a CD34$^+$ clonogenic progenitor (CFU-DC) of pure human dendritic cell colonies was discovered (Fig. 1) (Young *et al.*, 1995). c-*kit* Ligand supported about a 2-fold increase in primary cloning efficiency, but expanded CFU-DC almost 100-fold over 14 days as documented in secondary clonogenic assays. c-*kit* Ligand did not directly affect dendritic cell differentiation, however. The progeny recovered from CFU-DC-derived colonies were typical dendritic cells: nonadherent and motile when resuspended and transferred to liquid culture; pronounced cytoplasmic veil-like projections or lamellopodia; absent CD14 but intense expression of HLA-DR; and potent allostimulatory activity comparable to that effected by mature blood dendritic cells.

CFU-GM-derived colonies also developed when bone marrow CD34$^+$ progenitors were cultured with GM-CSF and TNF-α. These were in addition to CFU-DC-derived colonies. However, in contrast to GM colonies grown in the presence of GM-CSF only, which contained no dendritic cells, those GM colonies grown under conditions supporting CFU-DC expansion in the same cultures included 1% dendritic cells with the same features of CFU-DC progeny. These particular GM colonies were therefore similar to those identified in the mouse (Inaba *et al.*, 1993a). This trace representation of dendritic cells in mixed myeloid colonies is again comparable to their proportion among myeloid cells in most resident sites *in vivo*. This finding also supports a common ancestry for these particular dendritic cells and other myeloid populations. It further highlights the capacity of exogenous cytokines, TNF-α in this case, to alter the otherwise stochastic hematopoietic process. The solely dendritic cell-committed pathway may contribute dendritic cells to sites like the epidermis, afferent lymph, and T cell areas of lymphoid

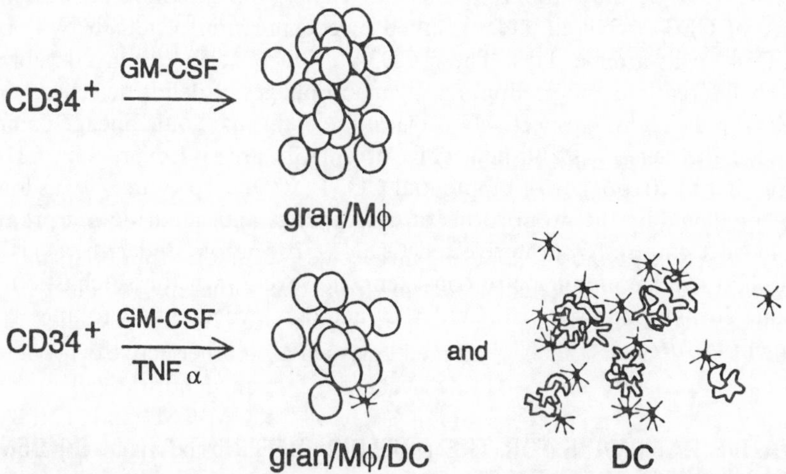

Fig. 1. The addition of TNF-α to GM-CSF supports the development of pure human dendritic cell colonies, in addition to typical GM colonies. Note the trace presence of dendritic cells in the GM colonies that develop in the presence of GM-CSF and TNF-α, alongside the pure dendritic cell colonies. The progeny developing in CFU-DC-derived colonies are maturing asynchronously, as illustrated by the variation in cell morphology. GM colonies that develop in GM-CSF alone, without TNF-α, contain no dendritic cells. Modified from Young *et al.* (1995).

organs where dendritic cells are the principal myeloid cell type, but this point remains hypothetical at this time.

Dendritic Cell Commitment at the Level of CD34⁺ Progenitors

Although hematopoiesis is a stochastic, or random process, ample evidence has already been presented that this process can be biased or frankly skewed by hematopoietic cytokines *in vitro*. Investigators have also usually considered different types of dendritic cells to represent no more than different stages of maturation. However, the definition of myeloid (Caux *et al.*, 1992; Szabolcs *et al.*, 1995; Strunk *et al.*, 1996; Grouard *et al.*, 1996) vs lymphoid dendritic cells (Galy *et al.*, 1995; Saunders *et al.*, 1996; Vremec and Shortman, 1997; Grouard *et al.*, 1997), epidermal/Langerhans vs dermal dendritic cells (Caux *et al.*, 1996a; Caux *et al.*, 1997; de Saint-Vis *et al.*, 1998), dendritic cells in germinal centers (Grouard *et al.*, 1996) vs those in the T cell-enriched parafollicular areas of secondary lymphoid tissues (Grouard *et al.*, 1997), and so on, all support very real heterogeneity within the dendritic cell lineage.

Accordingly, studies have recently searched for lineage commitment even at the level of $CD34^+$ progenitors. Strunk and colleagues demonstrated that $CD34^+$ cells in the circulation could be segregated into CLA^+, $CD45RA^+$, CD71 low vs CLA^-, CD45RA low, $CD71^+$ subsets (Strunk *et al.*, 1997). While both starting populations could develop into $CD1a^+$, HLA-DR bright dendritic cells when supplemented with GM-CSF and TNF-α, only those derived from the $CD34^+$, CLA^+ subset were continuously motile during culture, expressed Lag, and contained Birbeck granules of Langerhans cells.

Another group has recently reported that coexpression of CD86 by bone marrow $CD34^+$ precursors is regulated by TNF-α (Ryncarz and Anasetti, 1998). Without prior exposure to TNF-α, only about 3% of the $CD34^+$ precursors coexpressed CD86. Preculture of $CD34^+$ cells in TNF resulted in coexpression of CD86 by about 15% of the $CD34^+$ cells after 6 days. These $CD34^+$, $CD86^+$ cells displayed a bipotential capacity to differentiate into predominantly macrophages or dendritic cells in GM-CSF or GM-CSF plus TNFα, respectively, suggesting again that some lineage commitment toward dendritic cells is established while precursors are still expressing CD34. It is interesting that the frequency of bipotential $CD34^+$, $CD86^+$ precursors was lower than would be predicted by the proportions of macrophage and dendritic cell progeny that develop in bulk cultures from unselected $CD34^+$ progenitors under the aegis of GM-CSF and TNF-α. The findings are consistent, however, with the stochastic nature of steady-state hematopoiesis *in vivo* and the fact that exogenous cytokines can skew development *in vitro*.

ALTERNATIVE PATHWAYS FOR THE MYELOID DIFFERENTIATION OF DENDRITIC CELLS FROM CD34⁺ PRECURSORS

Macrophages and Dendritic Cells (Fig. 2A)

Two groups, one using bone marrow (Szabolcs *et al.*, 1996) and the other using cord blood (Caux *et al.*, 1996a), have independently defined two pathways by which dendritic cells may develop. After 4–5 days', and certainly by 6 days' culture of bone marrow CD34$^+$ cells in exogenous c-*kit* ligand, GM-CSF, TNF-α, and FCS-based medium, HLA-DR$^+$ populations could be distinguished based on the presence or absence of CD14. Cells that coexpressed CD14, HLA-DR, and CD115 (c-*fms* or M-CSF receptor), ordinarily a macrophage phenotype, persisted despite depletion of already matured macrophages. Whereas the CD14$^-$, HLA-DR bright cells were typical dendritic cells in morphology, phenotype, and function, the other population of CD14$^+$, HLA-DR$^+$, c-*fms*$^+$ cells exhibited mixed stimulatory, phagocytic, and phenotypic properties characteristic of a sort of *forme fruste* for both macrophages and dendritic cells. Reculture of the CD14$^+$ HLA-DR$^+$ intermediates in GM-CSF and TNF-α terminally differentiated these cells into CD14$^-$, HLA-DR bright, c-*fms*$^-$, CD86 bright dendritic cells. Reculture of the same cells in M-CSF or medium alone without cytokines generated CD14$^+$ macrophages. This CD14$^+$ HLA-DR$^+$ intermediate cell therefore had bipotential differentiation capacity, dependent on the subsequent cytokine milieu. Terminal differentiation could not be reversed, and cells of the same CD14$^+$ HLA-DR$^+$ phenotype isolated beyond 6–7 days of culture were already macrophage-committed and no longer bipotential.

Caux and colleagues used the mutually exclusive expression of CD1a and CD14 to define a bipotential intermediate that developed by day 5 from cord blood CD34$^+$ precursors which were also cultured in FCS-based medium with GM-CSF, TNF-α, and c-*kit* ligand (Caux *et al.*, 1996a). GM-CSF, but not TNF-α, proved critical in this system to the subsequent differentiation of both CD1a$^-$, CD14$^+$ and CD1a$^+$, CD14$^-$ intermediates. Both populations recultured in GM-CSF generated CD1a$^+$, CD14$^-$ progeny. However, the progeny of each type of intermediate precursor could be distinguished from the other. Those that arose from CD1a$^-$, CD14$^+$ intermediates lacked Birbeck granules and expressed other markers typical of dermal dendritic cells (factor XIIIa, CD2, CD9, CD68), whereas those arising from CD1a$^+$, CD14$^-$ intermediates were typical epidermal dendritic/Langerhans cells with Birbeck granules, the Lag antigen, and E-cadherin.

This group further distinguished these two types of progeny functionally (Caux *et al.*, 1997). CD14-derived dermal dendritic cells maintained efficient antigen capture via receptors for mannose polymers, and this activity corresponded to expression of nonspecific esterase. In contrast, the phagocytic activity of dendritic cells derived from CD14$^-$, CD1a$^+$ intermediates was restricted to the immature stage, and these progeny never expressed nonspecific esterase. Furthermore, only the CD14-derived dermal dendritic cells could induce resting B cells to secrete IgM in response to IL-2 and activation via CD40. The two types of dendritic cells also had different patterns of cytokine expression, as well as distinct activation pathways for inducing cytokine secretion (de Saint-Vis *et al.*, 1998). A notable finding was that only the dermal dendritic cells derived from CD14$^+$ intermediates secreted IL-10, an important immunoregulatory cytokine (see below), in response to activation through CD40.

It is likely that the CD14$^+$ immunostimulatory progeny originally reported by Egner and Hart in 7-day bone marrow cultures (Egner and Hart, 1995) may have corresponded to the CD14$^+$ intermediates described above (Szabolcs *et al.*, 1996; Caux *et al.*, 1996a). However, the bipotential differentiation capacity and relation to other myeloid progeny, specifically macrophages, were not investigated. It is also plausible that the nondividing mononuclear cell precursor in peripheral blood, which is responsive to GM-CSF and IL-4

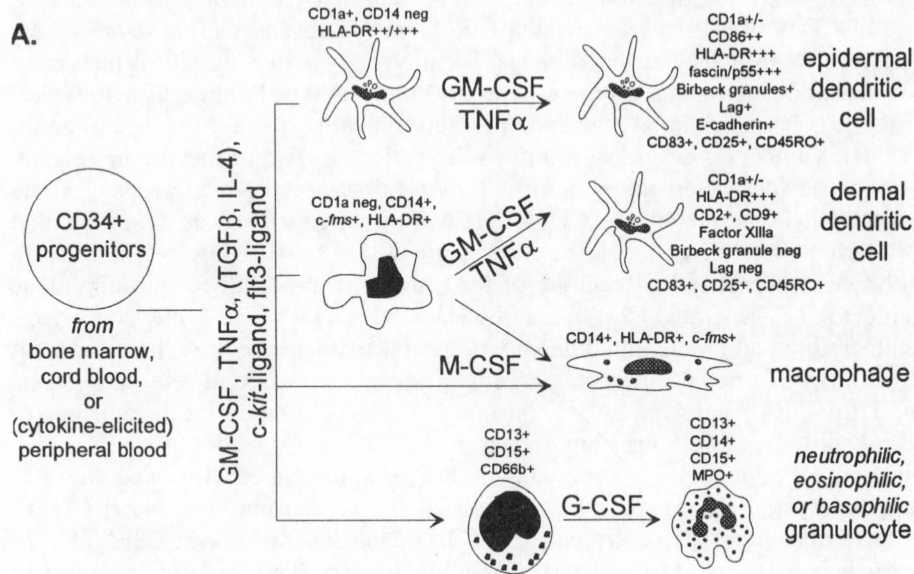
A.
CD34+
progenitors
from
bone marrow,
cord blood,
or
(cytokine-elicited)
peripheral blood
GM-CSF, TNFα, (TGFβ, IL-4), c-kit-ligand, flt3-ligand
CD1a+, CD14 neg
HLA-DR++/+++
GM-CSF
TNFα
CD1a+/-
CD86++
HLA-DR+++
fascin/p55+++
Birbeck granules+
Lag+
E-cadherin+
CD83+, CD25+, CD45RO+
epidermal
dendritic
cell
CD1a neg, CD14+,
c-fms+, HLA-DR+
GM-CSF
TNFα
CD1a+/-
HLA-DR+++
CD2+, CD9+
Factor XIIIa
Birbeck granule neg
Lag neg
CD83+, CD25+, CD45RO+
dermal
dendritic
cell
M-CSF
CD14+, HLA-DR+, c-fms+
macrophage
CD13+
CD15+
CD66b+
G-CSF
CD13+
CD14+
CD15+
MPO+
neutrophilic,
eosinophilic,
or basophilic
granulocyte

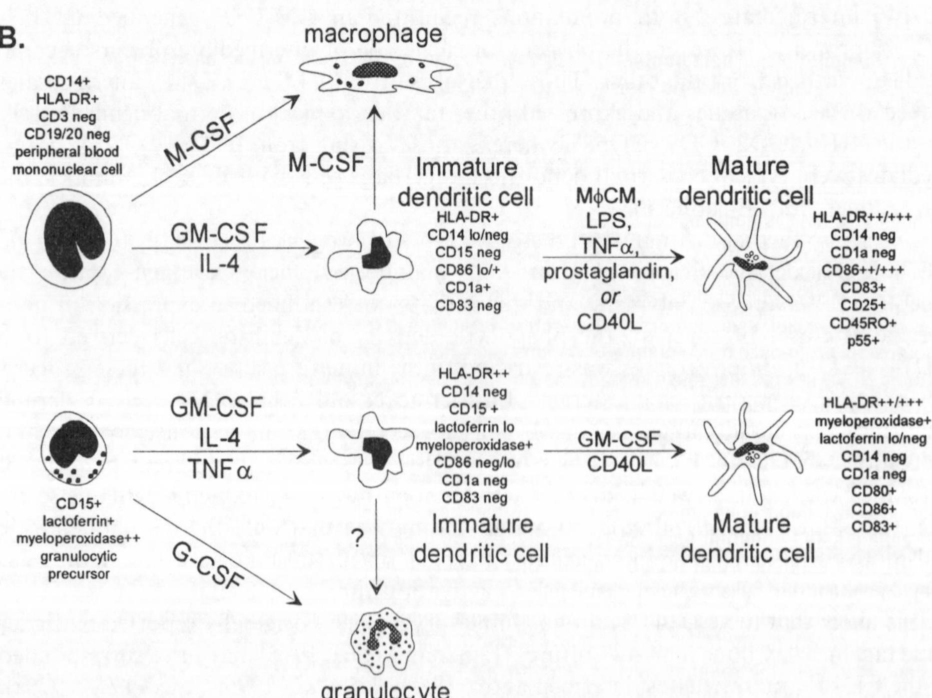
B.
CD14+
HLA-DR+
CD3 neg
CD19/20 neg
peripheral blood
mononuclear cell
M-CSF
macrophage
M-CSF
GM-CSF
IL-4
Immature
dendritic cell
HLA-DR+
CD14 lo/neg
CD15 neg
CD86 lo/+
CD1a+
CD83 neg
MφCM,
LPS,
TNFα,
prostaglandin,
or
CD40L
Mature
dendritic cell
HLA-DR++/+++
CD14 neg
CD1a neg
CD86++/+++
CD83+
CD25+
CD45RO+
p55+
CD15+
lactoferrin+
myeloperoxidase++
granulocytic
precursor
GM-CSF
IL-4
TNFα
HLA-DR++
CD14 neg
CD15 +
lactoferrin lo
myeloperoxidase+
CD86 neg/lo
CD1a neg
CD83 neg
GM-CSF
CD40L
HLA-DR++/+++
myeloperoxidase+
lactoferrin lo/neg
CD14 neg
CD1a neg
CD80+
CD86+
CD83+
Immature
dendritic cell
Mature
dendritic cell
?
G-CSF
granulocyte

in generating dendritic cells (Sallusto and Lanzavecchia, 1994; Romani *et al.*, 1994; Bender *et al.*, 1996; Romani *et al.*, 1996; see below) corresponds to these $CD14^+$ intermediates. In fact, Bender and colleagues noted that the $CD14^+$ fraction of fresh peripheral blood mononuclear cells was relatively enriched in precursors responsive to GM-CSF and IL-4 (Bender *et al.*, 1996), and CD14 and c-*fms* expression were lost with dendritic cell differentiation (Bender *et al.*, 1996; Romani *et al.*, 1996). Experiments are in progress to define more precisely the relationships between intermediate cells and terminally differentiated progeny with respect to clonogenic progenitors, and to determine the extent to which the frequency of these CFUs, especially CFU-DCs, varies between umbilical cord and placental blood, bone marrow, and cytokine-elicited peripheral blood.

Granulocytes and Dendritic Cells (Fig. 2B)

In all of these culture systems, granulocytes are the principal other myeloid cells that develop, especially eosinophilic precursors reflecting the influence of GM-CSF. Pertinent to the granulocytes that develop in these cultures is a recent report by Knapp and colleagues demonstrating a reversal in the maturation of polymorphonuclear leukocytes (PMNs) to become candidate dendritic cells instead (Oehler *et al.*, 1998). By isolating $CD15^+$, lactoferrin-positive, proximate precursors to PMNs obtained from patients with chronic myelogenous leukemia or infection-induced leukocytosis, and

---

Fig. 2. Compilation of hematopoietic pathways for the development of human dendritic cells: (A) from $CD34^+$ progenitors in bone marrow, peripheral blood, or placental and umbilical cord blood; or (B) from peripheral blood, nondividing precursors. This schematic representation is intended to summarize the starting populations, intermediate precursors, critical cytokines, and progeny that develop in *ex vivo* cultures for the generation of dendritic cells, recognizing that there is not complete concordance between the results reported by all groups. Although there is some overlap with rodent models, the human system is emphasized here.

In (A) note that the two pathways for generation of dendritic cells have been defined both in bone marrow (Szabolcs *et al.*, 1996) and in cord blood (Caux *et al.*, 1996a), although the dendritic cell progeny have been more readily distinguished from each other in studies using cord blood (Caux *et al.*, 1997; de Saint-Vis *et al.*, 1998). Investigators have reported variations in the degree of maturation reported for the dendritic cell progeny in these cultures. Markers like CD83, CD25, and CD45RO increase with maturation, whereas CD1a decreases; these phenotypic changes can be asynchronous. Terminal maturation signals, such as those provided via CD40L:CD40 interactions (Caux *et al.*, 1994b; Flores-Romo *et al.*, 1997), may be necessary under some conditions. In bulk cultures of $CD34^+$ precursors, dendritic cells develop alongside macrophages and granulocytes, especially eosinophilic precursors owing to the effects of GM-CSF, the receptor for which shares a common β chain with the IL-5-R. CD34 subsets have also been reported that exhibit commitment toward epidermal Langerhans cells (Strunk *et al.*, 1997), or toward macrophages and dendritic cells via the bipotential, $CD14^+$ intermediate (Ryncarz and Anasetti, 1998).

In (B), note especially that terminal maturation is necessary to achieve stable and irreversible differentiation of dendritic cells from peripheral blood mononuclear cells. To date, in the absence of fetal calf serum, this maturation is best driven by macrophage-conditioned medium. Single factors like TNF-α have not been adequate to support terminal maturation in the absence of fetal calf serum-containing medium. Also note the recently described pathway from granulocytic precursors (Oehler *et al.*, 1998). The bipotential capacity of this intermediate or immature dendritic cell has not been definitively proven, nor have any similarities been established between this intermediate and that which develops from $CD34^+$ progenitors. Modified from Sallusto and Lanzavecchia (1994); Romani *et al.*, 1994; Zhou and Tedder 1996; Romani *et al.*, 1996; Bender *et al.* (1996); Oehler *et al.* (1998).

then culturing in GM-CSF, IL-4, and TNF-α, these investigators were able to generate cells with allostimulatory function and some phenotypic characteristic of dendritic cells. Terminal differentiation and expression of CD83, as well as increased expression of CD80, CD86, and HLA-DR, however, required stimulation by CD40L. This is the first report of yet another myeloid differentiation pathway by which dendritic cells can develop, in this case in relation to granulocytes. The extent to which this pathway is physiologically operative in normal humans, however, is unknown.

IMMATURE, CYTOKINE-RESPONSIVE DENDRITIC CELL PRECURSORS IN HUMAN PERIPHERAL BLOOD (Fig. 2B)

Studies of murine epidermal Langerhans cells first clarified that dendritic cells were not simply a widely distributed system of active antigen-presenting cells (APCs). These experiments demonstrated that typical mature, immunostimulatory dendritic cells could develop from immature precursors under the influence of keratinocyte-conditioned medium, and more specifically GM-CSF (Witmer-Pack *et al.*, 1987; Heufler *et al.*, 1988). IL-1 could further enhance maturation when used in combination with GM-CSF (Heufler *et al.*, 1988). Comparable maturation events occur *in vivo*. For example, when skin is transplanted, the Langerhans cells leave the skin to enter the afferent lymph (Larsen *et al.*, 1990; Lukas *et al.*, 1996). Human skin explant cultures have also demonstrated that Langerhans cell emigrate from the skin into the medium, upregulating MHC products, adhesion molecules, and costimulatory ligands in the process (Demarchi *et al.*, 1992). This has led to the concept that Langerhans cells first capture and process antigens while actively synthesizing MHC molecules. Large numbers of MHC–peptide complexes therefore form during dendritic cell maturation, entry into the afferent lymph, and eventual deposition in the T cell areas of secondary lymphoid tissue where dendritic cells select and expand T cells with specificity for the presented Ag (Kampgen *et al.*, 1991; Pure *et al.*, 1990; Stossel *et al.*, 1990).

O'Doherty and colleagues first described subsets of immature dendritic cells circulating in human peripheral blood that expressed CD4, but not other lineage-specific markers (O'Doherty *et al.*, 1993). These cells morphologically resembled monocytes but did not express CD14 (O'Doherty *et al.*, 1993), and they could be further segregated according to the presence or absence of CD11c expression. Maturation required culture in macrophage-conditioned medium, although the specific, active cytokines were not identified (O'Doherty *et al.*, 1994). The $CD4^+$, $CD11c^-$, $CD45RA^+$ precursor may be the counterpart of the recently described human lymphoid dendritic cell isolated from secondary lymphoid tissue by Liu and colleagues (Grouard *et al.*, 1997), whereas the $CD4^+$, $CD11c^+$, $CD45RO^+$ cell likely corresponds to the typical myeloid dendritic cell. Regardless, the essential features of myeloid maturation have continued to be the upregulation of MHC products, costimulatory molecules, and MLR stimulatory capacity, as was seen in the earlier studies of Langerhans cells.

In addition to GM-CSF, IL-4 has been extensively evaluated because of its known suppression of macrophage development, even at the clonogenic level (Jansen *et al.*, 1989). With the support of GM-CSF and IL-4, candidate dendritic cells developed from unselected mononuclear cell precursors in human peripheral blood (Sallusto and Lanzavecchia, 1994; Romani *et al.*, 1994), many of which were initially adherent to tissue culture plastic in vitro and expressed CD14. Together with GM-CSF, IL-4 also supported the capacity of immature dendritic cells to present soluble antigen, a process further enhanced by endocytosis of immune complexes via FcR-mediated binding to the immature cells (Sallusto and Lanzavecchia, 1994). Addition of TNF-α halted antigen capture and presentation by this mechanism (Sallusto and Lanzavecchia, 1994), but concomitantly led to upregulation of MHC products, accessory molecules, and T cell stimulatory capacity (Sallusto and Lanzavecchia, 1994; Zhou and Tedder, 1996).

Bender, Romani, and their respective colleagues demonstrated in companion reports that GM-CSF and IL-4 in non-FCS-containing medium could only prime peripheral blood mononuclear cells to develop into dendritic cells. However, phenotype, function, and morphology were unstable when cytokines were removed (Bender *et al.*, 1996; Romani *et al.*, 1996). Human plasma or serum was less supportive than fetal calf serum-based medium of dendritic cell differentiation, and the resulting cells failed to express additional markers of terminal maturation, e.g., CD83 (Zhou and Tedder, 1995a,b) and p55 (Mosialos *et al.*, 1996). It had previously been shown that a single factor like TNF-α could induce terminal maturation after GM-CSF and IL-4 priming in the presence of FCS (Sallusto and Lanzavecchia, 1994; Zhou and Tedder, 1996). However, undefined cytokines present in macrophage-conditioned medium proved essential to the irreversible and terminal maturation of dendritic cells after an initial 7 days' culture in GM-CSF and IL-4 without FCS (Bender *et al.*, 1996; Romani *et al.*, 1996), reminiscent of the earlier studies of immature blood dendritic cells by O'Doherty and colleagues (O'Doherty *et al.*, 1994). Attempts to define the operative cytokines in

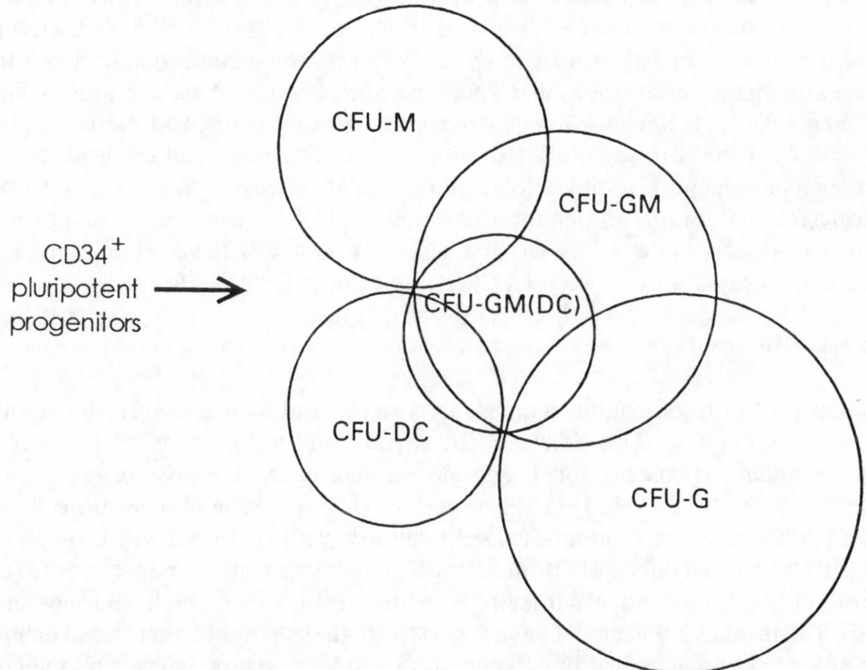

Fig. 3. Venn diagram representing the stochastic hematopoietic development of myeloid dendritic cells, and the relationship of CFU-DC to both earlier, less differentiated, progenitor populations, as well as the progeny of committed CFUs like CFU-Gs and CFU-Ms.

macrophage-conditioned medium have identified TNF-α, IL-1β, IL-6, and IFN-α as important but inadequate to substitute for macrophage-conditioned medium, either alone or in combination (Reddy *et al.*, 1997). Other inflammatory stimuli, like LPS (Sallusto and Lanzavecchia, 1995; Verhasselt *et al.*, 1997; De Smedt *et al.*, 1996) or prostaglandins (Jonuleit *et al*, 1997; Rieser *et al.*, 1997), can induce terminal maturation, as can activated T cells via CD40L:CD40 interactions (Cella *et al.*, 1996; Caux *et al.*, 1994b). TRANCE (Wong *et al.*, 1997), or RANKL (Anderson *et al.*, 1997), which is a newly described member of the TNF family expressed especially by T lymphocytes, can also prolong dendritic cell survival and thereby enhance function.

OTHER CYTOKINES ACTIVE IN THE DIFFERENTIATION OF DENDRITIC CELLS

TNF Family of Cytokines

TNF homologues like gp39/CD40L/CD154 can substitute for and/or augment many of the effects attributed to TNF-α in the human system (Sallusto and Lanzavecchia, 1994). Caux and colleagues first demonstrated high expression of CD40 by human dendritic cells generated from CD34$^+$ cord blood cells; and in this context, CD40:CD40L interactions maintained dendritic cell viability, upregulated CD80 and CD86, and enhanced cytokine secretion (Caux *et al.*, 1994b). Ligation of CD40 on human CD34$^+$ progenitors has even been shown to result in the generation of dendritic cells (Flores-Romo *et al.*, 1997). Recently, another member of the TNF family, known as either TRANCE (TNF-related activation induced cytokine; Wong *et al.*, 1997) or RANKL (receptor activator of NF-κB ligand; Anderson *et al.*, 1997), which enhances dendritic cell function by prolonging survival, has also been described by two different groups. CD40L, TNF, and TRANCE/RANKL are expressed by lymphoid tissue, and more specifically by T cells, and the corresponding receptors are expressed by myeloid dendritic cells. These findings support a physiologic, intercellular dialogue that fosters terminal dendritic cell maturation and continued stimulation of T cells. This is analogous to the cross-talk between dendritic cells and T cells mediated by the costimulatory ligand and receptor interactions between CD28/CTLA4 and CD80/CD86.

Interleukin-10

IL-10 has proved to be another important cytokine, but with respect to its immunosuppressive properties. The effects of IL-10 on dendritic cells result in decreased immunostimulatory capacity for T cells (Macatonia *et al.*, 1993; Caux *et al.*, 1994a; Peguet-Navarro *et al.*, 1994). IL-10 also prevents the generation of dendritic cells from human peripheral blood mononuclear cells cultured with GM-CSF and IL-4 (Buelens *et al.*, 1997a). Interestingly, IL-10 differentially interferes with terminal dendritic cell maturation, depending on whether the stimulus is LPS or CD40L (Buelens *et al.*, 1997b). The results of this model have suggested that IL-10 could alter initial dendritic cell maturation *in vivo* caused by inflammatory stimuli in the periphery and mimicked by LPS *in vitro*. Subsequent maturation and function when interacting with CD40L-expressing, activated T cells would be less affected, or more specifically limited to an inhibitory effect on IL-12 synthesis, which may in turn skew toward T_H2-type responses. Fully mature and terminally differentiated dendritic cells seem to be resistant to the immunosuppressive effects of IL-10 (Enk *et al.*, 1993), whereas immature dendritic cells can be rendered tolerogenic in the presence of IL-10 (Steinbrink *et al.*, 1997).

Interleukin-3 and Interleukin-13

Cytokine redundancy is sometimes seen in the hematopoietic system. With respect to dendritic cells, this is exemplified by overlapping activities of IL-3 with GM-CSF, and IL-13 with IL-4. The heterodimeric receptors for IL-3 and GM-CSF, as well as IL-5, share a common β subunit, although each cytokine receptor has a unique α chain (Miyajima *et al.*, 1992). This common β chain is presumably pertinent to the mechanism through which IL-3 mediates its effects. In conjunction with TNF-α, IL-3 has been demonstrated to have activity similar to that of GM-CSF in generating dendritic cells from $CD34^+$ precursors in cord blood (Caux *et al.*, 1996b). Along these lines, it has also been reported that GM-CSF deficient mice maintain apparently normal hematopoiesis, including normal numbers of splenic dendritic cells (Dranoff *et al.*, 1994). Here again, IL-3 can likely substitute for GM-CSF, the requirement for which is apparently not always absolute in dendritic cell differentation. Redundancy has also been documented with IL-13, which can substitute for IL-4 (Zurawski and de Vries, 1994) in the differentiation of dendritic cells from peripheral blood mononuclear leukocytes (Romani *et al.*, 1996).

TGF-β

TGF-β is another important cytokine in the differentiation of dendritic cells. Udey and colleagues reported the absence of epidermal Langerhans cells in mice that were null homozygotes for TGF-β1 (Borkowski *et al.*, 1996). Almost simultaneously in the human, Strobl and colleagues demonstrated a requirement for TGF-β1 in generating $CD1a^+$, Lag^+, Birbeck granule-containing candidate dendritic cells from $CD34^+$ progenitors, together with c-*kit* ligand, GM-CSF, and TNF-α, but in serum- and plasma-free medium (Strobl *et al.*, 1996). The mechanism was at least in part attributed to reduced expression of CD95/FAS/Apo-1 by $CD34^+$ progenitors cultured for as few as 72 h in the presence of these exogenous cytokines, which in turn was associated with protection from apoptosis (Riedl *et al.*, 1997). This same group has further shown a requirement for TGF-β1 in supporting the enhanced growth of epidermal dendritic, or Langerhans cells mediated by flt3 ligand, when added to the combination of GM-CSF, TNF-α, and c-*kit* ligand in serum- and plasma-free medium (Strobl *et al.*, 1997). This was also the case at the clonogenic level with respect to CFU-DC growth under serum- and plasma-free conditions (Strobl *et al.*, 1997). One of the issues raised by these studies, however, is the incomplete maturation of these cells based on the critical test of stimulatory function in the mixed leukocyte reaction. These progeny have stimulated substantially less T cell proliferation than should be observed with mature dendritic cells. The lack of intense expression of CD86, or even clearly positive expression of CD83 and CD80, further indicates that these progeny have not fully matured. This is not unlike resident populations of epidermal Langerhans cells, however, which undergo maturation to express a fully differentiated phenotype and become highly immunostimulatory.

Flt3 Ligand

Flt3 ligand is another early-acting cytokine like c-*kit* ligand, which works in synergy with other hematopoietic cytokines, but seems to be only additive with respect to c-*kit* ligand. The receptors for flt3 ligand, c-*kit* ligand, and M-CSF (c-*fms*) are similar and linked to tyrosinase kinase (Lyman and Jacobsen, 1998). The receptor for flt3 ligand was cloned before the ligand itself, and its similarity to the M-CSF receptor led to the name flt3, (*fms*-like tyrosine kinase 3) (Rosnet *et al.*, 1991a,b). Another group isolated the receptor using murine fetal liver stem cells, bestowing the name flk-2 (fetal liver kinase 2) (Matthews *et al.*, 1991). Unlike c-*kit* ligand, the mouse and human flt3 ligands are interchangeable and fully active on cells bearing either the murine or human receptors (Lyman *et al.*, 1994). Also unlike c-*kit* ligand, which is critical to erythropoiesis (Galli *et al.*, 1994), flt3 is absent from erythroid progenitors, and its ligand therefore plays no role here. Like c-*kit*, however, flt3 is expressed by most GM progenitors among $CD34^+$ cord blood and bone marrow cells (Rappold *et al.*, 1997); and at least 60% of $flt3^+$ bone marrow precursors coexpress the myeloid epitope CD33 (Rosnet *et al.*, 1996).

Flt3 ligand treatment of mice *in vivo* has been shown to increase substantially the numbers of both myeloid and lymphoid dendritic cells in all tissues examined (Maraskovsky *et al.*, 1996). Preclinical phase I studies in normal volunteers have also shown a 30-fold increase in circulating dendritic cells after flt3 ligand administration (Lebsack *et al.*, 1997). Flt3 ligand in combination with GM-CSF and TNF-α increased the yield of myeloid-type dendritic cells derived *in vitro* from mobilized peripheral blood $CD34^+$ progenitors, similar to that effected by c-*kit* ligand; together these early-acting cytokines were additive (Siena *et al.*, 1995). Flt3 ligand, like c-*kit* ligand, seems primarily to affect expansion, rather than differentiation per se; but further studies are underway to clarify this with respect to dendritic cells.

RELATIONSHIP BETWEEN LINEAGE, MATURATION, AND FUNCTION

The characterization and use of intermediate or immature dendritic cell precursors have been addressed in several models. Only immature dendritic cells in the mouse can phagocytose particulate antigen (Inaba *et al.*, 1993b), as can immature human dendritic cells (Szabolcs *et al.*, 1996; Caux *et al.*, 1996a; Romani *et al.*, 1996). Human dendritic cells can also capture and present soluble antigen, a process that is enhanced by endocytosis of immune complexes via FcR-mediated binding to the immature cells (Sallusto and Lanzavecchia, 1994). Dendritic cells that develop from $CD14^+$, $CD1a^-$ intermediates maintain efficient antigen capture and even express some nonspecific esterase, whereas those that arise from $CD14^-$, $CD1a^+$ intermediates never express nonspecific esterase and limit their phagocytic activity to the intermediate precursor stage (Caux *et al.*, 1997).

Investigators have also recently discovered an important mechanism whereby dendritic cells can charge MHC molecules with peptides by active uptake of antigens from apoptotic cells (Albert *et al.*, 1998; Inaba *et al.*, submitted). This has been delineated for class II MHC-restricted antigen in the mouse (Inaba *et al.*, submitted) and for class I MHC-restricted antigen in the human (Albert *et al.*, 1998), where immature dendritic cells are even more efficient. The uptake of antigen via mechanisms like this may prove to be more physiologically relevant than phagocytosis of indigestible particulates. This highlights the fact that myeloid dendritic cells always capture, process, retain, and present antigen for the purpose of interacting with T cells, whereas other myeloid cells (e.g., macrophages and PMNs) phagocytose antigen primarily for clearance and disposal. Functional counterparts to maturation *in vitro* and *in vivo* have been more extensively studied in the context of class II MHC-restricted T cell responses stimulated by Langerhans cells (Romani *et al.*, 1989; Koch *et al.*, 1995; Witmer-Pack *et al.*, 1987; Heufler *et al.*, 1988), although there are some corresponding data regarding class I MHC-restricted responses (Porgador and Gilboa, 1995).

The recurring theme in all of these models is that immaturity is associated with a lower stimulatory capacity but a greater ability to capture and present intact antigens that require processing. As this function declines with maturity, dendritic cells become highly stimulatory but present antigens like peptides and alloantigens that do not require processing. Similarly, some of these functions are beginning to be segregated between different types of dendritic cell progeny (Caux *et al.*, 1997), which may prove to be substantially different in the manner in which they handle antigen and traffic *in vivo* to initiate cell-mediated immune responses.

CONCLUSION

At the most reductive level, human dendritic cells share a common progenitor with all other myeloid cells, and even with lymphoid populations under certain conditions. However, *a propos* of this chapter's emphasis on cell fate development in myeloid differentiation, is the fact that at various levels in development from $CD34^+$ progenitors, dendritic cells share a common ancestry with granulocytes and macrophages, the principal other myeloid populations (Fig. 3). Although the process of steady-state differentiation *in vivo* is stochastic, cell fate decisions in hematopoietic lineage selection can be substantially altered, or skewed, by exposure to selected cytokines. Furthermore, with increasing differentiation comes greater commitment toward a specific cell type, and a decreasing probability of developing along alternative lineages. The ongoing refinement of the definition and functional characterization of progenitors, intermediates, and terminally differentiated dendritic cells, as well as the operative cytokines, are collectively providing basic and clinical investigators with multiple control points for the manipulation of T cell immune responses.

ACKNOWLEDGMENTS

The author thanks especially Ralph Steinman and Malcolm Moore for their early instruction, mentorship, and encouragement in this field, as well as the contribution of many colleagues, including Paul Szabolcs, Kayo Inaba, Gerold Schuler, Nikolaus Romani, Nina Bhardwaj, Alan Houghton, David Ciocon, Jiri Trcka, and Christel Buelens. The author's laboratory is supported by R01 AI26875, P01 CA23766, and

P01 CA59350 from the National Institutes of Health, and by the DeWitt Wallace Clinical Research Institute Fund for Memorial Sloan-Kettering Cancer Center.

REFERENCES

Albert, M.L., Sauter, B. and Bhardwaj, N. (1998). Dendritic cells acquire antigen from apoptotic cells and induce class I-restricted CTLs. *Nature* **392**, 86–89.

Anderson, D.M., Maraskovsky, E., Billingsley, W.L., Dougall, W.C., Tometsko, M.E., Roux, E.R., Teepe, M.C., DuBose, R.F., Cosman, D. and Galibert, L. (1997). A homologue of the TNF receptor and its ligand enhance T cell growth and dendritic-cell function. *Nature* **390**, 175–179.

Banchereau, J. and Steinman, R.M. (1998). Dendritic cells and the control of immunity. *Nature* **392** 245–252.

Bender, A., Sapp, M., Schuler, G., Steinman, R.M. and Bhardwaj, N. (1996). Improved methods for the generation of dendritic cells from nonproliferating progenitors in human blood. *J. Immunol. Methods* **196**, 121–135.

Borkowski, T.A., Letterio, J.J., Farr, A.G. and Udey, M.C. (1996). A role for endogenous transforming growth factor β1 in Langerhans cell biology: the skin of transforming growth factor β1 null mice is devoid of epidermal Langerhans cells. *J. Exp. Med.* **184**, 2417–2422.

Buelens, C., Verhasselt, V., De Groote, D., Thielemans, K., Goldman, M. and Willems, F. (1997a). Interleukin-10 prevents the generation of dendritic cells from peripheral blood mononuclear cells cultured with interleukin-4 and granulocyte/macrophage-colony-stimulating factor. *Eur. J. Immunol.* **27**, 756–762.

Buelens, C., Verhasselt, V., De Groote, D., Thielemans, K., Goldman, M. and Willems, F. (1997b). Human dendritic cell responses to LPS and CD40 ligation are differentially regulated by IL-10. *Eur. J. Immunol.* **27**, 1848–1852.

Caux, C., Saeland, S., Favre, C., Duvert, V., Mannoni, P. and Banchereau, J. (1990). Tumor necrosis factor-alpha strongly potentiates interleukin-3 and granulocyte-macrophage colony-stimulating factor-induced proliferation of human CD34$^+$ hematopoietic progenitor cells. *Blood* **75**, 2292–2298.

Caux, C., Favre, C., Saeland, S., Duvert, V., Durand, I., Mannoni, P. and Banchereau, J. (1991). Potentiation of early hematopoiesis by tumor necrosis factor-α is followed by inhibition of granulopoietic differentiation and proliferation. *Blood* **78**, 635–644.

Caux, C., Dezutter-Dambuyant, C., Schmitt, D. and Banchereau, J. (1992). GM-CSF and TNF-α cooperate in the generation of dendritic Langerhans cells. *Nature* **360**, 258–261.

Caux, C., Durand, I., Moreau, I., Duvert, V., Saeland, S. and Banchereau, J. (1993). Tumor necrosis factor-α cooperates with interleukin 3 in the recruitment of a primitive subset of human CD34$^+$ progenitors. *J. Exp. Med.* **177**, 1815–1820.

Caux, C., Massacrier, C., Vanbervliet, B., Barthelemy, C., Liu, Y.-J. and Banchereau, J. (1994a). Interleukin 10 inhibits T cell alloreaction induced by human dendritic cells. *Int. Immunol.* **6**, 1177–1185.

Caux, C., Massacrier, C., Vanbervliet, B., Dubois, B., Van Kooten, C., Durand, I. and Banchereau, J. (1994b). Activation of human dendritic cells through CD40 cross-linking. *J. Exp. Med.* **180**, 1263–1272.

Caux, C., Vanbervliet, B., Massacrier, C., Dezutter-Dambuyant, C., de Saint-Vis, B., Jacquet, C., Yoneda, K., Imamura, S., Schmitt, D. and Banchereau, J. (1996a). CD34$^+$ hematopoietic progenitors from human cord blood differentiate along two independent dendritic cell pathways in response to GM-CSF + TNF α. *J. Exp. Med.* **184**, 695–706.

Caux, C., Vanbervliet, B., Massacrier, C., Durand, I. and Banchereau, J. (1996b). Interleukin-3 cooperates with tumor necrosis factor alpha for the development of human dendritic/langerhans cells from cord blood CD34$^+$ hematopietic progenitor cells. *Blood* **87**, 2376–2385.

Caux, C., Massacrier, C., Vanbervliet, B., Dubois, B., Durand, I., Cella, M., Lanzavecchia, A. and Banchereau, J. (1997). CD34$^+$ hematopoietic progenitors from human cord blood differentiate along two independent dendritic cell pathways in response to granulocyte-macrophage colony-stimulating factor plus tumor necrosis factor α: II. Functional analysis. *Blood* **90**, 1458–1470.

Cella, M., Scheidegger, D., Palmer-Lehmann, K., Lane, P., Lanzavecchia, A. and Alber, G. (1996). Ligation of CD40 on dendritic cells triggers production of high levels of interleukin-12 and enhances T cell stimulatory capacity: T-T help via APC activation. *J. Exp. Med.* **184**, 747–752.

Civin, C.I. (1990). Human monomyeloid cell membrane antigens. *Exp. Hematol.* **18**, 461–467.

de Saint-Vis, B., Fugier-Vivier, I., Massacrier, C., Vanbervliet, B., Ait-Yahia, S., Banchereau, J., Liu, Y.-J., Lebecque, S., and Caux, C. (1998). The cytokine profile expressed by human dendritic cells is dependent on cell subtype and mode of activation. *J. Immunol.* **160**, 1666–1676.

De Smedt, T., Pajak, B., Muraille, E., Lespagnard, L., Heinen, E., De Baetselier, P., Urbain, J., Leo, O. and Moser, M. (1996). Regulation of dendritic cell numbers and maturation by lipopolysaccharide in vivo. *J. Exp. Med.* **184**, 1413–1424.

Demarchi, F., D'Agaro, P., Falaschi, A. and Giacca, M. (1992). Probing protein–DNA interactions at the long terminal repeat of human immunodeficiency virus type 1 by in vivo footprinting. *J. Virol.* **66**, 2514–2518.

Dranoff, G., Crawford, A.D., Sadelain, M., Ream, B., Rashid, A., Bronson, R.T., Dickersin, G.R., Bachurski, C.J., Mark, E.L., Whitsett, J.A. and Mulligan, R.C. (1994). Involvement of granulocyte-macrophage colony-stimulating factor in pulmonary homeostasis. *Science* **264**, 713–716.

Egner, W. and Hart, D.N.J. (1995). The phenotype of freshly isolated and cultured human bone marrow allostimulatory cells: possible heterogeneity in bone marrow dendritic cell populations. *Immunology* **85**, 611–620.

Enk, A.H., Angeloni, V.L., Udey, M.C. and Katz, S.I. (1993). Inhibition of Langerhans cell antigen-presenting function by IL-10. *J. Immunol.* **151**, 2390–2398.

Flechner, E.R., Freudenthal, P.S., Kaplan, G. and Steinman, R.M. (1988). Antigen-specific T lymphocytes efficiently cluster with dendritic cells in the human primary mixed-leukocyte reaction. *Cell. Immunol.* **111**, 183–195.

Flores-Romo, L., Bjorck, P., Duvert, V., Van Kooten, C., Saeland, S. and Banchereau, J. (1997). CD40 ligation on human $CD34^+$ hematopoietic progenitors induces their proliferation and differentiation into functional dendritic cells. *J. Exp. Med.* **185**, 341–349.

Freudenthal, P.S. and Steinman, R.M. (1990). The distinct surface of human blood dendritic cells, as observed after an improved isolation method. *Proc. Natl Acad. Sci. USA* **87**, 7698–7702.

Galli, S.J., Zsebo, K.M. and Geissler, E.N. (1994). The kit ligand, stem cell factor. *Adv. Immunol.* **55**, 1–96.

Galy, A., Travis, M., Cen, D. and Chen, B. (1995). Human T, B, natural killer, and dendritic cells arise from a common bone marrow progenitor cell subset. *Immunity* **3**, 459–473.

Grouard, G., Durand, I., Filgueira, L., Banchereau, J. and Liu, Y.-J. (1996). Dendritic cells capable of stimulating T cells in germinal centres. *Nature* **384**, 364–367.

Grouard, G., Rissoan, M.-C., Filgueira, L., Durand, I., Banchereau, J. and Liu, Y.-J. (1997). The enigmatic plasmacytoid T cells develop into dendritic cells with IL-3 and CD40-ligand. *J. Exp. Med.* **185**, 1101–1111.

Hart, D.N.J. (1997). Dendritic cells: unique leukocyte populations which control the primary immune response. *Blood* **90**, 3245–3287.

Heufler, C., Koch, F. and Schuler, G. (1988). Granulocyte/macrophage colony-stimulating factor and interleukin 1 mediate the maturation of murine epidermal Langerhans cells into potent immunostimulatory dendritic cells. *J. Exp. Med.* **167**, 700–705.

Inaba, K., Young, J.W. and Steinman, R.M. (1987). Direct activation of $CD8^+$ cytotoxic T lymphocytes by dendritic cells. *J. Exp. Med.* **166**, 182–194.

Inaba, K., Inaba, M., Romani, N., Aya, H., Deguchi, M., Ikehara, S., Muramatsu, S. and Steinman, R.M. (1992a). Generation of large numbers of dendritic cells from mouse bone marrow cultures supplemented with granulocyte/macrophage colony-stimulating factor. *J. Exp. Med.* **176**, 1693–1702.

Inaba, K., Steinman, R.M., Witmer-Pack, M., Aya, H., Inaba, M., Sudo, T., Wolpe, S. and Schuler, G. (1992b). Identification of proliferating dendritic cell precursors in mouse blood. *J. Exp. Med.* **175**, 1157–1167.

Inaba, K., Inaba, M., Deguchi, M., Hagi, K., Yasumizu, R., Ikehara, S., Muramatsu, S. and Steinman, R.M. (1993a). Granulocytes, macrophages, and dendritic cells arise from a common major histocompatibility complex class II-negative progenitor in mouse bone marrow. *Proc. Natl. Acad. Sci. USA* **90**, 3038–3042.

Inaba, K., Inaba, M., Naito, M. and Steinman, R.M. (1993b). Dendritic cell progenitors phagocytose particulates, including Bacillus Calmette-Guerin organisms, and sensitize mice to mycobacterial antigens in vivo. *J. Exp. Med.* **178**, 479–488.

Jacobsen, S.E.W., Ruscetti, F.W., Dubois, C.M. and Keller, J.R. (1992). Tumor necrosis factor α directly and indirectly regulates hematopoietic progenitor cell proliferation: role of colony-stimulating factor receptor modulation. *J. Exp. Med.* **175**, 1759–1772.

Jansen, J.H., Wientjens, G.-J.H.M., Fibbe, W.E., Willemze, R. and Kluin-Nelemans, H.C. (1989). Inhibition of human macrophage colony formation by interleukin 4. *J. Exp. Med.* **170**, 577–582.

Jonuleit, H., Kuhn, U., Muller, G., Steinbrink, K., Paragnik, L., Schmitt, E., Knop, J. and Enk, A.H. (1997). Pro-inflammatory cytokines and prostaglandins induce maturation of potent immunostimulatory dendritic cells under fetal calf serum-free conditions. *Eur. J. Immunol.* **27**, 3135–3142.

Kampgen, E., Koch, N., Koch, F., Stoger, P., Heufler, C., Schuler, G. and Romani, N. (1991). Class II major histocompatibility complex molecules of murine dendritic cells: synthesis, sialylation of invariant chain, and antigen processing capacity are down-regulated upon culture. *Proc. Natl Acad. Sci. USA* **88**, 3014–3018.

Kampgen, E., Koch, F., Heufler, C., Eggert, A., Gill, L.L., Gillis, S., Dower, S.K., Romani, N. and Schuler, G. (1994). Understanding the dendritic cell lineage through a study of cytokine receptors. *J. Exp. Med.* **179**, 1767–1776.

Kasinrerk, W., Baumruker, T., Majdic, O., Knapp, W. and Stockinger, H. (1993). CD1 molecule expression on human monocytes induced by granulocyte-macrophage colony-stimulating factor. *J. Immunol.* **150**, 579–584.

Katz, S.I., Tamaki, K. and Sachs, D.H. (1979). Epidermal Langerhans cells are derived from cells originating in bone marrow. *Nature* **282**, 324–326.

Koch, F., Trockenbacher, B., Kampgen, E., Grauer, O., Stossel, H., Livingstone, A.M., Schuler, G. and Romani, N. (1995). Antigen processing in populations of mature murine dendritic cells is caused by subsets of incompletely matured cells. *J. Immunol.* **155**, 93–100.

Larsen, C.P., Steinman, R.M., Witmer-Pack, M., Hankins, D.F., Morris, P.J. and Austyn, J.M. (1990). Migration and maturation of Langerhans cells in skin transplants and explants. *J. Exp. Med.* **172**, 1483–1493.

Lebsack, M.E., McKenna, H.J., Hoek, J.A., Hanna, R., Feng, A., Maraskovsky, E. and Hayes, F.A. (1997). Safety of FLT3 ligand in healthy volunteers. *Blood* **90**, 170a.

Lukas, M., Stoessel, H., Hefel, L., Imamura, S., Fritsch, P., Sepp, N.T., Schuler, G. and Romani, N. (1996). Human cutaneous dendritic cells migrate through dermal lymphatic vessels in a skin organ culture model. *J. Invest. Dermatol.* **106**, 1293–1299.

Lyman, S.D. and Jacobsen, S.E.W. (1998). c-kit ligand and flt3 ligand: Stem/progenitor cell factors with overlapping yet distinct activities. *Blood* **91**, 1101–1134.

Lyman, S.D., Brasel, K., Rousseau, A.M. and Williams, D.E. (1994). The flt3 ligand: a hematopoietic stem cell factor whose activities are distinct from steel factor. *Stem Cells* **12**, 99–110.

Macatonia, S.E., Doherty, T.M., Knight, S.C. and O'Garra, A. (1993). Differential effect of IL-10 on dendritic cell-induced T cell proliferation and IFN-gamma production. *J. Immunol.* **150**, 3755–3765.

Maraskovsky, E., Brasel, K., Teepe, M., Roux, E.R., Lyman, S.D., Shortman, K. and McKenna, H.J. (1996). Dramatic increase in the numbers of functionally mature dendritic cells in Flt3 ligand-treated mice: Multiple dendritic cell subpopulations identified. *J. Exp. Med.* **184**, 1953–1962.

Matthews, W., Jordan, C.T., Wiegand, G.W., Pardoll, D. and Lemischka, I.R. (1991). A receptor tyrosine kinase specific to hematopoietic stem and progenitor cell-enriched populations. *Cell* **65**, 1143–1152.

Miyajima, A., Kitamura, T., Harada, N., Yokota, T. and Arai, K. (1992). Cytokine receptors and signal transduction. *Annu. Rev. Immunol.* **10**, 295–331.

Moore, M.A.S. (1991). The clinical use of colony stimulating factors. *Annu. Rev. Immunol.* **9**, 159–191.

Mosialos, G., Birkenbach, M., Ayehunie, S., Matsumura, F., Pinkus, G.S., Kieff, E. and Langhoff, E. (1996). Circulating human dendritic cells differentially express high levels of a 55-kd actin-bundling protein. *Am. J. Pathol.* **148**, 593–600.

O'Doherty, U., Steinman, R.M., Peng, M., Cameron, P.U., Gezelter, S., Kopeloff, I., Swiggard, W.J., Pope, M. and Bhardwaj, N. (1993). Dendritic cells freshly isolated from human blood express CD4 and mature into typical immunostimulatory dendritic cells after culture in monocyte-conditioned medium. *J. Exp. Med.* **178**, 1067–1078.

O'Doherty, U., Peng, M., Gezelter, S., Swiggard, W.J., Betjes, M., Bhardwaj, N. and Steinman, R.M. (1994). Human blood contains two subsets of dendritic cells, one immunologically mature, and the other immature. *Immunology* **82**, 487–493.

Oehler, L., Majdic, O., Pickl, W.F., Stockl, J., Riedl, E., Drach, J., Rappersberger, K., Geissler, K. and Knapp, W. (1998). Neutrophil granulocyte committed cells can be driven to acquire dendritic cell characteristics. *J. Exp. Med.* **187**, 1019–1028.

Ogawa, M. (1995). Differentiation and proliferation of hematopoietic stem cells (Review). *Blood* **81**, 2844–2853.

Peguet-Navarro, J., Moulon, C., Caux, C., Dalbiez-Gauthier, C., Banchereau, J. and Schmitt, D. (1994). Interleukin-10 inhibits the primary allogeneic T cell response to human epidermal Langerhans cells. *Eur. J. Immunol.* **24**, 884–891.

Porgador, A. and Gilboa, E. (1995). Bone marrow-generated dendritic cells pulsed with a class I-restricted peptide are potent inducers of cytotoxic T lymphocytes. *J. Exp. Med.* **182**, 255–260.

Pugh, C.W., MacPherson, G.G. and Steer, H.W. (1983). Characterization of nonlymphoid cells derived from rat peripheral lymph. *J. Exp. Med.* **157**, 1758–1779.

Pure, E., Inaba, K., Crowley, M.T., Tardelli, L., Witmer-Pack, M.D., Ruberti, G., Fathman, G. and Steinman, R.M. (1990). Antigen processing by epidermal Langerhans cells correlates with the level of biosynthesis of major histocompatibility complex class II molecules and expression of invariant chain. *J. Exp. Med.* **172**, 1459–1469.

Rappold, I., Ziegler, B.L., Kohler, I., Marchetto, S., Rosnet, O., Birnbaum, D., Simmons, P.J., Zannettino, A.C., Hill, B., Neu, S., Knapp, W., Alitalo, R., Alitalo, K., Ullrich, A., Kanz, L. and Buhring, H.J. (1997). Functional and phenotypic characterization of cord blood and bone marrow subsets expressing FLT3 (CD135) receptor tyrosine kinase. *Blood* **90**, 111–125.

Reddy, A., Sapp, M., Feldman, M., Subklewe, M. and Bhardwaj, N. (1997). A monocyte conditioned medium is more effective than defined cytokines in mediating the terminal maturation of human dendritic cells. *Blood* **90**, 3640–3646.

Reid, C.D.L., Fryer, P.R., Clifford, C., Kirk, A., Tikerpae, J. and Knight, S.C. (1990). Identification of hematopoietic progenitors of macrophages and dendritic Langerhans cells [DL-CFU] in human bone marrow and peripheral blood. *Blood* **76**, 1139–1149.

Reid, C.D.L., Stackpoole, A., Meager, A. and Tikerpae, J. (1992). Interactions of tumor necrosis factor with granulocyte-macrophage colony-stimulating factor and other cytokines in the regulation of dendritic cell growth in vitro from early bipotent $CD34^+$ progenitors in human bone marrow. *J. Immunol.* **149**, 2681–2688.

Reis e Sousa, C., Stahl, P.D. and Austyn, J.M. (1993). Phagocytosis of antigens by Langerhans cells in vitro. *J. Exp. Med.* **178**, 509–519.

Riedl, E., Strobl, H., Majdic, O. and Knapp, W. (1997). TGF-β1 promotes in vitro generation of dendritic cells by protecting progenitor cells from apoptosis. *J. Immunol.* **158**, 1591–1597.

Rieser, C., Bock, G., Klocker, H., Bartsch, G. and Thurnher, M. (1997). Prostaglandin E2 and tumor necrosis factor α cooperate to activate human dendritic cells: synergistic activation of interleukin 12 production. *J. Exp. Med.* **186**, 1603–1608.

Romani, N., Koide, S., Crowley, M., Witmer-Pack, M., Livingstone, A.M., Fathman, C.G., Inaba, K. and Steinman, R.M. (1989). Presentation of exogenous protein antigens by dendritic cells to T cell clones: intact protein is presented best by immature, epidermal Langerhans cells. *J. Exp. Med.* **169**, 1169–1178.

Romani, N., Gruner, S., Brang, D., Kampgen, E., Lenz, A., Trockenbacher, B., Konwalinka, G., Fritsch, P.O., Steinman, R.M. and Schuler, G. (1994). Proliferating dendritic cell progenitors in human blood. *J. Exp. Med.* **180**, 83–93.

Romani, N., Reider, D., Heuer, M., Ebner, S., Eibl, B., Niederwieser, D. and Schuler, G. (1996). Generation of mature dendritic cells from human blood: An improved method with special regard to clinical applicability. *J. Immunol. Methods* **196**, 137–151.

Rosnet, O., Marchetto, S., de Lapeyriere, O. and Birnbaum, D. (1991a). Murine Flt3, a gene encoding a novel tyrosine kinase receptor of the PDGFR/CSF1R family. *Oncogene* **6**, 1641–1650.

Rosnet, O., Mattei, M.-G., Marchetto, S., and Birnbaum, D. (1991b). Isolation and chromosomal location of a novel fms-like tyrosine kinase gene. *Genomics* **9**, 380–385.

Rosnet, O., Buhring, H.J., Marchetto, S., Rappold, I., Lavagna, C., Sainty, D., Arnoulet, C., Chabannon, C., Kanz, L., Hannum, C. and Birnbaum, D. (1996). Human FLT3/FLK2 receptor tyrosine kinase is expressed at the surface of normal and malignant hematopoietic cells. *Leukemia* **10**, 238–248.

Ryncarz, R.E. and Anasetti, C. (1998). Expression of CD86 on human marrow $CD34^+$ cells identifies immunocompetent committed precursors of macrophages and dendritic cells. *Blood*, **91**, 3892–3900.

Sallusto, F. and Lanzavecchia, A. (1994). Efficient presentation of soluble antigen by cultured human dendritic cells is maintained by granulocyte/macrophage colony-stimulating factor plus interleukin 4 and downregulated by tumor necrosis factor α. *J. Exp. Med.* **179**, 1109–1118.

Sallusto, F. and Lanzavecchia, A. (1995). Dendritic cells use macropinocytosis and the mannose receptor to concentrate antigen in the MHC class II compartment. Downregulation by cytokines and bacterial products. *J. Exp. Med.* **182**, 389–400.

Santiago-Schwarz, F., Belilos, E., Diamond, B. and Carsons, S.E. (1992). TNF in combination with GM-CSF enhances the differentiation of neonatal cord blood stem cells into dendritic cells and macrophages. *J. Leukocyte Biol.* **52**, 274–281.

Saunders, D., Lucas, K., Ismaili, J., Wu, L., Maraskovsky, E., Dunn, A. and Shortman, K. (1996). Dendritic cell development in culture from thymic precursor cells in the absence of granulocyte/macrophage colony-stimulating factor. *J. Exp. Med.* **184**, 2185–2196.

Shieh, J.-H., Peterson, R.H.F., Warren, D.J. and Moore, M.A.S. (1989). Modulation of colony-stimulating factor-1 receptors on macrophages by tumor necrosis factor. *J. Immunol.* **143**, 2534–2539.

Shieh, J.-H., Peterson, R.H.F. and Moore, M.A.S. (1991). Modulation of granulocyte colony-stimulating factor receptors on murine peritoneal exudate macrophages by tumor necrosis factor-α. *J. Immunol.* **146**, 2648–2653.

Siena, S., Di Nicola, M., Bregni, M., Mortarini, R., Anichini, A., Lombardi, L., Ravagnani, F., Parmiani, G. and Gianni, A.M. (1995). Massive ex vivo generation of functional dendritic cells from mobilized $CD34^+$ blood progenitors for anticancer therapy. *Exp. Hematol.* **23**, 1463–1471.

Steinbrink, K., Wolfl, M., Jonuleit, H., Knop, J. and Enk, A.H. (1997). Induction of tolerance by IL-10-treated dendritic cells. *J. Immunol.* **159**, 4772–4780.

Steinman, R.M. (1991). The dendritic cell system and its role in immunogenicity. *Annu. Rev. Immunol.* **9**, 271–296.

Steinman, R.M. (1997). Dendritic cells. In: *Fundamental Immunology* (ed. W.E. Paul), Lippincott-Raven, Philadelphia.

Steinman, R.M., Lustig, D.S. and Cohn, Z.A. (1974). Identification of a novel cell type in peripheral lymphoid organs of mice. III. Functional properties in vivo. *J. Exp. Med.* **139**, 1431–1445.

Stossel, H., Koch, F., Kampgen, E., Stoger, P., Lenz, A., Heufler, C., Romani, N. and Schuler, G. (1990). Disappearance of certain acidic organelles (endosomes and Langerhans cell granules) accompanies loss of antigen processing capacity upon culture of epidermal Langerhans cells. *J. Exp. Med.* **172**, 1471–1482.

Strobl, H., Riedl, E., Scheinecker, C., Bello-Fernandez, C., Pickl, W.F., Rappersberger, K., Majdic, O. and Knapp, W. (1996). TGF-β1 promotes in vitro development of dendritic cells from $CD34^+$ hemopoietic progenitors. *J. Immunol.* **157**, 1499–1507.

Strobl, H., Bello-Fernandez, C., Riedl, E., Pickl, W.F., Majdic, O., Lyman, S.D. and Knapp, W. (1997). FLT3 ligand in cooperation with transforming growth factor-beta1 potentiates in vitro development of Langerhans-type dendritic cells and allows single cell dendritic cell cluster formation under serum-free conditions. *Blood* **90**, 1425–1434.

Strunk, D., Rappersberger, K., Egger, C., Strobl, H., Kromer, E., Elbe, A., Maurer, D. and Stingl, G. (1996). Generation of human dendritic cells/Langerhans cells from circulating $CD34^+$ hematopoietic progenitor cells. *Blood* **87**, 1292–1302.

Strunk, D., Egger, C., Leitner, G., Hanau, D. and Stingl, G. (1997). A skin homing molecule defines the Langerhans cells progenitor in human peripheral blood. *J. Exp. Med.* **185**, 1131–1136.

Sutherland, H.J., Eaves, C.J., Eaves, A.C., Dragowska, W. and Lansdorp, P.M. (1989). Characterization and partial purification of human marrow cells capable of initiating long-term hematopoiesis in vitro. *Blood* **74**, 1563–1570.

Szabolcs, P., Moore, M.A.S. and Young, J.W. (1995). Expansion of immunostimulatory dendritic cells among the myeloid progeny of human $CD34^+$ bone marrow precursors cultured with c-kit ligand, granulocyte-macrophage colony-stimulating factor, and TNF-α. *J. Immunol.* **154**, 5851–5861.

Szabolcs, P., Avigan, D., Gezelter, S., Ciocon, D.H., Moore, M.A.S., Steinman, R.M. and Young, J.W. (1996). Dendritic cells and macrophages can mature independently from a human bone marrow-derived, post-CFU intermediate. *Blood* **87**, 4520–4530.

Terstappen, L.W.M.M., Huang, S., Safford, M., Lansdorp, P.M. and Loken, M.R. (1991). Sequential generations of hematopoietic colonies derived from single nonlineage-committed $CD34^+$ $CD38^-$ progenitor cells. *Blood* **77**, 1218–1227.

Thomas, R., Davis, L.S. and Lipsky, P.E. (1993). Isolation and characterization of human peripheral blood dendritic cells. *J. Immunol.* **150**, 821–834.

Verhasselt, V., Buelens, C., Willems, F., De Groote, D., Haeffner-Cavaillon, N. and Goldman, M. (1997). Bacterial lipopolysaccharide stimulates the production of cytokines and the expression of costimulatory molecules by human peripheral blood dendritic cells. *J. Immunol.* **158**, 2919–2925.

Volc-Platzer, B., Stingl, G., Wolff, K., Hinterberg, W. and Schnedl, W. (1984). Cytogenetic identification of allogeneic epidermal Langerhans cells in a bone marrow graft recipient. *N. Engl. J. Med.* **310**, 1123–1124.

Vremec, D. and Shortman, K. (1997). Dendritic cells subtypes in mouse lymphoid organs. Cross-correlation of surface markers, changes with incubation, and differences among thymus, spleen, and lymph nodes. *J. Immunol.* **159**, 565–573.

Witmer-Pack, M.D., Olivier, W., Valinsky, J., Schuler, G. and Steinman, R.M. (1987). Granulocyte/macrophage colony-stimulating factor is essential for the viability and function of cultured murine epidermal Langerhans cells. *J. Exp. Med.* **166**, 1484–1498.

Wong, B.R., Josien, R., Lee, S.Y., Sauter, B., Li, H., Steinman, R.M. and Choi, Y. (1997). TRANCE (tumor necrosis factor [TNF]-related activation-induced cytokine), a new TNF family member predominantly expressed in T cells, is a dendritic cell specific survival factor. *J. Exp. Med.* **186**, 2075–2080.

Wright, S.D., Ramos, R.A., Tobias, P.S., Ulevitch, R.J. and Mathison, J.D. (1990). CD14, a receptor for complexes of lipopolysaccharide [LPS] and LPS binding protein. *Science* **249**, 1431–1433.

Young, J.W. and Steinman, R.M. (1988). Accessory cell requirements for the mixed leukocyte reaction and polyclonal mitogens, as studied with a new technique for enriching blood dendritic cells. *Cell. Immunol.* **111**, 167–182.

Young, J.W. and Steinman, R.M. (1990). Dendritic cells stimulate primary human cytolytic lymphocyte responses in the absence of $CD4^+$ helper T cells. *J. Exp. Med.* **171**, 1315–1332.

Young, J.W., Szabolcs, P. and Moore, M.A.S. (1995). Identification of dendritic cell colony-forming units among normal $CD34^+$ bone marrow progenitors that are expanded by c-kit-ligand and yield pure dendritic cell colonies in the presence of granulocyte/macrophage colony-stimulating factor and tumor necrosis factor α. *J. Exp. Med.* **182**, 1111–1120.

Zhou, L.-J. and Tedder, T.F. (1995a). HB15, a specific marker for human blood dendritic cells. In: *Leukocyte Typing V, White Cell Differentiation Antigens* (eds S.F. Schlossman, L. Boumsell, W. Gilks *et al.*), Oxford University Press Oxford, pp. 695–697.

Zhou, L.-J. and Tedder, T.F. (1995b). Human blood dendritic cells selectively express CD83, a member of the immunoglobulin superfamily. *J. Immunol.* **154**, 3821–3835.

Zhou, L.-J. and Tedder, T.F. (1996). $CD14^+$ blood monocytes can differentiate into functionally mature $CD83^+$ dendritic cells. *Proc. Natl. Acad. Sci. USA* **93**, 2588–2592.

Zurawski, G. and de Vries, J.E. (1994). Interleukin 13, an interleukin 4-like cytokine that acts on monocytes and B cells, but not on T cells. *Immunol. Today* **15**, 19–26.

CHAPTER 4
Origin of Follicular Dendritic Cells

John G. Tew[1], Zoher Kapasi[3], Dahui Qin[1], Jiuhua Wu[1], Stephen T. Haley[2] and Andras K. Szakal[2]

Departments of [1]Microbiology and Immunology and [2]Anatomy, Division of Immunobiology, Medical College of Virginia, Virginia Commonwealth University, Richmond, Virginia, USA; [3]Department of Rehabilitative Medicine, Division of Physical Therapy, Emory University School of Medicine, Atlanta, Georgia, USA.

INTRODUCTION

Follicular dendritic cells (FDC) are found in the B cell regions of all secondary lymphoid tissue and three FDC features are useful for distinguishing these cells from other immune system cells: (1) they exhibit a dendritic morphology; (2) these dendritic cells are restricted to the light zones of germinal centers in the lymphoid follicles; and (3) they trap and retain immune complexes on their surfaces for long periods of time (Tew *et al.*, 1990; Tew *et al.*, 1997). Germinal centers are characterized by rapidly proliferating somatically mutating B cells and FDC play an important role in regulating events in this special microenvironment. Most B cells in the germinal centers appear to die and are taken up by tingible body macrophages (Smith *et al.*, 1988); however, some germinal center B cells compete for and bind antigens on the FDC and emerge as antibody-forming cells (AFC) producing a high affinity antibody or as B memory cells with high affinity receptors (DiLosa *et al.*, 1991; Tew *et al.*, 1997; Tsiagbe *et al.*, 1996). The production of the specific high affinity antibody is thought to lead to affinity maturation in primary responses and upon secondary immunization this antibody rapidly converts the antigen into immune complexes which are transported to the FDC in germinal centers where the secondary response is initiated (Szakal *et al.*, 1983). The AFC formed in the germinal centers then home to the bone marrow where most of the antibodies in secondary responses are produced (DiLosa *et al.*, 1991). Other features which are generally accepted for FDC include: the lack of phagocytic activity, the presence of long highly convoluted dendrites, one or more euchromatic irregularly shaped nuclei, the presence of complement receptors CR1 and CR2, and adhesion molecules including ICAM-1 (CD54) (Petrasch *et al.*, 1990; Schriever *et al.*, 1989a,b; Sellheyer *et al.*, 1989; Gerdes *et al.*, 1983; Maeda *et al.*, 1992; Hanna, and Szakal, 1968; Szakal and Hanna, 1968). A number of names have been used for FDC, including dendritic reticular cell (DRC), antigen-retaining reticular cell, follicular immune complex-retaining cell, follicular antigen-binding dendritic cell, follicular dendritic reticulum cell, dendritic macrophage, and follicular reticular cell, but a committee on

Dendritic Cells: Biology and Clinical Applications
ISBN 0-12-455860-7

nomenclature recommended the name 'follicular dendritic cell' and abbreviation 'FDC' and this has been generally adopted (Tew *et al.*, 1982).

The features and functions of FDC described above contrast markedly with the other dendritic-type cells discussed in this book. Other dendritic-type cells may be found in virtually any area of the body and may be thought of as sentinels of the immune system (Ibrahim et al., 1995). Rather than presenting antigens to B cells, these dendritic-type cells typically interact with T cells and they process and present antigens to T cells in a highly efficient fashion (Cella *et al.*, 1997; Schuler *et al.*, 1997; Shortman *et al.*, 1997; Steinman, 1996). Recent data indicate that the T cell-associated dendritic-type cells may also be found in germinal centers and antigen presentation by these T cell-associated dendritic cells could occur in the germinal center (Grouard *et al.*, 1996). However, these dendritic cells appear throughout the light and dark zones of germinal centers and do not appear to form the 'antigen-retaining reticulum' typical of FDC, although there is evidence that they bear antigens on their surfaces (Grouard *et al.*, 1996).

Antigen trapping in the lymphoid follicles was reported as early as 1950 in studies with fluoresceinated carbohydrate antigens (Hill *et al.*, 1950). The interpretation of these early observations was that antigen was trapped in follicular lymphocytes (Kaplan *et al.*, 1950). In the mid-1960s, radiolabeled salmonella flagella was used as a model protein antigen, and autoradiography revealed that follicular trapping was restricted to the germinal centers and that specific antibody improved trapping (Ada *et al.*, 1964; Nossal *et al.*, 1964). The follicular antigen persists for a time in association with these germinal center cells and the initial interpretation was that this antigen was in a 'phagocytic reticulum' generated by a collection of phagocytic cells (Miller and Nossal, 1964). These early interpretations were rejected when ultrastructural studies indicated the antigen was not phagocytosed but was retained on the surface of long processes that interdigitated among the lymphocytes in the germinal centers (Nossal *et al.*, 1968; Szakal and Hanna, 1968; Hanna, Jr. and Szakal, 1968; Mitchell and Abbot, 1965). Mitchell and Abbot first observed the cells at the ultrastructural level in 1965 and reported that these cells were distinct from phagocytes and that an 'antigen-retaining reticulum' rather than a 'phagocytic reticulum' was present as the antigen was on the surface of long processes rather than inside the cells (Mitchell and Abbot, 1965). In 1968, Szakal and Hanna from the Oak Ridge National Laboratory, Tennessee, and Nossal and colleagues from the Walter and Eliza Hall Institute in Melbourne Australia, published the first detailed descriptions of these antigen-bearing cells. Both groups used ^{125}I-labeled antigens and examined autoradiographs of the follicles of rodent spleens or lymph nodes using the electron microscope. Both groups found that radiolabel persisted on or near the surface of highly convoluted fine cell processes of dendritic-type cells with irregularly shaped euchromatic nuclei. The fine cell processes formed an elaborate meshwork around passing lymphocytes which allowed for near maximal cell–cell contact.

The origin of FDC remains controversial. FDC have morphological similarities or critical markers in common with a variety of cell types including reticular cells, pericytes, some antigen-transporting cells, mononuclear cells, and endothelial cells (Ruco *et al.*, 1991; Parwaresch *et al.*, 1983a,b; Szakal *et al.*, 1983; Rademakers *et al.*, 1988; Dijkstra *et al.*, 1982; Dijkstra *et al.*, 1984; Imai *et al.*, 1986). These morphological similarities or common markers have prompted the suggestion that each of these cell types may represent an FDC precursor and may explain the origin of FDC. These relationships will be explained below, but our recent work favors the hypothesis that FDC are derived from bone marrow and this will be explained in detail below.

EVIDENCE FAVORING A NON-BONE-MARROW ORIGIN FOR FDC

FDC clearly have morphological similarities and have critical markers in common with a variety of cell types. In 1980 Heusermann and colleagues used light and electron microscopy and observed cells that appeared to represent transitional forms between FDC and reticular cells in rabbit spleens (Heusermann *et al.*, 1980). Dijkstra *et al.* (1982; 1984) studied lymph nodes and spleen and Imai *et al.* (1986) observed the draining lymph nodes of newborn rats and followed the ontological development of FDC. The initial trapping of immune complex appeared to take place on reticular cells in the stroma of primary follicles. In 1997 Kasajima and colleagues studied the ontogenetic development of human FDC and reported the appearance of cells with the FDC phenotype ($CD21^+$, $KiM4p^+$) in the cortical area of the fetal lymph node around the 20th gestational week and saw no indication that the cells were migrating into the site. In 1988 Rademakers and colleagues observed similarities in alkaline phosphatase activity between FDC and pericytes. In ultrastructural studies they also found some FDC around capillaries in the germinal center in direct contact by desmosome-like attachments with cells present in the perivascular space. These interrelationships suggested the possibility that pericytes were precursors of the FDC. In 1991 Ruco and colleagues observed expression of the DRC-1 antigen and endothelial leukocyte adhesion molecule-1 on FDC-like cells from lymph nodes of patients with Castleman's disease, prompting the suggestion that FDC might originate from endothelial cells.

An alternative experimental approach to establish origin is to carry out adoptive transplantation experiments to see whether FDC of the donor phenotype emerge in recipients of various cell types. In 1984 Humphrey and colleagues examined allogeneic bone marrow of irradiation chimeras and found FDC expressed the MHC molecules of the murine host for over one year after transplantation. The monocytes and lymphocytes in these animals were clearly of donor origin, indicating that the transplants were successful, and the results supported a non-bone-marrow origin for FDC. Similar results have been reported by Yoshida *et al.* (1995), who transplanted severe combined immunodeficient (SCID) mice with splenic B and T cells and found that the FDC were of host origin. The SCID mice lack mature FDC (Kapasi *et al.*, 1993) and are easily transplanted with a variety of donor cells. Again the fact that FDC were of host phenotype supports a non-bone-marrow origin. Similarly, in 1992 Imazeki and colleagues transplanted allogeneic spleen and observed that FDC in the regenerated splenic grafts were of donor origin while the host cells were clearly recirculating through the transplanted organ. The data supported the concept that the FDC were coming from stationary cells which were not in the recirculating population. In recent studies, Kapasi *et al.* (1997) also found FDC of host origin were present in SCID mice adoptively transplanted with bone marrow. However, as will be described in detail below, they also found some FDC of host origin. It is clear from all transplantation studies that bone marrow chimeras do have FDC of host origin and these FDC may be found for months to years after transplantation. This is in marked contrast to typical leukocytes which are recirculating and are restricted to the donor phenotype after a relatively short period of time. If FDC arise from bone marrow cells they must have characteristics that are very different from the typical hemopoeitic cells and the hypothesis that FDC are derived from a local non-bone-marrow origin would fit the morphological data and most of the transplantation data very well.

EVIDENCE SUPPORTING AN EXTRA-NODAL ORIGIN OF FDC

The Antigen-transporting Cells (ATC) and FDC

Our contention that FDC are of extra-nodal origin was suggested by multiple lines of evidence derived from morphological, kinetic, and phenotypic studies. The initial idea of extra-nodal origin came from the studies of antigen transport to FDC. In 1983 we described this cell-mediated mechanism of antigen transport to follicles (Szakal *et al.*, 1983). A group of cells, collectively termed antigen-transporting cells (ATC), was observed migrating from the afferent lymph to the subcapsular sinus and then to the follicles, carrying antigen in the form of immune complexes on their surfaces. This migration takes place during the first 24–36 h after antigenic challenge (Szakal *et al.*, 1983). Antigen transport is rapid and can be recognized by the histochemical staining of the path of immune complex-coated ATC as early as 1 min after antigen injection of immunized mice. This path fans out from narrow sections of the subcapsular sinus, where ATC cross the floor of the sinus through pores toward the follicles in the cortex. In tissue sections, the path appears as a triangular peroxidase-positive area when horseradish peroxidase (HRP) is used as the antigen or when labeling the ATC with monoclonal antibodies (Haley *et al.*, 1995; Szakal *et al.*, 1983). This mechanism is antibody dependent and primarily functional during the late phases of the primary and the secondary antibody responses.

An important finding that directly relates to the idea of extra-nodal origin of FDC was that, during antigen transport, the first cells with immune complexes on their surfaces were found in the afferent lymph of the subcapsular sinus (Szakal *et al.*, 1983). These cells had a monocyte-like morphology, an indented, relatively euchromatic nucleus, and small peroxidase-positive, cytoplasmic granules (primary lysosomes) associated with the Golgi apparatus (Szakal *et al.*, 1983). These nonphagocytic cells are quite distinct from the typical phagosome-rich sinusoidal macrophages that phagocytose the majority of immune complexes (Szakal *et al.*, 1983). There is always a distinct spatial separation between these veiled and dendritic ATC and the antigen-laden macrophages in the subcapsular sinus. This cell-mediated antigen transport pathway is focused on specific anatomical sites of the subcapsular sinus floor, typically located over follicles.

These ATC penetrate the subcapsular sinus floor through pores. This passage through a pore can be convincingly followed by electron microscopy (Szakal *et al.*, 1983). During this development of the antigen transport pathway, the initial ATC are morphologically transformed from veiled to dendritic cells. As these cells move below the sinus floor, their nuclei increase in size and number of lobes. At that time, ATC begin to develop long dendritic processes, which interdigitate with processes of other ATC in the antigen transport pathway. Thus, these ATC form a chain—a reticulum—which expands toward the nearby follicle in the cortex with the arrival of new ATC. ATC become increasingly more dendritic along this antigen transport chain and as the cells enter the follicles they take on the morphology of mature FDC. By 24 h after antigen injection, the FDC antigen-retaining reticulum is established at most sites through this mechanism.

In our original paper on antigen transport, we proposed three hypothetical mechanisms of antigen transport. According to one mechanism, ATC may be cells strictly concerned with the transport and transfer of antigen to FDC. According to the second hypothetical mechanism—by far the most attractive idea—ATC may be pre-FDC that mature to become FDC (as described above) and thus no transfer of the transported antigen would take place. A third alternative might be the combination of these two mechanisms. More recently, we reasoned that if ATC were pre-FDC, then their antigenic phenotype should be either very similar to or identical to that of mature FDC. To determine this, we phenotyped ATC in situ between 1 and 15 min after antigen injection, during the initial phase of development of the transport path. As controls, we phenotyped mature FDC at 3 days after antigen injection. The results revealed that ATC and FDC bear the same phenotype (Table 1).

From this phenotyping and the observed maturation of ATC in the transport chain as indicated by light- and electron-microscopic morphology, we concluded that ATC are pre-FDC. Furthermore, since the first monocyte-like, veiled ATC were seen in the afferent lymph of the subcapsular sinus, we proposed that FDC originate outside of the lymph node from monocyte-like, veiled cells.

The recognition of this cell-mediated, antibody-dependent mechanism of antigen transport to lymph node follicles prompted some pertinent questions. For example: Are there enough ATC to transport the antigen? Can the amount of antigen transported by ATC account for the amount of antigen retained by FDC networks? What happens when new immune complexes are transported to an existing FDC network? Are the new ATC added to the reticulum? Would not that eventually make the reticulum too large? What happens when an antigen of different specificity is transported to follicles already occupied by an immune complex-bearing FDC network? For a detailed discussion of these questions, the reader is referred to Szakal *et al.* (1995).

Table 1. Antigen transport cell (ATC) vs follicular dendritic cell (FDC) phenotype *in situ*

Monoclonal antibodies	Rat isotype	Anti-mouse reactivity	ATC 1–15 min post Ag	FDC 3 days post Ag
FDC-M1	IgG	FDC and TBM	+++	+++
MK-1	IgG2a	ICAM-1	+++	+++
2.4G2	IgG1	Low affinity FcγRII	+++	+++
8C12	IgG	CR1	+++	+++
F4/80	IgG2b	Mo, Mϕ, and LC	+	+
Mac-2	IgG2a	Mϕ subset	−	−
MOMA-2	IgG2b	Mo, Mϕ, and LDC ±	+	+
MIDC-8	IgG2a	DC cytoplasm, VC, LC	+	+
NLDC-145	IgG2a	Cytoplasm and membrane IDC, VC, LC	+	+
Anti-CD45: clones:	IgG	Ly-5 (T200); LCA		
30F11.1		All 3 isoforms	−	−
M1/9.3		Only isoform on T and B cells	++	++

In short, it appears that the cell-mediated antigen transport mechanism can account for the transport of an adequate amount of antigen to follicles. Concomitantly, this antigen transport mechanism also provides pre-FDC (ATC) of an identical phenotype with FDC. The pre-FDC mature in transit from the afferent lymph to the follicles and ultimately form the FDC antigen-retaining reticulum. While new ATC transporting additional complexes may be added to the existing FDC reticulum, a relatively steady state in the size of FDC networks may be achieved in concert with the mechanisms of iccosome formation and dispersion that result in a partial or complete dissipation of FDC networks. Antigen transport, as it exists in the lymph node, supports the extranodal FDC derivation theory.

Putative FDC Precursors in the Blood and Bone Marrow

Since the initial SCID mouse/bone marrow chimera studies suggested that FDC precursors come from the bone marrow, we reasoned that FDC precursors must be present in the blood as well as in the bone marrow. In fact, Parwaresch *et al.* (1983a,b), using the monoclonal antibody KiM4 specific for human FDC, identified KiM4$^+$ cells in human blood. We also found similarly sized (14–16 μm diameter) cells in mouse blood with the aid of the mouse FDC-specific mAb, FDC-M1 (Haley *et al.*, 1995). Furthermore, these cells also proved to be highly positive for complement receptors just like ATC and mature FDC. Using FDC-M1, we also located FDC-M1$^+$ cells in the bone marrow. A definite identification of the FDC-M1$^+$ cells in the bone marrow was not possible by electron microscopy. However, the finding of these potential FDC precursors in the blood and bone marrow made an encouraging connection between the bone marrow, a source of the precursors, and the tissues drained by the lymph nodes.

SCID MOUSE/BONE MARROW CHIMERAS STUDIES SUPPORTING A BONE MARROW ORIGIN FOR FDC

We were prompted to use SCID mice for the construction of chimeras because SCID mice lack mature FDC (Kapasi *et al.*, 1993). Concern about preexisting mature FDC developed as a consequence of studies of bone marrow chimeras using normal mice. We confirmed the findings of Humphrey *et al.* (1984), who found FDC of host origin for long periods after constructing bone marrow chimeras in wild-type mice. However, in our studies a critical control failed—irradiation did not destroy the preexisting FDC. In our hands, FDC are resistant to even very high doses of radiation, (i.e., 1600 rads (Burton *et al.*, unpublished); 18.5 Gy (Nettesheim and Hanna, 1969)). If host FDC were not eliminated from the system by radiation, then it is not surprising that host FDC are present after reconstitution with donor bone marrow. We know that antigen-bearing FDC are present in murine hosts for over a year and we suspect that these are very long-lived cells. Consequently, we are not surprised that FDC of host origin may persist for months to years and the presence of these host cells may make it difficult to detect FDC of donor origin.

To circumvent this FDC radioresistance problem, we turned to the SCID mouse model where the absence of FDC was shown by the lack of antigen localization on FDC in lymph node and splenic follicles of passively immunized mice, and by the lack of labeling with the monoclonal antibody FDC-M1 (Kapasi *et al.*, 1993). However, reconstitution of SCID mice with B and T cells results in the rapid development of FDC networks, indicating that SCID mice have FDC precursors (Kapasi *et al.*, 1993). In ontogeny, FDC do not appear until about 3 weeks after birth (Holmes *et al.*, 1984; Dijkstra *et al.*, 1982; Dijkstra *et al.*, 1984). We reasoned that transferring bone marrow or fetal liver cells to newborn SCID mice would be advantageous as it would allow donor pre-FDC to expand and compete with host FDC precursors throughout development. Recipients of F_1 (Balb/c × C57BL/6) mouse bone marrow were evaluated 6 months after cell transfer for donor phenotype FDC, using monoclonal antibodies against C57BL/6 class I antigens (Kapasi *et al.*, 1994; Kapasi *et al.*, 1997). As expected, FDC bearing host class I molecules were present. However, cells were also present in the germinal center light zones that double-labeled for donor class I and FDC-MI, indicating that FDC of donor phenotype were also present.

We sought to confirm the presence of donor FDC in bone marrow chimeras using a system where we could use a mAb that was uniquely specific for donor FDC. SCID mice accept xenogeneic transplants (Surh and Sprent, 1991) and this prompted us to reconstitute SCID mice with rat bone marrow or rat fetal liver cells. We then evaluated the recipients for rat donor phenotype FDC 6–8 weeks after rat bone marrow or rat fetal liver cell transfers, using the mouse-anti-rat FDC-specific monoclonal antibody, ED5. Of 7 rat bone marrow reconstituted SCID mice, 3 mice clearly showed the presence of $ED5^+$ FDC networks in lymph nodes and spleens (Kapasi *et al.*, 1997). Similarly, 1 out of 5 recipients of rat fetal liver also had rat FDC in the lymphoid organs (Kapasi *et al.*, 1997). It should be noted that $FDC\text{-}M1^+$ FDC were not reactive with ED5, indicating that the monoclonal antibody ED5, as reported (Jeurissen and Dijkstra, 1986), does not cross-react with mouse FDC. Similarly, the $ED5^+$ cells did not cross-react with the monoclonal antibody FDC-M1. Again, murine FDC were present in the recipients and that is not surprising, considering that SCID mice have FDC precursors. However, the presence of rat-FDC networks can only be explained on the basis of FDC precursors in the transferred rat bone marrow (Kapasi *et al.*, 1994; Kapasi *et al.*, 1997). These observations also give further credence to the pre-FDC nature of ATC and to the extra-nodal origin of FDC.

Further confirmation of the presence of FDC precursors in the bone marrow was obtained using flow cytometric analysis and the *lacZ* mouse model (Sanes *et al.*, 1986). Rosa-26 mice transfected with the *lacZ* gene express the gene product, β-galactosidase, in all cells. Through the action of this gene product, the fluoresceinated substrate, fluorescein-di-β-galactopyranoside (FDG) (Roederer *et al.*, 1991) is cleaved and the fluorescein is released into the cytoplasm. As a result, the cell becomes fluorescent and detectable by flow cytometry. Using the same protocol for the construction of chimeras as above, newborn (3-day-old) SCID mice received bone marrow cell transfers from Rosa-26 mice. We reasoned that if the SCID mice were repopulated by Rosa-26 bone marrow FDC precursors, then donor FDC would be identifiable through the presence of the *lacZ* gene product. For flow cytometry, FDC were isolated and labeled with FDC-M1. As indicated in Fig. 1D, about half of the $FDC\text{-}M1^+$ cells obtained from these chimeric mice also labeled with FDG, indicating the presence of the *lacZ* gene product representing-donor derived FDC. Incubating these preparations without the fluoresceinated substrate or streptavidin–PE provided the background level of labeling (Fig. 1A). An FDC-enriched preparation obtained from normal BALB/cBy mice treated with the FDC-M1 mAb and the fluoresceinated substrate (Fig. 1B) is

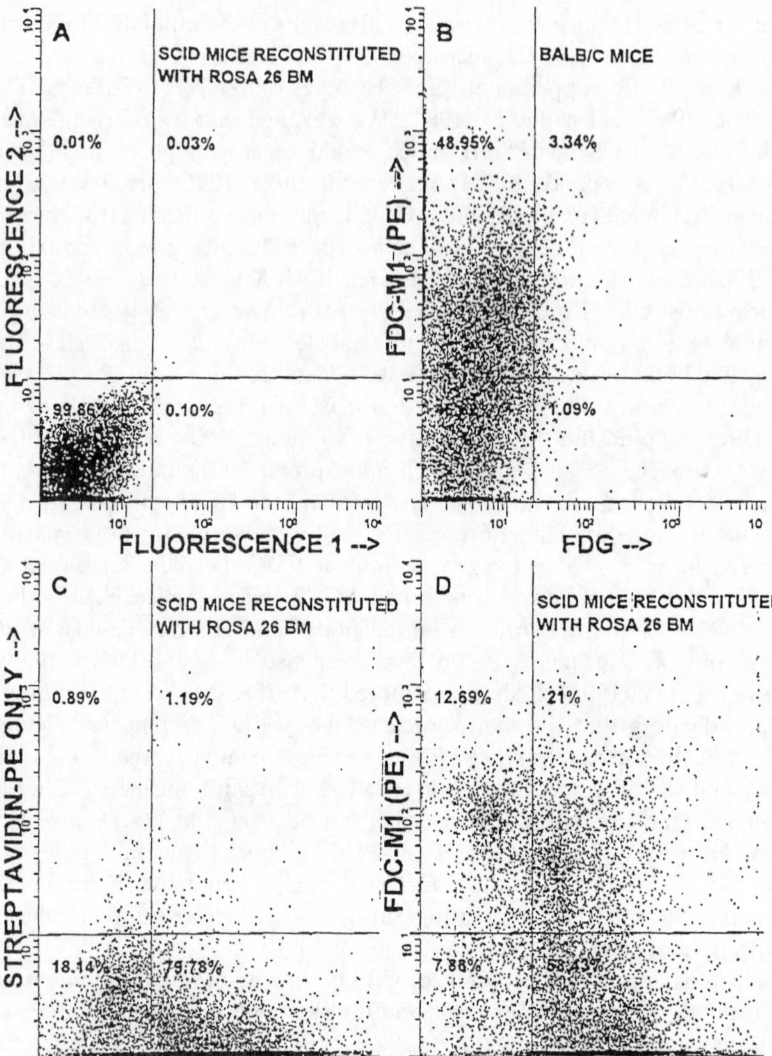

Fig. 1. FDC exhibit the *lacZ* gene product, β-galactosidase, when isolated from SCID mice reconstituted with ROSA BL/6 F1 bone marrow cells. FDC were identified by the mouse FDC-specific monoclonal antibody FDC-M1 and β-galactosidase activity was indicated by incubation with FDG, a fluorogenic substrate which releases fluorescein when cleaved. Newborn SCID mice were chosen to minimize the potential for host FDC precursors to become established before the donor FDC precursors. In this experiment, 6 months after injecting donor bone marrow the FDC were isolated and the cells were tested for β-galactosidase activity. Panel A represents the background control. These FDC were incubated without the fluoresceinated substrate or streptavidin–PE. Panel B represents results from an FDC preparation obtained from normal BALB/cBy mice treated with the FDC-M1 mAb and the fluoresceinated substrate isolated at the same time as those in panels A, C, & D. Panel C illustrates results from the FDC preparation from chimeric mice incubated without the FDC-M1 mAb. Panel D indicates that over half of the FDC-M1$^+$ cells obtained from these chimeric mice also labeled with FDG, indicating the presence of the *lacZ* gene product and therefore of donor-derived FDC. These data are typical of 3 experiments of this type. From Kapasi *et al.* (1998). Copyright © 1998 The American Association of Immunologists.

included for comparison, as is an FDC-enriched preparation from chimeric mice incubated without the FDC-M1 mAb (Fig. 1C) (Kapasi *et al.*, 1997).

Lymphocytes are often intimately associated with FDC and thus could contribute to the *lacZ*-positive FDC population detected by flow cytometry. Irradiation eliminates most lymphocytes and minimizes this problem. However, to rule out the possibility that *lacZ*-positive lymphocytes were responsible for the labeling, FDC in the preparations were identified by morphology using a microscope equipped with Nomarski optics (Schnizlein *et al.*, 1985). The results confirmed the presence of the *lacZ* gene product in cells with FDC morphology. These results support the results of the SCID mouse–F1 and SCID mouse–rat chimeras and we conclude that FDC precursors *can* come from the bone marrow.

Recently, Yoshida *et al.* (1995) showed the presence of host FDC in the spleen of SCID mice after transferring allogeneic lymphocytes. This is in agreement with our data showing the development of mouse FDC in SCID mice reconstituted with rat bone marrow and fetal liver cells. It appears that FDC precursors in SCID mice can develop in the presence of syngeneic, allogeneic, or even xenogeneic lymphocytes as shown in the study with rat bone marrow. Additionally, they also noted the presence of FDC-M1-positive cells that did not appear to bear the host phenotype. These authors indicate that FDC-M1 reacts with two FDC populations of different origin (Yoshida *et al.*, 1995). It is possible that heterogeneous populations of FDC may have different origin. However, the fact that they used 6-week-old SCID mice in contrast to newborn SCID mice for reconstitution, and splenic cells enriched for T and B lymphocytes in contrast to bone marrow cells, may have minimized the development of FDC of donor origin in their study. Moreover, these authors examined the spleens 5–6 weeks after reconstitution in contrast to 3–6 months in most of our experiments. We believe that owing to slow turnover of FDC (Tew *et al.*, 1990) long-term reconstitution (3–6 months) allows time for donor precursors to be recruited in the formation of FDC networks.

CONCLUDING COMMENTS

Clearly, FDC represent a unique cell type and they have morphological and physiological features that are at variance with those of the known leukocytes. However, we suspect that many of these unusual features, like the resistance to irradiation and long half-life, relate to the unique function in trapping and retaining immune complexes for long periods of time. Cells with the FDC phenotype may be found in the bone marrow and the blood as well as on cells which transport immune complexes into the follicles where germinal centers will develop. Given the phenotypic and morphological similarities between ATC and FDC, we have hypothesized that ATC are FDC precursors that are derived from the bone marrow. This view is further advanced by studies, reviewed here, indicating that bone marrow contains FDC precursors. The conclusion that FDC may be derived from bone marrow is supported by results obtained in three different systems: (1) FDC in F_1 bone marrow reconstituted SCID mice bear donor class I molecules; (2) FDC in SCID mice reconstituted with rat bone marrow bear the rat FDC specific marker ED5; and (3) FDC in SCID mice reconstituted with ROSA BL/6 F1 bone marrow are $LacZ^+$ indicating donor origin. Clearly, FDC can be derived from primary lymphoid tissue and need not develop from local stromal cells originating in the local secondary lymphoid tissue. However, our data do not prove that the FDC precursor is the hematopoietic bone marrow precursor and this is a critical issue. We have transplanted lymphoid/myeloid precursor cells (c-kit$^+$ and negative for lymphocyte and monocyte markers) from bone marrow of *lacZ* mice into newborn SCID mice and the results are being evaluated at the present time.

ACKNOWLEDGMENT

This work was supported by National Institutes of Health Grant AI-17142.

REFERENCES

Ada, G.L., Nossal, G.J.V. and Austin, C.M. (1964). Antigens in immunity V. The ability of cells in lymphoid follicles to recognize foreignness. *Aust. J. Exp. Biol. Med. Sci.* **42**, 331–346.

Cella, M., Sallusto, F. and Lanzavecchia, A. (1997). Origin, maturation and antigen presenting function of dendritic cells. *Curr. Opin. Immunol.* **9**, 10–16.

Dijkstra, C.D., van Tilburg, N.J. and Dopp, E.A. (1982). Ontogenetic aspects of immune-complex trapping in the spleen and popliteal lymph nodes of the rat. *Cell Tissue Res.* **223**, 545–552.

Dijkstra, C.D., Kamperdijk, E.W.A. and Dopp, E.A. (1984). The ontogenetic development of the follicular dendritic cell. An ultrastructural study by means of intravenously injected horseradish peroxidase (HRP)-anti-HRP complexes as marker. *Cell Tissue Res.* **236**, 203–206.

DiLosa, R.M., Maeda, K., Masuda, A., Szakal, A.K. and Tew, J.G. (1991). Germinal center B cells and antibody production in the bone marrow. *J. Immunol.* **1460**, 4071–4077.

Gerdes, J., Stein, H., Mason, D.Y. and Ziegler, A. (1983). Human dendritic reticulum cells of lymphoid follicles: their antigenic profile and their identification as multinucleated giant cells. *Virchows Arch (Cell Pathol.)* **42**, 161.

Grouard, G., Durand, I., Filgueira, L., Banchereau, J. and Liu, Y.J. (1996). Dendritic cells capable of stimulating T cells in germinal centres. *Nature* **384**, 364–367.

Haley, S.T., Tew, J.G. and Szakal, A.K. (1995). The monoclonal antibody FDC-M1 recognizes possible follicular dendritic cell precursors in the blood and bone marrow. *Adv. Exp. Med. Biol.* **378**, 289–291.

Hanna, M.G. Jr. and Szakal, A.K. (1968). Localization of ^{125}I-labeled antigen in germinal centers of mouse spleen: histologic and ultrastructural autoradiographic studies of the secondary immune reaction. *J. Immunol.* **101**, 949–962.

Heusermann, U., Zuborn, K., Schroeder, L. and Sutte, H. (1980). The origin of the dendritic reticulum cell. *Cell Tissue Res.* **209**, 279.

Hill, A.G.S., Deane, H.W., and Coons, A.H. (1950). Localization of antigen in tissue cells V. Capsular polysaccharide of Friedlaner Bacillus, type B, in the mouse. *J. Exp. Med.* **92**, 35–44.

Holmes, K.L., Schnizlein, C.T., Perkins, E.H. and Tew, J.G. (1984). The effect of age on antigen retention in lymphoid follicles and in collagenous tissue of mice. *Mech. Age. Dev.* **25**, 243–255.

Humphrey, J.H., Grennan, D. and Sundaram, V. (1984). The origin of follicular dendritic cells in the mouse and the mechanism of trapping of immune complexes on them. *Eur. J. Immunol.* **14**, 859–864.

Ibrahim, M.A., Chain, B.M. and Katz, D.R. (1995). The injured cell: the role of the dendritic cell system as a sentinel receptor pathway. *Immunol. Today* **16**, 181–186.

Imai, Y., Dobashi, M. and Terashima, K. (1986). Postnatal development of dendritic reticulum cells and their immune complex trapping ability. *Histol. Histopathol.* **1**, 19–26.

Imazeki, N., Senoo, A. and Fuse, Y. (1992). Is the follicular dendritic cell a primarily stationary cell? *Immunology* **76**, 508–510.

Jeurissen, S.H.M. and Dijkstra, C.D. (1986). Characteristics and functional aspects of non-lymphoid cells in rat germinal centers, recognized by two monoclonal antibodies ED5 and ED6. *Eur. J. Immunol.* **16**, 562.

Kapasi, Z.F., Burton, G.F., Shultz, L.D., Tew, J.G. and Szakal, A.K. (1993). Induction of functional follicular dendritic cell development in severe combined immunodeficiency mice. Influence of B and T cells. *J. Immunol.* **150**, 2648–2658.

Kapasi, Z.F., Kosco-Vilbois, M.H., Shultz, L.D., Tew, J.G. and Szakal, A.K. (1994). Cellular origin of follicular dendritic cells. *Adv. Exp. Med. Biol.* **355**, 231–235.

Kapasi, Z.F., Qin, D., Kerr, W.G., Kosco-Vilbois, M., Shultz, L.D., Tew, J.G. and Szakal, A.K. (1998). Follicular dendritic cells (FDC) precursors in primary lymphoid tissues. *J. Immunol.* **160**, 1078–1084.

Kaplan, M.H., Coons, A.H. and Deane, H.W. (1950). Localization of antigen in tissue cells III. Cellular distribution of pneumococcal polysaccharides types II and III in the mouse. *J. Exp. Med.* **91**, 15–29.

Kasajima, N., Maeda, K., Liu, D., Matsuda, M., Fuyama, S., Ito, M., Arai, S. and Imai, Y. (1997). Origin and maturation of follicular dendritic cells (FDCs)—literature review and our preliminary observations on the ontogenesis of human FDCs. *Dendritic Cells* **7**, 53–58.

Maeda, K., Matsuda, M., Imai, Y., Szakal, A.K. and Tew, J.G. (1992). An immunohistochemical study of the phenotype of murine follicular dendritic cells (FDC). *Dendritic Cells* **1**, 23–30.

Miller, J.J. and Nossal, G.J. (1964). Antigens in immunity VI. The phagocytic reticulum of lymph node follicles. *J. Exp. Med.* **120**, 1075–1086.

Mitchell, J. and Abbot, A. (1965). Ultrastructure of the antigen-retaining reticulum of lymph node follicles as shown by high resolution autoradiography. *Nature* **208**, 500–502.

Nettesheim, P. and Hanna, M.G. Jr. (1969). Radiosensitivity of the antigen-trapping mechanism and its relation to the suppression of immune response. *Adv. Exp. Med. Biol.* **5**, 167.

Nossal, G.J., Ada, G.L. and Austin, C.M. (1964). Antigens in immunity IV. Cellular localization of ^{125}I-labelled flagella in lymph nodes. *Aust. J. Exp. Biol. Med. Sci.* **42**, 311–330.

Nossal, G.J.V., Abbot, A., Mitchell, J. and Lummus, Z. (1968). Antigens in immunity XV. Ultrastructural features of antigen capture in primary and secondary lymphoid follicles. *J. Exp. Med.* **127**, 277–290.

Parwaresch, M.R., Radzun, H.J., Feller, A.C., Peters, K.P. and Hansmann, M.L. (1983a). Peroxidase-positive mononuclear leukocytes as possible precursors of human dendritic reticulum cells. *J. Immunol.* **131**, 2719.

Parwaresch, M.R., Radzun, H.J., Hansmann, M.L. and Peters, K.P. (1983b). Monoclonal antibody Ki-M4 specifically recognizes human dendritic reticulum cells (follicular dendritic cells) and their possible precursor in blood. *Blood* **62**, 585–590.

Petrasch, S., Perez, A.C., Schmitz, J., Kosco, M.H. and Brittinger, G. (1990). Antigenic phenotyping of human follicular dendritic cells isolated from nonmalignant and malignant lymphatic tissue. *Eur. J. Immunol.* **20**, 1013–1018.

Rademakers, L.H., de Weger, R.A. and Roholl, P.J. (1988). Identification of alkaline phosphatase positive cells in human germinal centres as follicular dendritic cells. *Adv. Exp. Med. Biol.* **237**, 165–169.

Roederer, M., Fiering , S. and Herzenberg, L.A. (1991). FACS-Gal: flow cytometric analysis and sorting of cells expressing reporter gene constructs. *Methods.* **2**, 248–260.

Ruco, L.P., Gearing, A.J., Pigott, R., Pomponi, D., Burgio, V.L., Cafolla, A., Baiocchini, A. and Baroni, C.D. (1991). Expression of ICAM-1, VCAM-1 and ELAM-1 in angiofollicular lymph node hyperplasia (Castleman's disease): evidence for dysplasia of follicular dendritic reticulum cells. *Histopathology* **19**, 523–528.

Sanes, J.R., Rubenstein, J.L. and Nicolas, J.F. (1986). Use of a recombinant retrovirus to study post-implantation cell lineage in mouse embryos. *EMBO J.* **5**, 3133–3142.

Schnizlein, C.T., Kosco, M.H., Szakal, A.K. and Tew, J.G. (1985). Follicular dendritic cells in suspension: identification, enrichment, and initial characterization indicating immune complex trapping and lack of adherence and phagocytic activity. *J. Immunol.* **134**, 1360–1368.

Schriever, F., Freedman, A.S., Freeman, G., Messner, E., Lee, G., Daley, J. and Nadler, L.M. (1989a). Isolated human follicular dendritic cells display a unique antigenic phenotype. *J. Exp. Med.* **169**, 2043.

Schriever, F., Freedman, A.S., Freeman, G., Messner, E., Lee, G., Daley, J. and Nadler, L.M. (1989b). Isolated human follicular dendritic cells display a unique antigenic phenotype. *J. Exp. Med.* **169**, 2043–2058.

Schuler, G., Thurner, B. and Romani, N. (1997). Dendritic cells: from ignored cells to major players in T-cell-mediated immunity. *Int. Arch. Allergy Immunol.* **112**, 317–322.

Sellheyer, K., Schwarting, R. and Stein, H. (1989). Isolation and antigenic profile of follicular dendritic cells. *Clin . Exp. Immunol.* **78**, 431–436.

Shortman, K., Wu, L., Suss, G., Kronin, V., Winkel, K., Saunders, D. and Vremec, D. (1997). Dendritic cells and T lymphocytes: developmental and functional interactions. *Ciba Found. Symp.* **204**, 130–138.

Smith, J.P., Kosco, M.H., Tew, J.G. and Szakal, A.K. (1988). Thy-1 positive tingible body macrophages (TBM) in mouse lymph nodes. *Anat. Rec.* **222**, 380–390.

Steinman, R.M. (1996). Dendritic cells and immune-based therapies. *Exp. Hematol.* **24**, 859–862.
Surh, C.D. and Sprent, J. (1991). Long-term xenogeneic chimeras. Full differentiation of rat T and B cells in SCID mice. *J. Immunol.* **147**, 2148–2154.
Szakal, A.K. and Hanna, M.G. Jr. (1968). The ultrastructure of antigen localization and virus-like particles in mouse spleen germinal centres. *Exp. Mol. Pathol.* **8**, 75–89.
Szakal, A.K., Holmes, K.L. and Tew, J.G. (1983). Transport of immune complexes from the subcapsular sinus to lymph node follicles on the surface of nonphagocytic cells, including cells with dendritic morphology. *J. Immunol.* **131**, 1714–1727.
Szakal, A.K., Kapasi, Z.F., Haley, S.T. and Tew, J.G. (1995). A theory of follicular dendritic cell origin. *Curr. Top. Microbiol. Immunol.* **201**, 1–13.
Tew, J.G., Thorbecke, G.J. and Steinman, R.M. (1982). Dendritic cells in the immune response: characteristics and recommended nomenclature. *J. Reticuloendothel. Soc.* **31**, 371–380.
Tew, J.G., Kosco, M.H., Burton, G.F. and Szakal, A.K. (1990). Follicular dendritic cells as accessory cells. *Immunol. Rev.* **117**, 185–211.
Tew, J.G., Wu, J., Qin, D., Helm, S., Burton, G.F. and Szakal, A.K. (1997). Follicular dendritic cells and presentation of antigen and costimulatory signals to B cells. *Immunol. Rev.* **156**, 39–52.
Tsiagbe, V.K., Inghirami, G. and Thorbecke, G.J. (1996). The physiology of germinal centers. *Crit. Rev. Immunol.* **16**, 381–421.
Yoshida, K., Kaji, M., Takahashi, T., Van den Berg, T.K. and Dijkstra, C.D. (1995). Host origin of follicular dendritic cells induced in the spleen of SCID mice after transfer of allogeneic lymphocytes. *Immunology* **84**, 117–126.

CHAPTER 5
Developmental Pathways of Human Myeloid Dendritic Cells

Christophe Caux[1], Serge Lebecque[1], Yong-Jun Liu[2] and Jacques Banchereau[3]
[1]Schering-Plough, Laboratory for Immunological Research, Dardilly, France;
[2]DNA Research Institute, Palo Alto, California, USA;
[3]Baylor Research Institute, Dallas, Texas, USA

INTRODUCTION

Dendritic cells (DC) are bone marrow-derived professional antigen-presenting cells (APC) which are required for initiation of immune responses. They represent a trace population of cells, expressing high levels of MHC class II antigens, with a characteristic dendritic shape. They comprise a system that occupies: (1) discrete areas of non-lymphoid tissues with the Langerhans cells of epithelium (skin, mucosa, lung) and the interstitial DC of heart, kidney as well as virtually all other organs; (2) the circulation with the afferent lymph veiled cells and the peripheral blood DC; (3) the T cell-rich areas within secondary lymphoid organs where they are the interdigitating cells (IDC); (4) the thymic medulla; and (5) the B cell follicles of secondary lymphoid organs (Grouard *et al.,* 1996) where they are the germinal center DC (GCDC) (for review see Caux and Banchereau, 1996; Hart, 1997; Knight and Stagg, 1993; Shortman and Caux, 1997; Steinman, 1991; Steinman *et al.*, 1997). Although the relationship between the various DC populations is not yet fully understood, they are thought to represent different steps of maturation interconnected by defined pathways of circulation (Steinman, 1991). In the periphery, DC such as Langerhans cells (LC) capture antigens, then migrate via the lymphatics or blood vessels and home to the T cell-rich areas of secondary lymphoid organs (IDC) (Austyn *et al.*, 1988; De Smedt *et al.*, 1996; Fossum, 1988; Kudo *et al.*, 1997; Larsen *et al.*, 1990; Macatonia *et al.*, 1987). There, they present processed antigen to naive T cells and generate an antigen-specific primary T cell response (Inaba *et al.*, 1990; Liu and MacPherson, 1993; Sornasse *et al.*, 1992). This T cell priming is then followed by the extrafollicular primary B cell response (Inaba and Steinman, 1985; Sornasse *et al.*, 1992). During their migration, from periphery to draining lymph nodes, DC undergo modulations of phenotype and functions including loss of antigen uptake and processing and acquisition of accessory function (Romani *et al*, 1989; Sallusto *et al.*, 1995; Schuler and Steinman, 1985; Streilein *et al.*, 1990).

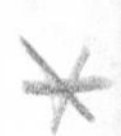

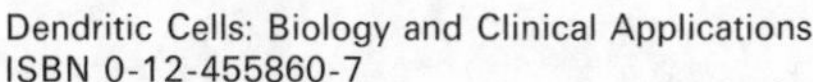

Dendritic Cells: Biology and Clinical Applications
ISBN 0-12-455860-7

Defining the mechanisms of DC action is important as it may ultimately permit understanding of how T cells are primed. This knowledge should allow the manipulation of the immune responses at the early sensitization phase of immunity: downregulation in the case of autoimmunity or transplantation and enhancement in the case of infectious diseases or cancer. In addition, understanding of DC physiology has implications in the context of viral infections, inasmuch as DC appear to be targets for viruses such as HIV, HTLV-1, measles virus, influenza virus, and HSV, and might be involved in virus spreading and general immune suppression (for reviews see Bhardwaj, 1997; Cameron *et al.*, 1996; Knight and Patterson, 1997).

While the bone marrow origin of DC was recognized 20 years ago, it is only recently that the conditions that direct their growth and differentiation have been deciphered. GM-CSF appears to act as a central factor for DC development both in mice and in humans. As DC are difficult to isolate from tissues, their *in vitro* generation represents an important step toward the understanding of DC physiology and their potential use in immunotherapy.

We will first illustrate with Langerhans cells the cell cycle of myeloid DC and next concentrate our attention on the pathways of myeloid DC development *in vitro*. Lastly, the functional properties of these *in vitro* generated cells will be detailed.

LANGERHANS CELLS AS A MODEL OF DENDRITIC CELLS' LIFE CYCLE

Epithelial Langerhans Cells

Epidermal LC are the best-characterized nonlymphoid DC. LC are localized in basal and suprabasal layers of the epidermis (Birbeck *et al.*, 1961). LC are the only cell type in the healthy epidermis that express MHC class II. Those cells have also been described in other stratified epithelia such as mouth, esophagus, and lung (de Fraissinette *et al.*, 1989; Holt *et al.*, 1990; McWilliam *et al.*, 1995; Schon-Hegrad *et al.*, 1991). In humans, 460–1000 LC are found per cm^2 of skin (Rowden, 1981). LC have a multilobulated nucleus and are characterized by cytoplasmic structures formed by double membrane joins, termed the Birbeck granules (Birbeck *et al.*, 1961; Sagebiel and Reed, 1968; Wolff, 1967).

Human LC are characterized by the expression of the CD1a antigen (Fithian *et al.*, 1981; van de Rijn *et al.*, 1984), which is otherwise found only on thymocytes. CD1a is a nonpolymorphic class I-like molecule associated with the β_2-microglobulin (Terhorst *et al.*, 1981), of unknown function. However, recent studies have described $CD4^-CD8^-$ $\alpha\beta$ T cell clones recognizing mycolic acid, a lipid from *Mycobacterium tuberculosis* cell wall, presented by the CD1b or CD1c molecules (for review see Maher and Kronenberg, 1997; see also Beckman *et al.*, 1994). This suggests that the function of the CD1 family (CD1a to CD1e) might be to present to $CD4^-CD8^-$ T cell clones nonpeptidic antigenic determinants specifically borne by some pathogens.

Bone Marrow Origin of Dendritic Cells

The fact that DC express the leukocyte common antigen (CD45) argues for their hematopoietic origin, but direct evidence comes from irradiation reconstitution experiments following bone marrow transplantation. DC from mouse spleen (Steinman *et al.*,

1974), mouse epidermis (Katz *et al.*, 1979), rat lymph (Pugh *et al.*, 1983), and human epidermis (Pelletier *et al.*, 1984; Volc-Platzer *et al.*, 1984) are derived from bone marrow progenitors, as shown by their expression of donor MHC molecules in recipients of marrow transplants. Since epidermal Langerhans cells express myeloid antigens such as CD13, CD33, CD11 and are present in *Ikaros* mutant mice which lack all lymphoid cells (Georgopoulos *et al.*, 1994), the precursor of Langerhans cells is likely to be of myeloid origin.

Migration of Dendritic Cells

From the Bone Marrow to the Periphery

Newly generated DC migrate, presumably through the bloodstream, from the bone marrow to the nonlymphoid tissues (Fig. 1). In particular, in the lung, following inhalation of *Moraxella catarrhalis* organisms, DC accumulate rapidly ($\leq$1 h) into the airway epithelium (McWilliam *et al.*, 1994; McWilliam *et al.*, 1996). Also, in the skin, intradermal injection of GM-CSF induces local accumulation of LC within 48–72 h

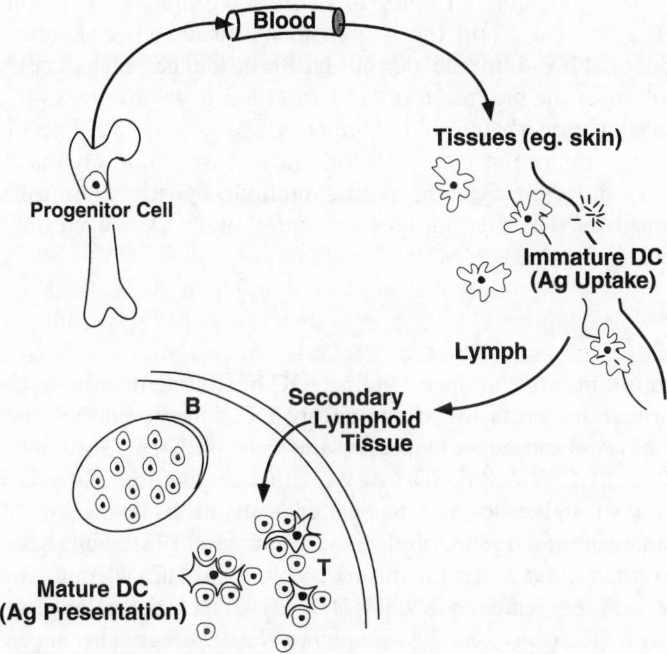

Fig. 1. Life cycle of dendritic cells. Newly generated dendritic cells migrate from the bone marrow to the nonlymphoid tissues presumably through the bloodstream (peripheral blood dendritic cells). During an injury, immature dendritic cells (such as Langerhans cells in the epidermis) capture the antigen and then, under microenvironmental signals (such as TNF-α production in the dermis) leave the nonlymphoid tissues through the afferent lymph (veiled cells) and undergo maturation. Then, mature dendritic cells enter into lymph nodes where they home to the T cell-rich area (interdigitating cells) and induce an antigen-specific primary T cell response. Few dendritic cells exit lymph nodes, possibly because they may be programmed to die after antigen presentation or are destroyed by the efferent immune response.

(Kaplan *et al.*, 1992). These accumulations of DC are thought to represent recruitment of circulating DC precursors. The precursor that enters the epidermis has not been characterized, but culture studies indicate that it could be a $CD34^+$ cell bearing the skin homing cutaneous-associated antigen (CLA), and that it is already committed to Langerhans cell development (Strunk *et al.*, 1997).

From the Periphery to the Secondary Lymphoid Organs

DC enter the spleen from circulating blood (Austyn *et al.*, 1988; Kupiec-Weglinski *et al.*, 1988). DC administered intravenously migrate through the liver, then proceed via the afferent lymphatics to the celiac lymph nodes (Fossum, 1988; Kudo *et al.*, 1997), but few, if any, enter the lymph nodes directly from blood. Several experiments suggest that DC leave the nonlymphoid organs through the afferent lymph. First, during intestinal *Salmonella* infection, specific antigens are present on DC in lymph draining the intestines (Mayrhofer *et al.*, 1986). Second, after subcutaneous injection of antigen, DC in lymph draining the site of injection could present the antigen to sensitized T cells (Bujdoso *et al.*, 1989). Finally, allogeneic skin transplantation models (Kripke *et al.*, 1990; Larsen *et al.*, 1990; Macatonia *et al.*, 1987), as well as injection of labeled DC (Barratt-Boyes *et al.*, 1997; Fossum, 1988) or *Leishmania*-infected LC (Moll *et al.*, 1993) demonstrated that DC enter into the lymph nodes through the afferent lymph. The local production of TNF-α in the dermis has been suggested as representing one mechanism involved in the migration of epidermal LC to lymph nodes (Cumberbatch and Kimber, 1992; Cumberbatch and Kimber, 1995). Also, LPS injection has been shown to induce DC migration into the T cell area of lymphoid organs (De Smedt *et al.*, 1996; Roake *et al.*, 1995). Few DC exit lymph nodes, possibly because they may be either programmed to die after antigen presentation or destroyed by the efferent immune response.

Maturation

During their migration, after antigen loading, DC are thought to undergo changes in phenotype and function. Fresh LC are immature DC that can capture native proteins with great efficiency and subsequently present the processed peptides to memory T cells. Conversely, cultured LC as well as IDC of lymphoid organs are relatively inefficient in antigen uptake but strongly efficient in naive T cell activation (Inaba *et al.*, 1986; Larsen *et al.*, 1990; Romani *et al.*, 1989; Schuler and Steinman, 1985; Shimada *et al.*, 1987; Streilein and Grammer, 1989). In this respect, epidermal LC, when compared to cultured LC or IDC, express relatively low levels of MHC class II molecules and accessory molecules such as B7 (Larsen *et al.*, 1992; Inaba *et al.*, 1994; Larsen *et al.*, 1994; Romani *et al.*, 1989; Teunissen *et al.*, 1990). The maturation of LC that occurs *in vitro* in culture is viewed as a counterpart to the physiological events that occur *in vivo* during migration of LC from skin to draining lymph nodes (Larsen *et al.*, 1990).

The mechanisms involved in this functional maturation have recently been explored using *in vitro* generated DC (see below) both in human and mice. It has been shown that factors known to induce DC migration (i.e. LPS, TNF-α) trigger DC maturation (De Smedt *et al.*, 1996; Sallusto *et al.*, 1995; Sallusto *et al.*, 1996). During the maturation process, the antigen uptake capacity is lost and MHC class II molecules undergo coordinated regulation (rapid and transient boost of synthesis, increase of protein half-life) (Cella *et al.*, 1997; Pierre *et al.*, 1997). These changes result in the rapid accumulation of large numbers of long-lived peptide-loaded MHC class II molecules.

PROPAGATION OF MYELOID DENDRITIC CELLS *IN VITRO*

Progress in the generation of DC from mouse and human precursors has been accomplished recently (for technical review see Caux *et al.*, 1998), allowing the *in vitro* production of high numbers of DC.

From Mouse Precursor Cells

While it was known early that DC arise from proliferating precursors *in vivo* (Fossum, 1989), it has been difficult to identify progenitors in culture. Inaba and colleagues found that aggregates of growing DC develop in cultures of mouse blood that are supplemented with GM-CSF but not with other CSFs (Inaba *et al.*, 1992b). The DC precursors derive from the Ia-negative and nonadherent cell fraction. Comparable culture systems have also been applied to bone marrow cells (Inaba *et al.*, 1992; Scheicher *et al.*, 1992a). The starting population is composed of MHC class II negative precursors and the majority of nonadherent, newly formed granulocytes are removed by gentle washes during the first 2–4 days of culture. The proliferating clusters that are loosely attached remain in culture. At day 4–6, clusters can be resuspended and, upon reculturing, by about 2 weeks large numbers of single, MHC class II-rich DC are being released into the medium. Cells, which proliferate within the aggregates, lack certain antigenic markers that are found on mature DC. However, in pulse chase protocols, the [^{3}H]TdR-labeled progeny exhibit many typical DC features, including abundant MHC class II. Culturing blood or bone marrow progenitors for 2 weeks in semisolid culture medium permitted identification of DC in 1–2% of the colonies in association with granulocytes and monocytes. This demonstrates that granulocytes, monocytes, and DC can develop from a common MHC class II$^-$ progenitor under the aegis of GM-CSF (Inaba *et al.*, 1993).

Marrow progenitors represent a major source of DC since more than 5×10^6 DC can develop within 1 week from precursors present in the large hind limb bones of a single animal.

From Human Peripheral Blood Monocytes

A decade ago, Knight *et al.*, (1986) described monocytes that had acquired a veiled and dendritic appearance after separation. More recently, monocytes were induced to express CD1a after treatment with GM-CSF+IL-4 (Porcelli *et al.*, 1992) or GM-CSF alone (Kasinrerk *et al.*, 1993). This phenomenon was observed only with monocytes and only with GM-CSF (Kasinrerk *et al.*, 1993). It is now well established that monocytes can be induced, without any proliferation, to differentiate into CD1a$^+$ DC, upon culture with GM-CSF and IL-4 (Cella *et al.*, 1997b; Chapuis *et al.*, 1997; Pickl *et al.*, 1996; Romani *et al.*, 1994; Romani *et al.*, 1996; Sallusto and Lanzavecchia, 1994; Zhou and Tedder, 1996) or IL-13 (Piemonti *et al.*, 1995). The monocyte-derived DC display a phenotype of immature DC including low levels of CD80, CD86, CD58, expression of MHC class II within intracytoplasmic compartments, and presence of monocyte markers (CD11b, CD36, CD68, CD115). The cells display an efficient antigen uptake by macropinocytosis or by receptor-mediated endocytosis through the mannose-receptor, and a weak capacity to prime naive T cells. These DC can undergo maturation when stimulated by signals activating ceramide mediators such as LPS, TNF-α, IL-1 (signals also inducing DC migration) or by T cell signals such as CD40L (Sallusto *et al.*, 1995; Sallusto *et al.*, 1996; Sallusto and Lanzavecchia, 1994). Then DC display a mature phenotype including a typical morphology with extended dendrites, a loss of monocyte markers, a loss of antigen uptake, an upregulation of accessory molecules (CD80, CD86, CD58), a translocation of MHC class II onto the cell surface, and a strong capacity to prime naive T cells.

From Human CD34$^+$ Hematopoietic Progenitor Cells

TNF-α in Association with GM-CSF or IL-3 Induces Development of Dendritic Cells from CD34$^+$ Cells

Tumor necrosis factors (α or β) strongly potentiate the proliferation induced by either IL-3 or GM-CSF of CD34$^+$ hematopoietic progenitor cells (HPC), isolated from cord blood or bone marrow mononuclear cells (Backx *et al.*, 1991; Caux *et al.*, 1990; Jacobsen *et al.*, 1992; Reid *et al.*, 1992). In these culture conditions the cooperation between TNF-α and GM-CSF/IL-3 is critical for the development of DC from CD34$^+$ HPC (Caux *et al.*, 1992; Reid *et al.*, 1992; Rosenzwajg *et al.*, 1996; Santiago-Schwarz *et al.*, 1992; Strunk *et al.*, 1996; Szabolcs *et al.*, 1995). Within 8 days in liquid cultures of CD34$^+$ HPC, addition of TNF-α to GM-CSF leads to a 6–8-fold increase in cell number (Caux *et al.*, 1990; Caux *et al.*, 1992). At day 12, 50–80% of cells express CD1a, thus yielding 10–30 $\times$ 10^6 CD1a$^+$ cells from 10^6 CD34$^+$ HPC. Moreover, SCF or FLT3-L increase by 3–6-fold the yield of CD1a$^+$ cells (Saraya and Reid, 1996; Siena *et al.*, 1995; Strobl *et al.*, 1997; Young *et al.*, 1995). These CD1a$^+$ cells are DC according to (1) a typical morphology (Fig. 2); (2) a phenotype of DC (expression of high MHC class II, CD4, CD40, CD54, CD58, CD80, CD86, CD83, and lack of CD64/FcγRI and CD35/CR1); (3) the presence of Birbeck granules (characteristic of LC) in 20% of cells; (4) a high capacity to stimulate proliferation of naive T cells and to present soluble antigen to CD4$^+$ T cell clones (Caux *et al.*, 1992; Caux *et al.*, 1995; Caux *et al.*, 1996a, b). CD1a$^+$ cells are CD45RO$^+$ and express the myeloid markers CD13 and CD33. In this culture system, the effect of TNF-α on the development of DC seems to be mediated through the TNF-R1 (Lardon *et al.*, 1997).

Recently, in cultures performed under serum-free conditions, TGF-β was shown to be required for the development of DC with characteristics of LC (Birbeck granules and Lag molecule) (Riedl *et al.*, 1997; Strobl *et al.*, 1996; Strobl *et al.*, 1997).

Using semisolid cultures, DC were shown to arise within single colonies together with monocytes/macrophages, suggesting the existence of a common precursor cell (Reid *et al.*, 1992; Santiago-Schwarz *et al.*, 1992; Young *et al.*, 1995).

Although GM-CSF or IL-3 (Caux *et al.*, 1996b), in association with TNF-α or TNF-β, appear critical to support DC development from CD34$^+$ progenitors, other pathways of development have been reported. In this respect, *in vivo* injection of FLT3-L in

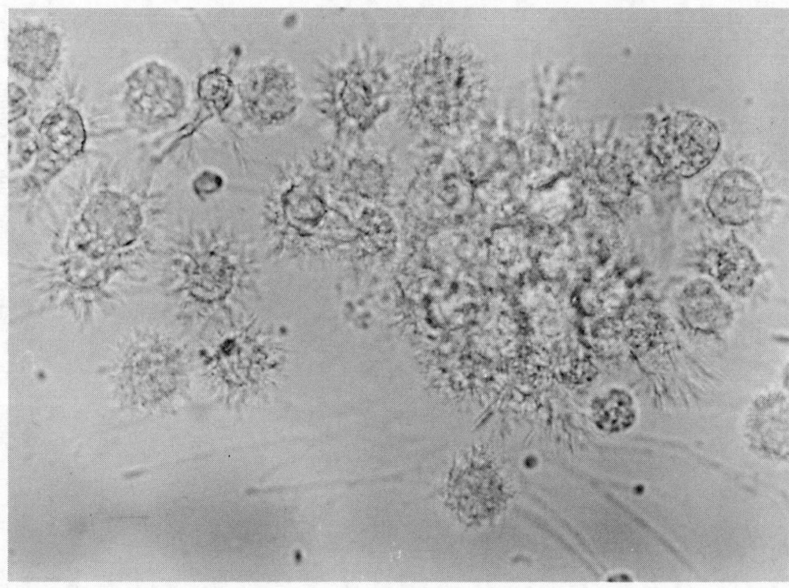

Fig. 2. Morphology of cells generated from CD34⁺ HPC in response to GM-CSF and GM-CSF+TNF-α. $CD34^+$ HPC were cultured for 12 days with GM-CSF+TNF-α. FACS-sorted $CD1a^+$ DC were examined under phase-contrast microscopy. Original magnification ×400.

mice induces a dramatic increase in the number of mature DC in lymphoid organs (Maraskovsky *et al.*, 1996; Pulendran *et al.*, 1997; Shurin *et al.*, 1997). Also, CD40L induces a GM-CSF-independent development of DC from $CD34^+$ HPC (Florès-Romo *et al.*, 1997).

Identification of Two Pathways of Dendritic Cell Development

While most cells are $CD1a^+CD14^-$ after 12 days of culture, at early time points (days 5–7) of the culture, two subsets of DC precursors, identified by the exclusive expression of CD1a and CD14, emerge independently (Caux *et al.*, 1996a) (Fig. 3). Both precursor subsets mature at days 12–14 into DC with typical morphology, phenotype (CD80, CD83, CD86, CD58, high HLA class II) and function. $CD1a^+$ precursors give rise to cells with Langerhans cell characteristics (Birbeck granules, Lag antigen and E-cadherin). In contrast, the $CD14^+$ precursors mature into $CD1a^+$ DC lacking Birbeck granules, E-cadherin and Lag antigen but expressing CD2, CD9, CD69 and the coagulation factor XIIIa described in dermal DC. Interestingly, the $CD14^+$ precursors, but not the $CD1a^+$ precursors, represent bipotent cells that can be induced to differentiate, in response to M-CSF, into macrophage-like cells, lacking accessory function for T cells. Furthermore, CD14- but not CD1a-derived DC express IL-10 mRNA and protein (de Saint-Vis *et al.*, 1998).

Addition of exogenous TGF-β favors the development of DC with characteristics of Langerhans cells such as the expression of E-cadherin, Birbeck granules and the Lag molecule (Caux *et al.*, in preparation). Furthermore TGF-β induces the expression of

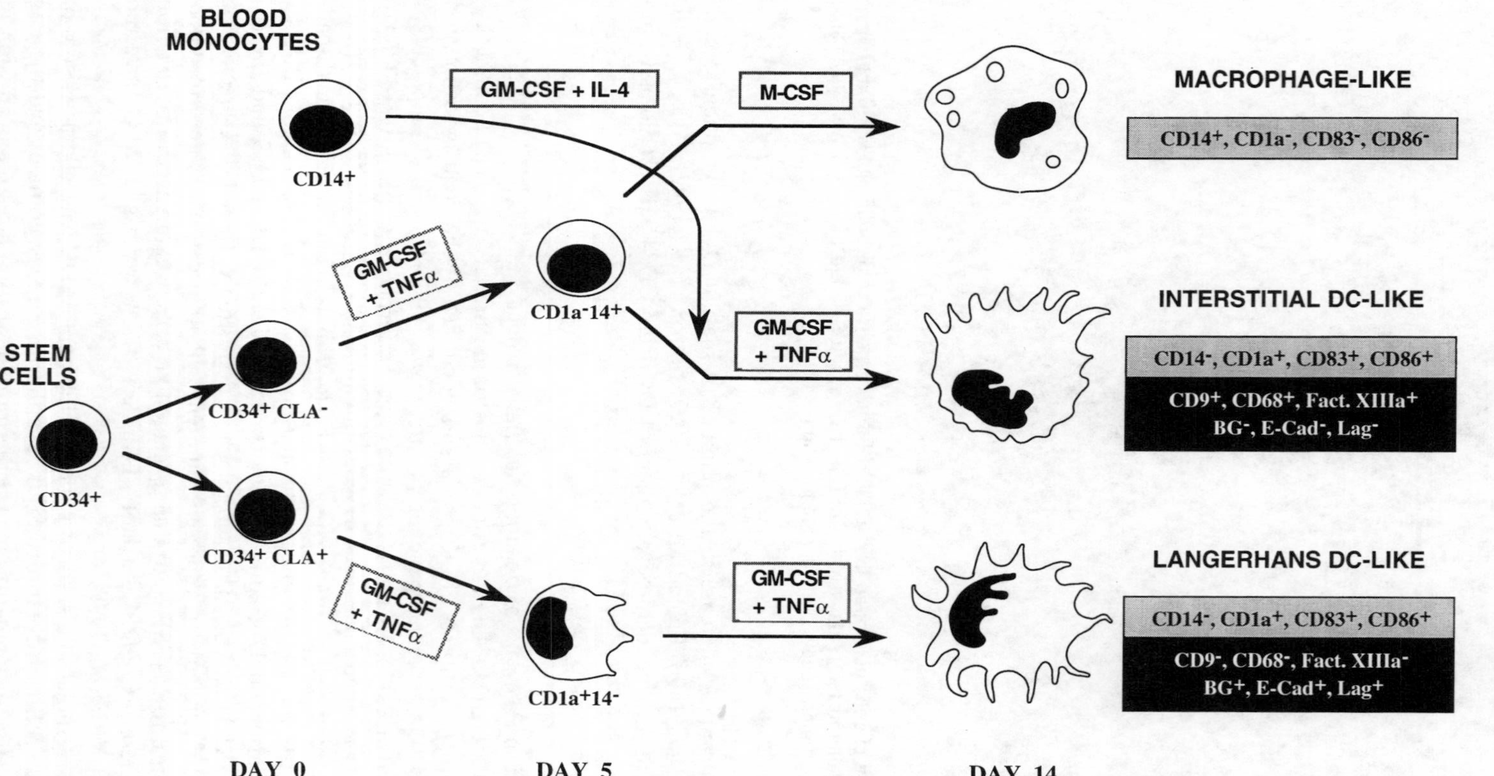

Fig. 3. Pathways of myeloid dendritic cell development. *In vitro* studies in humans suggest that several dendritic cell subsets may originate from different progenitors. A progenitor cell common for granulocytes, monocytes, and dendritic cells (myeloid progenitor), identified in semisolid medium, further differentiates into several lineage-specific precursors. DC-specific precursors ($CLA^+/CD1a^+$) lead to Langerhans cell type DC. In the presence of GM-CSF, $CLA^-/CD14^+$ cells lead to interstitial type DC related to monocyte-derived DC (GM-CSF+IL-4). The same precursor $CLA^-/CD14^+$ cells differentiate into macrophage-like cells in the presence of M-CSF.

molecules recognized by the antibody DCGM4 which stains specifically Langerhans cells *in vivo* (IDC and GCDC from lymphoid organs are negative) (Valladeau *et al.*, in preparation).

These two pathways of development have been documented and further characterized by others. In particular, the commitment into either pathway has already occurred at the level of $CD34^+$ cells (Strunk *et al.*, 1997). Peripheral blood $CD34^+$ which express CLA (cutaneous lymphocyte-associated antigen) differentiate in response to GM-CSF+TNF-α into $CD1a^+$, Birbeck $granule^+$, Lag^+ Langerhans cells, while, CLA^- progenitors differentiate into $CD1a^+$ Birbeck $granule^-$, Lag^- interstitial DC.

While the two populations are equally potent in stimulating naive CD45RA cord blood T cells, each also displays specific activities (Caux *et al.*, 1997). In particular CD14-derived DC demonstrate a potent and long-lasting (from day 8 to day 13) antigen uptake activity (FITC-dextran or peroxidase) that is about 10-fold higher than that of $CD1a^+$ cells. The antigen capture is exclusively mediated by receptors for mannose polymers. The high efficiency of antigen capture of CD14-derived cells is coregulated with the expression of nonspecific esterase activity, a tracer of the lysosomal compartment. In contrast, the $CD1a^+$ population never expresses nonspecific esterase activity. A striking difference between the two populations is the unique capacity of CD14-derived DC to induce naive B cells to differentiate into IgM-secreting cells, in response to CD40 triggering and IL-2. Thus, while T cell priming is borne by both DC populations, initiation of humoral responses might be preferentially regulated by the CD14-derived DC.

Therefore, two different pathways of DC development might produce two populations of DC: (1) the Langerhans cell type which might be mainly involved in cellular immune responses, and (2) the CD14-derived DC related to dermal DC or circulating blood DC, which may be more dedicated to the development of humoral immune responses.

Regulation of Myeloid Dendritic Cell Development and Maturation

While GM-CSF appears to be a key factor required for DC development *in vitro*, other molecules are involved in this process (Fig. 4). TNF-α is mandatory for the recruitment of $CD34^+$ progenitors by GM-CSF (Caux *et al.*, 1992; Reid *et al.*, 1992; Rosenzwajg *et al.*, 1996; Santiago-Schwarz *et al.*, 1992; Strunk *et al.*, 1996; Szabolcs *et al.*, 1995). SCF and FLT3-L act in synergy with GM-CSF and TNF-α to increase the yield of DC (Saraya and Reid, 1996; Siena *et al.*, 1995; Strobl *et al.*, 1997; Young *et al.*, 1995). TGF-β is a required component of bovine serum involved in Langerhans cell development (Riedl *et al.*, 1997; Strobl *et al.*, 1996; Strobl *et al.*, 1997).

Other molecules interfere with DC development. IL-10 prevents the differentiation of monocytes into DC and drives them into macrophage-like cells (Buelens *et al.*, 1997a,b, De Smedt *et al.*, 1997). These effects of IL-10 are also observed during CD34 progenitor differentiation (unpublished observations). Also, M-CSF can interfere with GM-CSF by skewing the differentiation toward the monocyte/macrophage lineage. Similarly, and in synergy with M-CSF, IL-6 blocks DC differentiation and favors macrophage development. These last two molecules appear to be involved in the suppression of DC

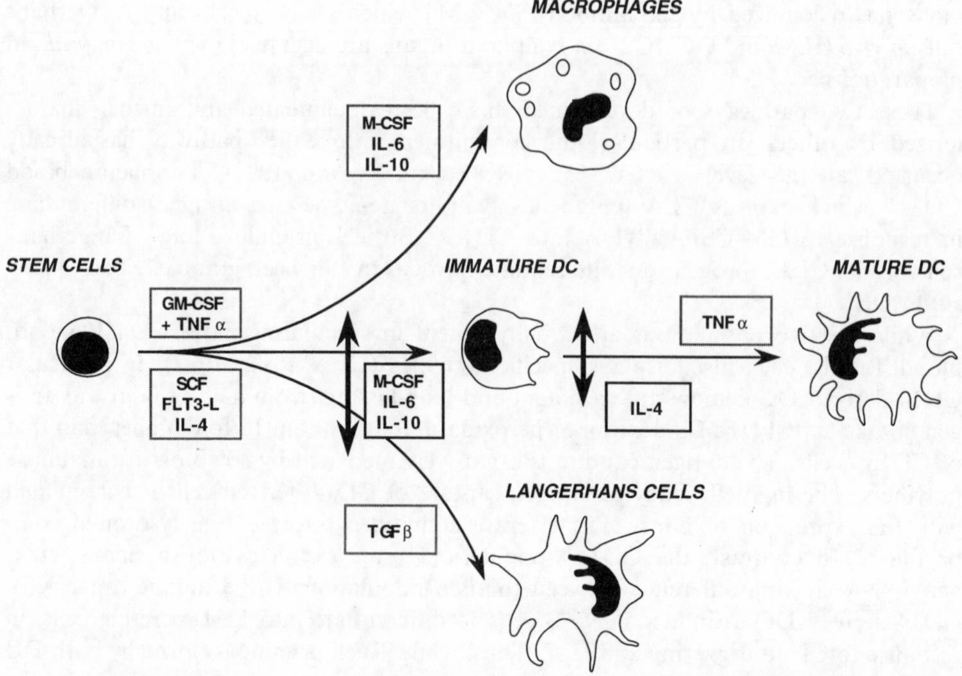

Fig. 4. Regulation of myeloid DC development and maturation. For the development of CD34+ HPC into myeloid DC, GM-CSF and TNF-α are mandatory factors. SCF and FLT3-L act in synergy with GM-CSF+TNF-α. The differentiation into Langerhans cells is dependent on TGF-β. IL-10, IL-6 and M-CSF block the differentiation into DC and induce the development of monocytes/macrophages. IL-4 favors the development of DC but blocks the differentiation at the immature stage. TNF-α in addition to its involvement in progenitor recruitment, induces DC maturation.

development by tumors (Menetrier-Caux *et al.*, submitted). VEGF has also been proposed to be involved in this phenomenon (Gabrilovich *et al.*, 1996).

Regarding DC maturation, IL-4, which is required for differentiation of monocytes into DC, appears to block DC maturation when added to CD34 progenitor cultures. IL-4 blocks upregulation of accessory (CD58, CD80, CD83, CD86) and MHC class II molecules. TNF-α, in addition to its involvement in progenitor recruitment, induces DC maturation (Sallusto *et al.*, 1995; Sallusto and Lanzavecchia, 1994). The TNF-α effect is particularly evident on monocyte-derived DC, whose maturation is also induced by LPS or CD40L: all three molecules signal through the ceramide pathway (Sallusto *et al.*, 1996). The effects of IL-4 on maturation seem to be dominated by those of TNF-α.

A LYMPHOID PATHWAY OF DENDRITIC CELL DEVELOPMENT

The DC propagated in the presence of GM-CSF are of myeloid origin: they express myeloid markers such as CD13, CD33, and CD11c and share origin with monocytes and granulocytes. In contrast, the existence of a population of DC of lymphoid origin has been suggested in mice.

Thymic Dendritic Cells in Mice

One tissue where the Langerhans cell model of DC development seems inappropriate is the thymus. The function of thymic DC is not to initiate a T cell response to foreign antigens, but rather to induce the death of the developing T cells with self-reactive potential (Ardavin, 1997; Brocker *et al.*, 1997). An endogenous DC precursor was identified in the adult mouse thymus by Ardavin *et al.* (1993). In transfer studies this endogenous precursor generated DC and T cells in the same ratio as found in normal thymus, suggesting that it was the major if not the exclusive source of thymic DC (Wu *et al.*, 1995). Such DC would be more likely to present only locally synthesized self-antigens to T cells, rather than presenting foreign antigens collected in the periphery as in the Langerhans cell model.

Origin of Thymic Dendritic Cells in Mice

Mouse thymic DC, and a subgroup of DC in spleen (50%) and lymph nodes, express several markers usually associated with lymphoid cells, including CD8 ($\alpha\alpha$ homodimer), CD2, BP-1, and CD25 (Vremec *et al.*, 1992; Wu *et al.*, 1995). In cell transfer studies, the earliest T cell precursor population in the adult mouse thymus, 'the low CD4 precursor', is unable to produce detectable macrophages and granulocytes. This lymphoid-restricted progenitor was shown to be an efficient precursor of DC (Ardavin *et al.*, 1993). The capacity to differentiate into DC appeared to be the last developmental alternative to be lost as precursors became fully committed to the T lineage (Wu *et al.*, 1996). This attests to a tight linkage between T cell and DC development in the thymus. In reconstitution experiments, this early thymic precursor produces only CD8α^+ DC, in thymus and in spleen, whereas multipotent bone marrow precursors produced both CD8α^- and CD8α^+ DC (Wu and Shortman, 1996). This suggests that the CD8α marks a lymphoid-related DC lineage and that the CD8α^- DC represent myeloid-derived DC.

The early thymic precursor population could be induced to differentiate into DC in culture, with a cloning efficiency of 70% (Saunders *et al.*, 1996). The cytokine requirement for maximal development of DC was complex and included TNF-α, IL-1, IL-3, IL-7, SCF, FLT3-L and CD40L (Saunders *et al.*, 1996).

Putative Function of Lymphoid Dendritic Cells

The function of lymphoid DC is thought to differ from that of myeloid DC. Thymic lymphoid DC are involved in the deletion of developing T cells with self-reactive potential (Ardavin, 1997; Brocker *et al.*, 1997). Regarding their function on mature T cells, it is suggested that lymphoid DC might be involved in the maintenance of peripheral tolerance (reviewed in Shortman and Caux, 1997; Steinman *et al.*, 1997). Indeed, CD8α^+ DC might kill CD4$^+$ T cells via a Fas-mediated apoptosis mechanisms (Süss and Shortman, 1996). Furthermore, CD8α^+ DC, in contrast to CD8α^- DC, have been shown to induce T cell proliferation without inducing concomitant cytokine production such as IL-2, IL-3, GM-CSF, IFN-γ (Kronin *et al.*, 1996; Shortman and Caux, 1997). Along this line, lymphoid DC have recently been shown to express high levels of

MHC class II/self-peptide complex in the T cell areas of lymph nodes (Inaba *et al.*, 1997).

Dendritic Cells in Mutant Mice

Recent experiments with mice whose Rel-B, TGF-β1 or Ikaros genes have been disrupted further illustrate the different origin/relationship of DC subsets and lend support to the concept of lymphoid-related DC in mice. Rel-B−/− animals display epidermal LC but no DC in their thymus and spleen (Burkly *et al.*, 1995; Weih *et al.*, 1995). In contrast, TGFβ−/− mice lack Langerhans cells but display CD11c$^+$ DC in lymph nodes (Borkowski *et al.*, 1996). Ikaros−/− mice lacking T, B, and NK cells display a deficiency in CD11c$^+$ splenic DC. In contrast, epidermal Langerhans cells as well as myeloid lineages (granulocytes, monocytes) are not affected (Georgopoulos *et al.*, 1994; Wu *et al.*, 1997).

CD11c$^-$ Dendritic Cell Precursors in Human

In human tonsils, which are part of mucosal-associated lymphoid tissues, different subsets of DCs and DC precursors have been identified, including CD1a$^+$ Langerhans cells in mucosal epidermis, CD40$^+$ CD80$^+$ CD83$^+$ CD86$^+$ interdigitating cells (IDC), CD4$^+$ CD3$^-$ CD11c$^-$ plasmacytoid DC precursors within the T cell-rich areas, and CD4$^+$ CD3$^-$ CD11c$^+$ DCs in germinal centers (GCDC).

A subset of CD4$^+$ CD11c$^-$ CD3$^-$ blood cells was recently shown to develop into DC when cultured with monocyte conditioned medium (O'Doherty *et al.*, 1994). These cells correspond to the so-called plasmacytoid T cells, an obscure cell type that has long been observed by pathologists within secondary lymphoid tissues. They express CD45RA, but no markers specific for known lymphoid- or myeloid-derived cell types. They undergo rapid apoptosis in culture, unless rescued by IL-3. Further, addition of CD40-Ligand results in their differentiation into dendritic cells that express low levels of myeloid antigens CD13 and CD33. These cells may represent the precursors of lymphoid DCs in humans (Grouard *et al.*, 1997).

Interestingly, and in contrast with other DC populations, the CD11c$^-$ precursors undergo appoptosis in the presence of IL-4 (Soumelis *et al.*, submitted).

DIFFERENT PATHWAYS OF DENDRITIC CELL DEVELOPMENT

In vitro and *in vivo* studies in mice and humans indicate that several DC subsets may originate from at least three different progenitors (Plate 5.5). A progenitor cell common for granulocytes, monocytes and dendritic cells (G-M-DC), identified in semisolid medium, further differentiates into several lineage-specific precursors (Cella *et al.*, 1997; Peters *et al.*, 1996; Young and Steinman, 1996). CD1a$^+$ precursors give rise to Langerhans cells characterized by the expression of Birbeck granules, the Lag antigen and E-cadherin. In contrast, the CD14$^+$ progenitors mature into CD1a$^+$ DC lacking Langerhans cell antigens but expressing CD1lb, CD9, CD68, and the coagulation factor XIIIa described in dermal DC. These characteristic features of CD14$^+$-derived DC are also shared with a population of blood DC (CD11c$^+$, CD13$^+$, CD33$^+$), that has been shown to home, at least in part, within germinal center (GCDC) of human tonsils (de Saint-Vis *et al.*, 1997; Grouard *et al.*, 1996). Interestingly, the CD14$^+$ precursors, but not the CD1a$^+$ precursors, represent bipotent cells that can be induced to differentiate, in response to M-CSF, into macrophage-like cells.

Following maturation signal, monocyte-derived DC display a full DC phenotype and may be closest to dermal DC, germinal center DC, or CD14 precursor-derived DC in view of the lack of Birbeck granules and expression of CD11b and CD68. Indeed, it is tempting to speculate that dermal DC may originate from monocytes that have entered tissues and been activated by IL-4 or IL-13 released by tissular mast cells. Like CD14$^+$ precursors, monocytes can differentiate into macrophages in the presence of M-CSF (Chapuis *et al.*, 1997). As mentioned above, the Langerhans cell type might be mainly involved in cellular immune responses, while the monocyte-derived DC could also be involved in humoral immune responses.

A thorough analysis of cellular populations within the mouse thymus has permitted the identification of progenitors that can differentiate into either T cells or DC when injected into thymic lobes or into B cells following homing into the spleen after i.v. injection (Ardavin *et al.*, 1993; Saunders *et al.*, 1996; Wu *et al.*, 1996). In no case have these progenitors been found to differentiate into the myeloid pathway. Such T-B-DC progenitors might have been identified in humans (Galy *et al.*, 1995; Res *et al.*, 1996) but their function remains undetermined.

FUNCTIONS OF MYELOID DENDRITIC CELLS

Antigen Uptake

Although described as professional APC, DC were until recently considered as displaying poor endocytic and phagocytic capacities (Austyn, 1996; Steinman and Swanson, 1995). Yet LC were shown to perform all steps of receptor-mediated endocytosis (Hanau *et al.*, 1987), and to phagocytose relatively large particles such as latex beads (Matsuno *et al.*, 1996), apoptotic bodies (Rubartelli *et al.*, 1997) viruses (Barfoot *et al.*, 1989), bacteria (Reis e Sousa *et al.*, 1993), and intracellular parasites such as *Leishmania major* (Moll, 1993). DC efficiently concentrate extracellular solutes into vacuoles through macropinocytosis (Sallusto *et al.*, 1995). Antigen uptake by afferent lymph DC can also occur in the form of immune complexes (Harkiss *et al.*, 1990). Lastly, DC express lectins with multiple lectin domains such as the mannose receptor and DEC-205 (Jiang *et al.*, 1995; Sallusto *et al.*, 1995). Such molecules mediate through specific glycan recognition, efficient antigen uptake, and delivery to MHC class II compartment allowing optimal antigen presentation to CD4$^+$ T cell clones (Engering *et al.*, 1997; Tan *et al.*, 1997). These membrane lectins are likely to contribute to the uptake of antigens from bacteria that display glycosylation patterns different from those of mammals, and might therefore represent a first line of discrimination between self and non-self.

Migration

Although factors inducing DC migration *in vivo* have been characterized (LPS, TNF-α), very little is known regarding the regulation of DC trafficking from the blood to the

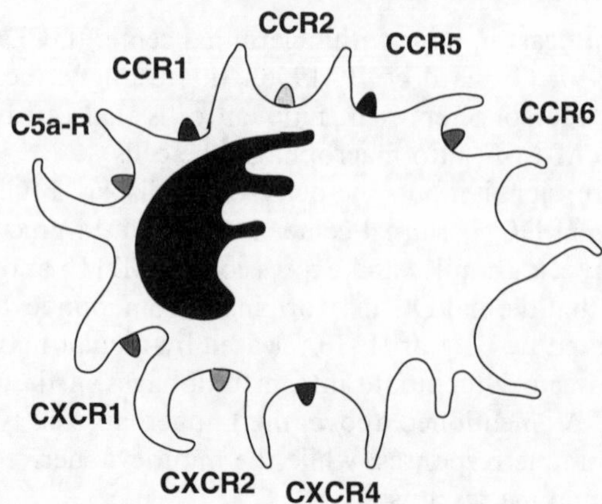

Fig. 6. Human myeloid DC express several chemokine receptors. This scheme is a compilation from studies performed on Langerhans cells, monocyte-derived DC and CD34-derived DC. DC expressed CCR1, CCR2, CCR5, CCR6 (CD34 derived), CXCR1, CXCR2, CXCR4 and C5aR.

tissue and from the tissues to the lymphoid organs. The *in vitro* generated DC have been recently used to characterize the response of DC to various chemokines (Fig. 6).

In vitro generated DC express the chemokine receptors C5aR, CCR1, CCR2, CCR5, CCR6, CXCR1, CXCR2, and CXCR4 (Sozzani *et al.*, 1997). They migrate *in vitro* in response to the CC chemokines MCP-3, MCP-4, Rantes, MIP-1α, MIP-1β, and MIP-5 and to the CXC chemokine SDF-1 (Morelli *et al.*, 1996; Sozzani *et al.*, 1995; Sozzani *et al.*, 1997). In contrast, they do not respond to the C-C chemokine eotaxin, nor to the C-X-C chemokines IL-8, IP10 and Groß, and nor to the C chemokine lymphotactin (Sozzani *et al.*, 1997). The response to MCP-1 and MCP-2 is controversial (Nakamura *et al.*, 1995; Sozzani *et al.*, 1995; Xu *et al.*, 1996). DC respond to C5a, formyl peptides and platelet activating factor (Sozzani *et al.*, 1995; Sozzani *et al.*, 1997). DC migrate in response to a recently identified C-C chemokine MDC, produced by macrophages and DC (Godiska *et al.*, 1997). Recently, a novel C-C chemokine receptor CCR6 has been cloned and demonstrated to be specifically expressed in CD34-derived DC and not in monocyte-derived DC (Greaves *et al.*, 1997; Power *et al.*, 1997). A ligand for this receptor MIP-3α induces the migration of CD34-derived DC but not that of monocyte-derived DC (Power *et al.*, 1997 and personal observation). Also, a C-C chemokine specifically expressed by thymic DC (TECK) has been reported to support migration of DC in mice (Vicari *et al.*, 1997).

The chemokine receptors CCR5 and CXCR4 have been shown to be involved in infection by HIV (Ayehunie *et al.*, 1997; Granelli-Piperno *et al.*, 1996).

It appears that many chemokines can induce DC migration *in vitro*. However, determination of the stage of maturation of the DC, the source of production, and the signals regulating the secretion of the various chemokines will be required to understand the control of DC trafficking (Dieu *et al.*, 1998). Moreover, DC trafficking is also controlled by expression of adhesion molecules. Several molecules have been suggested to participate in the regulation of Langerhans cell migration including E-cadherin (Tang *et al.*, 1993), CLA (Strunk *et al.*, 1997), and CD44 isoforms (Weiss *et al.*,

1997). During their migration, DC have to cross barriers such as basal membrane and endothelial cell wall, processes that should require specific enzymatic activities. Indeed, DC express several metalloproteinases potentially involved in matrix degradation such as interstitial collagenase (MMP-1), stromelysin-2 (MMP-10), human macrophage elastase (MMP-12), as well as newly identified members of the MT-MMP family. Some of these metalloproteinases appear to be DC restricted, suggesting a specific role in their unique migratory capacities (personal observations).

Interactions between Dendritic Cells and T Cells

The capacity of DC for priming T cells *in vivo* has been directly demonstrated in cell transfer experiments. Thus, upon reinjection into foot-pad or blood, or upon intratracheal instillation, mouse DC pulsed *in vitro* with protein antigen induce MHC-restricted antigen-specific T cell responses (Inaba *et al.*, 1990; Levin *et al.*, 1993; Liu and MacPherson, 1993). Furthermore, mouse DC pulsed with HIV envelope-derived or tumor-restricted peptides have been shown to induce $CD8^+$ cytotoxic responses *in vivo*, leading to virus elimination or tumor clearance, respectively (Celluzzi *et al.*, 1996; Mayordomo *et al.*, 1995; Mayordomo *et al.*, 1997; Zitvogel *et al.*, 1996).

Recently, mice expressing transgenic T cell receptors have allowed the quantitative analysis of the capacity of DC to induce a primary T cell response to soluble antigens *in vitro*. In such conditions, DC turned out to be 100- to 300-fold more efficient than any other APC (Croft *et al.*, 1992; Macatonia *et al.*, 1993).

The most common assessment of DC function relates to their remarkable ability to drive allogeneic mixed lymphocyte reaction (MLR). In such asays, DC are about 100-fold more efficient than any other APC populations, including B cells and monocytes (Crow and Kunkel, 1982; Steinman and Witmer, 1978; Van Voorhis *et al.*, 1983). DC can also stimulate allogeneic $CD8^+$ T cells, although higher numbers of DC are required (Inaba *et al.*, 1987; Young and Steinman, 1990). The use of superantigens has further demonstrated the efficiency of DC in primary T cell activation (Bhardwaj *et al.*, 1992; Bhardwaj *et al.*, 1993).

DC generated *in vitro* from $CD34^+$ HPC induce a strong proliferation of allogeneic naive $CD4^+$ T cells and of syngeneic naive $CD4^+$ T cells in the presence of low concentration of superantigens (Caux *et al.*, 1992; Caux *et al.*, 1995). The proliferation of allogeneic $CD8^+$ T cells is weaker than that of $CD4^+$ T cells when cultured with DC alone, but reaches comparable levels in the presence of cytokines such as IL-2, IL-4, or IL-7. Accordingly, allospecific $CD4^+$ or $CD8^+$ T cell lines can be generated by repeated cultures of T cells on DC, and the $CD8^+$ T cell lines are highly cytotoxic in an MHC-restricted manner (Caux *et al.*, 1995; Wettendorff *et al.*, 1995). DC generated from $CD34^+$ HPC or monocytes are able to present efficiently soluble antigen to MHC-matched tetanus toxoid-specific T cell clones (Caux *et al.*, 1995; Sallusto and Lanzavecchia, 1994).

Role of CD40/CD40L in DC–T Cell Interactions (Fig. 7)

The CD40 antigen, which is of critical importance in T cell-dependent B cell growth, differentiation and isotype switch, is also functional on other cell types (Banchereau *et al.*, 1994; van Kooten and Banchereau, 1997). In particular, CD40 is expressed on LC,

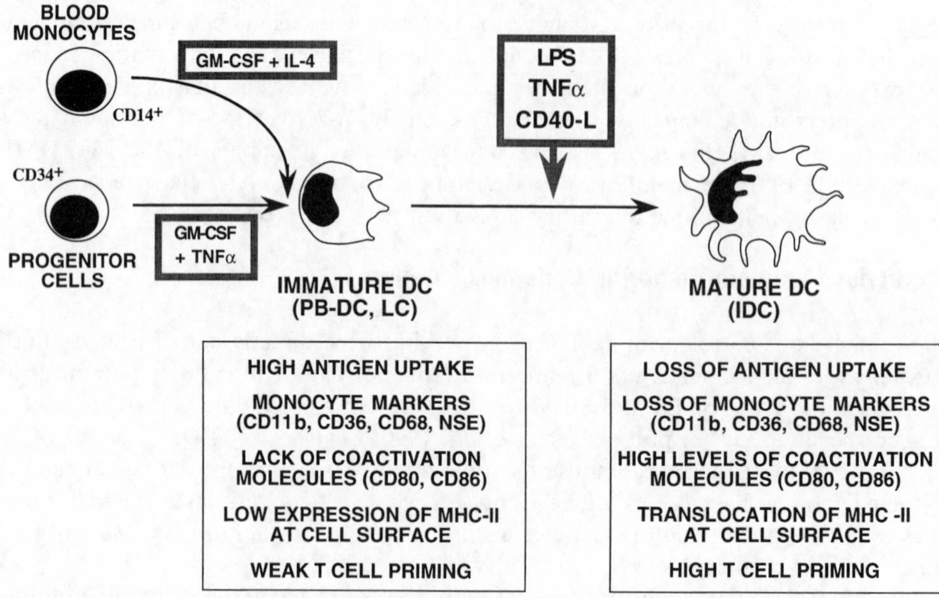

Fig. 7. CD40 activation regulates DC maturation and functions. CD40 engagement on immature DC induces changes in morphology, phenotype and functions. CD40 triggering allows DC survival and induces loss of antigen uptake capacity, upregulation of coactivation molecules, secretion of regulatory cytokines (IL-10, IL-12) and chemokines, translocation of MHC class II at the cell surface and upregulation of the capacity to activate naive T cells. TNF-α and LPS induce similar changes in DC functions. The immature stage of DC corresponds to peripheral DC such as Langerhans cells. The mature stage of DC corresponds to interdigitating cells of secondary lymphoid organs.

blood DC, and interdigitating cells as well as *in vitro* generated DC (Björck *et al.*, 1997; Caux *et al.*, 1994; Lenz *et al.*, 1993; Nestle *et al.*, 1993; O'Doherty *et al.*, 1994). Transferring *in vitro* generated DC into a medium depleted of GM-CSF results in their prompt death unless their CD40 antigen is engaged. In addition, CD40 triggering induces changes in DC morphology, phenotype, and function. Thus, CD40-activated DC upregulate accessory molecules such as CD58, CD80 and CD86 and secrete cytokines (IL-10, TNF-α) and chemokines (IL-8, MIP-1α). CD40 engagement also turns on DC maturation as illustrated by upregulation of CD25 and downregulation of CD1a mimicking the maturation of LC/veiled cells when they enter secondary lymphoid organs to become interdigitating dendritic cells (Larsen *et al.*, 1990; Romani *et al.*, 1989). Moreover, CD40 triggering abolishes antigen uptake capacity, in line with the disappearance of endocytic receptors such as the mannose receptor (personal observation).

In addition, CD40 activation induces the upregulation of newly identified human DC-restricted molecules whose functions remain to be determined. In particular, CD40 engagement induces the expression of a novel disintegrin proteinase belonging to the family of TNF-α and Fas-L processing enzymes (Mueller *et al.*, 1997). Also, a newly identified DC-restricted lysomal associated membrane protein, homologous to CD68, is induced upon maturation by CD40L and is detected *in vivo* only on mature IDC within T cell areas (de Saint-Vis, in preparation). The expression of a diubiquitin molecule, the gene of which has been localized in the MHC class I locus, is upregulated by CD40-L

(Bates *et al.*, 1997). In contrast, and in line with the loss of antigen uptake capacity occurring during maturation, CD40 triggering induces downregulation of newly identified putative endocytic receptors (Garrone and Saeland, personal communication).

As T cells that are activated by DC upregulate CD40-L (Caux *et al.*, 1994), it is likely that CD40 activation of DC represents an important physiological interaction between DC and T cells. The role of CD40 engagement on DC activation/maturation has also been clearly demonstrated using monocyte-derived DC (Sallusto *et al.*, 1995; Sallusto *et al.*, 1996). CD40 triggering on GM-CSF+IL-4-derived DC induces the loss of antigen uptake capacities, upregulation of costimulatory molecules, translocation of MHC class II from intracellular compartments to the cell surface, and, importantly, secretion of IL-12 (Cella *et al.*, 1996; Koch *et al.*, 1996). So far, CD40 engagement appears to be the only stimulus for IL-12 production by DC which results, after interaction with T cells, in the production of IFN-γ by the primed T cells (Macatonia *et al.*, 1995; and Blanchard, personal communication).

CD40 triggering also induced maturation of epidermal LC (Péguet-Navarro *et al.*, 1995), Peyer's patch DC (Ruedl and Hubele, 1997), and CD11c precursors (Grouard *et al.*, 1997). In keeping with this, T cell alloreaction induced by blood DC (Zhou and Tedder, 1995) and epidermal LC (Péguet-Navarro *et al.*, 1995) is inhibited by antibodies interrupting CD40/CD40-L interactions. Indeed, X-linked hyper-IgM patients who have nonfunctional CD40-L present a major T cell defect (impaired IL-12/IFN-γ production) resulting in frequent *Pneumocystis carinii* infections (Grewal *et al.*, 1995; Kamanaka *et al.*, 1996; Notarangelo *et al.*, 1992). Finally, *in vivo* administration of CD40/CD40-L antagonists has been shown to block the development of T cell-dependent collagen-induced arthritis (Durie *et al.*, 1993) as well as graft-versus-host disease (Durie *et al.*, 1994). Taken together, these data can be interpreted as reflecting the interruption of a CD40/CD40-L interaction between T cells and DC rather than between T cells and B cells. A cell type-specific disruption of the CD40 gene would clarify the role of CD40 on the various cell types.

Production of Chemokines (Fig. 8)

Following antigen uptake and migration, DC have to interact with T cells and B cells with the right antigen specificity. These interactions are likely to be favored by the production of chemokines by DC. Indeed, DC secrete many chemokines following CD40 activation such as MIP-1α, MIP-1β, and IL-8 (Caux *et al.*, 1994) and express mRNA for many others (Rantes, I-309, lymphotactin, MIP-3α, MIP-3β, MIP-1γ, MIG) (Mohamadzadeh *et al.*, 1996; Zlotnik, 1996; de Saint Vis, in preparation).

Very recently, several new chemokines have been identified whose expression is restricted to DC: MDC (macrophages and DC) (Godiska *et al.*, 1997), Tarc (essentially DC) (personal observation), DC-CK1 (high levels in DC) (Adema *et al.*, 1997), Teck (mouse thymic DC) (Vicari *et al.*, 1997). Most of these DC-specific chemokines (Teck, Tarc, DC-CK1) induce migration of T cells (Adema *et al.*, 1997; Imai *et al.*, 1996; Vicari *et al.*, 1997) and are most likely involved in T cell attraction in the paracortical area of lymphoid organs during initiation of primary immune responses.

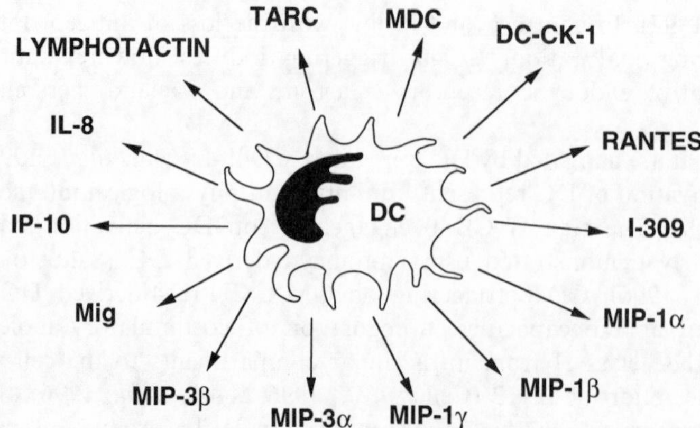

Fig. 8. Human myeloid DC secrete a large array of chemokines. This scheme is a compilation from studies performed with monocyte-derived DC and CD34-derived DC.

Interactions between Dendritic Cells and B Cells

Although the T cell-dependent primary B cell activation requires DC (Flamand *et al.*, 1994; Francotte and Urbain, 1985; Inaba and Steinman, 1985; Inaba *et al.*, 1983; Inaba *et al.*, 1984; Sornasse *et al.*, 1992), and occurs in the extrafollicular area of secondary lymphoid organs, little information is presently available regarding potential interactions between DC and B cells. In a culture system, where the T cell signal is mimicked by CD40-L-transfected L cells, $CD34^+$ HPC-derived DC directly modulate B cell growth and differentiation (Dubois *et al.*, 1997; see Chapter 15). In particular, DC induce a 3–6-fold enhancement of CD40-L-dependent B cell proliferation in the absence of exogenous cytokines. Furthermore, DC considerably enhance (10–100-fold increase) the secretion of IgG, IgA, and IgM by CD40-activated memory B cells, in the absence of exogenous cytokines. Importantly, in the presence of DC, naive $sIgD^+$ B cells produce very large amounts of IgM, in response to IL-2. This latter effect is dependent on the release by DC of soluble mediators after CD40 engagement, in particular IL-12 and gp80 (sIL-6-R) (Dubois *et al.*, 1998). In addition, in the presence of IL-10, DC stimulate CD40-activated naive $sIgD^+$ B cells to express surface IgA and secrete large amounts of both IgA subclasses (Fayette *et al.*, 1997).

POTENTIAL PHYSIOLOGICAL RELEVANCE

DC form a heterogenous family of cells with characteristic features. Their heterogeneity in terms of lineages and functions is not yet fully elucidated. At least three independent pathways of differentiation yielding different DC populations have been identified in human and mouse (Fig. 5). In human, two pathways of development yielding DC of myeloid origin have been documented *in vitro*. Langerhans cells can be generated from $CD34^+$ HPC when cultured in the presence of GM-CSF+TNF-α. In the same culture conditions, another population of DC can be generated from $CD34^+$ HPC; this population lacks the characteristics of Langerhans cells and is probably related to the monocyte-derived DC. Although this cell type displays phenotypic similarities with interstitial DC and CD11c$^+$ circulating DC or tonsil germinal center DC, its *in vivo* counterpart is not yet clearly established. Based on the effect of CD14-derived DC (also borne by monocyte-derived DC) on naive B cell differentiation it is tempting to speculate that this population might be related to CD11c$^+$ DC located within B cell follicules in tonsils.

Thus, these two different pathways of DC development might also exist *in vivo*. The Langerhans cell type might be mainly involved in cellular immune responses as illustrated by their involvement in delayed type hypersensitivity reactions observed after hapten application on the epidermis (Larsen *et al.*, 1990; Macatonia *et al.*, 1987; Sullivan *et al.*, 1986). In contrast, CD14-derived DC, related to monocyte-derived DC, potentially located into tissues such as dermis or blood, might after antigen capture migrate through the blood stream (or lymph) into the T cell-rich area and/or the B cell follicules where they could be involved in the regulation of primary B cell responses.

In mice, the lymphoid origin of thymic DC and of one subset of splenic DC has been demonstrated by K. Shortman and collaborators. Although this pathway of DC development has not yet been clearly demonstrated in humans, the CD11c$^-$ CD13$^-$ DC precursors identified in blood and in tonsils might be related to mouse lymphoid DC. The work of Shortman (Kronin *et al.*, 1996; Süss and Shortman, 1996) suggests that this lymphoid population might be involved in the negative regulation of T cell activation, and might play a role in the maintenance of peripheral tolerance.

The remarkable ability of DC to elicit immune responses and the availability of DC culture systems will allow their use in cancer immunotherapy. Indeed, the induction of therapeutic anti-tumor responses based on DC immunotherapy has been achieved successfully in several mouse models (reviewed in Mayordomo *et al.*, 1997; Schuler and Steinman, 1997). Different strategies for loading DC with tumor-associated antigens have been used to elicit therapeutic anti-tumor responses: tumor-derived peptide-pulsed DC (Celluzzi *et al.*, 1996; Mayordomo *et al.*, 1995; Zitvogel *et al.*, 1996), DC/tumor fusion (Gong *et al.*, 1997), recombinant virus-transduced DC (Song *et al.*, 1997; Specht *et al.*, 1997), tumor RNA-transfected DC (Ashley *et al.*, 1997; Boczkowski *et al.*, 1996). All these strategies were based on expansion and manipulation of DC *in vitro*, followed by their reinjection into animals. A better understanding of the DC system should allow *in vivo* manipulation of DC to achieve anti-tumor immunity, as recently illustrated by the use of FLT3-L *in vivo* in mice (Chen *et al.*, 1997; Lynch *et al.*, 1997).

Similarly, appropriate manipulation of the DC system might allow the induction of tolerance instead of immunity, opening new avenues for therapeutic interventions in autoimmunity, transplantation, and allergy.

ACKNOWLEDGMENTS

We thank our many collaborators over the past three years who permitted us through their work and discussions to write this chapter. S. Ait-Yahia, C. Barthélémy, E. Bates, N. Bendriss, D. Blanchard, F. Brière, J.M. Bridon, L. Chalus, V. Clair, O. de Bouteiller, S. Denépoux, B. de Saint-Vis, M.C. Dieu, O. Djossou, B. Dubois, I. Durand, V. Duvert, J. Fayette, F. Fossiez, N. Fournier, C. Gaillard, E. Garcia, P. Garrone, G. Grouard, S. Ho, C. Massacrier, C. Muller, C. Péronne, J.J. Pin, O. Ravel, M.C. Rissoan, S. Saeland, B. Salinas, V. Soumelis, J. Valladeau, B. Vanbervliet, and S. Vandenabeele have greatly contributed to the most recent experiments. We thank O. Clear and L. Saitta for wonderful daily organization, S. Bourdarel for outstanding help, and D. Lepot and M. Vatan for invaluable assistance.

REFERENCES

Adema, G.J., Hartgers, F., Verstraten, R., de Vries, E., Marland, G., Menon, S., Foster, J., Xu, Y., Nooyen, P., McClanahan, T., Bacon, K.B. and Figdor, C.G. (1997). A dendritic-cell-derived CC chemokine that preferentially attracts naive T cells. *Nature* **387**, 713–717.

Ardavin, C. (1997). Thymic dendritic cells. *Immunol. Today* **18**, 350–361.

Ardavin, C., Wu, L., Li, C.L. and Shortman, K. (1993). Thymic dendritic cells and T cells develop simultaneously in the thymus from a common precursor population. *Nature* **362**, 761–763.

Ashley, D.M., Faiola, B., Nair, S., Hale, L.P., Bigner, D.D. and Gilboa, E. (1997). Bone marrow-generated dendritic cells pulsed with tumor extracts or tumor RNA induce antitumor immunity against central nervous system tumors. *J. Exp. Med.* **186**, 1177–1182.

Austyn, J. D. (1996). New insights into the mobilization and phagocytic activity of dendritic cells. *J. Exp. Med.* **183**, 1287–1292.

Austyn, J.M., Kupiec-Weglinski, J.W., Hankins, D.F. and Morris, P.J. (1988). Migration patterns of dendritic cells in the mouse. Homing to T cell-dependent areas of spleen, and binding within marginal zone. *J. Exp. Med.* **167**, 646–651.

Ayehunie, S., Garcia-Zepeda, E.A., Hoxie, J.A., Horuk, R., Kupper, T.S., Luster, A.D. and Ruprecht, R.M. (1997). Human immunodeficiency virus-1 entry into purified blood dendritic cells through CC and CXC chemokine coreceptors. *Blood* **90**, 1379–1386.

Backx, B., Broeders, L., Bot, F.J. and Lowenberg, B. (1991). Positive and negative effects of tumor necrosis factor on colony growth from highly purified normal marrow progenitors. *Leukemia* **5**, 66–70.

Banchereau, J., Bazan, F., Blanchard, D., Brière, F., Galizzi, J.P., van Kooten, C., Liu, Y.J., Rousset, F. and Saeland, S. (1994). The CD40 antigen and its Ligand. *Annu. Rev. Immunol.* **12**, 881–922.

Barfoot, R., Denham, S., Gyure, L.A., Hall, J.G., Hobbs, S.M., Jackson, L.E. and Robertson, D. (1989). Some properties of dendritic macrophages from peripheral lymph. *Immunology* **68**, 233–239.

Barratt-Boyes, S M., Watkins, S.C. and Finn, O.J. (1997). *In vivo* migration of dendritic cells differentiated *in vitro:* a chimpanzee model. *J. Immunol.* **158**, 4543–4547.

Bates, E.E.M., Ravel, O., Dieu, M.C., Ho, S., Guret, C., Bridon, J.M., Ait-Yahia, S., Brière, F., Caux, C., Banchereau, J. and Lebecque, S. (1997). Identification and analysis of a novel member of the ubiquitin family expressed in dendritic cells and mature B cells. *Eur. J. Immunol.* **27**, 2471–2477.

Beckman, E.M., Porcelli, S.A., Morita, C.T., Behar, S.M., Furlong, S.T. and Brenner, M.B. (1994). Recognition of a lipid antigen by CD1-restricted $\alpha\beta^+$ T cells. *Nature* **372**, 691–694.

Bhardwaj, N. (1997). Interactions of viruses with dendritic cells: a double-edged sword. *J. Exp. Med.* **186**, 795–799.

Bhardwaj, N., Friedman, S.M., Cole, B.C. and Nisanian, A.J. (1992). Dendritic cells are potent antigen-presenting cells for microbial superantigens. *J. Exp. Med.* **175**, 267–273.

Bhardwaj, N., Young, J.W., Nisanian, A.J., Baggers, J. and Steinman, R.M. (1993). Small amounts of superantigen, when presented on dendritic cells, are sufficient to initiate T cell responses. *J. Exp. Med.* **178**, 633–642.

Birbeck, M.S., Breathnach, A.S. and Everall, J.D. (1961). An electron microscopic study of basal melanocytes and high level clear cells (Langerhans' cells) in vitiligo. *J. Invest. Dermatol.* **37**, 51–64.

Björck, P., Banchereau, J. and Florès-Romo, L. (1997). CD40 ligation counteracts Fas-induced apoptosis of human dendritic cells. *Int. Immunol.* **9**, 365–372.

Boczkowski, D., Nair, S.K., Snyder, D. and Gilboa, E. (1996). Dendritic cells pulsed with RNA are potent antigen-presenting cells *in vitro* and *in vivo. J. Exp. Med.* **184**, 465–472.

Borkowski, T.A., Letterio, J.J., Farr, A.G. and Udey, M.C. (1996). A role for endogenous transforming growth factor β1 in Langerhans cell biology: the skin of transforming growth factor β1 null mice is devoid of epidermal Langerhans cells. *J. Exp. Med.* **184**, 2417–2422.

Brocker, T., Riedinger, M. and Karjalainen, K. (1997). Targeted expression of major histocompatibility complex (MHC) class II molecules demonstrates that dendritic cells can induce negative but not positive selection of thymocytes *in vivo*. *J. Exp. Med.* **185**, 541–550.

Buelens, C., Verhasselt, V., De Groote, D., Thielemans, K., Goldman, M. and Willems, F. (1997a). Human dendritic cell responses to lipopolysaccharide and CD40 ligation are differentially regulated by interleukin-10. *Eur. J. Immunol.* **27**, 1848–1852.

Buelens, C., Verhasselt, V., de Groote, D., Thielemans, K., Goldman, M. and Willems, F. (1997b). Interleukin-10 prevents the generation of dendritic cells from human peripheral blood mononuclear cells cultured with interleukin-4 and granulocyte/macrophage-colony-stimulating factor. *Eur. J. Immunol.* **27**, 756–762.

Bujdoso, R., Hopkins, J., Dutia, B.M., Young, P. and McConnell, I. (1989). Characterization of sheep afferent lymph dendritic cells and their role in antigen carriage. *J. Exp. Med.* **170**, 1285–1301.

Burkly, L., Hession, C., Ogata, L., Reilly, C., Marconi, L.A., Olson, D., Tizard, R., Cate, R. and Lo, D. (1995). Expression of *relB* is required for the development of thymic medulla and dendritic cells. *Nature* **373**, 531–536.

Cameron, P., Pope, M., Granelli-Piperno, A. and Steinman, R.M. (1996). Dendritic cells and the replication of HIV-1. *J. Leukocyte Biol.* **59**, 158–171.

Caux, C. and Banchereau, J. (1996). *In vitro* regulation of dendritic cell development and function. In: *Blood Cell Biochemistry* (eds T. Whetton and J. Gordon), Plenum Press, London, pp. 263–301.

Caux, C., Saeland, S., Favre, C., Duvert, V., Mannoni, P. and Banchereau, J. (1990). Tumor necrosis factor-alpha strongly potentiates interleukin-3 and granulocyte-macrophage colony-stimulating factor-induced proliferation of human CD34$^+$ hematopoietic progenitor cells. *Blood* **75**, 2292–2298.

Caux, C., Dezutter-Dambuyant, C., Schmitt, D. and Banchereau, J. (1992). GM-CSF and TNF-α cooperate in the generation of dendritic Langerhans cells. *Nature* **360**, 258–261.

Caux, C., Massacrier, C., Vanbervliet, B., Dubois, B., van Kooten, C., Durand, I. and Banchereau, J. (1994). Activation of human dendritic cells through CD40 cross-linking. *J. Exp. Med.* **180**, 1263-1272.

Caux, C., Massacrier, C., Dezutter-Dambuyant, C., Vanbervliet, B., Jacquet, C., Schmitt, D. and Banchereau, J. (1995). Human dendritic Langerhans cells generated *in vitro* from CD34$^+$ progenitors can prime naive CD4$^+$ T cells and process soluble antigen. *J. Immunol.* **155**, 5427–5435.

Caux, C., Vanbervliet, B., Massacrier, C., Dezutter-Dambuyant, C., de Saint-Vis, B., Jacquet, C., Yonada, K., Imamura, S., Schmitt, D. and Banchereau, J. (1996a). CD34$^+$ hematopoietic progenitors from human cord blood differentiate along two independent dendritic cell pathways in response to GM-CSF+TNF-α. *J. Exp. Med.* **184**, 695–706.

Caux, C., Vanbervliet, B., Massacrier, C., Durand, I. and Banchereau, J. (1996b). Interleukin-3 cooperates with tumor necrosis factor α for the development of human dendritic/Langerhans cells from cord blood CD34$^+$ hematopoietic progenitor cells. *Blood* **87**, 2376–2385.

Caux, C., Massacrier, C., Vanbervliet, B., Dubois, B., Durand, I., Cella, M., Lanzavecchia, A. and Banchereau, J. (1997). CD34$^+$ hematopoietic progenitors from human cord blood differentiate along two independent dendritic cell pathways in response to GM-CSF+TNF-α: II. Functional analysis. *Blood* **90**, 1458–1470.

Caux, C., Dezutter-Dambuyant, C., Liu, Y.J. and Banchereau, J. (1998). Isolation and propagation of human dendritic cells. In: *Methods in Microbiology: Immunological Methods* (eds D. Kabelitz and K. Ziegler), Academic Press, London.

Cella, M., Engering, A., Pinet, V., Pieters, J. and Lanzavecchia, A. (1997a). Inflammatory stimuli induce accumulation of MHC class II complexes on dendritic cells. *Nature* **388**, 782–787.

Cella, M., Sallusto, F. and Lanzavecchia, A. (1997b). Origin, maturation and antigen presenting function of dendritic cells. *Curr. Opin. Immunol.* **9**, 10–16.

Cella, M., Scheidegger, D., Palmer-Lehmann, K., Lane, P., Lanzavecchia, A. and Alber, G. (1996). Ligation of CD40 on dendritic cells triggers production of high levels of interleukin-12 and enhances T cell stimulatory capacity: T-T help via APC activation. *J. Exp. Med.* **184**, 747–752.

Celluzzi, C.M., Mayordomo, J.I., Storkus, W.J., Lotze, M.T. and Falo, L.D. (1996). Peptide-pulsed dendritic cells induce antigen-specific, CTL-mediated protective tumor immunity. *J. Exp. Med.* **183**, 283–287.

Chapuis, F., Rosenzwajg, M., Yagello, M., Ekman, M., Biberfield, P. and Gluckman, J.C. (1997). Differentiation of human dendritic cells from monocytes *in vitro*. *Eur. J. Immunol.* **27**, 431–441.

Chen, K., Braun, S., Lyman, S., Fan, Y., Traycoff, C.M., Wiebke, E.A., Gaddy, J., Sledge, G., Broxmeyer, H.E. and Cornetta, K. (1997). Antitumor activity and immunotherapeutic properties of Flt3-ligand in a murine breast cancer model. *Cancer Res.* **57**, 3511–3516.

Croft, M., Duncan, D.D. and Swain, S.L. (1992). Response of naive antigen-specific CD4$^+$ T cells *in vitro*: characteristics and antigen-presenting cell requirements. *J. Exp. Med.* **176**, 1431–1437.

Crow, M.K. and Kunkel, H.G. (1982). Human dendritic cells: major stimulators of the autologous and allogeneic mixed leucocyte reactions. *Clin. Exp. Immunol.* **49**, 338–346.

Cumberbatch, M. and Kimber, I. (1992). Dermal tumour necrosis factor-alpha induces dendritic cell migration to draining lymph nodes, and possibly provides one stimulus for Langerhans' cell migration. *Immunology* **75**, 257–263.

Cumberbatch, M. and Kimber, I. (1995). Tumour necrosis factor-α is required for accumulation of dendritic cells in draining lymph nodes and for optimal contact sensitization. *Immunology* **84**, 31–35.

de Fraissinette, A., Schmitt, D. and Thivolet, J. (1989). Langerhans cells of human mucosa. *J. Dermatol.* **16**, 255–262.

de Saint-Vis, B., Fugier-Vivier, I., Massacrier, C., Vanbervliet, B., Aït-Yahia, S., Banchereau, J., Liu, Y.J., Lebecque, S. and Caux, C. (1998). The cytokine profile expressed by human dendritic cells is dependent on cell subtype and mode of activation. *J. Immunol.*, **160**, 1666–1676.

De Smedt, T., Pajak, B., Muraille, E., Lespagnard, L., Heinen, E., De Baetselier, P., Urbain, J., Leo, O and Moser, M. (1996). Regulation of dendritic cell numbers and maturation by lipopolysaccharide *in vivo*. *J. Exp. Med.* **184**, 1413–1424.

De Smedt, T., van Mechelen, M., De Becker, G., Urbain, J., Leo, O. and Moser, M. (1997). Effect of interleukin-10 on dendritic cell maturation and function. *Eur. J. Immunol.* **27**, 1229–1235.

Dieu, M.C., Vanbervliet, B., Vicari, A., Bridon, J.M., Oldham, E., Aït-Yahia, S., Brière, F., Zlotnik, A., Lebecque, S. and Caux, C. (1998). Selective recruitment of immature and mature dendritic cells by distinct chemokines expressed in different anatomic sites. *J. Exp. Med.* **188**, 1–4.

Dubois, B., Vanbervliet, B., Fayette, J., Massacrier, C., van Kooten, C., Brière, F., Banchereau, J. and Caux, C. (1997). Dendritic cells enhance growth and differentiation of CD40-activated B lymphocytes. *J. Exp. Med.* **185**, 941–951.

Dubois, B., Massacrier, C., Vanbervliet, B., Fayette, J., Brière, F., Banchereau, J. and Caux, C. (1998). Critical role of IL-12 in dendritic cell-induced differentiation of naive B lymphocytes. *J. Immunol.*, in press.

Durie, F.H., Fava, R.A., Foy, T.M., Aruffo, A., Ledbetter, J.A. and Noelle, R.J. (1993). Prevention of collagen-induced arthritis with an antibody to gp39, the ligand for CD40. *Science* **261**, 1328-1330.

Durie, F. H., Aruffo, A., Ledbetter, J., Crassi, K.M., Green, W.R. and Fast, L.D. (1994). Antibody to the ligand of CD40, gp39, blocks the occurrence of the acute and chronic forms of graft-vs-host disease. *J. Clin. Invest.* **94**, 1333–1338.

Engering, A.J., Cella, M., Fluitsma, D.M., Hoefsmit, E.C., Lanzavecchia, A. and Pieters, J. (1997). Mannose receptor mediated antigen uptake and presentation in human dendritic cells. *Adv. Exp. Med. Biol.* **417**, 183–187.

Fayette, J., Dubois, B., Vandenabeele, S., Bridon, J.M., Vanbervliet, B., Durand, I., Banchereau, J., Caux, C. and Brière, F. (1997). Human dendritic cells skew isotype switching of CD40-activated naive B cells towards IgA1 and IgA2. *J. Exp. Med.* **185**, 1909–1918.

Fithian, E., Kung, P., Goldstein, G., Rubenfeld, M., Fenoglio, C. and Edelson, R. (1981). Reactivity of Langerhans cells with hybridoma antibody. *Proc. Natl Acad. Sci. USA* **78**, 2541–2544.

Flamand, V., Sornasse, T., Thielemans, K., Demanet, C., Bakkus, M., Bazin, H., Tielemans, F., Leo, O., Urbain, J. and Moser, M. (1994). Murine dendritic cells pulsed *in vitro* with tumor antigen induce tumor resistance *in vivo*. *Eur. J. Immunol.* **24**, 605–610.

Florès-Romo, L., Björck, P., Duvert, V., van Kooten, C., Saeland, S. and Banchereau, J. (1997). CD40 ligation on human CD34$^+$ hematopoietic progenitors induces their proliferation and differentation into functional dendritic cells. *J. Exp. Med.* **185**, 341–349.

Fossum, S. (1988). Lymph-borne dendritic leucocytes do not recirculate, but enter the lymph node paracortex to become interdigitating cells. *Scand. J. Immunol.* **27**, 97–105.

Fossum, S. (1989). The life history of dendritic leukocytes (DL). In: *Current Topics in Pathology* (ed. O. H. Ivessen), (Springer-Verlag, Berlin), pp. 101–124.

Francotte, M. and Urbain, J. (1985). Enhancement of antibody responses by mouse dendritic cells pulsed with tobacco mosaic virus or with rabbit antiidiotypic antibodies raised against a private rabbit idiotype. *Proc. Natl Acad. Sci. USA* **82**, 8149–8152.

Gabrilovich, D.I., Chen, H.L., Girgis, K.R., Cunningham, H.T., Meny, G.M., Nadaf, S., Kavanaugh, D. and Carbone, D.P. (1996). Production of vascular endothelial growth factor by human tumors inhibits the functional maturation of dendritic cells. *Nature Medicine,* **2**, 1096–1103.

Galy, A., Travis, M., Cen, D. and Chen, B. (1995). Human T, B, natural killer, and dendritic cells arise from a common bone marrow progenitor cell subset. *Immunity* **3**, 459–473.

Georgopoulos, K., Bigby, M., Wang, J.H., Molnar, A., Wu, P., Winandy, S. and Sharpe, A. (1994). The Ikaros gene is required for the development of all lymphoid lineages. *Cell* **79**, 143–156.

Godiska, R., Chantry, D., Raport, C.J., Sozzani, S., Allavena, P., Levitin, D., Mantovani, A. and Gray, P.W. (1997). Human macrophage-derived chemokine (MDC), a novel chemoattractant for monocytes, monocyte-derived dendritic cells, and natural killer cells. *J. Exp. Med.* **185**, 1595-1604.

Gong, J., Chen, D., Kashiwaba, M. and Kufe, D. (1997). Induction of antitumor activity by immunization with fusions of dendritic and carcinoma cells. *Nature Medicine,* **3**, 558–561.

Granelli-Piperno, A., Moser, B., Pope, M., Chen, D., Wei, Y., Isdell, F., O'Doherty, U., Paxton, W., Koup, R., Mojsov, S., Bhardwaj, N., Clark-Lewis, I., Baggioloni, M. and Steinman, R. M. (1996). Efficient interaction of HIV-1 with purified dendritic cells via multiple chemokine coreceptors. *J. Exp. Med.* **184**, 2433–2438.

Greaves, D.R., Wang, W., Dairaghi, D.J., Dieu, M.C., de Saint-Vis, B., Franz-Bacon, K., Rossi, D., Caux, C., McClanahan, T., Gordon, S., Zlotnik, A. and Schall, T.J. (1997). CCR6, a CC chemokine receptor that interacts with macrophage inflammatory protein alpha and is highly expressed in human dendritic cells. *J. Exp. Med.* **186**, 837-844.

Grewal, I.S., Xu, J. and Flavell, R.A. (1995). Impairment of antigen-specific T-cell priming in mice lacking CD40 ligand. *Nature* **378**, 617–620.

Grouard, G., Durand, I., Filgueira, L., Banchereau, J. and Liu, Y.J. (1996). Dendritic cells capable of stimulating T cells in germinal centers. *Nature* **384**, 364–367.

Grouard, G., Rissoan, M.C., Filgueira, L., Durand, I., Banchereau, J. and Liu, Y.J. (1997). The enigmatic plasmacytoid T cells develop into dendritic cells with IL-3 and CD40-ligand. *J. Exp. Med.* **185**, 1101–1111.

Hanau, D., Fabre, M., Schmitt, D.A., Stampf, J.-L., Garaud, J.-C., Bieber, T., Grosshans, E., Benezra, C. and Cazenave, J.-P. (1987). Human epidermal Langerhans cells internalize by receptor-mediated endocytosis T6 (CD1 "NA1/34") surface antigen. Birbeck granules are involved in the intracellular traffic of the antigen. *J. Invest. Dermatol.* **89**, 172–177.

Harkiss, G.D., Hopkins, J. and McConnell, I. (1990). Uptake of antigen by afferent lymph dendritic cells mediated by antibody. *Eur. J. Immunol.* **20**, 2367–2373.

Hart, D.N.J. (1997). Dendritic cells: unique leukocyte populations which control the primary immune response. *Blood* **90**, 3245–3287.

Holt, P.G., Schon-Hegrad, M.A. and McMenamin, P.G. (1990). Dendritic cells in the respiratory tract. *Int. Rev. Immunol.* **6**, 139–149.

Imai, T., Yoshida, T., Baba, M., Nishimura, M., Kakisaki, M. and Yoshie, O. (1996). Molecular cloning of a novel T cell-directed CC chemokine expressed in thymus by signal sequence trap using Epstein–Barr virus vector. *J. Biol. Chem.* **271**, 21514-21521.

Inaba, K. and Steinman, R.M. (1985). Protein-specific helper T lymphocyte formation initiated by dendritic cells. *Science* **229**, 475–479.

Inaba, K., Granelli-Piperno, A. and Steinman, R.M. (1983). Dendritic cells are critical accessory cells for thymus-dependent antibody responses in mouse and man. *Proc. Natl Acad. Sci. USA* **80**, 6041–6045.

Inaba, K., Witmer, M.D. and Steinman, R.M. (1984). Clustering of dendritic cells, helper T lymphocytes, and histocompatible B cells, during primary antibody responses *in vitro*. *J. Exp. Med.* **160**, 858–876.

Inaba, K., Schuler, G., Witmer, M.D., Valinksy, J., Atassi, B. and Steinman, R.M. (1986). Immunologic properties of purified epidermal Langerhans cells. *J. Exp. Med.* **164**, 605–613.

Inaba, K., Young, J.W. and Steinman, R.M. (1987). Direct activation of $CD8^+$ cytotoxic T lymphocytes by dendritic cells. *J. Exp. Med.* **166**, 182–194.

Inaba, K., Metlay, J.P., Crowley, M.T. and Steinman, R.M. (1990). Dendritic cells pulsed with protein antigens *in vitro* can prime antigen-specific, MHC-restricted T cells *in situ*. *J. Exp. Med.* **172**, 631–640.

Inaba, K., Inaba, M., Romani, N., Aya, H., Deguchi, M., Ikehara, S., Muramatsu, S. and Steinman, R.M. (1992a). Generation of large numbers of dendritic cells from mouse bone marrow cultures supplemented with granulocyte/macrophage colony-stimulating factor. *J. Exp. Med.* **176**, 1693–1702.

Inaba, K., Steinman, R.M., Pack, M.W., Aya, H., Inaba, M., Sudo, T., Wolpe, S. and Schuler, G. (1992b). Identification of proliferating dendritic cell precursors in mouse blood. *J. Exp. Med.* **175**, 1157–1167.

Inaba, K., Inaba, M., Deguchi, M., Hagi, K., Yasumizu, R., Ikehara, S., Muramatsu, S. and Steinman, R. M. (1993). Granulocytes, macrophages, and dendritic cells arise from a common major histocompatibility complex class II-negative progenitor in mouse bone marrow. *Proc. Natl Acad. Sci. USA* **90**, 3038–3042.

Inaba, K., Witmer-Pack, M., Inaba, M., Hathcock, K.S., Sakuta, H., Azuma, M., Yagita, H., Okumura, K., Linsley, P.S., Ikehara, S., Muramatsu, S., Hodes, R.J. and Steinman, R.M. (1994). The tissue distribution of the B7-2 costimulator in mice: abundant expression on dendritic cells *in situ* and during maturation *in vitro*. *J. Exp. Med.* **180**, 1849–1860.

Inaba, K., Pack, M., Inaba, M., Sakuta, H., Isdell, F. and Steinman, R.M. (1997). High levels of a major histocompatibility complex II–self peptide complex on dendritic cells from the T cells areas of lymph nodes. *J. Exp. Med.* **186**, 665–672.

Jacobsen, S.E. W., Ruscetti, F.W., Dubois, C.M. and Keller, J.R. (1992). Tumor necrosis factor α directly and indirectly regulates hematopoietic progenitor cell proliferation: role of colony-stimulating factor receptor modulation. *J. Exp. Med.* **175**, 1759–1772.

Jiang, W., Swiggard, W.J., Heufler, C., Peng, M., Mirza, A., Steinman, R.M. and Nussenzweig, M.C. (1995). The receptor DC-205 expressed by dendritic cells and thymic epithelial cells is involved in antigen processing. *Nature* **375**, 151–155.

Kamanaka, M., Yu, P., Yasui, T., Yosha, K., Kawabe, T., Horii, T., Kishimoto, T. and Kikutani, H. (1996). Protective role of CD40 in *Leishmania major* infection at two distinct phases of cell-mediated immunity. *Immunity* **4**, 275–281.

Kaplan, G., Walsh, G., Guido, L.S., Meyn, P., Burkhardt, R.A., Abalos, R.M., Barker, J., Frindt, P.A., Fajardo, T.T., Celona, R. and Cohn, Z.A. (1992). Novel responses of human skin to intradermal recombinant granulocyte/macrophage-colony-stimulating factor: Langerhans cell recruitment, keratinocyte growth, and enhanced wound healing. *J. Exp. Med.* **175**, 1717–1728.

Kasinrerk, W., Baumruker, T., Majdic, O., Knapp, W. and Stockinger, H. (1993). CD1 molecule expression on human monocytes induced by granulocyte-macrophage colony-stimulating factor. *J. Immunol.* **150**, 579–584.

Katz, S.I., Tamaki, K. and Sachs, D.H. (1979). Epidermal Langerhans cells are derived from cells originating in bone marrow. *Nature* **282**, 324–326.

Knight, S.C. and Patterson, S. (1997). Bone marrow-derived dendritic cells, infection with human immunodeficiency virus, and immunopathology. *Annu. Rev. Immunol.* **15**, 593–615.

Knight, S.C. and Stagg, A.J. (1993). Antigen-presenting cell types. *Curr. Opin. Immunol.* **5**, 374–382.

Knight, S.C., Farrant, J. and Bryan, A. (1986). Non-adherent, low density cells from human peripheral blood contain dendritic cells and monocytes, both with veiled morphology. *Immunology* **57**, 595–603.

Koch, F., Stanzl, U., Jennewein, P., Janke, K., Heufler, C., Kämpgen, E., Romani, N. and Schuler, G. (1996). High level IL-12 production by murine dendritic cells: upregulation via MHC class II and CD40 molecules and downregulation by IL-4 and IL-10. *J. Exp. Med.* **184**, 741–746.

Kripke, M.L., Munn, C.G., Jeevan, A., Tang, J.-M. and Bucana, C. (1990). Evidence that cutaneous antigen-presenting cells migrate to regional lymph nodes during contact sensitization. *J. Immunol.* **145**, 2833–2838.

Kronin, V., Winkel, K., Süss, G., Kelso, A., Heath, W., Kirberg, J., von Boehmer, H. and Shortman, K. (1996). A subclass of dendritic cells regulates the response of naive CD8 T cells by limiting their IL-2 production. *J. Immunol.* **157**, 3819–3827.

Kudo, S., Matsuno, K., Ezaki, T. and Ogawa, M. (1997). A novel migration pathway for rat dendritic cells from the blood: hepatic sinusoid–lymph translocation. *J. Exp. Med.* **185**, 777–784.

Kupiec-Weglinski, J.W., Austyn, J.M., and Morris, P.J. (1988). Migration patterns of dendritic cells in the mouse. Traffic from blood, and T cell-dependent and independent entry to lymploid tissues. *J. Exp. Med.* **167**, 632–645.

Lardon, F., Snoeck, H.W., Berneman, Z.N., van Tendeloo, V.F., Nijs, G., Lenjou, M., Henckaerts, E., Boeckxtaens, C.J., Vandenabeele, P., Kestens, L.L., van Bockstaele, D.R. and Vanham, G.L. (1997).

Generation of dendritic cells from bone marrow progenitors using GM-CSF, TNF-alpha, and additional cytokines: antagonistic effects of IL-4 and IFN-gamma and selective involvement of TNF-alpha receptor-1. *Immunology* **91**, 553–559.

Larsen, C.P., Steinman, R.M., Witmer-Pack, M.D., Hankins, D.F., Morris, P.J. and Austyn, J.M. (1990). Migration and maturation of Langerhans cells in skin transplants and explants. *J. Exp. Med.* **172**, 1483–1494.

Larsen, C.P., Ritchie, S.C., Pearson, T.C., Linsley, P.S. and Lowry, R.P. (1992). Functional expression of the costimulatory molecule, B7/BB1, on murine dendritic cell populations. *J. Exp. Med.* **176**, 1215–1220.

Larsen, C.P., Ritchie, S.C., Hendrix, R., Linsley, P.S., Hathcock, K.S., Hodes, R.J., Lowry, R.P. and Pearson, T.C. (1994). Regulation of immunostimulatory function and costimulatory molecule (B7-1 and B7-2) expression on murine dendritic cells. *J. Immunol.* **152**, 5208–5219.

Lenz, A., Heine, M., Schuler, G. and Romani, N. (1993). Human and murine dermis contain dendritic cells. *J. Clin. Invest.* **92**, 2587–2596.

Levin, D., Constant, S., Pasqualini, T., Flavell, R. and Bottomly, K. (1993). Role of dendritic cells in the priming of $CD4^+$ T lymphocytes to peptide antigen *in vivo. J. Immunol.* **151**, 6742–6750.

Liu, L.M. and MacPherson, G.G. (1993). Antigen acquisition by dendritic cells: intestinal dendritic cells acquire antigen administered orally and can prime naive T cells *in vivo. J. Exp. Med.* **177**, 1299–1307.

Lynch, D.H., Andreasen, A., Maraskovsky, E., Whitmore, J., Miller, R.E. and Schuh, J.C. (1997). Flt3 ligand induces tumor regression and antitumor immune responses *in vivo. Nature Medicine* **3**, 625–631.

Macatonia, S.E., Knight, S.C., Edwards, A.J., Griffiths, S. and Fryer, P. (1987). Localization of antigen on lymph node dendritic cells after exposure to the contact sensitizer fluorescein isothiocyanate. *J. Exp. Med.* **166**, 1654–1667.

Macatonia, S.E., Hsieh, C.-S., Murphy, K.M. and O'Garra, A. (1993). Dendritic cells and macrophages are required for Th1 development of $CD4^+$ T cells from $\alpha\beta$ TCR transgenic mice: IL-12 substitution for macrophages to stimulate IFN-γ production is IFN-γ-dependent. *Int. Immunol.* **5**, 1119–1128.

Macatonia, S.E., Hosken, N.A., Litton, M., Vieira, P., Hsieh, C.-S., Culpepper, J.A., Wysocka, M., Trinchieri, G., Murphy, K.M. and O'Garra, A. (1995). Dendritic cells produce interleukin-12 and direct the development of Th1 cells from naive $CD4^+$ T cells. *J. Immunol.* **154**, 5071–5079.

Maher, J.K. and Kronenberg, M. (1997). The role of CD1 molecules in immune responses to infection. *Curr. Opin. Immunol.* **9**, 456–461.

Maraskovsky, E., Brasel, K., Teepe, M., Roux, E.R., Lyman, S.D., Shortman, K. and McKenna, H.J. (1996). Dramatic increase in the numbers of functionally mature dendritic cells in Flt3 ligand-treated mice: multiple dendritic cell subpopulations identified. *J. Exp. Med.* **184**, 1953–1962.

Matsuno, K., Ezaki, T., Kudo, S. and Uehara, Y. (1996). A life stage of particle-laden rat dendritic cells *in vivo*: their terminal division, active phagocytosis, and translocation from the liver to the draining lymph. *J. Exp. Med.* **183**, 1865–1878.

Mayordomo, J.I., Zorina, T., Storkus, W.J., Zitvogel, L., Celulzzi, C., Faldo, L.D., Melief, C.J., Ildstad, S.T., Martin Kast, W., DeLeo, A.B. and Lotze, M.T. (1995). Bone marrow-derived dendritic cells pulsed with synthetic tumour peptides elicit protective and therapeutic antitumour immunity. *Nature Medicine* **1**, 1297–1302.

Mayordomo, J.I., Zorina, T., Storkus, W.J., Zitvogel, L., Garcia-Prats, M.D., DeLeo, A.B. and Lotze, M.T. (1997). Bone marrow-derived dendritic cells serve as potent adjuvants for peptide-based antitumor vaccines. *Stem Cells* **15**, 94–103.

Mayrhofer, G., Holt, P.G. and Papadimitriou, J.M. (1986). Functional characteristics of the veiled cells in afferent lymph from the rat intestine. *Immunology* **58**, 379–387.

McWilliam, A.S., Nelson, D., Thomas, J.A. and Holt, P.G. (1994). Rapid dendritic cell recruitment is a hallmark of the acute inflammatory response at mucosal surfaces. *J. Exp. Med.* **179**, 1331–1336.

McWilliam, A.S., Nelson, D.J. and Holt, P.G. (1995). The biology of airway dendritic cells. *Immunol. Cell. Biol.* **179**, 405–413.

McWilliam, A.S., Napoli, S., Marsh, A.M., Pemper, F.L., Nelson, D.J., Pimm, C.L., Stumbles, P.A., Wells, T.N. and Holt, P.G. (1996). Dendritic cells are recruited into the airway epithelium during the inflammatory response to a broad spectrum of stimuli. *J. Exp. Med.* **184**, 2429–2432.

Mohamadzadeh, M., Poltorak, A.N., Bergstressor, P.R., Beutler, B. and Takashima, A. (1996). Dendritic cells produce macrophage inflammatory protein-1 gamma, a new member of the CC chemokine family. *J. Immunol.* **156**, 3102–3106.

Moll, H. (1993). Epidermal Langerhans cells are critical for immunoregulation of cutaneous leishmaniasis. *Immunol. Today* **14**, 383–387.

Moll, H., Fuchs, H., Blank, C. and Rollinghoff, M. (1993). Langerhans cells transport *Leishmania major* from the infected skin to the draining lymph node for presentation to antigen-specific T cells. *Eur. J. Immunol.* **23**, 1595–1601.

Morelli, A., Larregina, A., Chuluyan, I., Kolkowski, E. and Fainboim, L. (1996). Expression and modulation of C5a receptor (CD88) on skin dendritic cells. Chemotactic effect of C5a on skin migratory dendritic cells. *Immunology* **89**, 126–134.

Mueller, C.G.F., Rissoan, M.C., Salinas, B., Ait-Yahia, S., Ravel, O., Bridon, J.M., Lebecque, S. and Liu, Y.J. (1997). PCR selects a novel disintegrin-proteinase from CD40-activated germinal center dendritic cells. *J. Exp. Med.* **186**, 655–663.

Nakamura, K., Williams, I.R. and Kupper, T.S. (1995). Keratinocyte-derived monocyte chemoattractant protein 1 (MCP-1): analysis in a transgenic model demonstrates MCP-1 can recruit dendritic and Langerhans cells to skin. *J. Invest. Dermatol.* **105**, 635–643.

Nestle, F.O., Zheng, X.-G., Thompson, C.B., Turka, L.A. and Nickoloff, B.J. (1993). Characterization of dermal dendritic cells obtained from normal human skin reveals phenotypic and functionally distinctive subsets. *J. Immunol.* **151**, 6535–6545.

Notarangelo, L.D., Duse, M. and Ugazio, A.G. (1992). Immunodeficiency with hyper-IgM (HIM). *Immunodef. Rev.* **3**, 101–122.

O'Doherty, U., Peng, M., Gezelter, S., Swiggard, W.J., Betjes, M., Bhardwaj, N. and Steinman, R.M. (1994). Human blood contains two subsets of dendritic cells, one immunologically mature and the other immature. *Immunology* **82**, 487–493.

Péguet-Navarro, J., Dalbiez-Gauthier, C., Rattis, F.M., van Kooten, C., Banchereau, J. and Schmitt, D. (1995). Functional expression of CD40 antigen on human epidermal Langerhans cells. *J. Immunol.* **155**, 4241–4247.

Pelletier, M., Perreaut, C., Landry, D., David, M. and Montplaisir, S. (1984). Ontogeny of human epidermal Langerhans cells. *Transplantation* **38**, 544–546.

Peters, J.H., Gieseler, R., Thiele, B. and Steinbach, F. (1996). Dendritic cells: from ontogenetic orphans to myelomonocytic descendants. *Immunol. Today* **17**, 273–278.

Pickl, W. F., Majdic, O., Kohl, P., Stöckl, J., Riedl, E., Scheinecker, C., Bello-Fernandez, C. and Knapp, W. (1996). Molecular and functional characteristics of dendritic cells generated from highly purified $CD14^+$ peripheral blood monocytes. *J. Immunol.* **157**, 3850–3859.

Piemonti, L., Bernasconi, S., Luini, W., Trobonjaca, Z., Minty, A., Allavena, P. and Mantovani, A. (1995). IL-13 supports differentiation of dendritic cells from circulating precursors in concert with GM-CSF. *Eur. Cytokine Netw.* **6**, 245–252.

Pierre, P., Turley, S.J., Gatti, E., Hull, M., Meltzer, J., Mirza, A., Inaba, K., Steinman, R.M. and Mellman, I. (1997). Developmental regulation of MHC class II transport in mouse dendritic cells. *Nature* **388**, 787–792.

Porcelli, S., Morita, C.T. and Brenner, M.B. (1992). CD1b restricts the response of human CD4-8-T lymphocytes to a microbial antigen. *Nature* **360**, 593–597.

Power, C.A., Church, D.J., Meyer, A., Alouani, S., Proudfoot, A.E., Clark-Lewis, I., Sozzani, S., Mantovani, A. and Wells, T.N. (1997). Cloning and characterization of a specific receptor for the novel CC chemokine MIP-3alpha from lung dendritic cells. *J. Exp. Med.* **186**, 825–835.

Pugh, C.W., MacPherson, G.G. and Steer, H.W. (1983). Characterization of nonlymphoid cells derived from rat peripheral lymph. *J. Exp. Med.* **157**, 1758–1779.

Pulendran, B., Lingappa, J., Kennedy, M.K., Smith, J., Teepe, M., Rudensky, A., Maliszewski, C.R. and Maraskovsky, E. (1997). Developmental pathways of dendritic cells *in vivo*: distinct function, phenotype, and localization of dendritic cell subsets in Flt3 ligand-treated mice. *J. Immunol.* **159**, 2222–2231.

Reid, C.D.L., Stackpoole, A., Meager, A. and Tikerpae, J. (1992). Interactions of tumor necrosis factor with granulocyte-macrophage colony-stimulating factor and other cytokines in the regulation of dendritic cell growth *in vitro* from early bipotent $CD34^+$ progenitors in human bone marrow. *J. Immunol.* **149**, 2681–2688.

Reis e Sousa, C., Stahl, P.D. and Austyn, J.M. (1993). Phagocytosis of antigens by Langerhans cells *in vitro*. *J. Exp. Med.* **178**, 509–519.

Res, P., Martinez-Caceres, E., Jaleco, A.C., Staal, F., Noteboom, E., Weijer, K. and Spits, H. (1996). $CD34^+$ $CD38^{dim}$ cells in the human thymus can differentiate into T, natural killer, and dendritic cells but are distinct from pluripotent stem cells. *Blood* **87**, 5196–5206.

Riedl, E., Strobl, H., Majdic, O. and Knapp, W. (1997). TGF-beta 1 promotes *in vitro* generation of dendritic cells by protecting progenitor cells from apoptosis. *J. Immunol.* **158**, 1591–1597.

Roake, J.A., Rao, A.S., Morris, P.J., Larsen, C.P., Hankins, D.F. and Austyn, J.M. (1995). Dendritic cell loss from nonlymphoid tissues after systemic administration of lipopolysaccharide, tumor necrosis factor, and interleukin 1. *J. Exp. Med.* **181**, 2237–2247.

Romani, N., Lenz, A., Glassl, H., Stossel, H., Stanzl, U., Majdic, O., Fritsch, P. and Schuler, G. (1989). Cultured human Langerhans cells resemble lymphoid dendritic cells in phenotype and function. *J. Invest. Dermatol.* **93**, 600–609.

Romani, N., Gruner, S., Bran D., Kämpgen, E., Lenz, A., Trockenbacher, B., Konwalinka, G., Fritsch, P.O., Steinman, R.M. and Schuler, G. (1994). Proliferating dendritic cell progenitors in human blood. *J. Exp. Med.* **180**, 83–93.

Romani, N., Reider, D., Heuer, M., Ebner, S., Kämpgen, E., Eibl, B., Niederwieser, D. and Schuler, G. (1996). Generation of mature dendritic cells from human blood an improved method with special regard to clinical applicability. *J. Immunol. Methods* **196**, 137–151.

Rosenzwajg, M., Canque, B. and Gluckman, J.C. (1996). Human dendritic cell differentiation pathway from $CD34^+$ hematopoietic precursor cells. *Blood* **87**, 535–544.

Rowden, G. (1981). The Langerhans cells. *Crit. Rev. Immunol.* **3**, 94–180.

Rubartelli, A., Poggi, A. and Zocchi, M.R. (1997). The selective engulfment of apoptotic bodies by dendritic cells is mediated by the $\alpha v\beta 3$ integrin and requires intracellular and extracellular calcium. *Eur. J. Immunol.* **27**, 1893–1900.

Ruedl, C. and Hubele, S. (1997). Maturation of Peyer's patch dendritic cells *in vitro* upon stimulation via cytokines or CD40 triggering. *Eur. J. Immunol.* **27**, 1325–1330.

Sagebiel, R.W. and Reed, T.H. (1968). Serial reconstruction of the characteristic granule of the Langerhans cell. *J. Cell. Biol.* **36**, 595–608.

Sallusto, F. and Lanzavecchia, A. (1994). Efficient presentation of soluble antigen by cultured human dendritic cells is maintained by granulocyte/macrophage colony-stimulating factor plus interleukin 4 and downregulated by tumor necrosis factor alpha. *J. Exp. Med.* **179**, 1109–1118.

Sallusto, F., Cella, M., Danieli, C. and Lanzavecchia, A. (1995). Dendritic cells use macropinocytosis and the mannose receptor to concentrate macromolecules in the major histocompatibility complex class II compartment: down-regulation by cytokines and bacterial products. *J. Exp. Med.* **182**, 389–400.

Sallusto, F., Nicolo, C., de Maria, R., Corinti, S. and Testi, R. (1996). Ceramide inhibits antigen uptake and presentation by dendritic cells. *J. Exp. Med.* **184**, 2411–2416.

Santiago-Schwarz, F., Belilos, E., Diamond, B. and Carsons, S.E. (1992). TNF in combination with GM-CSF enhances the differentiation of neonatal cord blood stem cells into dendritic cells and macrophages. *J. Leukocyte Biol.* **52**, 274–281.

Saraya, K. and Reid, C.D. (1996). Stem cell factor and the regulation of dendritic cell production from $CD34^+$ progenitors in bone marrow and cord blood. *Br. J. Haematol.* **93**, 258–264.

Saunders, D., Lucas, K., Ismaili, J., Wu, L., Maraskovsky, E., Dunn, A. and Shortman, K. (1996). Dendritic cell development in culture from thymic precursor cells in the absence of granulocyte/macrophage colony-stimulating factor. *J. Exp. Med.* **184**, 2185–2196.

Scheicher, C., Mehlig, M., Zecher, R. and Reske, K. (1992). Dendritic cells from mouse bone marrow: *in vitro* differentiation using low doses of recombinant granulocyte-macrophage colony-stimulating factor. *J. Immunol. Methods* **154**, 253–264.

Schon-Hegrad, M.A., Oliver, J., McMenamin, P.G. and Holt, P.G. (1991). Studies on the density, distribution, and surface phenotype of intraepithelial class II major histocompatability complex antigen (Ia)-bearing dendritic cells (DC) in the conducting airways. *J. Exp. Med.* **173**, 1345–1356.

Schuler, G. and Steinman, R.M. (1985). Murine epidermal Langerhans cells mature into potent immunostimulatory dendritic cells *in vitro*. *J. Exp. Med.* **161**, 526–546.

Schuler, G. and Steinman, R.M. (1997). Dendritic cells as adjuvants for immune-mediated resistance to tumors. *J. Exp. Med.* **186**, 1183–1187.

Shimada, S., Caughman, S.W., Sharrow, S.O., Stephany, D. and Katz, S.I. (1987). Enhanced antigen-presenting capacity of cultured Langerhans cells is associated with markedly increased expression of Ia antigen. *J. Immunol.* **139**, 2551–2555.

Shortman, K. and Caux, C. (1997). Dendritic cell development: multiple pathways to Nature's adjuvants. *Stem Cells* **15**, 409–419.

Shurin, M.R., Pandharipande, P.P., Zorina, T.D., Haluszczak, C., Subbotin, V.M., Hunter, O., Brumfield, A., Storkus, W.J., Maraskovsky, E. and Lotze, M.T. (1997). Flt3 ligand induces the generation of functionally active dendritic cells in mice. *Cell. Immunol.* **179**, 174–184.

Siena, S., Di Nicola, M., Bregni, M., Mortarini, R., Anichini, A., Lombardi, L., Ravagnani, F., Parmiani, G. and Gianni, A.M. (1995). Massive *ex vivo* generation of functional dendritic cells from mobilized $CD34^+$ blood progenitors for anticancer therapy. *Exp. Hematol.* **23**, 1463–1471.

Song, W., Kong, H.L., Carpenter, H., Torii, H., Granstein, R., Rafii, S., Moore, M.A.S. and Crystal, R.G. (1997). Dendritic cells genetically modified with an adenovirus vector encoding the cDNA for a model antigen induce protective and therapeutic antitumor immunity. *J. Exp. Med.* **186**, 1247–1256.

Sornasse, T., Flamand, V., de Becker, G., Bazin, H., Tielemans, F., Thielemans, K., Urbain, J., Oberdan. L. and Moser, M. (1992). Antigen-pulse dendritic cells can efficiently induce an antibody response *in vivo*. *J. Exp. Med.* **175**, 15–21.

Sozzani, S., Sallusto, F., Luini, W., Zhou, D., Piemonti, L., Allavena, P., van Damme, J., Valitutti, S., Lanzavecchia, A. and Mantovani, A. (1995). Migration of dendritic cells in response to formyl peptides, C5a, and a distinct set of chemokines. *J. Immunol.* **155**, 3292-3295.

Sozzani, S., Luini, W., Borsatti, A., Polentarutti, N., Zhou, D., Piemonti, L., D'Amico, G., Power, C.A., Wells, T.N., Gobbi, M., Allavena, P. and Mantovani, A. (1997). Receptor expression and responsiveness of human dendritic cells to a defined set of CC and CXC chemokines. *J. Immunol.* **159**, 1993–2000.

Specht, J.M., Wang, G., Do, M. T., Lam, J.S., Royal, R.E., Reeves, M.E., Rosenberg, S.A. and Hwu, P. (1997). Dendritic cells retrovirally transduced with a model antigen gene are therapeutically effective against established pulmonary metastases. *J. Exp. Med.* **186**, 1213–1221.

Steinman, R.M. (1991). The dendritic cell system and its role in immunogenicity. *Annu. Rev. Immunol.* **9**, 271–296.

Steinman, R.M. and Swanson, J. (1995). The endocytic activity of dendritic cells. *J. Exp. Med.* **182**, 283–288.

Steinman, R.M. and Witmer, M.D. (1978). Lymphoid dendritic cells are potent stimulators of the primary mixed leukocyte reaction in mice. *Proc. Natl Acad. Sci. USA* **75**, 5132–5136.

Steinman, R.M., Lustig, D.S. and Cohn, Z.A. (1974). Identification of a novel cell type in peripheral lymphoid organs of mice. III. Functional properties *in vivo*. *J. Exp. Med.* **139**, 1431–1445.

Steinman, R.M., Pack, M. and Inaba, K. (1997). Dendritic cells in the T-cell areas of lymphoid organs. *Immunol. Rev.* **156**, 25–37.

Streilein, J. W. and Grammer, S. F. (1989). *In vitro* evidence that Langerhans cells can adopt two functionally distinct forms capable of antigen presentation to T lymphocytes. *J. Immunol.* **143**, 3925–3933.

Streilein, J.W., Grammer, S.F., Yoshikawa, T., Demidem, A. and Vermeer, M. (1990). Functional dichotomy between Langerhans cells that present antigen to naive and memory/effector T lymphocytes. *Immunol. Rev.* **117**, 159–184.

Strobl, H., Riedl, E., Scheinecker, C., Bello-Fernandez, C., Pickl, W.F., Rappersberger, K., Majdic, O. and Knapp, W. (1996). TGF-β1 promotes *in vitro* development of dendritic cells from $CD34^+$ hemopoietic progenitors. *J. Immunol.* **157**, 1499–1507.

Strobl, H., Bello-Fernandez, C., Riedl, E., Pickl, W.F., Majdic, O., Lyman, S.D. and Knapp, W. (1997). Flt3 ligand in cooperation with transforming growth factor-beta1 potentiates *in vitro* development of Langerhans-type dendritic cells and allows single-cell dendritic cell cluster formation under serum-free conditions. *Blood* **90**, 1425–1434.

Strunk, D., Rappersberger, K., Egger, C., Strobl, H., Krömer, E., Elbe, A., Maurer, D. and Stingl, G. (1996). Generation of human dendritic cells/Langerhans cells from circulating $CD34^+$ hematopoietic progenitor cells. *Blood* **87**, 1292–1302.

Strunk, D., Egger, C., Leitner, G., Hanau, D. and Stingl, G. (1997). A skin homing molecule defines the Langerhans cell progenitor in human peripheral blood. *J. Exp. Med.* **185**, 1131–1136.

Sullivan, S., Bergstresser, P.R., Tigelaar, R.E. and Streilein, J.W. (1986). Induction and regulation of contact hypersensitivity by resident bone marrow derived, dendritic epidermal cells: Langerhans cells and Thy-1^{+} epidermal cells. *J. Immunol.* **137**, 2460–2467.

Süss, G. and Shortman, K. (1996). A subclass of dendritic cells kills CD4 T cells via Fas/Fas-Ligand-induced apoptosis. *J. Exp. Med.* **183**, 1789–1796.

Szabolcs, P., Moore, M.A.S. and Young, J.W. (1995). Expansion of immunostimulatory dendritic cells among the myeloid progeny of human CD34^{+} bone marrow precursors cultured with c-kit-ligand, GM-CSF, and TNFα. *J. Immunol.* **154**, 5851–5861.

Tan, M.C., Mommaas, A.M., Drijfhout, J.W., Jordens, R., Onderwater, J.J., Verwoerd, D., Mulder, A.A., van der Heiden, A.N., Ottenhoff, T.H., Cella, M., Tulp, A., Neefjes, J.J. and Koning, F. (1997). Mannose receptor mediated uptake of antigens strongly enhances HLA-class II restricted antigen presentation by cultured dendritic cells. *Adv. Exp. Med. Biol.* **417**, 171–174.

Tang, A., Amagai, M., Granger, L.G., Stanley, J.R. and Udey, M.C. (1993). Adhesion of epidermal Langerhans cells to keratinocytes mediated by E-cadherin. *Nature* **361**, 82–85.

Terhorst, C., Van Agthoven, A., Le Clair, K., Stanley, J.R. and Udey, M.C. (1981). Biochemical studies of the human thymocyte cell-surface antigens T6, T9 and T10. *Cell* **23**, 771–780.

Teunissen, M.B.M., Wormeester, J., Krieg, S.R., Peters, P.J., Vogels, I.M.C., Kapsenberg, M.L. and Bos, J.D. (1990). Human epidermal Langerhans cells undergo profound morphological and phenotypical changes during *in vitro* culture. *J. Invest. Dermatol.* **94**, 166–173.

van de Rijn, M., Lerch, P.G., Bronstein, B.R., Knowles, R.W., Bhan, A.K. and Terhost, C. (1984). Human cutaneous dendritic cells express two glycoproteins T6 and M241 which are biochemically identical to those found on cortical thymocytes. *Hum Immunol.* **9**, 201–210.

van Kooten, C. and Banchereau, J. (1997). Functions of CD40 on B cells, dendritic cells and other cells. *Curr. Opin. Immunol.* **9**, 330–337.

Van Voorhis, W.C., Valinsky, J., Hoffman, E., Luban, J., Hair, L.S. and Steinman, R.M. (1983). Relative efficacy of human monocytes and dendritic cells as accessory cells for T cell replication. *J. Exp. Med.* **158**, 171–191.

Vicari, A.P., Figueroa, D.J., Hedrick, J.A., Foster, J.S., Singh, K.P., Menon, S., Copeland, N.G., Gilbert, D.J., Jenkins, N.A., Bacon, K.B. and Zlotnik, A. (1997). TECK: a novel CC chemokine specifically expressed by thymic dendritic cells and potentially involved in T cell development. *Immunity* **7**, 291–301.

Volc-Platzer, B., Stingl, G., Wolff, K., Hinterberg, W. and Schnedl, W. (1984). Cytogenetic identification of allogeneic epidermal Langerhans cells in a bone-marrow-graft recipient. *N. Engl. J. Med.* **310** (Abst), 1123–1124.

Vremec, D., Zorbas, M., Scollay, R., Saunders, D.J., Ardavin, C.F., Wu, L. and Shortman, K. (1992). The surface phenotype of dendritic cells purified from mouse thymus and spleen: investigation ot the CD8 expression by a subpopulation of dendritic cells. *J. Exp. Med.* **176**, 47–58.

Weih, F., Carrasco, D., Durham, S.K., Barton, D.S., Rizzo, C.A., Ryseck, R.-P., Lira, S.A. and Bravo, R. (1995). Multiorgan inflammation and hematopoietic abnormalities in mice with a targeted disruption of RelB, a member of the NFκ/Rel family. *Cell* **80**, 331–340.

Weiss, J.M., Sleeman, J., Renkl, A.C., Dittmar, H., Termeer, C.C., Taxis, S., Howells, N., Hofmann, M., Kohler, G., Schopf, E., Ponta, H., Herrlich, P. and Simon, J.C. (1997). An essential role for CD44 variant isoforms in epidermal Langerhans cell and blood dendritic cell function. *J. Cell. Biol.* **137**, 1137–1147.

Wettendorff, M., Massacrier, C., Vanbervliet, B., Urbain, J., Banchereau, J. and Caux, C. (1995). Activation of primary allogeneic CD8^{+} T cells by dendritic cells generated *in vitro* from CD34^{+} cord blood progenitor cells. In: *Dendritic Cells in Fundamental and Clinical Immunology* (eds J. Banchereau and D. Schmitt), Plenum Press, London, pp. 371–374.

Wolff, K. (1967). The fine structure of the Langerhans cell granule. *J. Cell. Biol.* **35**, 1484–1498.

Wu, L., Li, C. L. and Shortman, K. (1996). Thymic dendritic cell precursors: relationship to the T-lymphocyte lineage and phenotype of the dendritic cell progeny. *J. Exp. Med.* **184**, 903–911.

Wu, L., Vremec, D., Ardavin, C., Winkel, K., Suss, G., Georgiou, H., Maraskovsky, E., Cook, W. and Shortman, K. (1995). Mouse thymus dendritic cells: kinetics of development and changes in surface markers during maturation. *Eur. J. Immunol.* **25**, 418–425.

Wu, L., Nichogiannopoulou, A., Shortman, K. and Georgopoulos, K. (1997). Cell-autonomous defects in dendritic cell populations of Ikaros mutant mice point to a developmental relationship with the lymphoid lineage. *Immunity* **7**, 483–492.

Xu, L.L., Warren, M.K., Rose, W.L., Gong, W. and Wang, J.M. (1996). Human recombinant monocyte chemotactic protein and other CC chemokines bind and induce directional migration of dendritic cells *in vitro*. *J. Leukocyte Biol.* **60**, 365–371.

Young, J.W. and Steinman, R.M. (1990). Dendritic cells stimulate primary human cytolytic lymphocyte responses in the absence of CD4$^+$ helper T cells. *J. Exp. Med.* **171**, 1315–1332.

Young, J.W. and Steinman, R.M. (1996). The hematopoietic development of dendritic cells: a distinct pathway for myeloid differentiation. *Stem Cells* **14**, 376–387.

Young, J.W., Szabolcs, P. and Moore, M.A.S. (1995). Identification of dendritic cell colony-forming units among normal human CD34$^+$ bone marrow progenitors that are expanded by c-*kit*-ligand and yield pure dendritic cell colonies in the presence of granulocyte/macrophage colony-stimulating factor and tumor necrosis factor α. *J. Exp. Med.* **182**, 1111–1120.

Zhou, L.J. and Tedder, T.F. (1995). Human blood dendritic cells selectively express CD83, a member of the immunoglobulin superfamily. *J. Immunol.* **154**, 3821–3835.

Zhou, L.-J. and Tedder, T.F. (1996). CD14$^+$ blood monocytes can differentiate into functionally mature CD83$^+$ dendritic cells. *Proc. Natl Acad. Sci USA* **93**, 2588–2592.

Zitvogel, L., Mayordomo, J.I., Tjandrawan, T., DeLeo, A.B., Clarke, M.R., Lotze, M.T. and Storkus, W.J. (1996). Therapy of murine tumors with tumor peptide pulsed dendritic cells: dependence on T cells, B7 costimulation, and Th1-associated cytokines. *J. Exp. Med.* **183**, 87–97.

Zlotnik, A. (1996). The expression by dendritic cells of a new CC or beta family chemokine. *J. Immunol.* **157**, 2736.

CHAPTER 6
Lymphoid-Related Dendritic Cells

Eugene Maraskovsky[1], Bali Pulendran[1] and Ken Shortman[2]
[1]Department of Immunobiology, Immunex Corporation, Seattle, Washington, USA; [2]The Walter and Eliza Hall Institute of Medical Research, Melbourne, Victoria, Australia

... If it isn't a dendritic cell, then its a waste of cytoplasm ... .

Mark Teepe, 1995

INTRODUCTION

Dendritic cells (DC) are rare, hematopoietically derived leukocytes that form a cellular network involved in immune surveillance, antigen capture, and antigen presentation (Steinman, 1991; Steinman *et al.*, 1997). DC are predominantly found in the T cell-dependent areas of lymphoid tissue (Metlay *et al.*, 1990; Steinman, 1991; Steinman *et al.*, 1997), as well as in other tissues and organs. In mouse spleen, DC express high levels of class I and class II major histocompatibility complex (MHC) proteins, CD11c (Metlay *et al.*, 1990), the mannose-receptor-like protein DEC-205 (Jiang *et al.*, 1995; Kraal *et al.*, 1986) as well as adhesion (CD11a and CD54) and accessory molecules (CD40, CD80 and CD86) (Caux and Banchereau, 1996; Steinman *et al.*, 1997). Furthermore, a distinct subset of thymic and splenic DC also express the lymphocyte antigen, CD8, as an $\alpha\alpha$ homodimer (Vremec *et al.*, 1992). DC acquire antigens in peripheral tissues, migrate to lymphoid organs and present these antigens as processed peptides to T cells in the context of MHC antigens (Austyn, 1996; Caux and Banchereau, 1996; Steinman *et al.*, 1997). This initiates a cascade of events that results in an antigen-specific immune response. In addition, a subpopulation of DC which reside within the B cell areas of lymphoid tissue may induce B cell differentiation (Caux and Banchereau, 1996; Grouard *et al.*, 1996). In this way, DC are key regulators of immune responses. Not only can DC process and present foreign or altered self-antigens to induce immunity (Steinman, 1991; Steinman *et al.*, 1997), but certain DC subsets are also capable of negatively regulating the course of T cell immunity (Inaba *et al.*, 1991; Kronin *et al.*, 1996; Matzinger and Guerder, 1989; Mazda *et al.*, 1991; Steinman *et al.*, 1997; Süss and Shortman, 1996). In this respect, certain DC subsets may also be responsible for T cell cytokine repertoire development during the induction of immunity (Macatonia *et al.*, 1993).

Dendritic Cells: Biology and Clinical Applications
ISBN 0-12-455860-7

This capacity to initiate or regulate immunity has led to the study of DC as cellular vaccine adjuvants for the immunotherapy of cancer or infectious disease, or as inducers of transplantation tolerance (Mayordomo *et al.*, 1995; Thomson *et al.*, 1995; Young and Inaba, 1996). However, the extremely small numbers of DC found in the peripheral blood of normal individuals and the uncertainty as to which DC subsets are the most appropriate for the induction or regulation of immunity *in vivo* limits their clinical use.

THE GROWING HETEROGENEITY IN DC POPULATIONS

Ontogenic Heterogeneity

The most rapidly evolving aspect of DC biology is the striking diversity of phenotypes that have been described from both *in vitro* and *in vivo* murine and human studies. However, while the number of seemingly distinct DC subsets appears to be growing, the developmental relationships between these distinct DC subsets remain largely undefined. More importantly, the identification of functional differences between these distinct DC phenotypes is relatively sparse.

DC from Myeloid-committed Precursors

Recent work suggests that there are at least two distinct ontogenic pathways for DC development (see earlier chapters on myeloid DC and thymic DC) (Fig. 1). DC can be derived from either myeloid- or lymphoid-committed hematopoietic precursors. Myeloid-committed precursors which give rise to granulocytes and monocytes can also differentiate into Langerhans cells of the skin (LC) and myeloid-related DC in secondary lymphoid tissue (Caux and Banchereau, 1996; Caux *et al.*, 1992; Inaba *et al.*, 1992b; Romani *et al.*, 1994; Sallusto and Lanzavecchia, 1994; Steinman *et al.*, 1997; Young *et al.*, 1995). The myeloid origin of DC predominantly comes from *in vitro* studies in which DC can be grown from either bone marrow (BM) or cord blood progenitors, or from peripheral blood mononuclear cells (PBMC) using granulocyte/macrophage colony-stimulating factor (GM-CSF) (Caux *et al.*, 1992; Inaba *et al.*, 1992a, b; Inaba *et al.*, 1993; Romani *et al.*, 1994; Sallusto and Lanzavecchia, 1994; Szabolcs *et al.*, 1995; Young *et al.*, 1995).

DC from Lymphoid-committed Precursors

DC can also be derived from lymphoid-committed hematopoietic progenitors. In particular, the DC of the adult mouse thymus appear to be derived from the early, lymphoid-committed precursor (Ardavin *et al.*, 1993; Caux and Banchereau, 1996; Saunders *et al.*, 1996; Steinman *et al.*, 1997; Vremec *et al.*, 1992; Wu *et al.*, 1996) (see chapter 2 on thymic DC). In those studies, transfer of purified thymic lymphoid precursors into irradiated hosts resulted in the development of T cells, B cells, NK cells and $CD8\alpha^+$ DC, but not cells of the myeloid lineage (Ardavin *et al.*, 1993; Wu *et al.*, 1996). Interestingly, DC-producing potential, but not B or NK cell capacity, was maintained even by the downstream $CD44^+CD25^+$ pre-T cell population, suggesting that DC are more closely related to T cells than to B or NK cells (Wu *et al.*, 1996). These early thymic precursors can also generate thymic DC *in vitro* when cultured with a

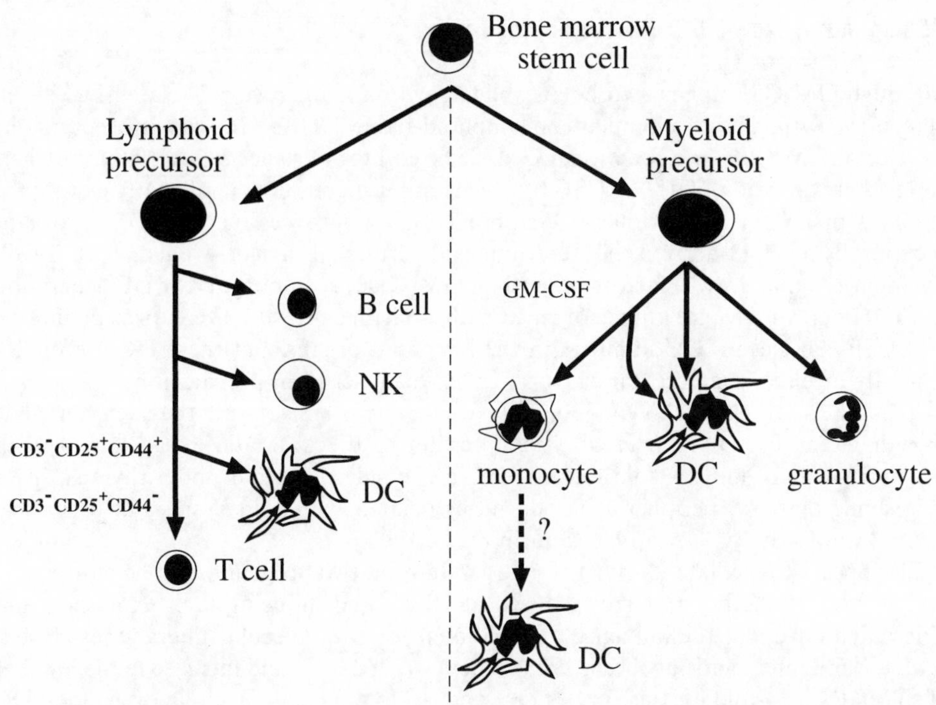

Fig. 1. Schematic of lineage derivation of DC from bone marrow progenitors. Myeloid-committed progenitors can give rise to granulocytes, monocytes, and myeloid-precursor-derived DC. Monocytes can also transiently transform into cells that appear morphologically, phenotypically and functionally DC-like. Lymphoid-committed progenitors which eventually seed the thymus have the capacity to generate B cells, NK cells, T cells, and lymphoid-precursor-derived DC.

combination of cytokines such as IL-1β, IL-3, IL-7, TNF-α, Flt3 ligand (FL), c-kit ligand (KL) and CD40 ligand (CD40-L) (Saunders *et al.*, 1996). The conspicuous absence of GM-CSF, a cytokine which is essential for the *in vitro* development of myeloid-precursor-derived DC, suggests that GM-CSF is not required for lymphoid-precursor-derived DC development (Saunders *et al.*, 1996). Although the lymphoid origin of DC has only been demonstrated for CD8α^+ thymic DC, the similarity in surface phenotype of CD8α^+ splenic and lymph node (LN) DC to that of thymic DC suggests that these peripheral tissue DC are also of lymphoid origin. We will therefore refer to CD8α^+ spleen and LN DC as lymphoid-related DC.

Studies performed with human BM progenitors have also demonstrated a lymphoid origin for DC *in vitro* (Galy *et al.*, 1995) and DC have also been cultured from thymic precursors (Res *et al.*, 1996). However, these putative human lymphoid-related DC are phenotypically indistinguishable from their putative myeloid-related counterparts (expressing CD1a$^+$, CD1b/c$^+$, CD2$^+$, CD4$^+$, CD14$^-$, CD33$^+$, HLA-DR$^+$, CD80$^{+/-}$, CD83$^+$, CD86$^+$) (also see chapters on myeloid DC and thymic DC). Furthermore, unlike in murine studies, human thymic DC do not express high levels of surface CD8 (but rather are CD4$^+$) (Sotzik *et al.*, 1994; Winkel *et al.*, 1994). To date, it has not been possible to discriminate phenotypically between human DC of myeloid and lymphoid origin.

Flt3 Ligand: A Novel DC Growth Factor *in vivo*

Although GM-CSF appears to be an obligate cytokine for myeloid-related DC development *in vitro*, the development of lymphoid-tissue DC *in vivo* can proceed in the absence of GM-CSF or a functional GM-CSF receptor (Vremec *et al.*, 1997). Furthermore, overexpression of a GM-CSF transgene in mice does not significantly elevate the numbers of DC in the peripheral lymphoid organs but does increase DC in organs occupied by myeloid-derived cells (e.g. lung and peritoneal cavity) (Metcalf *et al.*, 1996). This suggests that growth factors other than GM-CSF are important for DC generation *in vivo*. Interestingly, treatment of mice with a chemically stabilized form of murine GM-CSF can elevate DC numbers in the lymphoid organs, but these DC are predominantly myeloid-related (Maraskovsky *et al.*, manuscript in preparation).

It has been recently shown that daily treatment of mice with the hematopoietic growth factor FL (Lyman *et al.*, 1993) results in the dramatic expansion of both lymphoid-related and myeloid-related DC in the spleen, lymph node, thymus, liver, lung, bone marrow, peripheral blood, gut-associated lymphoid tissue and peritoneal cavity (Maraskovsky *et al.*, 1996; Shurin *et al.*, 1997).

FL appears to mediate its effects by targeting primitive progenitors in hematopoietic organs such as the bone marrow, spleen and liver and inducing their expansion and differentiation under the influence of additional *in vivo* molecular interactions (Brasel *et al.*, 1996; Lyman and Jacobsen, 1998). There was a 20–30-fold increase in the number of spleen DC, a 4-fold increase in LN DC, and a 6-fold increase in circulating blood DC (Maraskovsky *et al.*, 1996). Both myeloid-related and lymphoid-related DC appear to be equally expanded by FL administration. This discovery has allowed for a more in-depth examination of DC development and their ontogenic derivation. It now provides biologists with a means of expanding sufficient numbers of DC subsets *in vivo* to more thoroughly identify ontogenic and functional differences between the various DC subsets and establish their distinct clinical utility.

Identification of Lymphoid-related DC in Peripheral Lymphoid Organs

Lymphoid-related versus Myeloid-related DC Phenotype

The distinct origins of DC should be reflected by differences in the expression of cell surface molecules. This has been used in the mouse system to discriminate between DC of myeloid-precursor and lymphoid-precursor origin. In the mouse, myeloid-related DC constitutively express high levels of CD11b, but not CD8α (Maraskovsky *et al.*, 1996; Pulendran *et al.*, 1997; Vremec and Shortman, 1997). In contrast, the putative lymphoid-related DC constitutively coexpress CD8α and the multi-lectin receptor DEC-205, with only low to negligible levels of CD11b (Ardavin *et al.*, 1993; Kronin *et al.*, 1997; Maraskovsky *et al.*, 1996; Pulendran *et al.*, 1997; Saunders *et al.*, 1996; Vremec and Shortman, 1997; Wu *et al.*, 1995). Although there is a strict correlation between CD8α and DEC-205 expression for lymphoid-derived thymic and the related splenic DC subset (Kronin *et al.*, 1997; Vremec and Shortman, 1997), a third subset has also been described in the LN, which is CD8α^- DEC-205$^+$ CD11b$^-$ (Salomon *et al.*, 1998; Vremec and Shortman, 1997). It is not clear whether this subset is lymphoid-related or of myeloid origin, but recent evidence suggests that it may be derived from loco-regional DC which include Langerhans cells of the skin (Salomon *et al.*, 1998).

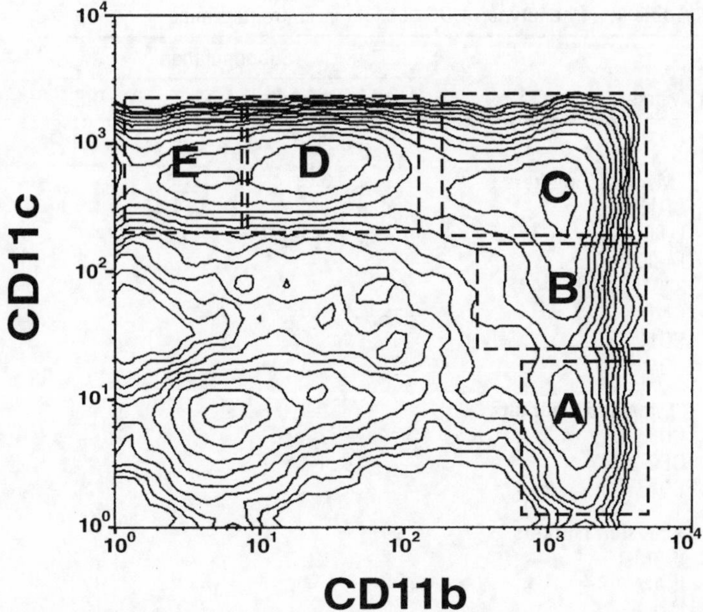

Fig. 2. Flow cytometric analysis of spleen cells from mice treated with FL for 9 days. The distribution of CD11c and CD11b on spleen cells after depletion with anti-B220, anti-Thy1, anti-NK1.1 and anti-Ter119 mAb. Populations A, B, C, D, and E are defined as shown. The probability contours represent logarithmic plots derived from files of 50 000 events.

Interestingly, expression of the CD8α homodimer by lymphoid-related DC does not appear to be required for their biological function (Kronin *et al.*, 1997).

In FL-treated mice, three populations of splenic DC were reported. These were referred to as populations C (CD11c$^+$ CD11b^{bright} CD8α^-), D (CD11c$^+$ CD11b^{dull} CD8α^+) and E (CD11c$^+$ CD11b$^-$ CD8α^+) (Maraskovsky *et al.*, 1996; Pulendran *et al.*, 1997) (Fig. 2). Two additional cell populations were also described; populations A (CD11c$^-$ CD11b^{bright} CD8α^-) and B (CD11c^{dull} CD11b^{bright} CD8α^-), which were found to be myeloid cells and myeloblasts, respectively. These latter two populations appear to also contain myeloid-related DC precursors.

Population C was reported to represent myeloid-related DC, whereas populations D and E were described as lymphoid-related DC. Interestingly, only 60% of DC within population D were CD8α^+ DEC-205$^+$, whilst almost all DC within population E were CD8α^+ DEC-205$^+$. The relationship of the CD8α^- DEC-205$^-$ DC within population D to either the lymphoid or myeloid lineage is, as yet, not known. DC within population C expressed the highest levels of the myeloid antigens F4/80, Gr-1, and Ly6c while a subset also expressed the marginal zone marker, 33D1 and the T cell antigen, CD4 (Pulendran *et al.*, 1997) (Table 1). This phenotype has also been described for myeloid-related DC in LN (Salomon *et al.*, 1998). In contrast, only DC within populations D and E expressed DEC-205 and CD1d and the highest levels of CD13, HSA and c-kit (Pulendran *et al.*, 1997) (Table 1). The expression of HSA and c-kit on lymphoid-derived thymic DC and the related splenic DC subset has been previously described

Table 1. Phenotype of DC subsets in FL-treated mice

Marker	Subpopulation A	B	C	D/E
CD11c	−	+	+++	+++
"Myeloid" markers				
CD11b	+++	+++	+++	+
Ly6C	+++	++	+	+/−
F4-80	++	+	+	+/−
33D1	−	+	+	−
Gr-1	+++	++	−	−
CD14	−	−	−	−
CD4	−	−	+	−
"Lymphoid" markers				
CD8α	−	−	−	++
DEC-205	−	−	−/+	+++
CD1d	−	−	−	++
Adhesion markers				
ICAM-1	+	+	++	+++
ICAM-2	+	+	+	+
LFA-1	++	++	+++	+++
VCAM-1	−	−	−/+	+/−
Activation markers				
CD40	−	−	+	+
Fas	−	−	−	−
B7-1	−	−	−	−
B7-2	−	−	+	+
Miscellaneous				
CD9	++	++	++	++
CD13	−	+	++	+++
CD16/32	++	++	++	++
CD23	−	−	−	++
Flt3-receptor	−	−	−	−
c-*fms*-receptor	−	−	−	−
c-*kit*	−	−	+/−	+
Class II MHC	−	−/+	++	++
CD24 (HSA)	+	+	++	++

(Salomon *et al.*, 1998; Vremec and Shortman, 1997; Wu *et al.*, 1995). Interestingly, several surface molecules displayed a gradient of expression from populations A to E (e.g. class II MHC, CD11a, CD11b, CD11c, CD13, CD40, CD54, CD86, F4/80, Gr-1, Ly6c, HSA, c-kit) (see Table 1). This raises the question whether the gradient of antigen expression from A to E represents the developmental progression of the various populations along a single maturation pathway or whether two distinct ontogenic pathways are simultaneously developing (Pulendran *et al.*, 1997).

Both CD8α^+ and CD8α^- DC subsets express equivalent levels of CD11c, class I and class II MHC, the costimulatory molecules CD40, CD80, and CD86, and the adhesion receptors CD11a and CD54, suggesting that they should be equally efficient at stimulating T cell proliferation *in vitro* (Maraskovsky *et al.*, 1996; Pulendran *et al.*, 1997;

Vremec and Shortman, 1997). However, $CD8\alpha^+$ DC also express the highest levels of the apoptosis-inducing molecule Fas ligand (Fas-L) which suggests that their function may be distinct from that of stimulatory $CD8\alpha^-$ DC (Süss and Shortman, 1996).

Modulation of Lymphoid-related and Myeloid-related Antigens during in vitro Culture

Although in mice, CD11b and $CD8\alpha$ and the multi-lectin receptor DEC-205 have been used to distinguish between DC of myeloid and lymphoid origin, respectively, these antigens can be coexpressed on the same DC or can be induced during culture or by contact with T cells or cytokines (Vremec and Shortman, 1997). For example, although $CD8\alpha^+$ lymphoid-precursor-derived DC normally express low to negligible levels of the myeloid marker, CD11b, this molecule can be upregulated during *in vitro* culture. Similarly, DEC-205 (a putative lymphoid-related DC marker), which is not detected on $CD11b^+$ myeloid-related DC, is also upregulated during culture although the difference in the levels of DEC-205 between the subpopulations appears to be maintained (Vremec and Shortman, 1997). In addition, mouse DC generated *in vitro* from purified thymic precursors fail to express $CD8\alpha$ (Saunders *et al.*, 1996). However, the expression of these molecules on freshly isolated DC continues to be a useful means of discriminating DC according to their putative lineage derivation. Support for the correlation of expression of these markers and their distinct lineage derivation comes from recent studies where normal mice are treated with a chemically stabilized form of murine GM-CSF or when GM-CSFR deficient mice are treated with FL (Maraskovsky *et al.*, manuscript in preparation). It was found that treatment of mice with GM-CSF induced significant myelopoiesis as well as DC expansion *in vivo*. Interestingly, the type of DC that were expanded were indistinguishable phenotypically from the myeloid-related DC (population C) generated during FL treatment of mice (i.e. $CD11c^+$ $CD11b^+$ $CD8\alpha^-$ $DEC\text{-}205^+$). In contrast, no significant increase in the putative lymphoid-related DC subset (populations D and E) was observed ($CD11c^+$ $CD11b^{low/-}$ $CD8\alpha^+$ $DEC\text{-}205^+$). In addition, treatment of mice lacking a functional GM-CSFR with FL resulted in deficient expansion of the putative myeloid-related DC (population C) but normal expansion of the putative lymphoid-related DC subset (populations D/E) (Maraskovsky *et al.*, manuscript in preparation). Taken together, these studies indicate that the myeloid cytokine, GM-CSF, preferentially expands myeloid cells and myeloid-related DC *in vivo* and signaling through its receptor is required for their optimal FL-mediated expansion. In contrast, the putative lymphoid-related subset is not significantly influenced by systemic GM-CSF and their expansion does not require GM-CSFR signaling. This also supports the premise that DC within population C are, in fact, ontogenically distinct from those within populations D and E and that these populations represent DC development along two distinct maturation pathways (Pulendran *et al.*, 1997).

Geographical Location of Lymphoid-related DC

The striking diversity in DC subsets raises the question of their geographical localization within secondary lymphoid tissues. In spleen (Metlay *et al.*, 1990) and within Peyer's patch (Kelsall and Strober, 1996), there is evidence that phenotypically heterogenous DC subsets occur in distinct microenvironments. However, it is not known whether these phenotypically distinct DC subsets differ in their function. In an attempt to correlate DC phenotype and function to their localization, we used two-color immunohistology to examine the occurrence of the various DC subsets in FL-treated (and in normal) mice within splenic microenvironments (Plate 6.3). In both sets of mice, $CD11c^+$ cells were found in the T cell-rich areas of the periarteriolar-lymphatic sheaths (PALS), as well as in the marginal zones (MZ). However, $CD11b^+$ cells could only be detected in MZ and in the red pulp. Furthermore, $CD8\alpha^+$ staining was largely confined to the PALS. Taken together, this suggests that the $CD11c^+$ $CD11b^{dull/-}$ $CD8\alpha^+$ DEC-205^+ DC (lymphoid-related populations D/E) are localized in the T cell areas, whereas the $CD11c^+$ $CD11b^{bright}$ $CD8\alpha^-$ DEC-205^- DC (myeloid-related population C) are localized in the MZ (Plate 6.3). This is consistent with previous reports (Inaba *et al.*, 1995; Jiang *et al.*, 1995; Witmer-Pack *et al.*, 1995), demonstrating the presence of DEC-205^+ DC only in the T cell areas. In addition, it has also been shown that 33D1, a marker which is expressed on populations C and B, is confined to the MZ (Metlay *et al.*, 1990). Thus, the different subsets of mature DC are localized in distinct microenvironments in the spleen (Pulendran *et al.*, 1997). In addition, Inaba and colleagues show that the DEC-205^+ interdigitating cells that normally reside within the T cell areas of lymphoid tissue predominantly express $CD8\alpha^+$ (Inaba *et al.*, 1997). Taken together, these data indicate that the $CD8\alpha^+$ lymphoid-related DC primarily reside within the T cell areas while the myeloid-related DC are found in the MZ.

Functional Differences of Lymphoid-related DC

Phagocytosis

The presence of phenotypically distinct DC subsets in distinct microenvironments raises the question whether these subsets have functional differences. One criterion that has been used to distinguish between mature and immature DC is the capacity to phagocytose particulate antigens (Inaba *et al.*, 1993). Immature DC and Langerhans cells are known to be very efficient at phagocytosis, and this property is known to decline with maturation (Matsuno *et al.*, 1996; Sallusto *et al.*, 1995; Winzler *et al.*, 1997). When the various splenic populations from FL-treated mice were sorted by flow cytometry, and assayed for their relative phagocytic capacities by uptake of FITC-zymosan, there were significant differences between them (Pulendran *et al.*, 1997). The myeloid cells within population A were highly phagocytic, comparable to peritoneal macrophages. At the other extreme, the lymphoid-related DC (populations D/E) were poorly phagocytic. In contrast, the myeloid-related DC within population C showed significantly higher levels of phagocytosis than the lymphoid-related DC within populations D/E. Furthermore, according to recent findings (Salomon *et al.*, 1998), only myeloid-related DC within the LN were found to have ingested the intravenously administered macromolecule, FITC-dextran. In contrast, few lymphoid-related DC expressed FITC fluorescence (Salomon *et al.*, 1998). Both these studies indicate that lymphoid-related DC are poor at phagocytosing macromolecules, whereas myeloid-related DC are more efficient in this function. Taken together with the marginal zone location of myeloid-related DC (a primary entry point for particulate antigen trafficking from the circulation), these data suggest that myeloid-related DC may play an important role in the control of blood pathogens and particulate antigens, a function that may not be as efficiently expressed by lymphoid-related DC.

T Cell Activation

Lymphoid-related DC Regulation of T Cell Activation. As mentioned earlier, the CD8α^+ lymphoid-related DC express the highest levels of Fas-L suggesting a distinct regulatory function of this DC subset. Indeed, the functional examination of splenic CD8α^+ DC from normal mice revealed that they do not interact with T cells in the classic stimulatory manner observed with CD8α^- DC. Rather, these CD8α^+ DC appear to play a regulatory role during T cell interactions, which can ultimately result in diminished T cell responses (Kronin *et al.*, 1997; Süss and Shortman, 1996). The mechanism of this regulation seems to differ for CD4$^+$ and CD8$^+$ T cells.

CD4$^+$ T cells. In vitro studies have shown that CD8α^+ splenic DC are less efficient at stimulating the proliferation of alloreactive and hemagglutinin-specific CD4$^+$ T cells (Süss and Shortman, 1996). This was also confirmed when comparing the allostimulatory activity and KLH-presenting capacity of the DC generated in FL-treated mice, where the predominantly CD8α^+ lymphoid-related DC (population E) was found to be less efficient at stimulating the proliferation of alloreactive or KLH-specific CD4$^+$ T cells (Maraskovsky *et al.*, 1996). Furthermore, Süss and Shortman (1996) found that the apparent deficit in T cell-stimulating capacity of CD8α^+ DC was actually due to their ability to directly induce the apoptotic death of the CD4$^+$ T cells during *in vitro* stimulation. This effect was obviated when using either DC from *gld* (Fas-L−/−) mice or CD4$^+$ T cells from *lpr* (Fas−/−) mice, implicating a direct role for Fas-L expressed on the CD8α^+ DC (Süss and Shortman, 1996). This suggests that Fas-L expressing CD8α^+ DC can negatively regulate T cell activation via a programmed cell death pathway.

CD8α^+ T cells. In the case of CD8$^+$ T cells, the CD8α^+ DC were initially efficient at stimulating CD8$^+$ T cells to proliferate, but T cell proliferation was significantly reduced later in culture (Kronin *et al.*, 1996). Studies performed with *lpr* or *gld* mice indicated that Fas-induced apoptosis was not involved, suggesting that the mechanism was distinct from that observed for CD4$^+$ T cells (Süss and Shortman, 1996). The reduced proliferation was rescued only when high levels of IL-2 were added to the cultures (Kronin *et al.*, 1996). The requirement for exogenous IL-2 was directly correlated with the significantly reduced IL-2 production by the CD8$^+$ T cells. This indicated that CD8α^+ DC were actually not deficient in their ability to induce T cell proliferation but did not induce adequate cytokine production in the responding CD8$^+$ T cells, with IL-2 being the most limiting cytokine for the CD8$^+$ T cells. This indicates that CD8α^+ DC are not only capable of killing activated CD4$^+$ T cells via a Fas-mediated pathway but are also capable of regulating CD8$^+$ T cell proliferation by controlling T cell cytokine production.

The regulatory nature of CD8α^+ DC is further demonstrated by Inaba *et al.* (1997), who show that the CD8α^+ DC which are localized in the T cell areas of secondary lymphoid tissue predominantly express MHC molecules occupied by self-peptides. Furthermore, these CD8α^+ DC induced the initial proliferation and then death of self-peptide reactive T cell clones *in vitro*. These findings indicate that CD8α^+ DC are functionally specialized to regulate the course of T cell activation and may play a critical role in the maintenance of peripheral tolerance to self-reactive T cells as well as regulating the development of the T cell cytokine repertoire.

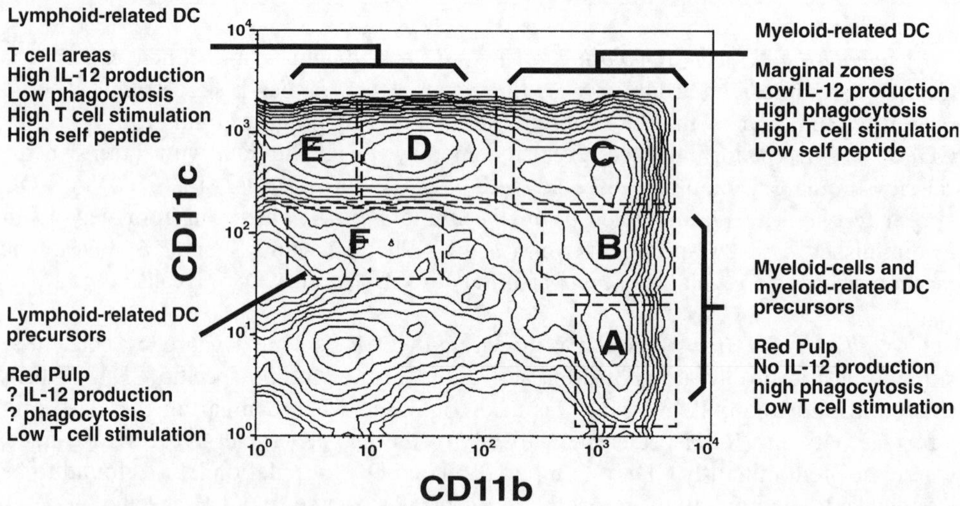

Fig. 4. A model for the maturation pathways of DC lineages in the spleen of FL-treated mice. Figure 2 is represented with a current hypothesis of the lineage derivation of the spleen cell subpopulations composed from data from Maraskovsky *et al.* (*J. Exp. Med.* **184**, 1953–1962), Pulendran *et al.* (*J. Immunol.* **159**, 2222–2231) and Inaba *et al.* (*J. Exp. Med.* **186**, 665–672).

Lymphoid-related DC and Inducible IL-12 Production. It has been demonstrated that biologically active IL-12 can be produced by DC upon triggering through CD40 (Cella *et al.*, 1996; Koch *et al.*, 1996), stimulation with SAC (Kang *et al.*, 1996; Scheicher *et al.*, 1995), or interaction with T cells (Cella *et al.*, 1996; Koch *et al.*, 1996; Trinchieri, 1995). We examined whether spleen DC derived from FL-treated mice secreted biologically active IL-12 upon stimulation and whether the levels of IL-12 produced differed between the myeloid-related and lymphoid-related DC populations in FL-treated mice. Equivalent numbers of DC from populations C, D, or E were stimulated with SAC in the presence of GM-CSF and IFN-γ. It was found that the CD8α^+ lymphoid-related DC (populations D and E) were induced to secrete much higher levels of biologically active IL-12 than the myeloid-related DC (population C) (Pulendran *et al.*, 1997). Interestingly, there was no significant difference in IL-12 secretion between the CD8α^+ and CD8α^- DC subpopulations within D and E.

Figure 4 presents a model summarizing what is known about the various spleen populations generated in FL-treated mice. We have also included the data from Inaba *et al.* (1997) showing that DC within the T cell areas express a higher proportion of MHC–self-peptide complexes than DC in the MZ. The figure correlates the differences found in phenotype and function of the various splenic subpopulations with their geographical localization.

Physiological Relevance of Lymphoid-related DC

The implications of the difference in location, phagocytosis, stimulatory capacity, and IL-12 production by the different DC subsets for T cell immunity has yet to be fully elucidated. However, IL-12 is known to induce IFN-γ production by T cells and appears to be an important cytokine for the development of type 1 cytokine production by T cells (Macatonia *et al.*, 1993; Trinchieri, 1995). Therefore, the DC producing the highest levels of biologically active IL-12 are the most likely to induce the highest IFN-γ production from the interacting T cells. Indeed, preliminary experiments *in vitro*, and *in vivo*, suggest that although the CD8α^+ lymphoid-related (populations D and E) and the myeloid-related (population C) DC subsets are equally able to prime naive (CD62L^{high}) ovalbumin-specific TcR-transgenic T cells, they induce different amounts of IFN-γ by the activated T cells, with lymphoid-related DC inducing greater IFN-γ and IL-2 production than the myeloid-related DC (Pulendran *et al.*, manuscript in preparation).

Interestingly, IFN-γ and IL-2 producing type 1 T cell clones are more susceptible to activation-induced cell death via a Fas/Fas-L pathway (Ramsdell *et al.*, 1994; Varadhachary *et al.*, 1997; Zhang *et al.*, 1997). The development of these cytokine-producing T cells is likely regulated by IL-12-producing APC. If CD8α^+ lymphoid-related DC produce the highest levels of IL-12, which stimulates the development of type 1 cytokine secreting T cells and CTL effectors, then they may also be the most likely to regulate the inappropriate or chronic expansion of these same T cells. Their strategic position in the T cell-rich areas of secondary lymphoid tissues not only allows them to initiate T cell immune responses which require type 1-secreting T helper and effector cells but also allows them to monitor the trafficking of sanctioned self-reactive T cells into this region (Inaba *et al.*, 1997) or chronically activated T cells that may persist long after the clearance of a pathogen-mediated infection (Ramsdell *et al.*, 1994; Varadhachary *et al.*, 1997; Zhang *et al.*, 1997). In this way, the CD8α^+ lymphoid-related DC may be a critical component to both the development and regulation of effective immunity.

It is not clear how the lymphoid-related DC can discriminate T cells that require positive stimulation from those that need to be negatively regulated. One possibility is that previously activated T cells express a different molecular repertoire on their surface that can be recognized by CD8α^+ DC. Indeed, it has been reported that previously activated or memory T cells express high levels of surface CTLA4 (a competitive receptor to CD28 for binding to CD80 and CD86 costimulatory molecules) and engagement of this molecule has been shown to negatively regulate T cells via an unknown pathway (Krummel and Allison, 1995; Krummel *et al.*, 1996; Linsley, 1995; Walunas *et al.*, 1994). The affinity of CTLA4 for CD80 and CD86 costimulatory molecules is 20-fold higher than that of CD28 (Linsley *et al.*, 1994). It is possible that CD8α^+ DC will preferentially engage CTLA4 on activated T cells, which in turn triggers the initiation of a regulatory rather than stimulatory program within the DC, resulting in the death of the T cell via Fas or other TNFR family members (in the case CD4$^+$ T cells) or in reduced cytokine production and perhaps death by neglect (in the case of CD8$^+$ T cells). In contrast, myeloid-related DC situated in the marginal zones may be more specialized to ingest blood-borne pathogens and macromolecules prior to trafficking into the T cell areas and interacting with T cells. These myeloid-related DC may instruct those T cells in a distinct way from lymphoid-related DC. Thus, functional differences between the various DC subsets are slowly emerging, and it now remains a challenge to investigate the physiological relevance of such differences in *in vivo* models and systems.

CONCLUSIONS: 'THE DC SYSTEM'

We are currently witnessing a paradigm shift in the biology of DC. Many new subsets of DC in mice and in humans are being identified. The notion of DC simply being immunostimulatory cells no longer seems be an accurate description of this leukocyte family. It may be more physiologically and clinically relevant to view DC as a 'system', consisting of many phenotypically and functionally diverse cells, located in distinct parts of the body. The location, state of maturity, ontogenic derivation and quality of the DC interaction with T or B cells will ultimately dictate the outcome of the immune response generated. The greatest challenge now lies in exploiting these differences for the purposes of immunotherapy of cancer, autoimmunity, and infectious diseases.

REFERENCES

Ardavin, C., Wu, L., Li, C.L. and Shortman, K. (1993). Thymic dendritic cells and T cells develop simultaneously in the thymus from a common precursor population. *Nature* **362**, 761–763.

Austyn, J.M. (1996). New insights into the mobilization and phagocytic activity of dendritic cells. *J. Exp. Med.* **183**, 1287–1292.

Brasel, K., McKenna, H.J., Morrissey, P.J., Charrier, K., Morris, A.E., Lee, C.C., Williams, D.E. and Lyman, S.D. (1996). Hematological effects of Flt3 ligand *in vivo* in mice. *Blood* **88**, 2004–2012.

Caux, C. and Banchereau, J. (1996). In vitro regulation of dendritic cell development and function. In : *Blood Cell Biochemistry, vol. 7: Hemopoietic Growth Factors and Their Receptors* (eds A. Whetton and J. Gordon). Plenum Press, London, p. 263.

Caux, C., Dezutter-Dambuyant, C., Schmitt, D. and Banchereau, J. (1992). GM-CSF and TNF-α cooperate in the generation of dendritic Langerhans cells. *Nature* **360**, 258–261.

Cella, M., Scheidegger, D., Palmer-Lehmann, K., Lane, P., Lanzavecchia, A. and Alber, G. (1996). Ligation of CD40 on dendritic cells triggers production of high levels of interleukin-12 and enhances T cell stimulatory capacity: T-T help via APC activation. *J. Exp. Med.* **184**, 747–752.

Galy, A., Travis, M., Cen, D. and Chen, B. (1995). Human T, B, natural killer, and dendritic cells arise from a common bone marrow progenitor cell subset. *Immunity* **3**, 459–473.

Grouard, G., Durand, I., Filgueira, L., Banchereau, J. and Liu, Y.J. (1996). Dendritic cells capable of stimulating T cells in germinal centres. *Nature* **384**, 364–367.

Inaba, M., Inaba, K., Hosono, M., Kumamoto, T., Ishida, T., Muramatsu, S., Masuda, T. and Ikehara, S. (1991). Distinct mechanisms of neonatal tolerance induced by dendritic cells and thymic B cells. *J. Exp. Med.* **173**, 549–559.

Inaba, K., Inaba, M., Romani, N., Aya, H., Deguchi, M., Ikehara, S., Muramatsu, S. and Steinman, R.M. (1992a). Generation of large numbers of dendritic cells from mouse bone marrow cultures supplemented with granulocyte/macrophage colony-stimulating factor. *J. Exp. Med.* **176**, 1693–1702.

Inaba, K., Steinman, R.M., Pack, M.W., Aya, H., Inaba, M., Sudo, T., Wolpe, S. and Schuler, G. (1992b). Identification of proliferating dendritic cell precursors in mouse blood. *J. Exp. Med.* **175**, 1157–1167.

Inaba, K., Inaba, M., Naito, M. and Steinman, R.M. (1993). Dendritic cell progenitors phagocytose particulates, including Bacillus Calmette-Guerin organisms, and sensitize mice to mycobacterial antigens *in vivo*. *J. Exp. Med.* **178**, 479–488.

Inaba, K., Swiggard, W.J., Inaba, M., Meltzer, J., Mirza, A., Sasagawa, T., Nussenzweig, M.C. and Steinman, R.M. (1995). Tissue distribution of the DEC-205 protein that is detected by the monoclonal antibody NLDC-145. I. Expression on dendritic cells and other subsets of mouse leukocytes. *Cell. Immunol.* **163**, 148–156.

Inaba, K., Pack, M., Inaba, M., Sakuta, H., Isdell, F. and Steinman, R.M. (1997). High levels of a major histocompatibility complex II–self peptide complex on dendritic cells from the T cell areas of lymph nodes. *J. Exp. Med.* **186**, 665–672.

Jiang, W., Swiggard, W.J., Heufler, C., Peng, M., Mirza, A., Steinman, R.M. and Nussenzweig, M.C. (1995). The receptor DEC-205 expressed by dendritic cells and thymic epithelial cells is involved in antigen processing. *Nature* **375**, 151–155.

Kang, K., Kubin, M., Cooper, K.D., Lessin, S.R., Trinchieri, G. and Rook, A.H. (1996). IL-12 synthesis by human Langerhans cells. *J. Immunol.* **156**, 1402–1407.

Kelsall, B.L. and Strober, W. (1996). Distinct populations of dendritic cells are present in the subepithelial dome and T cell regions of the murine Peyer's patch. *J. Exp. Med.* **183**, 237–247.

Koch, F., Stanzl, U., Jennewein, P., Janke, K., Heufler, C., Kampgen, E., Romani, N. and Schuler, G. (1996). High level IL-12 production by murine dendritic cells: upregulation via MHC class II and CD40 molecules and downregulation by IL-4 and IL-10. *J. Exp. Med.* **184**, 741–746.

Kraal, G., Breel, M., Janse, M. and Bruin, G. (1986). Langerhans' cells, veiled cells, and interdigitating cells in the mouse recognized by a monoclonal antibody. *J. Exp. Med.* **163**, 981–997.

Kronin, V., Winkel, K., Süss, G., Kelso, A., Heath, W., Kirberg, J., von Boehmer, H. and Shortman, K. (1996). A subclass of dendritic cells regulates the response of naive CD8 T cells by limiting their IL-2 production. *J. Immunol.* **157**, 3819–3827.

Kronin, V., Vremec, D., Winkel, K., Classon, B.J., Miller, R.G., Mak, T.W., Shortman, K. and Süss, G. (1997). Are $CD8^+$ dendritic cells (DC) veto cells? The role of CD8 on DC in DC development and in the regulation of CD4 and CD8 T cell responses. *Int. Immunol.* **9**, 1061–1064.

Krummel, M.F. and Allison, J.P. (1995). CD28 and CTLA-4 have opposing effects on the response of T cells to stimulation. *J. Exp. Med.* **182**, 459–465.

Krummel, M.F., Sullivan, T.J. and Allison, J.P. (1996). Superantigen responses and co-stimulation: CD28 and CTLA-4 have opposing effects on T cell expansion *in vitro* and *in vivo*. *Int. Immunol.* **8**, 519–523.

Linsley, P.S. (1995). Distinct roles for CD28 and cytotoxic T lymphocyte-associated molecule-4 receptors during T cell activation. *J. Exp. Med.* **182**, 289–292.

Linsley, P.S., Greene, J.L., Brady, W., Bajorath, J., Ledbetter, J.A. and Peach, R. (1994). Human B7-1 (CD80) and B7-2 (CD86) bind with similar avidities but distinct kinetics to CD28 and CTLA-4 receptors. *Immunity* **1**, 793–801.

Lyman, S.D. and Jacobsen, S.E.W. (1998). c-*kit* ligand and Flt3 ligand: stem/progenitor cell factors with overlapping yet distinct activities. *Blood* **91**, 1101–1134.

Lyman, S.D., James, L., VandenBos, T., de Vries, P., Brasel, K., Gliniak, B., Hollingsworth, L.T., Picha, K.S., McKenna, H.J., Splett, R.R., Fletcher, F.A., Maraskovsky, E., Farrah, T., Foxworthe, D., Williams, D.E. and Beckmann, M.P. (1993). Molecular cloning of a ligand for the flt3/flk-2 tyrosine kinase receptor: a proliferative factor for primitive hematopoietic cells. *Cell* **75**, 1157–1167.

Macatonia, S.E., Hsieh, C.-S., Murphy, K.M. and O'Garra, A. (1993). Dendritic cells and macrophages are required for Th1 development of $CD4^+$ T cells from $\alpha\beta$ TCR transgenic mice: IL-12 substitution for macrophages to stimulate IFN-γ production is IFN-γ-dependent. *Int. Immunol.* **5**, 1119–1128.

Maraskovsky, E., Brasel, K., Teepe, M., Roux, E.R., Lyman, S.D., Shortman, K. and McKenna, H.J. (1996). Dramatic increase in the numbers of functionally mature dendritic cells in Flt3 ligand-treated mice: multiple dendritic cell subpopulations identified. *J. Exp. Med.* **184**, 1953–1962.

Matsuno, K., Ezaki, T., Kudo, S. and Uehara, Y. (1996). A life stage of particle-laden rat dendritic cells *in vivo*: their terminal division, active phagocytosis, and translocation from the liver to the draining lymph. *J. Exp. Med.* **183**, 1865–1878.

Matzinger, P. and Guerder, S. (1989). Does T-cell tolerance require a dedicated antigen-presenting cell? *Nature* **338**, 74–76.

Mayordomo, J.I., Zorina, T., Storkus, W.J., Zitvogel, L., Celluzzi, C., Falo, L.D., Melief, C.J., Ildstad, S.T., Kast, W.M., Deleo, A.B. and Lotze, M.T. (1995). Bone marrow-derived dendritic cells pulsed with synthetic tumour peptides elicit protective and therapeutic antitumour immunity. *Nature Medicine* **1**, 1297–1302.

Mazda, O., Watanabe, Y., Gyotoku, J.-I. and Katsura, Y. (1991). Requirement of dendritic cells and B cells in the clonal deletion of Mls-reactive T cells in the thymus. *J. Exp. Med.* **173**, 539–547.

Metcalf, D., Shortman, K., Vremec, D., Mifsud, S. and Di Rago, L. (1996). Effects of excess GM-CSF levels on hematopoiesis and leukemia development in GM-CSF/max 41 double transgenic mice. *Leukemia* **10**, 713–719.

Metlay, J.P., Witmer-Pack, M.D., Agger, R., Crowley, M.T., Lawless, D. and Steinman, R.M. (1990). The distinct leukocyte integrins of mouse spleen dendritic cells as identified with new hamster monoclonal antibodies. *J. Exp. Med.* **171**, 1753–1771.

Pulendran, B., Lingappa, J., Kennedy, M.K., Smith, J., Teepe, M., Rudensky, A., Maliszewski, C.R. and Maraskovsky, E. (1997). Developmental pathways of dendritic cells *in vivo*. Distinct function, phenotype and localization of dendritic cell subsets in FLT3 ligand-treated mice. *J. Immunol.* **159**, 2222–2231.

Ramsdell, F., Seaman, M.S., Miller, R.E., Picha, K.S., Kennedy, M.K. and Lynch, D.H. (1994). Differential ability of T_h1 and T_h2 T cells to express Fas ligand and to undergo activation-induced cell death. *Int. Immunol.* **6**, 1545–1553.

Res, P., Martínez-Cáceres, E., Jaleco, A.C., Staal, F., Noteboom, E., Weijer, K. and Spits, H. (1996). $CD34^+CD38^{dim}$ cells in the human thymus can differentiate into T, natural killer, and dendritic cells but are distinct from pluripotent stem cells. *Blood* **87**, 5196–5206.

Romani, N., Gruner, S., Brang, D., Kämpgen, E., Lenz, A., Trockenbacher, B., Konwalinka, G., Fritsch, P.O., Steinman, R.M. and Schuler, G. (1994). Proliferating dendritic cell progenitors in human blood. *J. Exp. Med.* **180**, 83–93.

Sallusto, F. and Lanzavecchia, A. (1994). Efficient presentation of soluble antigen by cultured human dendritic cells is maintained by granulocyte/macrophage colony-stimulating factor plus interleukin 4 and downregulated by tumor necrosis factor α. *J. Exp. Med.* **179**, 1109–1118.

Sallusto, F., Cella, M., Danieli, C. and Lanzavecchia, A. (1995). Dendritic cells use macropinocytosis and the mannose receptor to concentrate macromolecules in the major histocompatibility complex class II compartment: downregulation by cytokines and bacterial products. *J. Exp. Med.* **182**, 389–400.

Salomon, B., Cohen, J.L. and Klatzmann, D. (1998). Three populations of mouse lymph node dendritic cells with different origins and dynamics. *J. Immunol.*, **160**, 708–717.

Saunders, D., Lucas, K., Ismaili, J., Wu, J., Maraskovsky, E., Dunn, A. and Shortman, K. (1996). Dendritic cell development in culture from thymic precursor cells in the absence of granulocyte/macrophage colony-stimulating factor. *J. Exp. Med.* **184**, 2185–2196.

Scheicher, C., Mehlig, M., Dienes, H.-P. and Reske, K. (1995). Uptake of microparticle-adsorbed protein antigen by bone marrow-derived dendritic cells results in up-regulation of interleukin-1α and interleukin-12 p40/p35 and triggers prolonged, efficient antigen presentation. *Eur. J. Immunol.* **25**, 1566–1572.

Shurin, M.R., Pandharipande, P.P., Zorina, T.D., Haluszczak, C., Subbotin, V.M., Hunter, O., Brumfield, A., Storkus, W.J., Maraskovsky, E. and Lotze, M.T. (1997). FLT3 ligand induces the generation of functionally active dendritic cells in mice. *Cell. Immunol.* **179**, 174–184.

Sotzik, F., Rosenberg, Y., Boyd, A.W., Honeyman, M., Metcalf, D., Scollay, R., Wu, L. and Shortman, K. (1994). Assessment of CD4 expression by early T precursor cells and by dendritic cells in the human thymus. *J. Immunol* **152**, 3370–3377.

Steinman, R.M. (1991). The dendritic cell system and its role in immunogenicity. *Annu. Rev. Immunol.* **9**, 271–296.

Steinman, R.M., Pack, M. and Inaba, K. (1997). Dendritic cells in the T-cell areas of lymphoid organs. *Immunol. Rev.* **156**, 25–37.

Süss, G. and Shortman, K. (1996). A subclass of dendritic cells kills CD4 T cells via Fas/Fas-ligand-induced apoptosis. *J. Exp. Med.* **183**, 1789–1796.

Szabolcs, P., Moore, M.A.S. and Young, J.W. (1995). Expansion of immunostimulatory dendritic cells among the myeloid progeny of human $CD34^+$ bone marrow precursors cultured with c-*kit* ligand, granulocyte-macrophage colony-stimulating factor, and TNF-α. *J. Immunol.* **154**, 5851–5861.

Thomson, A.W., Lu, L., Murase, N., Demetris, A.J., Rao, A.S. and Starzl, T.E. (1995). Microchimerism, dendritic cell progenitors and transplantation tolerance. *Stem Cells* **13**, 622–639.

Trinchieri, G. (1995). Interleukin-12: a proinflammatory cytokine with immunoregulatory functions that bridge innate resistance and antigen-specific adaptive immunity. *Annu. Rev. Immunol.* **13**, 251–276.

Varadhachary, A.S., Perdow, S.N., Hu, C., Ramanarayanan, M. and Salgame, P. (1997). Differential ability of T cell subsets to undergo activation-induced cell death. *Proc. Natl Acad. Sci. USA* **94**, 5778–5783.

Vremec, D. and Shortman, K. (1997). Dendritic cell subtypes in mouse lymphoid organs. Cross-correlation of surface markers, changes in incubation, and differences among thymus, spleen, and lymph nodes. *J. Immunol.* **159**, 565–573.

Vremec, D., Zorbas, M., Scollay, R., Saunders, D.J., Ardavin, C.F., Wu, L., and Shortman, K. (1992). The surface phenotype of dendritic cells purified from mouse thymus and spleen: investigation of the CD8 expression by a subpopulation of dendritic cells. *J. Exp. Med.* **176**, 47–58.

Vremec, D., Lieschke, G.J., Dunn, A.R., Robb, L., Metcalf, D. and Shortman, K. (1997). The influence of granulocyte/macrophage colony-stimulating factor on dendritic cell levels in mouse lymphoid organs. *Eur. J. Immunol.* **27**, 40–44.

Walunas, T.L., Lenschow, D.J., Bakker, C.Y., Linsley, P.S., Freeman, G.J., Green, J.M., Thompson, C.B. and Bluestone, J.A. (1994). CTLA-4 can function as a negative regulator of T cell activation. *Immunity* **1**, 405–413.

Winkel, K., Sotzik, F., Vremec, D., Cameron, P.U. and Shortman, K. (1994). CD4 and CD8 expression by human and mouse thymic dendritic cells. *Immunol. Lett.* **40**, 93–99.

Winzler, C., Rovere, P., Rescigno, M., Granucci, F., Penna, G., Adorini, L., Zimmermann, V.S., Davoust, J. and Ricciardi-Castagnoli, P. (1997). Maturation stages of mouse dendritic cells in growth factor-dependent long-term cultures. *J. Exp. Med.* **185**, 317–328.

Witmer-Pack, M.D., Swiggard, W.J., Mirza, A., Inaba, K. and Steinman, R.M. (1995). Tissue distribution of the DEC-205 protein that is detected by the monoclonal antibody NLDC-145. II. Expression *in situ* in lymphoid and nonlymphoid tissues. *Cell. Immunol.* **163**, 157–162.

Wu, L., Li, C.-L. and Shortman, K. (1996). Thymic dendritic cell precursors: relationship to the T lymphocyte lineage and phenotype of the dendritic cell progeny. *J. Exp. Med.* **184**, 903–911.

Wu, L., Vremec, D., Ardavin, C., Winkel, K., Süss, G., Georgiou, H., Maraskovsky, E., Cook, W. and Shortman, K. (1995). Mouse thymus dendritic cells: kinetics of development and changes in surface markers during maturation. *Eur. J. Immunol.* **25**, 418–425.

Young, J.W. and Inaba, K. (1996). Dendritic cells as adjuvants for class I major histocompatibility complex-restricted antitumor immunity. *J. Exp. Med.* **183**, 7–11.

Young, J.W., Szabolcs, P. and Moore, M.A.S. (1995). Identification of dendritic cell colony-forming units among normal human $CD34^+$ bone marrow progenitors that are expanded by c-kit-ligand and yield pure dendritic cell colonies in the presence of granulocyte/macrophage colony-stimulating factor and tumor necrosis factor α. *J. Exp. Med.* **182**, 1111–1120.

Zhang, X., Brunner, T., Carter, L., Dutton, R.W., Rogers, P., Bradley, L., Sato, T., Reed, J.C., Green, D. and Swain, S.L. (1997). Unequal death in T helper cell (Th)1 and Th2 effectors: Th1, but not Th2, effectors undergo rapid Fas/FasL-mediated apoptosis. *J. Exp. Med.* **185**, 1837–1849.

II DENDRITIC CELLS IN THE PERIPHERY

CHAPTER 7
Dendritic Cells in the Context of Skin Immunity

Dieter Maurer and Georg Stingl
Division of Immunology, Allergy and Infectious Diseases, Department of Dermatology, University of Vienna Medical School, Vienna, Austria

INTRODUCTION

An intact immune system is required for all higher organisms to detect and destroy invading microorganisms (viruses, bacteria, fungi, and parasites) and to eliminate cells that undergo malignant transformation. Anatomically, the first barrier to microbiological invasion is the skin, an organ that for many years was considered only a passive barrier against this invasion. Over the last two decades, however, concepts of a previously unrecognized role for skin have unfolded, a role in which dendritic leukocytes of the epidermis (i.e., Langerhans cells; LC) and dermis (i.e., dermal dendritic cells; DDC), initiate immune responses that protect the integrity of this organ.

In 1868, the medical student Paul Langerhans, driven by his interest in the anatomy of skin nerves, discovered in the suprabasal regions of the epidermis a population of dendritic cells which now bear his name. While he was uncertain about their histogenetic nature (original quotation: 'Epithelzellen können sie nach ihrer Gestalt nicht sein; es handelt sich somit um die Frage: bindegewebig oder nervös?'), their reactivity with gold salts made him believe that 'his cells' represented sensory nerve endings [1]. Today, we know that LC are dendritic leukocytes which reside mainly within stratified squamous epithelia and constitute approximately 2–4% of all epithelial cells (see [2] for review). In the epidermis, they are usually located at a suprabasal position and attach to neighboring keratinocytes via an E-cadherin- and Ca^{2+}-dependent mechanism [3]. LC cannot be easily identified on routine H&E sections. Their visualization and quantification *in situ* therefore requires the use of appropriate histochemical and/or immunolabeling techniques. Using adenosine triphosphatase (ATPase) histochemistry, Chen *et al.* [4] determined a LC density range within human epidermis of $\sim$200/mm^2 (palms, soles) to $\sim$970/mm^2 (face, neck). On electron microscopy, LC exhibit unique trilaminar cytoplasmic structures (Birbeck granules, BG) that allow their identification (reviewed in [2]; Fig. 1). Using this organelle as a marker, it became clear that histiocytosis X represents a LC neoplasm [5], which is now referred to as Langerhans cell histiocytosis (see Chapter 19). In adults, the disease is mostly localized to skin and bone and usually runs a rather benign and protracted course. In children, it may also affect multiple internal organs and, thus, represents a life-threatening condition (reviewed in [6]).

Dendritic Cells: Biology and Clinical Applications
ISBN 0-12-455860-7

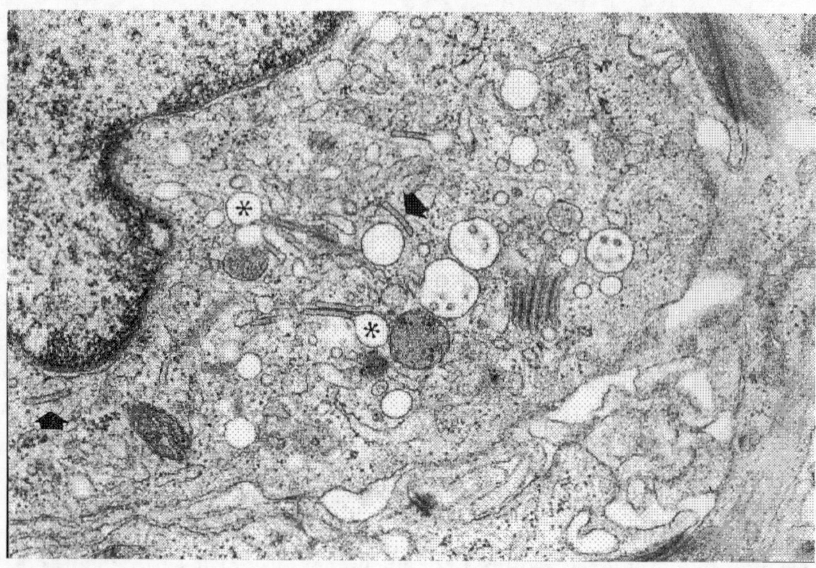

Fig. 1. Electron micrograph of a Langerhans cell within the human epidermis. Depending on the plane of sectioning, Birbeck granules appear as either rod-shaped (arrowheads) or tennis racket-shaped structures (stars). (Original magnification × 40 000.)

Langerhans cells are a mobile cell population with a relatively slow turnover [7, 8]. Epidermal residence is only one step in their life cycle. They originate from bone marrow precursors which, upon circulation in the peripheral blood, populate the skin. Upon receipt of appropriate activating stimuli (e.g., antigenic challenge), they can leave the cutaneous compartment and migrate to peripheral lymphoid organs where they initiate T cell responses. Having accomplished this task, they initiate events which finally result in their own demise (reviewed in [2] and [9]) (see Plate 7.2).

At each stage of their development, phenotype and function of LC are determined by their cellular and molecular microenvironment. Within skin, keratinocytes (KC) are the major symbionts of LC. They are capable of producing and secreting various mediators of the inflammatory reaction and of the immune response such as eicosanoids and cytokines. KC-derived cytokines include IL-1, IL-6, IL-7, IL-8 and other chemokines, IL-10, IL-12, GM-CSF, tumor necrosis factor (TNF)-α as well as some of the factors regulating the growth of epithelial and/or mesenchymal cells, e.g., transforming growth factors (TGF)-α and -β, platelet-derived growth factor (PDGF), and basic fibroblast growth factor (bFGF) (reviewed in [10]). It should be kept in mind that—with the notable exception of IL-1, IL-7, and TGF-β—most of these mediators are not produced constitutively by KC but only after perturbation of the epidermal homeostasis, for example, by hypoxia as well as chemical (e.g., haptens) and physical (ultraviolet radiation (UV), cell dissociation) injury [11–13]. This is also true for those cytokines (i.e., GM-CSF and TNF-α) which, together with IL-1α, initiate major phenotypic and functional changes in the LC population [14].

Resident LC display nonspecific esterase and ATPase activity, and are the only cells within the normal epidermis to express Fc-IgG receptors type II (FcγRII, CD32), Fc-IgE receptors type I (FcεRI), C3bi receptors (CD11b–CD18), and major histocompatibility complex (MHC)-encoded class II antigens (Table 1). Although having only a limited potency for stimulating naive resting T cells, they possess the machinery for uptake and processing of large protein antigens [15]. Upon cytokine activation, certain features (e.g., FcγRII, FcεRI, ATPase activity, Birbeck granules) slowly disappear, whereas the expression of other molecules becomes more apparent, for example, MHC class I and II, CD24, CD25, CD40, CD54, CD58, CD80, CD83, and CD86 (Table 1). These cytokine-activated LC, while no longer capable of effective antigen processing, secrete biologically active IL-1β, IL-6, and IL-12, and act as powerful inducers of both primary and secondary MHC class I- or class II-restricted T cell responses [16–18].

Dermal dendritic cells are located primarily in the perivascular areas of the superficial plexus. They have a folded nucleus and a highly ruffled, irregular surface. Their cytoplasm is relatively dark, contains the organelles needed for an active cellular metabolism, but is devoid of BG. Phenotypic features of DDC include ATPase and nonspecific esterase activity as well as the expression of CD45, CD11b, CD11c, CD36, FcεRI, and MHC class II antigens and of the subunit A of the clotting proenzyme factor XIII (factor XIIIa). DDC express low amounts of CD1a and are CD14$^-$ and CD15$^-$ [19, 20]. Recent studies indicate that their immunostimulatory capacity is similar to that of cells of the LC lineage [19, 20].

DEVELOPMENT OF LC AND DDC-LIKE CELLS FROM CD34$^+$ HEMATOPOIETIC PRECURSORS

A major breakthrough in the understanding of LC development came from the observation that the exposure of CD34$^+$ hematopoietic stem cells to GM-CSF and TNF-α gives rise to a progeny of CD1a$^+$, E-cadherin$^+$, BG-containing cells with immunostimulatory properties strikingly resembling those of LC isolated from human skin [21, 22] (Plate 7.2). Subsequent studies have tried to delineate the phenotype of LC progenitors at their various states of maturation/differentiation. It is now quite clear that, already at the CD34$^+$ precursor stage, cells exist which are committed to the LC lineage. An apparently useful marker to identify these cells is the cutaneous leukocyte homing antigen (CLA) which is abundantly expressed by LC precursors rather than by cells giving rise to non-LC DC [23] (Plate 7.2). It has still to be determined whether and when this fucosylated PSGL-1 moiety [24] with affinity for vascular E- and P-selectin can mediate skin homing of LC/LC progenitors. Around days 4–6 of *in vitro* culture in GM-CSF- and TNF-α-supplemented medium, LC precursors acquire CD1a expression and, upon prolongation of the culture until days 12–14, develop into typical DC displaying all the features found in and on epidermal LC. Besides the CD1a$^+$ LC precursor, CD14$^+$ CD1a$^-$ cells emerge early during the culture. The lineage commitment of these cells is apparently less restricted as they can give rise to a monocyte/macrophage phenotype when exposed to M-CSF while differentiating into non-LC DC in the presence of GM-CSF and TNF-α [25] (Plate 7.2). Phenotypically, these non-LC DC are characterized by abundant expression of factor XIIIa, CD1a, CD68, CD11b, and CD36, and the virtual absence of E-cadherin and BG and, thus, display striking

Table 1. Phenotype of resident vs. cytokine-activated human epidermal Langerhans cells

Property	Resident LC	Cytokine-activated LC
Morphology		
Birbeck granules	+++	+/−
Cytoplasmic veils	++	+++
Enzyme profiles		
Adenosine triphosphatase	+++	+/−
Nonspecific esterase	+	−
Antigenic profiles		
MHC class I	+	++
MHC class II	++	+++
CD1a	+++	+
CD1b	−	+
CD1c	+	−
CD3-TCR	−	−
CD4	+	?
CD8	−	−
CD14	−	−
CD15	−	−
CD19	−	−
CD20	−	−
FcγRI (CD64)	−	−
FcγRII (CD32)	+	−
FcγRIII (CD16)	−	−
FcεRI	+	−
Adhesion molecules		
β_1-integrins	+ or ++	? (α 4↑, α 6↓)
β_2-integrins	+ or +/−	?
CD44		
pan	+	++
v7/v8	+	−
v4-v6, v9	+/−	++
E-cadherin	++	+/−
CLA	+	+ or ++
Costimulatory molecules/activation markers		
CD24	−	++
CD40	+/−	+
CD54	+/−	++
CD58	+	++
CD69	+	−
CD80	−	+
CD83	−	+
CD86	+	++
Cytokine receptors		
GM-CSFRα (CD116)	+	++
GM-CSFRβ (CD131)	+/−	++
M-CSFR (CD115)	−	−
TNF-RII (75 kD) (CD120b)	+	+/−
IL-1RI (CD121a)	+	+/−
IL-1RII (CD121b)	+	++
IL-2Rα (CD25)	−	++
IL-2Rβ (CD122)	−	+
IFN-γR (CDw119)	+	+
CXCR4/fusin	+/−	+
CCR6	+	−
CCR7	−	+

similarities to DDC. The dichotomy of LC and non-LC DC emerging from distinct precursors is reflected not only at the phenotypic but, more importantly, at the functional level. Non-LC DC, in contrast to LC, are macropinocytotic and can induce maturational events in pre-activated B cells [26].

Still, the exact relationship between LC and other members of the DC family is not entirely understood. Although prevailing opinion holds that DC residing within the T cell zones of skin-draining lymph nodes originate, at least partly, from a pool of antigen-laden LC, it was somewhat surprising to learn that mice lacking the transcription factors relB and Ikaros harbor essentially no DC within their lymphoid organs, but contain a phenotypically normal-appearing LC population [27–29].

Additional factors governing the development of LC/DC from $CD34^+$ progenitors have been identified. The DC maturation-promoting effect of GM-CSF can apparently be replaced by IL-3, a finding that is consistent with the observations that the skin of GM-CSF gene-targeted knockout mice harbors LC and that IL-3 and GM-CSF receptors display similarities in structure and function [30]. Interestingly enough, other stimuli (i.e., stem cell factor [SCF] and Flt3-L), amplify the DC differentiation pathways initiated by GM-CSF and TNF-α without any apparent selectivity for LC or non-LC DC development (Plate 7.2). In contrast, TGF-β_1 seems to be of unique importance in LC ontogeny (Plate 7.2). This is evidenced by the lack of LC in TGF-β_1 – /– mice [31] and by the preferential development of $CD1a^+$, BG^+ cells in GM-CSF- and TNF-α-containing, TGF-β_1-supplemented serum-free stem cell cultures [32, 33]. It is not yet entirely clear which cell types serve as the biologically relevant source of TGF-β_1 in LC differentiation. Cell transfer studies in mice suggest that radiation-resistant host cells other than keratinocytes are important in this regard [34]. Recent data from our laboratory indicate that TGF-β_1 may have a LC-promoting effect at the $CD14^+$ DC precursor stage and, perhaps even, at the level of peripheral blood monocytes. When appropriately stimulated in the presence of bioactive TGF-β_1, these cells massively upregulate E-cadherin along with CD1a and display BG-like cytoplasmic structures (S. Jaksits, G. Stingl and D. Maurer, unpublished observations) (Plate 7.2).

RECEPTORS AND CYTOKINES PRESUMABLY INVOLVED IN THE SELECTIVE TISSUE-HOMING PROPERTIES OF LC/LC PRECURSORS

The mechanisms leading to tissue-specific homing of LC/LC precursors are poorly understood, and the exact maturational stage at which LC enter the skin *in vivo* is still unknown. Recent attention has focused on the impact of the chemokine (CK) system, a multipartite superfamily of chemoattractant cytokines that induce the directional migration of leukocytes and other cells, and on the superfamily of G-protein-coupled CK receptor proteins, which contain seven transmembrane domains [35, 36]. It is well established that monocyte-derived DC and $CD34^+$ cord blood-derived LC/DC are chemotactically responsive to the C-C chemokines RANTES, macrophage inflammatory protein (MIP)-1, monocyte chemotactic protein (MCP)-1, and macrophage-derived CK (MDC) [37–39]. More recently, it has been shown that MIP-3α/Exodus/LARC (liver activation-related CK) via the expression of a specific receptor (i.e., CCR6) can execute DC migration [40, 41]. Interestingly, this receptor is apparently expressed by $CD34^+$ cord blood-derived LC/DC but not by monocyte-derived DC [40]. Although this expression pattern suggests a specific role for MIP-3α in LC recruitment to the skin, one should not forget that this CK is also expressed in many other tissues such as fetal lung, liver, and pancreatic islets [41, 42]. Data from our laboratory show that CCR6 mRNA expression actually starts early during LC development (before day 6 of culture) and can be detected in both the $CD1a^+CD14^-$ and, perhaps to a lesser extent, in the $CD1a^-CD14^+$ progenitor populations indicating that MIP-3α could exert its chemotactic activity even at the LC/DC precursor level (A.S. Charbonnier, unpublished observations). Other CK expressed by *in vitro* generated LC/DC and LC resident in human skin include the HIV-1 coreceptors CCR5 and CXCR4/fusin which are receptors for RANTES, MIP-1α/β and stromal cell-derived factor (SDF)-1, respectively [43]. Interestingly, resident LC display anti-CCR5-reactive moieties at the cell surface and are susceptible to infection with M-tropic HIV-1 strains in a CCR5-dependent fashion, whereas CXCR4/fusin occurs mainly in the cytoplasm of these cells. For reasons not entirely understood, purified LC, upon prolonged *in vitro* culture/cytokine activation, shuffle CXCR4 protein to the cell surface where it can be targeted by T-tropic HIV-1 [43].

EMIGRATION AND MATURATION OF LANGERHANS CELLS

Evidence exists that perturbation of the cutaneous microenvironment leads to phenotypic and functional changes in the LC population which are similar to those seen in epidermal single cell cultures (Plate 7.3). A few hours after skin transplantation, LC begin to enlarge and to exhibit increased amounts of surface-bound MHC class II molecules. Subsequently, a marked reduction in the number of epidermal LC occurs concomitantly with the appearance of strongly Ia^+ cells in the dermis of the transplants [44]. Other investigators found that 24 h after application of a contact sensitizer LC appear larger than normal, exhibit more intense anti-Ia staining, and are several-fold more potent in their T cell stimulatory capacity than LC from nontreated or vehicle-treated animals [45]. Further, it was possible to identify antigen-bearing LC/DC in draining lymph nodes after the application of contact sensitizers [46, 47] and to demonstrate antigen-specific T cell activation by these cells. Thus, it appears likely that LC function involves two components: antigen uptake and processing by 'immature' cutaneous LC and, in the regional lymphoid organs, actual antigen presentation by mature skin-derived LC.

At the ultrastructural level, LC in their resident, immature state display MHC class II antigens in cytoplasmic vesicles and, to a much lesser extent, on the cell surface [48]. Certain paracrine and/or autocrine stimuli, e.g., GM-CSF, TNF-α, IL-1β and/or ligation of CD40, induce a transient accumulation of MHC class II-related gene products in multilamellar/multivesicular compartments of DC [49, 50]. It appears that these *de novo* synthesized, nascent moieties are efficiently loaded by peptides derived from external antigens. The concomitant export of peptide-loaded MHC class II as stable dimers and downregulation of MHC class II neosynthesis are, at least partly, responsible for the switch of LC from the processing/loading to the presentation mode. This dynamic molecular model of LC maturation is in good agreement with previous observations showing that freshly isolated, but not cultured, LC are capable of processing large protein antigens [15], while cultured LC are far superior to freshly isolated LC in their capacity to stimulate naive resting T cells [51]. LC maturation is further accompanied by a massive upregulation of costimulatory molecule

(CD54, CD58, CD80, CD86, HSA) expression as well as by an increased secretion of effector T cell-promoting cytokines (e.g., IL-12), while receptors involved in antigen/allergen uptake (FcεRI, FcγRII) are clearly diminished (Table 1). Thus, matured LC are essentially indistinguishable from certain MHC class II-bearing DC of lymphoid tissues which are potent stimulators of primary and secondary T cell responses [52].

Recent studies have also identified a role for epidermal cell-derived cytokines in regulating LC migration from the skin into draining lymph nodes. Antibodies to TNF-α and IL-1β prevent the early migration of LC from the epidermis, the accumulation of DC in lymph nodes, and the development of optimal contact sensitization. In keeping with these observations is the finding that the intradermal injection of TNF-α or IL-1β stimulates the migration of LC out of the epidermis and the accumulation of DC in draining lymph nodes [53–55]. The effect of TNF-α is apparently mediated by the 75 kDa TNF-RII as LC migration in TNF-RI gene-targeted knockout mice is unchanged but still sensitive to TNF-α neutralization [56]. The further sequence of events occurring in LC emigration includes the loosening of the E-cadherin-dependent attachment of LC to neighboring KC which can, at least partly, be explained by a LC maturation-related downregulation of this molecule [57]. Other yet poorly investigated conditions may include changes in the ligand binding avidity of LC-expressed E-cadherin and/or the modification of the E-cadherin anchoring to cytoskeletal elements, perhaps resulting in enhanced lateral mobility of this moiety. Recently, two additional LC surface receptors have been implicated as being essential for LC emigration to occur. One is CD44, a hyaluronic acid receptor putatively involved in the tissue homing of leukocytes and certain cancer cells. Antibody blocking studies suggest that an N-terminal epitope of CD44 is involved in LC emigration, while the differentiation-related expression of the CD44 splice variant v6 allows for LC binding to T cell rather than to B cell areas of lymph nodes [58]. It will be important to determine which skin-bound and lymph node-bound ligands of CD44 and of its different splice variants are responsible for the observed phenomena. The other LC-bound receptor structure involved in tissue emigration is a heterodimer composed of the integrin chains α_6/β_1 or α_6/β_4 [59]. Importantly, the prototype cell expressing the latter moiety is the KC. These cells express this receptor in the hemidesmosome where it mediates KC attachment to laminin, a major constituent of the basement membrane. It is conceivable that *in vivo* stimulated LC loosen their KC-binding sites, and use α_6-containing integrin receptors to specifically recognize basement membrane components. The antigenic stimulus itself, stimulation-induced KC products, or the receptor-mediated interaction with extracellular matrix proteins may then induce LC to secrete proteolytic activity (e.g., type IV collagenase (MMP-9) [60]), allowing them to penetrate the basement membrane and to pave their route through the dense dermal network into the lymphatic system.

CUTANEOUS DC AS SENSITIZING AND TOLERIZING ELEMENTS IN SKIN-INDUCED IMMUNE RESPONSES

One can assume that the major *in vivo* function of LC is to provide a sensitizing signal in the induction of an immune response against antigens introduced into the skin (e.g., contactants, microorganisms) or newly generated in the skin (e.g., tumor antigens). The validity of this assumption is supported by several *in vivo* experiments: (1) While the application of a contact sensitizer to a skin area with high LC density leads to the induction of contact hypersensitivity, the application of the same contactant to a skin area deficient in LC results in antigen-specific nonresponsiveness [61]. (2) Antigen-bearing LC induce sensitization even when administered via routes (e.g., intravenously) that favor the induction of tolerance [62]. (3) CD4-bearing T cells that have been sensitized *in vitro* with hapten-modified LC act as effector cells of contact hypersensitivity [63]. (4) Compared to transplants with high LC density (body skin), transplants devoid of LC (central portion of cornea) or subtotally depleted of LC (tape-stripped skin) enjoy a prolonged survival on MHC class II-disparate recipients [64]. (5) GM-CSF-activated, LC-containing epidermal cells, but not LC-depleted epidermal cells, are capable of presenting tumor antigens for the generation of protective anti-tumor immunity *in vivo* [65]. Thus, the development of protein/peptide-based and, importantly, DNA-based immunization strategies to optimize antigen presentation by skin dendritic cells is a rational approach to anti-cancer and anti-microbial vaccine design. Recently, it has been demonstrated that cutaneous genetic immunization with naked DNA results in the transfection of and/or uptake of DNA-encoded proteins by skin DC which migrate to draining lymph nodes and efficiently elicit antigen-specific, cytotoxic and helper T cell responses [66, 67]. Alternatively, strategies aiming at introducing tumor or microbial antigen-derived peptides or cancer cell-derived RNA selectively into skin DC are certainly worth pursuing.

Recent evidence suggests that the immunoregulatory cytokine IL-10 [68–71], and presumably also certain neuropeptides such as calcitonin gene-related peptide [72] and α-MSH (melanocyte-stimulating hormone) [73] can convert immature DC into antigen-presented cells capable of tolerizing T cells and, perhaps, even of inducing regulatory/suppressor T cells [74]. The hypothesis that similar tolerization phenomena can occur also within the skin *in vivo* appears not to be too far-fetched as IL-10 is massively produced by UV-exposed KC and can be detected in progressing metastases from melanoma cells [75]. In fact, melanoma-derived factors can convert tumor-infiltrating DC into potent tolerogens and hapten-specific tolerance induced by UVB radiation of skin is mediated via KC-derived IL-10 [75, 76].

These findings imply that cutaneous DC can subserve a dual function in skin-derived immune responses which is apparently determined by the cellular and molecular composition of their microenvironment. Under conditions which favor their terminal maturation, LC/DDC will provide the skin with unique immune surveillance mechanisms, i.e., the capacity to generate protective responses against exogenous and endogenous pathogens [77]. On the other hand, stimuli which interfere with the acquisition of maturation-related immunostimulatory molecules and/or endow LC/DDC with tolerizing/anergizing properties would not only render the skin more vulnerable toward potentially harmful invaders but also prevent exaggerated tissue responses to innocuous moieties, e.g., autoantigens and certain haptens.

An understanding of the mechanisms that maintain the delicate balance between sensitization- and tolerization-promoting signals should provide a clue to the role of the skin immune system in the maintenance of cutaneous homeostasis and integrity and, at the same time, provide the basis for re-establishing it when perturbed.

ACKNOWLEDGMENTS

This work was supported, in part, by grants S06702-MED and P10797-MED from the Austrian Science Foundation, and by a grant from the Federal Ministry of Science and Transport, Vienna, Austria.

We thank S. Wichlas, MD and E. Csinády, MD for technical assistance, and Mrs Barbara Wibmer for carefully typing the manuscript.

REFERENCES

1. Langerhans, P. (1868). Über die Nerven der menschlichen Haut. *Virchows Arch. (Pathol. Arch.)* **44**, 325–337.
2. Schuler, G. (ed.). (1991). *Epidermal Langerhans Cells.* CRC Press, Boca Raton, FL.
3. Tang, A., Amagai, M., Granger, L.R., Stanley, J.R. and Udey, M.C. (1993). Adhesion of epidermal Langerhans cells to keratinocytes mediated by E-cadherin. *Nature* **361**, 82–85.
4. Chen, H., Yuan, J., Wang, Y. and Silvers, W.K. (1985). Distribution of ATPase-positive Langerhans cells in normal adult human skin. *Br. J. Dermatol.* **113**, 707–711.
5. Basset, F. and Nezelof, C. (1966). Présence en microscopie électronique de structures filamenteuses originales dans les lesions pulmonaires et osseuses de l'histiocytose X. Etat actuel de la question. *Soc. Med. Hop.* **117**, 413–426.
6. Gadner, H. and Grois, N. (1993). The histiocytosis syndromes. In: *Dermatology in General Medicine* (eds T.B. Fitzpatrick, A.Z. Eisen, K. Wolff, I.M. Freedberg, and K.F. Austen), vol. II. McGraw-Hill, New York, pp. 2003–2017.
7. Krueger, G.G., Daynes, R.A. and Emam, M. (1982). Biology of Langerhans cells: selective migration of Langerhans cells into allogeneic and xenogeneic grafts on *nude* mice. *Proc. Natl Acad. Sci. USA* **80**, 1650–1654.
8. Holt, P.G., Haining, S., Nelson, D.J. and Sedgwick. J.D. (1994). Origin and steady-state turnover of class II MHC-bearing dendritic cells in the epithelium of the conducting airways. *J. Immunol.* **153**, 256–261.
9. Schuler, G., Thurner, B. and Romani, N. (1997). Dendritic cells: from ignored cells to major players in T cell-mediated immunity. *Int. Arch. Allergy Immunol.* **112**, 317–322.
10. Luger, T.A., Bhardwaj, R.S., Grabbe, S. and Schwarz, T. (1996). Regulation of the immune response by epidermal cytokines and neurohormones. *J. Dermatol. Sci.* **13**, 5–10.
11. Kilgus, O., Payer, E., Schreiber, S., Elbe, A., Strohal, R. and Stingl, G. (1993). In vivo cytokine expression in normal and perturbed skin. Analysis by competitive quantitative polymerase chain reaction. *J. Invest. Dermatol.* **100**, 674–680.
12. Enk, A.H., Angeloni, V.L., Udey, M.C. and Katz, S.I. (1991). Early molecular events in the induction phase of contact sensitivity. *Proc. Natl Acad. Sci. USA* **89**, 1398–1402.
13. Luger, T.A. and Schwarz, T. (1995). Effects of UV light on cytokines and neuroendocrine hormones. In: *Photoimmunology* (eds J. Krutmann and C.A. Elmets), Part 1. Blackwell Science, Oxford, 55–76.
14. Heufler, C., Koch, F. and Schuler, G. (1988). Granulocyte-macrophage colony-stimulating factor and interleukin-1 mediate the maturation of murine epidermal Langerhans cells into potent immunostimulatory dendritic cells. *J. Exp. Med.* **167**, 700–705.
15. Romani, N., Koide, S., Crowley, M., Witmer-Pack, M., Livingstone, A.M., Fathman, C.G., Inaba, K. and Steinman, R.M. (1989). Presentation of exogenous protein antigens by dendritic cells to T cell clones. Intact protein is presented best by immature, epidermal Langerhans cells. *J. Exp. Med.* **169**, 1169–1178.
16. Schuler, G. and Steinman, R.M. (1985). Murine epidermal Langerhans cells mature into potent immunostimulatory dendritic cells in vitro. *J. Exp. Med.* **161**, 526–546.
17. Schreiber, S., Kilgus, O., Payer, E., Kutil, R., Elbe, A., Mueller, C. and Stingl, G. (1992). Cytokine pattern of Langerhans cells isolated from murine epidermal cell cultures. *J. Immunol.* **149**, 3524–3534.
18. Kang, K., Kubin, M., Cooper, K.D., Lessin, S.R., Trinchieri, G. and Rook, A.H. (1996). IL-12 synthesis by human Langerhans cells. *J. Immunol.* **156**, 1402–1407.

19. Lenz, A., Heine, M., Schuler, G. and Romani, N. (1993). Human and murine dermis contain dendritic cells. Isolation by means of a novel method and phenotypical and functional characterization. *J. Clin. Invest.* **92**, 2587–2596.
20. Meunier, L., Gonzalez-Ramos, A. and Cooper K.D. (1993). Heterogeneous populations of MHC class II$^+$ cells in human dermal suspensions. Identification of a small subset responsible for potent dermal antigen-presenting cell activity with features analogous to Langerhans cells. *J. Immunol.* **151**, 4067–4080.
21. Caux, C., Dezutter-Dambuyant, C., Schmitt, D. and Banchereau, J. (1992). GM-CSF and TNF-α cooperate in the generation of dendritic Langerhans cells. *Nature* **360**, 258–261.
22. Strunk, D., Rappersberger, K., Egger, C., Strobl, H., Krömer, E., Elbe, A., Maurer, D. and Stingl, G. (1996). Generation of human dendritic cells/Langerhans cells from circulating CD34$^+$ hematopoietic progenitor cells. *Blood* **87**, 1292–1302.
23. Strunk, D., Egger, C., Leitner, G., Hanau, D. and Stingl, G. (1997). A skin homing molecule defines the Langerhans cell progenitor in human peripheral blood. *J.Exp. Med.* **185**, 1131–1136.
24. Fuhlbrigge, R.C., Kieffer, J.D., Armerding, D. and Kupper, T.S. (1997). Cutaneous lymphocyte antigen is a specialized form of PSGL-1 expressed on skin-homing T cells. *Nature* **389**, 978–981.
25. Caux, C., Vanbervliet, B., Massacrier, C., Dezutter-Dambuyant, C., de Saint-Vis, B., Jacquet, C., Yoneda, K., Imamura, S., Schmitt, D. and Banchereau, J. (1996). CD34$^+$ hematopoietic progenitors from human cord blood differentiate along two independent dendritic cell pathways in response to GM-CSF + TNF-α. *J. Exp. Med.* **184**, 695–706.
26. Caux, C., Massacrier, C., Vanbervliet, B., Dubois, B., Durand, I., Cella, M., Lanzavecchia, A. and Banchereau, J. (1997). CD34$^+$ hematopoietic progenitors from human cord blood differentiate along two independent dendritic cell pathways in response to granulocyte-macrophage colony-stimulating factor plus tumor necrosis factor alpha: II. Functional analysis. *Blood* **90**, 1458–1470.
27. Burkly, L., Hession, C., Ogata, L., Relly, C., Marconi, L.A., Olson, D., Tizard, R., Cate, R. and Lo, L. (1995). Expression of RelB is required for the development of thymic medulla and dendritic cells. *Nature* **373**, 531–536.
28. Georgopoulos, K., Bigby, M., Wang, J.H., Molnar, A., Wu, P., Winandy, S. and Sharpe, A. (1994). The Ikaros gene is required for the development of all lymphoid lineages. *Cell* **79**, 143–156.
29. Wu, L., Nichogiannopoulou, A., Shortman, K. and Georgopoulos, K. (1997). Cell-autonomous defects in dendritic cell populations of Ikaros mutant mice point to a developmental relationship with the lymphoid lineage. *Immunity* **7**, 483–492.
30. Caux, C., Vanbervliet, B., Massacrier, C., Durand, I. and Banchereau, J. (1996). Interleukin-3 cooperates with tumor necrosis factor alpha for the development of human dendritic/Langerhans cells from cord blood CD34$^+$ hematopoietic progenitor cells. *Blood* **87**, 2376–2385.
31. Borkowski, T.A., Letterio, J.J., Farr, A.G. and Udey, M.C. (1996). A role for endogenous transforming growth factor beta 1 in Langerhans cell biology: the skin of transforming growth factor-β1 null mice is devoid of epidermal Langerhans cells. *J. Exp. Med.* **184**, 2417–2422.
32. Strobl, H., Riedl, E., Scheinecker, C., Bello-Fernandez, C., Pickl, W.F., Rappersberger, K., Majdic, O. and Knapp, W. (1996). TGF-β1 promotes in vitro development of dendritic cells from CD34$^+$ hemopoietic progenitors. *J. Immunol.* **157**, 1499–1507.
33. Strobl, H., Bello-Fernandez, C., Riedl, E., Pickl, W.F., Majdic, O., Lyman, S.D. and Knapp, W. (1997). Flt3 ligand in cooperation with transforming growth factor-β1 potentiates in vitro development of Langerhans-type dendritic cells and allows single-cell dendritic cell cluster formation under serum-free conditions. *Blood* **90**, 1425–1434.
34. Borkowski, T.A., Letterio, J.J., Mackall, C.L., Saitoh, A., Wang, K.J., Roop, D.R., Gress, R.E. and Udey, M.C. (1997). A role for TGF-β1 in Langerhans cell biology. Further characterization of the epidermal Langerhans cell defect in TGF-β1 null mice. *J. Clin. Invest.* **100**, 575–581.
35. Premarck, B.D. and Schall, T.J. (1996). Chemokine receptors: gateways to inflammation and infection. *Nature Medicine* **2**, 1174–1178.
36. Adams, D.H. and Lloyd, A.R. (1997). Chemokines: leukocyte recruitment and activation cytokines. *Lancet* **349**, 490–494.
37. Sozzani, S., Sallusto, F., Luini, W., Zhou, D., Pietmontli, L., Allavena, P., VanDamme, J., Valitutti, S., Lanzavecchia, A. and Mantovani, A. (1995). Migration of dendritic cells in response to formyl peptides, C5a and a distinct set of chemokines. *J. Immunol.* **155**, 3292–3296.

38. Godiska, R., Chantry, D., Raport, C.J., Sozzani, S., Allavena, P., Leviten, D., Mantovani, A. and Gray, P.W. (1997). Human macrophage-derived chemokine (MDC), a novel chemoattractant for monocytes, monocyte-derived dendritic cells, and natural killer cells. *J. Exp. Med.* **185**, 1595–1604.
39. Xu, L.L., Warren, M.K., Rose, W.I.L., Gong, W.H. and Wang, J.M. (1996). Human monocyte chemotactic protein and other C-C chemokines bind and induce directional migration of dendritic cells in vitro. *J. Leukocyte Biol.* **60**, 365–371.
40. Greaves, D.R., Wang, W., Dairaghi, D.J., Dieu, M.C., de Saint-Vis, B., Franz-Bacon, K., Rossi, D., Caux, C., McClanahan, T., Gordon, S., Zlotnik, A. and Schall, T. (1997). CCR6, a CC chemokine receptor that interacts with macrophage inflammatory protein 3α and is highly expressed in human dendritic cells. *J. Exp. Med.* **186**, 837–844.
41. Power, C.A., Church, D.J., Meyer, A., Aluani, S., Proudfoot, A.E.I., Clark-Lewis, I., Sozzani, S., Mantovani, A. and Wells, T.N.C. (1997). Cloning and characterization of a specific receptor for the novel CC chemokine MIP-3α from lung dendritic cells. *J. Exp. Med.* **186**, 825–835.
42. Rossi, D.L., Vicari, A.P., Franz-Bacon, K., McClanahan, T. and Zlotnik, A. (1997). Identification through bioinformatics of two new macrophage proinflammatory human chemokines MIP-3α and MIP-3β. *J. Immunol.* **158**, 1033–1036.
43. Zaitseva, M., Blauvelt, A., Lee, S., Lapham, C.K., Klaus-Kovtun, V., Mostowski, H., Manischewitz, J. and Golding, H. (1997). Expression and function of CCR5 and CXCR4 on human Langerhans cells and macrophages: implications for HIV primary infection. *Nature Medicine* **3**, 1369–1375.
44. Larsen, C.P., Steinman, R.M., Witmer-Pack, M., Hankins, D.P., Morris, D.P. and Austyn, J.M. (1990). Migration and maturation of Langerhans cells in skin transplants and explants. *J. Exp. Med.* **172**, 1483–1493.
45. Aiba, S. and Katz, S.I. (1990). Phenotypic and functional characteristics of in vivo-activated Langerhans cells. *J. Immunol.* **145**, 2791–2796.
46. Macatonia, S.E., Knight, S.C., Edwards, A.J., Griffiths, S. and Fryer, P. (1987). Localization of antigen on lymph node dendritic cells after exposure to the contact sensitizer fluorescein isothiocyanate. Functional and morphological studies. *J. Exp. Med.* **166**, 1654–1667.
47. Silberberg-Sinakin, I., Thorbecke, G.J., Baer, R.L., Rosenthal, S.A. and Berezowsky, V. (1976). Antigen-bearing Langerhans cells in skin, dermal lymphatics and in lymph nodes. *Cell. Immunol.* **25**, 137–151.
48. Mommaas, A.M., Mulder, A.A., Out, C.J., Girolomoni, G., Koerten, H.K., Vermeer, B.J. and Koning, F.D. (1995). Distribution of HLA class II molecules in epidermal Langerhans cells in situ. *Eur. J. Immunol.* **25**, 520–525.
49. Cella, M., Engering, A., Pinet, V., Pieters, J. and Lanzavecchia, A. (1997). Inflammatory stimuli induce accumulation of MHC class II complexes on dendritic cells. *Nature* **388**, 782–786.
50. Sallusto, F., Cella, M., Danielli, C. and Lanzavecchia, A. (1995). Dendritic cells use macropinocytosis and the mannose receptor to concentrate antigen in the MHC II compartment. Downregulation by cytokines and bacterial products. *J. Exp. Med.* **182**, 389–400.
51. Inaba, K., Schuler, G., Witmer, M.D., Valinksy, J., Atassi, B. and Steinman, R.M. (1986). Immunologic properties of purified epidermal Langerhans cells. Distinct requirements for stimulation of unprimed and sensitized T lymphocytes. *J. Exp. Med.* **164**, 605–613.
52. Steinman, R.M. (1991). The dendritic cell system and its role in immunogenicity. *Annu. Rev. Immunol.* **9**, 271–296.
53. Cumberbatch, M., Fielding, I. and Kimber, I. (1994). Modulation of epidermal Langerhans cell frequency by tumour necrosis factor-α. *Immunology* **81**, 395–401.
54. Cumberbatch, M., Dearman, R.J. and Kimber, I. (1997). Langerhans cells require signals from both tumour necrosis factor-α and interleukin-1β for migration. *Immunology* **92**, 388–395.
55. Rambukkana, A., Pistoor, F.H., Bos, J.D., Kapsenberg, M.L. and Das, P.K. (1996). Effects of contact allergens on human Langerhans cells in skin organ culture: migration, modulation of cell surface molecules, and early expression of interleukin-1β protein. *Lab. Invest.* **74**, 422–436.
56. Wang, B., Kondo, S., Shivji, G.M., Fujisawa, H., Mak, T.W. and Sauder, D.N. (1996). Tumour necrosis factor receptor II (p75) signalling is required for the migration of Langerhans cells. *Immunology* **88**, 284–288.
57. Schwarzenberger, K. and Udey, M.C. (1996). Contact allergens and epidermal proinflammatory cytokines modulate Langerhans cell E-cadherin expression in situ. *J. Invest. Dermatol.* **106**, 553–558.

58. Weiss, J.M., Sleeman, J., Renkl, A.C., Dittmar, H., Termeer, C.C., Taxis, S., Howells, N., Hofmann, M., Köhler, K., Schöpf, E., Ponta, H., Herrlich, P. and Simon, J.C. (1997). An essential role for CD44 variant isoforms in epidermal Langerhans cell and blood dendritic cell function. *J. Cell Biol.* **137**, 1137–1147.
59. Price, A.A., Cumberbatch, M., Kimber, I. and Ager, A. (1997). α_6 integrins are required for Langerhans cell migration from the epidermis. *J. Exp. Med.* **186**, 1725–1735.
60. Kobayashi, Y. (1997). Langerhans cells produce type IV collagenase (MMP-9) following epicutaneous stimulation with haptens. *Immunology* **90**, 496–501.
61. Toews, G.B., Bergstresser, P.R. and Streilein, J.W. (1980). Epidermal Langerhans cell density determines whether contact hypersensitivity or unresponsiveness follows skin painting with DNFB. *J. Immunol.* **124**, 445–453.
62. Sullivan, S., Bergstresser, P.R. and Streilein, J.W. (1985). Intravenously injected, TNP-derivatized, Langerhans cell-enriched epidermal cells induce contact hypersensitivity in Syrian hamsters. *J. Invest. Dermatol.* **84**, 249–252.
63. Hauser, C. (1990). Cultured epidermal Langerhans cells activate effector T cells for contact sensitivity. *J. Invest. Dermatol.* **95**, 436–440.
64. Streilein, J.W., Toews, G.B. and Bergstresser, P.R. (1979). Corneal allografts fail to express Ia antigens. *Nature* **282**, 326–327.
65. Grabbe, S., Bruvers, S., Gallo, R.L., Knisely, T.L., Nazareno, R. and Granstein, R.D. (1991). Tumor antigen presentation by murine epidermal cells. *J. Immunol.* **146**, 3656–3661.
66. Condon, C., Watkins, S.C., Celluzzi, C.M., Thompson, K. and Falo, L.D. Jr. (1996). DNA-based immunization by in vivo transfection of dendritic cells. *Nature Medicine* **2**, 1122–1128.
67. Casares, S., Inaba, K., Brumeanu, T.D., Steinman, R.M. and Bona, C.A. (1997). Antigen presentation by dendritic cells after immunization with DNA encoding a major histocompatibility complex class II-restricted viral epitope. *J. Exp. Med.* **186**, 1481–1486.
68. Enk, A.H., Angeloni, V.L., Udey, M.C. and Katz, S.I. (1993). Inhibition of Langerhans cell antigen-presenting function by IL-10. A role for IL-10 in induction of tolerance. *J. Immunol.* **151**, 2390–2398.
69. Enk, A.H., Saloga, J., Becker, D., Mohamadzadeh, M. and Knop, J. (1994). Induction of hapten-specific tolerance by interleukin 10 in vivo. *J. Exp. Med.* **179**, 1397–1402.
70. Ozawa, H., Aiba, S., Nakagawa, N. and Tagami, H. (1996). Interferon-γ and interleukin-10 inhibit antigen presentation by Langerhans cells for T helper type 1 cells by suppressing their CD80 (B7-1) expression. *Eur. J. Immunol.* **26**, 648–652.
71. Steinbrink, K., Wölfl, M., Jonuleit, H., Knop, J. and Enk, A.H. (1997). Induction of tolerance by IL-10-treated dendritic cells. *J. Immunol.* **159**, 4772–4780.
72. Hosoi, J., Murphy, G.F., Egan, C.L., Lerner, E.A., Grabbe, S., Asahina, S. and Granstein, R.D. (1993). Regulation of Langerhans cell function by nerves containing calcitonin gene-related peptide. *Nature* **363**, 159–163.
73. Grabbe, S., Bhardwaj, R.S., Mahnke, K., Simon, M.M., Schwarz, T. and Luger, T.A. (1996). alpha-Melanocyte-stimulating hormone induces hapten-specific tolerance in mice. *J. Immunol.* **156**, 473–478.
74. Groux, H., O'Garra, A., Bigler, M., Rouleau, M., Antonenko, S., deVries, J.E. and Roncarolo, M.G. (1997). A $CD4^+$ T-cell subset inhibits antigen-specific T-cell responses and prevents colitis. *Nature* **389**, 737–742.
75. Enk, A.H., Jonuleit, H., Saloga, J. and Knop, J. (1997). Dendritic cells as mediators of tumor-induced tolerance in metastatic melanoma. *Int. J. Cancer* **73**, 309–316.
76. Niizeki, H. and Streilein, J.W. (1997). Hapten-specific tolerance induced by acute, low-dose ultraviolet B radiation of skin is mediated via interleukin-10. *J. Invest. Dermatol.* **109**, 25–30.
77. Streilein, J.W. (1983). Skin-associated lymphoid tissues (SALT): origins and functions. *J. Invest. Dermatol.* **80**, S12–16.

CHAPTER 8
Dendritic Cells in the Lung

A.S. McWilliam, P.A. Stumbles and P.G. Holt
Division of Cell Biology, TVW Telethon Institute for Child Health Research, West Perth, Western Australia, Australia

INTRODUCTION

The epithelial surfaces of the conducting airways and the deep lung are continuously exposed to inert and pathogenic antigens present in inspired air. The maintenance of local immunological homeostasis requires efficient sampling of these antigens, and rapid transmission of processed immunogens to T cells in the central immune system. The intensity of antigenic stimulation at these sites necessitates the presence in respiratory tract tissues of a highly dynamic antigen-presenting cell (APC) system. As discussed below, local networks of dendritic cells appear specialized for these functions, and exhibit several distinctive attributes which equip them uniquely for this task.

DISTRIBUTION AND SURFACE PHENOTYPE OF RESPIRATORY TRACT DENDRITIC CELLS

Rat

In laboratory animals, dendritic cells (DC) have now been identified in sections of parenchymal lung tissue, and airway mucosa (Simecka *et al.*, 1986; Holt and Schon Hegrad, 1987; Holt *et al.*, 1988; Kradin *et al.*, 1991). However, the relatively large size and pleiomorphic morphology of DC have posed significant problems in their accurate determination and quantification within sections of lung and airway tissue. Thus, sections cut either transversely or parallel to the lumen of the airway and subsequently immunostained for the presence of MHC class II (Ia) antigen either fail to show the presence of Ia antigen or merely succeed in sectioning isolated portions of the arborizing processes of the 'dendritic' cells. Consequently this has created a false impression of the position, morphology, and number of these cells within the airway mucosa.

Studies from our laboratory have therefore concentrated on this problem of visualizing and quantifying the DC population present within the airway epithelium of the rat. Sections which have been cut along the length of the rat trachea and immunostained for the presence of Ia antigen using the mAb OX6 are shown in Figs 1A and 1B. These

Dendritic Cells: Biology and Clinical Applications
ISBN 0-12-455860-7

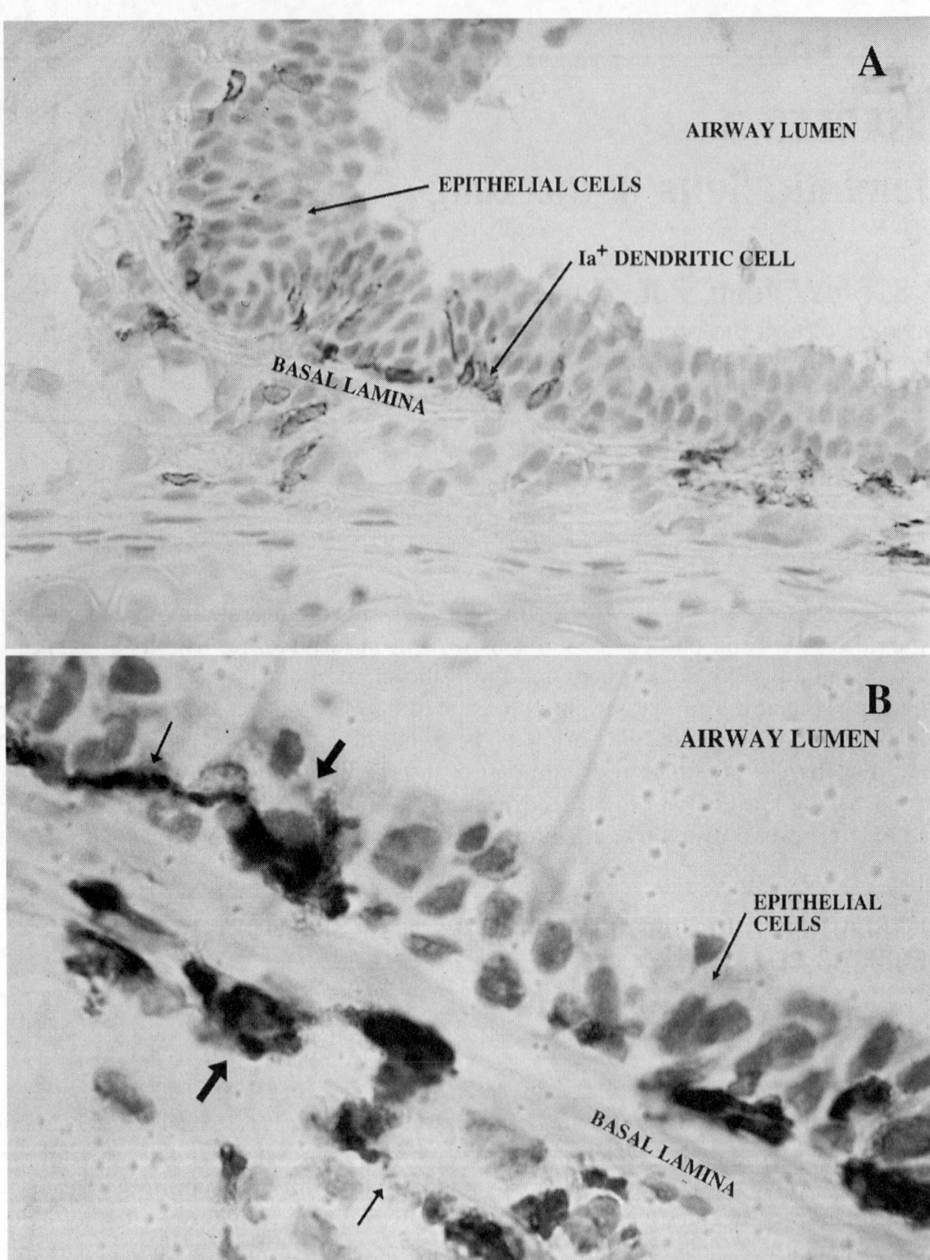

Fig. 1. Photomicrographs of longitudinal sections of rat trachea immunohistochemically stained with the mAb OX6, recognizing rat dendritic cells expressing MHC class II antigen (Ia). In (A) several DC bodies can be seen in close association with the basal lamina. Dendritiform processes from these cells can be seen to extend upwards from the basal lamina, interdigitating between the epithelial cells as they progress towards the lumen. The association between the DC and the basal lamina is illustrated in (B), where the cell body of an individual DC can be seen straddling the basal lamina (thick arrow) and the extended dendriform processes of the same cell can also be seen (thin arrow).

sections clearly demonstrate that Ia-positive cells are present and appear to maintain contact with the basal lamina at the base of the epithelium. Ia-positive processes can be seen to extend out from these cells and interdigitate between the individual epithelial cells. At present it is not clear whether these processes extend to the base of the inter-epithelial junctions or onto the luminal surface, nor is the nature and extent of the attachment to the basal lamina understood. Detailed electron-microscopic studies are needed to answer these important questions.

It was reasoned that, for isolated airway segments, a tangential plane of section would produce some sections passing through the epithelium in a plane parallel to the underlying basal lamina. Staining of these sections would then, in theory, provide a 'view from above' of the intraepithelial cell population and should illustrate the overall distribution of this population, analogous to the picture obtained after staining of epidermal sheets for Ia on Langerhans cells.

Immunoperoxidase staining of these tangential airway sections for Ia reveals an extensive network of intraepithelial DC similar to that found in the epidermis of both rat and human skin tissue (Holt *et al.*, 1990; Holt *et al.*, 1992). A schematic representation of the distribution of the tracheal epithelial DC population is presented in Fig. 2a. This allows an appreciation of how tangential sectioning of airway tissue results in a 'plan view' of DC distribution. Figure 2a also shows a representative tangential section of tracheal epithelium immunostained for Ia with the mAb OX6 and depicts the interlocking network formed by these arborizing cells. Within epithelial sections from animals taken under steady-state noninflammatory conditions, we have found few if any ED2-positive macrophages and no B cells; hence it is thought that virtually 100% of the intraepithelial Ia staining is restricted to the DC population.

The technique of tangential sectioning has also provided an excellent means of visualizing and quantifying cellular changes occurring within the epithelium during inflammatory reactions. Thus, a detailed analysis of the numbers of DC within the epithelium of rat airways, analysed under steady-state conditions in animals born and housed in an environment in which there is minimum exposure to respirable dust, has consistently found a higher density of DC on the dorsal surface of the airways compared with the ventral surfaces (881/mm^2, cf. 675/mm^2) (Holt *et al.*, 1992). If the supposition that these epithelial DC are critical to the processing and ultimate presentation of antigens impinging on the airways is correct, then a greater density on the dorsal airway surface may not be unexpected and may reflect the greater amount of material likely to be deposited on the dorsal surface of the airway as a result of the aerodynamics of inhalation.

This contention was further supported when epithelial DC densities within each airway generation were compared (Holt *et al.*, 1992). Again, densities of DC were highest in the upper airways (600–800/mm^2) and decreased with progression down the respiratory tree, reaching lower limits of 75/mm^2 in the peripheral lung.

In an extension of this study, exposure of rats to an aerosol of LPS resulted in a transient increase of tracheal DC numbers from 600/mm^2 to approximately 1000/mm^2 after 24 h. These studies of rat airway DC suggested, for the first time, that DC may be a more dynamic population than was previously thought and may be active players in the pathogenesis of the airway inflammatory response.

(a)

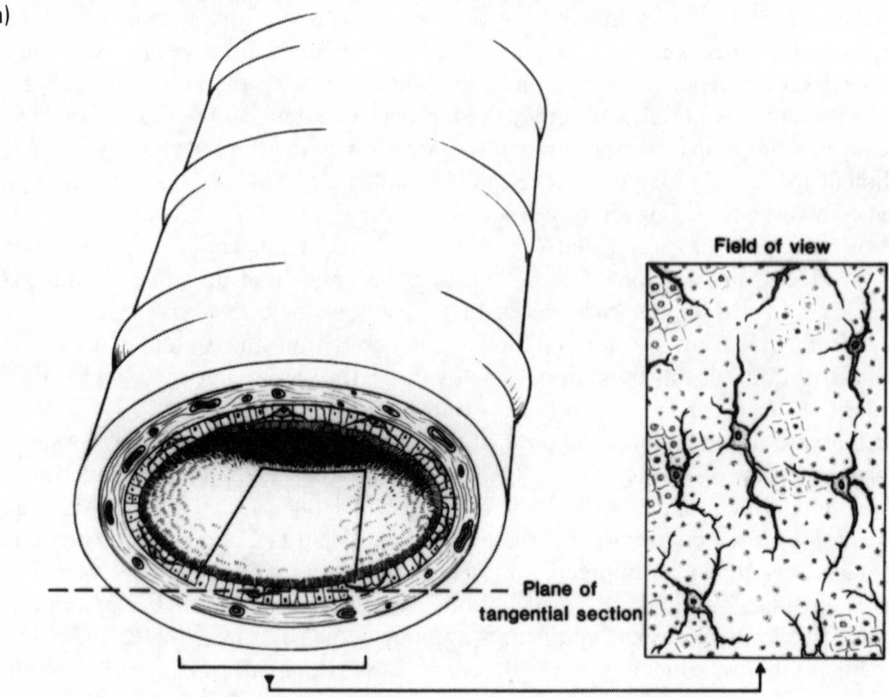

Fig. 2. Schematic representations of the location and distribution of DC within the epithelial lining of the upper airways (a) and the parenchyma of the lung (b). Part (a) depicts how intraepithelial dendritic cells are pictured after tangential sectioning of rat tracheal tissue. The insert shows the interlocking network formed by these cells which permeates throughout the epithelial lining of the upper respiratory tract. The spatial relationship between alveolar macrophages and interstitial lung dendritic cells is illustrated schematically in (b). The alveolar macrophage can be seen located at the interseptal junction and is adherent to part of the membrane of a type I epithelial cell which forms most of the lining of the alveolar spaces. Lying immediately beneath this, and separated by a gap of approximately 0.2–1 μm, is a putative dendritic cell with a typical indent nucleus.

Rat Lung Parenchymal DC

The location of DC within the tissue of the lung has been examined both at a light-microscopic and electron-microscopic level (Holt *et al.*, 1992; Holt *et al.*, 1993). In these studies care was taken to ensure that fixation was performed by intravascular perfusion so that the alveolar macrophages would be adequately fixed *in situ* and hence allow an appreciation of the spatial relationship between pulmonary alveolar macrophages (PAM) and interstitial DC. A schematic representation of the relative positions of these two cells types is depicted in Fig. 2b. The PAM occupy a position at the alveolar junctional zones and are spread out upon a bed composed of the thin attenuated lining created by the type I epithelial cell membrane. The DC appear to lie within the underlying interstitium near to the PAM. Indeed, the separation between the PAM and the DC would be in the order of 0.2–1.0 μm. A separation of this

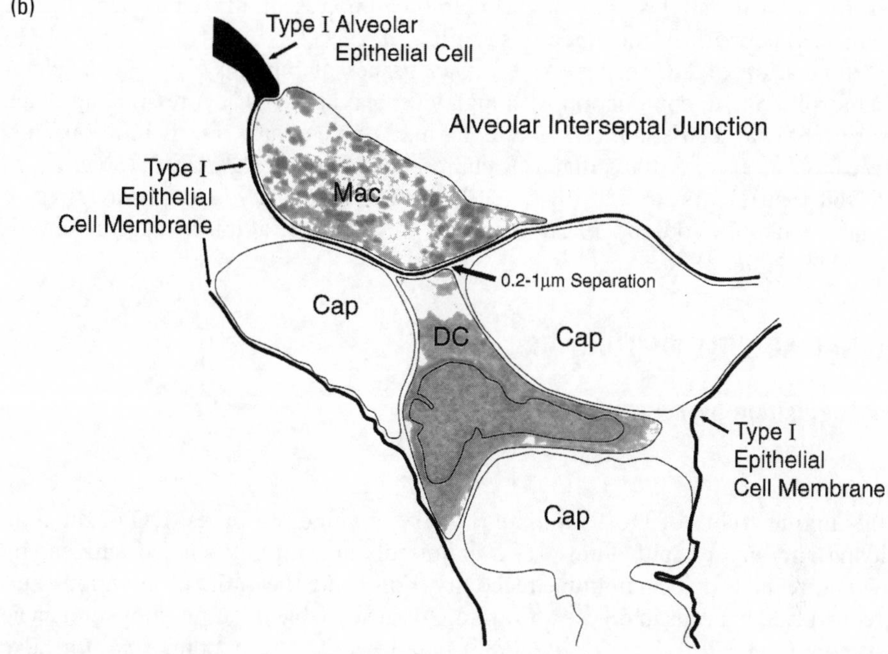

Fig. 2. (*Continued*)

magnitude allows for the possibility of a functional interaction between these cell types and would explain the downregulation of APC function attributed to alveolar macrophages which will be discussed in more detail later in this chapter. This close juxtaposition of PAM and DC may also allow for the suggestion (MacLean *et al.*, 1996) that PAM function to remove inhaled particulate material from the immediate environment of the DC and thus prevent unwanted inflammatory responses which may impair the antigen-specific function of the DC.

Distribution and Surface Phenotype of Human Respiratory Tract DC

The presence of DC in human respiratory tract tissues was first noted in the context of diseases such as histiocytosis X (Soler *et al.*, 1985), carcinoma (Hammar *et al.*, 1986), and various granulomatous disorders (Webber *et al.*, 1985; Munro *et al.*, 1987). However, further investigation revealed their presence in normal airway epithelium (Richard *et al.*, 1987; van Nieuwkerk *et al.*, 1991) and lung parenchyma (Sertl *et al.*, 1986). In addition, variable numbers of DC are found on the epithelial surfaces of the lower respiratory tract (Casolaro *et al.*, 1988; van Haarst *et al.*, 1994).

The use of a tangential sectioning technique developed in our laboratories has provided insight into the distribution of DC within the epithelium of the conducting airways. These cells are distributed as a tightly meshed network within the epithelium, at a density of 600–700 DC per mm^2 of epithelium, essentially equivalent to the Langerhans cell network in the epidermis (Holt *et al.*, 1989).

The identification of DC in lung and airway tissues of humans is based on pleiomorphic morphology in conjunction with high level class II MHC expression, and lack of expression of characteristic B cell, T cell and macrophage markers. In addition, they express variable levels of S-100 antigen (Richard *et al.*, 1987), CD1a/CD1c (Soler *et al.*, 1989), CD68 (van Haarst *et al.*, 1994), RFD1 (van Haarst *et al.*, 1994), a range of adhesion molecules (Nicod and El Habre 1992), and the low affinity receptor for IgE (Tunon-de-lara *et al.*, 1996).

FUNCTIONAL ACTIVITY OF LUNG DC

Antigen Acquisition by Lung DC

Antigen Uptake in situ

Given the unique ability of DC to initiate primary immune responses, DC of the lung parenchyma and airway epithelium play a major role in sampling inhaled antigens by initiating and regulating local immune reactivity. Following the initial observations that DC were the principal cells in digests of rat lung tissue capable of stimulating allogeneic T cell responses *in vitro* (Holt *et al.*, 1985), studies on antigen uptake *in situ* have demonstrated that DC isolated from the lung parenchyma or airway epithelium of rats exposed to aerosolized soluble protein antigen are able to activate antigen-specific T cell responses *in vitro* (Holt *et al.*, 1988; Holt *et al.*, 1992). These observations have been repeated in separate studies in rats and extended to show that primary airway challenge with soluble antigen leads to a mobilization of antigen-bearing DC to the draining lymph nodes (Gong *et al.*, 1992; Xia *et al.*, 1995). Thus, lung and airway DC are clearly capable of uptake of inhaled soluble antigen *in situ* and traffic to regional lymph nodes for initiation of primary immunity.

Antigen uptake in vitro

To date, the endocytic activity of lung DC has not been well characterized. Endocytosis, via pinocytosis or cell surface receptors, represents the primary mechanism for cellular uptake of soluble antigens and has been extensively studied in DC from a number of sites including blood, bone marrow and peripheral tissues (Steinman and Swanson, 1995). Recent studies from our laboratory have shown that approximately one-third of highly purified DC freshly isolated from rat lung digests by cell sorting are capable of endocytosing high amounts of soluble antigen *in vitro* (Fig. 3A). Microscopically, fluorescently labelled vesicles can be seen clearly and these appear to be localized peripherally to submembranal regions of the cell and, although not formally proven, it is likely that these correspond to the MHC class II-rich vesicles described for DC isolated from the peripheral blood of humans (Sallusto *et al.*, 1995). The observation that at any given time point lung DC are heterogeneous in terms of endocytic activity, with a significant proportion of fresh lung DC not actively endocytic (Fig. 3A),

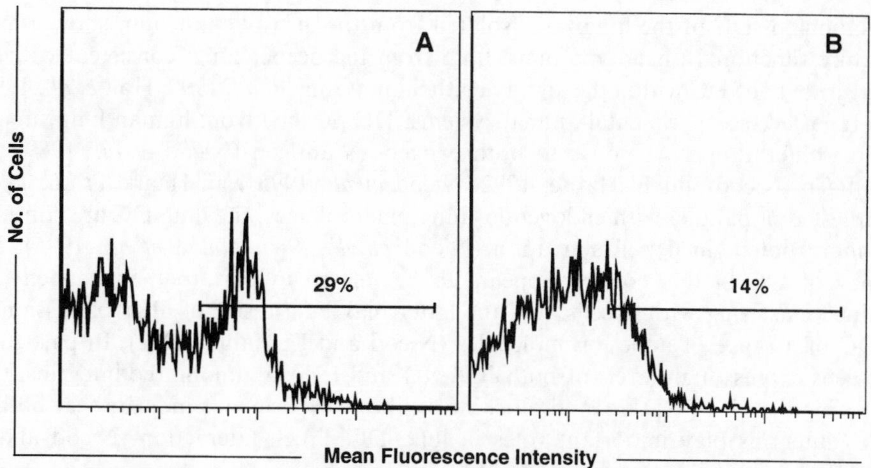

Fig. 3. Downregulation of soluble antigen uptake in lung DC by GM-CSF. Highly purified rat lung DC were incubated with FITC-labelled dextran (FITC-DX) for 90 min at 37°C either fresh (A) or after overnight culture in 10 ng/ml GM-CSF (B) and mean fluorescence intensity was determined by flow cytometry. Curve (A) demonstrates FITC-DX uptake by a proportion (30%) of lung DC, which is downregulated by exposure to GM-CSF (B).

may reflect the relative maturational states of airway versus deep lung DC and, in turn, the rapid turnover of DC at the airway mucosa (Holt *et al.*, 1994).

Rapid downregulation of the ability to acquire soluble antigen following *in vitro* exposure to maturation factors such as GM-CSF or inflammatory stimuli such as LPS or TNF-α is a hallmark of tissue DC and is thought to mimic the functional maturation that occurs *in vivo* prior to migration to regional lymph nodes (Steinman, 1991). Again, recent studies from our laboratory have confirmed that the endocytic activity of freshly isolated lung DC is rapidly and markedly inhibted by overnight maturation in the presence of GM-CSF (Fig. 3B). As previous studies have shown, this maturation process also corresponds with an upregulation of the ability to present antigen to presensitized antigen-specific T cells (see below).

Antigen Presentation by Lung DC

Antigen Presentation in vitro

As referred to above, studies on collagenase digests of rat parenchymal lung tissue were the first to identify DC as the primary APC of the lung (Holt *et al.*, 1985) and subsequent studies have extended these observations to both mouse and human (Nicod *et al.*, 1990; Pollard and Lipscomb, 1990). Further studies also showed that these DC were able to present protein antigen to primed T cells and, moreover, that this presenting capacity was markedly upregulated by maturation in GM-CSF, corresponding with an increase in surface Ia expression (Holt *et al.*, 1992). Thus, it is clear that lung DC behave in a similar fashion to DC from other tissue sites, requiring a maturational signal in the form of cytokines or inflammatory stimuli in order to become efficient APC for T cell activation. However, it is also clear that heterogeneity exists among populations of DC in the lung: DC isolated from the airway epithelium show a more immature functional phenotype than those from the deeper lung, consistent with the rapid turnover of DC within the airway epithelium (Gong *et al.*, 1992; Holt *et al.*, 1994).

As reported in experimental animal systems, DC purified from human lung support T cell proliferation in response to both exogenous antigen (Nicod *et al.*, 1989) and alloantigen (Nicod and El Habre, 1992; Nicod *et al.*, 1995; van Haarst *et al.*, 1996). When tested in parallel with endogenous lung macrophages, the lung DC are considerably more potent in T cell activation (Nicod *et al.*, 1989; Nicod *et al.*, 1995). The potency of DC in this context appears to be related in part to their capacity for sustained clustering with T cells, and the latter may be a result of high expression on the DC of a range of adhesion molecules (Nicod and El Habre, 1992). In particular, these cells express high levels of both ICAM-1 and LFA-3; among the integrins, they express high levels of CD11c, and blocking antibody experiments indicate that both β_1 and β_2 integrins play important roles in lung DC–T cell interaction (Nicod and El Habre, 1992).

APC Activity in vivo

Although the *in vivo* APC activity of lung DC has not been studied extensively, recent adoptive transfer studies from our laboratory have demonstrated the potent ability of lung DC to initiate antigen-specific immune reactivity. Recipients of antigen-pulsed, GM-CSF-matured lung DC produced high levels of antigen-specific IgG antibody and *in vitro* T cell reactivity when re-challenged with soluble antigen, while freshly isolated DC showed poor APC activity *in vivo*. Moreover, analysis of IgG subclass production indicated a tendency for fresh DC to weakly prime for T_H2-dependent subclasses (IgG1, IgG2a), while GM-CSF-exposed DC primed strongly for both T_H1- and T_H2-dependent IgG subclasses (Table 1). Thus it appears that resident lung DC are able to efficiently acquire soluble antigen but remain poor inducers of primary antigen-specific immunity, inducing low-level, T_H2-biased responses which, we would postulate, under normal conditions act to protect the lung from locally activated and potentially damaging T_H1-dependent immune reactions. *In vitro* exposure to GM-CSF, however, markedly upregulated the capacity of these cells to prime for both T_H1 and T_H2-dependent responses, mimicking the functional maturation of DC that occurs *in vivo* prior to migration to secondary lymphoid organs (Steinman 1991).

Table 1. *In vivo* IgG subclass induction by fresh and GM-CSF-exposed lung DC*

	IgG subclass (μg/ml)		
Type of lung DC	IgG1	IgG2a	IgG2b
Fresh	7.2	7.1	0.08
GM-CSF-exposed	132	419	122

*1×10^5 purified rat lung DCs were pulsed with 500 μg/ml OVA and injected i.v. into syngeneic recipients after 90 min (fresh) or after overnight culture in GM-CSF. After 5 days, the animals were re-challenged with OVA i.v. and 15 days later serum OVA-specific, T_H1 (IgG2b) and T_H2 (IgG1, 2a)-dependent IgG subclass levels determined by ELISA.

Regulation of Lung DC Function

Regulation of the functional phenotype of lung and airway DC is a potentially important issue in relation to the pathogenesis of respiratory inflammatory diseases. The limited data available on cytokine modulation of *in vitro* human lung DC functions are consistent with that reported in animal systems, in particular with respect to the effects of GM-CSF, IL-4, IL-10 and TGF-β (Nicod *et al.*, 1995; van Haarst *et al.*, 1996). In addition, *in situ* cytohybridization studies have demonstrated colocalization of $CD1a^+$ DC and intraepithelial GM-CSF production, in both normal lung tissue and lung cancers (Tazi *et al.*, 1993), arguing for an important role for this cytokine in the maintenance of local DC population density in the respiratory tract.

Overexpression of T_H2-type cytokines and associated IgE production have been strongly implicated in the pathogenesis of allergic airway responses. Given their ability to activate naive T cells, DC are likely to play a key role in regulating the balance between T_H1- and T_H2-mediated immune reactions, although their exact role in this process is still unclear. Activation of T_H1 versus T_H2 responses by DC is likely to be dependent on several factors, including the expression of appropriate costimulatory molecules and production of T cell-activating cytokines. For naive T cell activation, expression of the B7 family of costimulatory molecules (B7-1 (CD80) and B7-2 (CD86)) has been shown to be critical for full T cell activation and IL-2 production (Schwartz, 1992). Lung DC have been shown to express both CD80 and CD86 (Masten *et al.*, 1997) and blocking the function of these molecules, particularly CD86, *in vivo* has been shown to inhibit eosinophil infiltration, IgE production and T_H2-cytokine production in response to airway allergen challenge (Tsuyuki *et al.*, 1997).

In terms of cytokine production, IL-12 is a potent promotor of T_H1-mediated immunity and inhibition of the production of IL-12 by DC has been implicated in promoting T_H2-dominated responses (Macatonia *et al.*, 1995). An important IL-12 inhibitor appears to be IL-10: pretreatment with this cytokine inhibited IL-12 production and promoted T_H2 responses induced by mouse splenic DC (De Smedt *et al.*, 1997), while for the lung IL-10 inhibited the upregulation of MHC class I and II on human lung DC and the ability of these cells to activate IFN-α and IFN-β production by allogeneic T cells (Nicod *et al.*, 1995). Thus, production of IL-12 by lung DC may play an important role in switching from T_H2-dominant (allergic) to T_H1-dominant (tolerant) responses to inhaled antigens.

In situ, DC function within the lung environment has been shown to be regulated by locally produced factors. Extensive studies in the rat have shown that PAM are potent inhibitors of lung DC function. *In vitro* coculture of lung DC with PAM across semipermeable membranes demonstrated a soluble factor that inhibited the APC activity and GM-CSF responsiveness of lung DC and identified this factor as nitric oxide (NO), as shown by the ability to inhibit the suppressive activity of PAM by *N*-monomethyl arginine, a competitive inhibitor of NO production (Holt *et al.*, 1993). Separate studies have also implicated TGF-β, prostaglandins, and direct cell–cell contact in the suppression of lung DC activity by bronchoalveolar cells (Lipscomb *et al.*, 1993). Furthermore, selective depletion of PAM *in vivo* markedly increased the APC activity of lung DC (Thepen *et al.*, 1992) and together these studies support the conclusion that the bronchoalveolar environment acts *in vivo* to regulate lung DC function under normal circumstances.

POPULATION DYNAMICS

DC are believed to arise from precursors in the peripheral circulation, and are recruited into tissues, via as yet undefined mechanisms, to replace mature resident DC which migrate principally to central lymphoid organs to complete their life cycle as interdigitating cells. The latter phase of this trafficking process has been formally demonstrated in the rat model for DC populations both in the airway mucosa (McWilliam *et al.*, 1994) and the lung parenchyma (Xia *et al.*, 1995). DC populations in quiescent peripheral tissues such as skin (Chen *et al.*, 1986) and muscle (Leszczynski *et al.*, 1985) turn over relatively slowly, exhibiting half-lives up to 30 days. However, as detailed below, respiratory tract DC appear considerably more dynamic, reflecting their important role in antigen surveillance at these mucosal surfaces in direct contact with the outside environment.

Turnover

The origin and turnover of respiratory tract DC have been studied in normal rats employing a radiation chimera model (Holt *et al.*, 1994). In this system, the supply of precursor DC from bone marrow is interrupted by X-irradiation of animals, with lead shielding the thoracic cavity to prevent local tissue damage, followed by transplantation of congenic bone marrow; host/donor DC can be discriminated in frozen tissue sections via appropriate pairs of monoclonal antibodies. By following the rate of decline in resident (host) DC numbers post-irradiation and pre-engraftment of congenic bone marrow, and the subsequent rate of replenishment of the tissue population with donor DC, a close approximation of population half-life can be estimated. These studies indicated that the steady-state half-life of airway intraepithelial DC is 2–3 days (Holt *et al.*, 1994). These rapid kinetics at the periphery are rivalled only by DC populations in the gut wall, the half-life of which has been estimated at 3 days (Fossum, 1989).

Within the same animals, half-lives of 7–10 and 21 days were estimated for lung parenchymal and skin DC, respectively (Holt *et al.*, 1994). The differences between DC turnover times at different levels of the respiratory tree mirror variations in the respective intensity of local antigenic and irritant stimulation, as the majority of inhaled particulates impact on the epithelium of the conducting airways and do not penetrate deep into the lung.

Despite these extremely rapid steady-state kinetics, the airway mucosal DC population is capable of further upregulation in response to both acute and chronic inflammatory stimulation. The most profound responses have been documented following challenge of rats with aerosols containing bacterial lipopolysaccharide (Schon-Hegrad *et al.*, 1991) or heat-killed bacteria (McWilliam *et al.*, 1994); in these models, DC influx occurs within 20 min of cessation of challenge (equivalent to neutrophils), and peaks within 2 h, at which time local airway intraepithelial DC numbers are up to 2.5 times baseline levels. The DC population remains at high levels for a further 24–48 h, prior to migration to regional lymph nodes (McWilliam *et al.*, 1994).

Similar 'inflammatory' DC responses have been observed following live virus infection of the tracheal epithelium (McWilliam *et al.*, 1996; McWilliam *et al.*, 1997), commencing concomitantly with the first expression of viral nucleoprotein within infected airway epithelial cells (McWilliam *et al.*, 1997), and also within 2–6 h of challenge of immune animals with an aerosol containing a soluble recall antigen (McWilliam *et al.*, 1997).

These findings are consistent with an essential surveillance role for DC in the acute airway mucosal response to all forms of exogenous challenge, and we hypothesize that they provide the link between the innate and adaptive arms of the immune system.

Chemotaxis

Recent studies have also provided insight into the mechanism(s) of recruitment of these cells. It is evident that they respond to a wide range of chemokines from the C-C family, but are unresponsive to C-X-C chemokines; in addition, they respond to the microbial peptide FMLP and (in particular) to complement cleavage products (McWilliam *et al.*, 1997).

It is also clear that the airway DC population upregulates in response to low-level chronic inflammatory challenge. Increases in density and surface expression of function-associated molecules have been observed on airway DC in rats exposed to dusts containing the chemical irritants abietic and pleicatic acids (Schon-Hegrad *et al.*, 1991), and in human atopics exposed to airborne environmental allergens (Godthelp *et al.*, 1996; Möller *et al.*, 1996; Tunon-de-lara *et al.*, 1996).

Steroid Modulation

It has been hypothesized (Holt, 1993; Semper and Hartley, 1996), but is as yet unproven, that *in situ* upregulation of the APC functions of these airway DC in chronically stimulated atopics may be an essential part of the pathogenesis of atopic asthma. In this context it is relevant to note the effects of topical and systemic anti-inflammatory steroids on these airway DC. Studies in the rat indicate that these drugs are capable of reducing steady-state DC numbers, and can also prevent their recruitment during acute implementation (Nelson *et al.*, 1995).

A recent study also suggests that inhaled steroids may control the expansion of the airway mucosal DC population which occurs in allergen-exposed atopic asthmatics (Möller *et al.*, 1996). However, experiments involving *in vitro* exposure of rat DC to high levels of dexamethasone demonstrate that steroids may not necessarily provide full protection against the potentially pro-inflammatory effects of upregulation of DC functions in the asthmatic airway. These studies demonstrated that GM-CSF confers partial 'protection' against the damping effects of steroids, conserving B7 and MHC class II expression and the capacity to present already processed antigen to T cells (Lim *et al.*, 1996; Holt and Thomas, 1997); however, steroid treated DC lose their capacity for uptake and processing of newly encountered antigen (Holt and Thomas, 1997). High level production of GM-CSF by airway epithelial cells is a consistent feature of atopic asthma (Poston *et al.*, 1992), and this may be a factor which limits the overall effectiveness of inhaled steroids in ameliorating immunoinflammatory airway tissue damage in this disease.

ONTOGENY

The ontogeny of lung and airway DC has been studied in detail only in the rat. In this species, cells expressing MHC class II (Ia) antigen are infrequent at birth, in marked contrast to the dense networks of Ia^{high} cells characteristic of the adult lung and airway mucosa of adults. Studies from our laboratory indicate that, at birth, the airway epithelium contains a sparse network of Ia^{low} DC precursors, which expand progressively in number until weaning (Nelson *et al.*, 1994). Contemporaneously, Ia expression on individual cells progressively upregulates, also approximating adult-equivalent levels by weaning (Nelson *et al.*, 1994). However, a small subset maintains a low level of Ia expression into adulthood (Nelson and Holt, 1995).

Examination of the distribution and surface phenotype of DC at different levels of the developing respiratory tree has identified marked differences in the kinetics of this process. Notably, DC density and Ia expression within the nasal turbinates approximates adult levels by approximately 1 week after birth, whereas the populations in the conducting airways and particularly within the lung parenchyma, develop much more slowly (Nelson *et al.*, 1994). This inverse relationship between depth within the respiratory tract and kinetics of postnatal maturation suggests that the process is driven by environmental stimuli present within inspired air. This suggestion is consistent with earlier findings on the role of airborne particulates (including those in bedding and animal cages) in upregulating numbers and Ia expression of adult airway DC (Schon-Hegrad *et al.*, 1991). It is also noteworthy that the developmental process can be stimulated by administration of the pro-inflammatory cytokine IFN-γ and slowed by repeated exposure to anti-inflammatory topical steroids (Nelson *et al.*, 1994).

During infancy, the functional capacity of respiratory tract DC also appears deficient relative to that of adults. In particular, their capacity to upregulate *in vitro* Ia expression and APC activity in response to GM-CSF, and their *in situ* Ia expression in response to intravenous administration of IFN-γ, remains low (Nelson and Holt, 1995). In addition, the capacity of this population for rapid local expansion in the face of microbial challenge, a hallmark of their adult counterparts (McWilliam *et al.*, 1994), does not attain adult equivalence until after 5 weeks of age (Nelson and Holt, 1995).

Parallel studies on epidermal Langerhans cells in the same animals indicate that the maturation of this network occurs with the first 7–10 days of postnatal life (Nelson *et al.*, 1994). Given that the epidermal and respiratory tract DC arise from a common precursor in peripheral blood, it appears likely that the slower maturation kinetics observed with the respiratory tract population may be secondary to local production of factor(s) that actively inhibit DC function. A possible candidate is TGF-β, which is produced at high levels in remodelling epithelial tissues such as those of the infant airways.

The relatively slow postnatal maturation of the respiratory tract DC networks may have significant implications in relation to immunological homeostasis during early life. In particular, this may be the basis for the heightened susceptibility of infants to respiratory infections (e.g. Wilson, 1986), and also to allergic sensitization to airborne environmental allergens, a process which may normally be downregulated via immune deviation mechanisms controlled by respiratory tract DC (Holt, 1996).

THE ROLE OF DENDRITIC CELLS IN INFLAMMATION AND INFECTION

Considering what is known regarding the functions of DC, very little work has been done on how DC function during inflammatory and infectious processes, particularly within the respiratory tract. This has been redressed somewhat by recent work highlighting the importance of DC in infections such as measles (Fugier-Vivier *et al.*, 1997; Grosjean *et al.*, 1997; Snorr *et al.*, 1997) and cytomegalovirus infections (Söderberg-Nauclér *et al.*, 1997).

Rat

Previous work from our laboratory has begun to examine the contribution of airway DC to inflammatory responses, in particular and in the first instance from the perspective of the epithelial DC population as a whole (McWilliam *et al.*, 1995a,b). Initial work involved normal rats exposed to an aerosol of heat-killed *Moraxella catarrhalis* bacteria, which was chosen as a result of its clinical association with acute purulent tracheitis in children and hence its ability to induce a rapid inflammatory response (McWilliam *et al.*, 1994). Using this model, it was apparent that one of the earliest detectable cellular changes within the inflamed tracheal mucosa is the recruitment of small, round, MHC class II-positive, putative DC precursors into the epithelium. These cells were detectable shortly before the influx of neutrophils, and while the inflammatory neutrophils pass through the epithelium and enter the lumen of the airway (presumably in response to chemotactic signals generated by macrophages), the DC remain within the epithelium. DC numbers within the epithelium reached a maximum within 1 h after exposure, numbers ultimately exceeding 3 times the steady state population. In contrast to neutrophil numbers, which remained high for approximately 8 h, DC numbers remained elevated for over 24 h. During this time the DC continued to differentiate morphologically into the typically dendritiform cells found in the steady state. The signal which induces this differentiation is unknown but is presumably derived from the local environment. Within 48 h after exposure it was possible to detect a 200% increase in the number of DC within the draining lymph nodes, reflecting the movement of DC from surface epithelium to T cell-rich lymph nodes.

In a series of related studies (McWilliam *et al.*, 1996) a number of different inflammatory stimuli were examined for their capacity to alter airway DC numbers. These stimuli included viral infection (Sendai) (McWilliam *et al.*, 1997), infection with a live bacterium (*Bordetella pertussis*), and a soluble recall antigen (ovalbumin) delivered by aerosol. The nature of the cellular influx generated within the airway epithelium was examined in detail in each of these models. The cellular influx was quite separate and distinct in each system; i.e. restricted to neutrophils in the *Moraxella* model; T cells plus eosinophils in the ovalbumin model; a mixed response comprising neutrophils, T cells, and NK cells in the Sendai model (Fig. 4). Despite the differing cellular profile associated with each inflammatory model, the common factor was the influx of DC, which in each case represented the first cell to appear within the airway epithelium. If recruitment of DC into the mucosa is a universal feature of the inflammatory response in these areas, this then suggests that the rapid amplification of antigen surveillance mechanisms at challenge sites may be an integral part of the innate immune response at mucosal surfaces, and hence may represent a form of 'early warning system' to signal the

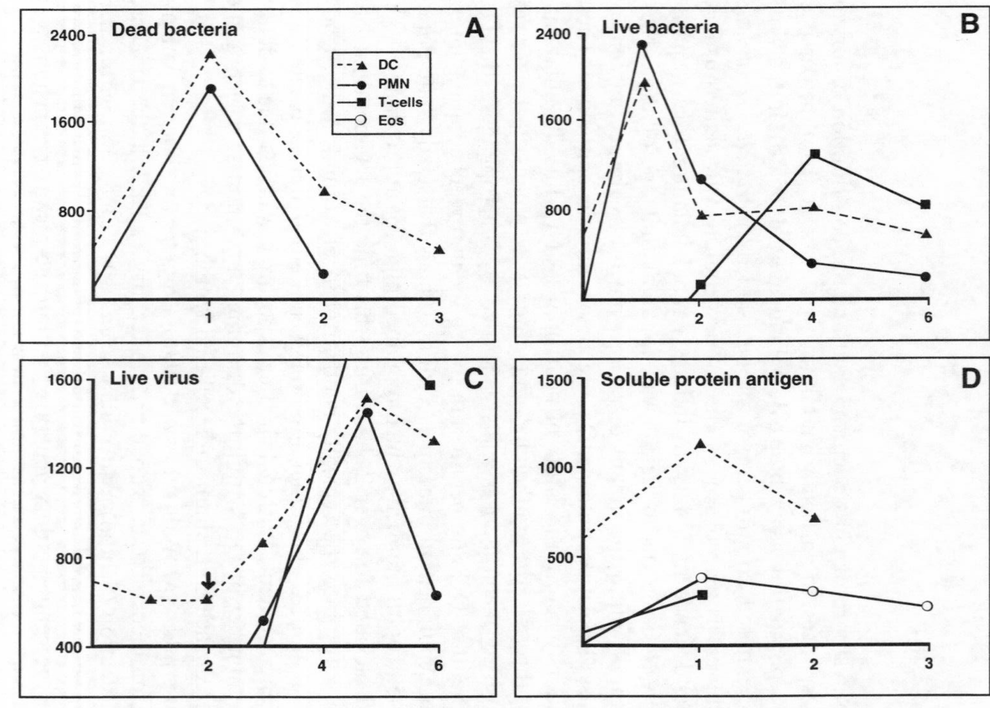

Fig. 4. Quantitative cellular responses within tracheal epithelium during inflammatory responses. (A) Inhalation of aerosolized heat-killed *Moraxella catarrhalis* produced an acute inflammatory reaction in which $Ox6^+$ DC and $RP3^+$ neutrophils were the only inflammatory cell type detected in the epithelium. (B) Live *Bordetella pertussis* organisms inoculated intratracheally resulted in an influx of $Ox6^+$ DC, $RP3^+$ neutrophils and $R73^+$ (rat TcR β) T cells. (C) Intranasal Sendai virus initiated a cellular response which commenced with an $Ox6^+$ DC influx shortly after the earliest detection of intraepithelial Sendai virus nucleoprotein immunostaining at day 2 and shortly before changes could be detected in other cell types. (D) Following i.p. priming with ovalbumin and $Al(OH)_6$, animals were challenged 14 days later with an aerosol of ovalbumin and cellular changes within the epithelium were measured. In this instance, $Ox6^+$ DC, endogenous peroxidase-positive eosinophils, and $R73^+$ T cells were detected.

adaptive or cognate arm of the immune system to incoming pathogens (McWilliam *et al.*, 1996).

In general we find very few DC within the lavage fluid obtained during these experiments and this must suggest that there are specific mechanisms in place to prevent egress of the DC into the alveolar space. Other studies (Havenith *et al.*, 1992) have, however, shown that in certain inflammatory situations such as BCG infection there is a 25-fold increase in the number of DC within the alveolar space, although in these systems the DC never comprise more than 2% of the overall cellular influx.

Human

There is increasing interest in the acute and chronic effects of local inflammation on human respiratory tract DC populations, given the potential contribution of these cells to local disease processes (Holt, 1993; Semper and Hartley, 1996).

The initial evidence for upregulation of lung and airway DC in response to chronic inflammatory stimuli came from comparative studies in smokers and non-smokers. Increased numbers of DC have been reported in smokers in bronchoalveolar lavage fluids (Casolaro *et al.*, 1988), and also in the airway mucosa (Soler *et al.*, 1989); additionally, smoking was associated with upregulation of CD1a expression or concomitant loss of CD1c (Soler *et al.*, 1989).

It is also evident that airway mucosal DC populations increase in number, and display changes in surface phenotype, as a consequence of local allergic reactions. In particular, nasal mucosal $CD1^+$ DC increase in grass pollen allergic subjects during the pollen season (Fokkens *et al.*, 1989) and following controlled allergen challenge (Godthelp *et al.*, 1996). In the latter study, surface IgE^+ DC also appeared in the tissue after challenge (Godthelp *et al.*, 1996), a finding consistent with a recent report indicating expression of $Fc\varepsilon R1$-α on the surface of airway mucosal DC in atopic asthmatics (Tunon-de-lara *et al.*, 1996).

The numbers of DC present in the airway mucosa of atopic asthmatics is also increased significantly over normal controls (Möller *et al.*, 1996; Tunon-de-lara *et al.*, 1996). As noted in earlier studies in experimental animals, treatment with topical steroids markedly suppresses the inflammation-induced upregulation of the airway mucosal DC network (Möller *et al.*, 1996).

REFERENCES

Casolaro, M.A., Bernaudin, J.F., Saltini, C., Ferrans, V.J. and Crystal, R.G. (1988). Accumulation of Langerhans' cells on the epithelial surface of the lower respiratory tract in normal subjects in association with cigarette smoking. *Am. Rev. Respir. Dis.* **137**, 406–411.

Chen, H.-D., Ma, C., Yuan, J.-T., Wang, Y.-K. and Silvers, W.K. (1986). Occurrence of donor Langerhans cells in mouse and rat chimeraes and their replacement in skin grafts. *J. Invest. Dermatol.* **86**, 630–633.

De Smedt, T., Van Mechelen, M., De Becker, G., Urbain, J., Leo, O. and Moser, M. (1997). Effect of interleukin-10 on dendritic cell maturation and function. *Eur. J. Immunol.* **27**, 1229–1235.

Fokkens, W.J., Vroom, T.M., Rijntjes, E. and Mulder, P.G. (1989). Fluctuation of the number of CD-1(T6)-positive dendritic cells, presumably Langerhans cells, in the nasal mucosa of patients with an isolated grass-pollen allergy before, during, and after the grass-pollen season. *J. Allergy Clin. Immunol.* **84**, 39–43.

Fossum, S. (1989). Dendritic leukocytes: features of their *in vivo* physiology. *Res. Immunol.* **140**, 883–891.

Fugier-Vivier, I., Servet-Delprat, C., Rivailler, P., Rissoan, M.-C., Liu, Y.-J. and Rabourdin-Combe, C. (1997). Measles virus suppresses cell-mediated immunity by interfering with the survival and functions of dendritic and T cells. *J. Exp. Med.* **186**, 813–823.

Godthelp, T., Fokkens, W.J., Kleinjan, A., Holm, A.F., Mulder, P.G.H., Prens, E.P. and Rijntes, E. (1996). Antigen presenting cells in the nasal mucosa of patients with allergic rhinitis during allergen provocation. *Clin. Exp. Allergy* **26**, 677–688.

Gong, J.L., McCarthy, K.M., Telford, J. Tamatani, T., Miyasaka, M. and Schneeberger, E.E. (1992). Intraepithelial airway dendritic cells: a distinct subset of pulmonary dendritic cells obtained by microdissection. *J. Exp. Med.* **175**, 797–807.

Grosjean, I., Caux, C., Bella, C., Berger, I., Wild, F., Banchereau, J. and Kaiserlian, D. (1997). Measles virus infects human dendritic cells and blocks their allostimulatory properties for $CD4^+$ T cells. *J. Exp. Med.* **186**, 801–812.

Hammar, S., Bockus, D., Remington, F. and Bartha, M. (1986). The widespread distribution of Langerhans cells in pathologic tissues. *Hum. Pathol.* **17**, 894–905.

Havenith, C.E., Breedijk, A.J. and Hoefsmit, E.C. (1992). Effects of Bacillus Calmette-Guerin inoculation on numbers of dendritic cells in bronchoalveolar lavages of rats. *Immunobiology* **184**, 336–347.

Holt, P.G. (1993). Macrophage:dendritic cell interaction in regulation of the IgE response in asthma (Editorial). *Clin. Exp. Allergy* **23**, 4–6.

Holt, P.G. (1996). Primary allergic sensitisation to environmental antigens: perinatal T-cell priming as a determinant of responder phentotype in adulthood. *J. Exp. Med.* **183**, 1297–1301.

Holt, P.G. and Schon Hegrad, M.A. (1987). Localization of T cells, macrophages and dendritic cells in rat respiratory tract tissue: implications for immune function studies. *Immunology* **62**, 349-356.

Holt, P.G. and Thomas, J.A. (1997). Steroids inhibit uptake and/or processing but not presentation of antigen by airway dendritic cells. *Immunology* **91**, 145–150.

Holt, P.G., Degebrot, A., O'Leary, C., Krska, K. and Plozza, T. (1985). T cell activation by antigen-presenting cells from lung tissue digests: suppression by endogenous macrophages. *Clin. Exp. Immunol.* **62**, 586–593.

Holt, P.G., Schon-Hegrad, M.A. and Oliver, J. (1988). MHC class II antigen-bearing dendritic cells in pulmonary tissues of the rat: regulation of antigen presentation activity by endogenous macrophage populations. *J. Exp. Med.* **167**, 262–274.

Holt, P.G., Schon-Hegrad, M.A., Phillips, M.J. and McMenamin, P.G. (1989). Ia-positive dendritic cells form a tightly meshed network within the human airway epithelium. *Clin. Exp. Allergy* **19**, 597–601.

Holt, P.G., Schon-Hegrad, M.A., Oliver, J., Holt, B.J. and McMenamin, P.G. (1990). A contiguous network of dendritic antigen-presenting cells within the respiratory epithelium. *Int. Arch. Allergy Appl. Immunol.* **91**, 155–159.

Holt, P.G., Oliver, J., McMenamin, C. and Schon-Hegrad, M.A. (1992). Studies on the surface phenotype and functions of dendritic cells in parenchymal lung tissue of the rat. *Immunology* **75**, 582–587.

Holt, P.G., Oliver, J., Bilyk, N., McMenamin, C., McMenamin, P.G., Kraal, G. and Thepen, T. (1993). Downregulation of the antigen presenting cell function(s) of pulmonary dendritic cells in vivo by resident alveolar macrophages. *J. Exp. Med.* **177**, 397–407.

Holt, P.G., Haining, S., Nelson, D.J. and Sedgwick, J.D. (1994). Origin and steady-state turnover of class II MHC-bearing dendritic cells in the epithelium of the conducting airways. *J. Immunol.* **153**, 256–261.

Kradin, R.L., McCarthy, K.M., Xia, W.J., Lazarus, D. and Schneeberger, E.E. (1991). Accessory cells of the lung. I. Interferon-gamma increases Ia^+ dendritic cells in the lung without augmenting their accessory activities. *Am. J. Respir. Cell Mol. Biol.* **4**, 210–218.

Leszcynski, R., Renkonen, R. and Hayry, P. (1985). Turnover of dendritic cells in rat heart. *Scand J. Immunol.* **22**, 351–355.

Lim, T.K., Chen, G. H., McDonald, R.A. and Toews, G.B. (1996). Granulocyte-macrophage colony-stimulating factor overrides the immunosuppressive function of corticosteroids on rat pulmonary dendritic cells. *Stem Cells* **14**, 292–299.

Lipscomb, M.F., Pollard, A.M. and Yates, J.L. (1993). A role for TGF-beta in the suppression by murine bronchoalveolar cells of lung dendritic cell initiated immune responses. *Region Immun.* **5**, 151–157.

Macatonia, S.E., Hosken, N.A., Litton, M., Vieira, P., Hsieh, C.S., Culpepper, J.A., Wysocka, M., Trinchieri, G., Murphy, K.M. and O'Garra, A. (1995). Dendritic cells produce IL-12 and direct the development of Th1 cells from naive $CD4^+$ T cells. *J. Immunol.* **154**, 5071–5079.

MacLean, J.A., Xia, W., Pinto, C.E., Zhao, L., Liu, H.-W. and Kradin, R.L. (1996). Sequestration of inhaled particulate antigens by lung phagocytes. *Am. J. Pathol.* **148**, 657–666.

Masten, B.J., Yates, J. L., Pollard Koga, A.M. and Lipscomb, M.F. (1997). Characterization of accessory molecules in murine lung dendritic cell function: roles for CD80, CD86, CD54, and CD40L. *Am. J. Respir. Cell. Mol. Biol.* **16**, 335–342.

McWilliam, A.S., Nelson, D., Thomas, J.A. and Holt, P.G. (1994). Rapid dendritic cell recruitment is a hallmark of the acute inflammatory response at mucosal surfaces. *J. Exp. Med. 179*, 1331–1336.

McWilliam, A.S., Bilyk, N. and Holt, P.G. (1995a). Macrophages and dendritic cell populations in the airways. In: *Asthma and Rhinitis* (eds W.W. Busse and S.T. Holgate). Blackwell Scientific, Oxford, pp. 474–490.

McWilliam, A.S., Nelson, D.J. and Holt, P.G. (1995b). The biology of airway dendritic cells. *Immunol. Cell Biol.* **73**, 405–413.

McWilliam, A.S., Napoli, S., Marsh, A.M., Pemper, F.L., Nelson, D.J., Pimm, C.L., Stumbles, P.A., Wells, T.N.C. and Holt, P.G. (1996). Dendritic cells are recruited into the airway epithelium during the inflammatory response to a broad spectrum of stimuli. *J. Exp. Med.* **184**, 2429–2432.

McWilliam, A.S, Marsh, A.M. and Holt, P.G. (1997). Inflammatory infiltration of the upper airway epithelium during Sendai virus infection: involvement of epithelial dendritic cells. *J. Virol.* **71**, 226–236.

Möller, G.M., Overbeek, S.E., Van Helden-Meeuwsen, C.G., Van Haarst, J.M.W., Prens, E.P., Mulder, P.G., Postma, D.S. and Hoogsteden, H.C. (1996). Increased numbers of dendritic cells in the bronchial mucosa of atopic asthmatic patients: downregulation by inhaled corticosteroids. *Clin. Exp. Allergy* **26**, 517–524.

Munro, C.S., Campbell, D.A., Du Bois, R.M., Mitchell, D.N., Cole, P.J. and Poulter, L.W. (1987). Dendritic cells in cutaneous, lymph node and pulmonary lesions of sarcoidosis. *Scand. J. Immunol.* **25**, 461–467.

Nelson, D.J. and Holt, P.G. (1995). Defective regional immunity in the respiratory tract of neonates is attributable to hyporesponsiveness of local dendritic cells to activation signals. *J Immunol.* **155**, 3517–3524.

Nelson, D.J., McMenamin, C., McWilliam, A.S., Brenan, M. and Holt, P.G. (1994). Development of the airway intraepithelial dendritic cell network in the rat from class II MHC (Ia) negative precursors: differential regulation of Ia expression at different levels of the respiratory tract. *J. Exp. Med.* **179**, 203–212.

Nelson, D.J., McWilliam, A.S., Haining, S. and Holt, P.G. (1995). Modulation of airway intraepithelial dendritic cells following exposure to steroids. *Am. J. Respir. Crit. Care Med.* **151**, 475–481.

Nicod, L.P. and El Habre, F. (1992). Adhesion molecules on human lung dendritic cells and their role for T-cell activation. *Am. J. Respir. Cell Mol. Biol.* **7**, 207–213.

Nicod, L.P., Lipscomb, M.F., Weissler, J.C., Lyons, C.R., Albertson, J. and Tocws, G.B. (1989). Mononuclear cells from human lung parenchyma support antigen-induced T lymphocyte proliferation. *J. Leukocyte Biol.* **45**, 336–344.

Nicod, L.P., Galve de Rochemonteix, B. and Dayer, J.M. (1990). Dissociation between allogeneic T cell stimulation and interleukin-1 or tumor necrosis factor production by human dendritic cells. *Am. J. Respir. Cell Mol. Biol.* **2**, 515–522.

Nicod, L.P., Habre, F.E., Dayer, J.-M. and Boehringer, N. (1995). Interleukin-10 decreases tumor necrosis factor α and β in alloreactions induced by human lung dendritic cells and macrophages. *Am. J. Respir. Cell Mol. Biol.* **13**, 83–90.

Pollard, A.M. and Lipscomb, M.F. (1990). Characterization of murine lung dendritic cells: similarities to Langerhans cells and thymic dendritic cells. *J. Exp. Med.* **172**, 159–167.

Poston, R.N., Chancz, P., Lacoste, J.Y., Litchfield, T., Lee, T.H. and Bousquet, J. (1992). Immunohistochemical characterisation of the cellular infiltration in asthmatic bronchi. *Am. Rev. Respir. Dis.* **145**, 918–921.

Richard, S., Barbey, S., Pfister, A., Scheinmann, P., Jaubert, F. and Nezelof, C. (1987). Demonstration of Langerhans cells in the human bronchial epithelium. *C.R. Acad. Sci. III* **305**, 35–39.

Sallusto, F., Cella, M., Danieli, C. and Lanzavecchia, A. (1995). Dendritic cells use macropinocytosis and the mannose receptor to concentrate macromolecules in the major histocompatibility complex class II compartment: downregulation by cytokines and bacterial products. *J. Exp. Med.* **182**, 389–400.

Schon-Hegrad, M.A., Oliver, J., McMenamin, P.G. and Holt, P.G. (1991). Studies on the density, distribution, and surface phenotype of intraepithelial class II major histocompatibility complex antigen (Ia)-bearing dendritic cells (DC) in the conducting airways. *J. Exp. Med.* **173**, 1345–1356.

Schwartz, R. (1992). Costimulation of T lymphocytes: the role of CD28, CTLA-4 and B7/BB1 in interleukin-2 production and immunotherapy. *Cell.* **71**, 1065–1068.

Semper, A.E. and Hartley, J.A. (1996). Dendritic cells in the lung: what is their relevance to asthma? *Clin. Exp. Allergy* **26**, 485–490.

Sertl, K., Takemura, T., Tschachler, E., Ferrans, V.J., Kaliner, M.A. and Shevach, E.M. (1986). Dendritic cells with antigen-presenting capability reside in airway epithelium, lung parenchyma, and visceral pleura. *J. Exp. Med.* **163**, 436–451.

Simecka, J.W, Davis, J.K. and Cassell, G.H. (1986). Distribution of Ia antigens and T lymphocyte subpopulations in rat lungs. *Immunology* **57**, 93–98.

Snorr, J.-J., Xanthakos, S., Keikavoussi, P., Kämpgen, E., Ter Muelen, V. and Schneider-Schaulies, S. (1997). Induction of maturation of human blood dendritic cell precursors by measles virus is associated with immunosuppression. *Proc. Natl Acad. Sci. USA.* **94**, 5326–5331.

Söderberg-Nauclér, C., Fish, K.N. and Nelson, J.A. (1997). Reactivation of latent human cytomegalovirus by allogeneic stimulation of blood cells from healthy donors. *Cell* **91**, 119–126.

Soler, P., Chollet, S., Jacque, C., Fukuda, Y., Ferrans, V.J. and Basset, F. (1985). Immunocytochemical characterization of pulmonary histiocytosis X cells in lung biopsies. *Am. J. Pathol.* **118**, 439–451.

Soler, P., Moreau, A., Basset, F. and Hance, A.J. (1989). Cigarette smoking-induced changes in the number and differentiated state of pulmonary dendritic cells/Langerhans cells. *Am. Rev. Respir. Dis.* **139**, 1112–1117.

Steinman, R.M. (1991). The dendritic cell system and its role in immunogenicity. *Annu. Rev. Immunol.* **9**, 271–296.

Steinman, R.M. and Swanson, J. (1995). The endocytic activity of dendritic cells. *J. Exp. Med.* **182**, 283–288.

Tazi, A., Bouchonnet, F., Grandsaigne, M., Boumsell, L., Hance, A.J. and Soler, P. (1993). Evidence that granulocyte macrophage-colony-stimulating factor regulates the distribution and differentiated state of dendritic cells/Langerhans cells in human lung and lung cancers. *J. Clin. Invest.* **91**, 566–576.

Thepen, T., McMenamin, C., Girn, B., Kraal, G. and Holt, P.G. (1992). Regulation of IgE production in presensitized animals: in vivo elimination of alveolar macrophages preferentially increases IgE responses to inhaled allergen. *Clin. Exp. Allergy* **22**, 1107–1114.

Tsuyuki, S., Tsuyuki, J., Einsle, K., Kopf, M. and Coyle, A.J. (1997). Costimulation through B7-2 (CD86) is required for the induction of a lung mucosal T helper cell 2 (TH2) immune response and altered airway responsiveness. *J. Exp. Med.* **185**, 1671–1679.

Tunon-de-lara, J.M., Redington, A.E., Bradding, P., Church, M.K., Hartley, J.A., Semper, A.E. and Holgate, S.T. (1996). Dendritic cells in normal and asthmatic airways: expression of the α subunit of the high affinity immunoglobulin E receptor (FcεRI-α). *Clin. Exp. Allergy* **26**, 648–655.

van Haarst, J.M.W., Hoogsteden, H.C., de Wit, H.J., Verhoeven, G.T., Havenith, C.E. and Drexhage, H.A. (1994). Dendritic cells and their precursors isolated from human bronchoalveolar lavage: immunocytologic and functional properties. *Am. J. Respir. Cell Mol. Biol.* **11**, 344–350.

van Haarst, J.M.W., Verhoeven, G.T., de Wit, H.J., Hoogsteden, H.C., Debets, R. and Drexhage, H.A. (1996). CD1a$^+$ and CD1a$^-$ accessory cells from human bronchoalveolar lavage differ in allostimulatory potential and cytokine production. *Am. J. Respir. Cell Mol. Biol.* **15**, 752–759.

van Nieuwkerk, E.B.J., Kamperdijk, E.W.A., Verdaasdonk, M.A.M., van der Baan, S. and Hoefsmit, E.C.M. (1991). Langerhans cells in the respiratory epithelium of the human adenoid. *Eur. J. Cell Biol.* **54**, 182–186.

Webber, D., Tron, V., Askin, F. and Churg, A. (1985). S-100 staining in the diagnosis of eosinophilic granuloma of lung. *Am. J. Clin. Pathol.* **84**, 447–453.

Wilson, C.B. (1986). Immunologic basis for increased susceptibility of the neonate to infection. *J. Pediatr.* **108**, 1–12.

Xia, W., Pinto, C.E. and Kradin, R.L. (1995). The antigen-presenting activities of Ia$^+$ dendritic cells shift dynamically from lung to lymph node after an airway challenge. *J. Exp. Med.* **181**, 1275–1283.

CHAPTER 9
Intestinal Dendritic Cells

G. Gordon MacPherson[1] and LiMing Liu[2]
[1]Sir William Dunn School of Pathology, University of Oxford, UK; [2]Center for Neurologic Diseases, Brigham and Women's Hospital, Harvard Medical School, Boston, Massachusetts, USA

INTRODUCTION

Intestinal Immune Responses

The gastrointestinal tract faces a continual immunological onslaught from antigens (Ag) in food, commensal bacteria, and on occasion, potentially pathogenic bacteria, viruses, parasites, and perhaps prions. Yet, for the most part, we are totally unaware of the immune responses that are occurring all the time in the gut. In other sites such responses would inevitably lead to local inflammation, but in the gut this outcome is happily a rare event. It does of course occur at times and many chronic inflammatory bowel diseases probably represent an inappropriate response to foreign antigens or self-antigens.

Part of the reason that we are unaware of intestinal immune responses is that they are often dichotomous, in that oral antigens can induce a protective local secretory IgA response but animals (and perhaps humans) may be hyporesponsive to the same antigens when challenged systemically following oral administration (oral tolerance). The cellular and molecular mechanisms underlying oral tolerance are complex and controversial (reviewed in Kagnoff, 1996; Garside and Mowat, 1997) and the roles of antigen presenting cells (APC) in the induction of oral tolerance are obscure. Immune responses to antigens in the intestinal lumen are initiated at two or possibly three sites: Peyer's patches (PP), mesenteric lymph nodes (MLN), and the lamina propria of intestinal villi (LP) (see Brandtzaeg, 1996; Kohne *et al.*, 1996; Heel *et al.*, 1997 for reviews of intestinal immunity). PP are the sites at which IgA responses are initiated; B cells activated in PP may undergo further differentiation in MLN and effector B cells released into the blood migrate to the lamina propria of mucosal tissues. Whether immune responses can be initiated in the lamina propria is controversial. Dendritic cells (DC) are certainly present and it is claimed they can activate naive T cells (Clarke *et al.*, 1991; Harper *et al.*, 1996), but the frequency of naive T cells in the LP is low, with most $CD4^+$ T cells expressing memory/activation markers (Zeitz *et al.*, 1990 ; Stokes *et al.*, 1996). It is possible that DC in the LP have two roles, the acquisition of enteric antigen and its

Dendritic Cells: Biology and Clinical Applications
ISBN 0-12-455860-7

transport to draining nodes, and the restimulation of memory T cells in the LP itself; this would correlate with the memory phenotype seen in LP $CD4^+$ T cells.

Dendritic Cells in the Gut

As in almost all tissues of the body, the gut wall and its associated lymphoid structures contain populations of DC. Study of these DC is, however, at present very limited, largely owing to the difficulty of extracting DC from tissues and, in humans, the difficulty of obtaining intestinal tissues other than the colon and rectum. Considerably more is known about the properties of DC in PP and MLN than of those in LP, and in humans, information is only available in any detail about colonic DC. In this chapter we consider DC present in PP, LP and MLN in terms of their phenotypes, properties, and functions in the initiation and regulation of immune responses to enteric antigens. Inevitably, we shall raise more questions than we have answers, but perhaps we shall stimulate increased efforts to unravel the functions of DC in these critical sites.

INTESTINAL DENDRITIC CELLS

Morphological Studies

Nonlymphoid Tissues

Dendritic cells, identified by morphological and immunocytochemical criteria, have been described in all regions of the gut that have been examined. There are, however, difficulties with the identification of DC by these criteria alone. *In situ*, DC can be tentatively identified by their irregular morphology in conjunction with immunostaining for MHC class II and other surface markers that are more or less specific for DC (it should be noted that there do not seem to be any monoclonal antibodies (mAb) that recognize all DC and only DC).

Expression of MHC class II and an irregular morphology are not, however, sufficient for DC identification. This is exemplified by our studies of LP DC in the rat. Immunostaining of cryosections shows that the LP contains a population of large cells that are irregular and MHC class II^+. Only a proportion of these are also MRC $OX62^+$ (OX62 recognizes an antigen, probably an integrin, that is present on all DC in lymph draining the small intestine; Brenan and Puklavec, 1992). When fluorescent antigen or latex particles are injected intraintestinally, some MHC class II^+ cells in the LP accumulate the marker, but double labelling shows that such cells are MRC $OX62^-$. These cells might represent immature DC in 'antigen capture mode', but we have never seen DC carrying the markers in intestinal pseudo-afferent lymph from such animals, suggesting strongly that the cells that accumulate the marker do not leave the LP and are thus very unlikely to be DC (L.M. Liu and G.G. MacPherson, unpublished observations). There may be alternative explanations for these observations, but the point is that identification of DC *in situ* is difficult and may be unreliable. The identification of DC in pathological conditions is even more difficult; in many inflammatory states, macrophages will be strongly MHC class II^+ and display irregular outlines.

Given these provisos, DC appear to relatively abundant in the gut. The majority of DC lie in the LP underlying the epithelium, but in the small intestine of the rat, lined by columnar epithelium, there is evidence for a population of DC that resides above the basement membrane, and there is also much evidence that DC below the basement membrane can extend processes up between epithelial cells (Maric *et al.*, 1996). It is not clear from these *in situ* studies whether phenotypic or functional differences exist between DC in different sites.

Peyer's Patches

Peyer's patches are the major portals by which antigen in the intestinal lumen is made available to the cells of the immune system. Antigen is transported across the epithelium by specialized epithelial cells, M cells, that possess relatively few microvilli and are capable of transcytosis of soluble molecules and particles. A number of pathogens have 'hi-jacked' this route to bypass the epithelial barrier (see Wolf and Bye, 1984; Gebert *et al.*, 1996 for reviews of M cells). DC have been described at two sites in PP, the T cell areas, in which DC are thought to correspond to interdigitating cells in lymph nodes, and in the subepithelial area underlying the dome. This is the region into which antigen is delivered by M cells, and it is an attractive hypothesis that DC in this area capture antigen and transport it to T areas for presentation to recirculating T cells. In the mouse, DC in the two sites differ in their expression of surface markers. Subdome DC are negative for NLDC145 and CD11c, whereas T area DC express both markers (Kelsall and Strober, 1996) (see below).

Isolation of DC from the Gut

Dendritic cells are a rare cell type in all tissues and their isolation is fraught with difficulties. Most techniques involve mincing the tissue, enzymatic digestion, differential adherence, and negative or positive selection. The yields are low (we routinely start with six or more whole intestines to prepare LP or PP DC; Liu and MacPherson, 1995a) and the proportion of DC that is recovered is unknown. The procedures used to isolate DC are associated with two major problems—they may be selective for subpopulations of DC and they may induce changes in the isolated DC that do not represent normal *in vivo* events. This is particularly true of procedures that involve overnight incubations at 37°C, as many studies have shown that such incubation induces changes analogous to maturation or differentiation, especially if cytokines are present in the incubation mixture.

An alternative approach to the study of intestinal DC has been in use in our laboratory for some years. Lymph DC are normally removed from the lymph in the first node they reach. Mesenteric lymphadenectomy in the rat, sheep and mouse (Pugh *et al.*, 1983; Rhodes, 1985; Mayrhofer *et al.*, 1986; Bujdoso *et al.*, 1989) has been used to remove this blockage to migration. After a period of weeks, the afferent and efferent lymphatics of the removed nodes join up, with the result that DC can be collected by cannulation of central lymphatics, in the rat thoracic duct. Such DC have recently left the intestine physiologically, can be collected in the cold, and can be concentrated by simple density gradient centrifugation with or without negative or positive selection. They are as close to a physiological population of DC as can be acquired at present. These L-DC are, however, difficult to collect in large numbers and represent DC at just one stage in their life history. In addition, we do not know whether these DC derive from the LP, PP or both. Nevertheless, their study has given a number of important insights into DC properties and functions.

Life History and Migratory Properties of Gut DC

Steady State

The ability of DC to act as APC depends on their migrating to the draining lymph nodes. We have studied the migration and turnover of DC in the rat small intestine (Pugh *et al.*, 1983). Dividing DC precursors in the bone marrow can be labelled by an intravenous (i.v.) injection of a DNA precursor, usually tritiated thymidine ([^{3}H]TdR) or bromodeoxyuridine (BrdU). As there is no evidence for significant DC division in the intestine, the minimal time taken for labelled DC to appear in pseudo-afferent intestinal lymph represents the time from the last division in the marrow and includes the time taken to traverse the intestine. Labelled DC appear in lymph within 48 h, with peak numbers arriving at 3–4 days. Thus DC spend a minimum of 48 h and a modal time of 3–4 days in the intestine before migrating to the nodes. We cannot accurately estimate the maximum time in the intestine because the rate of decline of labelled DC appearance in lymph is affected both by input into the gut of cells that were labelled early in their differentiation in marrow and by those that have spent longer periods in the gut. These data show that intestinal DC turn over much more rapidly than Langerhans cells (LC), but with similar kinetics to murine splenic DC (Steinman *et al.*, 1974).

In the respiratory tract of rats, a different approach, measuring the kinetics of DC reconstitution after depletion by corticosteroids or irradiation, suggests that the average half-life of DC is about 2 days (Holt *et al.*, 1994). Thus it appears that in the absence of any known stimulation, DC spend only short times in mucosae before migrating to draining nodes.

Stimulated Migration

A variety of nonspecific stimuli can affect DC migration dramatically, possibly acting via a final common pathway involving TNF-α and IL-1. Intravenous endotoxin induces a rapid increase in the numbers of DC migrating in rat intestinal lymph. This effect occurs within 6 h, peaks at 12–24 h, and is over by 48 h, resulting in an approximately 10-fold increase in the numbers of DC that can be collected over that period. The source of the migrating DC appears to be the LP, as at 24 h the numbers of OX62$^+$ cells in the LP were much reduced. It seems unlikely that the LPS was acting directly on DC, but we suspect that TNF-α is involved because an anti-TNF Ab markedly inhibited the effects of LPS. The DC released following LPS administration do not differ from steady-state DC in mixed leukocyte reaction (MLR) stimulation but other properties were not investigated (MacPherson *et al.*, 1995). In other models (murine heart and kidney; Roake *et al.*,1995), IL-1 is also involved in stimulating DC migration.

In addition to inducing migration of DC from mucosae, inflammatory stimuli also cause a rapid influx of DC and/or DC precursors. Thus Holt's group has shown that large numbers of DC precursors enter respiratory epithelium within hours of challenge with bacterial, viral, or protein antigen. These cells spend up to 48 h in the epithelium and then migrate to the draining nodes (McWilliam *et al.*, 1996). Interestingly, similar stimuli did not result in DC accumulation in the peritoneal cavity or epidermis.

Recent studies in the rat (Matsuno *et al.*, 1996; Kudo *et al.*, 1997) have identified a novel migratory pathway for DC. Following i.v. particle administration, DC endocytose particles within the blood (probably in hepatic sinusoids), and then translocate into hepatic lymph, ending up in the hepatic/coeliac nodes. This route has important implications for the understanding of the immune response to blood-borne pathogens.

Functional Properties of Isolated Gut DC

Lamina Propria and Peyer's Patch DC

Relatively few studies have examined the phenotypic and functional properties of DC isolated from the gut LP or PP. Pavli *et al.* (1990) isolated DC from murine PP and LP. They found that these cells resembled splenic DC in phenotype and function. We used similar approaches to isolate DC from rat LP and PP (Liu and MacPherson, 1995a). Yields were small and DC could not be enriched to more than 30–40% purity. DC freshly isolated expressed high levels of MHC class II and, in contrast to freshly isolated LC (Schuler and Steinman, 1985) and heart or kidney DC (Austyn *et al.*, 1994), gave intermediate levels of stimulation in a MLR compared to lymph DC. After overnight culture with GM-CSF, LP DC became as potent MLR stimulators as lymph DC (Liu and MacPherson, 1995a). APC have been isolated from human colon (Mahida *et al.*, 1988). These cells gave good stimulation in a MLR, but the authors considered that they had both macrophage and DC characteristics. In contrast, another study (Pavli *et al.*, 1993) showed that when macrophages and DC were separately isolated from human colon most MLR stimulation could be attributed to DC.

In a recent study (Ruedl *et al.*, 1996) it was shown that $CD11c^-$ PP DC were functionally immature in terms of T cell activation but were actively endocytic and could phagocytose latex particles. After culture with GM-CSF, TNF-α, or anti-CD40 mAb, the $CD11c^-$, $NLDC145^-$ DC expressed both markers, lost the ability to process native antigen, downregulated MHC class II and invariant chain synthesis, upregulated B7, and became potent stimulators of resting T cells, thus acquiring the properties of mature DC. It is suggested that the subdome DC migrate to T cell areas but there is no direct proof for this. This differentiation is similar to that described for LC in culture, but it is not known whether it represents normal maturation in the absence of inflammatory stimuli.

Lymph DC

Dendritic cells isolated from the thoracic duct lymph of mesenteric-lymphadenectomized rats have recently left the small intestine and represent DC actively involved in antigen transport (Pugh *et al.*, 1983; Liu and MacPherson, 1991; Liu and MacPherson, 1993). These cells appear to differ functionally from DC isolated either from peripheral tissues or from secondary lymphoid tissues. Thus they are fully mature in terms of MLR stimulation and their potency does not change for at least 72 h in culture but they retain the ability to process native antigen for the same period (Liu and MacPherson, 1995b). A partial explanation for these observations comes from recent experiments (Liu *et al.*, manuscripts submitted). We have shown that in rat intestinal lymph, DC subpopulations can be distinguished by their expression of CD4. $CD4^+$ DC are more effective APC for naive and sensitized T cells, survive better in culture, but do not lose the ability to process antigen in culture. CD4$^-$ DC are weak APC, contain phagolysosomes but do not express detectable FcR, survive poorly in culture, and in culture completely lose the ability to process native antigen while becoming as strong stimulators of a MLR as the CD4$^+$ cells. Thus functionally CD4$^-$ DC resemble LC whereas the CD4$^+$ DC do not. We do not know how these two populations relate to each other, but *in vivo* kinetic studies show that their life spans and turnover times are similar, suggesting that the CD4$^+$ DC are not precursors of CD4$^-$ cells. It is tempting to suggest that the CD4$^-$ DC, with their phagocytic past, are monocyte derived, but we have no direct evidence for this.

Uptake of Antigen by Gut DC

In order to stimulate an immune response, protein antigen needs to gain access to DC. The presence of DC and their processes within intestinal epithelia (Maric *et al.*, 1996) may facilitate this interaction, but at present it is not known whether these DC can migrate to central lymphoid tissues. Soluble macromolecules can enter subepithelial tissues via M cells in PP but can also gain access via intact epithelial surfaces (reviewed in Sanderson and Walker, 1993). Particulate antigens can similarly cross the epithelial barrier and can be found in PP and MLN. However the relative efficiency of uptake at the two sites and their relative importance in the induction of immune responses is unclear (see *Oral Tolerance*, 1996; Thomas *et al.*, 1996 for reviews).

Although mucosal DC are strategically placed to acquire antigen via mucosal surfaces, there is very little concrete evidence that they can do this, and even less that they do so with pathogenic organisms. We have shown that soluble antigen, given by gavage or intraintestinal injection, is acquired by DC in the intestinal wall, and that antigen-bearing DC appear in intestinal lymph within 6 h (Liu and MacPherson, 1991; Liu and MacPherson, 1993). We have not been able to demonstrate the presence of antigen directly, but DC from antigen-fed rats can stimulate sensitized T cells and, more importantly, can sensitize naive T cells following subcutaneous injection. It was important in these experiments to show that the injected DC were presenting antigen directly, and this was done by injecting parental strain antigen-bearing DC into an F1 recipient and showing that T cells were only sensitized to the MHC of the injected DC.

We could not determine from these experiments the origin of the antigen-bearing DC; they could have arisen from PP, LP or both. Recently, Kelsall and Strober (1996) have shown that CD11c$^+$ DC isolated from murine PP after feeding ovalbumin (OVA) are able to activate OVA-specific naive T cells *in vitro*. Thus, as expected, PP are clearly a route for delivery of antigen to mucosal DC, but a route via LP cannot be excluded.

In contrast to studies with soluble antigen, essentially nothing is known about the interaction of mucosal DC with particulate antigen or pathogens *in situ*. Mayrhofer *et al.* (1986) showed that in rats infected with *Salmonella typhimurium*, cells with DC characteristics in pseudo-afferent intestinal lymph contained *Salmonella* antigens. A preliminary report has shown that following infection of mice with *S. typhimurium* expressing green fluorescent protein, bacteria colocalize in PP with cells expressing DC characteristics (N418 expression, lack of macrophage markers) (S.A. Hopkins and J.P. Kraehenbuhl, 4th International Symposium on Dendritic Cells in Fundamental and Clinical Immunology, Venice, 1996).

Regulation of Immune Responses by Intestinal DC

Are DC Always Immunostimulatory?

All studies using isolated gut DC have shown that they are capable of activating naive or memory T cells. We have shown that oral antigen is acquired by DC in the intestinal wall and transported to mesenteric lymph nodes, and that these DC can activate naive T cells following adoptive transfer (Liu and MacPherson, 1993). Normally, however, oral antigen is tolerogenic and recent evidence suggests that even antigen targeted directly to DC may be tolerogenic (Finkelman *et al.*, 1996). It is an attractive hypothesis that under noninflamed 'nondangerous' conditions (Matzinger, 1994), DC transport antigen to lymph nodes, where it either may be ignored or may actively tolerize naive T cells, and that this may form part of normal immune regulation. It is suggested that only when DC are present in inflamed tissues do they receive the signals that are necessary for their 'activation'. The ability of DC to activate naive T cells following their isolation is explained because the procedures involved in their isolation are sufficient to deliver surrogate activation signals.

Now that it is becoming clear that different DC lineages exist, and that DC can be 'activated' in different ways, it is increasingly important to characterize different DC populations functionally. We are not aware of any experiments in which this has been done for DC activated *in vivo* and it is not known how the DC that accumulate in inflamed tissues relate to those that traffic through mucosae under steady-state conditions.

Role of DC in Modulation of Immune Responses in the Gut

Immune responses initiated in PP are characterized by activation of B cells to secrete IgA. Although it is clear that T cells are finally responsible for inducing B cells to switch from IgM to IgG, the local signals that determine the differentiation patterns of those T cells are still unclear, although a role for TGF-β has been suggested (Chen and Li, 1990; Kim and Kagnoff, 1990).

It is possible that DC may have a role in inducing the differentiation of T cells to a mucosal phenotype. In early studies (Spalding *et al.*, 1983) it was shown that cells with properties similar to those of splenic DC could be isolated from murine PP, and in further studies it was suggested that these DC could have important roles in determining the quality of immune responses initiated in PP. Thus, when mixtures of PP DC and T cells were isolated and added to sIgM$^+$ splenic B cells, polyclonal activation of the B cells led to IgA synthesis, whereas the use of splenic DC led only to IgM synthesis. It was suggested that it was the DC and not the T cells that were important in stimulating this isotype switch. Cebra's group (Schrader *et al.*, 1990) have shown that PP DC and splenic DC could both support IgA secretion by appropriately primed B cells.

Murine lamina propria (LP), PP, and splenic APC have been compared in terms of their ability to activate naive T cells *in vitro* (Harper *et al.*, 1996). Different patterns of cytokine secretion were induced by the different APC, with splenic cells inducing both T_H1 and T_H2 cytokines, PP DC inducing secretion of cytokines appropriate for the induction of IgA synthesis, but LP cells inducing only IFN-γ and TGF-β. However, as the APC populations contained only 1–2% DC but large numbers of T and B cells, it is difficult to be certain that the differences seen were due to the influence of the APC. Everson (1996) has evidence that suggests that cytokine secretion by mucosal DC may influence T cell activation. He showed that activation of T cells by mucosal DC induced a T_H2 pattern of cytokine secretion, whereas splenic DC induced T_H1 cytokines. Again, the mechanisms by which DC influence cytokine secretion by T cells are unknown. Little information is available on cytokine and chemokine secretion by mucosal DC, but it is an attractive hypothesis that they regulate B and T cell activation by a combination of cell surface and secreted molecules. The effects of TGF-β and other locally available factors on DC differentiation and function in mucosae are important areas for future research.

Recent work from Bancherau's group supports the concept that DC may have a direct role in isotype switching. They showed that polyclonal activation of 'naive', $sIgM^+$ human tonsillar B cells in the presence of CD40 ligand and blood-derived DC led to a skewing of the response towards IgA (Fayette *et al.*, 1997). The mechanisms by which DC influence B cell isotype switching are unknown but we have evidence that it may occur as a direct result of DC–B cell contact, prior to T cell involvement (M. Wykes, and G.G. MacPherson, manuscript submitted). This area of research is worthy of further exploration; the roles of DC and/or stromal cells in the generation of IgA switch and helper T cells, and in isotype switching in B cells, are quite obscure.

Intestinal DC and HIV

HIV is most often acquired through infection of mucosal surfaces and DC are strategically placed to encounter the virus, transport it to lymphoid tissues, and infect T cells. It is of course impossible to investigate the role of DC as HIV transporters in humans, but some important evidence has come from studies of SIV in rhesus macaques (Spira *et al.*, 1996). After intravaginal inoculation of SIV, viral DNA was detected by *in situ* PCR. Viral DNA was first detected in lamina propria cells with the characteristics of DC in both the vagina and the cervix. Within 2 days, infected cells were detected in the subcapsular sinus and paracortex (T cell area) of the draining nodes. Interestingly, no infected cells were seen in vaginal or cervical epithelium, even though many LC are present in these sites. It is possible that LC are binding or endocytosing virus without it replicating; this would prevent detection by PCR. This study provides very suggestive evidence that DC are the primary target of SIV (and HIV) in mucosal infection.

DC can clearly be infected in the mucosal lymphoid tissues of infected individuals. Thus Frankel *et al.* (1996) have shown that infected syncytia at the surface of the tonsil express DC markers, and that such syncytia can be present in patients without clinical AIDS.

There is also evidence that HIV infection can decrease numbers of DC in mucosal tissues. Thus Lim *et al.* (1993) showed a decrease in cells with DC phenotype in the duodenum and Spinillo *et al.* (1993) in the cervical epithelium of HIV-infected patients. This might lead to increased susceptibility to intercurrent infections.

Clearly there remains much uncertainty concerning the roles of DC in mucosal infections and there is currently much interest in the role of mucosal DC in HIV infection.

CONCLUSIONS AND FUTURE DIRECTIONS

The understanding of intestinal DC is in its infancy. Many studies are still descriptive relying—particularly in humans—on morphological and immunocytochemical identification of DC. We know a moderate amount about the distribution of DC in the gut and are starting to realize that DC represent complex populations of cells whose lineage and functional relationships to each other are largely unknown. We do not understand the roles of DC in nonperturbed states, and know very little about how the changes in DC properties and functions are induced by inflammation or other 'danger' stimuli.

The molecular basis of DC function is even more poorly understood. We know very little about the signals that inform DC to position themselves at particular sites or to leave those sites, or about the regulation of those signals by environmental stimuli. We do not know how far we can translate the properties of DC grown *in vitro* to those that exist in tissues. Despite these shortcomings, in reality we can at least define many of the problems that remain in understanding the roles of DC in intestinal immune responses, and the next few years will undoubtedly see answers to many of those problems.

REFERENCES

Austyn, J.M., Hankins, D.F., Larsen, C.P., Morris, P.J., Rao, A.S, Roake, J.A. (1994). Isolation and characterization of dendritic cells from mouse heart and kidney. *J. Immunol.* **152**, 2401–2410.

Brandtzaeg, P. (1996). History of oral tolerance and mucosal immunity. *Ann. N. Y. Acad. Sci.* **778**, 1–27.

Brenan, M. and Puklavec, M. (1992). The MRC OX-62 antigen: a useful marker in the purification of rat veiled cells with the biochemical properties of an integrin. *J. Exp. Med.* **175**, 1457–1465.

Bujdoso, R., Hopkins, J., Dutia, B.M., Young, P. and McConnell, I. (1989). Characterisation of sheep afferent lymph dendritic cells and their role in antigen carriage. *J. Exp. Med.* **170**, 1285–1302.

Chen, S.S. and Li, Q. (1990). Transforming growth factor-beta 1 (TGF-beta 1) is a bifunctional immune regulator for mucosal IgA responses. *Cell. Immunol.* **128**, 353–361.

Clarke, C.J., Wilson, A.D., Williams, N.A. and Stokes, C.R. (1991). Mucosal priming of T-lymphocyte responses to fed protein antigens using cholera toxin as an adjuvant. *Immunology* **72**, 323–328.

Everson, M.P., McDuffie, D.S., Lemak, D.G., Koopman, W.J., McGhee, J.R. and Beagley, K.W. (1996). Dendritic cells from different tissues induce production of different T cell cytokine profiles. *J. Leukocyte Biol.* **59**, 494–498.

Fayette, J., Dubois, B., Vandenabeele, S., Bridon, J.M., Vanbervliet, B., Durand, I., Banchereau, J., Caux, C. and Briere, F. (1997). Human dendritic cells skew isotype switching of CD40-activated naive B cells towards IgA1 and IgA2. *J. Exp. Med.* **185**, 1909–1918.

Finkelman, F.D., Lees, A., Birnbaum, R., Gause, W.C. and Morris, S.C. (1996). Dendritic cells can present antigen in vivo in a tolerogenic or immunogenic fashion. *J. Immunol.* **157**, 1406–1414.

Frankel, S.S., Wenig, B.M., Burke, A.P., Mannan, P., Thompson, L.D., Abbondanzo, S.L., Nelson, A.M., Pope, M. and Steinman, R.M. (1996). Replication of HIV-1 in dendritic cell-derived syncytia at the mucosal surface of the adenoid. *Science* **272**, 115–117.

Garside, P. and Mowat, A.M. (1997). Mechanisms of oral tolerance. *Crit. Rev. Immunol.* **17**, 119–137.

Gebert, A., Rothkotter, H.J. and Pabst, R. (1996). M cells in Peyer's patches of the intestine. *Int. Rev. Cytol.* **167**, 91–159.

Harper, H.M., Cochrane, L. and Williams, N.A. (1996). The role of small intestinal antigen-presenting cells in the induction of T-cell reactivity to soluble protein antigens: association between aberrant presentation in the lamina propria and oral tolerance. *Immunology* **89**, 449-456.

Heel, K.A., McCauley, R.D., Papadimitriou, J.M. and Hall, J.C. (1997). Review: Peyer's patches. *J. Gastroenterol. Hepatol.* **12**, 122–136.

Holt, P.G., Haining, S., Nelson, D.J. and Sedgwick, J.D. (1994). Origin and steady-state turnover of class II MHC-bearing dendritic cells in the epithelium of the conducting airways. *J. Immunol.* **153**, 256–261.

Kagnoff, M.F. (1996). Oral tolerance: mechanisms and possible role in inflammatory joint diseases. *Bailliére's Clin. Rheumatol.* **10**, 41–54.

Kelsall, B.L. and Strober, W. (1996). Distinct populations of dendritic cells are present in the subepithelial dome and T cell regions of the murine Peyer's patch. *J. Exp. Med.* **183**, 237–247.

Kim, P.H. and Kagnoff, M.F. (1990). Transforming growth factor-beta 1 is a costimulator for IgA production. *J. Immunol.* **144**, 3411–3416.

Kohne, G., Schneider, T. and Zeitz, M. (1996). Special features of the intestinal lymphocytic system. *Bailliére's Clin. Gastroenterol.* **10**, 427–442.

Kudo, S., Matsuno, K., Ezaki, T. and Ogawa, M. (1997). A novel migration pathway for rat dendritic cells from the blood: hepatic sinusoids–lymph translocation. *J. Exp. Med.* **185**, 777–784.

Lim, S.G., Condez, A. and Poulter, L.W. (1993). Mucosal macrophage subsets of the gut in HIV: decrease in antigen-presenting cell phenotype. *Clin. Exp. Immunol.* **92**, 442–447.

Liu, L.M. and MacPherson, G.G. (1991). Lymph-borne (veiled) dendritic cells can acquire and present intestinally administered antigens. *Immunology* **73**, 281-286.

Liu, L.M. and MacPherson, G.G. (1993). Antigen acquisition by dendritic cells: intestinal dendritic cells acquire antigen administered orally and can prime naive T cells *in vivo*. *J. Exp. Med.* **177**, 1299–1307.

Liu, L.-M. and MacPherson, G.G. (1995a). Rat intestinal dendritic cells: immunostimulatory potency and phenotypic characterisation. *Immunology* **85**, 88–93.

Liu, L.M. and MacPherson, G.G. (1995b). Antigen processing: cultured lymph-borne dendritic cells can process and present native protein antigens. *Immunology* **84**, 241–246.

MacPherson, G.G., Jenkins, C.D., Stein, M.J. and Edwards, C. (1995). Endotoxin-mediated dendritic cell release from the intestine. Characterization of released dendritic cells and TNF dependence. *J. Immunol.* **154**, 1317–1322.

Mahida, Y.R., Wu, K.C. and Jewell, D.P. (1988). Characterization of antigen-presenting activity of intestinal mononuclear cells isolated from normal and inflammatory bowel disease colon and ileum. *Immunology* **65**, 543–549.

Maric, I., Holt, P.G., Perdue, M.H. and Bienenstock, J. (1996). Class II MHC antigen (Ia)-bearing dendritic cells in the epithelium of the rat intestine. *J. Immunol.* **156**, 1408–1414.

Matsuno, K., Ezaki, T., Kudo, S. and Uehara, Y. (1996). A life stage of particle-laden rat dendritic cells *in vivo*: their terminal division, active phagocytosis, and translocation from the liver to the draining lymph [see comments]. *J. Exp. Med.* **183**, 1865–1878.

Matzinger, P. (1994). Tolerance, danger, and the extended family. *Annu. Rev. Immunol.* **12**, 991–1045.

Mayrhofer, G., Holt, P.G. and Papadimitriou, J.M. (1986). Functional characteristics of the veiled cells in afferent lymph from the rat intestine. *Immunology* **58**, 379–387.

McWilliam, A.S., Napoli, S., Marsh, A.M., Pemper, F.L., Nelson, D.J., Pimm, C.L., Stumbles. P.A., Wells, T.N. and Holt, P.G. (1996). Dendritic cells are recruited into the airway epithelium during the inflammatory response to a broad spectrum of stimuli. *J. Exp. Med.* **184**, 2429–2432.

Oral Tolerance: Mechanisms and Applications. Proceedings of a conference, New York, 1995. *Ann. N. Y. Acad. Sci.* **13**, 1–453.

Pavli, P., Woodhams, C., Doe, W. and Hume, D. (1990). Isolation and characterization of antigen presenting dendritic cells from the mouse intestinal lamina propria. *Immunology* **70**, 40–47.

Pavli, P., Hume, D.A., Van De Pol, E. and Doe, W.F. (1993). Dendritic cells, the major antigen-presenting cells of the human colonic lamina propria. *Immunology* **78**, 132–141.

Pugh, C.W., MacPherson, G.G. and Steer, H.W. (1983). Characterization of nonlymphoid cells derived from rat peripheral lymph. *J. Exp. Med.* **157**, 1758–1779.

Rhodes, J.M. (1985). Isolation of large mononuclear Ia-positive veiled cells from the mouse thoracic duct. *J. Immunol. Methods* **85**, 383–392.

Roake, J.A., Rao, A.S., Morris, P.J., Larsen, C.P., Hankins, D.F. and Austyn, J.M. (1995). Dendritic cell loss from nonlymphoid tissues after systemic administration of lipopolysaccharide, tumor necrosis factor, and interleukin 1. *J. Exp. Med.* **181**, 2237–2247.

Ruedl, C., Rieser, C., Bock, G., Wick, G. and Wolf, H. (1996). Phenotypic and functional characterization of CD11c$^+$ dendritic cell population in mouse Peyer's patches. *Eur. J. Immunol.* **26**, 1801–1806.

Sanderson, I.R. and Walker, W.A. (1993). Uptake and transport of macromolecules by the intestine: possible role in clinical disorders (an update). *Gastroenterology* **104**, 622–639.

Schrader, C., George, A., Kerlin, R. and Cebra, J. (1990). Dendritic cells support production of IgA and other non IgM isotypes in clonal microculture. *Int. Immunol.* **2**, 563–570.

Schuler, G. and Steinman, R.M. (1985). Murine epidermal Langerhans cells mature into potent immunostimulatory dendritic cells *in vitro*. *J. Exp. Med.* **161**, 526–546.

Spalding, D.M., Koopman, W.J., Eldridge, J.H., McGhee, J.R. and Steinman, R.M. (1983). Accessory cells in murine Peyers patch. I Identification and enrichment of a functional dendritic cell. *J. Exp. Med.* **157**, 1646–1659.

Spinillo, A., Tenti, P., Zappatore, R., De Seta, F., Silini, E. and Guaschino, S. (1993). Langerhans' cell counts and cervical intraepithelial neoplasia in women with human immunodeficiency virus infection. *Gynecol. Oncol.* **48**, 210–213.

Spira, A.I., Marx, P.A., Patterson, B.K., Mahoney, J., Koup, R.A., Wolinsky, S.M. and Ho, D.D. (1996). Cellular targets of infection and route of viral dissemination after an intravaginal inoculation of simian immunodeficiency virus into rhesus macaques. *J. Exp. Med.* **183**, 215–225.

Steinman, R.M., Lustig, D.S. and Cohn, Z.A. (1974). Identification of a novel cell type in peripheral lymphoid organs of mice III. Functional properties *in vivo*. *J. Exp. Med.* **139**, 1431–1435.

Stokes, C.R., Haverson, K. and Bailey, M. (1996). Antigen presenting cells in the porcine gut. *Vet. Immunol. Immunopathol.* **54**, 171–177.

Thomas, N.W., Jenkins, P.G., Howard, K.A., Smith, M.W., Lavelle, E.C., Holland, J. and Davis, S.S. (1996). Particle uptake and translocation across epithelial membranes. *J. Anat.* **189**, 487–490.

Wolf, J.L. and Bye, W.A. (1984). The membranous epithelial (M) cell and mucosal immune system (review). *Ann. Rev. Med.* **35**, 95–112.

Zeitz, M., Schieferdecker, H.L., James, S.P. and Riecken, E.O. (1990). Special functional features of T-lymphocyte subpopulations in the effector compartment of the intestinal mucosa and their relation to mucosal transformation. *Digestion* **2**, 280–289.

CHAPTER 10
Dendritic Cells in the Liver, Kidney, Heart and Pancreas

Raymond J. Steptoe[1] and Angus W. Thomson[1,2]
Thomas E. Starzl Transplantation Institute and Departments of [1]Surgery and [2]Molecular Genetics and Biochemistry, University of Pittsburgh, Pittsburgh, Pennsylvania, USA

That swift as quicksilver it courses
The natural gates and alleys of the body.

Hamlet
William Shakespeare, 1564–1616

INTRODUCTION

Many of the recent advances in our understanding of the biology of dendritic cells (DC) have come through the study of DC development pathways. This has been made possible by development of *in vitro* methods for either the propagation of DC from stem/progenitor cells, for example $CD34^+$ bone marrow cells, or the cytokine-mediated maturation of blood monocytes (reviewed elsewhere in this book). Formerly, studies aimed at elucidating the role of DC relied heavily on the use of lymphoid tissue-derived DC owing to the scarcity and difficulty of isolation of DC from nonlymphoid tissues. In nonlymphoid tissues, it has been Langerhans cells (which may exhibit distinct developmental differences from other nonlymphoid tissue DC) that have been studied most intensely. DC in the vascularized nonlymphoid organs remain less well understood. This review focuses on what is currently known of the basic biology of DC in the solid 'parenchymal' organs—liver, kidney, heart, and pancreas. Much of the impetus for the study of DC in these organs has come from the need to understand the immunological processes that underlie rejection (or acceptance) of these organs following transplantation. However, the desire to clarify the potential role that DC in nonlymphoid tissues may play in maintaining peripheral self-tolerance has inspired some interesting recent work. Knowledge is accumulating that also implicates DC as important participants in disease states within these organs. This is summarized to highlight that, *in vivo*, the role of these cells may extend beyond that of mere sentinel cells which traffic to regional lymphoid tissues, and that they may be important components in the process of tissue homeostasis.

Dendritic Cells: Biology and Clinical Applications
ISBN 0-12-455860-7

LIVER

Histological Location and Phenotype

The description of DC as a novel minor cell population in peripheral lymphoid tissue (Steinman and Cohn, 1973; Steinman and Cohn, 1974; Steinman *et al.*, 1974), and the subsequent elucidation of their involvement in the activation of T cells (Steinman and Witmer, 1979; Nussenzweig and Steinman, 1980) was the forerunner of what is today the burgeoning field of DC biology. While Langerhans cells described in epithelial sites, such as in the oral mucosa (Hutchens *et al.*, 1971) and epidermis (Stingl *et al.*, 1978; Silberberg-Sinakin *et al.*, 1978), had been shown to be related to DC, Hart and Fabre (1981a) provided a ground-breaking immunohistological demonstration of the presence of presumptive DC in interstitial connective tissue of many nonlymphoid solid organs, including the liver. Previously, Forsum *et al.* (1979) had demonstrated sparsely distributed individual MHC class II^+ cells in the liver of the guinea pig; however, staining had been attributed to Kupffer cells, the resident macrophage population of the liver.

Anti-MHC class II mAbs localize constitutively MHC class II^+ cells located primarily in the periportal area and around central veins, with few cells scattered throughout the parenchyma of rat (Hart and Fabre, 1981a; Spencer and Fabre, 1990; Steiniger *et al.*, 1984), mouse (Witmer-Pack *et al.*, 1993; Woo *et al.*, 1994) (see Plate 10.1), and human (Prickett *et al.*, 1988; Ballardini *et al.*, 1989) livers. The constitutive expression of MHC class II and the dendriform morphology of these cells led to their initial morphological classification as DC. While MHC class II antigens are also apparently expressed by human (Hart and Fabre, 1981a; Prickett *et al.*, 1988), but not rodent (Steiniger *et al.*, 1984) Kupffer cells, the distribution of DC allows them to be readily distinguished from Kupffer cells, which are distributed uniformly throughout the parenchyma (Hart and Fabre, 1981a; Spencer and Fabre, 1990, Witmer-Pack *et al.*, 1993). The presence of MHC class II^+ presumptive DC has also been reported in the liver capsule (Prickett *et al.*, 1988). Recent immunomorphological studies in this laboratory have indicated that while DC are sparsely distributed in the liver, and the density of cells per unit volume may be low compared to other solid organs, the total DC content of murine livers is high and is up to 5- to 10-fold that of other mouse parenchymal organs, such as heart and kidney (Steptoe, Patel and Thomson, manuscript in preparation). In mice, the β_2-integrin p150,90 (CD11c) is expressed by DC in a wide variety of lymphoid and nonlymphoid sites (Metlay *et al.*, 1990) and is widely used as a marker of DC in this species. When compared to mouse spleen, the total number of $CD11c^+$ cells (assessed by flow cytometry) per liver is roughly one-sixth that of the former ($\sim 0.7 \times 10^6$ vs approx. 4×10^6 $CD11c^+$ cells/organ, respectively) (Shaw, Maung, Steptoe, Thomson and Vujanovic, *J. Immunol.*, in press).

Unlike Kupffer cells, liver DC do not express nonspecific esterase or α-napthylacetate esterase activity (Hart and Fabre, 1981a; Lautenschlager *et al.*, 1988), facilitating distinction of these cell types. Additionally, double immunostaining studies, while limited to date, have indicated that there is minimal overlap between constitutively MHC II^+ cells and macrophages in the liver (Prickett *et al.*, 1988; Steiniger *et al.*, 1984). *In situ* examination of liver following intravenous (i.v.) administration of colloidal carbon (Hart and Fabre, 1981a; Steiniger *et al.*, 1984; Witmer-Pack *et al.*, 1993) or sheep red blood cells (SRBC) (Lautenschlager *et al.*, 1988) has led to the conclusion that, unlike Kupffer cells, liver DC do not phagocytose these particles *in vivo*. However, cell-mediated transfer of colloidal carbon to the celiac (liver-draining) lymph nodes has been observed following i.v. injection of this agent. While this finding was previously attributed to migrating Kupffer cells (Hardonk *et al.*, 1986; Matsuno *et al.*, 1990), more recent studies suggest it may be due to phagocytic DC progenitors translocating from blood to celiac lymph within the liver (Matsuno *et al.*, 1996; Kudo *et al.*, 1997) (see below). *In vitro* generated DC progenitors propagated from stem progenitor cells present in adult liver are able to phagocytose opsonized SRBC; however, this activity is lost following provision of 'maturational' signals by the extracellular matrix protein type-1 collagen (Lu *et al.*, 1994) that is spatially associated with liver DC *in vivo* (see below). Thus, these differences in the location, morphology, phenotype, and other characteristics underline the distinct and separate nature of DC and Kupffer cells in this organ.

Few reports are available detailing the location of cells immunoreactive with mAbs recognizing DC-associated antigens within liver. However, in the rat, the anti-DC mAb OX62 recognizes cells predominantly in the portal areas, with only low numbers of cells visualized in the sinusoids and around the central vein (Brenan and Puklavec, 1992; Matsuno *et al.*, 1996). In the mouse, CD11c$^+$ (Witmer-Pack *et al.*, 1993) and DEC-205$^+$ cells (Shurin *et al.*, 1997) are located predominantly periportally, as reported for MHC class II$^+$ cells. Extensive characterization of the *in situ* phenotype of rodent liver DC has not been performed. In the rat, MHC class II$^+$ DC appear to express variable levels of CD4 (Steiniger *et al.*, 1984; Stein-Oakley *et al.*, 1991), in common with DC in other peripheral tissue sites of this species (Steiniger *et al.*, 1984; Schon-Hegrad *et al.*, 1991; Darden *et al.*, 1990). The *in situ* phenotype of human liver DC has been more extensively examined and is summarized in Table 1.

Immunomorphological analysis of the expression of the costimulatory molecules CD80 (B7-1) and CD86 (B7-2) in normal mouse liver indicate that liver DC do not constitutively express detectable amounts of these molecules *in situ*—a phenotype characteristic of DC in peripheral tissue sites (Inaba *et al.*, 1994). Interestingly, CD86 expression is evident on Kupffer cells in mouse normal liver (Inaba *et al.*, 1994).

While detailed analysis of the *in situ* phenotype of rodent liver DC is lacking, more information is available on the phenotype of DC isolated from mouse liver (see Fig. 2). Mouse liver DC isolated by the procedure of selection of overnight nonadherent low-buoyant density cells (LBDC) do not express detectable levels of CD3, CD4, CD8, B220, or the antigen associated with lymphoid tissue DC recognized by the mAb 33D1. These cells do express moderate levels of CD11b (Mac-1), CD44, heat-stable antigen (HSA), and DEC-205 (Woo *et al.*, 1994). They also express high levels of CD45, MHC class II antigens, and CD11c (Woo *et al.*, 1994; Steptoe *et al.*, 1997). Woo *et al.* (1994) concluded that mouse liver DC resembled those of other tissue sites in their exhibition of upregulation of MHC class II expression and concomitant down-regulation of CD16/32 (FcγRII) and F4/80 following overnight culture (Woo *et al.*, 1994). Thus it appears that DC in mouse liver exist in an 'immature' or 'antigen-processing' phenotype, as described for DC in other nonlymphoid tissue sites, rather than the 'antigen-presenting' phenotype reported for DC in lymphoid tissue sites (reviewed in Steinman, 1991). The lack of CD8α expression by murine liver DC (Woo *et al.*, 1994) suggests that the lymphoid-related DC described in other (lymphoid)

Table 1. Human liver dendritic and Kupffer cell antigen expression determined by immunomorphology

mAb specificity	Liver interstitial DC	Kupffer cells
MHC class I	+	++
MHC class II		
HLA-DP	+++	++
HLA-DQ	+++	++
HLA-DR	+++	+
LCA (CD45)	++	++
FcR		
CD16	−	+
CD32	−	+/−
FcRI	−	+/−
Adhesins/complement receptors		
CD11a	+	+
CD11b	−	+
CD11c	−	+
CD18	+	+
Other		
CD4	−	+
CD14	+	+
CD39	−	+
CD40	−	+/−

Reprinted and modified with permission from Prickett *et al.* (1988).

organs (Ardavin *et al.*, 1993; Suss and Shortman, 1996; Maraskovsky *et al.*, 1996; Kronin et al., 1996) may be absent from liver (see below).

The location of DC associated predominantly with portal tracts is consistent with the notion that DC are found in locations where immune surveillance may be necessary. In the case of the liver, the portal system draining the mucosal surface of the gut is exposed to both food-borne immunogens and pathogens and to symbiotic eukaryotic organisms. Interestingly, the development of tolerance to antigen administered either orally or via the portal venous tract may be dependent on liver DC (Yang *et al.*, 1994; Gorczynski *et al.*, 1996). Their location is ideally suited for surveillance of the portal tract and would equip them well for this role.

Population Dynamics

Demonstration of the replacement of donor-derived DC in liver allografts with those of host origin confirms that this pool of cells is maintained at least in part from progenitor cells derived from the host's hematopoietic system (Valdivia *et al.*, 1993). While data are not available to indicate the population dynamics of these cells in humans, isolation of DC from lymph draining the liver following bromodeoxyuridine feeding indicates that, in rats, the DC migration rate from the liver is approximately 1×10^5 DC/h (Matsuno *et al.*, 1995; Matsuno *et al.*, 1996), and that approximately half the DC leaving the liver via lymph have arisen by division within the previous 5.5 days (Matsuno *et al.*,

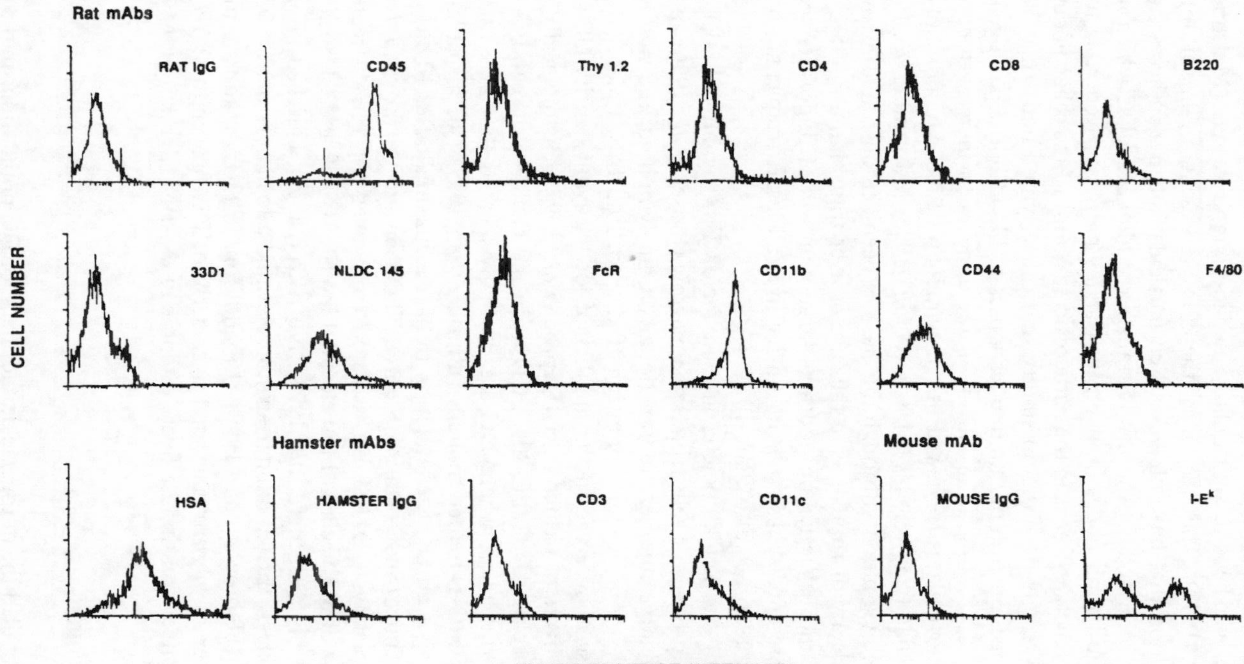

Fig. 2. DC in the liver. Flow cytometric profiles of overnight nonadherent low buoyant density cells prepared from liver nonparenchymal cells. Reprinted with permission from Woo *et al.* (1994).

1996). Additionally, DC bearing ingested latex particles appear quickly (within 1 h) in lymph draining the liver of rats administered latex particles i.v. (Matsuno *et al.*, 1996). It has been proposed that these particle-laden DC may not be derived from DC resident within the liver, but that they derive from a marginated pool in the circulation which rapidly translocates via hepatic sinusoids to hepatic lymph vessels (Matsuno *et al.*, 1996; Kudo *et al.*, 1997). The liver may therefore represent an important site in which DC in the blood that have phagocytosed particulates can gain access to lymph draining to celiac lymph nodes. Adoptively transferred allogeneic DC which migrated from blood to celiac lymph nodes (apparently via this pathway) were able to induce proliferation in alloreactive T cells in the paracortical regions of the celiac nodes (Kudo *et al.*, 1997). These results raise the possibility that celiac lymph nodes may represent an important site for induction of immune responses to blood-borne pathogens, particularly as the rate of DC migration via this route appears to increase following i.v. administration of particulates (reviewed in Austyn, 1996). Liver DC normally traffic, via lymph, to the celiac lymph nodes (Matsuno *et al.*, 1995; Matsuno *et al.*, 1996) and possibly to the spleen via blood (although this has not been demonstrated). However, if the lymphatic vessels are disrupted, as in the case of liver transplantation, DC migrate to both the spleen and celiac lymph nodes as large numbers of donor-derived MHC class II$^+$ cells are present in these sites in murine liver allograft recipients (Sun *et al.*, 1995; Bishop *et al.*, 1996; see also Plate 10.1).

Administration of the hematopoietic growth factor Flt3 ligand (Flt3-L) to mice mobilizes stem and progenitor cells from bone marrow (Brasel *et al.*, 1996) and results in accumulation of large numbers of functional DC in lymphoid and nonlymphoid tissues (Maraskovsky *et al.*, 1996). Following 10 days of Flt3-L treatment (10 μg/day) an ~90-fold increase is observed in the number of low-bouyant density CD11c$^+$ DC recovered from the livers of treated mice (Steptoe *et al.*, 1997). Histologically, clusters of infiltrating MHC class II$^+$, DEC-205$^+$, CD11c$^+$, and CD86$^+$ cells can be observed not only in the portal areas, where DC are normally located, but also throughout the parenchyma of Flt3-L-treated animals (Shurin *et al.*, 1997) (see also Plate 10.1). The influence of Flt3-L on DC accumulation in liver is maximal after 10 days of continuous treatment of mice (Shaw, Maung, Steptoe, Thomson and Vujanovic, *J. Immunol.*, in press). Phenotypically, CD11c$^+$ DC isolated from livers of Flt3-L-treated mice exhibit similar levels of MHC class II but elevated levels of CD80 and CD86 compared to those from controls (Steptoe *et al.*, 1997). Not surprisingly, enriched populations of liver DC from Flt3-L-treated animals exhibit elevated allostimulatory activity compared to controls (Steptoe *et al.*, 1997). In addition, Flt3-L treatment markedly increases the number of *in vitro* generated liver-derived 'DC progenitors' (see below) that can be propagated from mouse livers (Steptoe *et al.*, 1997; Drakes *et al.*, 1997a).

Ontogenic Development

Few reports have detailed the ontogenic development of DC populations in the liver. In humans, isolated HLA-DR$^+$ cells (of undefined histological type) have been reported in the liver of 8-week-old embryos; at this point the only other HLA-DR$^+$ cells that exist are DC in the thymus (Natali *et al.*, 1984). Development of an adult-equivalent distribution of HLA-DR$^+$ DC-like cells is attained in most human fetal tissues, including the liver, by 26 weeks of gestation (Natali *et al.*, 1984). In the rat, van Rees *et al.* (1988) demonstrated an absence of MHC class II$^+$ DC in the liver until after birth. Cell populations expressing the macrophage-associated antigens recognized by the mAbs ED1, ED2, and ED3, however, developed prenatally. A similar absence of MHC class II$^+$ cells in the liver prenatally has also been reported in mice (Natali *et al.*, 1981).

Function

DC Isolated from Liver Tissue

The functional capacity of liver DC has not been examined extensively, although studies indicate that these cells are able to acquire the potent allostimulatory capacity attributed to DC isolated from other tissue sites. Klinkert *et al.* (1982) provided evidence that the ability to act as accessory cells in periodate-induced mitogenesis was associated with DC-enriched populations from rat liver. Lautenschlager *et al.* (1988) demonstrated that rat liver DC, isolated as overnight nonadherent LBDC, when adoptively transferred, primed naive allogeneic recipients for accelerated allograft rejection. Interestingly, in these experiments, the DC-enriched preparations from liver contained approximately 80% DC but primed for accelerated allograft rejection only as efficiently as crude splenocytes which contained <5% DC (Lautenschlager *et al.*, 1988). This raises the question whether liver DC are as functionally competent as those from spleen. DC enriched from mouse liver using a similar technique of harvesting LBDC after overnight culture, either in the presence or the absence of granulocyte macrophage colony-stimulating factor (GM-CSF), effectively stimulate allogeneic mixed leukocyte responses (MLR) *in vitro* (Woo *et al.*, 1994; Steptoe *et al.*, 1997). It is unclear, however, how the relative allostimulatory ability of liver DC induced to mature by overnight culture *in vitro* compares with that of 'classical' immunostimulatory DC isolated from lymphoid tissues. The stimulatory capacity of freshly isolated unmanipulated liver DC has not been assessed, although the absence of CD80 and CD86 expression by these cells *in situ* (Inaba *et al.*, 1994) suggests that, in common with DC from other non-lymphoid tissue sites, these cells would exhibit weak stimulatory capacity when freshly isolated. It has been speculated that these donor-derived cells may remain 'immature' in liver allografts, or in host lymphoid tissues following migration, in allogeneic liver recipients treated with immunosuppressive therapy and could then constitute a population of cells that interact with alloreactive T cells in a potentially 'tolerogenic' fashion (Steinman *et al.*, 1993). It thus possible these cells could be important in contributing to the favorable outcome observed with liver allografts compared to other commonly transplanted organs. Interestingly, augmentation of not only the number of DC but also the functional capacity of these cells in murine donor livers by pretreatment with Flt3-L (see above) results in reversal of the spontaneous acceptance of allogeneic livers normally observed in this species and results in rapid rejection (Steptoe *et al.*, 1997). The authors concluded that these observations were consistent with the suggestion that, under normal circumstances, donor-derived liver DC may provide only a weak allostimulatory signal to allogeneic liver recipients, but that this may be altered by increasing the number and functional capacity of these cells in the liver.

Liver-derived DC collected from the thoracic duct of celiac lymphadenectomized rats possess allostimulatory activity in MLR assays equivalent to that of DC of intestinal origin collected in a similar manner from mesenteric lymphadectomized rats (Matsuno *et al.*, 1995; Matsuno *et al.*, 1996). DC of intestinal origin collected from mesenteric lymph have been characterized previously and, while able to stimulate MLR responses, they retain the capacity to ingest and process antigen (Liu and MacPherson, 1995a,b), suggesting that these cells may exhibit an intermediate form between 'antigen-processing' and 'antigen-presenting' stages. Whether liver-derived DC in celiac lymph are in a similar stage of development is unclear. In the studies of Kudo *et al.* (1997), however, DC bearing latex beads that were adoptively transferred and subsequently isolated from celiac lymph were unable to phagocytose further particulates *in vitro*. Therefore, the studies of Matsuno and co-workers (Matsuno *et al.*, 1995; Matsuno *et al.*, 1996) suggest that the DC which migrate from the liver via the lymphatics are either already 'mature' immunostimulatory cells or that they rapidly mature upon leaving the liver. The evidence provided by *in situ* studies of costimulatory molecule expression (Inaba *et al.*, 1994) suggest the latter alternative. This situation may, however, be altered when DC bearing particulates translocate from blood to celiac lymph as discussed above (Kudo *et al.*, 1997).

DC Progenitors Propagated in vitro from Adult Liver Hematopoietic Stem Cells

As with other tissue sites, one of the major difficulties of studying liver DC is the inability to readily obtain relatively large numbers of these cells. In an effort to overcome these shortcomings, Lu *et al.* (1994) developed a procedure whereby DC could be generated from stem/progenitor cells present within the nonparenchymal cell (NPC) population isolated from mouse liver, using a modification of the procedure described for GM-CSF-mediated propagation of DC from blood and bone marrow (Inaba *et al.*, 1992a,b). DC propagated in this manner expressed high levels of CD45, CD11b, HSA, and CD44, but only low to moderate levels of the macrophage marker F4/80, the antigen uptake-associated receptor CD16/32 (FcγRII), ICAM-1 (CD54), and the DC-restricted markers DEC-205, CD11c and 33D1 (Lu *et al.*, 1994). These cells exhibit the classic veiled morphology of DC, yet interestingly, exhibit only low levels of CD40 and the CD28/CTLA4 ligands CD80 and CD86 (Lu *et al.*, 1994; Drakes *et al.*, 1997a). These cells were therefore termed liver-derived 'DC progenitors'. Extended periods of culture or exposure to tumor necrosis factor-α (TNF-α), interferon-γ (IFN-γ), or bacterial lipopolysaccharide (LPS) are unable to induce high levels of MHC class II antigen expression, indicating that these cells exhibit a block in the ability to acquire fully 'mature' characteristics (Lu *et al.*, 1994). It was found, however, that incubation of these cells in the presence of collagen type-1, fibronectin, or laminin, extracellular proteins with which DC are spatially associated in liver, was able to provide a signal that induced 'maturation' (Lu *et al.*, 1994; Drakes *et al.*, 1997b). For example, in the absence of collagen type-1-mediated maturational signals, liver-derived DC progenitors were unable to effectively stimulate MLR responses, in contrast to those cultured in the presence of type-1 collagen for 3 days (Lu *et al.*, 1994). Likewise, phagocytic activity was also downregulated (Lu *et al.*, 1994). It is therefore interesting to speculate that contact with these extracellular matrix proteins during migration may provide signals which induce 'maturation' in DC. When the migratory potential of these cells was examined, they were found to home to the periarteriolar lymphoid sheath of the spleen and to express moderate to high levels of MHC class II when injected i.v. into allogeneic recipients (Lu *et al.*, 1994; Thomson *et al.*, 1995). The inability of these cells to stimulate allogeneic T cell proliferative responses led to speculation that they may possess the ability to act as 'tolerogenic' or anergy-inducing APC. This was examined by pretreatment of pancreatic islet allograft recipients with liver-derived DC progenitors of donor origin 7 days prior to islet cell transplantation, and was found to extend islet allograft survival (Rastellini *et al.*, 1995). The potential therapeutic role of these putative tolerogenic DC is discussed elsewhere in this volume.

Whether these DC propagated from liver NPC are developmentally identical to DC freshly isolated from liver tissue is unclear. To date, however, in all features examined these cells exhibit similar characteristics. As these DC progenitors are generated *in vitro* using GM-CSF, it is probable they arise from myeloid-lineage liver progenitor/stem cells. This is further evidenced by the inability to propagate cells resembling the *in vitro* generated lymphoid-related DC described by Saunders *et al.* (1996) from liver NPC using the cytokine cocktail interleukin (IL)-1, IL-3, IL-7, TNF-α, c-kit ligand, Flt3-L, which appears necessary for the development of these cells (R.J. Steptoe, unpublished observations).

Disease

In viral hepatitis, interdigitating DC have been identified by ultrastructural analysis (Bardadin and Desmet, 1984) and by immunohistochemical techniques (van den Oord *et al.*, 1990) in areas of piecemeal necrosis in human liver, and are often observed closely associated with CD8$^+$ T cells in the periphery of areas of piecemeal necrosis and in inflamed portal tracts (van den Oord *et al.*, 1990). Large numbers of HLA-DR$^+$ presumptive DC have also been observed in areas of 'spotty' inflammation. Additionally, HLA-DR$^+$ DC have been noted among CD4$^+$ T cells in severely inflamed portal tracts (van den Oord *et al.*, 1990). It has been suggested that within the central part of portal tracts, CD4$^+$ T cells were being activated by DC, whereas the periportal and centrilobular parenchyma apears to be the site where CD8$^+$ cells are mediating cytotoxic activity (van den Oord *et al.*, 1990).

DC may play a role in the development of primary biliary cirrhosis (PBC). They have been observed frequently within the bile duct in the early phases of PBC but are much less common in advanced disease where they may be more often located periductally (Demetris *et al.*, 1989; Ballardini *et al.*, 1989; Kaji *et al.*, 1997). This suggests a role for DC in the developing disease. In a transplant setting, Demetris *et al.* (1991) provided immunohistochemical evidence that donor-derived DC within rat liver allografts were clustering with, and possibly activating, CD4$^+$ and CD8$^+$ infiltrating T cells. Likewise, DC are found within the portal inflammatory infiltrate in obliterative arteriopathy (chronic allograft rejection) (Demetris *et al.*, 1989), and they have been observed interacting with T cells present within the cellular infiltrate (Oguma *et al.*, 1988; Oguma *et al.*, 1989).

KIDNEY

Histological Location and Phenotype

The presence of MHC class II$^+$ putative DC in the kidney was first demonstrated by Hart and Fabre (1981a) in specimens of rat tissue and then examined in more detail throughout the urinary tract (Hart and Fabre, 1981b). Subsequent reports have provided further details of MHC class II$^+$ DC in the kidney of rat (Steiniger *et al.*, 1984; Leszczynski *et al.*, 1985a), mouse (Austyn *et al.*, 1994), musk shrew (Kerschbaum *et al.*, 1995), and human (Hart *et al.*, 1981; Daar *et al.*, 1983; Hancock and Atkins, 1984). In humans, glomeruli apparently contain few MHC class II$^+$ DC; however, the intertubular areas are reportedly rich in these cells (Daar *et al.*, 1983; Hancock and Atkins, 1984), both in the cortex and medulla. In the rat, individual glomeruli contain a low number of DC (1–3 per glomerulus), with the majority of cells located in periglomerular and peritubular locations (Hart and Fabre, 1981a; Steiniger *et al.*, 1984; Leszczynski *et al.*, 1985a) with DC most numerous in the medullary region (Steiniger *et al.*, 1984). In addition, a cortico-medullary gradient in MHC class II expression by these cells has been reported in the rat, with the highest levels of expression observed in the cortex (Steiniger *et al.*, 1984). In our own studies of the mouse, the medullary rays of the kidney were observed to contain higher densities of MHC class II$^+$ dendriform cells than the cortex (Steptoe, Patel, Thomson, manuscript in preparation). Interestingly, in the bladder (Hart and Fabre, 1981b), MHC class II$^+$ DC are located beneath the epithelial layer, as in other epithelial surfaces (Schon-Hegrad *et al.*, 1991; Maric *et al.*, 1996). Despite expressing large quantities of MHC class II *in situ*, rat kidney DC, like those in heart and pancreas, express undetectable quantities of invariant chain (Ii), which is in contrast to the high expression of Ii by DC in lymphoid tissues (Saleem *et al.*, 1997). As Ii expression is related to expression of antigen-bearing MHC class II molecules, this may be an important mechanism regulating the expression of self-antigens by DC in peripheral nonlymphoid tissues. The regulation of Ii during maturation or responses to inflammatory stimuli by DC from solid organs has not been studied. Freshly isolated Langerhans cells have been reported to express high levels of Ii (Kampgen *et al.*, 1991; Puré *et al.*, 1991), but it is unclear whether this is a response to the isolation procedure.

Immunohistochemical studies have indicated that kidney DC phenotypically resemble those in other nonlymphoid sites, and do not express cell surface markers considered characteristic of macrophages (Daar *et al.*, 1983; Hancock and Atkins, 1984; Kaissling and Le Hir, 1994). Based on morphological criteria, DC are reported to outnumber the coexisting macrophages in the rat kidney (Kaissling and Le Hir, 1994). DC in the kidney also exhibit the characteristic ultrastructural features described for DC from other tissue sites, allowing them to be readily distinguished from macrophages and monocytes in electron micrographs (Gaudecker *et al.*, 1993). Austyn *et al.* (1994) reported that CD16/32 (FcγRII), CD11b and the macrophage antigen detected by the mAb F4/80 were present on freshly isolated MHC class II$^+$ presumptive DC from mouse kidney. However, following overnight culture, slight reductions in the expression of these markers was apparent (Austyn *et al.*, 1994). In contrast to DC from lymphoid tissues, the DC-associated markers DEC-205 and 33D1 were not expressed by these cells when freshly isolated; IL-2Rα (CD25) expression was also absent (Austyn *et al.*, 1994). These cells are therefore phenotypically similar to DC isolated from other nonlymphoid tissue sites. *In situ*, kidney DC also resemble those in other nonlymphoid tissue in their inability to phagocytose colloidal carbon injected i.v. (Hart and Fabre, 1981a). *In vitro*, MHC class II$^+$ presumptive kidney DC phagocytose zymosan particles, when freshly isolated, but with less avidity than freshly isolated mouse cardiac DC (Austyn *et al.*, 1994).

The location of DC lining the bladder and the ureter and in the vicinity of tubules within the kidney suggests a role for these cells in surveillance of these sites for invading pathogenic organisms. However, this suggestion has not been examined in experimental models of urinary tract infection.

Population Dynamics

The population dynamics of DC in the kidney appear similar to those of DC in other tissue sites. Irradiation and reconstitution studies have provided an estimate of population turnover in the order of 7–10 days in the rat (Leszczynski *et al.*, 1985a). Systemic treatment with IFN-γ is reported to result in an increase in the number MHC class II$^+$ DC in the kidneys of mice, with a 2–3-fold increase observed after 3 days of treatment, and a slow reduction to near normal levels within 2–3 weeks after cessation of treatment (Skoskiewicz *et al.*, 1985). A similar pattern has been reported in the rat; however, the degree of DC increase was not as dramatic (Leszczynski *et al.*, 1986). Conversely, treatment with IFN-α and IFN-β results in a reduction of the density of DC within the renal cortex of mice (Maguire *et al.*, 1990). It is unclear whether these effects are mediated by altered DC trafficking patterns. Systemic LPS administration has been shown to result in the mobilization of DC from kidney, with subsequent recruitment of MHC class II$^-$ DC progenitors (Roake *et al.*, 1995a,b). These effects of LPS administration have been attributed to mediation of DC migration by the cytokines TNF-α and IL-1α (Roake *et al.*, 1995a).

Ontogenic Development

Little detail is available of the ontogenic development of DC populations in the kidney. In the human, MHC class II$^+$ DC appear to develop first between 8 and 13 weeks gestational age, and increase in number between 12 and 21 weeks of gestation at a rate similar to that in other nonlymphoid sites (heart, lung, pancreas) (Natali *et al.*, 1984; Hofman *et al.*, 1984). Little is known of the ontogenic development of DC in the kidney of rodents other than mice, in which MHC class II$^+$ cells are not observed in this organ until after birth (Natali *et al.*, 1981).

Function

An extensive and demanding study of the functional capacity of murine kidney DC was performed by Austyn *et al.* (1994). The results indicated that MHC class II$^+$ DC in kidney possessed little capacity to stimulate resting allogeneic T cells in MLR assays, or to provide accessory cell activity in oxidative mitogenesis assays when freshly isolated. This capacity was acquired following overnight culture, in a fashion similar to that seen in skin-derived Langerhans cells (Schuler and Steinman, 1985; Inaba *et al.*, 1986; Romani *et al.*, 1989). These findings are consistent with the expectation that kidney DC exhibit features similar to those of DC in other nonlymphoid tissue sites thus far examined.

Depletion of DC from kidney by 'parking' in allogeneic hosts (Lechler and Batchelor, 1982) or a protocol of cyclophosphamide and irradiation treatment (McKenzie *et al.*,

1984a) prior to allografting has indicated that these cells are capable of providing a strong allogeneic immunostimulatory signal *in vivo*. Velasco and Hegre (1989) have provided similar data implying that the absence of DC from fetal rat kidneys renders these organs less immunogenic. These studies provide *in vivo* evidence complementary to that derived from *in vitro* studies, and indicate that kidney DC can acquire the immunostimulatory functional capacity characteristic of DC in other tissue sites. The role of DC in kidney allograft rejection has been utilized as a model system to demonstrate that *ex vivo* PUVA treatment (ultraviolet A irradiation of the donor organ in the presence of the photoactive substance 8-methoxypsoralen) may reduce the functional capacity of DC within the kidney allografts (Gaudecker *et al.*, 1993). Efforts to deplete kidney DC (e.g. by use of anti-CD45 mAbs) prior to human organ transplantation have not, however, led to significant improvement in graft survival.

HEART

Histological Location and Phenotype

As in other nonlymphoid tissues, MHC class II^+ presumptive cardiac DC are most closely associated with the endocardial blood vessels and connective tissue, and are generally aligned parallel to cardiac myocytes with their processes interdigitating between the myocytes (Hart and Fabre, 1981a; Steiniger *et al.*, 1984). Ultrastructural analysis indicates that Birbeck granules present in Langerhans cells of the epidermis are absent from cardiac DC (Zhang *et al.*, 1992). DC density in normal ACI rat heart has been estimated as 55–60 DC/mm^2 (Forbes *et al.*, 1986; Darden *et al.*, 1990) with a density range of approximately 10–75 DC/mm^2 between strains (Darden *et al.*, 1990). In addition to DC, a distinct population of resident tissue macrophages can be distinguished by expression of the macrophage-restricted antigens recognized by the mAbs BMAC-5 and ED2 in the rat (Spencer and Fabre, 1990) and also by the presence of nonspecific esterase activity (Hart and Fabre, 1981a). Rat cardiac DC express variable levels of CD4 and the CD68-like antigen recognized by the mAb ED1, but not CD8 or the resident-tissue macrophage antigen recognised by the mAb ED2 (Darden *et al.*, 1990; Zhang *et al.*, 1993; Suzuki, 1995), and are thus phenotypically similar to those in other peripheral tissues, such as lung (Schon-Hegrad *et al.*, 1991). Darden *et al.* (1990) suggested that a population of $CD4^+$/MHC II^- dendritiform cells present in the rat heart represented a precursor population from which the $CD4^+$/MHC II^+ tissue DC observed in this organ may arise. No efforts were made, however, to exclude the possibility that these cells represented $CD4^+$/MHC II^- macrophages. $CD4^+$/MHC class II^- precursors of DC have been described in human blood (O'Doherty *et al.*, 1994) and tonsils (Grouard *et al.*, 1997). Like DC in kidney (see above), rat cardiac DC do not express detectable quantities of invariant chain (Saleem *et al.*, 1997). In mice, cardiac DC express variable amounts of CD16/32 (FcγRII), CD11b, and the pan-macrophage marker recognized by the mAb F4/80, but not IL-2Rα (CD25) when freshly isolated, with little change observed in the phenotype of these cells following overnight culture (Austyn *et al.*, 1994). DEC-205 and 33D1 are reported to be absent from freshly isolated murine cardiac DC from normal animals (Austyn *et al.*, 1994), although CD11c has been reported on freshly isolated cells (Steptoe *et al.*, 1997). *In situ* immunohistochemistry has also revealed the expression of CD11a, CD44, and macrosialin on murine heart DC (Austyn *et al*., 1994). Little phenotypic information is available for cardiac DC in humans, but no differences were noted between these DC and those in other nonlymphoid sites (Daar *et al*., 1983; Hancock and Atkins, 1984).

While rat cardiac DC do not phagocytose colloidal carbon *in vivo* (Spencer and Fabre, 1990), freshly isolated mouse cardiac DC phagocytose zymosan particles *in vitro* with an avidity greater than that exhibited by MHC class II$^+$ DC freshly isolated from kidney (Austyn *et al*., 1994). Interestingly in these studies, there was little reduction in the phagocytic capacity of cardiac MHC class II$^+$ cells over 24 h of culture, which is in contrast with observations of the effects of culture on Langerhans cell phagocytic activity (Reis e Sousa *et al*., 1993).

Population Dynamics

The population turnover of heart DC appears rapid. Hart and Fabre (1981a) demonstrated that, following lethal irradiation, the presumptive DC population of the rat heart declined rapidly, and was virtually absent after 5 days. Consistent with this rapid turnover were observations that the MHC class II$^+$ DC population was rapidly reconstituted following bone marrow transplantation (Hart and Fabre, 1981a; Leszczynski *et al*., 1985b). The prolonged presence of donor MHC class II$^+$ cells in heart allografts parked in athymic nude rat recipients indicates that, like Langerhans cells (Czernielewski *et al*., 1985; Chen *et al*., 1986; Czernielewski *et al*., 1987), a long-lived or immobile population of DC may also be present in the heart (Burris *et al*., 1989). As macrophages are relatively immobile (Spencer and Fabre, 1990), it is possible the cells observed represent macrophages with induced MHC class II expression. Alternatively, it is possible that the presence of cytokine-secreting lymphocytes may be necessary to mediate DC migration in this model. Further work is required to clarify these alternatives.

The accumulation of donor-derived DC in the spleens of heart allograft recipients (Larsen *et al*., 1990) has demonstrated the ability of mouse cardiac DC to traffic to lymphoid tissue, and provided a model indicating the role of DC in central priming of anti-allograft immunity. Mobilization of DC from heart tissue can be very rapid, as donor-derived DC were detected in the spleens of recipient mice as early as 24 h after heart transplantation, but numbers were maximal between 2 and 4 days post-transplantation (Larsen *et al*., 1990). The rapid reduction in the number of donor-derived DC in recipient spleens 4 days post-transplantation indicated that DC are required only to initiate the allograft rejection response and not for a maintained anti-allograft response.

Systemic IFN-γ administration has been reported to result in rapid accumulation of DC in heart tissue of mice, with a 3–4-fold increase apparent after 3 days of treatment, and a continued increase when animals were treated for 9 days, with a time course resembling that observed in kidney (Skoskiewicz *et al*., 1985). Leszczynski *et al*. (1986) reported similar findings following 3 days of IFN-γ administration to rats, but also noted that the effect could be reversed by administration of the steroid methylprednisolone. Likewise, administration of the hematopoietic growth factor Flt3-L has been demonstrated to result in a 1.5-fold increase in the number of functionally mature DC in mouse cardiac tissue (Steptoe *et al*., 1997).

As in the kidney, systemic administration of LPS to mice results in the mobilization of DC from cardiac tissue and a subsequent accumulation, by recruitment, of MHC class II^- DC progenitors (Roake *et al.*, 1995a,b). It appears that this effect is mediated at least in part by TNF-α and IL-1α (Roake *et al.*, 1995a) as reported for DC in other tissue sites (Cumberbatch and Kimber, 1995; MacPherson *et al.*, 1995; Cumberbatch *et al.*, 1997).

Ontogenic Development

In the human, MHC class II^+ leukocyte populations appear to develop first in the heart between 13 and 17 weeks of gestation, relatively late compared to other nonlymphoid human tissues examined (Hofman *et al.*, 1984).

Function

Examination of the functional properties of murine cardiac DC reveals that similar to DC from other nonlymphoid sites, when freshly isolated these cells exhibit only a weak capacity to stimulate resting allogeneic T cells in MLR assays or to costimulate oxidative mitogenesis. The level of these activities is, however, markedly increased following overnight culture (Austyn *et al.*, 1994). Depletion of DC from heart tissue allografts by anti-MHC class II mAb (Faustman *et al.*, 1982) or from vascularized heart allografts by treatment with cyclophosphamide and total body irradiation (McKenzie *et al.*, 1984b) prior to transplantation extends allograft survival. Conversely, augmentation of the number of cardiac DC by Flt3-L pretreatment of donors exacerbates heart allograft rejection (Steptoe *et al.*, 1997). These results provide further evidence that these nonlymphoid tissue DC are able to acquire potent T cell-stimulating properties *in vivo*.

A key issue that has intrigued immunologists is whether DC can only prime responding T cells centrally in lymphoid tissue or whether they can also stimulate T cell activation in peripheral nonlymphoid tissues. Using a vascularized heart allograft model in the rat, Forbes *et al.* (1986) demonstrated cell–cell interaction of donor MHC class II^+ DC and graft-infiltrating T cells within the graft and the first apparent demonstration of peripheral T cell priming in an allograft. As the $CD4^+$:$CD8^+$ T cell ratio at day 4 post-transplantation was approximately 2:1, it is likely this represented an *in vivo* demonstration of DC–T cell clustering similar to that which has been demonstrated *in vitro* (Inaba and Steinman, 1986b; Inaba *et al.*, 1989) rather than cytotoxic T cell-mediated killing of DC. While further analysis is required to determine whether the interacting T cells are activated in these interactions, this observation may indicate that these DC possess the ability to prime T cell activation and proliferation peripherally, at least when provided with the 'activational' signals subsequent to transplantation.

Disease

The ability of cardiac DC to respond to tissue injury has been demonstrated in experimentally induced myocardial infarction lesions in rats (Zhang *et al.*, 1992; Zhang *et al.*, 1993). In this model, the accumulation of DC was maximal in the 'border zones' of the infarct site (796 DC/mm^2 vs 82/mm^2 in normal hearts) 7 days post-infarction, and clustering of these DC with CD4$^+$ T cells was prominent at this time. DC density then returned to relatively normal levels 21 days following the infarction event. Interestingly, within the center of the infarct lesion, only relatively minor changes occurred in the density of DC. The potential significance of DC–T cell interaction in mechanisms mediating the resolution of inflammation and scarring at this site of tissue damage is unclear. In an experimental model of actively induced experimental autoimmune myocarditis in rats, DC are the first leukocytes observed infiltrating around small blood vessels, and primary lesions are reported to form subsequently at these sites (Suzuki, 1995). It was suggested that in this model, DC mediated the initial anti-myocardial destructive events and that the subsequent macrophage infiltration was a response to the localized tissue necrosis induced by DC (Suzuki, 1995). The factors by which DC may mediate the proposed anti-myocardiocyte activity are unclear but may be similar to those proposed as mediating anti-β-cell activity in diabetes (see below).

PANCREAS

Histological Location and Phenotype

MHC class II$^+$ presumptive DC are distributed throughout both the exocrine and endocrine portions of the pancreas. In humans, individual islets of Langerhans contain 0–6 DC and these cells constitute only a small proportion (approximately 4%) of the total MHC class II$^+$ interstitial cells within normal human pancreata (Leprini *et al.*, 1987). When single-cell suspensions are prepared from isolated human pancreatic islets, DC comprise less than 1% of the total cell number (Lu *et al.*, 1996a). The location of presumptive DC within human islets is restricted predominantly to the periphery of the islets, where these cells exhibit a more extensive dendriform morphology than those in the exocrine portion of the pancreas (Leprini *et al.*, 1987). In other species examined, for example dog and pig (Shienvold *et al.*, 1986) and rat (Steiniger *et al.*, 1984; Lloyd *et al.*, 1987), the distribution of cells appears similar, although some predilection for blood vessels has been reported in the rat (Steiniger *et al.*, 1984). Likewise, the total number of DC per islet appears similar between species, at least in human, rat, and dog (Gebel *et al.*, 1983; Shienvold *et al.*, 1986; Leprini *et al.*, 1987).

In the rat, pancreatic DC express variable levels of CD4, with a population of CD4$^+$/MHC II$^-$ cells reminiscent of that reported in heart also present (Steiniger *et al.*, 1984; Darden *et al.*, 1990) (see above). In studies of human tissues reported by Hancock and Atkins (1984), no differences were noted for the phenotype of pancreatic DC compared with that of other nonlymphoid tissue DC. More detailed surface phenotype characterization by Leprini *et al.* (1987) suggested that MHC class II$^+$ cells in the pancreas of humans were composed of two phenotypically distinct subpopulations. One subset expressed numerous markers associated with macrophages and exhibited an ovoid morphology. The second subset was negative for surface and cytochemical markers of macrophages, exhibited more marked dendriform morphology, and comprised approximately 70% of all MHC class II$^+$ cells (Leprini *et al.*, 1987). Interestingly, it appears that some of the MHC class II$^+$ DC located within the islets express substantial levels of Leu7 (CD57) (Leprini *et al.*, 1987). Lu *et al.* (1996a) reported that in the human the majority of pancreatic MHC class II$^+$ cells were CD68$^+$, but that few were recognized by the anti-macrophage mAb MAC-387. These results suggest the existence of a small population of MHC class II$^+$ macrophages that coexist alongside DC in the human pancreas.

Population Dynamics

There have been no reports indicating the population kinetics of pancreatic DC.

Ontogenic Development

Examination of the development of MHC class II$^+$ leukocytes in the pancreata of rodents indicates that, as in many other nonlymphoid tissues, MHC class II$^+$ leukocytes are not observed until the time of parturition but that adult-equivalent populations are developed by 1 month postpartum (Fujiya *et al.*, 1985). However, in larger animals, DC development in the pancreas occurs at an earlier time. In adult pigs, MHC class II$^+$ cells are present in both endocrine and exocrine pancreatic tissues (Shienvold *et al.*, 1986) and rare MHC class II$^+$ leukocytes were observed in the exocrine portion as early as day 48 of gestation (Fujiya *et al.*, 1985). In humans, the presence of MHC class II$^+$ presumptive DC in the pancreas has been widely reported in fetuses between 14 and 20 weeks of gestation (Danilvos *et al.*, 1982; Hofman *et al.*, 1984; Oliver *et al.*, 1988; Koo Seen Lin *et al.*, 1991) but may develop as early as 8 gestational weeks, where the density of cells has been reported as 10 per × 100 microscope field (Koo Seen Lin *et al.*, 1991). The rate of DC development has been reported to undergo a rapid acceleration between 13 and 16 weeks of gestation where cell density increased from 10 per × 100 field to 30 per field (Hofman *et al.*, 1984; Koo Seen Lin *et al.*, 1991). The distinct populations of macrophages and DC described in adults have also been observed in fetal pancreata (Koo Seen Lin *et al.*, 1991; Jansen *et al.*, 1993).

Function

The functional activity of pancreatic DC has not been examined directly and it is unclear whether these cells express T cell-stimulatory activity equivalent to that of DC from other nonlymphoid tissue sites. A restriction on the interpretation of what little data are available is that many of the studies have been performed on diabetic or prediabetic rodents used as models of human disease. Enhanced DC–T cell clustering compared with control mice has been reported in the lymph nodes draining the pancreas of the nonobese diabetic (NOD) mouse (Clare-Salzler and Muller, 1992). The implications of this phenomenon are unclear, as DC derived *in vitro* from monocytes of humans with type 1 diabetes exhibit reduced maturational and functional potential (Jansen *et al.*, 1995). Similarly, macrophages generated *in vitro* from bone marrow of NOD mice are reported to exhibit defects in differentiation and function (Serreze *et al.*, 1993). Alternatively, following exposure to macrophage-derived factors, splenic DC from BB rats have been reported to exhibit enhanced stimulatory activity compared to those from nondiabetic WF rats (Tafuri *et al.*, 1993). Surprisingly, adoptive transfer of pancreatic lymph node DC from diabetic NOD mice to prediabetic NOD mice has been shown to limit the subsequent development of diabetes

(Clare-Salzler *et al.*, 1992). It is postulated that these findings are a consequence of interactions between antigen-specific T cells and adoptively transferred 'defective' DC bearing diabetogenic peptides which result in generation of regulatory T cells.

The strongest evidence that pancreatic DC of normal animals exhibit T cell stimulatory activity has been provided by transplantation studies. Depletion of MHC class II$^+$ presumptive DC from islets by anti-MHC class II mAb pretreatment (Faustman *et al.*, 1981; Lloyd *et al.*, 1987) or anti-DC mAb pretreatment (Faustman *et al.*, 1984; Faustman *et al.*, 1985) prior to allotransplantation extends the subsequent survival time of these pancreatic islet grafts. Likewise, when pancreatic islets were treated with UV irradiation (which inhibits the allostimulatory capacity of DC) prior to allotransplantation, the survival time of the grafts was extended (Lau *et al.*, 1984a,b).

Disease

DC have been described as a prominent cell type in the leukocytic infiltrate observed in pancreatic islets of rodent models of diabetes. In prediabetic BB rats, MHC class II$^+$ dendriform cells were observed to accumulate at the margins of islets of Langerhans in elevated numbers prior to the infiltration of this site by T lymphocytes and macrophages (Voorbij *et al.*, 1989; Ziegler *et al.*, 1992). Similar observations have been reported in NOD mice, where MHC class II$^+$ DC were the first hematopoietic cells to accumulate around and infiltrate into pancreatic islets during the early stages of insulitis (Jansen *et al.*, 1994) and cellular infiltrates may be organized around DEC-205$^+$ DC (Lo *et al.*, 1993). It has been suggested that the accumulation of DC around and within the islets may result in diabetogenic antigen transfer to the pancreas-draining lymph nodes, and that the subsequent stimulation of autoreactive T cells may be an important initiating mechanism of insulitis (Jansen *et al.*, 1994). Alternatively, DC could exhibit direct anti-β-cell activity mediated by IL-1 (Mandrup-Poulson *et al.*, 1986; Mandrup-Poulson *et al.*, 1989), nitric oxide (Stassi *et al.*, 1997), or Fas ligand (Itoh *et al.*, 1997), expressed or secreted by DC (Nagelkerken and van Breda Vriesman, 1986; Heufler *et al.*, 1992; Lu *et al.*, 1996b; Süss and Shortman, 1996, Lu *et al.*, 1997).

FUTURE DIRECTIONS

Further understanding of the unique aspects of DC within each of the solid organs discussed may aid in understanding of disease pathogenesis and in development of future strategies to combat disease or alleviate unwanted or inappropriate immunoinflammatory responses.

Evidence is accumulating of a key role for the liver in oral tolerance (Yang *et al.*, 1994). While the relative roles of Kupffer cells and liver DC are unclear (Roland *et al.*, 1993; Gorczynski *et al.*, 1996), there is evidence that DC may be important (Gorczynski *et al.*, 1996). Understanding of the potential of liver DC to selectively activate T cell subsets may be crucial to understanding the potential role of the liver in this phenomenon.

The effects of agents which cause accumulation of elevated numbers of DC in liver, heart, kidney, and pancreas may provide effective strategies for combating the problems of infectious and neoplastic diseases affecting these organs. Currently, a prime candidate here is Flt3-L which has been demonstrated to mediate antitumor activity *in vivo*, through as yet poorly understood mechanisms (Lynch *et al.*, 1997). Alternatively, in-depth understanding of the chemotactic signals, such as those provided by chemokines or other factors (Sozzani *et al.*, 1995; Sozzani *et al.*, 1997), that result in recruitment of DC progenitors to parenchymal organs may help identify signals that augment the DC content of individual organs while leaving others unaffected. Conversely, insight into the signals that activate or mobilize DC, or allow these cells to process and effectively present antigen in these tissues, may allow development of strategies which can alleviate autoimmune disorders or block the inherent allogeneic signals provided by transplanted organs via either the direct or indirect antigen presentation pathways.

It is therefore clear that while liver, kidney, heart, and pancreas present considerable challenges to workers investigating the nature of nonlymphoid tissue DC, they provide a repository from which many novel and useful findings may be drawn.

ACKNOWLEDGMENTS

These studies are supported by National Institutes of Health grants DK 49745 and AI 41011 to A.W.T. Much of the published information described relating to the liver has been contributed by our colleagues Drs Lina Lu and Maureen Drakes. We also acknowledge the contribution of Rajan Patel to the immunohistochemical and DC enumeration data presented.

REFERENCES

Ardavin, C., Wu., L., Li, C.L. and Shortman, K. (1993). Thymic dendritic cells and T-cells develop simultaneously in the thymus from a common precursor population. *Nature* **362**, 761–763.

Austyn, J.M. (1996). New insights into the mobilization and phagocytic activity of dendritic cells. *J. Exp. Med.* **183**, 1287–1292.

Austyn, J.M., Hankins, D.F., Larsen, C.P., Morris, P.J., Rao, A.S. and Roake, J.A. (1994). Isolation and characterization of dendritic cells from mouse heart and kidney. *J. Immunol.* **152**, 2401.

Ballardini, G., Fallani, M., Bianchi, F.B. and Pisi, E. (1989) Antigen presenting cells in liver biopsies from patients with primary biliary cirrhosis. *Autoimmunity* **3**, 135–144.

Bardadin, K.A. and Desmet, V.J. (1984) Interdigitating and dendritic reticulum cells in chronic active hepatitis. *Histopathology* **8**, 657–688.

Bishop, G.A., Sun, J., DeCruz, D.J., Rokahr, K.L., Sedgwick, J.D., Sheil, A.G.R., Gallagher, N.D. and McCaughan, G.W. (1996). Tolerance to rat liver allografts: III. Donor cell migration and tolerance-associated cytokine production in peripheral lymphoid tissues. *J. Immunol.* **156**, 4925–4931.

Brasel, K., McKenna, H.J., Morrissey, P.J., Charrier, K., Morris, A.E., Lee, C.C., Williams, D.E. and Lyman, S.D. (1996). Hematologic effects of flt3 ligand in vivo in mice. *Blood* **88**, 2004–2012.

Brenan, M. and Puklavec, M. (1992). The MRC OX-62 antigen; a useful marker in the purification of rat veiled cells with the biochemical properties of an integrin. *J. Exp. Med.* **175**, 1457–1465.

Burris, D.E., Gruel, S.M. and Rao, V.K. (1989). Persistence of dendritic cells and allograft antigenicity despite prolonged interim hosting of cardiac allografts in rats. *Transplantation* **47**, 1085–1087.

Chen, H.D., Ma, C.L., Yuan, J.T., Wang, Y.K. and Silvers, W.K. (1986) Occurrence of donor Langerhans cells in mouse and rat chimeras and their replacement in skin grafts. *J. Invest. Dermatol.* **86**, 630–633.

Clare-Salzler, M. and Mullen, Y. (1992). Marked dendritic cell–T cell cluster formation in the pancreatic lymph node of the non-obese diabetic mouse. *Immunology* **76**, 478–484.

Clare-Salzler, M.J., Brooks, J., Chai, A., Van Herle, K. and Anderson, C. (1992). Prevention of diabetes in nonobese diabetic mice by dendritic cell transfer. *J. Clin. Invest.* **90**, 741–748.

Cumberbatch, M. and Kimber, I. (1995). Tumour necrosis factor-alpha is required for accumulation of dendritic cells in draining lymph nodes and for optimal contact sensitization. *Immunology* **84**, 31–35.

Cumberbatch, M., Dearman, R.J. and Kimber, I. (1997). Interleukin 1 beta and the stimulation of Langerhans cell migration: comparisons with tumour necrosis factor alpha. *Arch. Dermatol. Res.* **289**, 277–284.

Czernielewski, J.M. and Demarchez, M. (1987). Further evidence for the self-reproducing capacity of Langerhans cells in human skin. *J. Invest. Dermatol.* **88**, 17–20.

Czernielewski, J., Vaigot, P. and Prunieras, M. (1985). Epidermal Langerhans cells—a cycling cell population. *J. Invest. Dermatol.* **84**, 424–426.

Daar, A.S., Fuggle, S.V., Hart, D.N.J., Dalchau, R., Abdulaziz, Z., Fabre, J.W., Ting, A. and Morris, P.J. (1983). Demonstration and phenotypic characterization of HLA-DR-positive interstitial dendritic cells widely distributed in human connective tissues. *Transplant. Proc.* **15**, 311–315.

Daar, A.S., Fuggle, S.V., Fabre, J.W., Ting, A. and Morris, P.J. (1984). The detailed distribution of MHC class II antigens in normal human organs. *Transplantation* **38**, 293–298.

Danilovs, J.A., Hofman, F.M., Taylor, C.R. and Brown, J. (1982). Expression of HLA-DR antigens in human fetal pancreas tissue. *Diabetes* **31** (Suppl.), 23–28.

Darden, A.G., Forbes, R.D.C., Darden, P.M. and Guttmann, R.D. (1990). The effects of genetics and age on expression of MHC class II and CD4 antigens on rat cardiac interstitial dendritic cells. *Cell. Immunol.* **126**, 322–330.

Demetris, A.J., Sever, C., Kakizoe, S., Oguma, S., Starzl, T.E. and Jaffe, R. (1989). S100 protein positive dendritic cells in primary biliary cirrhosis and other chronic inflammatory liver disease. Relevance to pathogenesis? *Am. J. Pathol.* **4**, 741–747.

Demetris, A.J., Qian, S., Sun, H., Fung, J.J., Yagihashi, A., Murase, N., Iwaki, Y., Gambrell, B. and Strazl, T.E. (1991). Early events in liver allograft rejection. Delineation of sites of simultaneous intragraft and recipient lymphoid tissue sensitization. *Am. J. Pathol.* **138**, 609–618.

Drakes, M.L., Lu, L., Subbotin, V.M. and Thomson, A.W. (1997a). In vivo administration of flt3 ligand markedly stimulates generation of dendritic cell progenitors from mouse liver. *J. Immunol.* **159**, 4268–4278.

Drakes, M.L., Lu, L., McKenna, H.J. and Thomson, A.W. (1997b). The influence of collagen, fibronectin and laminin on the maturation of dendritic cell progenitors propagated from normal or Flt3-ligand-treated mouse liver. *Adv. Exp. Biol. Med.* **417**, 115–120.

Faustman, D., Hauptfeld, V., Lacy, P. and Davie, J. (1981). Prolongation of murine islet allograft survival by pretreatment of islets with antibody directed to Ia determinants. *Proc. Natl Acad. Sci. USA* **78**, 5156–5159.

Faustman, D., Kraus, P., Lacy, P.E., Finke, E.H. and Davie, J.M. (1982) Survival of heart allografts in nonimmunosuppressed murine recipients by pretreatment of the donor tissue with anti-Ia antibodies. *Transplantation* **34**, 302–305.

Faustman, D.L., Steinman, R.M., Gebel, H.M., Hauptfeld, V., Davie, J.M. and Lacy, P.E. (1984). Prevention of rejection of murine islet allografts by pretreatment with anti-dendritic cell antibody. *Proc. Natl Acad. Sci. USA* **81**, 3864–3868.

Faustman, D.L., Steinman, R.M., Gebel, H.M., Hauptfeld, V., Davie, J.M. and Lacy, P.E. (1985) Prevention of mouse islet allograft rejection by elimination of intraislet dendritic cells. *Transplant. Proc.* **17**, 420–422.

Forbes, R.D.C., Parfrey, N.A., Gomersall, M., Darden, A.G. and Guttmann, R.D. (1986). Dendritic cell–lymphoid cell aggregation and major histocompatibility antigen expression during rat cardiac allograft rejection. *J. Exp. Med.* **164**, 1239–1258.

Forsum, U., Klareskog, L. and Peterson, P.A. (1979). Distribution of Ia-antigen-like molecules on non-lymphoid tissues. *Scand. J. Immunol.* **9**, 343–349.

Fujiya, H., Danilovs, J., Brown, J. and Mullen, Y. (1985). Species differences in dendritic cell distribution in pancreas during fetal development. *Transplant Proc.* **17**, 414–416.

Gaudecker, B.V., Petersen, R., Epstein, M., Kaden, J. and Oesterwitz, H. (1993). Down-regulation of MHC-expression on dendritic cells in rat kidney grafts by PUVA pretreatment. In: *Dendritic Cells in Fundamental and Clinical Immunology* (eds E.W.A. Kamperdijk, P. Niewenhuis, E.C.M. Hoefsmit). Plenum Press, New York, pp. 495–499.

Gebel, H.M., Yasunami, Y., Diekgraefe, B., Davie, J.M. and Lacy, P.E. (1983) IA-bearing cells within isolated canine islets. *Transplantation* **36**, 346–348.

Gorczynski, R.M., Cohen, Z., Fu, X.-M., Hua, Z., Sun, Y. and Chen, Z. (1996). Interleukin-13, in combination with anti-interleukin-12, increases graft prolongation after portal venous immunization with cultured allogeneic bone marrow-derived dendritic cells. *Transplantation* **62**, 1592–1600.

Grouard, G., Rissoan, M.C., Filgueira, L., Banchereau, J. and Liu, Y.J. (1997). The enigmatic plasmacytoid T cells develop into dendritic cells with interleukin (IL)-3 and CD40-ligand. *J. Exp. Med.* **185**, 1101–1111.

Hancock, W.W. and Atkins, R.C. (1984). Immunohistologic analysis of the cell surface antigens of human dendritic cells using monoclonal antibodies. *Transplant. Proc.* **16**, 963–967.

Hardonk, M.J., Dijkhuis, F.W.J., Grond, J., Koudstaal, J. and Poppema, S. (1986). Evidence for a migratory capability of rat Kupffer cells to portal tracts and hepatic lymph nodes. *Virchows Arch. B: Cell Pathol.* **51**, 429–442.

Hart, D.N.J. and Fabre, J.W. (1981a). Demonstration and characterization of Ia-positive dendritic cells in the interstitial connective tissues of rat heart and other tissues, but not brain. *J. Exp. Med.* **153**, 347–361.

Hart, D.N.J. and Fabre, J.W. (1981b). Major histocompatibility complex antigens in rat kidney, ureter, and bladder. *Transplantation* **31**, 318–325.

Hart, D.N.J. and McKenzie, J.L. (1990). Interstitial dendritic cells. *Int. Rev. Immunol.* **6**, 127–138.

Hart, D.N.J., Fuggle, S.V., Williams, K.A., Fabre, J.W., Ting, A. and Morris, P.J. (1981). Localization of HLA-ABC and DR antigens in human kidney. *Transplantation* **31**, 428–433.

Heufler, C., Topar, G., Koch, F., Trockenbacher, B., Kampgen, E., Romani, N. and Schuler, G. (1992). Cytokine gene expression in murine epidermal cell suspensions: interleukin 1 beta and macrophage inflammatory protein 1 alpha are selectively expressed in Langerhans cells but are differentially regulated in culture. *J. Exp. Med.* **176**, 1221–1226.

Hofman, F.M., Danilovs, J.A. and Taylor, C.R. (1984). HLA-DR (Ia)-positive dendritic-like cells in human fetal nonlymphoid tissues. *Transplantation* **37**, 590–594.

Hutchens, L.H., Sagebiel, R.W. and Clarke, M.A. (1971). Oral epithelial dendritic cells of the rhesus monkey. Histological demonstration, fine structure and quantitative distribution. *J. Invest. Dermatol.* **56**, 325–336.

Inaba, K. and Steinman, R.M. (1986). Accessory cell–T lymphocyte interactions. Antigen-dependent and -independent clustering. *J. Exp. Med.* **163**, 247–261.

Inaba, K., Schuler, G., Witmer, M.D., Valinksy, J., Atassi, B. and Steinman, R.M. (1986). Immunologic properties of purified epidermal Langerhans cells. Distinct requirements for stimulation of unprimed and sensitized T lymphocytes. *J. Exp. Med.* **164**, 605–613.

Inaba, K., Romani, N. and Steinman, R.M. (1989). An antigen-independent contact mechanism as an early step in T cell-proliferative responses to dendritic cells. *J. Exp. Med.* **170**, 527–542.

Inaba, K., Inaba, M., Romani, N., Aya, H., Deguchi, M., Ikehara, S., Muramatsu, S. and Steinman, R.M. (1992a). Generation of large numbers of dendritic cells from mouse bone marrow cultures supplemented with granulocyte/macrophage colony-stimulating factor. *J. Exp. Med.* **176**, 1693–1702.

Inaba, K., Steinman, R.M., Pack, M.W., Aya, H., Inaba, M., Sudo, T., Wolpe, S. and Schuler, G. (1992b). Identification of proliferating dendritic cell precursors in mouse blood. *J. Exp. Med.* **175**, 1157–1167.

Inaba, K., Witmer-Pack, M., Inaba, M., Hathcock, K.S., Sakuta, H., Azuma, M., Yagita, H., Okumura, K., Linsley, P.S., Ikehara, S., Muramatsu, S., Hodes, R.J. and Steinman, R.M. (1994). The tissue distribution of the B7-2 costimulator in mice: abundant expression on dendritic cells in situ and during maturation in vitro. *J. Exp. Med.* **180**, 1849–1860.

Itoh, N., Imagawa, A., Hanafusa, T., Waguri, M., Yamamoto, K., Iwahashi, H., Moriwaki M., Nakajima, H., Miyagawa, J., Namba, M., Makino, S., Nagata, S., Kono, N. and Matsuzawa, Y. (1997). Requirement of Fas for the development of autoimmune diabetes in nonobese diabetic mice. *J. Exp. Med.* **186**, 613–618.

Jansen, A., Voorbij, H.A.M., Jeucken, P.H.M., Bruining, G.J., Hooijkaas, H. and Drexhage, H.A. (1993). An immunohistochemical study on organized lymphoid cell infiltrates in fetal and neonatal pancreases. *Autoimmunity* **15**, 31–38.

Jansen, A., Homo-Delarche, F., Hooijkaas, H., Leenen, P.J., Dardenne, M. and Drexhage, H.A. (1994). Immunohistochemical characterization of monocytes-macrophages and dendritic cells involved in the initiation of the insulitis and β-cell destruction in NOD mice. *Diabetes* **43**, 667–675.

Jansen, A., van Hagen, M. and Drexhage, H.A. (1995). Defective maturation and function of antigen-presenting cells in type 1 diabetes. *Lancet* **345**, 491–492.

Kaissling, B. and Le Hir, M. (1994). Characterization and distribution of interstitital cell types in the renal cortex of rats. *Kidney Int.* **45**, 709–720.

Kaji, K., Nakanuma, Y., Harada, K., Tsuneyama, K., Kaneko, S. and Kobayashi, K. (1997). Dendritic cells in portal tracts in chronic hepatitis C and primary billiary cirrhosis with relevance to bile duct damage—an immunohistochemical study. *Hepatol. Res.* **8**, 1–12.

Kampgen, E., Koch, N., Koch, F., Stoger, P., Heufler, C., Schuler, G. and Romani, N. (1991). Class II major histocompatibility complex molecules of murine dendritic cells: synthesis, sialylation of invariant chain, and antigen processing capacity are down-regulated upon culture. *Proc. Natl Acad. Sci. USA* **88**, 3014–3018.

Kerschbaum, H.H., Singh, S.K. and Hermann, A. (1995). Lymphoid tissue in the kidney of the musk shrew, *Suncus murinus. Tissue & Cell* **27**, 421–424.

Klinkert, W.E.F., LaBadie, J.H. and Bowers, W.E. (1982). Accessory and stimulating properties of dendritic cells and macrophages isolated from various rat tissues. *J. Exp. Med.* **156**, 1–19.

Koo Seen Lin, L.C., Welsh, K.I., Koffman, C.G. and McColl, I. (1991). The immunology of the human foetal pancreas aged 8–13 gestational weeks. *Transplant Int.* **4**, 195–199.

Kronin, V., Winkel, K., Süss, G., Kelso, A., Heath, W., Kirberg, J., von Boehmer, H. and Shortman, K. (1996). A subclass of dendritic cells regulates the response of naive CD8 T cells by limiting their IL-2 production. *J. Immunol.* **157**, 3819–3827.

Kudo, S., Matsuno, K., Ezaki, T. and Ogawa, M. (1997). A novel migration pathway for rat dendritic cells from the blood: hepatic sinusoids–lymph translocation. *J. Exp. Med.* **185**, 777–784.

Larsen, C.P., Morris, P.J. and Austyn, J.M. (1990). Migration of dendritic leukocytes from cardiac allografts into host spleens: a novel pathway for initiation of rejection. *J. Exp. Med.* **171**, 307–314.

Lau, H., Reemtsma, K. and Hardy, M.A. (1984a). Prologation of rat islet allograft survival by direct ultraviolet irrradiation of the graft. *Science* **223**, 607–609.

Lau, H., Reemtsma, K. and Hardy, M.A. (1984b). The use of direct ultraviolet irradiation and cyclosporine in facilitating indefinite pancreatic islet allograft acceptance. *Transplantation* **38**, 566–569.

Lautenschlager, I., Halttunen, J. and Hayry, P. (1988). Characteristics of dendritic cells in rat liver. *Transplantation* **45**, 936–939.

Lechler, R.I. and Batchelor, J.R. (1982). Restoration of immunogenicity to passenger cell-depleted kidney allografts by the addition of donor strain dendritic cells. *J. Exp. Med.* **155**, 31–41.

Leprini, A., Valente, U., Celada, F., Fontana, I., Barocci, S. and Nocera, A. (1987). Morphology, cytochemical features, and membrane phenotype of HLA-DR$^+$ interstitial cells in the human pancreas. *Pancreas* **2**, 127–135.

Leszczynski, D., Renkonen, R. and Hayry, P. (1985a). Localization and turnover rate of rat renal 'dendritic' cells. *Scand. J. Immunol.* **21**, 355–360.

Leszczynski, D., Renkonen, R. and Hayry, P. (1985b). Turnover of dendritic cells in rat heart. *Scand. J. Immunol.* **22**, 351–355.

Leszczynski, D., Ferry, B., Schellekens, H., V.D. Meide, P. and Hayry, P. (1986). Antagonistic effects of γ interferon and steroids on tissue antigenicity. *J. Exp. Med.* **164**, 1470–1477.

Liu, L.M. and MacPherson, G.G. (1995a). Antigen processing: cultured lymph-borne dendritic cells can process and present native protein antigens. *Immunology* **84**, 241–246.

Liu, L.M. and MacPherson, G.G. (1995b). Rat intestinal dendritic cells: immunostimulatory potency and phenotypic characterization. *Immunology* **85**, 88–93.

Lloyd, D.M., Franklin, W., Buckingham, F., Buckingham, M., Rizzner, J.S., Stuart, F.P. and Thistlewaite, J.R., Jr. (1987). Ex vivo perfusion of the intact rat pancreas with anti-class II monoclonal antibody: labeling of dendritic cells. *Transplant. Proc.* **19**, 620–623.

Lo, D., Reilly, C.R., Scott, B., Liblau, R., McDevitt, H.O. and Burkly, L.C. (1993). Antigen-presenting cells in adoptively transferred and spontaneous autoimmune diabetes. *Eur. J. Immunol.* **23**, 1693–1698.

Lu, L., Woo, J., Rao, A.S., Li, Y., Watkins, S.C., Qian, S., Starzl, T.E., Demetris, A.J. and Thomson, A.W. (1994). Propagation of dendritic cell progenitors from normal mouse liver using granulocyte/macrophage colony-stimulating factor and their maturational development in the presence of type-1 collagen. *J. Exp. Med.* **179**, 1823–1834.

Lu, W.-G., Pipeleers, D.G., Kloppel, G. and Bouwens, L. (1996a). Comparative immunocytochemical study of MHC class II expression in human donor pancreas and isolated islets. *Virchows Arch.* **429**, 205–211.

Lu, L., Bonham, C.A., Chambers, F.D., Watkins, S.C., Hoffman, R.A., Simmons, R.L. and Thomson, A.W. (1996b). Induction of nitric oxide synthase in mouse dendritic cells by IFN-γ, endotoxin, and interaction with allogeneic T cells: nitric oxide production is associated with dendritic cell apoptosis. *J. Immunol.* **157**, 3577–3586.

Lu, L., Qian, S., Hershberger, P.A., Rudert, W.A., Lynch, D.H. and Thomson, A.W. (1997). Fas ligand (CD95L) and B7 expression on dendritic cells provide counter-regulatory signals for T cell survival and proliferation. *J. Immunol.* **158**, 5676–5684.

Lynch, D.H., Andreasen, A., Maraskovsky, E., Whitmore, J., Miller, R.E. and Schuh, J.C.L. (1997). Flt3 ligand induces tumor regression and antitumor immune responses in vivo. *Nature Medicine* **3**, 625–631.

MacPherson, G.G., Jenkins, C.D., Stein, M.J. and Edwards, C. (1995). Endotoxin-mediated dendritic cell release from the intestine. Characterization of released dendritic cells and TNF dependence. *J. Immunol.* **154**, 1317–1322.

Maguire, J.E., Gresser, I., Williams, A.H., Kielpinski, G.L. and Colvin, R.B. (1990). Modulation of expression of MHC antigens in the kidneys of mice by murine interferon-α/β. *Transplantation* **49**, 130–134.

Mandrup-Poulsen, T., Bendtzen, K., Nerup, J., Dinerello, C.A., Svenson, M. and Nielsen, J.H. (1986). Affinity purified human interleukin 1 is cytotoxic to isolated islets of Langerhans. *Diabetologia* **29**, 63–67.

Mandrup-Poulsen, T., Helqvist, S., Molvig, J., Wogensen, L.D. and Nerup, J. (1989). Cytokines as immune effector molecules in autoimmune endocrine diseases with special reference to insulin-dependent diabetes mellitus. *Autoimmunity* **4**, 191–218.

Maraskovsky, E., Brasel, K., Teepe, M., Roux, E.R., Lyman, S.D., Shortman, K. and McKenna, H.J. (1996). Dramatic increase in the numbers of functionally mature dendritic cells in Flt3 ligand-treated mice: multiple dendritic cell subpopulations identified. *J. Exp. Med.* **184**, 1953–1962.

Maric, I., Holt, P.G., Perdue, M.H. and Bienenstock, J. (1996). Class II MHC antigen (Ia)-bearing dendritic cells in the epithelium of the rat intestine. *J. Immunol.* **156**, 1408–1414.

Matsuno, K., Miyakawa, K., Ezaki, T. and Kotani, M. (1990) The liver lymphatics as a migratory pathway of macrophages from the sinusoids to the celiac lymph nodes in the rat. *Arch. Histol. Cytol.* **53** (Suppl.), 179–187.

Matsuno, K., Kudo, S., Ezaki, T. and Miyakawa, K. (1995). Isolation of dendritic cells in the rat liver lymph. *Transplantation* **60**, 765–768.

Matsuno, K., Ezaki, T., Kudo, S. and Uehara, Y. (1996). A life stage of particle-laden rat dendritic cells in vivo: their terminal division, active phagocytosis, and translocation from the liver to the draining lymph. *J. Exp. Med.* **183**, 1865–1878.

McKenzie, J.L., Beard, M.E. and Hart, D.N.J. (1984a). Depletion of kidney dendritic cells prolongs graft survival. *Transplant. Proc.* **16**, 948–951.

McKenzie, J.L., Beard, M.E.J. and Hart, D.N.J. (1984b). The effect of donor pretreatment on interstitial dendritic cell content and rat cardiac allograft survival. *Transplantation* **38**, 371–376.

Metlay, J.P., Witmer-Pack, M.D., Agger, R., Crowley, M.T., Lawless, D. and Steinman, R.M. (1990). The distinct leukocyte integrins of mouse spleen dendritic cells as identified with new hamster monoclonal antibodies. *J. Exp. Med.* **171**, 1753–1771.

Nagelkerken, L.M. and van Breda Vriesman, P.J.C. (1986). Membrane-associated IL 1-like activity on rat dendritic cells. *J. Immunol.* **136**, 2164–2170.

Natali, P.G., Nicotra, M.R., Giacomini, P., Pellegrino, M.A. and Ferrone, S. (1981). Ontogeny of murine I-A^k antigens in tissue of nonlymphoid origin. *Immunogenetics* **14**, 359–365.

Natali, P.G., Segatto, O., Ferrone, S., Tosi, R. and Corte, G. (1984). Differential tissue distribution and ontogeny of DC-1 and HLA-DR antigens. *Immunogenetics* **19**, 109–116.

Nussenzweig, M.C. and Steinman, R.M. (1980). Contribution of dendritic cells to stimulation of the murine syngeneic mixed lymphocyte reaction. *J. Exp. Med.* **152**, 1196–1212.

O'Doherty, U., Peng, M., Gezelter, S., Swiggrad, W.J., Betjes, M., Bhardwaj, N. and Steinman, R.M. (1994). Human blood contains two subsets of dendritic cells, one immunologically mature and the other immature. *Immunology.* **82**, 487–493.

Oguma, S., Banner, B., Zerbe, T., Starzl, T. and Demetris, A.J. (1988). Participation of dendritic cells in vascular lesions of chronic rejection of human allografts. *Lancet* **2** (8617), 933–935.

Oguma, S., Zerbe, T., Banner, B., Belle, S., Starzl, T.E. and Demetris, A.J. (1989). Chronic liver allograft rejection and obliterative arteriopathy: possible pathogenic mechanisms. *Transplant. Proc.* **21**, 2203–2207.

Oliver, A.M., Thomson, A.W., Sewell, H.F. and Abramovich, D.R. (1988). Major histocompatibility complex (MHC) class II antigen (HLA-DR, DQ, and DP) expression in human fetal endocrine organs and gut. *Scand. J. Immunol.* **27**, 731–737.

Prickett, T.C.R., McKenzie, J.L. and Hart, D.N.J. (1988). Characterization of interstitial dendritic cells in human liver. *Transplantation* **46**, 754–761.

Puré, E., Inaba, K., Crowley, M.T., Tardelli, L., Witmer-Pack, M.D., Ruberti, G., Fathman, G. and Steinman, R.M. (1990). Antigen processing by epidermal Langerhans cells correlates with the level of biosynthesis of major histocompatibility complex class II molecules and expression of invariant chain. *J. Exp. Med.* **172**, 1459–1469.

Rastellini, C., Lu, L., Ricordi, C., Starzl, T.E., Rao, A.S. and Thomson, A.W. (1995). Granulocyte/macrophage colony-stimulating factor-stimulated hepatic dendritic cell progenitors prolong pancreatic islet allograft survival. *Transplantation* **60**, 1366–1370.

Reis e Sousa, C., Stahl, P.D. and Austyn, J.M. (1993). Phagocytosis of antigens by Langerhans cells in vitro. *J. Exp. Med.* **178**, 509–519.

Roake, J.A., Rao, A.S., Morris, P.J., Larsen, C.P., Hankins, D.F. and Austyn, J.M. (1995a). Dendritic cell loss from nonlymphoid tissues after systemic administration of lipopolysaccharide, tumor necrosis factor, and interleukin 1. *J. Exp. Med.* **181**, 2237–2247.

Roake, J.A., Rao, A.S., Morris, P.J., Larsen, C.P., Hankins, D.F. and Austyn, J.M. (1995b). Systemic lipopolysaccharide recruits dendritic cell progenitors to nonlymphoid tissues. *Transplantation* **59**, 1319–1324.

Roland, C.R., Mangino, M.J., Duffy, B.F. and Flye, M.W. (1993). Lymphocyte suppression by Kupffer cells prevents portal venous tolerance induction: a study of macrophage function after intravenous gadolinium. *Transplantation* **55**, 1151–1158.

Romani, N., Koide, S., Crowley, M., Witmer-Pack, M., Livingstone, A.M., Fathman, C.G., Inaba, K. and Steinman, R.M. (1989). Presentation of exogenous protein antigens by dendritic cells to T cell clones. Intact protein is presented best by immature, epidermal Langerhans cells. *J. Exp. Med.* **169**, 1169–1178.

Saleem, M., Sawyer, G.J., Schofield, R.A., Seymour, N.D., Gustafsson, K. and Fabre, J.W. (1997). Discordant expression of major histocompatibility complex class II antigens and invariant chain in interstitial dendritic cells. *Transplantation* **63**, 1134–1138.

Saunders, D., Lucas, K., Ismaili, J., Wu, L., Maraskovsky, E., Dunn, A. and Shortman, K. (1996). Dendritic cell development in culture from thymic precursor cells in the absence of granulocyte/macrophage colony-stimulating factor. *J. Exp. Med.* **184**, 2185–2196.

Schon-Hegrad, M.A., Oliver, J., McMenamin, P.G. and Holt, P.G. (1991). Studies on the density, distribution, and surface phenotype of intraepithelial class II major histocompatibility complex antigen (Ia)-bearing dendritic cells (DC) in the conducting airways. *J. Exp. Med.* **173**, 1345–1356.

Schuler, G. and Steinman, R.M. (1985). Murine epidermal Langerhans cells mature into potent immunostimulatory dendritic cells in vitro. *J. Exp. Med.* **161**, 526–546.

Serreze, D.V., Gaskins, H.R. and Leiter, E.H. (1993). Defects in the differentiation and function of antigen presenting cells in NOD/Lt mice. *J. Immunol.* **150**, 2534–2543.

Shienvold, F.L., Alejandro, R. and Mintz, D.H. (1986). Identification of Ia-bearing cells in rat, dog, pig, and human islets of Langerhans. *Transplantation* **41**, 364–372.

Shurin, M.R., Pandharipande, P.P., Zorina, T.D., Haluszczak, C., Subbotin, V.M., Hunter, O., Brumfield, A., Storkus, W.J., Maraskovsky, E. and Lotze, M.T. (1997). Flt3 Ligand induces the generation of functionally active dendritic cells in mice. *Cell. Immunol.* **179**, 174–184.

Silberberg-Sinakin, I., Baer, R.L. and Thorbecke, G.J. (1978). Langerhans cells: a review of their nature with emphasis on their immunological function. *Progr. Allergy.* **24**, 268–294.

Skoskiewicz, M.J., Colvin, R.B., Schneeberger, E.F. and Russell, P.S. (1985). Widespread and selective induction of major histocompatibility complex-determined antigens in vivo by γ interferon. *J. Exp. Med.* **162**, 1645–1664.

Sozzani, S., Sallusto, F., Luini, W., Zhou, D., Piemonti, L., Allovena, P., Van Damme, J.V., Valitutti, S., Lanzavecchia, A. and Montovani, A. (1995). Migration of dendritic cells in response to formyl peptides, C5a, and a distinct set of chemokines. *J. Immunol.* **155**, 3292–3295.

Sozzani, S., Luini, W., Borsatti, A., Polentarutti, N., Zhou, D., Piemonti, L., D'Amico, G., Power, C.A., Wells, T.N.C., Gobbi, M., Allavena, P. and Mantovani, A. (1997). Receptor expression and responsiveness of human dendritic cells to a defined set of CC and CXC chemokines. *J. Immunol.* **159**, 1993–2000.

Spencer, S.C. and Fabre, J.W. (1990). Characterization of the tissue macrophage and the interstitial dendritic cell as distinct leukocytes normally resident in the connective tissue of rat heart. *J. Exp. Med.* **171**, 1841–1851.

Stassi, G., Demaria, R., Trucco, G., Rudert, W., Testi, R., Galluzzo, A., Giordano, C. and Trucco, M. (1997). Nitric oxide primes pancreatic beta cells for Fas-mediated destruction in insulin-dependent diabetes mellitus. *J. Exp. Med.* **186**, 1193–1200.

Steiniger, B., Klempnauer, J. and Wonigeit, K. (1984). Phenotype and histological distribution of interstitital dendritic cells in the rat pancreas, liver, heart, and kidney. *Transplantation* **38**, 169–175.

Steinman, R.M. (1991). The dendritic cell and its role in immunogenicity. *Annu. Rev. Immunol.* **9**, 271–296.

Steinman, R.M. and Cohn, Z.A. (1973). Identification of a novel cell type in peripheral lymphoid organs of mice. I. Morphology, quantitation, tissue distribution. *J. Exp. Med.* **137**, 1142–1162.

Steinman, R.M. and Cohn, Z.A. (1974). Identification of a novel cell type in peripheral lymphoid organs of mice. II. Functional properties in vitro. *J. Exp. Med.* **139**, 380–397.

Steinman, R.M., Lustig, D.S. and Cohn, Z.A. (1974). Identification of a novel cell type in peripheral lymphoid organs of mice. 3. Functional properties in vivo. *J. Exp. Med.* **139**, 1431–1435.

Steinman, R.M. and Witmer, M.D. (1979). Lymphoid dendritic cells are potent stimulators of the primary mixed leucocyte reaction in mice. *Proc. Natl Acad. Sci. USA* **75**, 5132–5136.

Steinman, R.M., Inaba, K. and Austyn, J.M. (1993). Donor-derived chimerism in recipients of organ transplants. *Hepatology* **17**, 1153–1156.

Stein-Oakley, A.N., Jablonski, P., Kraft, N., Biguzas, M., Howard, B.O., Marshall, V.C. and Thomson, N.M. (1991). Differential irradiation effects on rat interstitial dendritic cells. *Trans. Proc.* **23**, 632–634.

Steptoe, R.J., Fu, F., Li, W., Drakes, M.L., Lu, L., Demetris, A.J., Qian, S., McKenna, H.J. and Thomson, A.W. (1997). Augmentation of dendritic cells in murine organ donors by Flt3 ligand alters the balance between transplant tolerance and immunity. *J. Immunol.* **159**, in press.

Stingl, G., Katz, S.I., Clement, L., Green, I. and Shevach, E.M. (1978). Immunologic functions of Ia bearing epidermal Langerhans cells. *J. Immunol.* **121**, 2005–2013.

Sun, J., McCaughan, G.W., Gallagher, N.D., Sheil, A.G.R. and Bishop, G.A. (1995). Deletion of spontaneous rat liver allograft acceptance by donor irradiation. *Transplantation* **60**, 233–236.

Süss, G. and Shortman, K. (1996) A subclass of dendritic cells kills CD4 T cells via Fas/Fas-ligand-induced apoptosis. *J. Exp. Med.* **183**, 1789–1796.

Suzuki, K. (1995). A histological study on experimental autoimmune myocarditis with special reference to initiation of the disease and cardiac dendritic cells. *Virchows Arch.* **426**, 493–500.

Tafuri, A., Bowers, W.E., Handler, E.S., Appel, M., Lew, R., Greiner, D., Mordes, J.P. and Rossini, A.A. (1993). High stimulatory activity of dendritic cells from diabetes-prone biobreeding/worcester rats exposed to macrophage-derived factors. *J. Clin. Invest.* **91**, 2040–2048.

Thomson, A.W., Lu, L., Subbotin, V.M., Li, Y., Qian, S., Rao, A.S., Fung, J.J. and Starzl, T.E. (1995). In vitro propagation and homing of liver-derived dendritic cell progenitors to lymphoid tissues of allogeneic recipients. Implications for the establishment and maintenance of donor cell chimerism following liver transplantation. *Transplantation* **59**, 544–551.

Valdivia, L.A., Demetris, A.J., Langer, A.M., Celli, S., Fung, J.J. and Starzl, T.E. (1993). Dendritic cell replacement in long-surviving liver and cardiac xenografts. *Transplantation* **56**, 482–484.

Van Den Oord, J.J., De Vos, R., Facchetti, F., Delabie, J., De Wolf-Peeters, C. and Desmet, V.J. (1990). Distribution of nonlymphoid, inflammatory cells in chronic HBV infection. *J. Pathol.* **160**, 223–230.

Van Rees, E.P., Dijkstra, C.D., Van Der Ende, M.B., Janse, E.M. and Sminia, T. (1988). The ontogenetic development of macrophage subpopulations and Ia-positive non-lymphoid cells in gut-associated lymphoid tissue of the rat. *Immunology* **63**, 79–85.

Velasco, A.L. and Hegre, O.D. (1989). Decreased immunogenicity of fetal kidneys: the role of passenger leukocytes. *J. Pediatric Surg.* **24**, 59–63.

Voorbij, H.A.M., Jeucken, P.H.M., Kabel, P.J., De Haan, M. and Drexhage, H.A. (1989). Dendritic cells and scavenger macrophages in pancreatic islets of prediabetic BB rats. *Diabetes* **38**, 1623–1629.

Witmer-Pack, M.D., Crowley, M.T., Inaba, K. and Steinman, R.M. (1993). Macrophages, but not dendritic cells, accumulate colloidal carbon following administration in situ. *J. Cell Sci.* **105**, 965–973.

Woo, J., Lu, L., Rao, A.S., Li, Y., Subbotin, V., Starzl, T.E. and Thomson, A.W. (1994). Isolation, phenotype, and allostimulatory activity of mouse liver dendritic cells. *Transplantation* **58**, 484–491.

Yang, R., Liu, Q., Grosfeld, J.L. and Pescovitz, M.D. (1994). Intestinal venous drainage through the liver is a prerequisite for oral tolerance induction. *J. Pediatric Surg.* **29**, 1145–1148.

Zhang, J., Yu, Z.-X., Fujita, S., Yamaguchi, M.L. and Ferrans, V.J. (1992). Interstitial dendritic cells of the rat heart: quantitative and ultrastructural changes in experimental myocardial infarction. *Circulation* **87**, 909–920.

Zhang, J., Herman, E.H. and Ferrans, V.J. (1993). Dendritic cells in the hearts of spontaneously hypertensive rats treated with doxorubicin with or without ICRF-187. *Am. J. Pathol.* **142**, 1916–1926.

Ziegler, A.-G., Erhard, J., Lampeter, E.F., Nagelkerken, L.M. and Standl, E. (1992). Involvement of dendritic cells in early insulitis of BB rats. *J. Autoimmunity* **5**, 571–579.

CHAPTER 11
Dendritic Cells in Spleen and Lymph Node

Jonathan M. Austyn
Nuffield Department of Surgery, University of Oxford, John Radcliffe Hospital, Oxford, UK

Ce sont les microbes qui auront le dernier mot.
(The microbes will have the last word.)

Louis Pasteur

INTRODUCTION

The ultimate destination of all dendritic cells (DC) is the lymphoid tissues. Within spleen and lymph nodes, clear phenotypic heterogeneity of DC populations is evident, both as studied *in situ* and after isolation *in vitro*. The same is true for other secondary lymphoid tissues such as (mouse) Peyer's patch, lymphoepithelial sites such as (human) tonsil, and to a lesser extent the thymus. In part, this phenotypic heterogeneity can now be ascribed to developmentally distinct DC subsets, and different maturation stages of DC within lymphoid tissues.

This chapter focuses on the phenotype and functions of DC in spleen and lymph nodes. It will consider findings made from studies *in situ*, *in vitro*, and *in vivo*, and will attempt to provide a unifying hypothesis as to the origin and functions of different DC subsets in these tissues. Before considering these subsets, however, it is important to discuss some features of DC in peripheral, nonlymphoid tissues and the thymus.

DC SUBSETS IN THE PERIPHERY AND THYMUS

Studies of DC grown from progenitors cultured in the presence of various cytokine combinations have revealed distinct pathways for development of DC subsets including Langerhans cells (LC), myeloid DC, monocyte-derived DC, and lymphoid DC (reviewed in Austyn, 1998). After production in the bone marrow (or fetal liver) it seems likely that the *in vivo* counterparts of the first two subsets, and possibly the third, enter nonlymphoid tissues where they reside transiently before migrating to secondary lymphoid tissue. Their principal function appears to be the induction of immunity to foreign antigens (Cella *et al.*, 1997; Steinman, 1991; Young and Steinman, 1996). In contrast, cells of the lymphoid DC subset may enter lymphoid tissues directly

Dendritic Cells: Biology and Clinical Applications
ISBN 0-12-455860-7

from the blood. Lymphoid DC progenitors probably enter the thymus and develop into DC that play a crucial role in the induction of thymic (central) tolerance. Recent evidence also suggests that lymphoid DC may enter secondary lymphoid tissues directly from the blood and that these cells have regulatory functions that could conceivably be involved in the induction or maintenance of extrathymic (peripheral) tolerance to self-antigens (Shortman *et al.*, 1997).

An important difference between DC subsets in lymphoid tissues is whether or not they are derived from DC that resided transiently in nonlymphoid tissues. For convenience, these subsets will be described as 'nonlymphoid DC' (including LC, myeloid DC, and perhaps monocyte-derived DC) and 'lymphoid DC' respectively. In this section important features of DC in nonlymphoid tissues and the thymus will be described since they provide insights into the origin and function of DC in secondary lymphoid tissues including spleen and lymph nodes (see later sections).

Nonlymphoid Dendritic Cells

Dendritic Cells in Nonlymphoid Tissues

Localization and Functions. It is now reasonably well established that at least some DC can enter nonlymphoid tissues and develop into cells with specialized capacities for uptake and processing of foreign antigens and the production of peptide-MHC complexes that can be expressed at the cell surface. Cells with these properties can be termed 'immature' or 'processing' DC. They are localized in topologically external epithelial sites, such as skin epidermis and the mucosae of the respiratory, gastrointestinal, and urogenital tracts. Cells with similar functions are also present in the interstitial spaces of solid organs such as heart and kidney. However, in normal circumstances, DC are absent from 'immunologically privileged' sites such as central cornea, the bulk of the central nervous system (CNS), and the testis. With a few exceptions, the functions of DC in nonlymphoid tissues have been elucidated mainly after isolation of the cells and studies of their properties *in vitro*. For example, much information has come from studies of Langerhans cells (LC) from skin epidermis, and of DC isolated from interstitial spaces of vascularized organs such as heart and kidney (discussed in detail elsewhere in this volume).

In general, freshly isolated DC from nonlymphoid tissues can internalize foreign antigens by pinocytosis and macropinocytosis (soluble antigens) and phagocytosis (particles) (Austyn, 1992; Lanzavecchia, 1996; Steinman and Swanson, 1995). Receptor-mediated endocytosis of antigens may be mediated by pattern-specific recognition molecules that bind conserved microbial structures, such as mannose receptors and perhaps the DEC-205 molecule of mouse LC, and by Fc receptors (e.g. FcγRII, CD32); the cells also express integrins that can function as complement receptors (e.g. CD11b/CD18 or CR3, and perhaps CD11c). Freshly isolated LC have a developed endolysosomal system for generation of peptides from internalized proteins, and exhibit a high rate of biosynthesis of MHC class II and invariant chain molecules presumably for loading with antigenic peptides. These cells have been shown to process soluble native antigens for expression as peptide–MHC class II complexes at the plasma membrane. However, in general, DC isolated from nonlymphoid tissues have little or no expression of costimulatory molecules such as CD40, CD80, and CD86, and they have weak or little capacity to initiate responses of naive T cells *in vitro*.

Maturation in vitro. Profound phenotypic and functional changes can occur during culture of DC isolated from nonlymphoid tissues. For example, in the presence of GM-CSF, cultured LC lose the capacity to internalize and process antigens, and to synthesize MHC class II and invariant-chain molecules. In contrast, membrane expression of foreign peptide–MHC class II complexes is increased, the cells express higher levels of costimulatory molecules such as CD40, CD80, and CD86, and they can now initiate responses of naive T cells *in vitro*. Furthermore, they are capable of secreting cytokines such as IL-12 which promotes T_H1 type responses. In many respects these cells resemble DC that can be isolated from secondary lymphoid tissues such as spleen and lymph nodes. Cells with these properties can be termed 'mature' or 'costimulatory' DC; the process by which cells develop these capacities from the immature, processing stage can be referred to as 'maturation' or 'activation'. *In vivo*, maturation of DC in nonlymphoid tissues appears to be followed by their migration to secondary lymphoid tissues (see below).

Origin and Development

Mouse Bone Marrow-derived DC. DC can be grown from mouse bone marrow or blood cells cultured in GM-CSF (reviewed in Young and Steinman, 1996). Depending on culture conditions, the DC progeny can be relatively immature, and development into mature, costimulatory cells can be induced by subsequent exposure of the cells to TNF-α or LPS; it is also possible to generate mature DC by culturing mouse bone marrow in a combination of GM-CSF and IL-4. Yields of DC can be increased by inclusion in the cultures of Flk-2/Flt-3 ligand, which has been shown to increase the numbers of DC present in a wide variety of mouse tissues when administered on a daily basis (Maraskovsky *et al.*, 1996). Despite its use *in vitro*, GM-CSF does not seem to be required for differentiation of mouse DC *in vivo*, since GM-CSF cytokine or receptor knockout mice possess relatively normal subsets of DC (Vremec *et al.*, 1997). The *in vivo* conterparts of DC generated from bone marrow cultures may be cells that can enter nonlymphoid tissues, although this is not yet proven. The situation is clearer in human (see below).

Human Langerhans Cells and Myeloid DC. DC can be grown from human $CD34^+$ progenitors in fetal liver, cord blood, bone marrow, and adult peripheral blood (reviewed in Austyn, 1998; Reid, 1997; Young and Steinman, 1996). Growth and differentiation of DC can be induced by culture of these progenitors in GM-CSF and TNF-α, and yields can be increased by inclusion of c-kit ligand (stem cell factor; CSF) which expands the progenitor pool. Distinct $CD34^+$ progenitors have been identified according to whether or not they express the cutaneous lymphocyte-associated antigen (CLA) (Strunk *et al.*, 1997). $CD34^+$ CLA^+ progenitors give rise to $CD1a^+$ cells resembling LC via a committed $CD14^-$ $CD1a^+$ precursor. In contrast $CD34^+$ CLA^- progenitors give rise to $CD1a^+$ cells, lacking the characteristic features of LC, via a bipotential $CD14^+$ $CD1a^-$ precursor that can alternatively differentiate into macrophages in the presence of M-CSF (Caux *et al.*, 1996); the DC progeny of these progenitors have therefore been termed 'myeloid DC'. While the *in situ* counterparts of the $CD34^+$ CLA^+ derived progeny seem most likely to be epidermal LC, those of the $CD34^+$ CLA^- derived progeny are less clear, although cells with similar features have been described in the dermis of skin.

Further evidence for a distinct developmental pathway for LC has come from studies of mice lacking a functional TGF-β gene: DC are present in the lymphoid tissues of these mice, but LC are absent from the skin (Borkowski *et al.*, 1996a). There are indications that TGF-β is also required for generation of human DC from progenitors in culture (Strobl *et al.*, 1996). A converse phenotype to that in TGF-β knockout mice is seen in mice lacking relB or Ikaros transcription factors (Burkly *et al.*, 1995; Wang *et al.*, 1996; Wu, *et al.*, in press). The existence of a distinct progenitor for LC may reflect the fact that this subset needs to cross the dermal–epidermal junction (basement membrane) and enter a nonvascularized site (skin epidermis) from the blood.

Monocyte-derived DC. Culture of $CD14^+$ $CD1a^-$ human peripheral blood monocytes in GM-CSF and IL-4 or IL-13 induces the development of $CD14^{lo}$ $CD1a^+$ cells in the absence of significant proliferation (reviewed in Austyn 1998; Cella *et al.* 1997; Young and Steinman, 1996). The cells resemble immature, processing DC but they are not terminally differentiated and can develop into macrophages when they are cultured in M-CSF. Further development of these cells into mature, costimulatory $CD14^-$ $CD1a^+$ DC can be induced by culture in TNF-α, LPS, or monocyte-conditioned medium (MCM) which is produced by culture of monocytes on immobilized IgG. The active constituents of MCM are not yet well defined, but PGE2 seems to be involved in its function. A key question that has yet to be answered is whether or not monocytes that are recruited to tissues constitutively or in response to inflammatory stimuli (see below) can develop into DC *in situ*.

Recruitment, Maturation and Migration

Responses to Local Inflammatory Stimuli. It is becoming increasingly clear that inflammatory stimuli and infectious agents induce both the recruitment of DC to nonlymphoid tissues and their subsequent maturation and migration to secondary lymphoid tissues (reviewed in Austyn, 1996; Austyn, 1998; Cella *et al.*, 1997). DC recruitment to nonlymphoid tissues in response to acute inflammatory stimuli has been particularly well documented in the case of rat lung and airways (Chapter 8). For example, a wave of DC enters these sites in response to local challenge with a variety of agents, including bacterial, viral, and soluble protein antigens (McWilliam *et al.*, 1996; McWilliam *et al.*, 1997). Similar responses are likely to occur in other nonlymphoid tissues (e.g. Roake *et al.*, 1995b), and may also occur in the brain, from which DC are normally absent. For example, in rat brain, an infiltrate of cells resembling DC has been identified within CNS allografts (Lawrence *et al.*, 1990) and an influx of cells expressing the OX62 antigen (a marker of DC) has been described in certain inflammatory situations (Matyszak and Perry, 1996).

Certain DC subsets express counterligands for molecules expressed by inflamed endothelium. These include: PSGL-1 which binds E-selectin (CD62E) and P-selectin (CD62P) (Laszik *et al.*, 1996); VLA-4 and VLA-5 (CD49d/CD29, CD49e/CD29) which bind VCAM-1, CD62E, and/or fibronectin (Strunk *et al.*, 1997); and CLA which binds CD62E (Strunk *et al.*, 1997). Whether these molecules facilitate entry of DC into inflamed tissues is not yet clear. Expression by DC subsets of the neural cell adhesion molecule L1 which binds the $\alpha_v\beta3$ integrin, and gp40, the murine homologue of human epithelial cell adhesion molecule, has also been reported (Borkowski *et al.*, 1996b; Pancook *et al.*, 1997).

Microbial products, such as bacterial lipopolysaccharide (LPS), or cytokines elicited by this agent such as TNF-α or IL-1, play a central role in DC maturation and mobilization of DC populations (Austyn 1996; Jonuleit *et al.*, 1996). For example, systemic administration of LPS induces migration of DC from mouse heart and kidney and from rat gut, and recruits DC progenitors to the former tissues (MacPherson *et al.*, 1995; Roake *et al.*, 1995a, b). Interestingly, interstitial DC in rat heart express MHC class II but lack the invariant chain (Saleem *et al.*, 1997), suggesting that the cells *in situ* may not normally produce peptide–MHC complexes unless they are stimulated, e.g. by a local inflammatory response. Maturation of DC can also be induced by mycolic acid (K. Rigley, personal communication) and by exposure to mycobacteria and staphylococcal enterotoxin A, both of which induce TNF or IL-1 secretion (Shankar *et al.*, 1996; Thurnher *et al.*, 1997).

Molecular events during DC mobilization are becoming increasingly understood. For example, during maturation and/or migration, epidermal LC have been shown to downregulate E-cadherin, presumably to facilitate detachment from keratinocytes (Cumberbatch *et al.*, 1996); to secrete type IV collagenase, presumably to enable crossing of the basement membrane, (Kobayashi 1997); and to utilize α_6-integrin molecules, presumably for adhesion to laminin in the basement membrane (Price *et al.*, submitted) during egress from the epidermis.

Role of Chemokines. An increasing number of studies are addressing stimuli that induce chemotaxis of human DC *in vitro*. Leukocyte chemotaxis occurs in response to both classical chemoattractants, such as bacterial *N*-formyl peptides (fmlp) and complement components (C5a), and to a family of chemoattractant cytokines or chemokines. Most of the latter fall into one of two families, the C-C (β) and C-X-C (α) chemokines, although a single C chemokine (lymphotactin) and an unusual membrane-bound molecule with a terminal C-X-X-X-C domain (fractalkine) have been identified (Hedrick and Zlotnik, 1996; Schall, 1997; Schall and Bacon, 1994; Schluger and Rom, 1997).

Human monocyte-derived DC have been shown to undergo chemotaxis in transwell systems in response to fmlp, C5a, and a distinct set of chemokines. The latter include the C-C chemokines MIP-1α, MIP-1β and RANTES which can bind the CCR5 receptor, SDF-1 which binds CXCR4, and the macrophage-derived C-C chemokine MDC (Delgado *et al.*, in press; Godiska *et al.*, 1997; Sozzani *et al.*, 1995; Sozzani *et al.*, in press). CCR5 and CXCR4 are of particular interest, since they can function as coreceptors for HIV-1 (Moore *et al.*, 1997) and are required for viral entry to DC (Granelli-Piperno *et al.*, 1996). Maturation of monocyte-derived DC in MCM is accompanied by downregulation of CCR5 but no change in CXCR4 (Delgado *et al.*, in press); C5a receptors are also upregulated during maturation of LC (Morelli *et al.*, 1996). These observations indicate that different stages of DC may exhibit different chemotactic responses *in vivo*.

We have demonstrated (Lin *et al.*, submitted) that human monocyte-derived DC undergo chemotaxis as well as transendothelial migration *in vitro* (technique described in Rahdon *et al.*, 1997) in response to the CCR5-associated C-C chemokines and to SDF-1. Interestingly, maturation of the cells in LPS, TNF, or IL-1 was found to abolish chemotaxis in response to the C-C chemokines, but to enhance or induce the response to SDF-1. Hence production of C-C chemokines at sites of inflammation and infection may recruit immature DC that can internalize foreign antigens. Local exposure to LPS (e.g. on bacteria), IL-1 or TNF-α (e.g. produced by macrophages in response to LPS) is likely to downregulate CCR5 but to upregulate CXCR4 expression. The cells could presumably then migrate in response to SDF-1, which is reportedly produced by stromal cells in spleen, lymph nodes, and liver, key sites in DC migration (see below).

Additional evidence indicates that DC can produce chemokines that induce chemotaxis of T cells: mouse MIP-1γ that attracts naive and activated CD4$^+$ and CD8$^+$ T cells (Mohamadzadeh *et al.*, 1996), and human DCK1 that selectively attracts naive T cells (Adema *et al.*, 1997). Presumably these chemokines facilitate the interaction of DC with T cells and hence the induction of immune responses.

Lymphoid Dendritic Cells

DC in Thymus

DC have been identified in the medulla and perhaps the corticomedullary junction of thymus (Fairchild and Austyn, 1990). There is evidence that these cells can induce negative but not positive selection of developing thymocytes, and that they are required for induction of thymic (central) tolerance of T cells to self-antigens (e.g. Brocker, *et al.*, 1997). A major population of phenotypically homogeneous DC can be isolated from mouse thymus. The phenotype of these cells (CD11c$^+$ CD8α^+ DEC-205$^+$ HSA$^+$ CD11b$^-$ 33D1$^-$) is similar to DC subsets that can be isolated from spleen and thymus (see below), although trace levels of cells with different phenotypes can also be detected (e.g. Vremec and Shortman, 1997). An important characteristic of the major thymic DC subset is the expression of CD8 as $\alpha\alpha$ homodimers (see below). There is no evidence that DC can migrate from nonlymphoid tissues into the thymus, and it is probable that at least the majority of thymic DC originate from a distinct progenitor that seeds the thymus and generates cells of the lymphoid DC subset (see Chapter 2).

Lymphoid DC Progenitors

A CD34$^+$ CD10$^+$ CD45RA$^+$ progenitor has been isolated from human fetal and adult bone marrow that can generate T cells, B cells, NK cells, and DC (Galy *et al.*, 1995). Limiting dilution analysis appears to prove that this progenitor is truly multipotent. In addition, a CD34$^+$ CD38^{lo} progenitor isolated from thymus has the capacity to differentiate into T cells, NK cells, and DC, and is distinct from the pluripotent stem cell (Res *et al.*, 1996). These and other observations indicate that a developmentally distinct subset of lymphoid DC originates from bone marrow-derived progenitors that may seed the thymus.

A thymic lymphoid progenitor has also been isolated from mouse thymus that resembles the hematopoietic stem cell except for expression of the Sca-2 antigen and low levels of CD4 (Wu and Shortman, 1996). These CD4^{lo} cells can generate T cells, B cells, NK cells, and CD8α^+ DC when they are adoptively transferred to irradiated recipients. A downstream cell has also been isolated that resembles a pro-T cell and which gives rise to T cells and DC. Further downstream, at the pre-T cell stage, the capacity to generate DC appears to be lost and the cells become committed to the T cell lineage. In the absence of formal clonal proof, it is of course possible that distinct thymic progenitors that generate either DC or lymphoid cells may exist within the $CD4^{lo}$ subset, but heterogeneity has not been observed to date. The lymphoid origin of DC in the thymus may be supported by the finding that these cells are absent from mice lacking a functional Ikaros gene which encodes a transcription factor required for development of lymphoid cells (Wang *et al.*, 1996; Wu *et al.*, in press).

DC IN SPLEEN

DC Subsets in Spleen

A particularly good marker of most or all DC in mouse lymphoid tissues is the CD11c integrin, first defined using the N418 monoclonal antibody (Plate 11.1(a)). This antibody labels isolated cells in red pulp of spleen, interdigitating cells (IDC) in central white pulp (T cell areas), and 'nests' of DC which interrupt the marginal zone and extend into the T cell areas but not the B cell follicles (e.g. Steinman *et al.*, 1997). The latter have been termed 'marginal zone DC' (MZDC).

In contrast to CD11c, the DEC-205 antigen, defined by the NLDC-145 monoclonal antibody, is expressed on a subset(s) of DC in these tissues, and labelling appears to be confined largely to IDC (Plate 11.1(b)) (e.g. Steinman *et al.*, 1997). Molecular cloning of the DEC-205 molecule demonstrated the existence of ten contiguous C-type lectin domains, homologous to the eight domains found in the macrophage mannose receptor (MMR). Antibodies to DEC-205, acting as artificial ligands, have been shown to be endocytosed in coated pits, delivered to lysosomes, and subsequently presented efficiently to T cells. These findings suggest that DEC-205 may be a pattern-specific receptor molecule that could be used by DC to bind carbohydrate moieties on, for example, certain bacterial cell wall components. Nevertheless, the structures of the DEC-205 domains corresponding to the ligand-binding domains of the MMR are significantly different (P. Crocker, personal communication) and it is possible that this molecule could subserve some other function.

The first DC-restricted marker of mouse DC was defined by the complement-fixing antibody 33D1. Treatment of cell suspensions prepared from mouse spleen by mechanical disruption with 33D1 and complement was found to eliminate or reduce the stimulatory activity of these preparations in, for example, mixed leukocyte reactions and oxidative mitogenesis assays (Austyn, 1987). However, similar treatment of cell suspensions prepared by enzyme digestion was found to be less efficient. The residual activity in these preparations could be eliminated by treatment with the J11d antibody specific for the heat-stable antigen (HSA) and complement. This suggests that 33D1 and HSA are expressed on different subsets of DC, the former of which is more readily liberated from spleen by mechanical techniques. Although the 33D1 antibody labels very weakly in immunocytochemistry, it appears to bind to MZDC but not IDC.

An initially surprising observation was that a subset of DC in mouse lymphoid tissues expresses the CD8 molecule, as $\alpha\alpha$ homodimers. These cells also express a ligand for the Fas molecule, although at the time of writing it is not clear if this is FasL per se. Approximately equal numbers of $CD8\alpha^+$ and $CD8\alpha^-$ DC can be liberated from spleen by using enzyme digestion and calcium-free media (Vremec and Shortman, 1997).

The CD8α^+ subset has been shown to express DEC-205 and HSA, but lacks the myeloid-associated CD11b integrin, a phenotype that closely resembles the major population of DC that can be isolated from thymus (except that thymic DC also express BP-1). The CD8α^- subset has the converse phenotype. Traces of one or more DC subsets with different phenotypes have also been identified in these preparations.

Taken together, the preceding and other observations indicate the existence of two major subsets of DC in mouse spleen: CD11c$^+$ CD8α^+ DEC-205$^+$ HSA$^+$ CD11b$^-$ 33D1$^-$ cells seem to correspond to IDC, while CD11c$^+$ CD8α^- DEC-205$^-$ HSA$^-$ CD11b$^+$ 33D1$^+$ cells appear to represent MZDC. IDC express high levels of MHC class II and invariant-chain molecules together with CD40 and CD86 (Steinman *et al.*, 1997). In contrast, MZDC appear to be relatively immature. For example, they have low expression of 2A1 and M342 antigens (normally expressed by mature DC), and low expression of CD86; they also retain some antigen capture functions (e.g. Steinman *et al.*, 1997). Importantly, most or all CD8α^+ DC in mouse spleen express a ligand for Fas, perhaps FasL (see below).

It is currently thought that (immature) MZDC give rise to (mature) IDC *in vivo*. Some evidence for this idea comes from the observation that 6 h after systemic administration of LPS to mice, DC appear to move from marginal zone nests to the PALS, and to undergo functional maturation as assessed *in vitro* by their reduced ability to capture antigen but enhanced costimulatory activity (De Smedt *et al.*, 1996). However, phenotypic changes consistent with such a transition (e.g. increased CD8α and FasL but decreased CD11b expression) have not yet been observed *in vitro*.

While it seems reasonable to assume that similar DC subsets are also present in human spleen, the phenotypes of human splenic DC are not yet as well defined as in mouse. However, there are indications that human IDC express high levels of MHC class II molecules, CD4, S100 (a cytoplasmic protein), and p55 (fascin).

Entry of Nonlymphoid DC to Spleen

There is good evidence that DC can migrate from nonlymphoid tissues via the blood to the spleen. The evidence for a blood migration pathway is first summarized, before describing migration from interstitial spaces of solid organs. The latter route is presumably important for the induction of immunity to foreign antigens that gain access to interstitial spaces, although there is little direct evidence to support this assumption at present.

DC Migrate from Blood to Spleen

The capacity of DC to migrate from blood to spleen, and to home to distinct subcompartments of spleen, was first revealed from trafficking studies in mice (Austyn *et al.*, 1988; Kupiec-Weglinski *et al.*, 1988), and later in rats (Oluwole, *et al.*, 1991). DC isolated from mouse spleen and labelled with Indium-111 were injected intravenously into syngeneic recipients (Kupiec-Weglinski *et al.*, 1988). A substantial proportion of radiolabel was found to accumulate in spleen (and liver) by 3 h and to persist at similar levels at 24 h. Similar findings were made for radioabelled DC that had been isolated from lymph nodes, suggesting that the migration of DC into the spleen from the blood did not merely reflect homing back to the tissue of origin. This has also been confirmed in more recent studies showing that radiolabel accumulates to a similar extent in spleen (and liver) after intravenous injection of mouse bone marrow-derived DC labelled with technetium-99^{m} (R. Suri *et al.*, in preparation).

In localization studies, isolated spleen DC were labelled with a fluorochrome (Hoescht 33342) before intravenous administration, and frozen sections of recipient spleen were examined for the presence of labelled cells (Austyn *et al.*, 1988). At 3 h the majority of the labelled cells were found to be present in the red pulp, but by 24 h they were present in T cell areas (PALS) of white pulp and were clearly excluded from B cell follicles (Plate 11.2). The early appearance of DC in splenic red pulp remains an unexplained phenomenon, but presumably their capacity to home subsequently to T cell areas would normally be important for their ability to induce immune responses in spleen.

As with all labelling studies, one concern is whether the label detected *in situ* actually reflects that in live cells. Recently, mouse bone marrow-derived DC were labelled with a fluorochrome (such as CFDASE or PKH26) and label was localized to T cell areas of recipient spleens at 24 h following intravenous injection (R. Suri *et al.*, in preparation). Cell suspensions were then prepared from the spleens and labelled cells were recovered. FACS analysis confirmed that the label was associated with cells that expressed CD11c and DEC-205, but lacked markers of other cell types such as macrophages. These observations suggest (but still do not prove) that label is indeed associated with the administered, live cell population.

When isolated, fluorochrome-labelled spleen DC were incubated on frozen sections of spleen for 1 h at 37°C, they were found to attach specifically to the marginal zones (Austyn *et al.*, 1988). Hence it was proposed that DC initially entered the tissue from the blood via these regions. One explanation for DC adhesion to splenic marginal zone is that DC can adhere to cells such as marginal zone macrophages. A precedent for this comes from a more recent finding that rat DC, derived from celiac lymph, can adhere to Kupffer cells in frozen sections of liver (Kudo *et al.*, 1997). Furthermore, human monocyte-derived DC undergo chemotaxis in response to a macrophage-derived chemokine, MDC (Godiska *et al.*, 1997). Interestingly, DC within rat lung and airways are juxtaposed to macrophages *in situ*, and the macrophages appear to prevent or slow maturation of the DC, perhaps to facilitate their capacity to acquire and process antigens in these sites (see Chapter 8). Whether this might apply to DC within marginal zone of spleen is unclear, but at least some freshly isolated DC from spleen are able to internalize particulates and to process soluble antigens (Reis e Sousa *et al.*, 1993; Steinman *et al.*, 1997).

The entry of DC to spleen from the blood was found to be a T-dependent process (Kupiec-Weglinski *et al.*, 1988). When isolated splenic DC were labelled with indium-111 and administered intravenously to (syngeneic) nude mice, little or no radiolabel was detected in recipient spleen. In these mice there was a corresponding increase in label detected within the liver, suggesting that the cells that would normally have homed to the spleen had entered the liver instead. However, when nude mice were reconstituted with mature T cells before administering the DC, radiolabel now accumulated within the spleen to a similar extent as in euthymic recipients.

The mechanism for T-dependent entry of DC to spleen is not clear. Although chemokines such as MIP-1α, MIP-1β, and RANTES appear to be major products of cells such as T cells (Hedrick and Zlotnik, 1996), and can induce chemotaxis of DC *in vitro* (see above), one would normally expect these cytokines to be produced in significant quantities only after T cell activation, and the cells that were transferred in the above studies (Kupiec-Weglinski *et al.*, 1988) were, mostly, resting T cells. One possibility is that DC entering T cell areas of normal spleens adhere to naive T cells (i.e. in an antigen-independent manner) and are thereby retained in this compartment. In the absence of T cells their viability may be impaired, or they may even be actively killed.

An important question is at what stage DC acquire their capacity to migrate from blood to spleen. Recent studies indicate that relatively immature DC cultured from mouse bone marrow in the presence of GM-CSF, as well as the mature cells cultured in various combinations of GM-CSF, IL-4, TNFα, and/or LPS can enter spleen to a similar extent after intravenous administration and home to T cell areas (R. Suri *et al.*, in preparation). One report has also documented that immature (GM-CSF-cultured) bone marrow-derived DC home to splenic T cell areas after intravenous transfer to allogeneic recipients and that these cells upregulate costimulatory molecules (Fu *et al.*, 1996). It seems likely that such DC correspond to myeloid DC (or LC) but it is currently unclear whether lymphoid DC are also present in DC populations cultured from bone marrow, and if so to what extent these cells contribute to the splenic accumulation observed.

DC Migrate from Interstitial Spaces via Blood to Spleen

The physiological relevance of the blood migration pathway that was demonstrated in adoptive transfer studies (above) was first shown in transplantation settings, first in mice (Larsen *et al.*, 1990a) and later in rats (Codner *et al.*, 1990). It was found that following cardiac transplantation in the mouse, DC disappeared from allogeneic heart grafts over a period of 1–3 days. When recipient spleens were examined, small numbers of donor-derived cells were detected that expressed donor-specific polymorphisms of MHC class II and CD44 (Pgp-1) molecules (Plate 11.3(a) and (b)). Cells were first detectable 1 day after transplantation and maximum numbers were present between 2 and 4 days, but they were no longer detectable at day 6. Since the spleen lacks an afferent lymphatic supply, these cells were derived from the blood and presumably represented DC that had migrated from the transplants. Related observations were made in a rat limb transplantation model (Codner *et al.*, 1990).

An initially unexpected finding was that the donor-derived cells in spleens of mice that had received cardiac allografts were not localized within T cell areas at day 2 (Larsen *et al.*, 1990a). Instead, they were present in B cell areas of (peripheral) white pulp, or close to the border of B cell and T cell areas (Plate 11.3(c)). However, the DC were found to be associated primarily with $CD4^+$ but not $CD8^+$ T cells in these areas (Plate 11.3(d)–(f)). These observations suggested that movement of the allogeneic DC through the tissue might be retarded when they encountered alloreactive T cells, and that their asssociation with $CD4^+$ T cells in B cell areas might contribute to the generation of alloantibody responses. Later studies confirmed these observations and also revealed that donor-derived DC do in fact enter T cell areas, but only at later times (3–5 days) after transplantation (Roake *et al.*, 1995b). Presumably, these DC are then eliminated within recipient spleens, either because they are killed by alloreactive CTL they induce, or perhaps because they undergo Fas-dependent apoptosis when they interact with alloreactive (helper) T cells they activate, although this is not yet clear.

It seems most likely that the blood migration pathway revealed from studies of isolated and reinfused DC (above) and in transplantation settings (above) is physiologically important for the induction of immune responses against foreign antigens that gain access to interstitial spaces of solid organs. However, it seems probable that cells from these sites can also migrate via afferent lymph to regional lymph nodes (see below), and the relative importance of these respective pathways is at present unclear. DC from vascularized epithelial sites such as the dermis of skin may also migrate via blood to spleen (see below).

Lymphoid DC in Spleen

As noted earlier, a subset of CD8α^+ DC can be isolated from mouse spleen that closely resembles the major CD8α^+ subset in thymus. A lymphoid origin for these splenic DC is suggested from studies of mice with a dominant negative Ikaros gene (Wu *et al.*, in press) (Chapter 2). These mice have a profound deficiency of CD8α^+ DC in spleen and other lymphoid tissues (including lymph nodes) and their bone marrow cells are capable of generating myeloid cells but not DC or lymphoid cells after adoptive transfer to irradiated recipients. Surprisingly, CD8α^- DC are also absent from spleen and other lymphoid tissues of these mice. This suggests either that the Ikaros transcription factor is required for development of both lymphoid and myeloid DC subsets (but not LC, which are present in skin epidermis of these deficient mice), or that the proportion of myeloid DC in spleeen is considerably less than might have been expected (i.e. due to migration from nonlymphoid tissues). Whatever the case, there is good evidence that CD8α^+ DC isolated from spleens of normal mice have negative regulatory properties *in vitro* that are not exhibited by the CD8α^- subset (see below).

CD8α^- DC isolated from mouse spleen induce a vigorous proliferative response of allogeneic and antigen-specific (transgenic) CD4$^+$ T cells *in vitro*. In contrast, CD8α^+ DC induce a much lower response, and the activated T cells undergo apoptosis (Suss and Shortman, 1996). By using various mixtures of DC and T cells from Fas-deficient lpr/lpr mice and FasL-deficient gld/gld mice, it was shown that apoptosis is induced in CD4$^+$ T cells in a Fas-dependent manner. Moreover, CD8α^+ DC bind a Fas–Fc fusion protein, suggesting they express FasL, whereas most CD8α^- DC do not. Hence the CD8α^+ DC subset from mouse spleen has regulatory properties in addition to costimulatory activity for CD4$^+$ T cells.

Further evidence for regulatory properties of the splenic CD8α^+ subset was obtained from studies of CD8$^+$ T cell responses *in vitro*. CD8α^+ DC can activate allogeneic and antigen-specific (transgenic) CD8$^+$ T cells *in vitro*, but the T cell proliferative responses are markedly lower than those following stimulation with CD8α^- DC (Kronin *et al.*, 1996). IL-2 production was found to be very low in these cultures and the reduced T cell proliferative response could be completely reversed in the presence of exogenous IL-2. Hence, CD8α^+ DC can efficiently stimulate CD8$^+$ T cells into cell division but they are deficient in inducing IL-2 production and thereby limit T cell proliferation. The same findings were made when DC and T cells were used from lpr/lpr or gld/gld mice, indicating that Fas-mediated apoptosis is not involved. The molecular basis for this regulatory activity is not yet known.

The function of CD8a on DC is unclear. It does not seem to be required for development of the cells since all major subsets of DC (albeit lacking CD8 expression) appear to be present in spleen (and lymph nodes) of mice lacking a functional CD8α gene (Kronin *et al.*, 1997). Furthermore, addition of inhibitory anti-CD8 antibodies to cultures of DC and allogeneic or antigen-specific T cells does not alter the regulatory properties of the CD8α^+ DC.

DC in Germinal Centres of Spleen

For completenesss, we will note that a subset of CD4$^+$ CD11c$^-$ DC has been identified in germinal centres of human spleen (Grouard *et al.*, 1996). However, these cells are discussed later in relation to similar cells in tonsil from where they have been isolated and studied in most detail.

Correlation between Observations *in situ* and *in vivo*

A number of important gaps in our understanding will need to be filled before it is possible to correlate findings from different systems to explain the precise origin of the phenotypically distinct subsets of DC identified in spleen. The evidence outlined earlier indicates that adoptively transferred DC, and DC from allografts, can migrate via the blood to the spleen and home to distinct subcompartments of this tissue. Hence it is generally assumed that (nonlymphoid) DC migrating from the interstitial spaces of vascularized tissues in the blood enter the spleen via the marginal zone, perhaps become MZDC, and ultimately home to T cell areas where, as IDC, they induce immunity to foreign antigens. However, there are some apparent discrepancies that will need to be addressed before this scheme can be accepted with certainty.

First, in frozen section assays, DC appear to adhere evenly to the marginal zones of spleens rather than becoming attached to areas where DC appear to enter the T cell areas (i.e. 'nests' of MZDC) (Austyn *et al.*, 1988). In addition, no clear correlation was observed between the localization of donor-derived DC in spleens of cardiac allografts and CD11c$^+$ cells in these sites (Roake *et al.*, 1995b). These may not be major problems since the former observations were made in a relatively contrived system using isolated splenic DC, and DC could still enter at various points within the marginal zone before accumulating in these sites.

Second, it is difficult to identify DC within spleen or in isolated spleen cell suspensions that might correspond in phenotype to DC in nonlymphoid tissues. Certainly the phenotype of DC in tissues such as heart and kidney is not well established but, in mouse, at least some MHC class II$^+$ presumptive DC express the myeloid-associated molecules CD11b, CD32 (Fcγ receptor II) and F4/80 (which are also expressed by epidermal LC) (Austyn *et al.*, 1994), and there are essentially no cells in these tissues that express CD11c or DEC-205. By analogy with LC, one might anticipate that expression of the myeloid antigens would be downregulated during maturation and migration of these cells to spleen. If CD11c expression was induced at the same time, the phenotype of the cells would come to resemble that of splenic MZDC. There is some evidence for downregulation of myeloid-associated antigens during culture of isolated heart and kidney DC, but induction of CD11c has not been observed (Austyn *et al.*, 1994).

Third, the origin of DC in interstitial spaces of solid organs is not clear, but it is generally assumed that these cells are at least not lymphoid-derived. Hence, as noted above, the almost complete absence of DC in the spleen (including MZDC and IDC) of mice with a dominant negative Ikaros mutation is something of a surprise since one might expect to detect at least some DC that had migrated from nonlymphoid tissues. Clearly it will be important to establish whether these mice have DC in nonlymphoid tissues other than skin (where LC are present) and, if so, whether these cells can be detected in spleen after inducing their migration from the tissues in response to local inflammatory stimuli for example. An alternative explanation for their absence is that nonlymphoid DC in spleen could have a higher turnover rate than lymphoid DC. However, the half-life of (bulk) DC in spleen has been estimated to be of the order of 2–3 days, perhaps not so different from that of donor-derived DC in spleens of cardiac allografts (i.e. the latter cells are detectable 1–4 days after transplantation).

Finally, DC isolated from T cell areas of spleen (corresponding to IDC) appear to have negative regulatory properties (see above) that have not been associated with DC cultured from nonlymphoid tissues. Conceivably, these populations do contain both lymphoid and non-lymphoid DC, and the regulatory effects of the former subset could mask or obscure the (positive) costimulatory functions expected for the latter. However, the fact that negative effects predominate *in vitro* could suggest that the numbers of nonlymphoid DC in these sites are relatively low. Whatever the case, it seems reasonable to assume at present that both lymphoid and nonlymphoid DC ultimately enter T cell areas of spleen.

DC IN LYMPH NODES

DC Subsets in Lymph Nodes

Three populations of DC have been identified in mouse lymph node cell suspensions (Vremec and Shortman, 1997). A major CD8α^+ DEC-205$^+$ HSA$^+$ CD11b$^-$ subset resembles IDC of spleen and may correspond to IDC in paracortical regions (T cell areas) of lymph nodes. These cells appear to be relatively mature in that they express M342 and 2A1 antigens, and have costimulatory activity. A second subset of CD8α^- DEC-205$^-$ HSA$^-$ CD11b$^+$ cells resembles MZDC of spleen and could represent cells that have recently entered the subcapsular space of lymph nodes from nonlymphoid tissues via afferent lymph. A third subset, trace levels of which are also present in splenic DC suspensions, has the CD8α^- DEC-205$^+$ HSA$^+$ CD11b$^-$ phenotype. The origin of this subset is currently obscure.

Entry of Nonlymphoid DC to Lymph Nodes

Two migratory pathways have been defined for DC entering lymph nodes via afferent lymph that may be required for the induction of immunity to foreign antigens in distinct peripheral sites. First, DC have been shown to migrate from epithelial sites to regional lymph nodes, particularly LC from the epidermis of skin. Second, DC can be recruited to liver sinusoids before undergoing a blood–lymph translocation and entering celiac lymph nodes. The former pathway is presumably required for induction of immunity to antigens in epithelial tissues, while the latter may be a specialized pathway for induction of immunity to blood-borne antigens. A third route for migration of presumptive DC from vascularized organs via afferent lymph is suggested from early studies (for example, a flux of cells resembling DC was noted in afferent lymph draining sheep renal transplants; reviewed in Austyn and Larsen, 1990), but this route has been relatively little studied.

DC Migrate from Afferent Lymph to Lymph Nodes

A significant number of early studies demonstrated the presence of cells, most of which are now known to be DC, in afferent but not efferent lymph (reviewed in Austyn and Larsen, 1990). As described in more detail below, these cells, which have been termed veiled cells, were found not only in afferent lymph draining normal skin but also in lymph draining skin transplants and skin to which contact sensitizers had been applied. Furthermore, DC are absent from central lymph but can be isolated from the thoracic duct after mesenteric lymphadenectomy in the rat. These cells in pseudoafferent lymph represent DC that are migrating from the gut wall.

Following their entry to lymph nodes from nonlymphoid tissues, it is now reasonably well established that DC home to paracortical regions (T cell areas). When DC were isolated from mouse spleen, labelled with the H33342 fluorochrome, and injected into the footpads of syngeneic recipients, they could be detected in popliteal nodes (Austyn *et al.*, 1988). Entry of these cells, in contrast to that of DC migrating from blood to spleen, does not seem to be a T-dependent process since it appears to occur normally in nude mouse recipients. Localization of these cells to T cell areas of lymph nodes has been demonstrated in a number of studies. For example, DC have been identified in these regions of popliteal lymph nodes after footpad administration of radiolabelled DC isolated from rat pseudoafferent lymph (detected by autoradiography; Fossum, 1988), and of fluorochrome-labelled DC grown from mouse blood (Inaba *et al.*, 1992). Similar studies have also demonstrated homing of DC cultured from chimpanzee blood monocytes in GM-CSF and IL-4 into T cell areas of lymph nodes of this species (Barratt-Boyes *et al.*, 1997).

DC Migrate from Epithelial Sites to Regional Nodes

LC Migration after Skin Grafting. Early studies of skin allografts revealed the importance of intact afferent lymphatic connections for the induction of skin graft rejection (reviewed in Austyn and Larsen, 1990). Later studies of the behaviour of epidermal LC in mouse skin transplants and explants then provided a possible explanation for this requirement (Larsen *et al.*, 1990b). As early as 4 h after transplantation, or in organ culture, epidermal LC were observed to increase in size and to up-regulate MHC class II expression. After a day or so these cells then appeared to enter dermal lymphatics and 'cords' of cells could be observed in the deep dermis; similar observations have been made for human skin explants (Lukas *et al.*, 1996). In organ culture, when explants were floated on culture medium, DC could subsequently be recovered from the bottom of the culture wells. When the phenotype and function of these DC were compared to that of LC freshly isolated from skin epidermis, it became apparent that migration was accompanied by maturation. For example, the migratory cells had decreased or lost expression of CD32 and F4/80 antigens but increased stimulatory activity in allogeneic mixed leukocyte reactions and oxidative mitogenesis responses (Larsen *et al.*, 1990b).

The observations above suggest that, *in vivo*, epidermal LC can migrate from skin into afferent lymphatics and initiate transplantation rejection within regional nodes; hence the requirement for intact afferent lymphatics. Demonstrating this directly, however, has proved to be difficult. After skin grafting in mice and rats, very small numbers of donor-derived cells can indeed be detected in regional lymph nodes (Richters *et al.*, 1996; M. Liddington *et al.*, manuscript in preparation). Furthermore, adoptive transfer of cell suspensions from mouse lymph nodes draining skin allografts to which contact sensitizers were applied (see below) was found to induce donor-specific responses in the naive recipients (Kripke *et al.*, 1990). The assumption has therefore been made that donor-derived cells in recipient lymph nodes represent LC that originated from skin epidermis. An additional or alternative possibility is that they could be derived from the dermis.

To determine whether LC per se are actually capable of migrating from a skin graft into regional lymph nodes, a subcutaneous pocket model was developed (M. Liddington *et al.*, manuscript in preparation). This involved making a small incision in the skin and separating the skin from the underlying fascia to mimic the bed of a skin graft. When epidermal LC were isolated from mouse skin, labelled with a fluorochrome (DiI or PKH26), and administered into a skin pocket, labelled cells could be detected in regional lymph nodes 24 h later. These cells were, however, readily detected only after administration of at least 10^5 cells. Colocalization studies demonstrated that the bulk of the administered cells had homed to paracortical, T cell areas. Furthermore, rtPCR analysis demonstrated the presence of donor MHC (class I) in regional lymph nodes after administration of allogeneic LC into subcutaneous pockets, as well as after skin grafting.

One perhaps surprising observation was that rare donor-derived cells could be detected in recipient spleens after skin grafting (M. Liddington, manuscript in preparation). Such cells were not, however, demonstrable after injection of isolated LC into subcutaneous pockets, suggesting that they originated from the dermis. Overall, it seems most probable that LC can migrate from the epidermis of skin into dermal lymphatics and then to regional lymph nodes. There are also indications that DC can migrate from skin dermis into nodes. For example, when *Leishmania* parasites are injected into mouse skin they are internalized by presumptive dermal DC, and parasite-bearing DEC-205$^+$ cells can then be detected in T cell areas of regional lymph nodes where they appear to persist for long periods (Moll *et al.*, 1993; Moll *et al.*, 1995). In addition, it is possible that DC can migrate from the dermis of skin grafts (a fully vascularized tissue site) into the blood and then to spleen. The relative contribution of the latter route, if any, to the induction of skin graft rejection is unclear.

LC Migration in Response to Contact Sensitizers. The fact that maturation and migration of epidermal LC occurred in isolated skin explants suggested that these processes were induced by locally produced inflammatory mediators, even as early as 4 h after organ culture (or transplantation). TNF-α and IL-1 have been implicated as key mediators of these events (Cumberbatch and Kimber, 1992; Enk *et al.*, 1993). For example, injection of these recombinant cytokines into mouse skin leads to a reduction in the number of epidermal LC at 24 h, and culture of LC in exogenous IL-1 (but not TNF-α) promotes maturation *in vitro*. These and other cytokines are induced in skin following the application of contact sensitizers.

When contact sensitizers such as FITC were topically applied to mouse skin, many DC labelled with the contact sensitizing agent could be isolated from regional lymph nodes (Cumberbatch and Kimber, 1990; Kripke *et al.*, 1990; Macatonia *et al.*, 1987; van Wilsem *et al.*, 1994). These cells, and those isolated from lymph nodes draining skin sites to which sensitizers such as oxazolone or picryl chloride were applied, were found to induce anti-hapten responses after adoptive transfer to naive recipients (e.g. Kripke *et al.*, 1990). The interpretation of these and other related observations was that epidermal LC acquire the contact sensitizer locally before migrating to regional lymph nodes where they induce contact sensitivity reactions. This, in part, seems likely to be correct.

Other studies have shown that painting of skin grafts with FITC before or after restoration of lymphatic connections results in an accumulation of labelled cells within regional nodes, many of which express CD11c and DEC-205 (M. Liddington *et al*, manuscript in preparation). However, very few of these cells are donor-derived. This suggests that free FITC can travel from the skin to the draining lymph nodes, where it is acquired by (host) DC. An additional or alternative explanation is that the contact sensitizer is acquired by DC within the dermis (possibly recruited to or maturing within this site in response to inflammatory cytokines) and that these cells do not enter the epidermis but somehow gain access to dermal lymphatics. Moreover, increased numbers of DC can be isolated from lymph nodes draining skin sites that were injected with TNF-α (Cumberbatch and Kimber, 1992). Although it was thought that these cells represented epidermal LC that were induced to migrate, it now seems more likely that these cells were either recruited into the dermis before entry to lymphatics or recruited directly into the lymph nodes from the bloodstream.

In summary so far, observations from both (a) transplant models and (b) studies with contact sensitizers suggest that epidermal LC can migrate from skin to regional lymph nodes. However, it now seems likely that DC can also be recruited into the dermis (e.g. in response to GM-CSF) and perhaps directly into the lymph nodes from the blood (e.g. in response to TNF-α). The relative contribution of these DC of different (tissue) origin to the induction of immunity is unclear.

DC Migration from Gastrointestinal Epithelia. Following mesenteric lymphadenectomy of rats, DC that would normally migrate from the gut wall to the mesenteric lymph nodes can be isolated from central lymph by cannulation of the thoracic duct (Liu and MacPherson, 1995b). There is a continuous, low-level flux of such cells draining from the gut, probably from the lamina propria (Maric *et al.*, 1996). However, the cell output is markedly increased following systemic administration of LPS (MacPherson *et al.*, 1995). This indicates either that the resident population of DC is induced to leave the tissue or(and) that DC progenitors are recruited to the gut wall prior to exit in the mesenteric lymph.

The DC that enter normal mesenteric lymph have costimulatory activity for *in vitro* immune responses, but they also retain antigen uptake and processing activity. Hence these cells appear to represent an intermediate stage in the maturation process. Direct evidence that DC migrating from the gut wall can acquire and present foreign antigens delivered directly into the gut has been obtained (Liu and MacPherson, 1995a): DC isolated from the thoracic duct of mesenteric lymphadenectomized rats following delivery of antigens into the gut can induce antigen-specific responses after adoptive transfer to naive recipients.

DC Migration to Lymph Nodes in Transgenic Systems. Studies of the migration of antigen-pulsed DC into lymph nodes of transgenic mice have shed light on the subsequent fate of these cells. In one system, transgenic T cells specific for an ovalbumin peptide–MHC class II complex were injected into normal mice and were subsequently detected within secondary lymphoid tissues by using an anti-idiotypic antibody specific for the transgenic receptor (Ingulli *et al.*, 1997). Splenic DC were then isolated from syngeneic mice, pulsed with the ovalbumin peptide, and labelled with a fluorochome, before injection into the footpad of the chimeric mice. The DC were observed to home to paracortical regions and to cluster with the transgenic T cells, suggesting that antigen presentation could occur. Indeed, these findings were correlated with the induction of immune responses, including DTH responses in the chimeric mice. The antigen-pulsed DC persisted within the nodes for 2 days but then disappeared. In contrast, non-pulsed DC homed to the same regions, but did not associate with transgenic T cells, and persisted for at least 4 days. One possibility is that, after T cell activation, antigen-pulsed DC underwent apoptosis due to ligation of Fas on the mature DC with FasL on the activated T cells.

DC Migrate from Liver Sinusoids to Celiac Lymph Nodes. The celiac lymph nodes may be a specialized site for the induction of immune responses against blood-borne antigens (Austyn, 1996). The evidence for this has come from studies of rats that were injected intravenously with particulates after celiac lymphadenectomy had been performed (Kudo *et al.*, 1997; Matsuno *et al.*, 1996). A key finding was that particle-laden DC that would normally traffic in celiac lymph could be isolated from the central lymph of these rats, but these cells were not detected in mesenteric lymphadenectomized animals.

Following injection of particulates, DC are recruited to the liver sinusoids (Matsuno *et al.*, 1996). The signals for recruitment are not yet clear, but one possibility is that Kupffer cells (liver macrophages) phagocytose particles from the bloodstream and then elaborate cytokines or chemokines in response to the phagocytic load that attract DC progenitors; a precedent for this comes from the finding that DC from celiac lymph can adhere to Kupffer cells in frozen sections of liver (Kudo *et al.*, 1997). Within the liver sinusoids, the DC then appear to internalize the particles, before maturing and migrating into celiac lymph. At this stage, the DC are unable to phagocytose further particulates *in vitro*, but express costimulatory activity that would enable them to initiate immune responses within the celiac nodes.

Movement of DC from the liver sinusoids into celiac lymph involves a blood–lymph translocation, presumably via the space of Disse. This translocation has been demonstrated directly following intravenous injection of DC isolated from celiac lymph (Kudo *et al.*, 1997). When cells that had phagocytosed particles *in vivo* were injected into the blood, they could subsequently be detected within the celiac lymph nodes and were observed to home to paracortical regions (Plate 11.4). Furthermore, when allogeneic DC were injected they were found to be associated with proliferating T cells which they had presumably activated in these sites. Whether DC originating from other tissues, such as the interstitial spaces of vascularized organs, can also undergo such a blood–lymph translocation is not yet known. An early study demonstrated that mesenteric lymph DC can migrate from the blood into the celiac nodes (Fossum, 1988), although the physiological significance of this route is unclear.

Lymphoid DC in Lymph Nodes

Evidence for a distinct subset of lymphoid DC with regulatory properties in mouse spleen was discussed earlier. A similar subset is also present in mouse lymphoid tissues. While studies of the regulatory properties of these DC are not yet as advanced as those of the cells in spleen, CD8α^+ DC isolated from mouse lymph nodes have been shown to express high levels of a self-peptide MHC complex, and to induce apoptosis after antigen presentation to an antigen-specific T cell hybridoma (Inaba *et al.*, 1997).

Further evidence for a distinct subset of DC in lymph nodes has come from studies in humans. For many years an unusual cell type has been described within paracortical regions of human lymph nodes that has the cytology of a plasma cell and expresses CD4 but not intracellular immunoglobulin. These so-called 'plasmacytoid T cells' express CD45RA but not most other markers of known lymphoid or myeloid cell types (Plate 11.5). After isolation from human tonsils, these CD4$^+$ CD11c$^-$ CD3$^-$ cells underwent rapid apoptosis unless they were rescued with IL-3 (Grouard *et al.*, 1997). Remarkably, the addition of CD40 ligand was then shown to result in their differentiation into DC that express low levels of myeloid antigens CD13 and CD33. The freshly isolated cells were found to express MHC class II molecules (HLA-DR), low levels of CD40, and CD54, but not CD58, CD80, or CD86. Expression of all these molecules was upregulated or induced during culture with IL-3 and further increased on CD40 ligation.

A subset of CD4$^+$ CD11c$^-$ CD3$^-$ CD45RA$^+$ cells has also been identified in human blood (O'Doherty *et al.*, 1994) that develops into DC when cultured with monocyte-conditioned medium, a potent DC maturation stimulus (see above); this subset may be the same as one identified on the basis of different markers (Thomas and Lipsky, 1994). It is therefore possible these cells in blood give rise to the 'plasmacytoid T cells', now known to be DC, in tonsil, spleen, and lymph nodes. The fact that these cells can be detected (Grouard *et al.*, 1997) within the lumen and walls of high endothelial venules (HEV) within lymph nodes (Plate 11.5) strongly suggests that they enter the tissue directly from the bloodstream, rather than via the subcapsular space as for DC entering from nonlymphoid tissues. It also seems likely that the same precursors can enter the marginal zone of spleen from the blood. Possible regulatory functions of this presumptive DC subset have not been reported at the time of writing.

DC in Germinal Centres of Lymph Nodes and Other Secondary Lymphoid Tissues

As reviewed elsewhere (Chapter 4) follicular dendritic cells (FDC) within germinal centres (GC) retain immune complexes on the cell surface and are involved in affinity maturation of B cells. A distinct subset of CD4$^+$ CD11c$^+$ CD3$^-$ DC has also been identified in these sites (Grouard *et al.*, 1996). These germinal centre DC (GCDC) are present in both the dark and light zones of germinal centres in human tonsils, spleen, and lymph nodes, and are associated with GC T cells (Plate 11.6). Unlike IDC within T cell areas of these tissues, these leukocytes do not express CD1a and have low expression of CD40 *in situ*. However, after isolation, GCDC underwent spontanous maturation (as opposed to apoptosis seen for 'plasmacytoid T cells'; see above) and rapidly upregulated CD40, together with CD80, CD86, and MHC class II molecules.

It seems most likely that GCDC can induce or sustain the response of memory T cells in GC, and maintain the GC reaction during secondary T cell-dependent responses of B cells. Whether these DC enter the tissues directly from the blood or from nonlymphoid tissues is not yet clear. However, a subset of $CD4^+$ $CD11c^+$ $CD3^-$ $CD45RO^+$ DC has been identified in human peripheral blood, and it has been suggested that these cells represent functionally more mature cells that have migrated from nonlymphoid tissues (O'Doherty *et al.*, 1994). One (highly speculative) possibility is that the migration pathways of nonlymphoid DC might be altered during secondary responses, for example after ligation of Fc receptors on DC by pre-formed antibodies or immune complexes, so that these cells are diverted into GC.

Correlation between Observations *in situ* and *in vivo*

As for the situation in spleen, it is rather difficult to explain the precise origin of the phenotypically distinct subsets of DC identified in lymph nodes.

As outlined above, there is reasonably clear evidence for migration of (nonlymphoid) DC from skin to peripheral lymph nodes after transplantation, application of contact sensitizers, and injection of *Leishmania* parasites; from the gut wall to mesenteric lymph nodes; and from liver sinusoids to celiac lymph nodes. It seems reasonable to assume that DC migrating from nonlymphoid tissues in afferent lymph would enter lymph nodes via the subcapsular sinus and in most cases these cells have been shown to home to paracortical regions. However, as for DC in spleen, there are discrepancies relating to the phenotype of LC in skin ($CD11c^-$ DEC-205^+ $CD11b^+$) for example, and DC subsets observed in regional lymph nodes *in situ*, and questions arising over the absence of DC in lymph nodes of mice with a dominant negative Ikaros mutation despite the presence of LC in the epidermis of these mutants.

There is suggestive evidence that a subset of (lymphoid) DC may enter human lymph nodes via high endothelial venules, and that cells of this subset probably home to paracortical regions. It seems reasonable, therefore, to assume that both nonlymphoid and lymphoid DC coexist within T cell areas of lymph nodes. However, despite some indications that the latter cells may have negative regulatory properties *in vitro*, it is not yet clear whether these are involved in the induction or maintenance of tolerance to self-antigens or in homeostasis during immune responses to foreign antigens. Finally, a phenotypically distinct subset of DC has been identified in germinal centres of human lymph nodes and spleen, but the origin and function of these cells are unclear.

CONCLUSIONS

Summary

In situ studies have demonstrated at least three phenotypically distinct subsets of DC within spleen and lymph nodes (similar subsets have also been identified in Peyer's patches; Kelsall and Strober, 1996). In spleen, these subsets are situated close to the marginal zones at the periphery of the white pulp (MZDC), deep in the central white pulp within the T cell areas or PALS (IDC), and within germinal centres (GCDC). The corresponding subsets in lymph nodes appear to be situated close to the subcapsular sinus, deep in the paracortical areas within T cell zones (IDC), and within germinal centres (GCDC), respectively. The freshly isolated DC subsets differ in function: the former subset (e.g. splenic MZDC) seems to be relatively immature and capable of antigen uptake and processing, while the latter (i.e. IDC) appears to be relatively mature with costimulatory activity. Since the former subset matures in culture and comes to resemble the latter, there may be a precursor–product relationship between these cells *in situ*. An additional subset of DC is represented by 'plasmacytoid T cells' in T cell zones of tonsils.

In vitro studies have provided evidence for three, and perhaps four, developmental pathways that can generate distinct subsets of human DC: LC, myeloid DC, monocyte-derived DC, and lymphoid DC. LC originate from a $CD34^+$ CLA^+ progenitor; myeloid DC originate from a $CD34^+$ CLA^- progenitor via a bipotential intermediate that can alternatively produce macrophages; monocytes that can develop into DC may or may not represent a precursor in the latter (myeloid) pathway; and lymphoid DC originate from a distinct progenitor that can also generate lymphoid but not myeloid cells. A similar situation is likely to pertain in mice; for example, a distinct origin for LC versus many DC in lymphoid tissues is suggested from studies in knockout mice, and a distinct progenitor that appears able to generate DC and lymphoid but not myeloid cells has also been identified. From *in vitro* studies, the lymphoid DC subset isolated from spleen and thymus has regulatory properties that are not exhibited by other subsets.

In vivo studies have exposed three migration pathways that may be required for the induction of immune responses to foreign antigens in different anatomical compartments. DC can migrate from epithelia via afferent lymph into regional lymph nodes (e.g. from skin to peripheral nodes, and from gut to mesenteric nodes); from interstitial spaces of vascularized organs (e.g. heart, kidney) via blood into spleen; and from liver sinusoids via a blood–lymph translocation into celiac lymph nodes. These routes may be required, respectively, for the initiation of responses against foreign antigens that gain access to topologically external epithelial sites, topologically internal interstitial spaces, and the bloodstream.

Further Observations

Within different tissues, local specializations of DC may favour the generation of particular types of immune response. For example, at least as generated from progenitors *in vitro*, myeloid DC can influence B cell responses directly whereas LC may not (Caux *et al.*, in press). Hence myeloid DC may be primarily involved in humoral reponses whereas LC may generate cell-mediated responses. Possibly this relates to the capacity of circulating antibodies to access interstitial spaces of vascularized tissues, where they can directly effect elimination of certain antigens, versus their relative inaccessibility to sites such as skin epidermis. Clearly it will be important to define the *in vivo* conterparts of myeloid DC generated *in vitro*, and to investigate their homing properties. There is also evidence that DC within different lymphoid tissues may induce different types of immune response. In particular, DC isolated from spleen and Peyer's patch seem preferentially to induce T_H1 and T_H2 type responses, respectively (Everson *et al.*, 1996). The molecular basis for these apparent specializations is unknown. However, it seems likely that DC do not just induce immune reponses to foreign antigens; they also bias the response along certain pathways.

It seems probable that DC that have acquired foreign antigens in nonlymphoid tissues can initiate immune responses after migration into spleen or lymph nodes. However, soluble antigens injected directly into the blood may bypass this route, and can induce tolerance instead of immunity. While details are still not clear, there is evidence that such antigens can be presented by nearly all B cells as well as by DC in spleen (Zhong *et al.*, 1997). Because there are many more B cells than dendritic cells in lymphoid tissues, it has been suggested that in such circumstances the B cells may interact first or more frequently with naive T cells and induce (peripheral) T cell tolerance or immune deviation. Of course these observations need to be viewed in the light of evidence that DC can be recruited to liver sinusoids in response to blood-borne particulates prior to their migration into celiac lymph nodes, apparently for the induction of immunity; possibly the latter pathway does not operate, or is relatively ineffective, in the case of soluble antigens. Whatever the case, the balance between immunity and tolerance is likely to be controlled both by the relative contributions of different types of antigen-presenting cells *in vivo* and, conceivably, by different subsets of DC in secondary lymphoid tissues.

Hypothesis

An emerging concept is that DC within spleen and thymus could be involved in both the generation of immunity to foreign antigens and the induction of peripheral tolerance to self-antigens. Clearly, integrating our current and incomplete knowledge of the origin, migration, and localization of DC is difficult. However, we currently favour the following hypothesis.

Induction of Immunity to Foreign Antigens

(a) Bone marrow-derived ‘non-lymphoid DC’ progenitors (e.g. LC and myeloid DC progenitors in human) constitutively seed nonlymphoid tissues and develop locally into immature, processing DC in these sites. This pathway could maintain a basal level of DC within nonlymphoid tissues that are capable of acquiring foreign antigens that gain access to these sites. Inflammatory stimuli and/or microbial products such as LPS then induce the maturation of these cells and their migration into spleen and/or lymph nodes for the initiation of T-independent and T-dependent antigen-specific responses.

(b) Although there is no direct evidence for this pathway at present, monocytes may be rapidly recruited from the blood into inflamed tissues. Depending on the local environment, these cells could then develop into immature, processing DC and acquire antigens, before maturing and migrating to spleen and/or lymph nodes for initiation of immune responses as above. This pathway could ensure a rapid response to infection prior to mobilization of other DC progenitors from the bone marrow.

Induction of Tolerance to Self-antigens

(a) Bone marrow-derived ‘lymphoid DC’ progenitors enter the thymus and develop into DC that induce central tolerance to self-antigens. Tolerance of T cells is induced, in whole or in part, because the DC may interact with developing thymocytes, and their costimulatory and other properties that would activate mature T cells lead instead to clonal deletion or anergy of the immature T cells.

(b) The same lymphoid DC progenitors, or later intermediates in the developmental pathway, may seed secondary lymphoid tissues including spleen and lymph nodes directly from the blood. These cells develop into mature, regulatory cells that induce peripheral tolerance to self-antigens. Tolerance of T cells is induced, in whole or in part, because these DC express molecules (e.g. FasL) that are not expressed on 'non-lymphoid DC' and which deliver negative regulatory (e.g. apoptotic) signals to mature T cells after activation.

REFERENCES

Adema, G.J., Hartgers, F., Verstraten, R., de Vries, E., Marland, G., Menon, S., Foster, J., Xu, Y., Nooyen, P., McClanahan, T., Bacon, K.B. and Figdor, C.G. (1997). A dendritic-cell-derived C-C chemokine that preferentially attracts naive T cells. *Nature* **387**, 713–717.

Austyn, J.M. (1987). Lymphoid dendritic cells. *Immunology* **62**, 161–170.

Austyn, J.M. (1992). Antigen uptake and presentation by dendritic leukocytes. *Semin. Immunol.* **4**, 227–236.

Austyn, J.M. (1996). New insights into the mobilization and phagocytic activity of dendritic cells [comment]. *J. Exp. Med.* **183**, 1287–1292.

Austyn, J.M. (1998). Dendritic cells. *Curr. Opin. Hematol.* **9**, 3–15.

Austyn, J.M. and Larsen, C.P. (1990). Migration patterns of dendritic leukocytes. Implications for transplantation. *Transplantation* **49**, 1–7.

Austyn, J.M., Kupiec-Weglinski, J.W., Hankins, D.F. and Morris, P.J. (1988). Migration patterns of dendritic cells in the mouse. Homing to T cell-dependent areas of spleen, and binding within marginal zone. *J. Exp. Med.* **167**, 646–651.

Austyn, J.M., Hankins, D.F., Larsen, C.P., Morris, P.J., Rao, A.S. and Roake, J.A. (1994). Isolation and characterization of dendritic cells from mouse heart and kidney. *J. Immunol.* **152**, 2401–2410.

Barratt-Boyes, S.M., Watkins, S.C. and Finn, O.J. (1997). In vivo migration of dendritic cells differentiated in vitro: a chimpanzee model. *J. Immunol.* **158**, 4543–4547.

Borkowski, T.A., Letterio, J.J., Farr, A.G. and Udey, M.C. (1996a). A role for endogenous transforming growth factor β1 in Langerhans cell biology: the skin of transforming growth factor β1 null mice is devoid of epidermal Langerhans cells. *J. Exp. Med.* **184**, 2417–2422.

Borkowski, T.A., Nelson, A.J., Farr, A.G. and Udey, M.C. (1996b). Expression of gp40, the murine homologue of human epithelial cell adhesion molecule (Ep-CAM), by murine dendritic cells. *Eur. J. Immunol.* **26**, 110–114.

Brocker, T., Riedinger, M. and Karjalainen, K. (1997). Targeted expression of major histocompatibility complex (MHC) class II molecules demonstrates that dendritic cells can induce negative but not positive selection of thymocytes in vivo. *J. Exp. Med.* **185**, 541–550.

Burkly, L., Hession, C., Ogata, L., *et al.*, (1995). Expression of relB is required for the development of thymic medulla and dendritic cells. *Nature* **373**, 531–536.

Caux, C., Vanbervliet, B., Massacrier, C., *et al.* (1996). $CD34^+$ hematopoietic progenitors from human cord blood differentiate along two independent dendritic cell pathways in response to GM-CSF^+TNF-α. *J. Exp. Med.* **184**, 695–706.

Caux, C., Massacrier, C., Vanbervliet, B. *et al.* (1997). $DC34^+$ hematopoietic progenitors from human cord blood differentiate along two independent dendritic cell pathways in response to GM-CSF^+ TNF-α. II. Functional analysis. *Blood* **90**, 1458–1470.

Cella, M., Sallusto, F. and Lanzavecchia, A. (1997). Origin, maturation and antigen presenting function of dendritic cells. *Curr. Opin. Immunol.* **9**, 10–16.

Codner, M.A., Shuster, B.A., Steinman, R.M., Harper, A.D., La, T.G. and Hoffman, L.A. (1990). Migration of donor leukocytes from limb allografts into host lymphoid tissues. *Ann. Plast. Surg.* **25**, 353–359.

Cumberbatch, M. and Kimber, I. (1990). Phenotypic characteristics of antigen-bearing cells in the draining lymph nodes of contact sensitized mice. *Immunology* **71**, 404–410.

Cumberbatch, M. and Kimber, I. (1992). Dermal tumour necrosis factor-α induces dendritic cell migration to the draining lymph nodes, and possibly provides one stimulus for Langerhans cell migration. *Immunology* **75**, 257–263.

Cumberbatch, M., Dearman, R.J. and Kimber, I. (1996). Adhesion molecule expression by epidermal Langerhans cells and lymph node dendritic cells: a comparison. *Arch. Dermatol. Res.* **288**, 739–744.

De Smedt, T., Pajak, B., Muraille, E. *et al.* (1996). Regulation of dendritic cell numbers and maturation by lipopolysaccharide in vivo. *J. Exp. Med.* **184**, 1413–1424.

Delgado, E., Finkel, V., Baggiolini, M., Clark-Lewis, I., Mackay, C.R., Steinman, R.M. and Granelli-Piperno, A. (1998). Mature dendritic cells response to SDF-1, but not to several β-chemokines. *Immunobiology*, in press.

Enk, A.H., Angeloni, V.L., Udey, M.C. and Katz, S.I. (1993). An essential role for Langerhans cell-derived IL-1β in the initiation of primary immune responses in skin. *J. Immunol.* **150**, 3698–3704.

Everson, M.P., McDuffie, D.S., Lemak, D.G., Koopman, W.J., McGhee, J.R. and Beagley, K.W. (1996). Dendritic cells from different tissues induce production of different T cell cytokine profiles. *J. Leukocyte Biol.* **59**, 494–498.

Fairchild, P.J. and Austyn, J.M. (1990). Thymic dendritic cells: phenotype and function. *Int. Rev. Immunol.* **6**, 187–196.

Fossum, S. (1988). Lymph-borne dendritic leukocytes do not recirculate, but enter the lymph node paracortex to become interdigitating cells. *Scand. J. Immunol.* **27**, 97–105.

Fu, F., Li, Y., Qian, S., Lu, L., Chambers, F., Starzl, T.E., Fung, J.J. and Thomson, A.W. (1996). Costimulatory molecule-deficient dendritic cell progenitors (MHC class II^+, $CD80^{dim}$, $CD86^-$) prolong cardiac allograft survival in nonimmunosuppressed recipients. *Transplantation* **62**, 659–665.

Galy, A., Travis, M., Cen, D. and Chen, B. (1995). Human T, B, natural killer, and dendritic cells arise from a common bone marrow progenitor cell subset. *Immunity* **3**, 459–473.

Godiska, R., Chantry, D., Raport, C.J., Sozzani, S., Allavena, P., Leviten, D., Mantovani, A. and Gray, P.W. (1997). Human macrophage-derived chemokine (MDC), a novel chemoattractant for monocytes, monocyte-derived dendritic cells, and natural killer cells. *J. Exp. Med.* **185**, 1595–1604.

Granelli-Piperno, A., Moser, B., Pope, M., Chen, D., Wei, Y., Isdell, F., O'Doherty, U., Paxton, W., Koup, R., Mojsov, S., Bhardwaj, N., Clark, L.I., Baggiolini, M. and Steinman, R.M. (1996). Efficient interaction of HIV-1 with purified dendritic cells via multiple chemokine coreceptors. *J. Exp. Med.* **184**, 2433–2438.

Grouard, G., Durand, I., Filgueira, L., Banchereau, J. and Liu, Y.J. (1996). Dendritic cells capable of stimulating T cells in germinal centres. *Nature* **384**, 364–367.

Grouard, G., Rissoan, M.C., Filgueira, L., Durand, I., Banchereau, J. and Liu, Y.J. (1997). The enigmatic plasmacytoid T cells develop into dendritic cells with interleukin (IL)-3 and CD40-ligand. *J. Exp. Med.* **185**, 1101–1111.

Hedrick, J.A. and Zlotnik, A. (1996). Chemokines and lymphocyte biology. *Curr. Opin. Immunol.* **8**, 343–347.

Inaba, K., Steinman, R.M., Pack, M.W. *et al.* (1992). Identification of proliferating dendritic cell precursors in mouse blood. *J. Exp. Med.* **175**, 1157–1167.

Inaba, K., Pack, M., Inaba, M., Sakuta, H., Isdell, F. and Steinman, R.M. (1997). High levels of a major histocompatibility complex II-self peptide complex on dendritic cells from the T cell areas of lymph nodes. *J. Exp. Med.* **186**, 665–672.

Ingulli, E., Mondino, A., Khoruts, A. and Jenkens, M.K. (1997). In vivo detection of dendritic cell antigen presentation to CD4(+) T cells. *J. Exp. Med.* **185**, 2133–2141.

Jonuleit, H., Knop, J. and Enk, A.H. (1996). Cytokines and their effects on maturation, differentiation and migration of dendritic cells. *Arch. Dermatol. Res.* **289**, 1–8.

Kelsall, B.L. and Strober, W. (1996). Distinct populations of dendritic cells are present in the subepithelial dome and T cell regions of the murine Peyer's patch. *J. Exp. Med.* **183**, 237–247.

Kobayashi, Y. (1997). Langerhans' cells produce type IV collagenase (MMP-9) following epicutaneous stimulation with haptens. *Immunology* **90**, 496–501.

Kripke, M.L., Munn, C.G., Jeevan, A., Tang, J.-M. and Bucana, C. (1990). Evidence that cutaneous antigen-presenting cells migrate to regional lymph nodes during contact sensitization. *J. Immunol.* **145**, 2833–2838.

Kronin, V., Winkel, K., Suss, G., Kelso, A., Heath, W., Kirberg, J., von, B.H. and Shortman, K. (1996). A subclass of dendritic cells regulates the response of naive CD8 T cells by limiting their IL-2 production. *J. Immunol.* **157**, 3819–3827.

Kronin, V., Vremec, D., Winkel, K., Classon, B.J., Miller, R.G., Mak, T.W., Shortman, K. and Suss, G. (1997). Are CD8$^+$ dendritic cells (DC) veto cells? The role of CD8 on DC in DC development and in the regulation of CD4 and CD8 T cell responses. *Int. Immunol.* **9**, 1061–1064.

Kudo, S., Matsuno, K., Ezaki, T. and Ogawa, M. (1997). A novel migration pathway for rat dendritic cells from the blood: hepatic sinusoids–lymph translocation. *J. Exp. Med.* **185**, 777–784.

Kupiec-Weglinski, J.W., Austyn, J.M. and Morris, P.J. (1988). Migration patterns of dendritic cells in the mouse. Traffic from the blood, and T cell-dependent and -independent entry to lymphoid tissues. *J. Exp. Med.* **167**, 632–645.

Lanzavecchia, A. (1996). Mechanisms of antigen uptake for presentation. *Curr. Opin. Immunol.* **8**, 348–354.

Larsen, C.P., Morris, P.J. and Austyn, J.M. (1990a). Migration of dendritic leukocytes from cardiac allografts into host spleens. A novel pathway for initiation of rejection. *J. Exp. Med.* **171**, 307–314.

Larsen, C.P., Steinman, R.M., Witmer, P.M., Hankins, D.F., Morris, P.J. and Austyn, J.M. (1990b). Migration and maturation of Langerhans cells in skin transplants and explants. *J. Exp. Med.* **172**, 1483–1493.

Laszik, Z., Jansen, P.J., Cummings, R.D., Tedder, T.F., McEver, R.P. and Moore, K.L. (1996). P-selectin glycoprotein ligand-1 is broadly expressed in cells of myeloid, lymphoid, and dendritic lineage and in some nonhematopoietic cells. *Blood* **88**, 3010–3021.

Lawrence, J.M., Morris, R.J., Wilson, D.J. and Raisman, G. (1990). Mechanisms of allograft rejection in the rat brain. *Neuroscience* **37**, 431–462.

Lin, C.-L., Suri, R.M., Rahdon, R.A., Morris, P.J., Austyn, J.M. and Roake, J.A. (1998). Dendritic cell chemotaxis and transendothelial migration is induced by distinct chemokines and is regulated on maturation. *Eur. J. Immunol.*, in press.

Liu, L.M. and MacPherson, G.G. (1995a). Antigen processing: cultured lymphborne dendritic cells can process and present native protein antigens. *Immunology* **84**, 241–246.

Liu, L.M. and MacPherson, G.G. (1995b). Rat intestinal dendritic cells: immunostimulatory potency and phenotypic characterization. *Immunology* **85**, 88–93.

Lukas, M., Stossel, H., Hefel, L., Imamura, S., Fritsch, P., Sepp, N.T., Schuler, G. and Romani, N. (1996). Human cutaneous dendritic cells migrate through dermal lymphatic vessels in a skin organ culture model. *J. Invest. Dermatol.* **106**, 1293–1299.

Macatonia, S.E., Knight, S.C., Edwards, A.J., Griffiths, S. and Fryer, P. (1987). Localization of antigen on lymph node dendritic cells after exposure to the contact sensitizer fluorescein isothiocyanate. Functional and morphological studies. *J. Exp. Med.* **166**, 1654–1667.

MacPherson, G.G., Jenkins, C.D., Stein, M.J. and Edwards, C. (1995). Endotoxin-mediated dendritic cell release from the intestine. Characterization of released dendritic cells and TNF dependence. *J. Immunol.* **154**, 1317–1322.

Maraskovsky, E., Brasel, K., Teepe, M., Roux, E.R., Lyman, S.D., Shortman, K. and McKenna, H.J. (1996). Dramatic increase in the numbers of functionally mature dendritic cells in Flt3 ligand-treated mice: multiple dendritic cell subpopulations identified. *J. Exp. Med.* **184**, 1953–1962.

Maric, I., Holt, P.G., Perdue, M.H. and Bienenstock, J. (1996). Class II MHC antigen (Ia)-bearing dendritic cells in the epithelium of the rat intestine. *J. Immunol.* **156**, 1408–1414.

Matsuno, K., Ezaki, T., Kudo, S. and Uehara, Y. (1996). A life stage of particle-laden rat dendritic cells in vivo: their terminal division, active phagocytosis, and translocation from the liver to the draining lymph node. *J. Exp. Med.* **183**, 1865–1878.

Matyszak, M.K. and Perry, V.H. (1996). The potential role of dendritic cells in immune-mediated inflammatory diseases in the central nervous system. *Neuroscience* **74**, 599–608.

McWilliam, A.S., Napoli, S., Marsh, A.M., Pemper, F.L., Nelson, D.J., Pimm, C.L., Stumbles, P.A., Wells, T.N. and Holt, P.G. (1996). Dendritic cells are recruited into the airway epithelium during the inflammatory response to a broad spectrum of stimuli. *J. Exp. Med.* **184**, 2429–2432.

McWilliam, A.S., Marsh, A.M. and Holt, P.G. (1997). Inflammatory infiltration of the upper airway epithelium during Sendai virus infection: involvement of epithelial dendritic cells. *J. Virol.* **71**, 226–236.

Mohamadzadeh, M., Poltorak, A.N., Bergstressor, P.R., Beutler, B. and Takashima, A. (1996). Dendritic cells produce macrophage inflammatory protein-1γ, a new member of the CC chemokine family. *J. Immunol.* **156**, 3102–3106.

Moll, H., Fuchs, H., Blank, C. and Rollinghof, M. (1993). Langerhans cells transport *Leishmania major* from the infected skin to the draining lymph node for presentation to antigen-specific T cells. *Eur. J. Immunol.* **23**, 1595–1601.

Moll, H., Flohe, S. and Rollinghof, M. (1995). Dendritic cells in *Leishmania major*-immune mice harbor persistent parasites and mediate an antigen-specific T cell immune response. *Eur. J. Immunol.* **25**, 693–699.

Moore, J.P., Trkola, A. and Dragic, T. (1997). Co-receptors for HIV-1 entry. *Curr. Opin. Immunol.* **9**, 551–562.

Morelli, A., Larregina, A., Chuluyan, I., Kolkowski, E. and Fainboim, L. (1996). Expression and modulation of C5a receptor (CD88) on skin dendritic cells. Chemotactic effect of C5a on skin migratory dendritic cells. *Immunology* **89**, 126–134.

O'Doherty, U., Peng, M., Gezelter, S., Swiggard, W.J., Betjes, M., Bharwaj, N. and Steinman, R.M. (1994). Human blood contains two subsets of dendritic cells, one immunologically mature and the other immature. *Immunology* **82**, 487–493.

Oluwole, S.F., Engelstad, K., De, R.C., Wang, T.S., Fawwaz, R.A., Reemtsma, K. and Hardy, M.A. (1991). Migration patterns of dendritic cells in the rat: comparison of the effects of γ and UV-B irradiation on the migration of dendritic cells and lymphocytes. *Cell Immunol.* **133**, 390–407.

Pancook, J.D., Reisfeld, R.A., Varki, N., Vitiello, A., Fox, R.I. and Montgomery, A.M. (1997). Expression and regulation of the neural cell adhesion molecule L1 on human cells of myelomonocytic and lymphoid origin. *J. Immunol.* **158**, 4413–4421.

Price, A.A., Cumberbatch, M., Kimber, I. and Ager, A. Alpha 6 integrin–laminin interactions are required for Langerhans cell migration from the epidermis. *J. Exp. Med.* **186**, 1725–1735.

Rahdon, R.A., Lin, C.L., Suri, R.M., Morris, P.J., Austyn, J.M. and Roake, J.A. (1997). An endothelial cell-derived chemotactic factor promotes transendothelial migration of human dendritic cells. *Transplant. Proc.* **2**, 1121–1122.

Reid, C.D. (1997). The dendritic cell lineage in haemopoiesis. *Br. J. Haematol.* **96**, 217–223.

Reis e Sousa, C., Stahl, P.D. and Austyn, J.M. (1993). Phagocytosis of antigens by Langerhans cells in vitro. *J. Exp. Med.* **178**, 509–519.

Res, P., Martinez, C.E., Cristina, J.A., Staal, F., Noteboom, E., Weijer, K. and Spits, H. (1996). $CD34^{+}CD38^{dim}$ cells in the human thymus can differentiate into T, natural killer, and dendritic cells but are distinct from pluripotent stem cells. *Blood* **87**, 5196–5206.

Richters, C.D., van Pelt, A.M., van Geldrop, E., Hockstra, M.J., van Baare, J., du Pont, J.S. and Kamperdijk, E.W. (1996). Migration of rat skin dendritic cells. *J. Leukocyte Biol.* **60**, 317–322.

Roake, J.A., Rao, A.S., Morris, P.J., Larsen, C.P., Hankins, D.F. and Austyn, J.M. (1995a). Dendritic cell loss from nonlymphoid tissues after systemic administration of lipopolysaccharide, tumor necrosis factor, and interleukin 1. *J. Exp. Med.* **181**, 2237–2247.

Roake, J.A., Rao, A.S., Morris, P.J., Larsen, C.P., Hankins, D.F. and Austyn, J.M. (1995b). Systemic lipopolysaccharide recruits dendritic cell progenitors to nonlymphoid tissues. *Transplantation* **59**, 1319–1324.

Saleem, M., Sawyer, G.J., Schofield, R.A., Seymour, N.D., Gustafsson, K. and Fabre, J.W. (1997). Discordant expression of major histocompatibility complex class II antigens and invariant chain in interstitial dendritic cells. Implications for self-tolerance and immunity. *Transplantation* **63**, 1134–1138.

Schall, T. (1997). Fractalkine—a strange attractor in the chemokine landscape. *Immunol. Today* **18**, 147.

Schall, T.J. and Bacon, K.B. (1994). Chemokines, leukocyte trafficking, and inflammation. *Curr. Opin. Immunol.* **6**, 865–873.

Schluger, N.W. and Rom, W.N. (1997). Early responses to infection: chemokines as mediators of inflammation. *Curr. Opin. Immunol.* **9**, 504–508.

Shankar, G., Pickard, E.S. and Burnham, K. (1996). Superantigen-induced Langerhans cell depletion is mediated by epidermal cell-derived IL-1α and TNF-α. *Cell. Immunol.* **171**, 240–245.

Shortman, K., Wu, L., Suss, G., Kronin, V., Winkel, K., Saunders, D. and Vremec, D. (1997). Dendritic cells and T lymphocytes: developmental and functional interactions. *Ciba Found. Symp.* **204**, 130–138.

Sozzani, S., Sallusto, F., Luini, W., Zhou, D., Piemonti, L., Allavena, P., Van, D.J., Valitutti, S., Lanzavecchia, A. and Mantovani, A. (1995). Migration of dendritic cells in response to formyl peptides, C5a, and a distinct set of chemokines. *J. Immunol.* **155**, 3292–3295.

Sozzani, S., Luini, W., Borsatti, A., Polentarutti, N., Zhou, D., Piemonti, L., D'Amico, G., Power, C.A., Wells, T.N.C., Gobbi, M., Allavena, P. and Mantovani, A. (1997). Receptor expression and responsiveness of human dendritic cells to a defined set of CC and CXC chemokines. *J. Immunol.* **159**, 1993–2000.

Steinman, R.M. (1991). The dendritic cell system and its role in immunogenicity. *Annu. Rev. Immunol.* **9**, 271–296.

Steinman, R.M. and Swanson, J. (1995). The endocytic activity of dendritic cells [comment]. *J. Exp. Med.* **182**, 283–288.

Steinman, R.M., Pack, M. and Inaba, K. (1997). Dendritic cells in the T-cell areas of lymphoid organs. *Immunol. Rev.* **156**, 25–37.

Strobl, H., Riedl, E., Scheinecker, C., Bello, F.C., Pickl, W.F., Rappersberger, K., Majdic, O. and Knapp, W. (1996). TGF-β1 promotes in vitro development of dendritic cells from CD34$^+$ hemopoietic progenitors. *J. Immunol.* **157**, 1499–1507.

Strunk, D., Egger, C., Leitner, G., Hanau, D. and Stingl, G. (1997). A skin homing molecule defines the Langerhans cell progenitor in human peripheral blood. *J. Exp. Med.* **185**, 1131–1136.

Suss, G. and Shortman, K. (1996). A subclass of dendritic cells kills CD4 T cells via Fas/Fas-ligand-induced apoptosis. *J. Exp. Med.* **183**, 1789–1796.

Thomas, R. and Lipsky, P.E. (1994). Human peripheral blood dendritic cell subsets. Isolation and characterization of precursor and mature antigen-presenting cells. *J. Immunol.* **153**, 4016–4028.

Thurnher, M., Ramoner, R., Gastl, G., Radmayr, C., Bock, G., Herold, M., Klocker, H. and Bartsch, G. (1997). Bacillus Calmette-Guerin mycobacteria stimulate human blood dendritic cells. *Int. J. Cancer* **70**, 128–134.

van Wilsem, E.J.G., Breve, J., Kleijmeer, M. and Kraal, G. (1994). Antigen-bearing Langerhans cells in skin draining lymph nodes. Phenotype and kinetics of migration. *J. Invest. Dermatol.* **103**, 217–220.

Vremec, D. and Shortman, K. (1997). Dendritic cell subtypes in mouse lymphoid organs. Cross-correlation of surface markers, changes with incubation, and differences among thymus, spleen, and lymph nodes. *J. Immunol.* **159**, 565–573.

Vremec, D., Lieschke, G.J., Dunn, A.R., Robb, L., Metcalf, D. and Shortman, K. (1997). The influence of granulocyte/macrophage colony-stimulating factor on dendritic cell levels in mouse lymphoid organs. *Eur. J. Immunol.* **27**, 40–44.

Wang, J.H., Nichogiannopoulou, A., Wu, L., Sun, L., Sharpe, A.H., Bigby, M. and Georgopoulos, K. (1996). Selective defects in the development of the fetal and adult lymphoid system in mice with an Ikaros null mutation. *Immunity* **5**, 537–549.

Wu, L., Li, C.L. and Shortman, K. (1996). Thymic dendritic cell precursors: relationship to the T lymphocyte lineage and phenotype of the dendritic cell progeny. *J. Exp. Med.* **184**, 903–911.

Wu, L., Nichogiannopoulou, A., Shortman, K. and Georgopoulos, K. (1997). Cell autonomous defects in dendritic cell populations of Ikaros mutant mice point to a developmental relationship with the lymphoid lineage. *Immunity* **7**, 483–492.

Young, J.W. and Steinman, R.M. (1996). The hematopoietic development of dendritic cells: a distinct pathway for myeloid differentiation. *Stem Cells* **14**, 376–387.

Zhong, G., Reis e Sousa, C. and Germain, R.N. (1997). Antigen-unspecific B cells and lymphoid dendritic cells both show extensive surface expression of processed antigen–major histocompatibility complex class II complexes after soluble protein exposure in vivo or in vitro. *J. Exp. Med.* **186**, 673–682.

CHAPTER 12
Dendritic Cells in the Central Nervous System and Eye and Their Associated Supporting Tissues

P.G. McMenamin[1] and J.V. Forrester[2]
[1]Department of Anatomy and Human Biology, The University of Western Australia, Nedlands, Australia; [2]Department of Ophthalmology, University of Aberdeen, Medical School, Aberdeen, UK

INTRODUCTION

In this review we will discuss whether dendritic cells (DC) are present within the central nervous system (CNS). In this context we will consider not only the neural parenchyma of the brain, spinal cord and retina but also their surrounding tissues, namely the meninges and uveal tract of the eye respectively (see Figs 1 and 2). The first part of the review describes the organization of the CNS in relation to how immune responses are mediated via the meninges, the ventricular system, the choroid plexus and the uveal tract. The location and function of the blood–brain barrier (BBB) and blood–ocular barrier (BOB) in relation to regulation of trafficking of immune cells in the CNS and the concept of 'immune privileged sites' will be emphasized. A discussion of the likely candidates for antigen-presenting cells (APCs) in the CNS will centre on whether microglia are specialized macrophages or represent a type of DC. Other CNS macrophage populations (perivascular cells, intraventricular macrophages, meningeal macrophages, choroid plexus macrophages and uveal tract macrophages) will be discussed with relevance to their possible role as APCs. The identification and location of DC in the brain parenchyma, meninges, choroid plexus and the uveal tract of the eye will then be addressed. The factors which regulate DC function in the CNS and their supporting tissues will precede a discussion of why there appear to be no DC in the neural parenchymal microenvironment and how this fits with current concepts on immune responses and inflammation of the brain and retina.

The General Arrangement of the Brain, Meninges and Choroid Plexus

The brain and spinal cord are surrounded by three layers of meninges: an outer tough pachymeninx, the dura mater, and the inner leptomeninges consisting of the arachnoid

Dendritic Cells: Biology and Clinical Applications
ISBN 0-12-455860-7

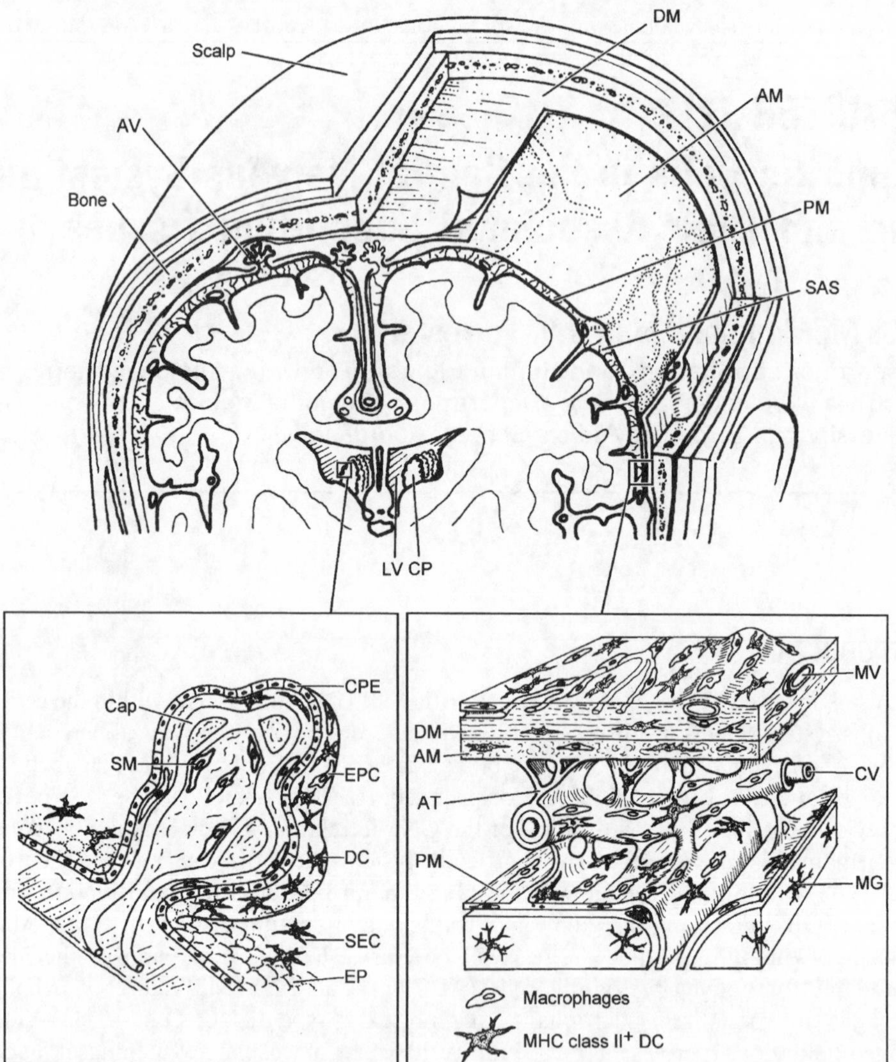

Fig. 1. The skull, choroid plexus and meninges. Upper: Schematic 3-D drawing (in the coronal plane) of the skull, cranial cavity, meninges, brain and ventricles containing the choroid plexus. Bottom left: The structure of the choroid plexus and distribution of macrophages and dendritic cells (DC). Bottom right: the distribution of macrophages and DC in the meninges. AV, Arachnoid villi; AM, arachnoid membrane; AT, arachnoid trabeculae; Cap, capillaries; CPE, choroid plexus epithelium; CV, cerebral vessel; DC, dendritic cell; EP, ependyma; EPC, epiplexus cell (type of macrophage); DM, dura mater; CP, choroid plexus; LV, lateral ventricle; MG, microglia; MV, meningeal vessel; PM, pia mater; SM, stromal macrophages; SEC, supraependymal cells; SAS, subarachnoid space.

(mater) and pia mater (pia-arachnoid). Between the arachnoid and pia is the subarachnoid space filled with cerebrospinal fluid (CSF) (Fig. 1).

The dura mater, a tough fibrous layer on the inner surface of the skull, forms the dural venous sinuses and dural folds (Fig. 1). The latter, together with the CSF, aids in providing physical support and protection for the brain. In the vertebral canal the dura forms a complete sleeve enclosing the spinal cord, and together these are surrounded by an epidural space (not present in the cranial cavity) containing connective tissue, fat and a plexus of veins.

The arachnoid is a delicate fibrocellular layer which bridges over the sulci and fissures on the brain surface, thus creating the subarachnoid cisterns (Fig. 1). The arachnoid is connected to the pia by numerous fibrocellular bands that cross the subarachnoid space (Fig. 1). These bands, lined by mesotheliocytes, form part of the cellular boundary of the subarachnoid space. This connection has led to leptomeninges being considered as a conjoined pia-arachnoid membrane. Specialized regions of arachnoid, the arachnoid villi and granulations, project into several of the dural venous sinuses (Fig. 1) and act as one-way pressure-sensitive valves allowing bulk drainage of CSF from the subarachnoid space into the venous blood in the dural sinuses. Structures passing to and from the brain to the skull or its foramina, such as cranial nerves or blood vessels, must traverse the subarachnoid space. Since the arachnoid fuses with the perineurium of spinal and cranial nerves, the CSF-containing subarachnoid space extends for a short distance around these nerves.

The pia mater is a vascular fibrocellular membrane covering the brain and spinal cord whose innermost cells lie upon a basal lamina which separates them from astrocytic foot processes. This is often called the 'pia-glia' or 'pia-intima'. The pia mater follows the surface contours of the brain and vessels entering or leaving the brain substance are surrounded by a pial sheath that is rich in astrocytes. There is debate as to the extent of the perivascular space (of 'Virchow-Robins') around these vessels. From an immunological perspective these spaces may allow communication between the CSF in the subarachnoid space and the brain parenchyma.

The choroid plexus arises where pia mater invaginates into the ventricles of the brain. They are vascular frond-like structures consisting of rich fenestrated capillary beds in a loose connective-tissue stroma covered by a modified secretory ependymal monolayer (Fig. 1). They are responsible for the constant secretion of CSF (2–4 μl/min) which fills the ventricular system and the subarachnoid space. The choroid plexus is present in the lateral ventricles, third ventricle and fourth ventricles of the brain, which are CSF-filled cavities in the cerebral hemispheres, midbrain and hindbrain respectively. The central nervous tissue itself consists of the cell bodies and processes of many classes of neurons and their supporting glial cells (astrocytes and oligodendrocytes). Other cell types associated with the vasculature are illustrated in Fig. 3.

Evolutionary Note

It is only in animals from reptiles and above that there exist true dura mater and leptomeninges with an intervening subarachnoid space. In animals from fishes and below there are no clearly defined layers of meninges and no subarachnoid space. Sharks and cyclostomes have large sac-like extensive expansions which cover the IV ventricle, midbrain and hindbrain and thus serve a similar function as the subarachnoid space. In some amphibians there are large endolymphatic sacs containing milky white proteinaceous fluid (≅lymph) that partially surround the brain and spinal cord and extend along the spinal nerves for a short distance.

It has been postulated for over 70 years that the CSF in the subarachnoid space and ventricles in mammals functions as the lymphatic fluid of the CNS (Kaper *et al.*, 1967).

The General Layout of the Retina and Uveal Tract of the Eye

The eye consists essentially of three layers: the inner neural retina surrounded by the uveal tract (choroid posteriorly and ciliary body–iris anteriorly), both protected by the fibrous corneoscleral envelope (Fig. 2). The structural, functional and embryological

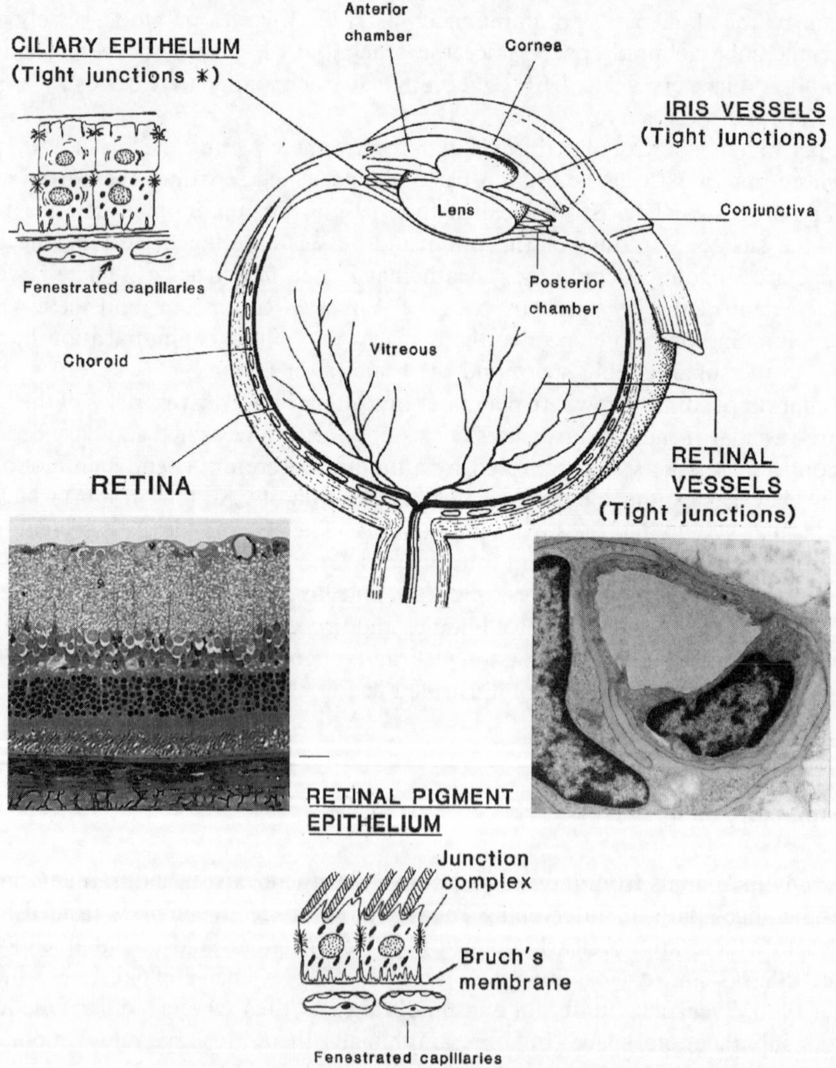

Fig. 2. Schematic summary of the anatomy of the eye and the sites of the blood–ocular barriers.

Table 1. Homologies between structures in the brain/spinal cord and those of the eye

Brain/spinal cord	Eye	Comments/shared function
Grey and white matter	Neural retina	The optic vesicle and optic stalk develop as outpouchings from the forebrain and differentiate to become the retina and optic nerve respectively.
Dura mater	Corneoscleral envelope	Both tough, dense, regular connective–collagenous tissues. Provide physical protection and support. Continuous at the optic nerve sheaths. Common embryological origin, namely condensed neural crest-derived mesenchyme.
Pia-arachnoid	Uveal tract	Fibrocellular vascular layers.
Cerebrospinal fluid (CSF)	Aqueous humour (AqH)	Both clear secretions with nutritive role. Responsible for intrinsic pressures (intracranial and intraocular pressures).
Choroid plexus	Ciliary processes	Both frond-like vascular structures covered by neuroepithelial layer(s). They actively secrete CSF and aqueous humour.
Ventricles (lateral, III and IV)	'Optic ventricle' or Subretinal space	Optic 'ventricle' obliterated during development, represented thereafter by 'potential' subretinal space.
Arachnoid villi (granulations)	Trabecular meshwork	Pressure sensitive one-way valves, drain CSF and aqueous humour into venous blood (dural venous sinuses and Schlemm's canal respectively).

basis of the homology between the various components of the eye and the brain is summarized in Table 1. An appreciation of the homologous structures in the eye and brain, particularly the blood–tissue barriers, is central to the discussions which follow on whether DC are present within the CNS.

The retina is the innermost of the three coats of the eye (Fig. 2) and consists of two primary layers—an inner neurosensory retina and an outer simple epithelium, the retinal pigment epithelium (RPE). Between the neural retina and RPE is a potential space, the subretinal space, across which the two layers must adhere. The retina consists of several cell types, of which neural cells, including photoreceptors, predominate. However, other cell types are also present such as glial cells, vascular endothelium, pericytes and microglia.

The choroid consists of vascular pigmented connective tissue with larger vessels externally and a rich bed of large fenestrated capillaries, the choriocapillaris, lying directly beneath the RPE (Fig. 4). The ciliary body (Fig. 2) of the eye consists of a smooth pars plana which extends from the cilio-retinal junction to the pars plicata anteriorly. The latter consists of 120 circumferentially arranged radial ridges, known as ciliary processes, which surround the lens (Fig. 2). The ciliary processes secrete aqueous humour (AqH) (2–4 μl/min), which circulates around the lens before it passes through the pupil into the anterior chamber from where it leaves via the aqueous outflow pathways. The ciliary processes consist of a connective-tissue stroma, rich in fenestrated capillaries, covered by a double layer of neuroepithelium which forms an important part of the blood–aqueous barrier (Fig. 2). The ciliary body is frequently the site of early inflammatory changes in both clinical anterior and posterior uveitis and the experimental models of these conditions (Forrester *et al.*, 1995; Nussenblatt, 1991).

The iris (Fig. 2) is the most anterior portion of the uveal tract and forms a perforated diaphragm between the anterior and posterior chambers and serves to regulate, via changes in pupil diameter, the amount of light entering the eye. Structurally it consists of an incomplete cellular anterior border layer, a highly vascularized and richly innervated connective-tissue stroma, a thin dilator pupillae muscle, the posterior iris pigment epithelium and a circumferential band of smooth muscle, the sphincter pupillae.

The 'Immune Privileged' Status of the CNS, the Blood–Brain and Blood–Ocular Barriers and Lymphatic Drainage

The normal CNS and interior compartments of the eye have been recognized for decades as possessing unusual immune status or 'privilege' (Barker and Billingham, 1977). It has been postulated that these tissues, vital for survival but without regenerative capacity, have evolved mechanisms to regulate the nature and magnitude of local immune responses. This contrasts with other tissues where 'bystander' damage and oedema that accompany acute inflammatory or cell-mediated immune responses may have no major functional consequences. Classically there have been a number of mechanisms proposed to underlie this immune privilege:

(1) The blood–brain barrier (BBB) and the blood–ocular barrier (BOB) (see Figs 1 and 2).
(2) The absence of specialized lymphatic drainage in the brain/spinal cord and eye.
(3) The absence or low expression of major histocompatability complex (class I and II) molecules.
(4) The absence of DC in the neural parenchyma.

(1) The BBB and BOB function to regulate the passage of macromolecules (drugs, hormones, high molecular mass proteins), microbial pathogens and intravascular leukocytes from the lumen of vessels in the neural parenchyma into the extravascular compartment. The restricted entry of leukocytes was considered a central tenet of the concept of 'immune privilege', namely that the neural environment was protected from surveillance by immune cells. These vascular-tissue barriers serve primarily to regulate the optimal extracellular environment facilitative of neural transmission (Rowland, 1985). The composition of CSF, and AqH in the eye, is a product or consequence of these barriers, and the CSF and the extracellular fluids in the brain, spinal cord and retina are at a critical equilibrium. The anatomical and physiological features of the BBB and BOB are summarized in Fig. 3 and Table 2.

There are a number of specialized regions in the brain adjacent to the III and IV ventricles, collectively referred to as the circumventricular organs, in which the BBB is not as highly developed or regulated. These include the median eminence, subforniceal organ, subcommisural organ adjacent to the III ventricle and the area postrema of the IV ventricle.

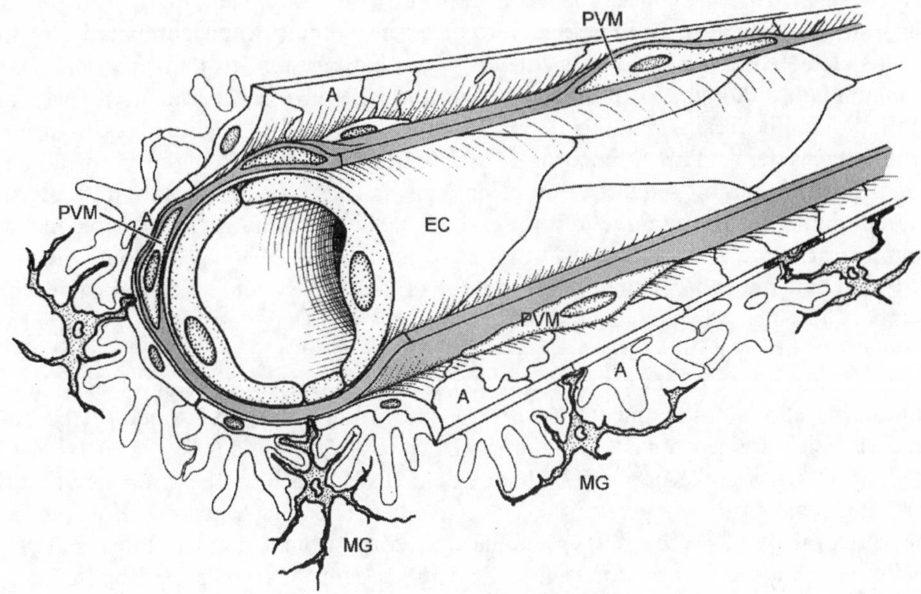

Fig. 3. Schematic diagram of a blood vessel in the brain parenchyma illustrating the components of the vessel wall that contribute to the blood–brain barrier. From the lumen outwards, these are the vascular endothelial cells (EC), basal lamina (shaded zone) and the glia limitans composed of astrocyte (A) foot processes. Note the relative position of perivascular microglia (MG) and perivascular macrophages (PVM).

Table 2. The anatomical and physiological basis of the blood–brain and blood–ocular barriers

Anatomical

1. Junctional complexes of the CNS parenchymal vascular endothelium, especially the zonulae occludentes.
2. Second barrier or 'glia limitans' consisting of pericytes and astrocytic foot processes external to endothelial basal lamina of brain parenchyma and retinal blood vessels.
3. Choroid plexus epithelium (modified ependyma) in the brain and ciliary epithelial bilayer in the eye are characterized by special junctional complexes which are essential to the secretion of CSF and AqH.
4. Arachnoid villi (brain) and trabecular meshwork (eye) act as routes for bulk flow of CSF and AqH into dural venous sinuses and Schlemm's canal respectively. These structures act as pressure-sensitive, one-way valves preventing reflux of blood back into subarachnoid space (brain) or anterior chamber (eye).
5. The pia mater on the brain/spinal cord surface acts to regulate the passage of macromolecules from the CSF in the subarachnoid space into the CNS parenchyma. In the eye the retinal pigment epithelium performs a similar function.

Physiological

The internal plasma membrane actively regulates, via specialized carrier-mediated transporter mechanisms, the nature of the peptides which cross the endothelium.

(2) The fluid-filled extracellular environment of the brain, spinal cord and retina is markedly smaller as a proportion of total tissue volume when compared to other organs. This reduces the requirement for a lymphatic system to remove excess extracellular fluid, although, as discussed above, the CSF in the subarachnoid space and ventricles of the brain and the AqH in the eye are widely regarded as a form of 'lymphatic system'. The absence of a lymphatic drainage within the brain and eye was thought to permit sequestration of antigens in these organs, thereby blocking the afferent limb of the immune response thus partly explaining the phenomenon of 'immune privilege' (Medawar, 1948). However, it has been known for some time that CSF can exit the subarachnoid space in the cranial cavity and vertebral canal via a number of routes. Physiological and anatomical studies have estimated that approximately 50% of brain interstitial fluid and CSF in the rat drains through the connective-tissue sheaths of the olfactory nerves which pierce the cribriform plate of the ethmoid bone. This allows communication with the interstitial connective tissue of the nasal mucosa which drains via nasal lymphatics to cervical lymph nodes (Weed, 1914; Weller *et al.*, 1992; Cserr and Knopf, 1992; Kida *et al.*, 1993). It is also likely some CSF in the vertebral canal drains via perineural connective tissue around spinal nerves as they exit the vertebral canal (Weed, 1914). In the eye, conventional dogma states that AqH drains via the iridocorneal angle into Schlemm's canal (or sinus venosus sclerae in most nonprimates), and thence into collector channels and episcleral veins. Antigens, either soluble or perhaps associated with ocular DC, leaving the anterior chamber via this route travel to the spleen where they elicit antigen-specific immune deviant responses (for review, see Streilein, 1993). However, there is recent evidence from

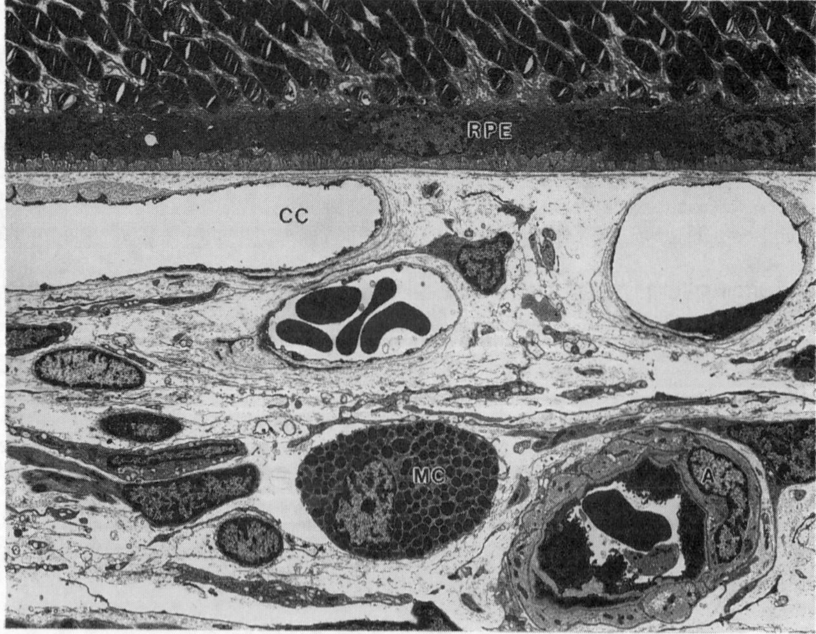

Fig. 4. The outer retina. Transmission electron micrograph of the outer retina, retinal pigment epithelium (RPE) and choroid. CC, choriocapillaris; MC, mast cell; A, arteriole.

studies utilizing congenic mice that antigens placed in the anterior chamber (AC) stimulate antigen-specific T cell clones in the submandibular lymph nodes (Egan *et al.*, 1996), thus suggesting communication with lymphatic vessels. There have also been rare reports of lymph channels in the mammalian choroid (Krebs *et al.*, 1988), which seems plausible as there are extensive lacunae in the avian choroid which have the characteristics of lymphatic vessels (De Stefano and Mugnaini, 1997).

The phenomenon of anterior chamber-associated immune deviation (ACAID) which results following experimental instillation of antigen into the anterior chamber (AC) of the eye in a range of species (Streilein and Niederkorn, 1981; see review, Streilein 1993), has been proposed as a paradigm of immune deviation which underlies the immunological tolerance to antigens placed in the AC. It is proposed that, following antigen administration, an antigen-specific ACAID-inducing signal leaves the eye and traffics to the spleen, where regulatory T-lymphocyte responses are induced (Ferguson *et al.*, 1987). In mice receiving intracameral soluble antigen (viz. injected directly into the AC), this signal is reported to be cell-associated and depletion studies suggested the relevant antigenic signal was carried by F4/80$^+$ cells (presumptive macrophages) (Wilbanks *et al.*, 1991). However, it is unusual for macrophages to act in such a manner and it is more likely that ocular DC act as the sentinel cells carrying antigen-specific signals from the eye (see below).

(3) Until recently the apparent paucity of MHC class I and class II expression in the brain, neural retina and supporting tissues, including the tissues lining the AC (i.e. inner corneal surface, iris and trabecular meshwork), appeared to fit with the proposed mechanisms of immune privilege in the brain and eye, namely that T cells entering the neural environment would be unable to recognize endogenous or exogenous antigens and thus be prevented from entering a state of activation (see Sedgwick, 1997).

Despite the apparent specializations in the brain and eye described above, which would seem to impose limitations on the afferent and efferent limbs of the immune system, immune and inflammatory responses do occur to both endogenous autoantigens (e.g. brain—myelin components; eye—S-antigen, rhodopsin, interphotoreceptor binding protein, lens proteins) and exogenous antigens derived from infectious agents (viral, bacterial and protozoan). Thus antigen presentation must take place somewhere within the CNS.

(4) It has been proposed that DCs play little or no role in immune responses within the CNS (Steinman, 1991). This stands in marked contrast to the pivotal role of these cells in regulating immune responses in other tissues. The view that the brain/spinal cord and eye are devoid of MHC class II$^+$ DCs derives from earlier immunohistochemical investigations of class II expression in conventional tissue in a variety of species in which only rare scattered or isolated cells were reported (see reviews by Sedgwick and Hickey 1997; McMenamin, 1994; McMenamin, 1997). However, as we will discuss presently, recent findings raise doubts about previous notions that the CNS is lacking

or devoid of potential APCs (DCs and to a lesser extent macrophages) (see below). Thus it is probably more accurate to state that this 'deficiency' in the CNS is relative and that routes of interaction between the CNS and immune system do indeed exist and are more highly regulated than in other organs.

Factors that Regulate Entry of Immune Cells into the CNS

While the concepts of the BBB and the blood–retinal barrier (BRB) have been fashioned on the basis of exclusion of transport of large molecules from the bloodstream into the parenchymal tissue of the CNS (Rowland, 1985; Greenwood, 1992), the assumption has been that these barriers naturally extend to cells. As inflammatory processes frequently occur in the brain and retina, it would appear that these barriers are readily broken down. Furthermore, contrary to earlier notions, there is recent evidence that normal CNS tissue is 'patrolled' by lymphocytes (Sedgwick, 1997), although the low incidence of extravasated lymphocytes in the normal CNS parenchyma means that they are rarely likely to be encountered in histological sections. How such cells gain access to the brain and retina is not clear. During inflammation or pathological conditions affecting the CNS, alterations in the adhesion properties of the endothelium occur which facilitate leukocyte extravasation. This area has generated a lot of interest in light of the likelihood that trafficking lymphocytes and monocytes may act as 'Trojan horses' aiding the entry of HIV and CMV into the brain (and retina) (see reviews by Dickson *et al.*, 1991; Hurwitz *et al.*, 1994). There is good *in vitro* evidence that cells close to the CNS vessels, such as astrocytes and perivascular macrophages (Fig. 3), when activated, are capable of synthesizing cytokines, such as TNF, that may cause upregulation of adhesion molecules such as ICAM-1 and E-selectin (Joo, 1994). The fact that in autoimmune conditions, such as MS or uveitis, autoreactive T cells enter the CNS has lent support to the concept of regular T cell trafficking in the brain (for reviews see Sedgwick, 1995; Sedgwick, 1997).

During and indeed prior to overt inflammation in the CNS, several processes are entrained which ensure that there is access not only of lymphocytes but of several other subsets of inflammatory cells such as monocytes, neutrophils, NK cells and DC. Inflammatory cells are attracted to the site of damage by chemokines (e.g. MIP-1α) and other molecules released by tissue cells such as astrocytes, microglia and, in the eye, retinal pigment epithelial cells (Miyagishi *et al.*, 1997; Gourmala *et al.*, 1997; Crane *et al.*, 1998). Endothelial cells also participate in this process by releasing chemokines but more importantly by altering their adhesiveness for circulating leukocytes and also with significant loosening of the tight endothelial junctions characteristic of these barriers. This they achieve by expressing specific adhesion molecules for leukocyte integrin receptors such as ICAMs-1, 2 and 3, VCAM and E-selection (Mesri *et al.*, 1994). Morphological changes occur during this process which have been compared with the appearance of high endothelial venules (HEV) in lymph nodes (McMenamin *et al.* 1992a; McMenamin *et al.*, 1993). Considerable debate has centred on whether leukocyte emigration in CNS endothelium occurs transcellularly or paracellularly at the site of the disengaged tight junctions (Greenwood, 1992).

As stated above, under normal circumstances a few lymphocytes, albeit activated, appear to have access to the CNS tissue (Wekerle, 1986) which enables them to 'patrol' CNS tissue for organisms such as viruses and bacteria. Monocytes/macrophages also appear to be capable of locating extravascularly in the perivascular spaces in the brain and the retina. However, not all cells appear to have similar access to the CNS. In particular, DCs appear to be excluded from the CNS but clearly migrate freely into other tissues since they can be found in all other tissues including the meninges and the uveal tract (see below). The reason for their exclusion from the CNS and retinal tissue is not clear but may relate to their relative lack of integrin receptor expression in the resting state (Ruedl and Hubele, 1997).

The extent of T cell trafficking in the uveal tract with its less developed vascular barriers (including a 'leaky' choriocapillaris) would be expected to be greater than in neural tissues. However, lymphocytes (based on histological studies) were originally reported to be absent or rare in the normal uveal tract of rodents and in human iris biopsies (for review see McMenamin, 1994). However, recent immunohistochemical staining of ocular tissue wholemounts has revealed a consistent but low density of T cells (4 cells/mm^2 in the rat iris, 20 cells/mm^2 in the normal rat choroid) (McMenamin and Crewe, 1995; Butler and McMenamin, 1996). Newly emerging evidence has shown that many cells and tissues in the intraocular environment (retina, cornea) are Fas ligand-positive and there is good evidence that when Fas$^+$ lymphocytes infiltrate the eye and come into contact with the ligand they undergo apoptosis *in situ* (Griffith *et al.*, 1995). This may act as a powerful mechanism of regulating unwanted T cell infiltration in the intraocular environment.

When immune reactions do occur in the CNS, there is clear evidence of T cell activation and proliferation, but the nature of the APC is largely unknown. Candidate APCs in the CNS include parenchymal cells such as astrocytes, oligodendrocytes and endothelium and nonparenchymal haematogenous-derived immune cells including microglia, perivascular macrophages and other macrophage populations (for review see Sedgwick, 1995; Sedgwick, 1997). Only the nonparenchymal immune cells will be dealt with in detail in this review. The potential role of parenchymal cells as APCs has been discussed extensively by Sedgwick and Hickey (1997).

MICROGLIA

Current Concepts of Brain and Retinal Microglia (Phenotype, Distribution, Ontogeny)

Recent advances in our understanding of microglial cells have been derived largely from data in the brain parenchyma and retina. The retina, being an extracerebral portion of the brain and being flat, is comparatively accessible and lends itself to forms of experimental manipulation not possible with the brain. For example, retinal flatmount preparations aid in the display of the regular array of microglia (Fig. 5). Scholarly reviews of the history of the discovery, characterization, origin and nature of microglia have been published (Ling and Wong, 1993; Banati and Graeber, 1994; Thanos *et al.*, 1996).

Microglia are a stable population of highly ramified or dendriform cells of bone marrow origin with nonoverlapping territories with neighbouring microglia that are generally accepted to represent the resident macrophages of the brain (Fig. 4) owing to their many functional and phenotypic similarities (Dijkstra, 1985; Flaris, 1993; Cuzner, 1997) (Table 3). Until recently, several groups disputed the monocyte origin of

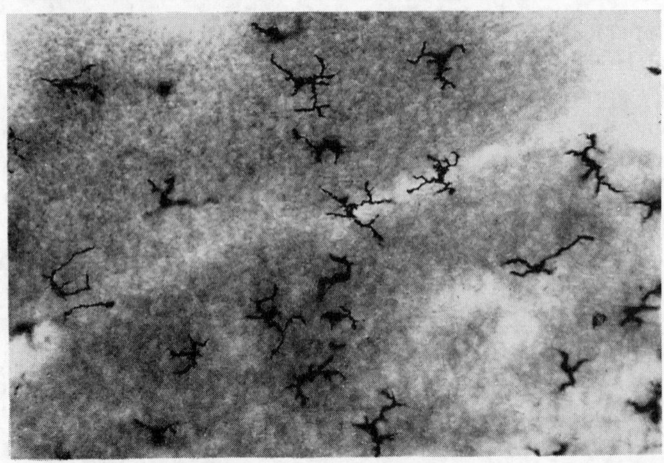

Fig. 5. 'Plan' view of microglia in retinal wholemount stained with the mAb Ox42. (Magnification × 250.)

microglia as they were negative for most conventional macrophage markers available at that time (Oechmichen, 1982; Sminia *et al.*, 1987) or they interpreted their low turnover as evidence of neuroectodermal origin (de Groot *et al.*, 1992). Most authors now agree that microglia form one class of CNS-resident haematopoietic cells together with perivascular macrophages, intraventricular macrophages, epiplexus cells, meningeal

Table 3. Summary of some of the literature on MHC class II expression by microglia (brain and retina)

	MHC class II$^+$	MHC class II$^-$
Human		
In vivo	Major subpopulation: Penfold *et al.* (1993); Mattiace *et al.* (1990) Fetal and adult: Lowe *et al.* (1989) Small subpopulation: Gerhmann *et al.* (1993); Lampson and Hickey (1986) White matter microglia: Hayes *et al.* (1987); Gehrmann (1993)	Hart (1981); Matsumoto *et al* (1986); Lampson and Hickey (1986)
In vitro	83%+ve (Ulvestad *et al.*, 1994)	
Rat		
In vivo	Brown Norway: Sedgewick *et al.* (1993); de Groot (1989) Wistar (mostly white matter, increase with age): Ogura *et al.* (1994); Lewis (30%): Cash *et al.* (1993) Several strains (retina): Zhang *et al.* (1997)	Lewis, Wistar, Sprague-Dawley, Long Evans and most other strains: Rao and Lund (1993); Mander and Morris (1995); Long *et al.* (1991); Xu and Ling (1994); and others Spinal: Kauer *et al.* (1993) Wistar Furth (retina): McMenamin *et al.* (1992) Lewis, minor subpopulation positive (retina): Dick *et al.* (1995)
In vitro		
Mouse		
In vivo		Frei *et al.* (1997)

Table 4. Phenotype of microglia compared with resident macrophages

	Microglia	Resident tissue macrophages
Histochemical markers		
Nonspecific esterase, chymotrypsin, trypsin, lysozyme	–	++
Enzyme histochemistry		
ATPase	+	+
NDPase	+	+
TPPase	+	+
Peroxidase		
IDPase	+	+
Phosphotyrosine	+	–/+
Vimentin	+/–	++
Lectins (bind to D-galactose) (see review by Thomas, 1992)		
Griffonia simplicifolia	+	+
K⁺ ion channels	Only inward K⁺ channels	Inward and outward K⁺ channels
Immunophenotype		
CD45 leukocyte common antigen	+ (subpopulations)	+
Complement receptor 3 (CR3) (Ox42 in rat; MAC-1, mouse)	+	++
Human EMBII	+	+
CD68 (EDI, rat)	Weakly + (juxtanuclear spot)	+
Amyloid precursor protein (APP)	+	ND[a]
CD4	+/–	+
CD14	–	+
Class I	+/–	++
Ox41	–	+/–
ED2	–	+++
ED3	–	+/–
F4/80	+/–	++
Fc receptor	+/–	++

[a]ND, not determined.

macrophages (brain, spinal cord), and uveal tract macrophages (eye). Within the parenchyma of the brain they express the complement receptor 3 antigens (CD11b in rat and CD11c in human) and are $CD45^{low}$ but in the rat do not express the pan-macrophage marker ED2. Studies on retinal microglia indicate that they are generally MHC class II negative at least in mice and most rat strains, but in humans retinal parenchymal and perivascular microglia appear to express some MHC class II (see below). The phenotype of mature resting microglia is summarized in Table 4.

In the brain, microglia are evenly distributed in the parenchyma of the grey and white matter of the CNS (Milligan *et al.*, 1991). Some make contact with the blood vessels as part of the glia limitans (Fig. 3) and are thus described as perivascular microglia. The latter are distinct from the perivascular macrophages which lie between the glia limitans and the basement membrane of the vessel or between the basement membrane and the endothelium (Fig. 3) (see next section). Microglia are estimated to constitute 20% of all

CNS glial cells or 13% of all cells in the human CNS white matter and between 5% and 12% of all mouse CNS cells (Thomas, 1992; Kreutzberg, 1996). Lawson *et al.* (1990) estimated that the mouse brain contained 3.5×10^6 microglial cells, a figure comparable to the number of macrophages in the liver.

The Function of Microglia

It has been suggested that in the resting state microglia have a constitutive role in 'cleansing' extracellular fluid in the CNS, for example by degradation of neurotransmitters and maintaining a state of 'vigilance' by monitoring changes in their extracellular milieu (Kreutzberg, 1996). Indeed pinocytosis is often used as a differential marker for microglia. When activated, microglia assume a more amoeboid form and actively phagocytose cell and tissue debris (Thanos *et al.*, 1996; Yao *et al.*, 1990; Thomas, 1992). This occurs in a number of situations ranging from normal development, where they phagocytose apoptotic neurons, to a variety of degenerative, traumatic or inflammatory conditions in the CNS (see Nakajima and Kohsaka, 1993; Thanos *et al.*, 1996 for review). In the eye, immunohistochemical and histochemical studies of retinal development suggest that monocytes enter the neural retina from the overlying developing vasculature to scavenge debris produced by neuronal cell death. They then differentiate to form a regularly spaced network of microglia in the plexiform layers (Hume *et al.*, 1983; Sanyal and De Ruiter, 1985; Thanos *et al.*, 1996). Elegant experiments and observations in which ganglion cells destined to die are labelled by retrograde transport of fluorescent lipophilic carbocyanine dyes injected into the superior colliculus have revealed labelled apoptotic ganglion cell debris within resident microglia. Adult animals with carbocyanine-labelled microglia (and the surviving ganglion cells) can be used to investigate the effects of procedures ranging from optic nerve lesions to retinal degeneration. In the latter experiments, prelabelled RCS rat retinae are used to visualize activated microglia removing degenerating photoreceptor cells (Thanos, 1991; Thanos 1992; Thanos *et al.*, 1996). Activated macrophages assume an amoeboid form, show enhanced migration capacity and phagocytic inclusions (see reviews, Thanos *et al.*, 1996; Kreutzberg, 1996) and upregulate the macrophage scavenger receptor (Bell *et al.*, 1994). Such features are strong evidence that resident microglia are active participants in repeated phagocytic events in the retina and brain and therefore represent a form of macrophage. There is, however, some speculation that they may also be a type of DC (see below).

Microglia secrete proteases and generate free radicals and nitric oxide species. Indeed, some have termed them the 'deadly' killers (Banati and Graeber, 1994) on the basis of evidence from *in vitro* cytotoxity studies of activated microglial interaction with tumour cells, neurons and oligodendria. It is possible that microglia, during ontogeny, may play a role beyond that of 'cellular undertakers' and may be more actively involved in mediating cell death similarly to the macrophages that remove the tunica vasculosis lentis surrounding the fetal lens (Lang and Bishop, 1993). It is clear that strict regulation of this cytotoxic function *in vivo* is crucial if these cells are to be effective and not cause unwanted damage to the CNS itself.

In certain inflammatory responses in the brain and retina microglia are likely candidates for the synthesis of pro-inflammatory cytokines. However their role in the steady state may be to downregulate or limit inflammatory responses via their recently demonstrated ability to induce apoptosis of activated T cells (see below). The function of microglial cells is currently an area of intense interest because, as weakly positive expressors of the CD4 molecule, they are also potential targets of infection by HIV.

Could Brain and Retinal Microglia be Considered as DCs or APCs in the CNS?

With the appreciation in the early 1980s that MHC class II expression was an essential feature of APCs, many authors investigated the expression of this molecule in the normal CNS and in diseased conditions with a suspected autoimmune aetiology, such as multiple sclerosis (MS). Since DC, currently considered to be the most potent APC in the immune system (Steinman, 1991), were reportedly absent from CNS and supporting tissues, considerable effort has been made to identify cells in the CNS which can act as APCs. One issue seemed to dominate for some time. Namely, do microglia act as APCs to infiltrating encephalitogenic T cells? The results were, and continue to be, controversial. Microglia, on the basis of their morphology and lineage, initially appear to be good candidates. There is evidence that human microglia can stimulate resting T cells (Ulvested *et al.*, 1994c; Williams *et al.*, 1994); however, studies with *ex vivo* rat brain microglia prepared using FACS technology by gating on a population of CD45^{low}, MHC class II^{-} cells have shown they are poor APCs in the presence of MBP-specific CD4^{+} T cells, as measured by T cell proliferation and IL-2 secretion (Ford *et al.*, 1995). Some authors have documented APC activity by microglia *in vitro*, although these have tended to require stimulation by interferon-γ or LPS (Cash *et al.*, 1993; Cash and Rott, 1994). It has recently been proposed that MHC class II expression on microglia is directed at cutting short T cell activation and proliferation and inducing apoptosis, thereby minimizing the inflammatory response in the CNS (Ford *et al.*, 1996). This apoptosis-promoting effect contrasts quite markedly with the recent data indicating that survival of mature T cells in the periphery, after leaving the thymus, is dependent specifically on lymphoid DC expression of MHC class II.

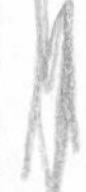

The extent of expression of MHC class II antigen by microglia is controversial (see Table 3). In summary, it appears that subpopulations of microglia, especially perivascular microglia, express MHC class II, albeit at low levels, in some species/strains. In addition, microglia have been reported to express accessory molecules B7/B7.1 (Williams *et al.*, 1994), although there is counterevidence that they lack these costimulatory molecules and B7.2 (Inaba *et al.*, 1995). *In vitro* evidence for microglia as APCs has been provided using myelin basic protein and antigen-specific T cell lines (Matsumoto *et al.*, 1993). However, the data from these rat studies have been challenged on the basis that the cell preparations of microglia were contaminated with meningeal APCs which can reportedly be distinguished in FACS analysis as a population of CD45^{high} MHC class II^{high} ED2^{+} (Sedgwick, 1997). More recent immunohistochemical studies have shown that the meninges also contain extensive populations of MHC class II^{+} Ox62^{+} DC (McMenamin *et al.*, unpublished data) (see below), which may represent the majority of the MHC class II^{high} cells in FACS analysis.

An important characteristic of DC is the migratory phase in their life cycle, which seems vital to their sentinel function. Their turnover varies from organ to organ from 3 days in mucosal sites (Pugh *et al.*, 1993; Holt *et al.*, 1994) to 10–14 days for Langerhans cells in the skin (Katz *et al.*, 1979). Therefore, if microglia were the equivalent of DC in the CNS one would predict some degree of turnover. A quantitative impression of the normal rate of turnover of CNS parenchymal microglia obtained using radiation chimera models indicates that turnover was very low (months) *in vivo* (Lassman *et al.*, 1993; Hickey *et al.*, 1992) and that microglia were 'radiation resistant'. This was recently confirmed for retinal microglia (Zhang *et al.*, 1997). On the basis of combined immunohistochemistry (F4/80 mAb) and autoradiography ([^{3}H]thymidine) it has been shown that resident microglia are capable of division *in situ* but that they are also replenished from the blood monocyte pool (Lawson *et al.* 1992). Thus, on the criteria of turnover, microglia do not appear to have a life cycle akin to DC.

In conclusion, functional studies have revealed that microglia purified from brain parenchyma (excluding the meninges) are very poor APCs in the presence of naive T cells. This evidence, combined with their immunophenotype, extremely low turnover rates and their phagocytic capacity, has led most authors to conclude that microglia represent specialized resident tissue macrophages of the CNS parenchyma and not DC.

The brain has several other resident populations of macrophages besides microglia (Table 5), however the eye has been studied in less detail and several analogous subpopulations have only recently been described.

Technical Note

In the normal CNS the overwhelming evidence seems to suggest that microglia are MHC class II negative, although on some strains of rat, such as Brown Norway (Sedgwick *et al.*, 1993), and in ostensibly 'normal' human neural parenchyma, MHC class I and II expression has been reported (see Table 3). However, one has to make a cautionary observation on some technical issues. The first is that isolation and flow cytometric analyses have often failed to consider the presence of rich populations of meningeal macrophages and DCs in their preparations. The second point is that in the case of human material the issue of post-mortem upregulation of MHC class II on microglia following ischaemia must be considered as a complicating factor (Graeber *et al.*, 1992). Furthermore, some authors have used intense amplification techniques (such as silver and nickel methods) during immunohistochemical procedures (Penfold *et al.*, 1993), which while allowing excellent visualization of the cells do not allow valid comment on the degree of MHC class II expression relative to other cells, such as lymphoid DC or skin Langerhans cells. Namely, all labelled cells appear black regardless of the intensity or degree of antigen expression and primary monoclonal antibody binding. Some authors (Lowe *et al.*, 1989) have commented that the level of MHC class II staining on microglia is a lot less than on other DC populations. The characteristic dendritic morphology of microglia and some indication of MHC class II staining has in our opinion misled some authors to conclude prematurely that microglia represent a form of DC (Lowe *et al.*, 1989; Penfold *et al.*, 1993; Gerhrmann *et al.*, 1993; Ulvestad *et al.*, 1994).

Table 5. Homology between the location and distribution of macrophage subpopulations in the brain and eye

Brain/spinal cord	Eye
Microglia in grey and white matter	Retinal microglia
Perivascular macrophages	Perivascular macrophages
Intraventricular macrophages	Subretinal macrophages (in 'optic ventricle' in fetus)
Epiplexus cells	Possibly macrophages on surface of ciliary processes
Choroid plexus stromal macrophages	Ciliary body stromal macrophages
Macrophages in meninges (pia mater, arachnoid, dura mater)	Macrophages in uveal tract (iris, ciliary body, choroid)
	Hyalocytes in vitreous (subhyaloid space)

PERIVASCULAR CELLS

Vessels in the CNS (brain and spinal cord parenchyma and neural retina) are characterized by a perivascular concentration of astrocytic foot processes which forms the 'glia limitans' external to the endothelium (Fig. 3). A small subpopulation of perivascular macrophages or 'perivascular cells' is associated with these vessels. Their phenotype indicates they are a less downregulated form of macrophage than microglia (Hickey and Kimura, 1988; Graeber *et al.*, 1989) with some of the characteristics of interstitial macrophages (ED2$^+$/class II$^-$ and ED2$^+$/class II$^+$) (Dick *et al.*, 1995). Some authors have reported expression of MHC class II on these cells, although this is not a universal finding (Sminia *et al.*, 1987). Around veins, the perivascular macrophages are believed to lie outside the basement membrane, between it and the foot process of the glial cells, or between layers of the basement membrane (Hickey *et al.*, 1992) (Fig. 3).

> As indicated above, perivascular macrophages in the rat are ED2 positive. ED2 is a monoclonal antibody which labels adherent macrophages, and *in vivo* specifically labels resident macrophages within most tissues studied (Damoiseaux *et al.*, 1989). The cell surface molecule bound by this antibody has recently been cloned and sequenced and appears to have a role in promoting cell–cell interactions (Dijkstra, personal communication).

Perivascular microglia, which some authors regard as a separate subpopulation from perivascular macrophages, also have processes which lie close to the glia limitans (Provis *et al.*, 1995). It appears that perivascular macrophages, along with microglia, may be the site of amyloid accumulation in the brain (Maat-Schieman *et al.*, 1997). Perivascular macrophages in the brain are derived, like other macrophages, from precursor cells in the bone marrow and, unlike microglia, have a relatively short turnover (Lassman *et al.*, 1993; Hickey *et al.*, 1992). No specific data are available on turnover of retinal perivascular macrophages, but it is likely they are similar to those in the brain. Brain and retinal perivascular macrophages have attracted interest as potential APC in the brain parenchyma and retina almost by default, since there is little evidence for such a role for retinal microglia (see above). In addition, in clinical and experimental

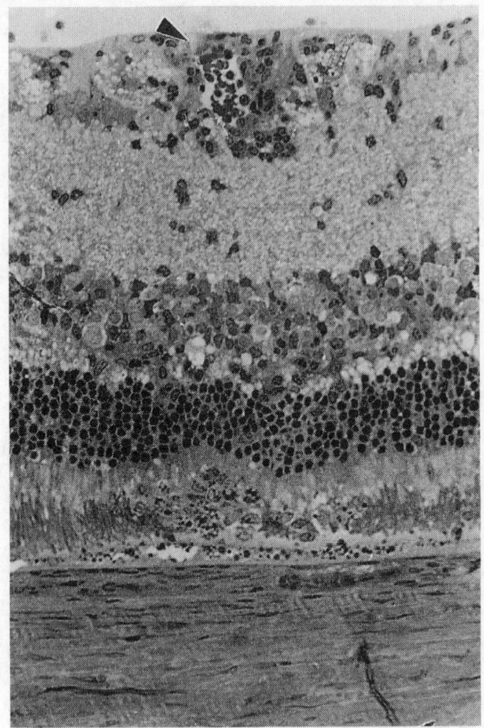

Fig. 6. Light micrograph of rat retina during active EAU (experimental autoimmune uveoretinitis). Note the perivascular inflammatory infiltrate and the subretinal accumulation of macrophages (arrowhead). (Magnification × 450.)

inflammation of the brain and retina, the initial site of lymphocyte accumulation in the parenchyma appears to be the perivascular space (Fig. 6) suggesting that this may be the initial site of antigen presentation for activated lymphocytes once they have crossed the blood–retinal or blood–brain barrier.

OTHER MACROPHAGE POPULATIONS ASSOCIATED WITH NONPARENCHYMAL TISSUE

In the Brain

Monocytes recruited to the CNS to phagocytose degenerating neurons persist not only as microglia, as discussed above, but also as other resident macrophage populations, including meningeal macrophages, supraependymal cells (SEC) and choroid plexus macrophages including epiplexus cells (Tseng *et al.*, 1983; Perry *et al.*, 1985; Perry and Gordon, 1987). The route of entry of these cells during development has been suggested as being via the meninges or the vasculature, or alternatively they may enter the ventricles via the choroidal epithelium (see review by Jordan and Thomas, 1988).

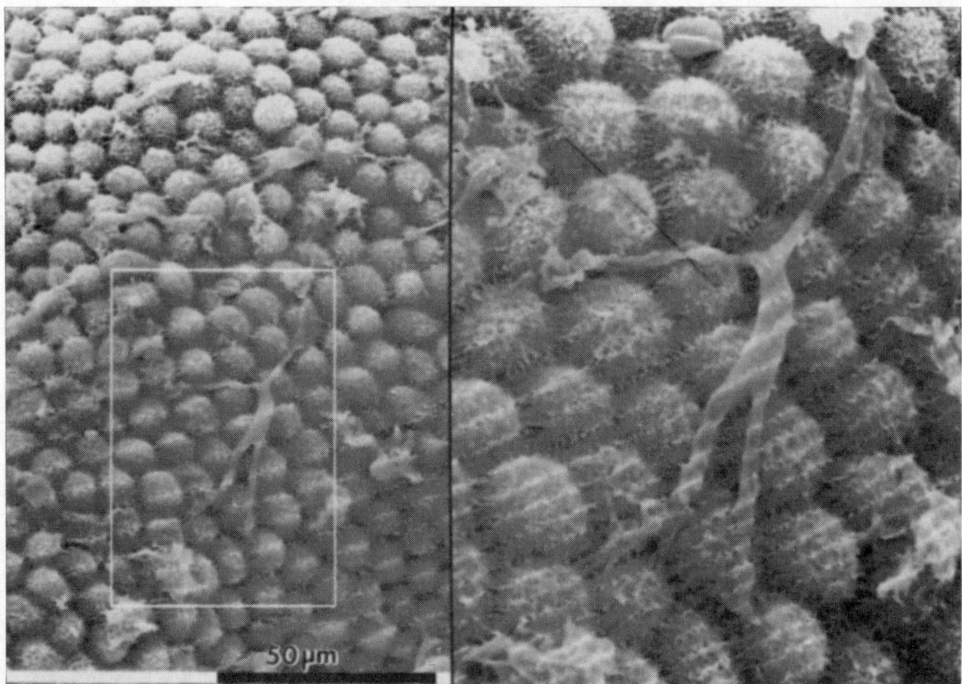

Fig. 7. Scanning electron micrograph of monkey choroid plexus. Note the morphology of the epiplexus cells upon the ventricular surface of the epithelium.

Choroid Plexus Macrophages

Since the descriptions in 1921 by Kolmer it has been known that a population of pleomorphic and dendriform phagocytic cells is located on the ventricular aspect of the choroid plexus epithelium (Fig. 1, Fig. 7). Since then, conventional histological or electron-microscopic studies have suggested these cells are a form of macrophage (Ling, 1983; Jordan and Thomas, 1988). Recent immunophenotypic analysis suggests that most are indeed F4/80^{+} (mouse) ED2^{+}, Ox42^{+} (rat) macrophages. The stromal macrophages of the choroid plexus in the mouse are of a similar phenotype (F4/80^{+} mouse) (Perry and Gordon, 1988; Matyszak *et al.*, 1992; McMenamin, unpublished observations), suggesting a common origin and function (see below).

Intraventricular Macrophages

These have been the subject of numerous investigations which have documented the great variety of morphological appearances of these cells in a wide range of species including mice, rats (Chamberlain, 1974; Peters, 1974), hamsters (Bleier and Albrecht, 1980), rabbits, dogs, monkeys (Ling, 1983), and in the developing human (Otani and Tanaka, 1988). The presence of numerous blebs, membrane ruffles, cytoplasmic pseudopodia and filopodia, and intracytoplasmic phagolysosomes has led to the generally accepted view that supraependymal cells are similar to epiplexus cells and constitute a population of resident motile mononuclear phagocytes of the ventricular surface

(Chamberlain, 1974; Bleier and Albrecht, 1980). There is supportive evidence for such a function from experimental models which have revealed that in adults of several species both epiplexus cells and supraependymal cells are capable of phagocytosing material on the ventricular surface ranging from haemorrhagic debris to latex particles (Maxwell and McGadey, 1988; Bleier and Albrecht, 1980; Ling *et al.* 1985).

Meningeal Macrophages

Despite the unquestioned importance of macrophages in a variety of neuropathological disorders and inflammatory/immune-mediated processes in the CNS, there have been only very limited immunophenotypic studies of resident macrophages within the meninges and choroid plexus (Sminia *et al.*, 1987; Matyszak *et al.*, 1992; Lassman *et al.*, 1993; Rinner *et al.*, 1995), although some authors investigating the immunopathological changes in human and experimental encephalomyelitis have made brief comments on occasional immunopositive cells in the meninges (Bauer *et al.*, 1994; McCombe *et al.*, 1994; and others). Milligin *et al.* (1991), in a study of the developing rat brain, observed $ED1^+$ $Ox42^+$ macrophages in the meninges and choroid plexus from P8 to adulthood. Studies performed using wholemount methods (McMenamin, unpublished observations) (Fig. 8) have compared macrophage populations in the normal rat dura mater, arachnoid, pia mater and choroid plexus. Wholemounts stained with ED2 revealed a high density of resident tissue macrophages, many of which displayed a longitudinal orientation and perivascular distribution (Plate 12.9). The mAb ED1

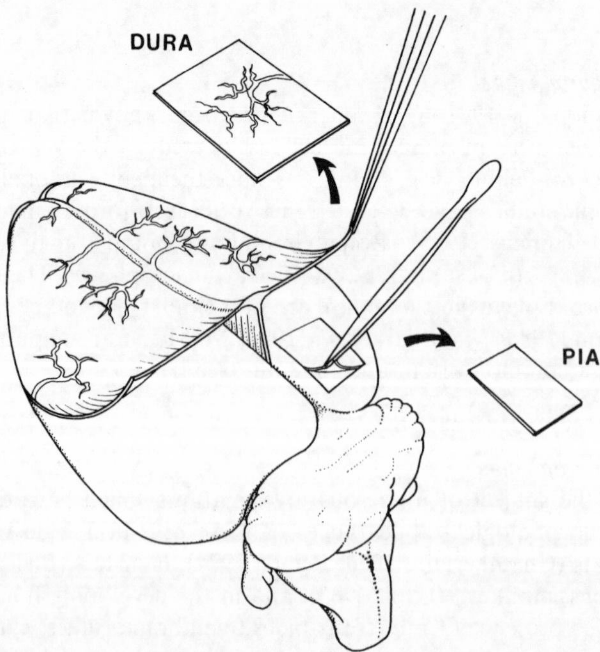

Fig. 8. Wholemounts of dura and pia mater. Schematic drawing illustrating the procedure used to remove dura mater and pia mater as wholemounts for immunohistochemical studies.

(anti-CD68) stained the same population of macrophages in the dura mater. Double immunostaining revealed that most resident tissue macrophages in the dura mater were $ED2^+/ED1^+$. Resident tissue macrophages in the dura mater were weakly $ED3^+$ and $Ox42^+$ (C3b receptor) (not illustrated). Perry and coworkers (Bell *et al.*, 1994) revealed that while choroid plexus and meningeal macrophages in the mouse expressed macrophage scavenger receptor in adults, expression was strongest in 4-day-old neonates.

There has been no indication to date that the pia mater contains networks of resident macrophages. However, immunostained wholemounts of pia mater or pial leptomeninges cut from the surface of the cerebral hemispheres (Fig. 8) revealed a moderately dense network of $ED1^+/ED2^+$ macrophages which displayed a variety of morphologies (McMenamin, unpublished observations).

Macrophages in the meninges and choroid plexus most likely perform a variety of functions in common with other tissue macrophages, such as removing effete or lysed erythrocytes or tissue debris from the CSF in the subarachnoid space which might otherwise cause obstruction to the CSF drainage pathways in the arachnoid villi. Secondly, they are likely, as in other tissues, to be involved in tissue repair, for example following trauma or inflammation. These cells are also a source of cytokines and prostaglandins in inflammatory situations. In this context it has recently been shown that cells, presumed but not proven to be macrophages, situated close to the ependyma and within the pia mater express IL-1β within hours of systemic endotoxin injection (Elmquist *et al.*, 1997). It is thus likely that this and other cytokines are released into the CSF and may affect areas of the brain (and spinal cord) distant from the major site of inflammation. If macrophages in the choroid plexus, ventricles and meninges possess CD14 receptors, they may act as a first line of detection of microbial invasion, particularly as the BBB is less regulated at these sites. This has, however, yet to be determined.

The role of macrophages as effector cells in the pathogenesis of EAE has been highlighted by experiments in which depletion of macrophages by mannosylated liposomes containing dichloromethylene diphosphonate results in amelioration of the disease (Huitinga *et al.*, 1990).

Evolutionary Note

The rapid accumulation of monocyte-derived cells at the site of injury is characteristic of mammalian peripheral nervous system and the CNS of lower vertebrates, namely, situations which are characterized by regenerative capacity such as the goldfish optic nerve (Battisti *et al.*, 1995). Interestingly, the parenchyma of the normal fish spinal cord contains very large numbers of leukocytes and macrophages (Dowding and Scholes, 1993). This contrasts with the situation in higher vertebrates, where the parenchyma is sparsely populated by microglia and regeneration is limited. It is tempting to speculate that the evolutionary trend towards lower numbers of immune cells in the CNS (and retina) may have a bearing on the apparent 'immune privilege' of these sites and their lack of regenerative capacity. Which of these has driven the evolutionary trend is uncertain.

Macrophage Subpopulations in the Eye Other than Retinal Microglia

Subretinal Macrophages

Since the cavity of the optic vesicle (ventricle) or subretinal space (SRS) is in continuity with the future third ventricle of the diencephalon during early morphogenesis, it is not surprising that a transient population of macrophages has been discovered within the peripheral subretinal space of fetal eyes in humans (McMenamin and Loffler, 1990; Loffler and McMenamin 1990) and other species (rabbit, mouse, rat and various marsupial species; McMenamin, unpublished observations) (Fig. 10). These cells possess phagocytic inclusions and bear strong morphological resemblance to intraventricular macrophages, indicating a shared function. The discovery of macrophages in the peripheral SRS in the developing eye led to the proposal that another route of entry for microglial precursors in the retina (besides the vessels at the optic nerve head) was the

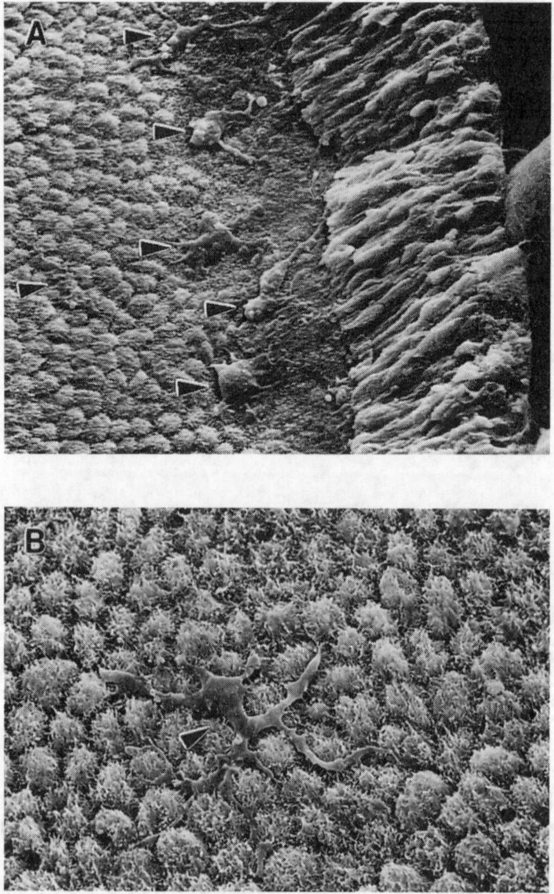

Fig. 10. Scanning electron micrographs of the peripheral subretinal space in the newborn rabbit eye. (A) low power; (B) high power. The neural retina has been removed to expose the surface of the RPE. Note the pleomorphic subretinal macrophages (arrowheads).

rich vascular bed of the developing ciliary body, which is homologous to the choroid plexus. This proposal was recently supported by immunohistochemical studies of human fetal retina (Diaz-Araya *et al.*, 1995).

Hyalocytes

A population of macrophages ($ED2^+$ in rat) is situated in the subhyaloid space (between the inner retinal surface and the vitreous 'membrane'). They are considered scavengers and probably arise from the population of macrophages that phagocytose the hyaloid vessels and tunica vasculosa lentis during development. It is worth noting that they may act as a source of contamination in 'retinal preparations' if all remnants of the vitreous are not carefully removed.

Macrophages in the Iris, Ciliary Body and Choroid

Conventional histological studies reveal macrophages in the human iris stroma close to the pupil margin and near the iris base. These phagocytose melanin shed from iris pigment epithelium throughout life, especially during movements of the iris where it comes into contact with the lens. More recently, studies of rat irides using wholemounts and specific anti-macrophage monoclonal antibodies (ED1, ED2 and ED3) have revealed that the normal rat iris contains a rich network (600–800 cells/mm^2) of resident tissue macrophages (Fig. 11) (McMenamin *et al.*, 1992b; McMenamin *et al.*, 1994). Preliminary immunofluorescence data and conventional immunohistological studies (McMenamin *et al.*, 1994) have confirmed the presence of a similar network of dendriform and pleomorphic resident tissue macrophages located throughout the human and mouse iris stroma.

Macrophages of a similar phenotype are also distributed in the connective-tissue stroma of the ciliary body and ciliary processes in the rat, mouse and human eye (McMenamin *et al.*, 1992b; McMenamin *et al.*, 1994). Like the anterior uveal tract, the connective-tissue stroma of the normal rodent choroid possesses a rich population of $ED1^+$, $ED2^+$ and $ED3^+$ (rat) or $F4/80^+$ $SER4^+$ (mouse) resident tissue macrophages (approximately 600 cells/mm^2) that display a largely perivascular distribution (Forrester *et al.*, 1993; Forrester *et al.*, 1994; Butler and McMenamin, 1996) (Fig. 12).

The distribution pattern of the resident tissue macrophages close to vascular beds suggests a sentinel or guardian role at the blood–tissue interface. It is known that uveal tract macrophages produce pro-inflammatory substances such as nitric oxide (McMenamin and Crewe, 1997) and cytokines (Yoshida *et al.*, 1994) following systemic administration of LPS (i.e. endotoxin-induced uveitis (EIU)). Whether uveal tract macrophages possess CD14 and thus the potential to bind LPS or LPS-binding protein is unknown. If this were the case, these macrophages could rapidly initiate the inflammatory cascade in the eye via subsequent cytokine release as a response to contact with bacteria or bacterial products leaking from ocular vessels.

While uveal tract macrophages are relatively poor APCs in comparison to DC in primary immune responses (Steptoe *et al.*, 1995), macrophages may in contrast be efficient local APCs to primed T cells in secondary immune responses. In the choroid, macrophages are poor APCs, but recent studies suggest that they may modify the primary MLR induced by DC (Forrester *et al.*, unpublished observations). This may

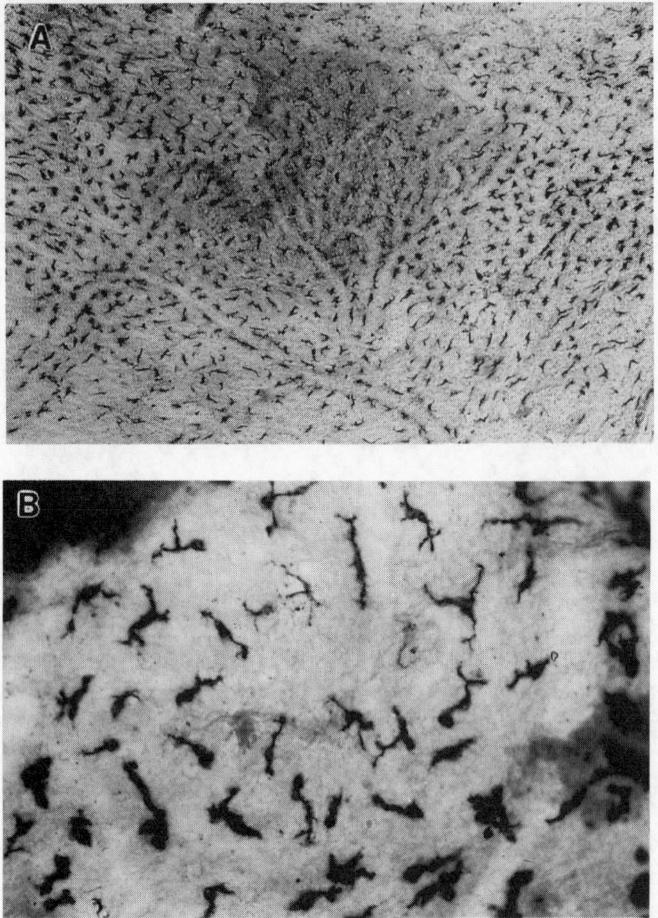

Fig. 11. Iris wholemounts (rat) stained with anti-macrophage mAb ED2. (A) low power (×90); (B) high power (×150).

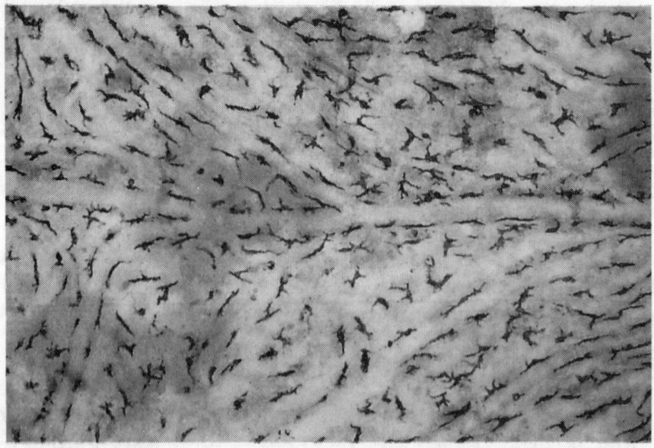

Fig. 12. Mouse choroid wholemount stained with mAb (SER4) to resident tissue macrophages. Note the largely perivascular distribution (×120).

be of particular importance in light of their location at the interface between the BOB and the fenestrated vascular beds of the choroid and ciliary processes where inflammatory infiltrates are frequently noted in clinical and experimental uveitis.

DENDRITIC CELLS IN THE CNS

DC in the Brain Parenchyma, Dura Mater, Arachnoid, Pia Mater and Choroid Plexus

The majority of studies which have aimed to elucidate the nature of the APC within the CNS environment have confirmed that the parenchyma of the brain, spinal cord and retina lack DC. In agreement with most other investigators we have consistently failed to detect any cells with the immunophenotypic profile (unpublished data), turnover, migration capacity and functional ability of DC within the rat brain parenchyma and the neural retina (McMenamin *et al.*, 1992b). There is a report of MHC class II^+ cells in the anterior pituitary, but whether they represent a subpopulation of folliculo-stellate cells or DC is still unclear (Allaerts *et al.*, 1996).

Studies of the dura mater, the leptomeninges and the choroid plexus in the ventricles have generally failed to detect DC-like cells with the exception of one study in which a few Ia^+ $F4/80^+$ cells were noted in the choroid plexus (Matyszak *et al.*, 1992). These authors later estimated in rats that $Ox62^+$ cells constituted only 1% of all MHC class II^+ cells (Matyszak and Perry, 1996a). However, recent observations indicate that the choroid plexus does contain extensive populations of MHC class II^+ dendriform cells in rats (Plate 12.13) (McMenamin, unpublished observations) and in humans (Serot *et al.*, 1997). The former observation was supported by Ox62 staining which revealed an extensive network of dendriform cells. Lu *et al.* (1994) have recently confirmed that occasional epiplexus cells are MHC class II^+ in adults and that the proportion of these cells increases with age and following injury. Confocal microscopic or immunoelectron-microscopic studies have yet to be performed to determine whether any of these cells are located on the ventricular aspect of the choroid plexus epithelium, although Serot *et al.* (1997) indicated that the DC-like cells they describe were located between the choroid plexus epithelial cells.

Studies of single and double immunostained wholemounts of rat dura have revealed a rich network of MHC class II $(Ia)^+$ cells whose dendriform and pleomorphic morphology and non-perivascular regular distribution strongly suggested they were of the DC lineage (Plate 12.14). These dural Ia^+ cells were generally $ED2^-/ED1^-$, although in some cells small perinuclear $ED1^+$ lysosomes were identified (not shown). A network of dendriform Ia^+ $ED2^-$ cells (Plate 12.15) which were also $Ox62^+$ were also identified in the pial preparations, suggesting that DC populated this meningeal layer close to the brain surface.

Technical Note

The successful demonstration of rich networks of DC in the dura mater, arachnoid, pia mater and choroid plexus (McMenamin, unpublished observations) is the result of the novel application of immunohistochemical techniques to tissue wholemounts (Fig. 8). Meningeal wholemounts provide 'plan' views of the tissue, allowing the observer a unique perspective of the pattern of distribution, density and morphology of immunopositive cells in semitransparent biological 'sheets' of tissue. Many adjacent serial histological sections would be required to obtain the same information. The cranial meningeal wholemount approach was a logical consequence of a previously described method (Kitz *et al.*, 1981) and our studies of DC networks in iris, ciliary body and choroid wholemounts (McMenamin *et al.*, 1994; Forrester *et al.*, 1994; Butler and McMenamin, 1996).

Minimal responses are elicited by placing a variety of antigens or inflammatory stimuli, such as endotoxin or pro-inflammatory cytokines, into the neural parenchyma. This contrasts with the rapid and typical neutrophilic and mononuclear cellular infiltrate response observed when these stimuli are placed in the ventricles or subarachnoid space (Matyszak and Perry, 1996b). These observations have been postulated to be due to differences in the nature of the endothelium, the lack of normal macrophage populations, and an immunosuppressive environment, possibly due to the influence of astrocytes, and a reduced ability to recruit neutrophils into the CNS parenchyma. The latter could be due to lack of adhesion molecule expression in neural endothelial cells. However, in light of the findings described above it would seem reasonable to postulate that DC (and resident tissue macrophages) in the vicinity of the ventricles and in tissues lining the subarachnoid space (dura and pia-arachnoid) could endow these sites with the potential to mount cell-mediated immune responses and inflammatory responses, unlike the CNS parenchyma which contains only microglia and perivascular cells.

Numerous immunopathological studies of MS and EAE have highlighted the appearance of the earliest inflammatory infiltrates in periventricular, leptomeningeal and perivascular sites. The involvement of the former two anatomical sites may be a consequence of the rich networks of MHC class II$^+$ DC which may act as APC of CNS antigens to trafficking autoreactive/activated T cells—the initiating events in the CNS of the characteristic pathology of EAE and MS lesions. It is likely that greater T cell traffic occurs in the meninges and choroid plexus as these areas lack the tight BBB of neural parenchymal vessels.

The demonstration of HIV within the choroid plexus of simians and humans infected with HIV (Lackner *et al.*, 1991) poses the important questions whether the virus is present within DC or macrophages in this site and whether the trafficking of these cells may be significant in disease spread to and from the CNS. Interestingly, combined in-situ hybridization and immunohistochemical studies of the brains revealed accumulations of HIV mRNA within cells of the monocyte/macrophage lineage in the pia and choroid plexus. The possibility exists that these cells represent DC.

Evolutionary Note

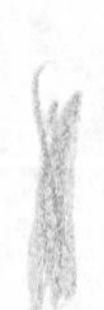

The numbers and density of macrophages (and DC) in the cranial meninges may surprise many observers. In a phylogenetic context it is not totally unexpected as the meninges of some primitive vertebrates (sharks, rays and urodeles) contain large accumulations of lymphohaematopoeitic tissue where macrophage and lymphocyte clusters extend from the meninges into the ventricles and choroid plexus (Torroba *et al.*, 1995). Collections of lymphoid cells have also been described in the chicken choroid plexus (Cogburn and Glick, 1987). Could the networks of DC and macrophages observed in the mammalian meninges and choroid plexus represent a similar but less well developed system of immune cells to that found in lower vertebrates? Teleologically it is possible that with increased encephalization and terrestrial life style, together with the evolution of a nonexpandable protective bony cranial cavity housing a functionally more developed brain, lymphoid sacs and expanding lymphoid tissue in the meningeal tissues and ventricles presented disadvantages. Thus evolutionary pressure may have led to the situation now present in most higher vertebrates where networks of DC and macrophages in these sites are the remnants of the more extensive intracranial lymphoid system seen in lower vertebrates.

DC in the Retina and Uveal Tract of the Eye

Distribution and Phenotype of Anterior Uveal Tract DC

Following the discovery that MHC class II expression was important to the outcome of transplantation and in the aetiology and pathogenesis of autoimmune and inflammatory-mediated diseases, many groups investigated the pattern of expression of this molecule in normal and diseased ocular tissues. Most of these studies, performed on conventionally sectioned tissue, either failed to reveal any MHC class II$^+$ cells or revealed only occasional, scattered cells in the normal eye (Abi-Hanna *et al.*, 1987; Bakker and Kijlstra, 1985; Bakker *et al.*, 1986; Lynch *et al.*, 1987; Latina *et al.*, 1988). More recently a contiguous network of MHC class II$^+$ DC has been described in the iris (Fig. 16A) and ciliary body (Fig. 16C) (McMenamin *et al.*, 1992b; McMenamin *et al.*, 1994). In all species examined, iris DC display a variety of forms from pleomorphic to the characteristic highly dendriform morphology with multiple, often branched, cytoplasmic processes and indented nucleus (Fig. 16B). The cells do not display as strong a perivascular orientation as resident tissue macrophages. In addition, the Ia$^+$ DCs form a network of similar density (400–600 cells/mm^2) to that of other well-recognized DC populations (e.g. skin 700–800/mm^2, tracheal epithelium 670–880/mm^2, oral mucosa 160–890/mm^2). Double colour immunohistochemical studies (Plate 12.17) have revealed that DC do not colocalize with anti-macrophage monoclonal antibodies. Immunoelectron microscopic and confocal studies have revealed that DC in the ciliary processes are intraepithelial on the vascular aspect of the tight junctions that form the blood–aqueous barrier. Thus they are ideally situated to sample intraocular antigens or blood-borne antigens arriving via the fenestrated vascular bed.

Low to moderate densities of MHC class II$^+$ dendriform cells have been identified in the rat (McMenamin and Holthouse, 1992) and human (Flügel *et al.*, 1992) trabecular meshwork and around episcleral vessels and collector channels which serve to drain AqH into the venous blood. Thus DC at these sites would be ideally located to sample antigens exiting the eye. Tracer studies have shown that proteins injected into the AC leak from limbal vessels (Sherman *et al.*, 1978), making it feasible that MHC class II$^+$

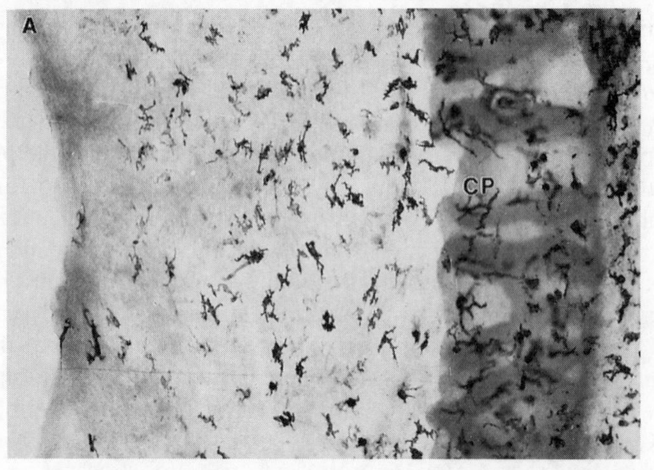
A
CP

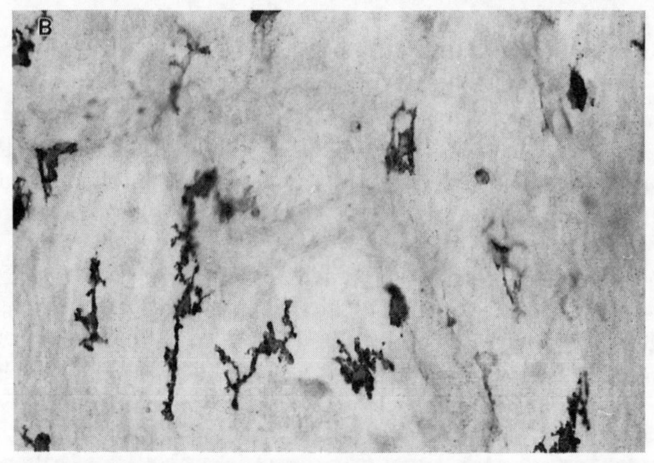
B

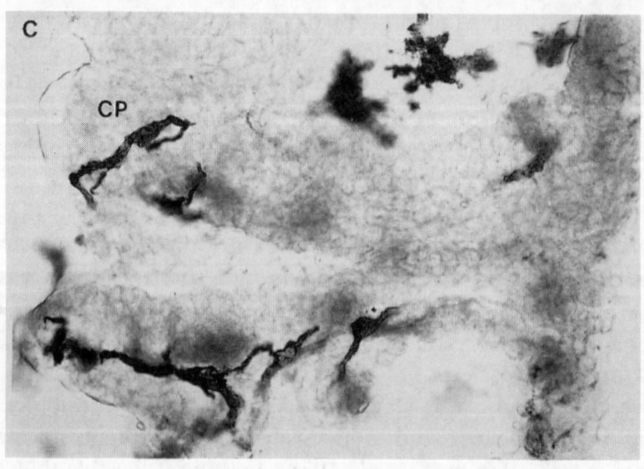
C
CP

cells around collector channels and episcleral vessels have access to intracameral antigens. These cells could then migrate, via conjunctival lymphatics, to draining submandibular lymph nodes, thus bypassing the 'camero-splenic axis'. Support for this postulated route has recently come from the elegant chimera experiments of Egan *et al.* (1996) in which antigen-specific T cells in the submandibular lymph nodes clonally expand following intracameral injections. This may represent another pathway, besides the spleen, whereby antigens in the eye become accessible to the systemic immune system.

Ontogeny, Migration Capacity and Function of Anterior Uveal Tract DC

The ontogeny of Ia^+ DC populations during fetal and postnatal development has been examined in a number of lymphoid and nonlymphoid tissues (Wilders *et al.*, 1983; van Rees *et al.*, 1988; Hsiao *et al.*, 1991; Nelson *et al.*, 1994). Following birth, DC populations in the rat attain adult-equivalent levels within 2–3 weeks postpartum in virtually all tissue sites examined to date. The development of Ia^+ DC in the aqueous outflow pathways (McMenamin and Holthouse, 1992) and the iris (Steptoe *et al.*, 1997) of the rat eye may occur more slowly than that observed in other tissue sites. It appears that DC infiltrate the iris primordium as $Ox62^+/Ia^-$ or Ia^{low} precursor cells, which subsequently develop *in situ* into DC bearing high levels of Ia antigen ($Ox62^+/Ia^+$) (Steptoe *et al.*, 1997). The mechanisms which induce DC maturation in nonlymphoid tissues are unclear at present. Although some studies suggest that exposure to environmental antigenic stimulation may provide the impetus for DC development (Romani, 1986; Elbe, 1994; Nelson *et al.*, 1994), it appears it is not essential for DC development (Mayrhofer *et al.*, 1983). In the eye the rate of development of Ia^+ iris DC was greatest between postnatal days 13 and 21, which coincides with eye-opening (day 14), a major event in the development of ocular function which may impinge on the intraocular environment via components of the photodetection cascades, via alteration in neuropeptide levels or via exposure of the globe to the external environment/exogenous antigens.

Bone marrow ablation studies have shown that iris DC have a half-life of 2–3 days in comparison to 10 days for epidermal Langerhans cells (LC) (Fig. 18). This rapid turnover of iris DC is comparable to DC populations in mucosal surfaces (Pugh *et al.*, 1983; Holt *et al.*, 1994).

Functional studies have shown that iris DC purified by positive immunomagnetic selection have the functional capacity to stimulate naive T cells in a mixed lymphocyte response (MLR) similar to conventional DC, such as LC (Steptoe *et al.*, 1995). Iris DC, like other 'immature' DC in peripheral tissues which are weak APCs, require appropriate cytokine maturational signals, such as GM-CSF, in order to display potent stimulatory capacity in an MLR assay (Fig. 19).

Do DC in the iris, ciliary body and outflow pathways have access to ocular autoantigens such as S-antigen or IRBP? There is evidence that S-Ag is detectable in human

Fig. 16. Wholemount of mouse iris and ciliary processes (CP) stained with M5/114 (anti-MHC class II). (A) low power (×90); (B) high power of individual DC in iris (×240); (C) high power of individual DC in ciliary processes (CP) (×600).

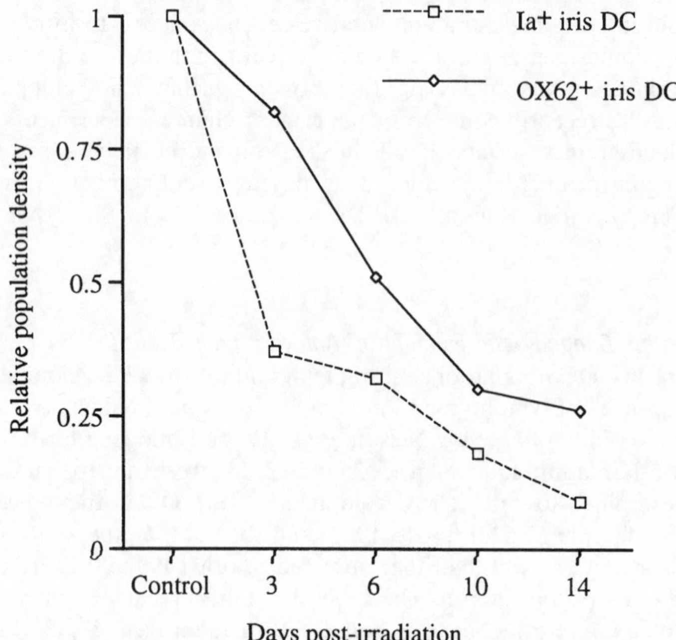

Fig. 18. Population kinetics of DC (Ia$^+$ and Ox62$^+$) in rat iris wholemounts following lethal X-irradiation (10 Gy). Data are presented as relative to normal control values for comparison (Steptoe *et al.* 1997).

AqH (Zaal *et al.*, 1986) and more recent in-situ hybridization evidence has shown that S-Ag cDNA is present in porcine iris and ciliary body (Singh *et al.*, 1996). Thus it seems plausible that local DC would have access to these autoantigens in addition to other endogenous antoantigens (e.g. lens proteins) or exogenous antigens derived from unicellular and multicellular pathogens which invade the intraocular compartments.

It appears that iris DC, like those in the respiratory and alimentary tracts (Schon-Hegrad *et al.*, 1991; MacPherson *et al.*, 1989), respond within 12–24 h to inflammatory signals by altering their phenotype, increasing their density (via immigration) and turnover time (McMenamin and Crewe, 1995). The net effect of this response is presumably to enhance the efficiency of immune surveillance at crucial times of viral or bacterial infection.

Dendritic Cells in the Normal Choroid and their Relevance to Ocular Autoimmune Disease

Dendritic cells in the choroid of the eye have mostly been studied in the rat (Forrester *et al.*, 1993; Butler and McMenamin, 1995). Subsequent investigations have confirmed that cells of the DC immunophenotype are present at similar densities in the mouse choroid (Plate 12.20A) (McMenamin, unpublished observations). In the rat, choroidal DCs (746 ± 37 cells/mm^2), like those in the iris, express MHC class II and in addition there is a small population of Ox62$^+$ round precursor cells, indicating that their turnover is likely to be similar to that in the iris (Steptoe *et al.*, 1996). Choroidal DC cells have at least two phenotypes: a very large, veiled cell with extensive ruffled membrane

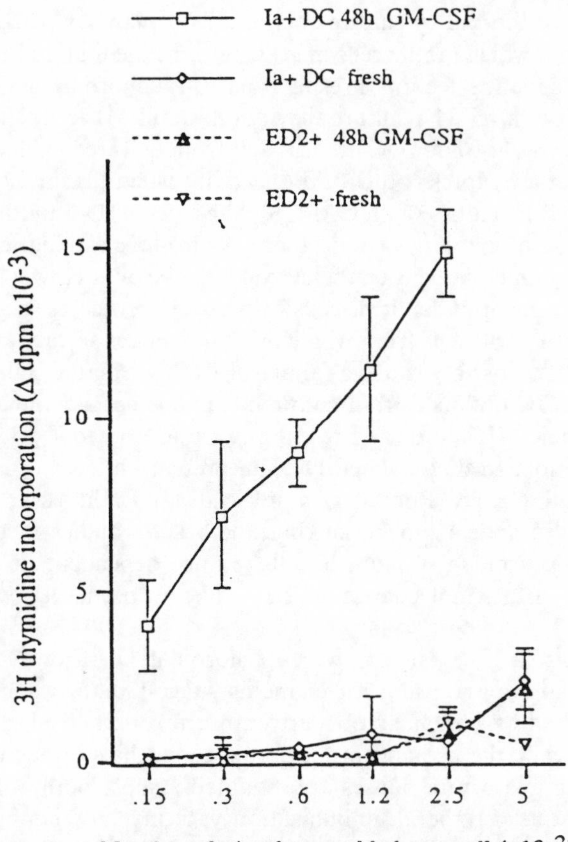

Fig. 19. Allostimulatory capacity of iris MHC class II-positive DC or ED2-positive iris macrophages either freshly isolated or following 48 h culture in GM-CSF. Data presented are [^{3}H]DNA synthesis by allogeneic MLR cultures in response to the addition of increasing numbers of iris DC, either freshly isolated or cultured for 48 h in GM-CSF and ED2$^+$ macrophages, either freshly isolated or cultured for 48 h in GM-CSF. Ordinate values represent mean (±SD) Δ dpm of triplicate cultures. The abscissa represents the number of Lewis stimulator cells added to each culture, 2×10^4 PVG responder cells were added to all cultures. Data are from a single experiment representative of a series of four. Purity of iris DC was 98% (fresh) and 91% (cultured), ED2$^+$ cell purity was 95% (fresh) and 98% (cultured). (From Steptoe *et al.*, 1995.)

and a smaller, more typical cell with dendritic processes and high levels of cell surface class II antigen (Forrester *et al.*, 1994). Both cell types are located perivascularly in the choroid, and immunoelectronmicroscopic studies have shown that they possess fine processes which lie directly adjacent to the basal aspect of the retinal pigment epithelial cells and Bruch's membrane (Plate 12.20B). This strategic location would be ideal to sample retinal proteins.

Functional studies of rat DC isolated from preparations of the entire posterior segment (retina, choroid and sclera) suggest that they are functionally similar to iris DC as assessed by mitogenesis assays and allostimulatory capacity in MLR assays (Choudhury *et al.*, 1994). Relatively pure populations of dendritic cells can be isolated from the rat and human choroid by culture of choroidal explants *in vitro* in the presence of fetal calf serum, from which motile cells migrate into the medium to be harvested and purified by immunomagnetic selection. Freshly isolated rat choroidal DC fail to present antigen in the MLR, but after 24 h culture they develop full MLR reactivity (Forrester *et al.*, in preparation). If choroidal DC are isolated from cultured explants rather than by enzyme digestion, they express potent APC activity when 'freshly' harvested. This activity is not increased by culture with GM-CSF, TNF-α or IL-4 and has been attributed to possible release of cytokines from other cells in the choroidal explant such as macrophages and/or retinal pigment epithelial cells (see below). However, it should be borne in mind that treatment of dendritic cells with certain proteases such as dispase, as done in many studies to purify DC from whole tissues, removes surface antigen activity, including MHC class II, possibly causing failure of freshly isolated cells to respond in the MLR. Choroidal DC obtained from cultured explants act as potent APC in both allogeneic and syngeneic MLR and can present antigen to primed T cells (Forrester, in preparation). In addition, freshly isolated DC can present antigen to naive T cells, as shown by the polarization assay (Forrester, in preparation). In this assay, a requirement for accessory molecules appears to be lacking and recent studies in a cluster assay suggest that this initial priming of naive T cells may be dependent on a recently discovered dendritic cell surface molecule with TNF-α-like properties, known as RANKL (Anderson *et al.*, 1997).

There are no data available on turnover of choroidal DC; however, preliminary observations in our laboratory using rat chimeras suggest that in common with iris DC they are replenished by bone marrow-derived precursors.

As stated earlier, while the eye and brain do appear to have a degree of immunological privilege, inflammatory responses are mounted against both autoantigens and infectious agents. Just as peripheral immunization with myelin components has been used as a paradigm for investigating the pathogenesis of multiple sclerosis (experimental allergic encephalomyelitis, EAE), similarly in the eye experimental immunization with retinal antigens at distant sites is used to mimic uveoretinitis or uveitis (experimental autoimmune uveitis, EAU). EAU is mediated by $CD4^{+}$ T cells, and both lymphocytes and macrophages constitute the earliest effector cells which initially infiltrate the retina and cause lysis of the photoreceptors, followed by phagocytosis and eventual destruction of the whole outer retina (for review see McMenamin *et al.*, 1994; Forrester, 1992). In many respects the disease that EAU most closely mimics is sympathetic ophthalmia, in which severe trauma or damage to one eye/retina can result in a consensual inflammatory response that may threaten the other undamaged eye, hence explaining why badly traumatized eyes are often enucleated to save the unaffected eye. Various candidates for the initial presentation of autoantigens in human endogenous uveitis (where both eyes were previously normal) have included vascular endothelium, retinal pigment epithelium and Müller cells; however, evidence for these cells as major activators of activated or naive T cells compares poorly with the evidence for macrophages or DC (Forrester *et al.*, 1995).

While several previous studies have reported MHC class II upregulation on retinal pigment epithelium and retinal vascular endothelium in EAU models (Chan *et al.*, 1986b; Baudouin *et al.*, 1988; Liversidge and Forrester, 1988; Liversidge *et al.*, 1988), sympathetic ophthalmia and uveitis (Chan *et al.*, 1986a), there have been only limited reports of MHC class II expression on cells of the choroid or retina in diseased states. It has recently been demonstrated that there is an obvious increase in the density of MHC class II$^+$ cells in the iris and choroid in the early stages of EAU (Butler and McMenamin, 1996). While some of the increase may be accounted for by MHC class II$^+$ activated T cells or macrophages, it probably represents enhanced recruitment of DC precursors from the circulation or an upregulation of Ia on previously Ia$^-$ DC. There is evidence that a population of DC precursors (OX62$^+$ Ia$^-$) exists within the choroid (Forrester *et al.*, 1994) and iris (see above). These may provide a rapidly recruitable source of DC in the event of local inflammatory episodes. The concurrent increase in density of Ia$^+$ DC and T cell infiltration in the uveal tract would provide the appropriate environment for local activation of uveitogenic T cells. The crucial importance of the interaction between the T cell receptor and peptide-bearing MHC class II molecule in induction of autoimmune disease has underpinned the rationale of experimental attempts to disrupt the complex using anti-Ia antibody therapy and therefore ameliorate diseases such as EAU (Rao *et al.*, 1989) and EAE (Gautam *et al.*, 1992; Jonker *et al.*, 1988) The partial success of such studies supports the concept that MHC class II expression is involved in induction and perpetuation of EAU.

FACTORS REGULATING DC FUNCTION IN THE EYE AND THE BRAIN

Despite the location and widespread distribution of DC in the meninges and the uveal tract, where they have the potential to cause damage to CNS and retinal tissue by initiating inflammatory responses, under normal circumstance little inflammation is induced. It is likely that meningeal and choroid plexus DC have access to CNS autoantigens such as MBP that have been detected in small quantities in the CSF (Warren *et al.*, 1983; Lowenthal *et al.*, 1984). This is so even though there is frequent non-CNS specific activation of circulating T cells which, as stated above, have the capacity to traffic across blood–CNS barriers and must therefore come into contact with meningeal and uveal DCs. The failure of DC to activate T cells in these circumstances may represent one aspect of so-called 'immune privilege' in the eye and brain but may more generally represent an illustration of how local microenvironmental factors modulate immune responses.

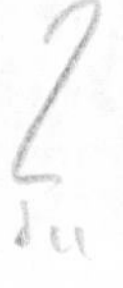

Little information is available on how meningeal DC function is affected by tissue cells, such as choroid plexus epithelium, but there is emerging evidence that ocular DC function is modified by other cells within that tissue. In other organs, macrophages can downregulate DC function, as is the case in the lung (Thepen *et al.*, 1992) and gut (Pavli *et al.*, 1990), possibly via production of TNF-α and nitric oxide. Alternatively, macrophages may act as APCs in their own right in secondary immune responses. Recent data suggest that ED2$^+$ iris macrophages lack lymphocytostatic activity (Steptoe *et al.*, manuscript submitted) and choroidal macrophages are poor APCs in isolation but may significantly augment, rather than downregulate, the MLR initiated by choroidal DCs (Forrester *et al.*, in preparation). Furthermore, cultured DCs appear to cluster with large macrophages, indicating that there is significant cross-talk between these two cell types.

In contrast, retinal pigment epithelium (RPE) cells appear to release factors which inhibit APC function. These factors include prostaglandins and nitric oxide (Liversidge *et al.*, 1994). Interestingly, both of these are also known to be released by brain microglia and thus may add to the immunoregulatory role of these cells in the brain parenchyma. Perivascular microglia synthesize cyclooxygenase and prostaglandins, which further supports their role as a type of downregulatory macrophage in the CNS. In support of this, systemic administration of prostaglandins inhibits the manifestation of EAE (Reder *et al.*, 1995); however, whether this specifically acts on APC is speculative.

In the eye, RPE cells are also known to release GM-CSF, which is a survival factor for DC (Vremec *et al.*, 1997; Crane *et al.*, 1998b). Production of GM-CSF by RPE cells is induced by other cytokines such as TGF-β, TNF-α and IL-1. GM-CSF may not only affect DC function in the choroid but if it were released into the retina or brain it might modulate the function of microglia since it has been shown to inhibit MHC class II expression by these cells (Hayashi and Abromson-Leeman, 1995). Thus it may have a pro-inflammatory effect on the CNS by blocking the recently discovered T cell apoptosis-inducing effect of microglia (see above).

Other chemokines released by RPE cells include IL-8 and RANTES, but these are produced only after exposure to pro-inflammatory cytokines such as IL-1 and IFN-γ (Kuppner *et al.*, 1995; Crane *et al.*, 1998a). In contrast, they preferentially release IL-6 when exposed to a combination of IL-1 and TGF-β (Kuppner *et al.*, 1995). This has led to the notion that RPE cells orchestrate the immune response at the blood–retinal barrier, promoting a T_H1 type response under certain circumstance and a T_H2 or even a null (?T_H3) type response when the immune response is being downregulated (Forrester *et al.*, 1995). It would be interesting to see whether similar events occurred at the choroid plexus epithelial layer.

RECRUITMENT OF DC AND MONONUCLEAR CELLS TO THE CNS DURING INFLAMMATION

Although DC and activated macrophages are absent from the CNS parenchyma under normal circumstances, large numbers of the latter type are found in inflammation, in which they appear to act as effector cells in tissue damage (Polman *et al.*, 1986). Recruitment of small numbers of DC into the neural parenchyma, namely behind the BBB, has also been reported in EAE and following local injection of heat-killed bacillus Calmette-Guerin (BCG) (Matyszak and Perry, 1996a). This recruitment probably depends on changes in adhesive interactions between leukocytes and the endothelium and on the release of specific chemokines which allow transendothelial cell migration of mononuclear cells. Recent studies have shown that population of damage sites with small numbers of antigen-specific T cells allows release of chemokines by tissue cells such as astrocytes (Barna *et al.*, 1994; Hurwitz *et al.*, 1995). Monocyte chemotactic protein-1 (MCP-1) has been detected in astrocytes in the acute phase of EAE (Hayashi *et al.*, 1995) and can be induced by release of T cell cytokines such as TNF-α. In contrast MIP-1α appears to be released from microglia rather than astrocytes. T-lymphocytes appear to secrete a further chemokine TCA3 which directly attracts macrophages and even induces chemotaxis in microglia. Other chemokines produced by these cells include RANTES and MIP-1β. In EAE, most of the RANTES produced appeared to be derived from T cells while some was produced by astrocytes and microglia. However, at the peak of disease all three chemokines appeared to be produced predominantly by perivascular cells (Miyagishi *et al.*, 1997).

Release of TNF by infiltrating T cells and macrophages also has a direct effect on the expression of adhesion molecules by the endothelium, thus adding a further dimension to the recruitment of inflammatory cells in CNS inflammation (Korner *et al.*, 1995). Interestingly, adhesion molecule expression commences prior to the onset of clinical disease, suggesting that the endothelium may regulate the traffic of T cells to the site of inflammation (Ma *et al.*, 1996). However, recent studies in EAU using direct observation of retinal vessels in the confocal scanning laser ophthalmoscope reveal that although nonspecifically activated T cells will adhere to a normal nonactivated endothelium in small numbers, both the endothelium and the T cells require to be activated before transendothelial migration and infiltration of the tissue occurs. Recent studies (Navratil *et al.*, 1997) indicate that the repertoire or combinations of adhesion molecules expressed by CNS endothelium does not differ from other endothelium, suggesting that the adaptation of the brain (and retinal) endothelium is due to expression of a few highly specific molecules, possibly yet to be discovered.

CONCLUSION AND FUTURE LINES OF RESEARCH

From the preceding discussions it is apparent that under normal conditions DC are excluded from the neural parenchyma; however, there is now recent evidence that they are well-represented in the tissues that physically and physiologically support the brain, spinal cord and retina. Despite the problems of isolating pure populations of DC from small ocular tissues, it has been shown that they are potent APCs capable of activating naive T cells. The use of tissue wholemount methods has also allowed extensive studies of phenotype, turnover and ontogeny that all support the proposal that the uveal tract of the eye is rich in DC. A similar approach should now prove invaluable in investigating similar features of the biology of DC within the choroid plexus and meninges. It will be crucial to ascertain whether purified DC from these sites are, as we have proposed, more likely candidate APCs in the CNS than microglia and perivascular cells, which have attracted most attention to date.

A pivotal question to be asked regarding DC in the supporting tissues of the eye and and CNS is whether they normally have access to and are capable of trapping and processing exogenous antigens and autoantigens, such as MBP (or retinal proteins in the eye), within the parenchyma or in the CSF. If so, are they 'mature' while resident in the brain and eye and therefore capable of acting as APCs *in situ*? Or do they, like most DC populations, mature under the influence of cytokine signals as they migrate to 'draining' lymphoid organs? The latter point raises the further question of migration route(s) and destiny of DC derived from the eye, brain and spinal cord, an important issue requiring further research, possibly utilizing prelabelled DC or congenic chimera models.

The heterogeneity of DC populations has attracted a lot of interest lately and is an area of potentially fruitful research with regard to uveal tract and meningeal DC. Namely, are subpopulations of DC responsible for presenting tolerogenic or immunogenic signals and, if so, could this knowledge be used in the prevention and treatment of autoimmune conditions affecting the eye and CNS? For example could some DC/antigen combinations be used to sensitize animals and prevent induction of EAE while another DC/antigen mixture might be used to induce disease? One problem likely to hamper the application of such approaches to the human condition is the difficulty of treating pre-existing conditions especially as the CNS and eye have poor reparative capacity. Perhaps strategies for the prevention and limitation of further tissue damage are a more realistic goal.

ACKNOWLEDGEMENTS

The authors thank Dr Raymond J. Steptoe for use of some material from his PhD thesis. P.G. McMenamin acknowledges support from the NH&MRC and ARC. J.V. Forrester thanks Lynne Lumsden for technical assistance in DC studies and Janet Liversidge, Isobelle Crane and Maria Kuppner for work with RPE cells.

REFERENCES

Abi-Hanna, D., Wakefield, D. and Watkins, S. (1987). HLA antigens in ocular tissue. I. In vivo expression in human eyes. *Transplantation* **45**, 610–613.

Allaerts, W., Fluitsma, D.M., Hoefsmit, E.C., Jeucken, P.H., Morreau, H., Bosman, F.T. and Drexhage, H.A. (1996) Immunohistochemical, morphological and ultrastructural resemblance between dendritic cells and folliculo-stellate cells in normal human and rat anterior pituitaries. *J. Neuroendocrinol.* **8**, 17–29.

Anderson, D.M., Maraskovsky, E., Billingsley, W.L., Dougall, W.C., Tometsko, M.E., Roux, E.R., Teepe, M.C., Dubose, R.F., Cosman, D. and Galibert, L. (1997). A homologue of the TNF receptor and its ligand enhance T cell growth and dendritic cell function. *Nature* **390** (6656), 175–177.

Bakker, M. and Kijlstra, A. (1985). The expression of HLA-antigens in the human anterior uvea. *Curr. Eye Res.* **4**, 599–604.

Bakker, M., Grumet, F.G., Feltkamp, T.E.W. and Kijlstra, A. (1986). HLA-antigens in the human uvea. *Doc. Opthalmol.* **61**, 271–279.

Barker, C.F. and Billingham, R.E. (1977). Immunologically privileged sites. *Adv. Immunol.* **25**, 1–54.

Banati, R.B. and Graeber, M.B. (1994). Surveillance, intervention and cytotoxicity: is there a protective role of microglia? *Dev. Neurosci.* **16**, 114–127.

Banati, R.B., Hoppe, D., Gottmann, K., Kreutzberg, G.W. and Kettenmann, H. (1991). A subpopulation of bone marrow-derived macrophage-like cells shares a unique ion channel pattern with microglia. *J. Neurosci. Res.* **30**, 593–600.

Banati, R.B., Gehrmann, J., Schubert, P. and Kreutzberg, G.W. (1993). Cytotoxicity of microglia. *Glia* **7**, 111–118.

Barna, B.P., Pettay, J., Barnett, G.H., Zhou, P., Iwaski, K. and Estes, M.L. (1994). Regulation of monocyte chemoattractant protein-1 expression in adult human non-neoplastic astrocytes is sensitive to tumor necrosis factor (TNF) or antibody to the 55-kDa TNF receptor. *J Neuroimmunol.* **50**(1), 101–107.

Battisti, W.P., Wang, J., Bozek, K. and Murray, M. (1995). Macrophages, microglia and astrocytes are rapidly activated after crush injury of the goldfish optic nerve: a light and electron microscopic analysis. *J. Comp. Neurol.* **354**, 306–320.

Baudouin, C., Fredj-Reygrobellet, D., Gastaud, P. and Lapalus, P. (1988). HLA DR and DQ distribution in normal ocular structures. *Curr. Eye Res.* **7**, 903–911.

Bauer, J., Sminia, T., Wouterlood, F.G. and Dijkstra, C.D. (1994). Phagocytic activity of macrophages and microglial cells during the course of acute and chronic relapsing experimental autoimmune encephalomyelitis. *J. Neurosci. Res.* **38**, 365–375.

Bell, M.D., Lopez-Gonzalez, R., Lawson, L., Hughes, D., Fraser, I., Gordon, S. and Perry, V.H. (1994). Upregulation of the macrophage scavenger receptor in response to different forms of injury in the CNS. *J. Neurocytol.* **23**, 605–613.

Bleier, R. and Albrecht, R. (1980). Supraependymal macrophages of third ventricle of hamster: morphological, functional and histochemical characterisation in situ and in culture. *J. Comp. Neurol.* **192**, 489.

Butler, T.L. and McMenamin, P.G. (1996). Immunohistochemical study of choroid and iris whole-mounts in the early and late stages of experimental autoimmune uveoretinitis. *Invest. Ophthalmol. Vis. Sci.* **37**, 2195–2210.

Cuadros, M.A., Martin, C., Coltey, P., Almendros, A. and Navascues, J. (1993). First appearance, distribution, and origin of macrophages in the early development of the avian central nervous system. *J. Comp. Neurol.* **330**, 113–129.

Cash, E. and Rott, O. (1994). Microglial cells qualify as the stimulators of unprimed $CD4^+$ and $CD8^+$ T lymphocytes in the central nervous system. *Clin. Exp. Immunol.* **98**, 313–318.

Cash, E., Zhang, Y. and Rott, O. (1993). Microglia present myelin antigens to T cells after phagocytosis of oligodendrocytes. *Cell. Immunol.* **147**, 129–138.

Chamberlain, J.G. (1974) Scanning electron microscopy of epiplexus cells (macrophages) in the fetal rat brain. *Am. J. Anat.* **139**, 443–448.

Chan, C-C., Detrick, B., Nussenblatt, R.B., Palestine, A., Fujikawa, L.S. and Hooks, J.J. (1986a). HLA-DR antigens on retinal pigment epithelial cells from patients with uveitis. *Arch. Ophthalmol.* **104**, 725.

Chan, C-C., Hooks, J.J., Nussenblatt, R.B. and Detrick, B. (1986b). Expression of Ia antigen on retinal pigment epithelium in experimental autoimmune uveoretinitis. *Curr. Eye Res.* **5**, 325–330.

Choudhury, A., Al Palkanis, V. and Bowers, W.E. (1994). Characterization and functional activity of dendritic cells from rat choroid. *Exp. Eye Res.* **59**, 297–304.

Cogburn, L.A. and Glick, B. (1987). Lymphopoeisis in the chicken pineal gland. *Am. J. Anat.* **162**, 1309–1321.

Crane, I., Kuppner, M.C., McKillop-Smith, S., Knott, R. and Forrester, J.V. (1998a). Cytokine regulation of RANTES production by human retinal pigment epithelium cells. *Cell. Immunol.* (in press).

Crane, I., Kuppner, S., McKillop-Smith, C.A., Wallace, C.A. and Forrester, J.V. (1998b). Production of granulocyte-macrophage colony stimulating factor by human retinal pigment epithelial cells. *Clin. Exp. Immunol.* in press.

Cserr, H.F. and Knopf, P.M. (1992). Cervical lymphatics, the blood–brain barrier and the immunoreactivity of the brain—a new view. *Immunol. Today* **13**, 507–512.

Cuzner, M.L. (1997). Microglia in health and disease. *Biochem. Soc. Trans.* **25**, 671-673.

Damoiseaux, J.G.M.C., Dopp, E.A., Neefjes, J.J., Beelen, R.H.J. and Dijkstra, C.D. (1989). Heterogeneity of macrophages in the rat evidenced by variability in determinants: two new anti-rat macrophage antibodies against a heterodimer of 160 and 95 kd (CD11/CD18). *J. Leukocyte Biol.* **46**, 556–564.

De Stefano, M.E. and Mugnaini, E. (1997). Fine Structure of the choroidal coat of the avian eye. *Invest. Ophthalmol. Vis. Sci.* **38**, 1241–1260.

de Groot, C.J.A., Huppes, W., Sminia, T., Kraal, G. and Dijkstra, C.D. (1992). Determination of the origin and nature of brain macrophages and microglial cells in mouse central nervous system, using non-radioactive in situ hybridization and immunoperoxidase techniques. *Glia* **6**, 301–309.

Dick, A.D., Ford, A.L., Forrester, J.V. and Sedgwick, J.D. (1995). Flow cytometric identification of a minority population of MHC class II positive cells in the normal rat retina distinct from $CD45^{low}CD11b/c^+CD4^{low}$ parenchymal microglia. *Br. J. Ophthalmol.* **79**, 834–840.

Dickson, D.W., Mattiace, L.A., Kure, K., Hutchins, K., Lyman, W.D. and Brosnan, C.F. (1991). Microglia in human disease, with an emphasis on acquired immune deficiency syndrome. *Lab. Invest.* **64**, 135–156.

Diaz-Araya, C.M., Provis, J.M. and Penfold, P.L. (1995). Ontogeny and cellular expression of MHC and leucocyte antigens in human retina. *Glia* **15**, 458–470.

Dijkstra, C.D., Dopp, E.A., Joling, P. and Kraal, G. (1985). The heterogeneity of mononuclear phagocytes in lymphoid organs: distinct macrophage subpopulations in the rat recognised by monoclonal antibodies ED1, ED2 and ED3. *Immunology* **54**, 589–599.

Dowding, A.J. and Scholes, J. (1993). Lymphoctes and macrophages outnumber oligodendrocytes in normal fish spinal cord. *Proc. Natl Acad. Sci. USA.* **90**, 10183–10187.

Egan, R.M., Yorkey, C., Black, R., Loh, W.K., Stevens, J.L. and Woodward, J.G. (1996). Peptide-specific T cell clonal expansion in vivo following immunization in the eye, an immune-privileged site. *J. Immunol.* **157**, 2262–2271.

Elbe, A., Schleischitz, S., Strunk, D. and Stingl, G. (1994). Fetal skin-derived MHC class I^+, MHC class II^- dendritic cells stimulate MHC class I-restricted responses of unprimed $CD8^+$ T cells. *J. Immunol.* **153**, 2878–2889.

Elmquist, J.K., Breder, C.D., Sherin, J.E., Scammell, T.E., Hickey, W.F., Dewitt, D. and Saper, C.B. (1997). Intravenous lipopolysaccharide induces cyclooxygenase 2-like immunoreactivity in rat brain perivascular microglia and meningeal macrophages. *J. Comp. Neurol.* **381**, 119–129.

Ferguson, T.A., Waldrep, J.C. and Kaplen, H.J. (1987). The immune response and the eye. II. The nature of T suppressor cell induction in anterior chamber-associated immune deviation (ACAID). *J. Immunol.* **139**, 352–357.

Flaris, N.A., Densmore, T.L., Molleston, M.C. and Hickey, W.F. (1993). Characterization of microglia and macrophages in the central nervous system of rats: definition of the differential expression of molecules using standard and novel monoclonal antibodies in normal CNS and in four models of parenchymal reaction. *Glia* **7**, 34–40.

Flügel, C., Kinne, R.W., Streilein, J.W. and Lutjen-Drecoll, E. (1992). Distinctive distribution of HLA class II presenting and bone marrow derived cells in the anterior segment of human eyes. *Curr. Eye Res.* **12**, 1173–1183.

Ford, A.L., Goodsall, A.L., Hickey, W.F. and Sedgwick, J.D. (1995). Normal adult ramified microglia separated from other central nervous sytem macrophages by flow cytometric sorting. *J. Immunol.* **154**, 4309–4321.

Ford, A.L., Foulcher, E., Lemckert, F.A. and Sedgwick, J.D. (1996). Microglia induce CD4 T lymphocyte final effector function and death. *J. Exp. Med.* **184**, 1737–1745.

Forrester, J.V. (1992). New concepts on the role of autoimmunity in the pathogenesis of uveitis. *Eye* **6**, 433–446.

Forrester, J.V., McMenamin, P.G., Liversidge, J. and Lumsden, L. (1993). Dendritic cells and 'dendritic' macrophages in the uveal tract. In *Dendritic Cells in Fundamental and Clinical Immunology* (eds Hoefsmit, E., Niewenhuis, P. and Kamperdiijk, E). Plenum Press, London.

Forrester, J.V., McMenamin, P.G., Holthouse, I., Lumsden, L. and Liversidge, J. (1994). Localisation and characterization of major histocompatibility complex class II-positive cells in the posterior segment of the eye: implications for induction of autoimmune uveoretinitis. *Invest. Ophthalmol. Vis. Sci.* **35**, 64–77.

Forrester, J.V., Lumsden, L., Liversidge, J., Kuppner, M. and Mesri, M. (1995). Immunoregulation of uveoretinal inflammation. *Prog. Ret. Eye Res.* **14**, 393–412.

Frei, K., Lins, H., Schwerdel, C. and Fontana, A. (1994). Antigen presentation in the central nervous system. The inhibitory effect of IL-10 on MHC class II expression and production of cytokines depends on the inducing signals and type of cell analyzed. *J. Immunol.* **152**, 2720–2728.

Gautam, A.M., Pearson, C.I., Sinha, A.A., Smilek, D.E., Stolnman, L. and McDevitt, H.O. (1992). Inhibition of experimental autoimmune encephalomyelitis by a nonimmunogenic non-self peptide that binds to I-A. *J. Immunol.* **148**, 3049–3054.

Gehrmann, J., Banati, R.B. and Kreutzberg, G.W. (1993). Microglia in the immune surveillance of the brain: Human microglia constitutively express HLA-DR molecules. *J. Neuroimmunol.* **48**, 189–198.

Graeber, M. B., Streit, W.J. and Kreutzberg, G.W. (1989). Identity of ED2-positive perivascular cells in the rat brain. *J. Neurosci. Res.* **22**, 103–106.

Graeber, M.B., Streit, W.J., Buringer, D.. Sparks, D.L. and Kreutzberg, G.W. (1992). Ultrastructural location of major histocompatibility complex (MHC) class II positive perivascular cells in histologically normal human brain. *J. Neuropathol. Exp. Neurol.* **51**, 303–311.

Greenwood, J. (1992). The blood–retinal barrier in experimental autoimmune uveitis (EAU): a review. *Curr. Eye Res.* **11**(suppl), 25–32.

Griffith, T.S., Brunner, T., Fletcher, S.M., Green, D.R. and Ferguson, T.A. (1995). Fas ligand-induced apoptosis as a mechanism of immune privilege. *Science* **270**, 1189–1192.

Gourmala, N.G., Buttini, M., Limonta, S., Sauter, A. and Boddeke, H.W. (1997). Differential and time-dependent expression of monocyte chemoattractant protein-1 mRNA by astrocytes and macrophages in rat brain: effects of ischemia and peripheral lipopolysaccharide administration. *J. Neuroimmunol.* **74**, 35–44.

Hart, D.N.J. and Fabre, J.W. (1981). Demonstration and characterization of Ia-positive dendritic cells in the interstitial connective tissues of rat heart and other tissues, but not brain. *J. Exp. Med.* **154**, 347–361.

Hayashi, M. and Abromson-Leeman, S. (1995). Granulocyte-macrophage colony stimulating factor inhibits class II major histocompatibility complex expression and antigen presentation by microglia. *J. Neuroimmunol.* **48**, 23–32.

Hayashi, M., Luo, Y., Laning, J., Strieter, R.M. and Dorf, M.E. (1995). Production and function of monocyte chemoattractant protein-1 and other beta-chemokines in murine glial cells. *J. Neuroimmunol.* **60**, 143–150.

Hayes, G.M., Woodruffe, M.N. and Cuzner, M.L. (1987). Microglia are the major cell type expressing MHC class II in human white matter. *J. Neurol. Sci.* **53**, 753–767.

Hickey, W.F. and Kimura, H. (1988). Perivascular microglial cells of the CNS are bone marrow-derived and present antigen in vivo. *Science* **239**, 290–292.

Hickey, W.F., Vass, K. and Lassmann, H. (1992). Bone marrow-derived elements in the central nervous system: an immunohistochemical and ultastructural survey of rat chimeras. *J. Neuropathol. Exp. Neurol.* **51**, 246–256.

Holt, P.G., Haining, S., Nelson, D.J. and Sedgwick, J.D. (1994). Origin and steady-state turnover of class II MHC-bearing dendritic cells in the epithelium of the conducting airways. *J. Immunol.* **153**, 256–261.

Hsiao, L., Takahashi, K., Takeya, M. and Arao, T. (1991). Differentiation and maturation of macrophages into interdigitating cells and their multicellular complex formation in the fetal and postnatal rat thymus. *Thymus* **17**, 219–235.

Huitinga, I., van Rooijen, N., de Groot, C., Uitdehaag, B.M.J. and Dijkstra, C.D. (1990). Suppression of experimental allergic encephalomyelitis in Lewis rats after elimination of macrophages. *J. Exp. Med.* **172**, 1025–1033.

Hume, D.A., Perry, V.H. and Gordon, S. (1983). Immunohistochemical localization of a macrophage-specific antigen in developing mouse retina: phagocytosis of dying neurons and differentiation of microglial cells to form a regular array in the plexiform layers. *J. Cell. Biol.* **97**, 253.

Hurwitz, A.A., Lyman, W.D. and Berman, J.W. (1995). Tumor necrosis factor alpha and transforming growth factor beta upregulate astrocyte expression of monocyte chemoattractant protein-1. *J. Neuroimmunol.* **57**, 193–198.

Inaba, K., Inaba, M.. Witmer-Pack, M., Hatchcock, K., Hodes, R. and Steinman, R.M. (1995). Expression of B7 costimulator molecules on mouse dendritic cells. *Adv. Exp. Med. Biol.* **378**, 65–70.

Joo, F. (1994). Insight into the regulation by second messenger molecules of the permeability of the blood–brain barrier. *Microsc. Res. Techn.* **27**(6), 507–515.

Jonker, M., van Lambalgen, R., Mitchell, D.J., Durham, S.K. and Steinman, L. (1988). Successful treatment of EAE in rhesus monkeys with MHC class II specific monoclonal antibodies. *J. Autoimmun.* **1**, 399–414.

Jordan, F.L. and Thomas, W.E. (1988). Brain macrophages: questions of origin and interrelationships. *Brain Res. Rev.* **13**, 165–178.

Kapers, C.U.A., Huber, C.G. and Crosby, E.C. (1967). *The Comparative Anatomy of the Nervous System of Vertebrates, Including Man.* Horner, New York, pp. 56–67.

Katz, S.I., Tamaki, K. and Sachs, D.H. (1979). Epidermal Langerhans cells are derived from cells originating in bone marrow. *Nature* **282**, 324–326.

Kaur, C. and Ling, E.A. (1995). Transient expression of transferrin receptors and localisation of iron in amoeboid microglia in postnatal rats. *J. Anat.* **186**, 165–173.

Kaur, C., Singh, J. and Ling, E.A. (1993). Immunohistochemical and lectin-labelling studies of the distribution and development of microglia in the spinal cord of postnatal rats. *Arch. Histol. Cytol.* **56**, 475–484.

Kida, S., Steart, P.V., Zhang, En-T. and Weller, R.O. (1993). Perivascular cells act as scavengers in the cerebral perivascular spaces and remain distinct from pericytes, microglia and macrophages. *Acta Neuropathol.* **85**, 646–652.

Kitz, K., Lassmann, H. and Wisniewski H.M. (1981). Isolated leptomeninges of the spinal cord: an ideal tool to study inflammatory reaction in EAE. *Acta Neuropathol (Berlin)* **Suppl VII**, 179–181.

Korner, H., Goodsall, A.L., Lemckert, F.A., Scallon, B.J., Ghreyeb, J., Ford, A.L. and Sedgwick, J.D. (1995). Unimpaired autoreactive T-cell traffic within the central nervous system during tumor necrosis factor receptor-mediated inhibition of experimental autoimmune encephalomyelitis. *Proc. Natl Acad. Sci. USA* **92**, 11066–11070.

Krebs, W., Ingeborg, P. and Krebs, P. (1988). Ultrastructural evidence for lymphatic capillaries in the primate choroid. *Arch. Ophthalmol.* **106**, 1615–1616.

Kreutzberg, G.W. (1996). Microglia: a sensor for pathological events in the CNS. *TINS* **19**, 312–318.

Kuppner, M.C., McKillop-Smith, S. and Forrester, J.V. (1995). Transforming growth factor b and IL-1 act in synergy to enhance IL6 and IL8 mRNA levels and IL6 production by human retinal pigment epithelial cells. *Immunology* **84**, 265–271.

Lackner, A.A., Smith, M.O., Munn, R.J., Martfeld, D.J., Gardner, M.B., Marx, P.A. and Dandekar, S. (1991). Localization of simian immunodeficiency virus in the central nervous system of Rhesus monkeys. *Am. J. Pathol.* **139**, 609–621.

Lampson, L.A. and Hickey, W.F. (1986). Monoclonal antibody analysis of MHC expression in human brain biopsies: tissue ranging from 'histogically normal' to that showing different levels of glial tumor involvement. *J. Immunol.* **136**, 4054–4062.

Lassmann, H., Schmied, M., Vass, K. and Hickey, W. (1993). Bone marrow derived elements and resident microglia in brain inflammation. *Glia* **7**, 19–24.

Latina, M., Flotte, T., Crean, E., Sherwood, M.E. and Granstein, R.D. (1988). Immunohistochemical staining of the human anterior segment. Evidence that resident cells play a role in immunologic responses. *Arch. Ophthalmol.* **106**, 95–99.

Lawson, L.J., Perry, V.H. and Gordon, S. (1992). Turnover of resident microglia in the normal adult mouse brain. *Neuroscience* **48**, 405–415.

Lang, R.A. and Bishop, J.M. (1993). Macrophages are required for cell death and tissue remodeling in the developing mouse eye. *Cell* **74**, 453–462.

Ling, E.A. (1983). Scanning electron microscopic study of epiplexus cells in the lateral ventricles of the monkey (*Macaca fascicularis*) *J. Anat.* **137**, 645–652.

Ling, E.-A. and Wong, W.-C. (1993). The origin and nature of ramified and amoeboid microglia: a historical review and current concepts. *Glia* **7**, 9–18.

Ling, E.A., Tseng C.Y. and Wong W.C. (1985). An electron microscopical study of epiplexus and supraependymal cells in the prenatal rat brain following a maternal injection of 6-aminonicotinamide. *J. Anat.* **140**, 119–129.

Ling, E.A., Kaur, C. and Wong, W.C. (1991). Expression of major histocompatibility complex and leukocyte common antigens in amoeboid microglia in postnatal rats. *J. Anat.* **177**, 117–126.

Liversidge, J.M. and Forrester, J.V. (1988). Experimental allergic uveitis (EAU) : immunophenotypic analysis of the inflammatory cells in chorioretinal lesions. *Curr. Eye Res.* **7**, 1231–1241.

Liversidge, J.M., Sewell, H.F. and Forrester, J.V. (1988). Human retinal pigment epithelial cells differentially express MHC class II (HLA DP, DR and DQ) antigens in response to in vitro stimulation with lymphokine or purified IFN-gamma. *Clin. Exp. Immunol.* **73**, 489–494.

Liversidge, J., Grabowski, P., Ralston, S., Benjamin, N. and Forrester, J.V. (1994). Rat retinal pigment epithelial cells express an inducible form of nitric oxide synthase and produce nitric oxide in response to inflammatory cytokines and activated T cells. *Immunology* **83**, 404–409.

Loffler, K. and McMenamin, P.G. (1990). Evaluation of subretinal macrophage-like cells in the human foetal eye. *Invest. Ophthalmol. Vis. Sci.* **31**, 1628–1636.

Lowe, J., MacLennan, K.A., Powe, D.G., Pound, J.D. and Palmer, J.B. (1989). Microglial cells in human brain have phenotypic characteristics related to possible function as dendritic antigen presenting cells. *J. Pathol.* **159**, 143–149.

Lowenthal, A., Crols, R., De Schutter, E., Gheuens, J., Karcher, D., Noppe, M. and Tasnier, A. (1984). Cerebrospinal fluid proteins in neurology. *Int. Rev. Neurobiol.* **25**, 95–138.

Lu, J., Kaur, C. and Ling, E.A. (1994). Immunophenotypic features of epiplexus cells and their response to interferon gamma injected intraperitoneally in postnatal rats. *J. Anat.* **185**, 75–84.

Lund, R.D., Banerjee, R. and Rao, K. (1994). Microglia, MHC expression and graft rejection. *Neuropathol. Appl. Neurobiol.* **20**, 202–203.

Lynch, M.G., Peeler, J.S., Brown, R.H. and Niederkorn, J.Y. (1987). Expression of HLA class I and II antigens on cells of the trabecular meshwork. *Ophthalmology* **94**, 851–857.

Ma, N., Hunt, N.H., Madigan, M.C. and Chan-Ling, T. (1996). Correlation between enhanced vascular permeability, up-regulation of cellular adhesion molecules and monocyte adhesion to the endothelium in the retina during the development of fatal murine cerebral malaria. *Am. J. Pathol.* **149**, 1745–1762.

Maat-Schieman, M.L.C., van Duinen, S.G., Rozemuller, A.J.M., Haan, J. and Roos, R.A.C. (1997). Association of vascular amyloid β and cells of the mononuclear phagocyte system in hereditary cerebral hemorrhage with amyloidosis (Dutch) and Alzheimer disease. *J. Neuropathol. Exp. Neurol.* **56**, 273–284.

MacPherson, G.G., Fossum, S. and Harrison, B. (1989). Properties of lymph borne (veiled) dendritic cells in culture—II. Expression of IL-2 receptor: role of GM-CSF. *Immunology.* **68**, 108–113.

Mander, T.H. and Morris, J.F. (1995). Immunophenotypic evidence for distinct populations of microglia in the rat hypothalamo-neurohypophysial system. *Cell Tissue Res.* **280**, 665–673.

Matsumoto, Y., Hara, N., Tanaka, R. and Fujiwara, M. (1986). Immunohistochemical analysis of the rat central nervous system during experimental allergic encephalomyelitis, with special reference to Ia-positive cells with dendritic morphology. *J. Immunol.* **136**, 3668–3676.

Matsumoto, Y., Hanawa, H., Tsuchida, M. and Abo, T. (1993). In situ inactivation of infiltrating T cells in the central nervous system with autoimmune encephalomyelitis. The role of astrocytes. *Immunology* **79**, 381–390.

Mattiace, L.A., Davies, P. and Dickson, D.W. (1990). Detection of HLA-DR on microglia in the human brain is a function of both clinical and technical factors. *Am. J. Pathol.* **136**, 1101–1114.

Matyszak, M.K. and Perry, V.H. (1996a). The potential role of dendritic cells in immune-mediated inflammatory diseases in the central nervous system. *Neuroscience* **74**, 599–608.

Matyszak, M.K. and Perry, V.H. (1996b). A comparison of leucocyte responses to heat-killed bacillus Calmette-Guerin in different CNS compartments. *Neuropathol. Appl. Neurobiol.* **22**, 44–53.

Matyszak, M.K., Lawson, J.L., Perry, V.H. and Gordon, S. (1992). Stromal macrophages of the choroid plexus situated at an interface between the brain and peripheral immune system constitutively express MHC class II antigens. *J. Neuroimmunol.* **40**, 173–182.

Maxwell, W.L. and McGadey, J. (1988). Response of intraventricular macrophages after a penetrant cerebral lesion. *J. Anat.* **160**, 145–155.

Mayrhofer, G., Pugh, C.W. and Barclay, A.N. (1983). The distribution, ontogeny and origin in the rat of Ia-positive cells with dendritic morphology and of Ia antigen in epithelia, with special reference to the intestine. *Eur. J. Immunol.* **13**, 112–122.

Medawar, P. (1948). Immunity to homologous grafted skin. III. The fate of skin homografts transplanted to the brain, to subcutaneous tissue, and to the anterior chamber of the eye. *Br. J. Exp. Pathol.* **29**, 58–69.

Mesri, M., Liversidge, J. and Forrester, J.V. (1994). ICAM-1/LFA-1 interactions in T-lymphocyte activation and adhesion to cells of the blood retina barrier in the rat. *Immunology* **83**, 52–57.

McCombe, P.A., de Jersey, J. and Pender, M.P. (1994). Inflammatory cells, microglia and MHC class II antigen-positive cells in the spinal cord of Lewis rats with acute and chronic relapsing experimental autoimmune encephalomyelitis. *J. Neuroimmunol.* **51**, 153–167.

McMenamin, P.G. (1994). Immunocompetent cells in the anterior segment. *Prog. Ret. Eye Res.* **13**, 555–589.

McMenamin, P.G. (1997). The distribution of immune cells in the uveal tract of the normal eye. *Eye* **11**, 183–193.

McMenamin, P.G. and Crewe, J. (1995). Endotoxin-induced uveitis: kinetics and phenotype of the inflammatory cell infiltrate and the response of the resident tissue macrophages and dendritic cells in the iris and ciliary body. *Invest. Ophthalmol. Vis. Sci.* **36**, 1949–1959.

McMenamin, P.G. and Crewe, J. (1997). The cellular localisation of nitric oxide synthase in the iris and ciliary body in the course of endotoxin-induced uveitis. *Exp. Eye Res.* **65**, 157–164.

McMenamin, P.G. and Holthouse, I. (1992). Immunohistochemical characterisation of dendritic cells and macrophages in the aqueous outflow pathways of the rat eye. *Exp. Eye Res.* **55**, 315–324.

McMenamin, P.G. and Loffler, K. (1990). Cells resembling intraventricular macrophages are present in the subretinal space of human foetal eyes. *Anat. Rec.* **227**, 245–253.

McMenamin, P.G. Forrester, J.V. Steptoe, R.J. and Dua, H.S. (1992a). Ultrastructural pathology of experimental autoimmune uveitis. Quantitative evidence of activation and possible high endothelial venule-like changes in retinal vascular endothelium. *Lab. Invest.* **67**, 42–55.

McMenamin, P.G, Holthouse, I. and Holt, P.G. (1992b). Class II MHC (Ia) antigen-bearing dendritic cells within the iris and ciliary body of the rat eye: distribution, phenotype, and relation to retinal microglia. *Immunology* **77**, 385–393.

McMenamin, P.G., Broekhuyse, R.M. and Forrester, J.V. (1993). Ultrastructural pathology of experimental autoimmune uveitis: a review. *Micron* **24**, 521–546.

McMenamin, P.G., Crewe, J.M., Morrison, S. and Holt, P.G. (1994). Immunomorphologic studies of macrophages and MHC class II-positive dendritic cells in the iris and ciliary body of the rat, mouse and human eye. *Invest. Ophthalmol. Vis. Sci.* **35**, 3234–3250.

Milligan, C.E., Cunningham, T.J. and Levitt, P. (1991). Differential immunochemical markers reveal the normal distribution of brain macrophages and microglia in the developing rat brain. *J. Comp. Neurol.* **314**, 125–135.

Miyagishi, R., Kikuchi, S., Takayama, C., Inoue, Y. and Tashiro, K. (1997). Identification of cell types producing RANTES, MIP-1 alpha and MIP-1 beta in rat experimental autoimmune encephalomyelitis by in situ hybridization. *J. Neuroimmunol.* **77**, 17–26.

Nakajima, K. and Kohsaka, S. (1993). Functional roles of microglia in the brain. *Neurosci. Res.* **17**, 187–203.

Navratil, E., Ouvelard, A., Rey, A. Henin, D. and Scoazec, J.Y. (1997). Expression of cell adhesion molecules by microvascular endothelial cells in the cortical and subcortical regions of the normal human brain: an immunohistochemical analysis. *Neuropathol. Appl. Neurobiol.* **23**, 68–80.

Nelson, D.J., McMenamin, C., McWilliam, A.S., Brenan, M. and Holt, P.G. (1994). Development of the airway intraepithelial dendritic cell network in the rat from class II major histocompatibility (Ia)-negative precursors—differential regulation of Ia expression at different levels of the respiratory tract. *J. Exp. Med.* **179**, 203–212.

Nguyen, K.B., McCombe, P.A. and Pender, M.P. (1997). Increased apoptosis of T lymphocytes and macrophages in the central and peripheral nervous systems fo Lewis rats with experimental autoimmune encephalomyelitis treated with dexamethasone. *J. Neuropathol. Exp. Neurol.* **56**, 58–69.

Nussenblatt, R.B. (1991). Experimental autoimmune uveitis: mechanisms of disease and clinical therapeutic indications. *Invest. Ophthalmol. Vis. Sci.* **32**, 3131–3141.

Oechmichen, M. (1982). Are resting and/or reactive microglia macrophages? *Immunobiology* **161**, 246–254.

Ogura, K., Ogawa, M. and Yoshida, M. (1994). Effects of ageing on microglia in the normal rat brain: immunohistochemical observations. *NeuroReport* **5**, 1224–1226.

Ohmori, K., Hong, Y., Fujiwara, M. and Matsumoto, Y. (1992). In situ demonstration of proliferating cells in the rat central nervous system during experimental autoimmune encephalomyelitis. Evidence suggesting that most infiltrating T cells do not proliferate in the target organ. *Lab. Invest.* **66**, 54–62.

Otani, H. and Tanaka, O. (1988). Development of the choroid plexus anlage and supraependymal structures in the fourth ventricular roof plate of human embryos: scanning electron microscopic observations. *Am. J. Anat.* **181**, 53–66.

Pavli, P., Woodhams, C.E., Doe, W.F. and Hume, D.A. (1990). Isolation and characterization of antigen-presenting dendritic cells from the mouse intestinal lamina propria. *Immunology* **70**, 40–47.

Penfold, P.L., Provis, J.M. and Liew, S.C.K. (1993). Human retinal microglia express phenotypic characteristics in common with dendritic antigen-presenting cells. *J. Neuroimmunol.* **45**, 183–192.

Perry, V.H. (1994). *Macrophages and the Nervous System.* Molecular Biology Intelligence Unit publication. R.G. Landes, Austin, TX, ch. 3, pp. 28–42.

Perry, V.H. and Gordon, S. (1987). Modulation of CD4 antigen on macrophages and microglia in rat brain. *J. Exp. Med.* **16**, 1138–1143.

Perry, V.H. and Gordon, S. (1988). Macrophages and microglia in the nervous system. *TINS* **11**, 273–277.

Perry, V.H., Hume, D.A. and Gordon, S. (1985). Immunohistochemical localisation of macrophages and microglia in the adult and developing mouse brain. *Neuroscience* **15**, 313–326.

Perry, V.H., Andersson, P.-B. and Gordon, S. (1993). Macrophages and inflammation in the central nervous system. *TINS,* **16**, (7).

Peters, A. (1974). The surface fine structure of the choroid plexus and ependymal lining of rat lateral ventricle. *J. Neurocytol.* **3**, 99–108.

Polman, C.H., Dijkstra, C.D., Sminia, T. and Koetsier, J.C. (1986). Immunohistological analysis of macrophages in the central nervous system of Lewis rats with acute experimental allergic encephalomyelitis. *J. Neuroimmunol.* **11**, 215–222.

Provis, J.M., Penfold, P.L., Edwards, A.J. and van Driel, D. (1995). Retinal microglia: expression of immune markers and relationship to the *glia limitans. Glia* **14**, 243–256.

Pugh, C.W., MacPherson, G.G. and Steer, H.W. (1983). Characterisation of nonlymphoid cells derived from rat peripheral lymph. *J. Exp Med.* **157**, 1758–1779.

Rao, K. and Lund, R.D. (1993). Optic nerve degeneration induces the expression of MHC antigens in the rat visual system. *J. Comp. Neurol.* **336**, 613–627.

Rao, N.A., Atalla, L., Linker-Israeli, M., Chen, F.Y., George, F.W. 4th, Martin, W.J. and Steinman, L. (1989). Suppression of experimental uveitis in rats by anti-I-A antibodies. *Invest. Ophthalmol. Vis. Sci.* **30**, 2348–2355.

Reder, A.T., Thapar, M., Sapugay, A.M. and Jensen, M.A. (1995). Prostaglandins and inhibitors of arachidonate metabolism suppress experimental allergic encephalomyelitis. *J. Neuroimmunol.* **54**, 117–127.

Rinner, W.A., Bauer, J., Schmidts, M., Lassmann, H. and Hickey, W.F. (1995). Resident microglia and hematogenous macrophages as phagocytes in adoptively transferred experimental autoimmune encephalomyelitis: an investigation using rat radiation bone marrow chimeras. *Glia* **14**, 257–266.

Rowland, L.P. (1985). Blood–brain barrier, cerebrospinal fluid, brain edema, and hydrocephalus. In *Principles of Neuroscience* (eds Kandel, E.R. and Schwartz, J.H). Elsevier, Amsterdam, pp. 837–844.

Romani, N., Schuler, G. and Fritsch, P. (1986). Ontogeny of Ia-positive and Thy-1-positive leukocytes of murine epidermis. *J. Invest. Dermatol.* **86**, 129–133.

Ruedl, C. and Hubele, S. (1997). Maturation of Peyer's patch dendritic cells in vitro upon stimulation via cytokines or CD40 triggering. *Eur. J. Immunol.* **27**, 1325–1330.

Sanyal, S. and DeRuiter, A. (1985). Inosinediphosphatase as a histochemical marker of retinal microvasculature, with special reference to transformation of microglia. *Cell Tissue Res* **241**, 291.

Schon-Hegrad, M.A., Oliver, J., McMenamin, P.G. and Holt, P.G. (1991). Studies on the density, distribution and surface phenotype of intraepithelial class II MHC (Ia)-bearing dendritic cells (DC) in the conducting airways. *J. Exp. Med.* **173**, 1345–1356.

Sedgwick, J.D. (1995). Immune surveillance and autoantigen recognition in the central nervous system. *Aust. NZ J. Med.* **25**, 784–792.

Sedgwick, J.D. (1997). T-Lymphocyte activation and regulation in the central nervous system. *Biochem. Soc. Trans.* **75**, 673–679.

Sedgwick, J.D. and Hickey, W.F. (1997). Antigen presentation in the central nervous system. In *Immunology of the Nervous System* (eds Keane, R.W. and Hickey W.F.). Oxford University Press, Oxford, pp. 364-418.

Sedgwick, J.D., Schwender, S., Gregersen, R., Dorries, R. and ter Meulen, V. (1993). Resident macrophages (ramified microglia) of the adult Brown Norway rat central nervous system are constitutively major histocompatibility complex class II positive. *J. Exp. Med.* **177**, 1145–1152.

Serot, J.M., Foliguet, B., Bene, M.C. and Faure G.C. (1997). Ultrastructural and immmunohistochemical evidence for dendritic-like cells within the human choroid plexus epithelium. *NeuroReport* **8**, 1995–1998.

Sherman, S.H., Green, K. and Laties, A.M. (1978). The fate of anterior chamber fluorescein in the monkey eye. 1. The anterior chamber outflow pathways. *Exp. Eye Res.* **27**, 159–173.

Singh, A.K., Kumar, G. Shinohara, T. and Shichi, H. (1996). Porcine S-antigen: cDNA sequence and expression in retina, ciliary epithelium and iris. *Exp. Eye Res.* **62**, 299–308.

Singh, C., Singh, J. and Ling, E.A. (1993). Immunohistochemical and lectin-labelling studies of the distribution and development of microglia in the spinal cord of postnatal rats. *Arch. Histol. Cytol.* **56**, 475–484.

Sminia, T., deGroot, C.J.A., Dijkstra, C.D., Koetsier, J.C. and Polman, C.H. (1987) Macrophages in the central nervous system of the rat. *Immunobiology* **174**, 43–50.

Steinman, R.M. (1991). The dendritic cell system and its role in immunogenicity. *Annu. Rev. Immunol.* **9**, 271–296.

Steptoe, R.J. and Thomson, A.W. (1996). Dendritic cells and tolerance induction. *Clin. Exp. Immunol.* **105**, 397–402.

Steptoe, R.J., Holt, P.G. and McMenamin, P.G. (1995). Functional studies of major histocompatability class II-positive dendritic cells and resident tissue macrophages isolated from the rat iris. *Immunology* **85**, 630–637.

Steptoe, R.J., Holt, P.G. and McMenamin, P.G. (1996). Origin and steady-state turnover of major histocompatibility complex class II-positive dendritic cells and resident-tissue macrophages in the iris of the rat eye. *J. Neuroimmunol.* **68**, 67–76.

Steptoe, R.J., Holt, P.G. and McMenamin, P.G. (1997). Major histocompatability complex class II-positive dendritic cells in the iris of the rat eye: in situ development from major histocompatability complex class II-negative precursors. *Invest. Ophthalmol. Vis. Sci.* **38**, 2639–2648.

Streilein, J.W. (1993). Immune privilege as the result of local tissue barriers and immunosuppressive microenvironments. *Curr. Opinion. Immunol.* **5**, 428–432.

Streilein, J.W. and Niederkorn, J.Y. (1981). Induction of anterior chamber associated immune deviation requires an intact, functional spleen. *J. Exp. Med.* **153**, 1058–1067.

Thanos, S. (1991). The relationship of microglial cells to dying neurons during natural neuronal cell death and axotomy-induced degeneration of the rat retina. *Eur. J. Neurosci.* **3**, 1189–1207.

Thanos, S. (1992). Sick photoreceptors attract activated microglia from the ganglion cell layer: a model to study the inflammatory cascades in rats with inherited retinal dystrophy. *Brain Res.* **588**, 21–28.

Thanos, S., Moore, S. and Hong, Y. (1996). Retinal microglia. *Prog Ret and Eye Res.* **15**, 331–361.

Thepen, T., McMenamin, C., Oliver, J., Kraal, G. and Holt, P.G. (1991). Regulation of immune responses to inhaled antigen by alveolar macrophages: differential effects of in vivo alveolar macrophage elimination on the induction of tolerance vs. immunity. *Eur. J. Immunol.* **21**, 2845–2850.

Thomas, W.E. (1992). Brain macrophages: evaluation of microglia and their functions. *Brain Res. Rev.* **17**, 61–74.

Torroba, M., Chiba, A., Vicente, A., Varas, A., Sacedon, R., Jimenez, E., Honma, Y. and Zapata, A.G. (1995). Macrophage-lymphocyte cell clusters in the hypothalamic ventricle of some elasmobranch fish: ultrastructural analysis and possible functional significance. *Anat. Rec.* **242**, 400–410.

Tripathi, R.C. (1977). The functional morphology of the outflow systems of ocular and cerebrospinal fluids. In *The Ocular and Cerebrospinal Fluids* (eds L.Z. Bito, H. Davson and J.D. Fenstermacher), pp. 65–116. London, Academic Press.

Tseng, C.Y., Ling, E.A. Wong, W.C. (1983). Light and electron microscopic and cytochemical identification of amoeboid microglial cells in the brain of prenatal rats. *J. Anat.* **136**, 837–849.

Ulvestad, E., Williams, K., Mork. S., Antel, J. and Nyland, H. (1994a). Phenotypic differences between human monocytes/macrophages and microglial cells studied *in situ* and *in vitro. J. Neuropathol. Exp. Neurol.* **53**, 492–501.

Ulvestad, E., Williams, K., Bø, L., Trapp, B., Antel, J. and Mork, S. (1994b). HLA class II molecules (HLA-DR, -DP, -DQ) on cells in the human CNS studied in situ and in vitro. *Immunology* **82**, 535–541.

Ulvestad, E., Williams, K., Bjerkvig, R., Tiekotter, K., Antel, J. and Matre, R. (1994c). Human microglial cells have phenotypic and functional characteristics in common with both macrophages and dendritic antigen-presenting cells. *J. Leuk. Biol.* **56**, 732–740.

van Dam, A-M. Bauer, J.,Tilders, F.J.H. and Berkenbosch, F. (1995). Endotoxin-induced appearance of immunoreactive interleukin-1β in ramified microglia in rat brain: alight and electron microscopic study. *Neuroscience* **65**, 815–826.

van Rees, E.P., Dijkstra, C.D., van der Ende, M.B., Janse, E.M. and Sminia, T. (1988). The ontogenic development of macrophage subpopulations and Ia-positive non-lymphoid cells in gut-associated lymphoid tissues of the rat. *Immunology* **63**, 79–85.

Vremec, D., Lieschko, G.J., Dunn, A.R., Robb, L., Metcalf, D. and Shortman, K. 1997. The influence of granulocyte-macrophage colony stimulating factor on dendritic cell levels in mouse lymphoid organs. *Eur. J. Immunol.* **27**, 40–44.

Warren, K.G., Catz, I. and McPherson, T.A. (1983). CSF myelin basic protein levels in acute optic neuritis and multiple sclerosis. *Can. J. Neurol. Sci.* **10**, 235–238.

Weed, L.H. (1914). The pathways of escape from the subarachnoid spaces with particular reference to the arachnoid villi. *J. Med. Res.* **31**(NS vol. 26), p. 51.

Wekerle, H., Linington, C., Lassman, H. and Meyermann, R. (1986). Cellular immune reactivity within the CNS. *Trends Neurosci.* **9**, 271–277.

Weller, R.O., Kida, S. and Zhang, E.T. (1992) Pathways of fluid drainage from the brain—morphological aspects and immunological significance in rats and man. *Brain Pathol.* **2**, 277–284.

Wilbanks, G.A., Mammolenti, M. and Streilein, J.W. (1991). Studies on the induction of anterior chamber-associated immune deviation (ACAID). II. Eye-derived cells participate in generating blood-borne signals that induce ACAID. *J. Immunol.* **146**, 3018–3024.

Wilders, M.M., Sminia, T. and Janse, E.M. (1983). Ontogeny of non-lymphoid and lymphoid cells in the rat gut with special reference to large mononuclear Ia-positive dendritic cells. *Immunology* **50**, 303–314.

Williams, K., Ulvestad, E. and Antel, J.P. (1994). B7/BB-1 antigen expression on adult human microglia studied in vitro and in situ. *Eur. J. Immunol.* **24**, 3031–3037.

Xu, J. and Ling, E.A. (1994). Upregulation and induction of major histocompatibility complex class I and II antigens on microglial cells in early postnatal rat brain following intraperitoneal injections of recombinant interferon-gamma. *Neuroscience* **60**, 959–967.

Yao, J., Harvath, L., Gilbert, D.L. and Colton, C.A. (1990). Chemotaxis by a CNS macrophage, the microglia. *J. Neurosci. Res.* **27**, 36–42.

Yoshida, M., Yoshimura, N., Hangai, M., Tanihara, H. and Honda, Y. (1994). Interleukin-1α, interleukin-1β, and tumor necrosis factor gene expression in endotoxin-induced uveitis. *Invest. Ophthalmol. Vis. Sci.* **35**, 1107–1113.

Zhang, J., Wu, G., Ishimoto, S., Pararajasegaram, G. and Rao, N.A. (1997). Expression of major histocompatibility complex molecules in rodent retina. *Invest Ophthalmol. Visual Sci.* **38**, 1848.

Zaal, J., Doekes, G., Breebaart, A.C. and Kijlstra, A. (1986). Quantitative determination of S-antigen in human ocular tissues, aqueous humour and serum. *Curr. Eye Res.* **5**, 763–775.

III DENDRITIC CELLS AND INTERACTION WITH OTHER CELLS

CHAPTER 13
The Role of Dendritic Cells in T Cell Priming: The Importance of Being Professional

Antonella Viola, Giandomenica Iezzi and Antonio Lanzavecchia
Basel Institute for Immunology, Basel, Switzerland

DIFFERENTIAL REQUIREMENTS FOR ACTIVATION OF NAIVE AND EFFECTOR T CELLS

Priming of naive T cells and activation of effector/memory T cells occur in different anatomical sites and involve different antigen-presenting cells (APC) (Sprent, 1997; Steinman, 1991; Zinkernagel *et al.*, 1996). On the one hand, naive T cells have been shown to have rather fastidious requirements for priming since they can be activated only by professional APC such as DC, which present high levels of antigen and express high levels of costimulatory molecules. On the other hand, effector T cells are known to be triggered easily since low doses of antigen displayed by any APC (including nonprofessional ones) are sufficient to trigger their effector function.

The existence of different thresholds for priming and effector function is a fundamental property of the immune system since it allows a tight control on the generation of T cell responses. A striking example is provided by cytotoxic T lymphocytes (CTL). Indeed, priming of naive CD8 T cells requires high doses of antigen, professional APC and, in some cases, even T cell help (De Bruijn *et al.*, 1992; Keene and Forman, 1982). In contrast, lysis of target cells by effector CTL can be triggered by recognition of a single peptide–MHC class I complex on essentially any target cell (Sykulev *et al.*, 1996).

We will review recent data that identify the distinct requirements for activation of naive and effector T cell responses and discuss them in the context of antigen presentation by professional and nonprofessional APC.

FROM SERIAL TCR TRIGGERING TO T CELL ACTIVATION

Recent evidence from our laboratory indicates that in living cells the interaction between T cell receptors (TCRs) and specific peptide–MHC complexes is a very dynamic process. T cells conjugated with antigen-pulsed APC undergo a sustained

Dendritic Cells: Biology and Clinical Applications
ISBN 0-12-455860-7

signalling that can be measured by increases in $[Ca^{2+}]_i$ or tyrosine phosphorylation of various molecules. We found that this signal, which otherwise lasts for several hours, can be terminated within 1–2 min by dissociating T cells from the APC, by adding antibodies that mask the MHC molecules recognized by the TCR, or by blocking the T cells' actin cytoskeleton (Valitutti *et al.*, 1995a). These results clearly rule out the possibility that signalling is sustained by the formation of a stable signaling complex and indicate that sustained signalling requires a continuous engagement of TCRs by peptide–MHC.

The observation that triggered TCRs undergo a time-dependent and antigen dose-dependent downregulation provided a means to measure the number of receptors triggered (Valitutti *et al.*, 1995b). In this way it was estimated that ~100 peptide–MHC complexes on an APC trigger and downregulate as many as 20 000 TCRs in a few hours. The striking difference between the number of ligands and receptors engaged provided the basis for the TCR serial triggering model (Valitutti and Lanzavecchia, 1997) that is illustrated in Plate 13.1.

TCR serial triggering is dependent on an optimal kinetics of TCR–ligand interaction. This kinetics must allow efficient triggering of the engaged TCRs as well as dissociation of the ligand once the TCR has been triggered in order to allow new engagements. Indeed strong agonists are characterized by rather fast kinetics with off rates of approximately 10 s (Lyons *et al.*, 1996; Matsui *et al*, 1994; Weber *et al.*, 1992). This optimal kinetics allows frequent engagement and triggering of TCRs, resulting in the delivery of a strong signal by few agonistic complexes. Deviation from this optimal kinetics results in all cases in a weaker agonist. On the one hand, altered peptide ligands with faster off rates trigger fewer TCRs (although probably engaging more) and are strictly dependent on the stabilizing effect of CD4 or CD8 coreceptors (Viola *et al.*, 1997). On the other hand, antibodies to the TCR/CD3 complex which are characterized by very slow off rates are inefficient because each antibody can trigger no more than one TCR (Viola and Lanzavecchia, 1996).

The above findings, indicating that a large number of TCRs are triggered over an extended period of time, raise the question of how T cells sense and respond to these signals. We have shown that T cells appear to 'count' the number of triggered TCRs since they respond only above an activation threshold (Viola and Lanzavecchia, 1996). This threshold is tunable by costimulation and consequently differs according to the nature of the APC. When APC express high levels of costimulatory molecules, the threshold is rather low (1000 TCR or less). In contrast, when the APC lack costimulatory molecules, the threshold is much higher (8000 or more depending on the APC). Such high levels of TCR triggering require extremely high doses of antigen and are therefore unlikely to be reached under physiological conditions. The tunable threshold explains the fact that presentation of antigen by nonprofessional APC does not result in T cell activation but only in sterile TCR triggering and downregulation (Cai *et al.*, 1997; Iezzi *et al.*, 1998).

Different thresholds of TCR engagement elicit different responses. For instance proliferation and cytokine production require higher levels of TCR occupancy than cytotoxicity, which has a much lower threshold (Valitutti *et al.*, 1996). This explains how CTL can kill any cell displaying minute amounts of antigen even in the absence of costimulation.

COMMITMENT OR DEATH: WHEN TIME MAKES THE DIFFERENCE

What is the significance of the tunable threshold? Do T cells really 'count' the number of triggered TCRs or does this number rather reflect a cumulative amount of signal delivered to the cell? Recent experiments indicate that a critical parameter that determines T cell response is the duration of stimulation. We found that while effector T cells are activated within 1 h of exposure to the antigen, naive T cells require a continuous stimulation for at least 12 h in the presence and even longer times (up to 30 h) in the absence of costimulation (Iezzi *et al.*, 1998). These results make sense if we consider that naive T cells are very small with a compact nucleus and, therefore, before being able to divide they first have to blast, a process that requires energy as well as time. This may explain both the long duration of signalling and the requirement for costimulation for priming of naive T cells. Indeed, the role of costimulation via CD28 may be to enhance the amount of second messengers produced by triggered TCRs or to activate parallel synergizing signal transduction pathways (Lenschow *et al.*, 1996), allowing a more rapid and effective stimulation of the cell and resulting in a more rapid commitment.

Interestingly, the long duration of signalling, essential for the activation of naive T cells, is detrimental for effector T cells (Iezzi *et al.*, 1998). In fact, effector cells, under conditions of prolonged TCR stimulation, undergo activation-induced cell death (AICD). This AICD is most prominent in the absence of costimulation, indicating that costimulation has a protective effect on T cell survival, most likely due to the upregulation of anti-apoptotic mechanisms (Boise *et al.*, 1995).

THE ROLE OF PROFESSIONAL APC IN THE IMMUNE RESPONSE

The differential requirements for activation of naive and effector T cells explain the different roles played by professional and nonprofessional APC in the course of the immune response (see Fig. 2). The long time of commitment of naive T cells determines the requirement for APC that are highly adhesive and costimulatory. On the one hand, adhesion molecules allow formation of stable APC–T cell conjugates that are essential to deliver the sustained TCR triggering. On the other hand, costimulation, by lowering the time required for commitment, increases the possibility that this time threshold is reached. Consequently, mature DC that express high levels of adhesion and costimulatory molecules can form stable clusters (Austyn *et al.*, 1988) and efficiently trigger T cells for enough time to reach commitment. In contrast, nonprofessional APC have low levels of adhesion molecules and therefore engage naive T cells only transiently. In addition, they lack costimulation, which further increases the requirement for longer contact times. Therefore, it is unlikely that commitment is reached when antigen is presented by nonprofessional APC.

Conversely, the short time of commitment of effector T cells decreases the need for adhesion and costimulation, allowing a productive interaction with nonprofessional APC as well. In this case a prolonged stimulation, especially if in the absence of costimulatory signals, may result in AICD (Critchfield *et al.*, 1994), thus explaining the rapid exhaustion of effector cells by massive antigenic stimulation *in vivo* (Moskophidis *et al.*, 1993).

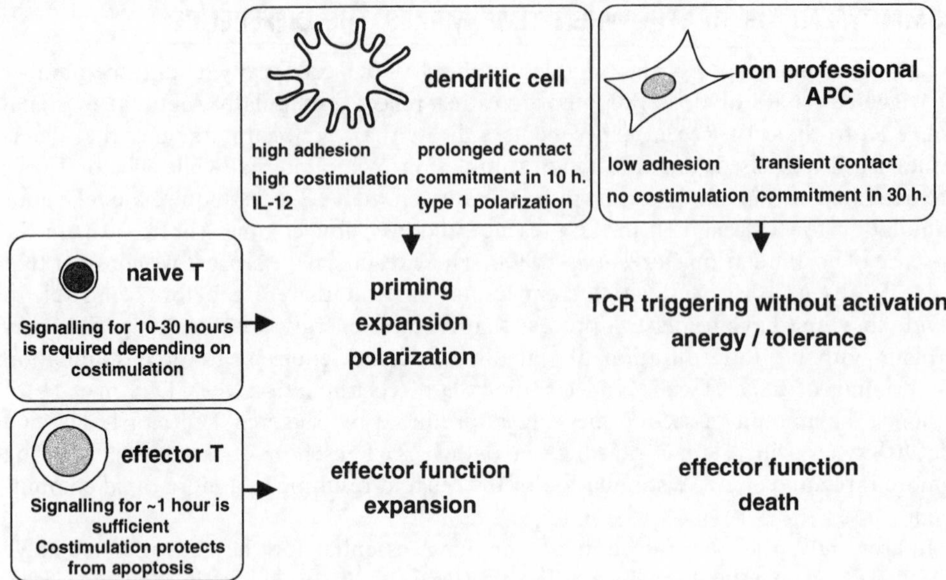

Fig. 2. T cell fate is determined by the type of APC. Naive T cells have strict requirements for activation. They need signalling sustained for at least 10 h in the presence of costimulation and of up to 30 h in its absence. These needs are met only by DC which express high levels of adhesion and costimulatory molecules. In contrast, nonprofessional APC can only interact transiently with naive T cells. They trigger and downregulate TCRs but fail to induce T cell activation. In addition to the requirements for a full T cell activation, DC can also deliver signals essential for T cell polarization to type 1 or type 2 effector cells. Effector cells have a shorter time of commitment and can be consequently activated by nonprofessional APCs to deliver their effector function. It is possible, however, that continuous stimulation by nonprofessional APC may lead to activation-induced cell death because the effector cells are not protected by stimulation of CD2B.

ACKNOWLEDGMENTS

We thank Klaus Karjalainen and Marco Colonna for critical reading and comments. The Basel Institute for Immunology was founded and is supported by F. Hoffmann La Roche Ltd, Basel, Switzerland.

REFERENCES

Austyn, J.M., Weinstein, D.E. and Steinman, R.M. (1988). Clustering with dendritic cells precedes and is essential for T-cell proliferation in a mitogenesis model. *Immunology* **63**, 691–696.

Boise, L.H., Minn, A.J., Noel, P.J., June, C.H., Accavitti, M.A., Lindsten, T. and Thompson, C.B. (1995). CD2B costimulation can promote T cell survival by enhancing the expression of Bcl-XL. *Immunity* **3**, 87–98.

Cai, Z., Kishimoto, H., Brunmark, A., Jackson, M.R., Peterson, P.A., and Sprent, J. (1997). Requirements for peptide-induced T cell receptor downregulation on naive CD8$^+$ T cells. *J. Exp. Med.* **185**, 641–651.

Critchfield, J.M., Racke, M.K., Zuniga-Pflucker, J.C., Cannella, B., Raine, C.S., Goverman, J. and Lenardo, M.J. (1994). T cell deletion in high antigen dose therapy of autoimmune encephalomyelitis. *Science* **263**, 1139–1143.

De Bruijn. M.L., Nieland, J.D., Schumacher, T.N., Ploegh, H.L., Kast, W.M. and Melief, C.J. (1992). Mechanisms of induction of primary virus-specific cytotoxic T lymphocyte responses. *Eur. J. Immunol.* **22**, 3013–3020.

Iezzi, G., Karjalainen, K. and Lanzavecchia, A. (1998). The duration of antigenic stimulation determines the fate of naive and effector T cells. *Immunity* **8**, 89–95.

Keene, J.A. and Forman, J. (1982). Helper activity is required for the *in vivo* generation of cytotoxic T lymphocytes. *J. Exp. Med.* **155**, 768–782.

Lenschow, D.J., Walunas, T.L. and Bluestone, J.A. (1996). CD2B/B7 system of T cell costimulation. *Annu. Rev. Immunol.* **14**, 233–258.

Lyons, D.S., Lieberman, S.A., Hampl, J., Boniface, J.J., Chien, Y., Berg, L.J. and Davis, M.M. (1996). A TCR binds to antagonist ligands with lower affinities and faster dissociation rates than to agonists. *Immunity* **5**, 53–61.

Matsui, K., Boniface, J.J., Steffner, P., Reay, P.A. and Davis, M.M. (1994). Kinetics of T-cell receptor binding to peptide/I-Ek complexes: correlation of the dissociation rate with T-cell responsiveness. *Proc. Natl Acad. Sci. USA* **91**, 12862–12866.

Moskophidis, D., Lechner, F., Pircher, H. and Zinkernagel, R.M. (1993). Virus persistence in acutely infected immunocompetent mice by exhaustion of antiviral cytotoxic effector T cells. *Nature* **362**, 758–761.

Sprent, J. (1997). Immunological memory. *Curr. Opin. Immunol.* **9**, 371–379.

Steinman, R.M. (1991). The dendritic cell system and its role in immunogenicity. *Annu. Rev. Immunol.* **9**, 271–296.

Sykulev, Y., Joo, M., Vturina, I., Tsomides, T.J. and Eisen, H.N. (1996). Evidence that a single peptide-MHC complex on a target U cell can elicit a cytolytic T cell response. *Immunity* **4**, 565–571.

Valitutti, S. and Lanzavecchia, A. (1977). Serial triggering of T-cell receptors: a basis for the sensitivity and specificity of T cell antigen recognition. *Immunol. Today* **18**, 299–304.

Valitutti, S., Dessing, M., Aktories, K., Gallati, H. and Lanzavecchia, A. (1995a). Sustained signaling leading to T cell activation results from prolonged T cell receptor occupancy. Role of T cell actin cytoskeleton. *J. Exp. Med.* **181**, 577–584.

Valitutti, S., Muller, S., Cella, M., Padovan, E. and Lanzavecchia, A. (1995b). Serial triggering of many T-cell receptors by a few peptide–MHC complexes. *Nature* **375**, 148–151.

Valitutti, S., Muller, S., Dessing, M. and Lanzavecchia, A. (1996). Different responses are elicited in cytotoxic T lymphocytes by different levels of T cell receptor occupancy. *J. Exp. Med.* **183**, 1917–1921.

Viola, A. and Lanzavecchia, A. (1996). T cell activation determined by T cell receptor number and tunable thresholds. *Science* **273**, 104–106.

Viola, A., Salio, M., Tuosto, L., Linkert, S., Acuto, A. and Lanzavecchia, A. (1997). Quantitative contribution of CD4 and CD8 to T cell antigen receptor serial triggering. *J. Exp. Med.* **186**, 1775–1779.

Weber, S., Traunecker, A., Oliveri, F., Gerhard, W. and Karjalainen, K. (1992). Specific low-affinity recognition of major histocompatibility complex plus peptide by soluble T-cell receptor. *Nature* **793**, 793–796.

Zinkernagel, R.M., Bachmann, M.F., Kundig, T.M., Oehen, S., Pirchet, H. and Hengartner, H. (1996). On immunological memory. *Annu. Rev. Immunol.* **14**, 333-367.

CHAPTER 14
NK Cells

Benedict J. Chambers and Hans-Gustaf Ljunggren
Microbiology and Tumor Biology Center, Karolinska Institute, Stockholm, Sweden

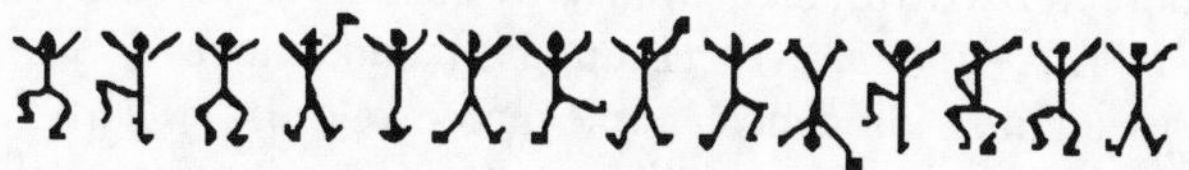

Sir Arthur Conan Doyle, from *The Adventure of the Dancing Men*

INTRODUCTION

In recent years, there has been an increased interest in dendritic cells (DC) as well as in natural killer (NK) cells. While DC have been appreciated for their role in T cell priming as well as for their ability to modulate B cell growth and differentiation, NK cells have been appreciated for their function in innate immunity. In contrast to the abundant information available about DC interaction with T cells (Steinman, 1991), and more recently also with B cells (Clark, 1997), there are as yet few reports on direct interactions between NK cells and DC. Indeed, a survey of the literature on this subject as well as the reports from recent DC and NK cell meetings reveals at most a handful of reports discussing direct interactions between DC and NK cells. Nonetheless, the few reports available suggest potentially interesting interactions between these cell types. In addition, NK cells and DC have also been found to share some common features. In this review, we aim to shed some light on these topics. However, before this a brief introduction to NK cells will be given as these cells have not been described elsewhere in this volume.

NK CELLS

Phenotype

Natural killer (NK) cells derive their name from their ability to kill certain tumor cell lines without prior sensitization (Kiessling *et al.*, 1975). These cells are now known to play a more general role in the host immune response (Trinchieri, 1989). NK cells

Dendritic Cells: Biology and Clinical Applications
ISBN 0-12-455860-7

represent a third lineage of bone marrow-derived lymphocytes that are distinct from T and B lymphocytes. Phenotypically, NK cells are currently characterized as much as by what cell surface molecules they do express as by the molecules they do not express (Gumperz and Parham, 1995; Lanier and Philips, 1996; Raulet, 1996). In contrast to T and B cells, NK cells are CD3-negative and lack expression of rearranged receptor genes, such as the T cell receptor and immunoglobulins. On the other hand, they do express a number of more or less specific cell surface molecules such as CD56 in man and NK1.1 in mice. Many NK cells have the characteristics of large granular lymphocytes (LGL), though not all NK cells share this phenotype, and conversely not all LGL are NK cells.

Function

Although well-characterized for their ability to mediate cytotoxic reactions to certain tumor cell lines *in vitro* and *in vivo* (Ljunggren and Kärre, 1990), and to mediate rejection responses against allogeneic bone marrow grafts *in vivo* (Yu *et al.*, 1992), the main function of NK cells probably lies in their contribution to the innate immune defense against certain viruses, intracellular bacteria and parasites (Bancroft, 1993; Scott and Trinchieri, 1995; Biron, 1997; Scharton-Kersten and Sher, 1997). NK cells secrete certain cytokines such as IFN-γ, GM-CSF, and TNF-α, and it is by their production of such cytokines as well as their cytotoxic potential that they act in the earliest stages of pathogen invasion. Moreover, NK cells are likely to influence the subsequent adaptive immune response. Exactly how this occurs is not known. It cannot be excluded that some of these steps may involve an interaction and/or interference with professional antigen-presenting cells (APC) such as DC.

Molecular Specificity

Recently, insights into the molecular specificity of NK cells have received increased attention. It is clear that several aspects of NK cell-mediated functions, such as their ability to mediate cytotoxic reactions and their secretion of cytokines, are under control of positive as well as negative signals transmitted via specific cell surface receptors (Gumperz and Parham, 1995; Lanier and Philips, 1996; Raulet, 1996). Initially, the specificity of NK cells was termed major histocompatibility complex (MHC) non-restricted. However, it is now evident that while NK cell-mediated lysis is not MHC-restricted, it is strongly influenced by MHC class I molecules. While T cells are triggered by the expression of MHC molecules loaded with non-self-peptides (or by allogeneic MHC molecules), NK cell activation is inhibited by MHC class I molecules (Ljunggren and Kärre, 1990). This has been explained by the identification of MHC class I specific receptors on NK cells, capable of transmitting a negative signal to NK cells that will turn off triggering signals (Long *et al.*, 1997; Lanier *et al.*, 1997). Significantly less is known about these 'triggering' signals, though some of those can probably be transmitted via the CD2, CD16, CD69, or NKR-P1 receptors (Raulet, 1996; Lanier *et al.*, 1997; Leibson, 1997; Long and Wagtmann, 1997). Although many of these signals have been identified through studies using tumor targets, many NK cell-mediated responses including recognition events and activation and effector phases are likely to be highly related to similar processes in NK cell-mediated innate immunity, and the regulation of immune responses by NK cells.

SHARED PROPERTIES BETWEEN NK CELLS AND DC

Common Progenitor

Several other chapters in this volume deals with the ontogeny of DC. Therefore, we shall only mention that thymic DC have been reported to be of lymphoid origin, and may share a common precursor with T and NK cells (Ardavin *et al.*, 1993; Res *et al.*, 1996; Reid, 1997; Mebius *et al.*, 1997; Márquez *et al.*, 1998). Furthermore, a common hematopoietic precursor for DC, B, T, and NK cells has also been described in humans (Galy *et al.*, 1995).

NK-like Activity by DC

Interestingly, rat thymus and spleen cell-derived DC were recently reported to express NKR-P1 (Josien *et al.*, 1997), a disulfide-linked homodimer expressed by all NK cells and a small subset of T cells in rodents (Yokoyama and Seaman, 1993). Furthermore, highly purified spleen DC, but not thymus DC, were shown to exhibit NK cell-like cytotoxicity *in vitro*, including the ability to kill YAC-1 cells. It was speculated that the latter function of DC might precede phagocytosis in some instances and facilitate antigen presentation to T cells. This mode of killing and subsequent antigen presentation may constitute a link between innate and adaptive immunity (Janeway, 1992; Josien *et al.*, 1997; see also discussion).

DC Function of NK Cells

DC have been characterized by their ability to process and present antigen, express costimulatory molecules, and stimulate naive T cells. Interestingly, several reports exist in which NK cells have been found to possess similar properties. Although freshly isolated NK cells have been reported not to express costimulatory molecules, expression of CD80 has been reported on NK cell lines (Azuma *et al.*, 1993). There are also several reports indicating that at least a subset of human LGL cells do express MHC class II molecules (Scala *et al.*, 1985; Brooks and Moore, 1986; Roncarolo *et al.*, 1991; D'Orazio and Stein-Streilein, 1996). One report has demonstrated that the presentation of soluble antigen by MHC class II$^+$ LGL cells was equivalent to that of macrophages (Scala *et al.*, 1985). However, another report failed to confirm the latter observations (Brooks and Moore, 1986). Nonetheless, both groups reported that the MHC class II$^+$ NK cells could stimulate T cells in allogeneic mixed lymphocyte reaction (Scala *et al.*, 1985; Brooks and Moore, 1986). Similar observations have also been made using NK cell clones (Roncarolo *et al.*, 1991). Furthermore, MHC class II$^+$ NK cells can present superantigens efficiently to T cells (D'Orazio and Stein-Streilein, 1996).

Flt3 Ligand

Another potential connection between NK cells and DC comes from studies of tumor rejection responses in mice treated with the flt3 ligand (flt3L). The flt3L has been shown to stimulate the proliferation of hematopoetic stem and progenitor cells, and in particular dramatically increase the generation of functionally mature DC (Lyman, 1995; Maraskovsky *et al.*, 1996). It was recently reported that the flt3L, when administered at the time of tumor inoculation in mice, led to a substantial reduction of tumor growth (Chen *et al.*, 1997; Lynch *et al.*, 1997). While the mechanisms for flt3L-mediated antitumor immune responses are under investigation, results using MHC class I-deficient tumors suggested a 'major role of NK cells' (Fernandez *et al.*, 1997). While the role of NK cells in these models needs to be substantiated and confirmed, it is not unlikely that future studies may demonstrate a direct effect of the flt3L on NK cells, or a tentative interference between activated DC and NK cells. Indeed, support for a direct influence of the flt3L on NK cells has come from recent studies in the human, indicating that flt3L is able to enhance NK cell expansion from $CD34^+$ hematopoietic precursor cells in the presence of IL-15 (Yu *et al.*, 1997). In relation to this, it was recently also reported that flt3L-treated mice had a moderate increase in $NK1.1^+$ NK cells in the spleens (Brasel *et al.*, 1996), indicating that the flt3L may affect NK cells in the mouse.

NK CELL INTERACTION WITH DC

Cytokines

NK cells play a primary role in the innate immune system. There has been limited work examining the role of DC in innate immunity, although, like macrophages, DC can be infected by certain bacteria, parasites, and viruses (Moll *et al.*, 1995; Bhardwaj, 1997; Knight and Patterson, 1997; Svensson *et al.*, 1997). A large body of work exists that examines the interaction between microbially infected macrophages and NK cells within the innate immune system. It is reasonable to speculate that at least some of the patterns of cross-talk between macrophages and NK cells via cytokines might also be true for DC and NK cells (Gorak *et al.*, 1998).

One of the key cytokines in innate immunity is interleukin-12 (IL-12) (Trinchieri and Gerosa, 1996). Both macrophages and DC can secrete IL-12, and this cytokine can activate NK cells to kill infected cells as well as to secrete cytokines such as interferons required in the early host defense (Biron, 1997; Scharton-Kersten and Sher, 1997; Unanue, 1997; Gorak *et al.*, 1998). Furthermore, there is a feedback stimulation loop in which IL-12 stimulates IFN-γ production by NK cells that in turn stimulates further IL-12 release by the APC (Trinchieri and Gerosa, 1996). Other cytokines released by APC, such as IL-1β, TNF-α, and IL-15, have also been shown to induce NK cell activation either by increasing the production of IL-12 or by directly affecting the NK cells (Hunter *et al.*, 1995a; Hunter *et al.*, 1997). It should be noted that some of the cytokines released by APC may also serve as chemotactic agents for NK cells (Allavena *et al.*, 1994). Thus, not only will they activate NK cells but they will also direct them to the site of inflammation.

It is interesting to note that some pathogens such as *Toxoplasma gondii* are able to evade detection by immune effectors as cells infected with such pathogens have been found to secrete TGF-β (Hunter *et al.*, 1995b). Both TGF-β and IL-10 have been shown to inhibit the production of IL-12 (Tripp *et al.*, 1993) and, presumably, NK activity. Thus, viruses and pathogens that possess homologous genes for these cytokines, or are able to trigger the release of the cytokines, can evade at least early detection by the innate immune system and so increase their chances of survival. Furthermore, IL-10-deficient mice die following treatment with LPS or infection with *Toxoplasma gondii* owing to the overwhelming release of IL-12 and IFN-γ (Berg *et al.*, 1995; Gazzanelli *et al.*, 1996), suggesting that this cytokine is critical in the control of the early immune response and potentially in the downregulation of the NK cell response.

Upon activation, NK cells will also secrete GM-CSF and TNF-α (Trinchieri, 1989). These cytokines affect the differentiation and maturation of DC (Cella *et al.*, 1997). NK cells are also capable of secreting chemotactic agents that may serve to recruit lymphocytes and potentially APC to a site of infection. Thus, it appears that, at the level of cytokine release, NK cells as well as DC have the ability to secrete soluble mediators that may affect their development, maturation, recruitment and final effector phases (Fig. 1). Perturbation of these reactions by pathogens or by gene disruption or antibody depletion demonstrates the fine balance that is required to keep an immune response under control.

NK Cell Targeting of DC

Although DC and NK cells appear to synergize with each other by their respective cytokine secretions, the role of NK cells in directly controlling DC is now under investigation. The first indication that NK cells could interfere with DC function came from experiments by Rowley and colleagues. In mixed lymphocyte cultures (MLC), they were unable to stimulate CD8$^+$ T cells when splenocytes from mice treated with the IFN-γ inducer poly I:C were added to the culture (Gilbertson *et al.*, 1986). However, the normal CD8$^+$ T cell response was restored when DC, but not macrophages, were added back into the culture (Shah, 1987). These results indicated not only that IFN-γ-stimulated splenocytes somehow affected the MLC, but also that DC were critical for the development of CD8$^+$ T cells responses *in vitro*. Unfortunately, in these studies, the authors were unable to demonstrate direct killing of DC by NK cells, nor were they able to demonstrate clearly that the effector cells from the poly I:C-induced splenocytes were indeed NK cells.

More direct evidence that APC could be targeted by NK cells was observed subsequently by Djeu and colleagues in the human system. In these studies, human monocytes treated with GM-CSF could be targeted by human lymphokine-activated killer (LAK) cells (Blanchard and Djeu, 1991). Interestingly, similar cells treated with IFN-γ were not susceptible to such killing. From these studies, triggering of the LAK cells appeared to be mediated through interactions with the CD11a/CD18 complex (Blanchard *et al.*, 1990). Antibodies to CD18 could inhibit in part the lysis of the GM-CSF stimulated monocytes without affecting the ability of the LAK cells and monocytes to adhere to each other.

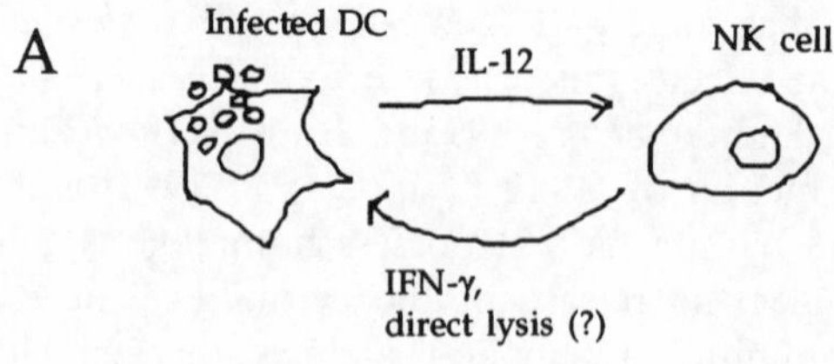

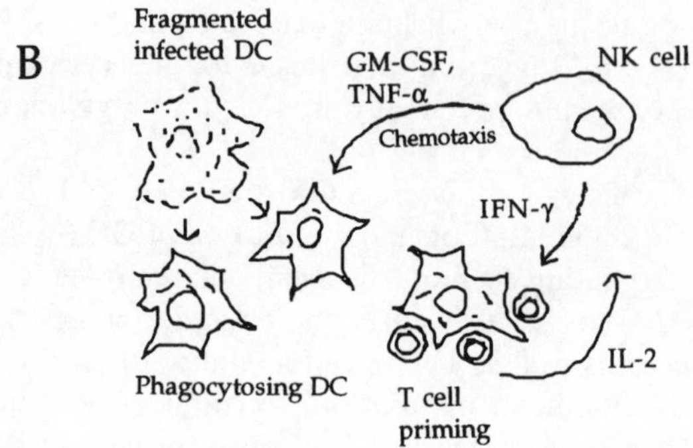

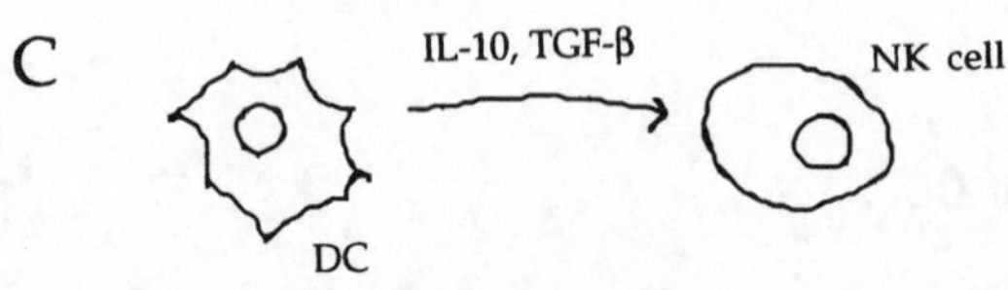

Fig. 1. Hypothetical DC/NK cell interactions *in vivo*. Infection of DC by a pathogen can induce the secretion of cytokines, such as IL-12. These cytokines can induce the activation of NK cells, which can lead to the secretion of IFN-γ, which induces more IL-12 to be released. Other cytokines released by the NK cells upon stimulation are GM-CSF and TNF-α, which may in turn stimulate more DC and act chemotactically in synergy with cytokines released by the infected DC. Cytokine activation of the NK cells may enhance the ability of the NK cell to lyse the infected DC, possibly owing to the recognition of increased levels of costimulatory and adhesion molecules expressed on the DC. Debris from the lysed cell as well as the cytokines being released might attract more DC to the inflammation area while the IFN-γ released by the NK cells can initiate T cell priming. Thus, newly arrived DC may take up the debris of the lysed DC. NK cell inhibitory cytokines such as IL-10 and TGF-β may prevent or inhibit further NK cell effector functions.

More recently, we and others have been able to demonstrate direct killing of DC by NK cells (Fig. 2). This has been possible owing to the identification of markers on both the NK cells and DC as well as improved techniques to isolate and culture DC *in vitro*. Our laboratory (Chambers *et al.*, 1996) found that mouse bone marrow-derived DC can be specifically lysed by NK1.1$^+$ cells *in vitro* (both IL-2 and IFN-γ induced) while Geldhof *et al.* (1998) have found that mouse splenic DC can also be targeted *in vitro* by both IL-2- and IL2/IL-12-stimulated NK cells. Furthermore, human CD1a$^+$ DC (our own observations and Carbone *et al.*, unpublished data) as well as CD83$^+$ (our own observations) can be targeted by CD56$^+$ CD16$^+$CD3$^-$ NK cell lines as well as CD56$^+$ LAK cells.

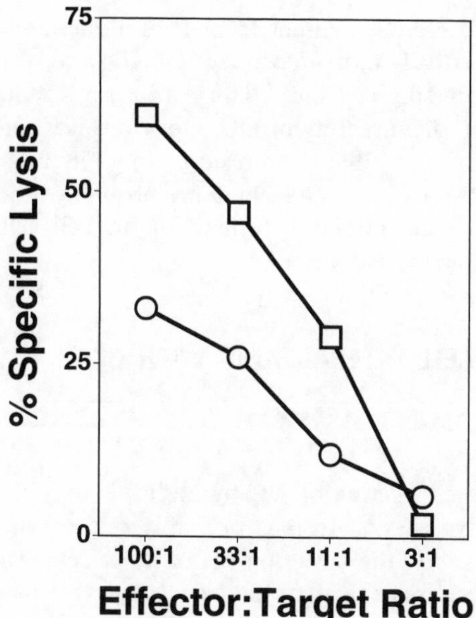

Fig. 2. NK cell killing of DC *in vitro*. NK cells activated *in vivo* with the interferon inducer tilorone (○) or *in vitro* with IL-2 (□) efficiently kill bone marrow-derived DC in a standard ^{51}Cr-release assay. For experimental procedures, see Chambers *et al.* (1996).

The nature of molecules on DC involved in the triggering of NK cells remains unclear. Activated APC express high levels of costimulatory and adhesion molecules and also upregulate the expression of other molecules such as MHC class II. Therefore, an interesting possibility is that some of these molecules may be involved in making DC sensitive to NK cell-mediated lysis. Indeed, we and others have observed that costimulatory molecules such as CD80 (Geldhof *et al.*, 1995; Chambers *et al.*, 1996), CD86 (Geldhof *et al.* 1998; and our unpublished observations), and CD40 (Carbone *et al.*, 1997), when transfected into NK cell-insensitive cell lines, make these lines sensitive to NK cell-mediated lysis. However, preliminary examination of lysis of DC from mice with the class II/CD40 or CD80/CD86 genes deleted revealed no significant differences in lysis compared to DC from wild-type mice, suggesting that none of these molecules is the sole contributor to the NK cell-sensitive phenotype of DC.

Molecules expressed by the NK cells that might be involved in the killing of DC have also been investigated, though to a limited extent. Interestingly, cytokines such as IL-12 and IL-15 have been found to induce the upregulation of CD28 on mouse NK cells (Hunter *et al.*, 1997; Geldhof *et al.*, 1998). Furthermore, the upregulation of CD28 on NK cells has also been related to activation of these cells and increased killing of the NK cell-sensitive target YAC-1 (Hunter *et al.*, 1997). In our hands, NK cells from CD28 and CTLA4 knockout mice lyse wild-type DC at levels comparable to wild-type effectors (Chambers *et al.*, 1996 and unpublished observations). However, another study has found that NK cells from CD28 knockout mice, when treated with IL-2/IL-12, were unable to efficiently lyse both splenic and bone marrow-derived DC (Geldhof *et al.*, 1997). One possible interpretation of these latter observations is that the IL-2/IL-12 stimulates NK cells in a different manner from IL-2 alone, and so IL-2/IL-12-stimulated NK cells became relatively more dependent on CD28 to recognize and kill CD80/CD86 transfected or expressing cell lines. Thus, it appears that under certain conditions, CD28 is involved in the targeting of DC. However, it would seem from our own published data (Chambers *et al.*, 1996) and results using NK cells from CD40L knockout mice (unpublished observations), that there are probably a host of receptor–ligand interactions ranging from costimulatory triggering to cell–cell adhesion molecules required for the NK cell-mediated lysis of DC.

SIGNIFICANCE OF NK CELL INTERACTIONS WITH DC

Evolution

One can speculate that the targeting of DC by NK cells may reflect an evolutionarily old response in immunity. Phagocytosis is probably one of the oldest forms of host defense mechanisms. Possibly, the development of killer cells was required to combat bacteria, parasites, and viruses that had evolved to survive in phagocytic cells. One possibility is that these early primitive killers (the NK cell ancestors?) were derived from the phagocytes themselves, and that they evolved to recognize infected cells including infected phagocytes. Recognition of infected phagocytes could hypothetically have been mediated via increased adhesion to integrins as well as by recognition of triggering molecules such as costimulatory molecules. Such a scenario would explain why NK cells on the one hand share certain features with DC, yet are able to kill DC under certain circumstances.

Infection Defense

In the previous sections, we have speculated that NK cell targeting of DC may play a role in the initial response against certain intracellular infections. It is already established that NK cells could be triggered by the release of cytokines from DC. NK cells could also stimulate DC maturation and differentiation through the production of cytokines (Fig. 1). However, we add that part of this response could also include the direct killing of DC by NK cells as possibly the first line of defense against infection. This could serve two functions: (1) killing 'freshly' infected cells would be more advantageous for the host than relying solely upon the adaptive immune response; (2) lysis of infected DC by the NK cells would create cellular debris, which has been reported to act as an adjuvant (Bevan, 1995). The debris, plus the cytokines released from both the NK cells and infected DC, would recruit more antigen-presenting cells to the infected area (Fig. 1). Such cells, we speculate, would be the actual cells that would then go to the lymph nodes and stimulate T cells as the innate/NK response is downregulated (Fig. 1).

Prevention of Autoimmunity

If NK cells *in vivo* do in fact target DC and other antigen-presenting cells, this may hypothetically have a beneficial side-effect by preventing autoimmunity. When the APC is stimulating the T cell, it must have a finite life span as one could speculate that tolerance might be broken by prolonged exposure to self-antigens emanating from the APC. Therefore, NK cell targeting of the DC could indeed serve as a mechanism for controlling normal immunohomeostasis along with programmed cell death of the DC and targeting by previously primed T cells.

CONCLUSION

As stated at the beginning of this review, this is a field with very little knowledge compared with those dealing with T cell and B cell interactions with DC. Indeed, our opening quotation indicates the puzzle which presently exists between NK cells and DC. We are faced with a number of characters, but the interpretation of these characters is unclear. These are: (1) the relationship in terms of the common origin of both NK and DC cells; (2) the role of NK cell and DC interaction in the immune system as a whole; (3) the possible implications for NK cell killing of DC; and (4) finally how the observations described can be beneficial in the physiological/pathological setting. Sherlock Holmes was able to solve the puzzle of the dancing men by first determining that the hieroglyphics represented single letters. Then he was able to determine which hieroglyphic was the letter ‘e’ and through a process of elimination break the code. Similarly we and others have begun to decipher parts of our interesting and complex puzzle and we hope that in time the mystery will be unraveled.

ACKNOWLEDGMENTS

We thank M.T. Bejarano, M. Salcedo, and J. Wilson as well as members of our group for collaborations and comments on the present manuscript; A. Schenyius, L. Heffler, C. Watts, C. Norbury, R. Harris, A. Sharpe, A. McAdam, J. Charo, R. Kiessling, A. Martin-Fontecha and K. Kärre for collaborations and discussions; and E. Carbone, C. Hunter, and A. Geldhof for providing unpublished results. H.G.L. is funded by the Swedish Cancer Foundation, The Swedish Medical Research Foundation, and the Karolinska Institute. B.J.C. is currently on a Scholarship awarded by the Swedish Society for Medical Research.

REFERENCES

Allavena, P., Paganin, C., Zhou, D., Bianchi, G., Sozzani, S. and Mantovani, A. (1994). Interleukin-12 is chemotactic for natural killer cells and stimulates their interaction with vascular endothelium. *Blood* **84**, 2261–2268.

Ardavin, C., Wu, L., Li., C.L. and Shortman, K. (1993). Thymic dendritic cells and T cells develop simultaneously in the thymus from a common precursor population. *Nature* **362**, 761–763.

Azuma, M., Yssel, H., Philips, J.H., Spits, H. and Lanier, L.L. (1993). Functional expression of B7/BB1 on activated T lymphocytes. *J. Exp. Med.* **177**, 845–850.

Bancroft, G.J. (1993). The role of natural killer cells in innate resistance to infection. *Curr. Opin. Immunol.* **5**, 503–510.

Berg, D.J., Kühn, R. Rajewsky, K., Müller, W., Menon, S., Davidson, N., Grünig, G. and Rennick, D. (1995). Interleukin-10 is a central regulator of the responses to LPS in murine models of endotoxic shock and the Schwartzman reaction but not endotoxin tolerance. *J. Clin. Invest.* **96**, 2339–2347.

Bevan, M.J. (1995). Antigen presentation to cytotoxic T lymphocytes in vivo. *J. Exp. Med.* **182**, 639–641.

Bhardwaj, N. (1997). Interactions of viruses with dendritic cells: a double edged sword. *J. Exp. Med.* **186**, 795–799.

Biron, C.A. (1997). Activation and function of natural killer cell responses during viral infections. *Curr. Opin. Immunol.* **9**, 24–34.

Blanchard, D.K. and Djeu, J.Y. (1991). Differential modulation of surface antigens on human macrophages by IFN-gamma and GM-CSF: effect on susceptibility to LAK lysis. *J. Leukocyte Biol.* **50**, 28–34.

Blandchard, D.K., Hall, R.E. and Djeu, J.Y. (1990). Role of CD18 in lymphocyte activated killer (LAK) cell-mediated lysis of human monocytes: comparison with other LAK targets. *Int. J. Cancer* **45**, 312–319.

Brasel, K., McKenna, H.J., Morrissey, P.J., Charrier, K., Morris, A.E., Lee, C.C., Williams, D.E. and Lyman, S.D. (1996). Hematologic effects of flt3 ligand in vivo in mice. *Cancer Res.* **88**, 2004–2012.

Brooks, C.F. and Moore, M. (1986). Presentation of a soluble bacterial antigen and cell surface alloantigens by large granular lymphocytes (LGL) in comparison with monocytes. *Immunol.* **58**, 343–350.

Carbone, E., Ruggiero, G., Terrazzano, G., Palomba, C., Manzo, C., Fontana, S., Spits, H., Kärre, K. and Zappacosta, S. (1997). A new mechanism of NK cell cytotoxicity activation: the CD40–CD40 ligand interaction. *J. Exp. Med.* **185**, 2053–2060.

Cella, M., Sallusto, F. and Lanzavecchia, A. (1997). Origin, maturation and antigen presenting function of dendritic cells. *Curr. Opin. Immunol.* **9**, 10–16.

Chambers, B.J., Salcedo, M. and Ljunggren, H.G. (1996). Triggering of natural killer cells by the costimulatory molecule CD80 (B7-1). *Immunity* **5**, 311–317.

Chen, K.Y., Braun, S., Lyman, S., Fan, Y., Traycoff, C.M., Wiebke, E.A., Gaddy, J., Sledge, G., Broxmeyer, H.E. and Cornetta, K. (1997). Anti-tumor activity and immunotherapeutic properties of flt3-ligand in a murine breast cancer model. *Cancer Res.* **57**, 3511–3516.

Clark, E.A. (1997). Regulation of B lymphocytes by dendritic cells. *J. Exp. Med.* **185**, 801–804.

D'Orazio, J.A. and Stein-Streilein, J. (1996). Human natural killer (NK) cells present staphylococcal enterotoxin B (SEB) to T lymphocytes. *Clin. Exp. Immunol.* **104**, 366–373.

Fernandez, N., Zitvogel, L., Maraskovsky, E., DiFalco, N., Opolon, P., Cordier, L., Perricaudet, M. and Haddada, H. (1997). Antitumor effects of Flt3L in poorly immunogenic mouse tumor models. *Immunol. Lett.* **56**, 224 [Abstract].

Galy, A., Travis, M., Cen, D. and Chen, B. (1995). Human T, B, natural killer and dendritic cells arise from a common bone marrow progenitor cell subset. *Immunity* **3**, 459–473.

Gazzanelli, R.T., Wysocka, M., Hieny, S., Scharton-Kersten, T., Cheever, A., Kähn, R., Müller,W., Trinchieri, G. and Sher, A. (1996). In the absence of endogenous IL-10, mice acutely infected with *Toxoplasma gondii* succumb to a lethal immune response dependent on $CD4^+$ T cells and accompanied by the overproduction of IL-12, IFN-γ and TNF-α. *J. Immunol.* **157**, 798–805.

Geldhof, A.B., Raes, G., Bakkus, M., Devos, S., Thielemans, K. and De Baetselier, P. (1995). Expression of B7-1 by highly metastatic mouse T lymphomas induces optimal natural killer cell-mediated cytotoxicity. *Cancer Res.* **55**, 2730–2733.

Geldhof, A.B., Moser, M., Lespagnard, L., Thielemans, K. and De Baetselier, P. (1998). IL-12-activated NK cells recognize B7 costimulatory molecules on tumor cells and autologous dendritic cells. *Blood* **91**, 196–206.

Gilbertson, S.M., Shah, P.D. and Rowley, D.A. (1986). NK cells suppress the generation of $lyt2^+$ cytolytic T cells by suppressing or eliminating dendritic cells. *J. Immunol.* **136**, 3567–3571.

Gorak, P.M.A., Engwenda, C.R. and Kaye, P.M. (1998). Dendritic cells, but not macrophages, produce IL-12 immediately following *Leishmania donovani* infection. *Eur. J. Immunol.* **28**, 687–695.

Gumperz, J.E. and Parham, P. (1995). The enigma of the natural killer cell. *Nature* **378**, 245–248.

Hunter, C.A., Chizzonite, R. and Remington, J.S. (1995a). IL-1β is required for IL-12 to induce production of IFN-γ by NK cells. *J. Immunol.* **155**, 4347–4354.

Hunter, C.A., Bermudez, L., Beernik, H., Waegell, W. and Remington, J.S. (1995b). Transforming growth factor-β inhibits interleukin-12-induced production of interferon-γ by natural killer cells: a role for transforming growth factor-β in the regulation of T cell-independent resistance to *Toxoplasma gondii. Eur. J. Immunol.* **25**, 994–1000.

Hunter, C.A., Ellis-Neyer, L., Gabriel, K.E., Kennedy, M.K., Grabstein, K.H., Linsley, P.S. and Remington, J.S. (1997). The role of the CD28/B7 interaction in the regulation of NK cell responses during infection with *Toxoplasma gondii. J. Immunol.* **158**, 2285–2293.

Janeway, C.A. (1992). The immune system evolved to discriminate infectious nonself from noninfectious self. *Immunol. Today* **13**, 11–16.

Josien, R., Heslan, M., Soulillou, J.P. and Cuturi, M.C. (1997). Rat spleen dendritic cells express natural killer cell receptor protein 1 (NKR-P1) and have cytotoxic activity to select targets via a Ca^{2+}-dependent mechanism. *J. Exp. Med.* **186**, 467–472.

Kiessling, R., Klein, E., Pross, H. and Wigzell, H. (1975). 'Natural' killer cells in the mouse. II. Cytotoxic cells with specificity for mouse Moloney leukemia cells. Characteristics of the killer cell. *Eur. J. Immunol.* **5**, 117–121.

Knight, S.C. and Patterson, S. (1997). Bone marrow-derived dendritic cells, infection with human immunodeficiency virus and immunopathology. *Annu. Rev. Immunol.* **15**, 593–615.

Lanier, L.L. and Philips, J.H. (1996). Inhibitory MHC class I receptors on NK cells and T cells. *Immunol. Today* **17**, 86–91.

Lanier, L.L., Corliss, B. and Philips, J.H. (1997). Arousal and inhibition of human NK cells. *Immunol. Rev.* **155**, 145–154.

Leibson, P.J. (1997). Signal transduction during natural killer cell activation: inside the mind of a killer. *Immunity* **6**, 655–661.

Ljunggren, H.G. and Kärre, K. (1990). In search of the 'missing self': MHC molecules and NK cell recognition. *Immunol. Today* **11**, 237–244.

Long, E.O. and Wagtmann, N. (1997). Natural killer cell receptors. *Curr. Opin. Immunol.* **9**, 344–350.

Long, E.O., Burshyn, D.N., Clark, W.P., Peruzzi, M., Rajagopalan, S., Rojo, S., Wagtmann, N. and Winter, C.C. (1997). Killer cell inhibitory receptors: diversity, specificity, and function. *Immunol. Rev.* **155**, 135–144.

Lyman, S.D. (1995). Biology of flt3 ligand and receptor. *Int. J. Hematol.* **62**, 63–73.

Lynch, D.H., Andreasen, A., Maraskovsky, E., Whitmore, J., Miller, R.E. and Schuh, J.C.L. (1997). Flt3 ligand induces tumor regression and antitumor immune responses in vivo. *Nature Medicine* **3**, 625–631.

Maraskovsky, E., Brasel, K., Teepe, M., Roux, E.R., Lyman, S.D., Shortman, K. and McKenna, H.J. (1996). Dramatic increase in the numbers of functionally mature dendritic cells in Flt3 ligand-treated mice: multiple dendritic cell subpopulations identified. *J. Exp. Med.* **184**, 1953–1963.

Marquez, C., Trigueros, C., Franco, J.M., Ramiro, A.R., Carrasco, Y.R., Lopez-Botet, M. and Toribio, M.L. (1998). Identification of a common developmental pathway for thymic natural killer cells and dendritic cells. *Blood* **91**, 2760–2771.

Mebius, R.E., Rennert, P. and Weissman, I.L. (1997). Developing lymph nodes collect $CD4^{+}CD3^{-}LT\beta^{+}$ cells that can differentiate to APC, NK cells and follicular cells but not T or B cells. *Immunity* **7**, 493–504.

Moll, H., Flohe, S. and Rollinghoff, M. (1995). Dendritic cells in *Leishmania major*-immune mice harbor persistent parasites and mediate an antigen-specific T cell immune response. *Eur. J. Immunol.* **25**, 693–696.

Raulet, D.H. (1996). Recognition events that inhibit and activate natural killer cells. *Curr. Opin. Immunol.* **8**, 372–377.

Reid, C.D.L. (1997). The dendritic cell lineage in haemopoiesis. *Br. J. Haematol.* **96**, 217–223.

Res, P., Martinez-Caceras, E., Jaleco, A.C., Staal, F., Noteboom, E., Weijer, K. and Spits, H. (1996). $CD34^{+}CD38^{dim}$ cells in the human thymus can differentiate into T, natural killer, and dendritic cells but are distinct from pluripotent stem cells. *Blood* **87**, 5196–5206.

Roncarolo, M.G., Bigler, M., Haanen, J.B., Yssel, H., Bacchetta, R., de Vries, J.E. and Spits, H. (1991). Natural killer cell clones can efficiently process and present protein antigens. *J. Immunol.* **147**, 781–787.

Scala, G., Allavena, P., Ortaldo, J.R., Herberman, R.B. and Oppenheim, J.J. (1985). Subsets of human large granular lymphocytes (LGL) exhibit accessory cell functions. *J. Immunol.* **134**, 3049–3055.

Scharton-Kersten, T.M. and Sher, A. (1997). Role of natural killer cells in innate resistance to protozoan infections. *Curr. Opin. Immunol.* **9**, 44–51.

Scott, P. and Trinchieri, G. (1995). The role of natural killer cells in host–parasite infections. *Curr. Opin. Immunol.* **7**, 34–40.

Shah, P.D. (1987). Dendritic cells but not macrophages are targets for immune regulation by natural killer cells. *Cell. Immunol.* **104**, 440–445.

Steinman, R.M. (1991). The dendritic cell system and its role in immunogenicity. *Annu. Rev. Immunol.* **9**, 271–296.

Svensson, M., Stockinger, B. and Wick, M.J. (1997). Bone marrow-derived dendritic cells can process bacteria for MHC-I and MHC-II presentation to T cells. *J. Immunol.* **158**, 4229–4236.

Trinchieri, G. (1989). Biology of natural killer cells. *Adv. Immunol.* **47**, 187–376.

Trinchieri, G. and Gerosa, F. (1996). Immunoregulation by interleukin-12. *J. Leukocyte Biol.* **59**, 505–511.

Tripp, C.S., Wolf, S.F. and Unanue, E.R. (1993). Interleukin 12 and tumor necrosis factor alpha are costimulators of interferon gamma production by natural killer cells in severe combined immunodeficiency mice with listeriosis and interleukin 10 is a physiologic antagonist. *Proc. Natl Acad. Sci. USA* **90**, 3725–3729.

Unanue, E.R. (1997). Inter-relationships among macrophages, natural killer cells and neutrophils in early stages of *Listeria* resistance. *Curr. Opin. Immunol.* **9**, 35–43.

Yokoyama, W.M. and Seaman, W.E. (1993). The Ly-49 and NKR-P1 gene families encoding lectin-like receptors on natural killer cells: the NK gene complex. *Annu. Rev. Immunol.* **11**, 613–635.

Yu, H., Carson, W.E. and Caligiuri, M.A. (1997). The Flt3 ligand combines with interleukin 15 for natural killer cell expansion from CD34$^+$ progenitor cells: evidence for redundancy with c-kit ligand. *Nat. Immun.* **15**, 170–171 [Abstract].

Yu, Y.Y.L., Kumar, V. and Bennet, M. (1992). Murine natural killer cells and marrow graft rejection. *Annu. Rev. Immunol.* **10**, 189–213.

CHAPTER 15
Interactions between Dendritic Cells and B-Lymphocytes

Francine Brière, Christophe Caux, Bertrand Dubois, Jérôme Fayette, Stéphane Vandenabeele and Jacques Banchereau[1]
Schering-Plough, Laboratory for Immunological Research, Dardilly, France;
[1]Baylor Research Institute, Dallas, Texas, USA

INTRODUCTION

Initially described in the skin by Langerhans in 1868, dendritic cells (DC) were identified as a critical element of the immune system by Steinman and Cohn in 1973. Since then, increasing work has underlined their key role in the initiation of immune responses and it is now well established that DC are the most potent antigen-presenting cells with the remarkable capacity of priming naive T cells. DC have since been identified as a persisting trace population in virtually every nonlymphoid tissue as well as in all lymphoid organs (for reviews see Banchereau and Steinman, 1998; Hart, 1997; Steinman *et al.*, 1997). Studies on DC have long been hampered by their low frequencies and the lack of specific markers allowing their isolation and purification. Those difficulties have been alleviated by the possibility of generating DC *in vitro*, for example from $CD34^+$ hematopoietic progenitors (Caux *et al.*, 1992) or from peripheral blood monocytes (Romani *et al.*, 1994; Sallusto and Lanzavecchia, 1994). Although several experiments strongly suggested the importance of DC in the establishment of humoral responses (Cebra *et al.*, 1994; Flamand *et al.*, 1994; Francotte and Urbain, 1985; Inaba and Steinman, 1985; Inaba *et al.*, 1983; Inaba *et al.*, 1984; Schrader and Cebra, 1993; Schrader *et al.*, 1990; Sornasse *et al.*, 1992; Spalding and Griffin, 1986), it is a common understanding that DC act to select and activate antigen-specific naive T cells which subsequently induce B cell responses. Upon priming with DC, activated T cells express CD40 ligand (CD40L), and not only interact with CD40-expressing B cells but also modulate DC functions through upregulation of costimulatory molecules (CD54, CD80, CD86) and secretion of cytokines (Caux *et al.*, 1994; Cella *et al.*, 1996; McLellan *et al.*, 1996). Activated T cells, through cytokines CD40L and CD70 (Jacquot *et al.*, 1997), promote B cell survival (Liu *et al.*, 1989) and proliferation (Banchereau *et al.*, 1991) as well as B cell differentiation and isotype switching (Defrance *et al.*, 1992; Jabara *et al.*, 1990; Malisan *et al.*, 1996; Rousset *et al.*, 1991). Thus among the signals involved in the triad composed of DC, T lymphocytes and B lymphocytes, CD40–CD40L

Dendritic Cells: Biology and Clinical Applications
ISBN 0-12-455860-7

interactions (Banchereau *et al.*, 1994) appear of critical importance as illustrated in the hyper-IgM syndrome (Callard *et al.*, 1993) or mice deficient for CD40 or CD40L (Kawabe *et al.*, 1994; Xu *et al.*, 1994). However, there is now evidence that DC directly interact with B cells and regulate humoral responses. This will represent the focus of the present review.

DC AND HUMORAL RESPONSES *IN VIVO*

In murine models, requirement for splenic adherent cells in primary antibody synthesis (Mosier, 1967) led to the discovery of a key role played by DC in such responses (Inaba *et al.*, 1983). In the case of hapten–carrier conjugates, DC sensitize carrier-specific T cells which can in turn have cognate interaction with hapten-specific B cells (Inaba and Steinman, 1985). Antigen-activated B cells then proliferate and differentiate in response to membrane molecules and cytokines. Furthermore, T cell priming (Inaba *et al.*, 1990a,b) was shown to be followed by the appearance of antigen-specific immunoglobulin in serum (Berg *et al.*, 1994; Flamand *et al.*, 1994; Francotte and Urbain, 1985; Sornasse *et al.*, 1992). Immunoglobulin levels become detectable after a second challenge with soluble antigen, a few days after DC injection (Liu and MacPherson, 1993; Sornasse *et al.*, 1992).

DC AND HUMORAL RESPONSES *IN VITRO*

In vitro Generation of DC

As DC are difficult to isolate from tissues, their *in vitro* generation represents an important step towards the understanding of DC physiology. Experiments detailed hereafter were performed using mostly DC generated *in vitro* by culturing cord blood-derived $CD34^+$ hematopoietic progenitors for 12 days in the presence of GM-CSF, TNF-α, and SCF (Caux *et al.*, 1992; see also Chapter 5). The high numbers of available DC allow a detailed molecular analysis of the observed biological effects.

DC Form Aggregates with B Cells

In order to determine the possible existence in the human of direct interactions between DC and B cells in a T cell-dependent context, *in vitro* generated DC were cocultured with allogeneic B cells using a CD40L-transfected cell line in order to partially mimic signals provided by T cells (Dubois *et al.*, 1997). In such cultures, clusters of DC and B cells were observed (Dubois *et al.*, 1997) (Plate 15.1) as had originally been described during DC and T cell interactions (Inaba and Steinman, 1985). Along with this observation, human tonsillar interdigitating DC of the T cell area have been colocalized with naive B cells *in situ* (Björck *et al.*, 1997). The molecules involved in DC–B cell interactions remain to be identified. Interestingly, such DC–B cell clusters have also been observed *in vivo* in rat lymph, where LFA-1/CD18 could be involved (Kushnir and MacPherson, 1996). In the mouse, clustering of DC, helper T lymphocytes, and histocompatible B cells has been obtained during primary antibody responses *in vitro* (Inaba *et al.*, 1984).

DC Enhance the Proliferation of Activated B Cells

Within a week, *in vitro* generated DC induce a 3–6-fold increase in number of viable human B cells activated solely through their CD40 antigen (in absence of T cells and any exogenous cytokines). This effect of DC is observed with naive or with memory B cells (Dubois *et al.*, 1997; Fayette *et al.*, 1997). B cells activated either through CD40 or using particles of *Staphylococcus aureus* Cowan I (unpublished observation) are capable of responding to DC stimulation.

DC can further enhance the considerable proliferation of CD40-activated B cells observed in response to IL-4, IL-13, and IL-10. Furthermore, DC allow CD40-activated B cells to proliferate in response to IL-2 (Dubois *et al.*, 1997; Fayette *et al.*, 1997). The mechanism by which DC induce B cell proliferation in the absence of exogeneous cytokines involves CD40-independent release of yet uncharacterized soluble mediators by DC, different from sgp80, IL-12, and IL-10. In contrast, induction by DC of IL-2-mediated B cell proliferation necessitates CD40 engagement of DC and involves both IL-12 and sgp80 (Dubois *et al.*, 1997; Dubois *et al.*, manuscript submitted).

DC Induce B Cell Differentiation

IL-2-dependent IgM Response by Naive B Cells

While CD40-activated naive B cells do not produce immunoglobulins in IL-2-supplemented cultures, addition of DC induces a dramatic production of IgM leading to the generation of 5–20% of IgM plasma cells at the end of the culture. Studies with neutralizing anti-cytokine antibodies have shown that IL-12 represents a critical DC-derived molecule, secreted upon CD40 engagement, that induces naive B cell differentiation into IgM plasma cells (Dubois *et al.*, manuscript submitted). In addition, DC induce not only a major IgM response by CD40-activated naive B cells but also high levels of IgG, suggesting a role of IL-2 in isotype switching in human (unpublished observation).

This finding complements other studies performed both in mice and humans that have reported biological effects of IL-12 on B-lymphocytes. In particular, IL-12 has been shown to enhance (1) the proliferation and polyclonal immunoglobulin secretion of BCR-activated human peripheral blood B cells cultured in the presence of IL-2 (Jelinek and Braaten, 1995; Li *et al.*, 1996); (2) the antigen-specific antibody response by peripheral blood mononuclear cells (Clerici *et al.*, 1993; Luzzati *et al.*, 1997; Uherova *et al.*, 1996). Furthermore, the primary humoral response to a microbial antigen in SCID mice engrafted with human PBL was shown to be IL-12-dependent (Westerink *et al.*, 1997). Finally, IL-12-treated mice display increased IgG2a antibody responses to protein and hapten antigens and suppressed IgG1 responses (Buchanan *et al.*, 1995; Germann *et al.*, 1995; McKnight *et al.*, 1994; Metzger *et al.*, 1996; Morris *et al.*, 1994). IL-12 would act on murine B cells by (1) inducing IFN-γ-dependent IgG2a isotype switch at the expense of IgG1 (Snapper, 1996) and (2) increasing immunoglobulin secretion of isotype-committed B cells through an IFN-γ-independent pathway as IL-12 leads to IgG1 and IgG2b anti-DNP antibody secretions in IFN-γ knockout mice (Metzger *et al.*, 1997).

Naive B cells have a low propensity to differentiate into plasma cells (Arpin *et al.*, 1997; Dubois *et al.*, 1997). However, addition of DC to experimental culture conditions allowing plasma cell differentiation to occur (Arpin *et al.*, 1995) strongly favors the generation of plasma cells from CD40-activated naive B cells. A majority of plasma cells is generated when DC are added in a first-step culture of CD40-activated naive B cells in the presence of IL-2, followed by a second-step culture requiring only the presence of IL-2 and IL-10. Addition of IL-10 to this culture system masks the contribution of endogenous IL-12 in DC-mediated plasma cell differentiation (Fayette *et al.*, manuscript submitted).

Thus DC, in addition to priming T cells toward T_H1 development, may through the production of IL-12 directly signal naive B cells during the initiation of the immune response. A pivotal role of IL-12 in controlling cell-mediated immunity (Afonso *et al.*, 1994; Hsieh *et al.*, 1993; Lamont and Adorini, 1996; Scott, 1993) and in regulating humoral responses provides an obvious advantage for immune intervention requiring both sides of the immune response.

Memory B Cell Differentiation without Cytokines

In the absence of exogenous cytokine, DC strongly potentiate the differentiation of CD40-activated memory B cells toward IgG- and IgA-secreting cells (Dubois *et al.*, 1997). Endogenous IL-6 appears as the major factor responsible for this differentiation, while IL-12 is clearly not involved (Dubois *et al.*, manuscript submitted). A contribution of IL-6 in B cell differentiation has been documented in culture systems devoid of DC (Akira *et al.*, 1993; Beagley *et al.*, 1989; Burdin *et al.*, 1996; Muraguchi *et al.*, 1988). However, through their secretion of soluble IL-6R α chain, gp80, DC may play a role in B cell differentiation (Dubois *et al.*, manuscript submitted). Indeed, IL-6/sgp80 complex has been demonstrated to bind with high affinity to the IL-6R-transducing chain, gp130, thus potentiating the biological activity of IL-6 (Peters *et al.*, 1996; Tamura *et al.*, 1993).

Skewing of Isotype Switching toward both IgA1 and IgA2

Provided that naive B cells are activated through CD40, DC induce isotype switching toward IgA, as measured by expression of surface IgA, in the absence of exogenous cytokine (Fayette *et al.*, 1997). Under these culture conditions, induction of surface IgA-expressing B cells is quantitatively comparable to that obtained with the combination of IL-10 and TGF-β, in a system devoid of DC, previously reported as the most potent combination for IgA switching (Defrance *et al.*, 1992). Induction of IgA-expressing B cells by DC is partially mediated by TGF-β (Fayette *et al.*, 1997), while IL-12 is not involved (Fig. 2).

In addition, DC provide another critical IgA-inducing signal that acts in concert with IL-10 and TGF-β to induce commitment toward IgA of one out of two naive B cells (Fayette *et al.*, 1997). While DC allow CD40-activated naive B cells to express surface IgA, IL-10 is necessary for their differentiation into IgA-secreting cells. However, in the presence of IL-10 and TGF-β, DC skewed immunoglobulin secretion toward IgA. Importantly, in the presence of DC, naive B cells can be induced to secrete both IgA1 and IgA2 subclasses (Fayette *et al.*, 1997). Of note, the presence of contaminating T cells was formally excluded in CD40-activated B cell and DC cocultures whatever combination of cytokine is used.

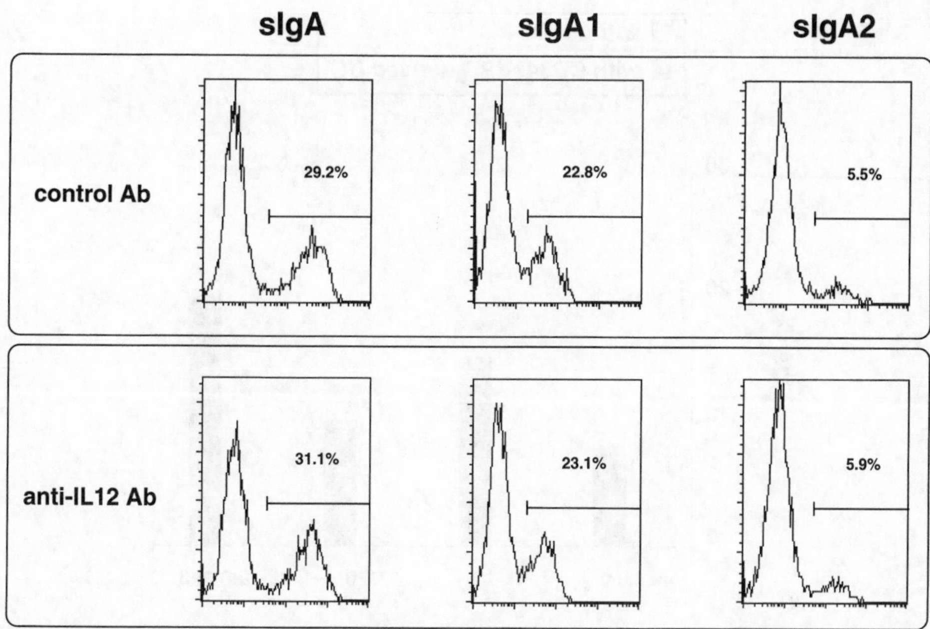

Fig. 2. Induction of surface IgA by DC is not IL-12-dependent. sIgD$^+$ naive B cells (5×10^4 cells) were cultured in a final volume of 1 ml in the presence of 5×10^4 CD34$^+$ HPC-derived DC over 1.25×10^4 irradiated CD40 ligand-transfected L cells with IL-10 (200 ng/ml) and TGF-β (0.3 ng/ml) with an isotype-matched control antibody or goat anti-IL-12 antibody. B cells were harvested after 7 days of culture and stained with rabbit polyclonal FITC-labeled anti-IgA or FITC-labeled anti-IgA1 or anti-IgA2 mAbs and analyzed by FACScan.

These results extend earlier studies with mouse Peyer's patch or splenic B cells (Cebra *et al.*, 1994; Schrader and Cebra, 1993; Schrader *et al.*, 1990) as well as pre-B cell lines (Spalding and Griffin, 1986) which were shown to secrete high levels of IgA with a combination of polyclonally activated T cells or T_H2 clones and DC. In contrast to the unique IgA isotype in mice, two IgA subclasses exist in humans whose differential *in vivo* expression suggests distinct regulation (Brandtzaeg, 1995). DC have been described in virtually all epithelia covering the mucosae (including epithelium of the oral and rectal cavities, epithelium of stomach, small and large bowel, lamina propria, and in the vagina and cervix) (Hart, 1997; see also Chapter 5). Here also heterogeneity of DC appears, at least in terms of phenotype (Kelsall and Strober, 1996). Thus, it is tempting to speculate that *in vitro* generated DC share properties with mucosal-associated DC involved in the regulation of mucosal humoral responses.

In summary, DC mediate their effect on B cell responses through IL-12-dependent and IL-12-independent pathways. Overall, DC are present in lymphoid organs where initiation of systemic responses occurs as well as in mucosal-associated lymphoid organs. DC of the respective compartments may participate in the outcome of those two pathways and thus contribute to the unique features of the systemic versus mucosal immune compartments. In this context, it has been reported in mice that in contrast to the T_H1-shift observed when IL-12 is delivered parenterally, oral administration of

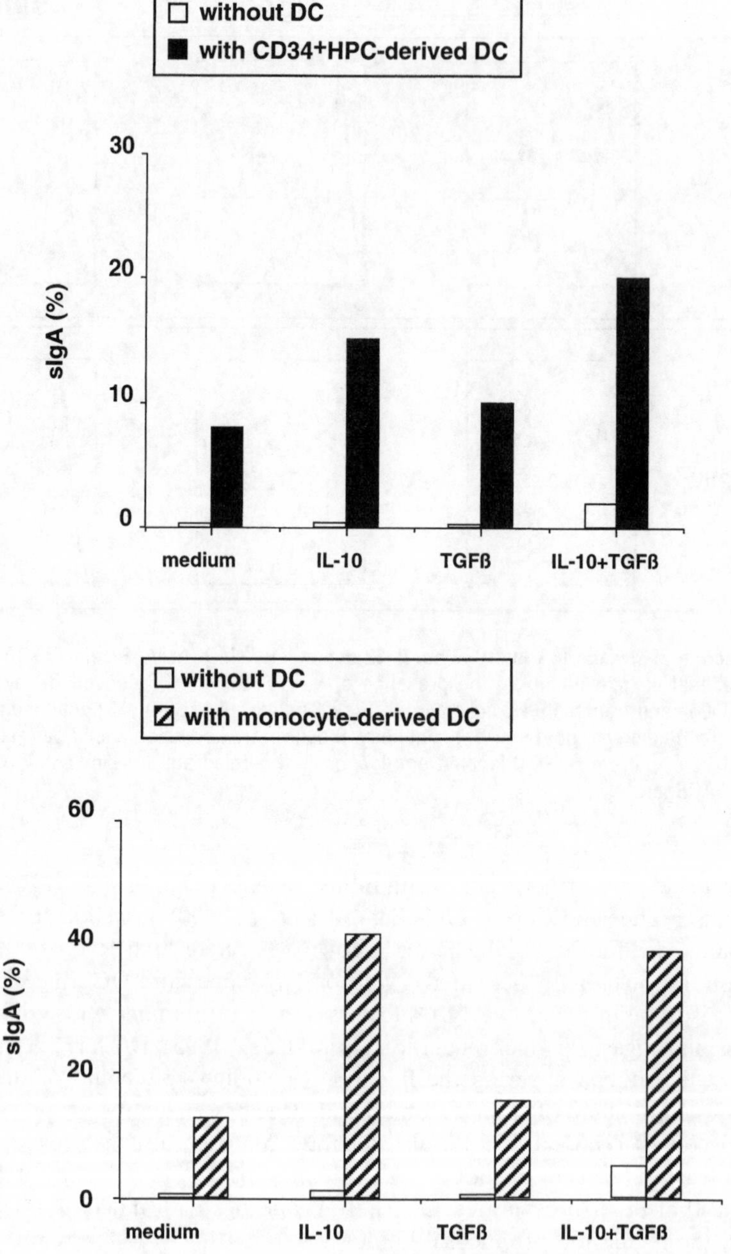

Fig. 3. Both monocyte-derived DC and CD34$^+$ HPC-derived DC induce IgA switch. sIgD$^+$ naive B cells (5×10^4 cells) were cultured in a final volume of 1 ml in the absence or presence of either 5×10^4 monocyte-derived DC or 5×10^4 CD34$^+$ HPC-derived DC over 1.25×10^4 irradiated CD40 ligand-transfected L cells without or with IL-10 (200 ng/ml), TGF-β (0.3 ng/ml) or both. B cells were harvested after 7 days of culture and stained with rabbit polyclonal FITC-labeled anti-IgA and analyzed by FACScan.

IL-12 induced secretion of T_H2-type cytokines without altering secretory IgA antibody responses (Marinaro *et al.*, 1997). This finding has important implications for the targeted induction of immune responses to mucosal vaccines.

Distinct Subpopulations of DC Differentially Regulate B Cell Responses

It is now well accepted that monocytes represent one of the precursor populations of DC (for reviews see Banchereau and Steinman, 1998; Caux *et al.*, 1998). In the context of B cell responses, DC and monocytes share an equal capability to enhance CD40-activated B cell proliferation, while DC are more efficient than monocytes in inducing memory B cells to secrete IgG and IgA in the absence of cytokines (Dubois *et al.*, 1997). In contrast, either $CD34^+$ hematopoietic progenitor-derived or monocyte-derived DC, but not monocytes, induce surface IgA expression on CD40-activated naive B cells in the absence of cytokines (Fig. 3).

DC derived from $CD34^+$ hematopoietic progenitors from cord blood differentiate along two independent DC pathways in response to GM-CSF and TNF-α (Caux *et al.*, 1996; see also Chapter 5). After 5–6 days two subsets, one $CD1a^+CD14^-$ and one $CD1a^-CD14^+$, can be observed, while after 12 days of culture all cells are $CD1a^+CD14^-$. These two subsets sorted at day 6 have no proliferating capacity, but mature at day 14 into $CD1a^+CD14^-$ cells that express high levels of MHC class II and accessory molecules (CD80, CD86, CD83, CD58). The $CD1a^+$ precursors differentiate into typical Langerhans cells that contain Birbeck granules (BG) and express E-cadherin, while the $CD14^+$ precursors lead to $CD1a^+$ DC, BG^-, that have the characteristics of interstitial (dermal) DC as shown by expression of CD68 and coagulation factor XIIIa (Caux *et al.*, 1996). While both DC subsets are able to enhance the proliferation of CD40-activated B cells and to induce the differentiation of memory B cells, only CD14-derived interstitial DC can induce naive B cells to differentiate into IgM-secreting cells in response to CD40 ligation and IL-2 (Caux *et al.*, 1997). This suggests that dermal-type DC rather than epidermal Langerhans cells could be critical in the launching of primary B cell responses (Chapter 5).

PHYSIOLOGICAL RELEVANCE

A cardinal feature of Langerhans cells or 'epithelial-DC' is to initiate immune responses by capturing foreign antigens following tissue injury. While migrating through the draining afferent lymph into the proximal secondary lymphoid organ, DC process the antigens. Within paracortical areas of the secondary lymphoid organs, DC, at this site referred to as interdigitating dendritic cells (IDC), have a strong capacity to stimulate antigen-specific naive T cells to proliferate, secrete cytokines, and express CD40L (Steinman *et al.*, 1997). IDC would thus allow the encounter of the rare antigen-specific T and B cells (Liu *et al.*, 1996; MacLennan *et al.*, 1997). In murine models, immunohistological studies have demonstrated that primary T cell-dependent B cell responses were initiated within the T cell/IDC-rich areas (Liu *et al.*, 1991). Activated T cells stimulate antigen-specific naive B cells to proliferate and to differentiate into germinal center founder cells or, in the majority, into short-lived plasma cells producing essentially IgM (Liu and Arpin, 1997). In view of the recent information obtained with *in vitro* generated DC, DC may play an important role at that stage, in the induction of an IL-2-dependent IgM plasma cell differentiation. Whether *ex vivo* purified human IDC (1) directly interact with antigen-specific B cells and (2) are responsible for the IgM plasma cell differentiation remains to be demonstrated. Germinal center formation starts with the colonization of GC founder cells in the primary follicles and depends on antigen transport onto follicular dendritic cells and on $CD40L^+CD57^+$ T cells producing cytokines such as IL-2, IL-4, and IL-10 (Liu and Arpin, 1997). One can hypothesize that antigen-specific T cells and antigen-transporting DC (Tew *et al.*, 1980) would migrate together with GC founder cells. Identification of a $CD3^-CD4^+CD11c^+$ DC population localized within germinal centers (GCDC) is a possible candidate for such a function (Grouard *et al.*, 1996; Liu and Arpin, 1997; Liu *et al.*, 1996). Although DC are key players in naive T cell activation, a role for DC in memory T cell maintenance has recently been emphasized (Brocker, 1997). Those GCDC could present processed antigens to memory T cells and could directly modulate GC-B cell responses. Accordingly, *ex vivo* purified GCDC rescue GC-B cells from spontaneous apoptosis and induce them to differentiate into plasma cells (B. Dubois, manuscript in preparation). The orphan chemokine receptor BLR1 is one of the first molecular mechanisms identified as being involved in follicular tropism of naive B cells and memory T cells (Förster *et al.*, 1994; Förster *et al.*, 1996). As DC do produce many chemokines, the possibility that GCDC may produce BLR1 ligand needs to be investigated. Finally, expression of several members of the TNF receptor family on DC, i.e. Ox40L (Ohshima *et al.*, 1997), RANK/TRANCE (Anderson *et al.*, 1997), and eventually their ligands, strongly encourages investigating the roles of such receptor–ligand pairs in the triad DC, T and B cell collaboration.

ACKNOWLEDGMENTS

A special acknowledgment to Sandrine Bourdarel for expert editorial assistance and to Daniel Lepot for his logistic support. We also thank Jean-Michel Bridon, Clarisse Barthélémy, Catherine Massacrier and Béatrice Vanbervliet for their continuous support.

REFERENCES

Afonso, L.C., Scharton, T.M., Vieira, L.Q., Wysocka, M., Trinchieri, G. and Scott, P. (1994). The adjuvant effect of interleukin-12 in a vaccine against *Leishmania major*. *Science* **263**, 235–237.

Akira, S., Taga, T. and Kishimoto, T. (1993). Interleukin-6 in biology and medicine. In: *Advances in Immunology* (ed. F.J. Dixon). Academic Press, San Diego.

Anderson, D.M., Maraskovsky, E., Billingsley, W.L., Dougall, W.C., Tometsko, M.E., Roux, E.R., Teepe, M.C., DuBose, R.F., Cosman, D. and Galibert, L. (1997). A homologue of the TNF receptor and its ligand enhance T-cell growth and dendritic-cell function. *Nature* **390**, 175–179.

Arpin, C., Déchanet, J., van Kooten, C., Merville, P., Grouard, G., Brière, F., Banchereau, J. and Liu, Y.J. (1995). Generation of memory B cells and plasma cells in vitro. *Science* **268**, 720–722.

Arpin, C., Banchereau, J. and Liu, Y.J. (1997). Memory B cells are biased towards terminal differentiation: a strategy that may prevent repertoire freezing. *J. Exp. Med.* **186**, 931–940.

Banchereau, J. and Steinman, R.M. (1998). Dendritic cells and the control of immunity. *Nature* **392**, 245–252.

Banchereau, J., de Paoli, P., Vallé, A., Garcia, E. and Rousset, F. (1991). Long term human B cell lines dependent on interleukin 4 and antibody to CD40. *Science* **251**, 70–72.

Banchereau, J., Bazan, F., Blanchard, D., Brière, F., Galizzi, J.P., van Kooten, C., Liu, Y.J., Rousset, F. and Saeland, S. (1994). The CD40 antigen and its ligand. *Annu. Rev. Immunol.* **12**, 881–922.

Beagley, K.W., Eldridge, J.H., Lee, F., Kiyono, H., Everson, M.P., Koopman, W.J., Hirano, T., Kishimoto, T. and McGhee, J.R. (1989). Interleukins and IgA synthesis. Human and murine interleukin 6 induce high rate IgA secretion in IgA-committed B cells. *J. Exp. Med.* **169**, 2133–2148.

Berg, S.F., Mjaaland, S. and Fossum, S. (1994). Comparing macrophages and dendritic leukocytes as antigen-presenting cells for humoral responses in vivo by antigen targeting. *Eur. J. Immunol.* **24**, 1262–1268.

Björck, P., Florès-Romo, L., and Liu, Y.J. (1997). Human interdigitating dendritic cells directly stimulate CD40-activated naive B cells. *Eur. J. Immunol.* **27**, 1266–1374.

Brandtzaeg, P. (1995). Basic mechanisms of mucosal immunity. *The Immunologist* **3**, 89–96.

Brocker, T. (1997). Survival of mature CD4 T lymphocytes is dependent on major histocompatibility complex class II-expressing dendritic cells. *J. Exp. Med.* **186**, 1223–1232.

Buchanan, J.M., Vogel, L.A., van Cleave, V.H. and Metzger, D.W. (1995). Interleukin 12 alters the isotype-restricted antibody response of mice to hen eggwhite lysozyme. *Int. Immunol.* **7**, 1519–1528.

Burdin, N., Galibert, L., Garrone, P., Durand, I., Banchereau, J. and Rousset, F. (1996). Inability to produce interleukin-6 is a functional feature of human germinal center B lymphocytes. *J. Immunol.* **156**, 4107–4113.

Callard, R.E., Armitage, R.J., Fanslow, W.C. and Spriggs, M.K. (1993). CD40 ligand and its role in X-linked hyper-IgM syndrome. *Immunol. Today* **14**, 559–564.

Caux, C., Dezutter-Dambuyant, C., Schmitt, D. and Banchereau, J. (1992). GM-CSF and TNF-α cooperate in the generation of dendritic Langerhans cells. *Nature* **360**, 258–261.

Caux, C., Vanbervliet, B., Massacrier, C., Azuma, M., Okumura, K., Lanier, L.L. and Banchereau, B. (1994). B70/B7-2 is identical to CD86 and is the major functional ligand for CD28 expressed on human dendritic cells. *J. Exp. Med.* **180**, 1841–1847.

Caux, C., Vanbervliet, B., Massacrier, C., Dezutter-Dambuyant, C., de Saint-Vis, B., Jacquet, C., Yoneda, K., Imamura, S., Schmitt, D. and Banchereau, J. (1996). $CD34^+$ hematopoietic progenitors from human cord blood differentiate along two independent dendritic cell pathways in response to GM-CSF + TNFα. *J. Exp. Med.* **184**, 695–706.

Caux, C., Massacrier, C., Vanbervliet, B., Dubois, B., Durand, I., Cella, M., Lanzavecchia, A. and Banchereau, J. (1997). $CD34^+$ hematopoietic progenitors from human cord blood differentiate along two independent dendritic cell pathways in response to GM-CSF + TNFα: II. Functional analysis. *Blood* **90**, 1458–1470.

Caux, C., Dezutter-Dambuyant, C., Liu, Y.J. and Banchereau, J. (1998). Isolation and propagation of human dendritic cells. In: *Methods in Microbiology: Immunological Methods* (eds D. Kabelitz and K. Ziegler). Academic Press, Orlando.

Cebra, J.J., Bos, N.A., Cebra, E.R., Cuff, C.F., Deenen, G.J., Kroese, F.G.M. and Shroff, K.E. (1994). Development of components of the mucosal immune system in SCID recipient mice. In *In Vivo Immunology* (ed. E. Heinen), Plenum Press, New York, pp. 255–259.

Cella, M., Scheidegger, D., Palmer-Lehmann, K., Lane, P., Lanzavecchia, A. and Alber, G. (1996). Ligation of CD40 on dendritic cells triggers production of high levels of interleukin-12 and enhances T cell stimulatory capacity: T–T help via APC activation. *J. Exp. Med.* **184**, 747–752.

Clerici, M., Lucey, D.R., Berzofsky, J.A., Pinto, L.A., Wynn, T.A., Blatt, S.P., Dolan, M.J., Hendrix, C.W., Wolf, S.F. and Shearer, G.M. (1993). Restoration of HIV-specific cell-mediated immune responses by interleukin-12 in vitro. *Science* **262**, 1721–1724.

Defrance, T., Vanbervliet, B., Brière, F., Durand, I., Rousset, F. and Banchereau, J. (1992). Interleukin 10 and transforming growth factor β cooperate to induce anti-CD40-activated naive human B cells to secrete immunoglobulin A. *J. Exp. Med.* **175**, 671–682.

Dubois, B., Vanbervliet, B., Fayette, J., Massacrier, C., van Kooten, C., Brière, F., Banchereau, J. and Caux, C. (1997). Dendritic cells enhance growth and differentiation of CD40-activated B lymphocytes. *J. Exp. Med.* **185**, 941–951.

Fayette, J., Dubois, B., Vandenabeele, S., Bridon, J.M., Vanbervliet, B., Durand, I., Banchereau, J., Caux, C. and Brière, F. (1997). Human dendritic cells skew isotype switching of CD40-activated naive B cells towards IgA1 and IgA2. *J. Exp. Med.* **185**, 1909–1918.

Flamand, V., Sornasse, T., Thielemans, K., Demanet, C., Bakkus, M., Bazin, H., Tielemans, F., Leo, O., Urbain, J. and Moser, M. (1994). Murine dendritic cells pulsed in vitro with tumor antigen induce tumor resistance in vivo. *Eur. J. Immunol.* **24**, 605–610.

Förster, R., Emrich, T., Kremmer, E. and Lipp, M. (1994). Expression of the G protein-coupled receptor BLR1 defines mature, recirculating B cells and a subset of T-helper memory cells. *Blood* **84**, 830–840.

Förster, R., Mattis, A.E., Kremmer, E., Wolf, E., Brem, G. and Lipp, M. (1996). A putative chemokine receptor, BLR1, directs B cell migration to defined lymphoid organs and specific anatomic compartments of the spleen. *Cell* **87**, 1037–1047.

Francotte, M. and Urbain, J. (1985). Enhancement of antibody responses by mouse dendritic cells pulsed with tobacco mosaic virus or with rabbit antiidiotypic antibodies raised against a private rabbit idiotype. *Proc. Natl Acad. Sci. USA* **82**, 8149–8152.

Germann, T., Bongartz, M., Dlugonska, H., Hess, H., Schmitt, E., Kolbe, L., Kolsch, E., Podlaski, F.J., Gately, M.K. and Rude, E. (1995). Interleukin-12 profoundly up-regulates the synthesis of antigen-specific complement-fixing IgG2a, IgG2b and IgG3 antibody subclasses in vivo. *Eur. J. Immunol.* **25**, 823–829.

Grouard, G., Durand, I., Filgueira, L., Banchereau, J. and Liu, Y.J. (1996). Dendritic cells capable of stimulating T cells in germinal centers. *Nature* **384**, 364–367.

Hart, D.N.J. (1997). Dendritic cells: unique leukocyte populations which control the primary immune response. *Blood* **90**, 3245–3287.

Hsieh, C.-S., Macatonia, S.E., Tripp, C.S., Wolf, S.F., O'Garra, A. and Murphy, K.M. (1993). Development of TH1 $CD4^+$ T cells through IL-12 produced by *Listeria*-induced macrophages. *Science* **260**, 547–549.

Inaba, K. and Steinman, R.M. (1985). Protein-specific helper T lymphocyte formation initiated by dendritic cells. *Science* **229**, 475–479.

Inaba, K., Granelli-Piperno, A. and Steinman, R.M. (1983). Dendritic cells are critical accessory cells for thymus-dependent antibody responses in mouse and man. *Proc. Natl Acad. Sci. USA* **80**, 6041–6045.

Inaba, K., Witmer, M.D. and Steinman, R.M. (1984). Clustering of dendritic cells, helper T lymphocytes, and histocompatible B cells, during primary antibody responses in vitro. *J. Exp. Med.* **160**, 858–876.

Inaba, K., Metlay, J.P., Crowley, M.T. and Steinman, R.M. (1990a). Dendritic cells pulsed with protein antigens in vitro can prime antigen-specific, MHC-restricted T cells in situ. *J. Exp. Med.* **172**, 631–640.

Inaba, K., Metlay, J.P., Crowley, M.T., Witmer-Pack, M. and Steinman, R.M. (1990b). Dendritic cells as antigen presenting cells in vivo. *Int. Rev. Immunol.* **6**, 197–206.

Jabara, H.H., Fu, S.M., Geha, R.S. and Vercelli, D. (1990). CD40 and IgE: synergism between anti-CD40 monoclonal antibody and interleukin 4 in the induction of IgE synthesis by highly purified human B cells. *J. Exp. Med.* **172**, 1861–1864.

Jacquot, S., Kobata, T., Iwata, S., Morimoto, C. and Schlossman, S.F. (1997). CD154/CD40 and CD70/CD27 interactions have different and sequential functions in T cell-dependent B cell responses. *J. Immunol.* **159**, 2652–2657.

Jelinek, D.F. and Braaten, J.K. (1995). Role of IL-12 in human B lymphocyte proliferation and differentiation. *J. Immunol.* **154**, 1606–1613.

Kawabe, T., Naka, T., Yoshida, K., Tanaka, T., Fujiwara, H., Suematsu, S., Yoshida, N., Kishimoto, T. and Kikutani, H. (1994). The immune response in CD40-deficient mice: impaired immunoglobulin class switching and germinal center formation. *Immunity* **1**, 167–178.

Kelsall, B.L. and Strober, W. (1996). Distinct populations of dendritic cells are present in the subepithelial dome and T cell regions of the murine Peyer's patch. *J. Exp. Med.* **183**, 237–247.

Kushnir, N. and MacPherson, G.G. (1996). B cell–dendritic cell clustering: role of LFA-1 and stimulation by cross-linking of MHC class II. In: *4th International Symposium on Dendritic Cells in Fundamental and Clinical Immunology*, Venice, pp. 284.

Lamont, A.G. and Adorini, L. (1996). IL-12: a key cytokine in immune regulation. *Immunol. Today* **17**, 214–217.

Li, L., Young, D., Wolf, S.F. and Choi, Y.S. (1996). Interleukin-12 stimulates B cell growth by inducing IFN-gamma. *Cell. Immunol.* **168**, 133–140.

Liu, Y.J. and Arpin, C. (1997). Germinal center development. *Immunol. Rev.* **156**, 111–126.

Liu, Y.J., Joshua, D.E., Williams, G.T., Smith, C.A., Gordon, J. and MacLennan, I.C.M. (1989). Mechanisms of antigen-driven selection in germinal centers. *Nature* **342**, 929–931.

Liu, Y.-J., Zhang, J., Lane, P.J.L., Chan, E.Y.-T. and MacLennan, I.C.M. (1991). Sites of specific B cell activation in primary and secondary responses to T cell-dependent and T cell-independent antigens. *Eur. J. Immunol.* **21**, 2951–2962.

Liu, L.M. and MacPherson, G.G. (1993). Antigen acquisition by dendritic cells: intestinal dendritic cells acquire antigen administered orally and can prime naive T cells in vivo. *J. Exp. Med.* **177**, 1299–1307.

Liu, Y.J., Grouard, G., de Bouteiller, O. and Banchereau, J. (1996). Follicular dendritic cells and germinal centers. In *International Review of Cytology* (ed. K.W. Jeon) Academic Press, San Diego, pp. 139–179.

Luzzati, A.L., Giordani, L. and Giacomini, E. (1997). Interleukin-12 up-regulates the induction of an antigen-specific antibody response in cultures of human lymphocytes. *Eur. J. Immunol.* **27**, 2696–2701.

MacLennan, I.C.M., Gulbranson-Judge, A., Toellner, K.M., Casamayor-Palleja, M., Chan, E., Sze, D.M.Y., Luther, S.A. and Orbea, H.A. (1997). The changing preference of T and B cells for partners as T-dependent antibody responses develop. *Immunol. Rev.* **156**, 53–66.

Malisan, F., Brière, F., Bridon, J.M., Harindranath, N., Mills, F.C., Max, E.E., Banchereau, J. and Martinez-Valdez, H. (1996). IL-10 induces IgG isotype switch recombination in human CD40-activated naive B lymphocytes. *J. Exp. Med.* **183**, 937–947.

Marinaro, M., Boyaka, P.N., Finkelman, F.D., Kiyono, H., Jackson, R.J., Jirillo, E. and McGhee, J.R. (1997). Oral but not parenteral Interleukin (IL)-12 redirects T helper 2 (Th2)-type responses to an oral vaccine without altering mucosal IgA responses. *J. Exp. Med.* **185**, 415–427.

McKnight, A.J., Zimmer, G.J., Fogelman, I., Wolf, S.F. and Abbas, A.K. (1994). Effects of IL-12 on helper T cell-dependent immune responses in vivo. *J. Immunol.* **152**, 2172–2179.

McLellan, A.D., Sorg, R.V., Williams, L.A. and Hart, D.N.J. (1996). Human dendritic cells activate T lymphocytes via a CD40:CD40 ligand-dependent pathway. *Eur. J. Immunol.* **26**, 1204–1210.

Metzger, D.W., Buchanan, J.M., Collins, J.L., Lester, T.L., Murray, K.S., van Cleave, V.H., Vogel, L.A. and Dunnick, W.A. (1996). Enhancement of humoral immunity by interleukin-12. *Ann. NY. Acad. Sci.* **795**, 100–115.

Metzger, D.W., McNutt, R.M., Collins, J.T., Buchanan, J.M., van Cleave, V.H. and Dunnick, W.A. (1997). Interleukin-12 acts as an adjuvant for humoral immunity through interferon-γ-dependent and -independent mechanisms. *Eur. J. Immunol.* **27**, 1958–1965.

Morris, S.C., Madden, K.B., Adamovicz, J.J., Gause, W.C., Hubbard, B.R., Gately, M.K. and Finkelman, F.D. (1994). Effects of IL-12 on in vivo cytokine gene expression and Ig isotype selection. *J. Immunol.* **152**, 1047–1056.

Mosier, D.E. (1967). A requirement for two cell types for antibody formation in vitro. *Science* **158**, 1573–1575.

Muraguchi, A., Hirano, T., Tang, B., Matsuda, T., Horii, Y., Nakajima, K. and Kishimoto, T. (1988). The essential role of B cell stimulatory factor 2 (BSF-2/IL-6) for the terminal differentiation of B cells. *J. Exp. Med.* **167**, 332–344.

Ohshima, Y., Tanaka, Y., Tozawa, H., Takahashi, Y., Maliszewski, C. and Delespesse, G. (1997). Expression and function of OX40 ligand on human dendritic cells. *J. Immunol.* **159**, 3838–3848.

Peters, M., Jacobs, S., Ehlers, M., Vollmer, P., Mullberg, J., Wolf, E., Brem, G., Meyer zum Buschenfelde, K.H. and Rose John, S. (1996). The function of the soluble interleukin 6 (IL-6) receptor in vivo: sensitization of human soluble IL-6 receptor transgenic mice towards IL-6 and prolongation of the plasma half-life of IL-6. *J. Exp. Med.* **183**, 1399–1406.

Romani, N., Gruner, S., Brang, D., Kämpgen, E., Lenz, A., Trockenbacher, B., Konwalinka, G., Fritsch, P.O., Steinman, R.M. and Schuler, G. (1994). Proliferating dendritic cell progenitors in human blood. *J. Exp. Med.* **180**, 83–93.

Rousset, F., Garcia, E. and Banchereau, J. (1991). Cytokine-induced proliferation and immunoglobulin production of human B lymphocytes triggered through their CD40 antigen. *J. Exp. Med.* **173**, 705–710.

Sallusto, F. and Lanzavecchia, A. (1994). Efficient presentation of soluble antigen by cultured human dendritic cells is maintained by granulocyte/macrophage colony-stimulating factor plus interleukin 4 and downregulated by tumor necrosis factor alpha. *J. Exp. Med.* **179**, 1109–1118.

Schrader, C.E. and Cebra, J.J. (1993). Dendritic cell dependent expression of IgA by clones in T/B microcultures. In *Dendritic Cells in Fundamental and Clinical Immunology* (ed. Kamperdijk, E.W.), Plenum Press, New York, pp. 59–64.

Schrader, C.E., Geroge, A., Kerlin, R.L. and Cebra, J.J. (1990). Dendritic cells support production of IgA and other non-IgM isotypes in clonal microculture. *Int. Immunol.* **2**, 563–570.

Scott, P. (1993). IL-12: initiation cytokine for cell-mediated immunity. *Science* **260**, 496–497.

Snapper, C.M. (1996). Interferon-gamma. In *Cytokine Regulation of Humoral Immunity. Basic and Clinical Aspects* (ed. C.M. Snapper). Wiley, Chichester, pp. 325–346.

Sornasse, T., Flamand, V., de Becker, G., Bazin, H., Tielemans, F., Thielemans, K., Urbain, J., Oberdan, L. and Moser, M. (1992). Antigen-pulse dendritic cells can efficiently induce an antibody response in vivo. *J. Exp. Med.* **175**, 15–21.

Spalding, D.M. and Griffin, J.A. (1986). Different pathways of differentiation of pre-B cell lines are induced by dendritic cells and T cells from different lymphoid tissues. *Cell* **44**, 507–515.

Steinman, R.M. and Cohn, Z.A. (1973). Identification of a novel cell type in peripheral lymphoid organs of mice. I. Morphology, quantitation, tissue distribution. *J. Exp. Med.* **137**, 1142–1162.

Steinman, R.M., Pack, M. and Inaba, K. (1997). Dendritic cells in the T-cell areas of lymphoid organs. *Immunol. Rev.* **156**, 25–37.

Tamura, T., Udagawa, N., Takahashi, N., Miyaura, C., Tanaka, S., Yamada, Y., Koishihara, Y., Ohsugi, Y., Kumaki, K. and Taga, T. (1993). Soluble interleukin-6 receptor triggers osteoclast formation by interleukin 6. *Proc. Natl Acad. Sci. USA* **90**, 11924–11928.

Tew, J.G., Phipps, R.P. and Mandel, T.E. (1980). The maintenance and regulation of the humoral immune response: persisting antigen and the role of follicular antigen-binding dendritic cells as accessory cells. *Immunol. Rev.* **53**, 175–201.

Uherova, P., Connick, E., MaWhinney, S., Schlichteimeier, R., Schooley, R.T. and Kuritzkes, D.R. (1996). In vitro effect of interleukin-12 on antigen-specific lymphocyte proliferative responses from persons infected with human immunodeficiency virus type 1. *J. Infect. Dis.* **174**, 483–489.

Westerink, M.A.J., Metzger, D.W., Hutchins, W.A., Adkins, A.R., Holder, P.F., Pais, L.B., Gheesling, L.L. and Carlone, G.M. (1997). Primary human immune response to *Neisseria meningitidis* serogroup C in interleukin-12-treated severe combined immunodeficient mice engrafted with human peripheral blood lymphocytes. *J. Infect. Dis.* **175**, 84–90.

Xu, J., Foy, T.M., Laman, J.D., Elliott, E.A., Dunn, J.J., Waldschmidt, T.J., Elsemore, J., Noelle, R.J. and Flavell, R.A. (1994). Mice deficient for the CD40 ligand. *Immunity* **1**, 423–431.

CHAPTER 16
Dendritic Cells and Cells of the Monocyte/Macrophage Lineage

Yasuo Yamaguchi and Michio Ogawa
Department of Surgery II, Kumamoto University Medical School, Kumamoto, Japan

INTRODUCTION

Dendritic cells (DC) are highly efficient antigen-presenting cells (APC) that are distributed widely throughout nonlymphoid and lymphoid tissue. APC can be categorized as professional or nonprofessional. While the latter are found predominantly in nonlymphoid organs, professional APC such as DC, macrophages, and B cells form an integral part of the immune system. DC are the most potent initiators of an immune response and, in particular, are responsible for the induction of primary antigen-specific immune reactions which prime naive T cells. Since the phenotypes of DC change during their life span, it is difficult to clearly establish individual phenotypes of DC through marker studies in order to determine ontogenetic derivation. DC can differentiate from both myeloid precursors and human peripheral blood monocytes. Thus, the relationship between macrophages and DC is made more complex by the potential of blood monocytes to become DC when appropriate cytokine signals are provided [1, 2].

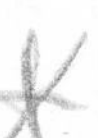

Studies of DC have been hampered greatly by difficulties in preparing reasonably pure DC in sufficient amounts. However, it has been shown that substantial numbers of functional DC can be generated by *in vitro* culture of blood or bone marrow precursors with appropriate cytokines. The ability to prepare pure, unstimulated DC is likely to provide novel and promising treatments of various immunological disorders. Accordingly, the concept of developmental plasticity not only has widespread implications for understanding immune defense and tolerance induction [3], but also promises to be of increasing value for future therapeutic applications [4]. In this chapter, we will discuss the relationships between DC and cells of the monocyte/macrophage lineage in terms of biology, development, and maturation, along with potential clinical implications.

CHARACTERISTICS OF DENDRITIC CELLS

DC develop from bone marrow myeloid lineage precursors and spread throughout tissue as interdigitating DC. The differentiation stages of DC are not well defined because of the lack of specific markers. In addition, DC and macrophages, long assumed to differentiate via separate pathways, are now believed to share transitional

Dendritic Cells: Biology and Clinical Applications
ISBN 0-12-455860-7

stages. In addition, the ability to derive DC from blood monocytes further complicates the separation of DC from monocytes [1].

The mechanisms that control the differentiation of DC during ontogeny, as well as the developmental stage at which DC precursors reach peripheral organs, have not been characterized. DC originate from major histocompatibility complex (MHC) class II-negative precursors and give rise to low MHC class II-positive cells (immature) which are poor stimulators in the primary mixed leukocyte reaction (MLR) assay, but are very efficient in antigen uptake and processing. It has been hypothesized that during this immature stage, in the absence of high levels of costimulatory molecules such as B7, DC may induce tolerance instead of immunity [5]. This hypothesis agrees with the two-signal theory in which activation of unprimed cells is achieved [6, 7] only when both signal 1 (antigenic signal) and signal 2 (costimulation signal) are delivered to T cells. In contrast, DC mature and acquire high MHC class II and B7 expression on their cell surface after activation, acquiring the ability to prime naive T cells and initiate a primary immune response. In fact, DC residing in unperturbed tissue efficiently capture and process antigen, but are poor activators of T cells. Differential functionality is found in DC isolated from blood and lymph nodes [8]. In response to tissue changes caused by infection, entrance of toxic chemicals, or necrosis, DC rapidly mature into cells with very potent APC properties [9].

Human DC are characterized by morphology, CD1a expression [10], high levels of MHC class II and accessory/costimulatory molecules, lack of CD14 expression and nonspecific esterase, and efficient elicitation of allogeneic MLR. The primary function of nonlymphoid DC is antigen uptake. Nonlymphoid DCs mature and migrate via the afferent lymphatics to T cell-rich regions of draining lymph nodes and the spleen where they develop antigen-presenting function [3, 11]. DC are more efficient than B cells and macrophages in the primary activation of naive T cells and antigen-pulsed DC, and can be administered *in situ* to prime T cells without additional adjuvants.

The precise role of APC in regulating the balance of T-helper type 1 (T_H1) and T-helper type 2 (T_H2) cytokine production is unclear. DC, the most potent activators of naive T cells, regulate T_H1 and T_H2 cytokine profiles in a fashion dependent on their tissue origin [12]. Splenic (systemic) DC primarily induce T_H1 cytokines, while Peyer's patch (mucosal) DC predominantly induce T_H2 cytokines. These observations support the concept that different tissues, each with a distinct microenvironment of cytokines, hormones, and cellular elements, are involved in the selection, promotion, and/or maintenance of different immune responses. The tissue from which DC originate determines the cytokines produced by T cells. DC derived from different tissues favor either cellular or humoral immune responses by influencing T-cell cytokine production. The tissue microenvironment may play an important role in controlling the development of immune responses. The balance of T_H1 and T_H2 cells, as well as the cytokine levels produced by these cells is important in determining whether protective or harmful sequelae result from T cell activation.

DC PROGENITORS

DC originate from a bone marrow $CD34^+$ precursor common to granulocytes and macrophages. A separate DC colony-forming unit (CFU-DC) that gives rise to pure DC colonies have been established in humans. $CD14^+$ blood monocytes can differentiate into functionally mature $CD83^+$ cells [13]. In addition, a post-CFU $CD14^+$ intermediate has been described which has the potential to differentiate along the DC or the macrophage pathway depending on the cytokine conditions [2]. This bipotential precursor is present in bone marrow, cord blood, and peripheral blood. Thus, blood monocytes can become DC when the appropriate cytokine signals are provided [1, 2]. The relationship between macrophages and DC is more complex in terms of ontogenicity.

DC can differentiate from myeloid precursors and human peripheral blood monocytes. The disruption of DC differentiation has been found to lead to enhanced production of macrophages and neutrophils [14], which supports the concept of a common lineage of DC and macrophages. Hence, DC and macrophages may be considered as polar representatives of one common regulatory system [1]. In addition, it remains difficult to identify true DC progenitors. DC may arise from committed stem cells common to monocytes and neutrophils [15], T cells, B cells, and/or NK cells [16]. They also may differentiate from monocytes.

Although human DC are derived from hematopoietic cells, their ontogeny is not entirely clear. Granulocyte-macrophage colony-stimulating factor (GM-CSF), tumor necrosis factor-α (TNF-α), and stem cell factor (SCF) have been shown to promote the growth of DC from $CD34^+$ haematopoietic progenitors *in vitro* [17–19]. Cells having the phenotypic and functional characteristics of DC have also been produced from fully differentiated human monocytes/macrophages using GM-CSF, interleukin-4 (IL-4), and serum [20–22].

There are two possible pathways of DC development. DC may originate from a myeloid precursor that is common to the monocyte/macrophage developmental pathway. DC may branch off early within this lineage to appear in the blood as immature-type DC which then fully differentiate after entering tissues.

Alternatively, DC and monocyte/macrophages may develop from a late monocyte or 'intermediate cell' which is poorly adherent, weakly phagocytic, and expresses low levels of nonspecific esterase and Fc receptors. Interconversion of DC and macrophages has not been clearly demonstrated [6].

DC MATURATION

Immature dendritic cells are recruited rapidly to sites of inflammation and are highly proficient in antigen uptake. The development and maturation of DC are dependent upon cytokines such as GM-CSF, TNF-α, and IL-1α *in vitro*. During the maturation process, they lose their ability to process and present soluble antigen and become extremely potent stimulators of T-lymphocytes [9, 23, 24].

The maturation of DC is completed only after they interact with T cells. The T cell-dependent maturation of DC is mediated by interactions between surface molecules (e.g. CD40 ligand (CD40L)–CD40) and by T cell-derived cytokines like IFN-γ [25, 26]. In addition, as yet unidentified factors released from activated monocytes can support the final stages of DC maturation [27, 28]. DC differentiate under the influence of broad microenvironmental factors and locally produced cytokines including GM-CSF, TNF-α, and IL-1β. These factors share properties with other inflammatory signals produced by bacteria, lipopolysaccharide (LPS), and lipotheicoic acid (LTA), which are all potent activators of DC. Activated DC are characterized by upregulation of MHC class II molecules and of the costimulatory molecules CD40 and B7-2. Upregulation of MHC class II mainly results from redistribution of molecules from intracellular vesicular compartments to the cell surface [29]. Immature DC appear loosely adherent to the surface of culture dishes, whereas mature DC detach from the plastic surface, develop larger veils and longer dendrites, and form large floating aggregates that phenotypically resemble bright class II FACS-sorted cells. DC that have encountered antigens have been shown to undergo a maturation process that renders them capable of migrating to regional lymph nodes and activating antigen-specific naive T cells [30].

DC MIGRATION

DC may migrate from epithelia exclusively via afferent lymph into regional nodes, and from solid organs via both afferent lymph and blood into regional nodes and the spleen [31, 32], respectively. Within afferent lymph, DC are often referred to as 'veiled cells' because of their distinctive cytological features, specifically the presence of sheet-like lamellipodia. Thus, there is continual movement of DC from peripheral tissue to lymph nodes via afferent lymphatics [33]. In fact, application of antigens to peripheral tissue can lead to increased DC release from tissue into lymph. Application of contact-sensitizing agents to skin causes a loss of Langerhans cells from the epidermis [34] and an increase in the number of DC that can be released from draining nodes. Skin transplantation or the maintenance of skin in organ culture alters the distribution of Langerhans cells in the epidermis [35].

The development and maturation of DC are certainly dependent on several cytokines, but little is known about the mediators of DC migration *in vivo* or the stimuli necessary to recruit DC progenitors to tissue. There is evidence that intradermal administration of GM-CSF leads to an increase in the number of DC within the dermis of human skin, and these DC may be the precursors of epidermal Langerhans cells [36]. In addition, GM-CSF produced by normal and inflamed tissue, and some carcinomas, within the human lung appears to recruit CD1a$^+$ Langerhans cells to local sites [37]. Additional information is provided by studies showing that DC are recruited into the epithelium of rat airways in response to LPS delivered in aerosol form to the lungs. The kinetics of the resulting transient influx of DC mirror those of the neutrophil component of an acute inflammatory response [38]. Thus, during acute inflammation, active DC 'surveillance' of the adjacent lining epithelium is amplified, resulting in an increase in the movement of these cells between the airway epithelium and regional lymph nodes [39].

APC have several mechanisms to internalize antigens. The best-characterized mechanisms are phagocytosis by macrophages and Langerhans cells [30], and receptor-mediated endocytosis by B cells [40, 41]. In monocyte-derived DC and Langerhans cells, the most efficient routes of antigen internalization have been attributed to macropinocytosis and mannose receptor-mediated endocytosis [42, 43]. DC found in nonlymphoid organs can internalize and process foreign antigens before migrating to secondary lymphoid tissue where they initiate primary immune responses. However, it is unclear which stimuli promote migration of DC from the tissue after antigen internalization.

Systemic administration of LPS leads to a reduction in the number of MHC class II-positive (Ia$^+$) leukocytes in mouse heart and kidney This response is due to migration of DC rather than to a loss of Ia expression or cytotoxic effects. DC from the gut (lamina propria), but not from lymph nodes, have been found to migrate into lymph after systemic LPS treatment [44]. Similarly, the number of Ia^+ epidermal Langerhans cells also was reduced after LPS administration in mice. Thus, with regard to the distribution and localization of APC, systemic LPS administration can increase migration of DC, especially from nonlymphoid tissue [44, 45]. DC migration appears to be controlled, at least in part, by cytokines like TNF-α and IL-1 which are probably produced by macrophages following endotoxin stimulation. Systemic administration of recombinant TNF-α results in a decrease in the number of Ia^+ cells in heart and kidney, as well as a decrease in epidermal Langerhans cells [46]. Administration of rhIL-1 causes a decrease in Ia^+ cells only in the renal medulla. rhIL-2 produces no obvious effects. The release of DC is almost totally blocked by a monoclonal anti-TNF-α antibody [33]. Therefore, TNF-α and IL-1α may promote DC migration from nonlymphoid tissue and may have differential effects on different DC populations. It is unclear whether these factors act directly or indirectly on DC [45].

CHEMOKINES AND DC

Chemokines comprise a family of secreted proteins that attract and activate a variety of cell types, and generally augment the immune response. The C-C chemokines usually act on monocytes, T-lymphocytes, and in some cases eosinophils, basophils, or mast cells. In contrast, the C-X-C chemokines generally act on neutrophils. Several C-C chemokines, including MCP-3, MIP-1α, and RANTES, are chemotactic for immature DC [47]. Recently, Godiska *et al.* [48] have described a novel human CC chemokine, macrophage-derived chemokine (MDC), which is highly expressed by fully differentiated macrophages and monocyte-derived DC, but it is not expressed by freshly isolated monocytes, granulocytic cells, or natural killer (NK) cells. Monocyte-derived DC and IL-2-activated NK cells migrate in response to MDC exposure in a dose-dependent manner. The activity and expression pattern of MDC may help explain the function of DC and may play an autocrine role in the accumulation of DC at sites of inflammation.

DC PROPAGATION

Over the past few years it has become possible to grow DC from bone marrow and blood progenitors and to control production of different stages of the lineage *in vitro*. Development of immature human DC is promoted by culture of bone marrow or blood progenitors in the presence of GM-CSF and IL-4 [20, 21, 49]. Further maturation can be induced by subsequent exposure to TNF-α [50], CD40 ligand, or to other agents such as LPS [42].

GM-CSF generally appears to be required for DC differentiation. Culture of monocytes in the presence of GM-CSF upregulates CD1a [51]. The incubation of monocytes with IL-4 causes the downregulation of CD14 [52–54]. Complete differentiation of DC can eventually be achieved when peripheral blood mononuclear cells [21], adherent blood cells [20], or monocytes [22] are incubated in culture media containing IL-4, GM-CSF, serum, and/or endogenous factors. In addition, other signals which upregulate expression of MHC class II, such as IFN-γ, synergize with IL-4 and GM-CSF to enhance the generation and functional potency of monocyte-derived DC (MODC) [55]. Their ability to capture soluble antigens, as well as the observation that their stimulatory capacity in MLR can be enhanced, suggests that human monocyte/macrophage DC derived with IL-4/GM-CSF are functionally more immature than DC derived from hematopoietic progenitors treated with TNF-α/GM-CSF [21]. Stem cell factor (SCF) enhances the proliferation of mixed colony-forming units (CFU)-DC/MO or pure CFU-DC [56, 57]. DC maturation may continue until they interact with T cells [58] through cross-linking of CD40 which upregulates expression of the costimulatory molecules CD80 (B7-1) and CD86 (B7-2) [59].

A large amount of information has been obtained by studying early CD34$^+$ stem cells in conjunction with monocytes. Triozzi *et al.* [60] have identified phenotypic and functional differences between human DC derived *in vitro* from hematopoietic progenitors and from monocytes/macrophages. Specifically, stem cells grown in the presence of TNF-α and GM-CSF give rise to CD14^{dim} cells that partially express Birbeck granules which are typical of Langerhans cells. After prolonged culture, stem cell-derived DC lose their characteristic morphology and the resulting colonies comprise macrophages and dendritic-like cells, suggesting that DC represent a transient state within the monocyte/macrophage lineage [61].

Transforming growth factor-β (TGF-β) is a pleiotropic 25 kDa homodimeric polypeptide produced by numerous cells. It has a variety of biological activities including the stimulation of cell proliferation and differentiation of many cell types [62]. The combination of GM-CSF and TNF-α, along with stem cell factor, commonly used for *in vitro* generation of DC in serum/plasma-supplemented medium, is very inefficient in inducing DC development in the absence of serum supplementation. However, supplementation with TGF-β1 is required for substantial DC development in the absence of serum [63]. Thus, TGF-β1 is an effective substitute for plasma and allows the development of DC from CD34$^+$ hematopoietic progenitors.

Recent advances in the ability to propagate large quantities of peripheral blood-derived DC using GM-CSF and IL-4 may provide the necessary tools for better understanding the role of DC in human disease [4, 64–66].

IMMUNOTHERAPY

One of the most important goals of DC research is the development of DC-based strategies for enhancing immune responses against tumors and infectious agents. Various studies using animal models have shown clearly that DC pulsed with tumor antigens *in vitro* and then reinjected *in vivo* induce protective immune responses that block tumor growth [67]. In addition, human studies have confirmed the value of such an approach [68].

Plasmid expression by invading professional APC is responsible for immune induction [69]. It is conceivable that DC with specific properties important for immune activation are crucially involved [11]. Indeed, an ever-increasing collection of proteins, peptides, and/or mRNA incorporated into DC *in vitro* subsequently enhances the level of immune induction achieved *in vivo* [70–75]. Cutaneous injection of naked DNA in mice can result in transfection of skin-derived DC which subsequently localize to draining lymph nodes [76]. Furthermore, the intramuscular delivery of naked plasmid DNA that encodes two proteins of herpes simplex virus (HSV) to DC leads to the induction of significantly enhanced resistance to viral challenge. Whereas DC transfected *in vitro* with DNA induce enhanced immunity, similarly transfected macrophages lack immunogenicity even though plasmid expression occurred *in vitro*. Enhanced immunity induced by DC-delivered DNA appears to be primarily associated with an increased T_H1 $CD4^+$ T cell response [77].

Girolomoni *et al.* [78] have indicated that the pulsing of DC with peptides may not be suitable for clinical application because of strict MHC restrictions of the immune response. Similarly, the use of unfractionated tumor-derived proteins may not be practical because tumor fragments of sufficient dimension are often unavailable, and there is a possibility of inducing immune responses against self-antigens. Interesting alternative approaches include DC pulsing with particulates carrying naive tumor protein antigens or innocuous bacteria engineered to express one or more tumor antigens. These methods can be effective in delivering exogenous proteins into the class I processing pathway. Other possibilities include the pulsing of DC *in vitro* with tumor-derived RNA, a procedure that generates large amounts of antigens from very small tumor fragments [71], or the transfection of DC with cDNA encoding tumor antigens [79, 80].

Other problems associated with immunotherapy using antigen-pulsed DC include the induction of sensitization or anergy. Antigen-specific $CD8^+$ cell responses are initiated by host immunization with P815AB, a self-peptide bearing CTL epitopes that are expressed by murine mastocytoma cells. The development of a T_H1-like response to P815-pulsed DC requires T-helper effects such as those mediated by coimmunization with MHC class II-restricted (helper) peptides or recombinant human IL-12. IL-12, a heterodimeric cytokine produced by activated monocytes and DC, plays a crucial role in regulating IFN-γ production and in generating IFN-γ-producing T_H1 cells [81]. The adjuvant effect of recombinant IL-12 (rIL-12) may involve improved recognition of class II-restricted epitopes of P815AB. IL-12 stimulates NK cells, mediates T_H1 development, and fosters CTL development [82]. Antigen-specific T cell anergy also is observed after neutralization of endogenous IL-12 at the time of priming with P185AB and helper peptide. All of these effects are reversed by rIL-12. Anergy induction thus may contribute to P815AB unresponsiveness *in vivo*. The induction of IL-12 responsiveness may be impaired in anergic T-lymphocytes [83]. IL-12 may act to prevent or revert anergy to tumor-associated and/or self-peptides [84]. Similarly, IL-12 initiates reactivity and prevents tolerance in a mouse model of contact sensitivity [85, 86]. Activated/memory T cells express CD40L and efficiently stimulate IL-12 production by DC, as well as further upregulating adhesion and costimulatory properties [87–89]. The importance of the CD40/CD40 ligand interaction for IL-12 induction in DC probably contributes to the recent finding that mice lacking the CD40 ligand have difficulty in mounting T_H1-type cell-mediated immune responses [90]. These observations have therapeutic implications if cultured DCs are used as adjuvants for immunization [91]. T cell tolerance also is induced in adult mice by the intravenous injection of soluble peptides [92, 93]. The responsible underlying mechanisms may involve ignorance to antigen or anergy to deletion [94, 95]. The nature of a self-peptide like P815AB might contribute to the low immunogenicity in a naive host via induction of T cell unresponsiveness [96].

One of the problems in the immunotherapy of cancer is that a tumor antigen exists but remains unidentified in most human cancers. Thus, DC have been pulsed with synthetic tumor peptides [97], tumor-associated antigen-derived epitopes [98], and

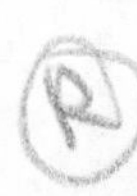

peptides eluted from class I MHC molecules or RNA from tumors [67]. In this context, Gong *et al.* [99] have reported that murine MC38 adenocarcinoma cells can be fused to bone marrow-derived DC and that immunization with the fusion cells induces rejection of established metastases. Vaccination with the fusion cells may be an alternative DC-based strategy for the immunotherapy of cancer.

SUMMARY

Cells of the monocyte/macrophage lineage are related closely to DC development, maturation, and migration, all of which are associated with cytokine production. In addition, there is considerable interest in using antigen-pulsed DC in the immunotherapy of infectious diseases, including human immunodeficiency virus-1, and cancer.

REFERENCES

1. Peters, J.H., Gieseler, R., Thiele, B. and Steinbach, F. (1996). Dendritic cells: from ontogenic orphans to myelomonocytic descendants. *Immunol. Today* **17**, 273–278.
2. Caux, C., Vanbervliet, B., Massacrier, C., Dezutter-Dambuyant, C., de Saint-Vis, B., Jacquet, C., Yoneda, K., Imamura, S., Schmit, D. and Banchereau, J. (1996) CD34$^+$ hematopoietic progenitors from human cord blood differentiate along two independent dendritic cell pathways in response to GM-CSF +TNF-α. *Blood* **184**, 695–706.
3. Ibrahim, M.A., Chain, B.M. and Katz, D.R. (1995).The injured cell: the role of the dendritic cell system as a sentinel receptor pathway. *Immunol. Today* **16**, 181–186.
4. Grabbe, S., Beissert, S., Schwarz, T. and Granstein, R.D. (1991). Dendritic cells as initiators of tumor immune response: a possible strategy for tumor immunotherapy? *Immunol. Today* **16**, 117–121.
5. Finkelman, F.D., Lees, A., Birbaum, R., Cause, W.C. and Morris, S.C. (1996). Dendritic cells can present antigen *in vivo* in a tolerogenic or immunogenic fashion. *J. Immunol.* **157**, 1406–1414.
6. Janeway, C.A. (1992). The immune system evolved to discriminate infectious nonself from noninfectious self. *Immunol. Today* **113**, 11–16.
7. Matzinger, P. (1994). Tolerance, danger, and the extended family. *Annu. Rev. Immunol.* **12**, 991–1045.
8. Hill, S., Coates, J.P., Kimber, I. and Knight, S.C. (1994). Differential function of dendritic cells isolated from blood and lymph nodes. *Immunology* **83**, 295–301.
9. Rescigno, M., Winzler, C., Delia, D., Mutini, C., Lutz, M. and Ricciardi-Castagnoli, P. (1997). Dendritic cell maturation is required for initiation of the immune response. *J. Leukocyte Biol.* **61**, 415–421.
10. Porcelli, S.A. (1995). The CD1 family: a third lineage of antigen-presenting molecules. *Adv. Immunol.* **59**, 1–98.
11. Steinman, R.M. (1991) The dendritic cell system and its role in immunogenicity. *Annu. Rev. Immunol.* **9**, 271–296.
12. Everson, M.P., McDuffie, D.S., Lemak, D.G., Koopman, W.J., McGhee, J.R. and Beagley, K.W. (1996). Dendritic cells from different tissues induce production of different T cell cytokine profiles. *J. Leukocyte Biol.* **59**, 494–498.
13. Zhou, L.-J. and Tedder, T.F. (1996). CD14$^+$ blood monocytes can differentiate into functionally mature CD83$^+$ dendritic cells. *Proc. Natl Acad. Sci. USA* **93**, 2588–2592.
14. Burkly, L., Hession, C., Ogata, L., Reilly, C., Marconi, L.A., Olsen, D., Tizard, R., Cate, R. and Lo, D. (1995). Expression of relB is required for the development of thymic medulla and dendritic cell. *Nature* **373**, 531–536.
15. Inaba, K., Inaba, M., Deguchi, M., Hagi, K., Yasumizu, R., Ikehara, S. and Muramatsu, S. (1993). Granulocytes, macrophages, and dendritic cells arise from a common major histocompatibility complex class II-negative progenitor in mouse bone marrow. *Proc. Natl Acad. Sci. USA* **90**, 3038–3042.
16. Galy, A., Travis, M., Cen, D. and Chen, B. (1995). Human T, B, natural killer, and dendritic cells arise from a common bone marrow progenitor cell subset. *Immunity* **3**, 459–473.

17. Bernhard, H., Disis, M.L., Heimfeld, S., Hand, S., Gralow, J.R. and Cheever, M.A. (1995). Generation of immunostimulatory dendritic cells from human $CD34^+$ hematopoietic progenitor cells of the bone marrow and peripheral blood. *Cancer Res.* **55**, 1099–1104.
18. Szabolcs, P., Moore, M.A. and Young, J.W. (1995). Expansion of immunostimulatory dendritic cells among the myeloid progeny of human $CD34^+$ bone marrow precursors cultured with c-kit ligand, granulocyte-macrophage colony-stimulating factors, and TNF-α. *J. Immunol.* **154**, 5851–5861.
19. Strunk, D., Rappersberger, K., Egger, C., Strobl, H., Kromer, E., Elbe, A., Maurer, D. and Sting, G. (1996). Generation of human dendritic cells/Langerhans cells from circulating $CD34^+$ hematopoietic progenitor cells. *Blood* **87**, 1292–1302.
20. Sallusto, F. and Lanzavecchia, A. (1994). Efficient presentation of soluble antigen by cultured human dendritic cells is maintained by granulocyte/macrophage colony-stimulating factor plus interleukin 4 and downregulated by tumor necrosis factor α. *J. Exp. Med.* **179**, 1109–1118.
21. Romani, N., Gruner, S., Brang, D., Kampgen, E., Lenz, A., Trockenbacher, B., Konwalinka, G., Fritsch, P.O., Steinman, R.M. and Schuler, G. (1994). Proliferating dendritic cell progenitors in human blood. *J. Exp. Med.* **180**, 83–93.
22. Steinbach, R., Krause, B. and Thiele, B. (1995). Monocyte derived dendritic cells (MODC) present phenotype and functional activities of Langerhans cell/dendritic cells. *Adv. Exp. Med. Biol.* **378**, 151–153.
23. Austyn, J.M. (1992). Antigen uptake and presentation by dendritic leukocytes. *Semin. Immunol.* **4**, 227–236.
24. Austyn, J.M. (1996). New insights into the mobilization and phagocytic activity of dendritic cells. *J. Exp. Med.* **183**, 1287–1292.
25. Cella, M., Scheidegger, D., Palmer-Lehmann, K., Lane, P., Lanzavecchia, A. and Albert, G. (1996). Ligation of CD40 on dendritic cells triggers production of high levels of interleukin-12 and enhances T cell stimulatory capacity: T–T help via APC activation. *J. Exp. Med.* **184**, 747–752.
26. Kitajima, T., Caceres-Dittmar, G., Tapia, F.J., Jester, J., Bergstresser, P.R. and Takashima, A. (1996). T cell-mediated terminal maturation of dendritic cells. *J. Immunol.* **157**, 2340–2347.
27. Bender, A., Sapp, M., Schuler, G., Steinman, R.M. and Bhardwaj, N. (1996). Improved methods for the generation of dendritic cells from nonproliferating progenitors in human blood. *J. Immunol. Methods* **196**, 121–135.
28. Romani, N., Reider, D., Heuer, M., Ebner, S., Kampgen, E., Eibl, B., Niederwieser, D. and Schuler, G. (1996). Generation of mature dendritic cells from human blood: an improved method with special regard to clinical applicability. *J. Immunol. Methods* **196**, 137–151.
29. Winzler, C., Rovere, P., Rescigno, M., Citterio, S., Cranucci, F., Mutini, C., Adorini, L., Penna, G., Delia, D., Zimmermann, V.S., Davoust, J. and Ricciardi-Castagnoli, P. (1997). Maturational stages of mouse dendritic cells in growth factor-dependent long-term cultures. *J. Exp. Med.* **185**, 317–328.
30. Reis e Sousa, C., Stahl, P.D. and Austyn, J.M. (1993). Phagocytosis of antigens by Langerhans cells *in vitro*. *J. Exp. Med.* **178**, 509-519.
31. Austyn, J.M. and Larsen, C.P. (1990). Migration patterns of dendritic leukocytes: implications for transplantation. *Transplantation* **49**, 1–7, 1990.
32. Larsen, C.P., Morris, P.J. and Austyn, J.M. (1990). Migration of dendritic leukocytes from cardiac allografts into host spleens. A novel pathway for initiation of rejection. *J. Exp. Med.* **171**, 307–314.
33. MacPherson, G.G., Jenkins, C.D., Stein, M.J., Edwards, C. (1995). Endotoxin-mediated dendritic cell release from the intestine. Characterization of released dendritic cells and TNF dependence. *J. Immunol.* **154**, 1317–1322.
34. Vermeer, M., Streilein, J.W. (1990). Ultraviolet B light-induced alterations in epidermal Langerhans cells are mediated in part by tumor necrosis factor-α. *Photodermatol. Photoimmunol. Photomed.* **7**, 258–265.
35. Larsen, C.P., Steinmann, R.M., Witmer-Pack, M., Hankins, D.F., Morris, P.J. and Austyn, J.M. (1990). Migration and maturation of Langerhans cells in skin transplants and explants. *J. Exp. Med.* **172**, 1483–1493.
36. Kaplan, G., Walsh, G., Guido, L.S., Meyn, P., Burkhardt, R.A., Abalos, R.M., Barker, J., Frindt, P.A., Fajardo, T.T., Celona, R. and Cohn, Z.A. (1992). Novel responses of human skin to intradermal recombinant granulocyte/macrophage colony-stimulating factor: Langerhans cell recruitment, keratinocyte growth, and enhanced wound healing. *J. Exp. Med.* **175**, 1717–1728.

37. Tazi, A., Bouchonnet, F., Grandsaigne, M., Boumsell, L., Hance, A.J. and Soler, P. (1993). Evidence that granulocyte macrophage-colony-stimulating factor regulates the distribution and differentiated state of dendritic cells/Langerhans cells in human and lung cancers. *J. Clin. Invest.* **91**, 556–576.
38. Schon-Hegard, M.A., Oliver, J., McMenamin, P.G. and Holt, P.G. (1991). Studies on the density, distribution, and surface phenotype of intraepithelial class II major histocompatibility complex antigen (Ia)-bearing dendritic cells (DC) in the conducting airway. *J. Exp. Med.* **173**, 1345–1356.
39. McWilliam, A.S., Nelson D., Thomas, J.A. and Holt, P.G. (1994). Rapid dendritic cell recruitment is a hallmark of the acute inflammatory response at mucosal surfaces. *J. Exp. Med.* **179**, 1331–1336.
40. Lamaze, C. and Schmidt, S.L. (1995). The emergence of clathrin-independent pinocytic pathways. *Curr. Opin. Cell Biol.* **7**, 573–580.
41. Robinson, M.S., Watts, C. and Zerial, M. (1996). Membrane dynamics in endocytosis. *Cell* **84**, 13–21.
42. Sallusto, F., Cella, M., Danieli, C. and Lanzavecchia, A. (1995). Dendritic cells use macropinocytosis and the mannose receptor to concentrate macromolecules in the major histocompatibility complex class II compartment: down-regulation by cytokines and bacterial products. *J. Exp. Med.* **182**, 389–400.
43. Lutz, M.B., Assmann, C.U., Girolomoni, G. and Ricciardi-Castagnoli, P. (1996). Different cytokines regulate antigen uptake and presentation of a precursor dendritic cell line. *Eur. J. Immunol.* **26**, 586–594.
44. MacPherson, G.C., Jenkins, C.D., Stein, M.J. and Edwards, C. (1995). Endotoxin-mediated dendritic cell release from the intestine: characterization of released dendritic cells and TNF dependence. *J. Immunol.* **154**, 1317–1322.
45. Roake, J.A., Rao, A.S., Morris, P.J., Larsen, C.P., Hankins, D.F. and Austyn, J.M. (1995). Dendritic cell loss from nonlymphoid tissues after systemic administration of lipopolysaccharide, tumor necrosis factor, and interleukin 1. *J. Exp. Med.* **181**, 2237–2247.
46. Cumberbatch, M. and Kimber, I. (1992). Dermal tumor necrosis factor-alpha induces dendritic cell migration to draining lymph nodes, and possibly provides one stimulus for Langerhans' cell migration. *Immunology* **75**, 257–263.
47. Sozzani, S., Sallusto, F., Luini, W., Zhou, D., Piemontli, L., Allavena, P., VanDamme, J., Valitutti, S., Lanzavecchia, A. and Mantovani, A. (1995). Migration of dendritic cells in response to formyl peptides, C5a and a distinct set of chemokines. *J. Immunol.* **155**, 3292–3295.
48. Godiska, R., Chantry, D., Raport, C.J., Sozzani, S., Allavena, P., Leviten, D., Mantovani, A. and Gray, P.W. (1997). Human macrophage-derived chemokine (MDC), a novel chemoattractant for monocyte-derived dendritic cells, and natural killer cells. *J. Exp. Med.* **185**, 1595–1604.
49. Kiertscher, A.M. and Roth, M.D. (1996). Human $CD14^+$ leukocytes acquire the phenotype and function of antigen-presenting dendritic cells when cultured in GM-CSF and IL-4. *J. Leukocyte Biol.* **59**, 208–218.
50. Caux, C, Vanbervliet, B., Massacrier, C., Dezutter-Dambuyant, C., de Saint-Vis, B., Jacquet, C., Yoneda, K., Imamura, S., Schmitt, D. and Banchereau, J. (1996). $CD34^+$ hematopoeitic progenitors from human cord blood differentiate along two independent dendritic cell pathways in response to GM-CSF+TNF-α. *Blood* **184**, 695–706.
51. Kasinrerk, W., Baumruker, T., Majdic, O., Knapp, W. and Stockinger, H. (1993). CD1 molecule expression on human monocytes induced by granulocyte-macrophage colony-stimulating factor. *J. Immunol* **150**, 579–584.
52. Peters, J.H., Ruppert, J., Gieseler, R.K., Najar, H.M. and Xu, H. (1991). Differentiation of human monocytes into CD14 negative accessory cells: do dendritic cells derive from the monocytic lineage? *Pathobiology* **59**, 122–126.
53. Ruppert, J., Friedrichs, D., Xu, H. and Peters, J.H. (1991). IL-4 decreases the expression of the monocyte differentiation marker CD14, paralleled by an increasing accessory potency. *Immunobiology* **182**, 449–464.
54. Lauener, R.P., Goyert, S.M., Geha, R.S. and Vercelli, D. (1990). Interleukin-4 down-regulates the expression of CD14 in normal human monocytes. *Eur. J. Immunol.* **20**, 2375–2381.
55. Xu, H., Kramer, M., Spengler, H.P. and Peters, J.H. (1995). Dendritic cells differentiated from human monocytes through a combination of IL-4, GM-CSF and IFN-gamma exhibit phenotype and function of blood dendritic cells. *Adv. Exp. Med. Biol.* **378**, 75–78.
56. Young, J.W., Szabolcs, P. and Moore, M.A.S. (1995). Identification of dendritic cell colony-forming units among normal human $CD34^+$ bone marrow progenitors that are expanded by c-kit-ligand and

yield pure dendritic cell colonies in the presence of granulocyte/macrophage colony-stimulating factor and tumor necrosis factor alpha. *J. Exp. Med.* **182**, 1111–1119.

57. Santiago-Schwartz, F., Laky, K. and Carsons, S.E. (1995) Stem cell factor enhances dendritic cell development. *Adv. Exp. Med. Biol.* **378**, 7–11.
58. Caux, C., Massacrier, C., Vanbervliet, B., Dubois, B., Van Kooten, C., Durand, I. and Banchereau, J. (1994). Activation of human dendritic cells through CD40 cross-linking. *J. Exp. Med.* **180**, 1263–1272.
59. Lanier, L.L., O'Fallon, S., Somoza, C., Phillips, J.H., Linsley, P.S., Okumura, K., Ito, D. and Azuma, M. (1995). CD80 (B7) and CD86 (B70) provide similar costimulatory signals for T cell proliferation, cytokine production, and generation of CTL. *J. Immunol.* **154**, 97–105.
60. Triozzi, P.L. and Aldrich, W. (1997). Phenotype and functional differences between human dendritic cells derived *in vitro* from hematopoietic progenitors and from monocytes/macrophages. *J. Leukocyte. Biol.* **61**, 600–608.
61. Santiago-Schwarz, F., Belilos, E., Diamond, B. and Carsons, S.E. (1992). TNF in combination with GM-CSF enhances the differentiation of neonatal cord blood stem cells into dendritic cells and macrophages. *J. Leukocyte Biol.* **52**, 274–281.
62. Massangue, J. (1990) The transforming growth factor-β family. *Annu. Rev. Cell. Biol.* **6**, 597–641.
63. Strobl, H., Riedl, E., Scheinecker, C., Bello-Fernandez, C., Pickl, W.F., Rappersberger, K. and Majdic, O. (1996). TGF-beta 1 promotes *in vitro* development of dendritic cells from $CD34^+$ hemopoietic progenitors. *J. Immunol.* **157**, 1499–1506.
64. Caux, S., Liu, Y.-J. and Banchereau, J. (1995). Recent advances in the study of dendritic cells and follicular dendritic cells. *Immunol. Today* **16**, 2–4.
65. Huang, A., Columbek, P., Ahmadzadeh, M., Jaffe, E., Pardoll, D. and Levitsky, H. (1994). Role of bone marrow-derived cells in presenting MHC class I-restricted tumor antigens. *Science* **264**, 961–965.
66. Weissman, D., Yuexia, L., Ananworanich, J., Zhou, L.-Z., Adelsberger, J., Tedder, T.F., Baseler, M. and Fauci, A.S. (1995). Three populations of cells with dendritic morphology exist in peripheral blood, only one of which is infectable with human immnodeficiency virus type I. *Proc. Natl Acad. Sci. USA* **92**, 826–830.
67. Young, J.W. and Inaba, K. (1996). Dendritic cells as adjuvants for class I major histocompatibility complex-restricted antitumor immunity. *J. Exp. Med.* **183**, 7–11.
68. Hsu, F.J., Benike, C., Fagnoni, F., Liles, T.M., Czerwinski, D., Taidi, B., Engleman, E.G. and Levy, R. (1996). Vaccination of patients with B-cell lymphoma using autologous antigen-pulsed dendritic cells. *Nature Medicine* **2**, 52–58.
69. Raz, E., Carson, D.A., Parker, S.E., Parr, T.B., Abai, A.M., Aichinger, G., Gromkowksi, S.H., Singh, M., Lew, D., Yankauckas, M.A., Baird, S.M. and Rhodes, G.H. (1994). Intradermal gene immunization: the possible role of DNA uptake in the induction of cellular immunity. *Proc. Natl Acad. Sci. USA* **91**, 9519–9523.
70. Grewal, I.S., Xu, J. and Flavell, R.A. (1995). Impairment of antigen-specific T-cell priming in mice lacking CD40 ligand. *Nature* **378**, 617–620.
71. Boczkowski, D., Nair, S.K., Snyder, D. and Gilboa, E. (1996). Dendritic cells pulsed with RNA are potent antigen presenting cells *in vitro* and *in vivo*. *J. Exp. Med.* **184**, 465–472.
72. Celluzzi, C.M., Mayordomo, J.I., Strokus, W.J., Lotze, M.T. and Falo, L.D. Jr. Peptide-pulsed dendritic cells induce antigen-specific CTL-mediated protective tumor immunity. *J. Exp. Med.* **183**, 283–287.
73. Paglia, P., Chidoni, C., Rodolfo, M. and Colombo, M.P. (1996). Murine dendritic cells loaded *in vitro* with soluble protein prime cytotoxic T lymphocytes against tumor antigen *in vivo*. *J. Exp. Med.* **183**, 317–322.
74. Porgador, A. and Gilboa, E. (1995). Bone marrow-generated dendritic cells pulsed with a class I-restricted peptide are potent inducers of cytotoxic T lymphocytes. *J. Exp. Med.* **182**, 255–260.
75. Zitvogel, L., Mayordomo, J.I., Tjandrawan, T., DeLeo, A.B., Clarke, M.R., Lotze, M.T. and Strokus, W.J. (1996). Therapy of murine tumors with tumor peptide-pulsed dendritic cells: dependence on T cells, B7 costimulation, and T helper cell 1-associated cytokines. *J. Exp. Med.* **183**, 87–97.
76. Condon, C., Watkins, S.C., Celluzzi, C.M., Thompson, K. and Falo, L.D. Jr. (1996). DNA-based immunization by *in vivo* transfection of dendritic cells. *Nature Medicine* **2**, 1122–1128.
77. Manickan, E., Kanagat, S., Rouse, R.J.D., Yu, Z. and Rouse, B.T. (1997). Enhancement of immune response to naked DNA vaccine by immunization with transfected dendritic cells. *J. Leukocyte Biol.* **61**, 125–132.

78. Girolomoni, G. and Ricciardi-Castagnoli, P. (1997). Dendritic cells hold promise for immunotherapy. *Immunol. Today* **18**, 102–104.
79. Alijagic, S., Moller, P., Artuc, M., Jurgovsky, K., Czarnetzki, B.M. and Schadendorf, D. (1995). Dendritic cells generated from peripheral blood transfected with human tyrosinase induce specific T cell activation. *Eur. J. Immunol.* **25**, 3100–3107.
80. Henderson, R.A., Nimgaonkar, M.T., Watkins, S.C., Robbins, P.D., Ball, E.D. and Finn, O.J. (1996). Human dendritic cells genetically engineered to express high levels of the human epithelial tumor antigen mucin (MUC-1). *Cancer Res.* **56**, 3763–3770.
81. Rogge, L., Barberis-Maino, L., Biffi, M., Passini, N., Presky, D.H., Gubler, U. and Sinigaglia, F. (1997). Selective expression of an interleukin-12 receptor component by human T helper 1 cells. *J. Exp. Med.* **185**, 825–831.
82. Trinchieri, G. (1995). Interleukin-12: a proinflammatory cytokine with immunoregulatory functions that bridge innate resistance and antigen-specific adaptive immunity. *Annu. Rev. Immunol.* **13**, 251–276.
83. Quill, H., Bhandoola, A., Trinchieri, G., Haluskey, J. and Peritt, D. (1994). Induction of interleukin 12 responsiveness is impaired in anergic T lymphocytes. *J. Exp. Med.* **179**, 1065–1070.
84. Grohmann, U., Bianchi, R., Ayroldi, E., Belladonna, M.L., Surace, D., Fioretti, M.C. and Puccetti, P. (1997). A tumor-associated and self antigen peptide presented by dendritic cells may induce T cell anergy *in vivo*, but IL-12 can prevent or revert the anergic state. *J. Immunol.* **158**, 3593–3602.
85. Muller, G., Saloga, J., Germann, T., Schuler, G., Knop, J. and Enk, A.H., (1995) IL-12 as mediator and adjuvant for the induction of contact sensitivity *in vivo*. *J. Immunol.* **155**, 4661–4668.
86. Riemann, H., Schwaz, A., Grabbe, S., Aragane, Y., Luger, T.A., Wysocka, M., Kubin, M., Trinchieri, G. and Schwarz, T. (1996). Neutralization of IL-12 *in vivo* prevents induction of contact hypersensitivity and induces hapten-specific tolerance. *J. Immunol.* **156**, 1799–1803.
87. Macatonia, S.E., Hosken, N.A., Litton, M., Vieira, P., Hsieh, C.S., Culpepper, J.A., Wysocka, M., Trinchieru, G., Murphy, K.M. and O'Garra, A. (1995). Dendritic cells produce IL-12 and direct the development of Th1 cells from naive $CD4^+$ T cells. *J. Immunol.* **154**, 5071-5079.
88. Scheicher, C., Mehlig, M., Dienes, H.P. and Reske, K. (1995). Uptake of microparticle-absorbed protein antigen by bone marrow dendritic cells results in upregulation of interleukin-1α and interleukin-12 p40/p35 and triggers prolonged, efficient antigen presentation. *Eur. J. Immunol.* **25**, 1566–1572.
89. Grewal, I.S., Xu, J. and Flavell, R.A. (1995). Impairment of antigen-specific T-cell priming in mice lacking CD40 ligand. *Nature* **378**, 617–620.
90. Koch, F., Stanzl, U., Jennewein, P., Janke, K., Heufler, C., Kampgen, E., Romani, N. and Schuler, G. (1996). High level of IL-12 production by murine dendritic cells: upregulation via MHC class II and CD40 molecules and downregulation by IL-4 and IL-10. *J. Exp. Med.* **184**, 741–746.
91. Cella, M., Scheidegger, D., Palmer-Lehmann, J.K., Lane, P., Lanzavecchia, A. and Albert, G. (1996). Ligation of CD40 on dendritic cells triggers production of high levels of interleukin-12 and enhances T cell stimulatory capacity: T–T help via APC activation. *J. Exp. Med.* **183**, 747–752.
92. Burstein, H.J. and Abbas, A.K. (1993). *In vivo* role of interleukin 4 in T cell tolerance induced by aqueous protein antigen. *J. Exp. Med.* **177**, 457–463.
93. Wraith, D.C. (1995). Induction of antigen-specific unresponsiveness with synthetic peptides: specific immunotherapy for treatment of allergic and autoimmune conditions. *Int. Arch. Allergy. Immunol.* **108**, 355–359.
94. Russell, J.H., (1995). Activation-induced death of mature T cells in the regulation of immune responses. *Curr. Opin. Immunol.* **7**, 328–388.
95. Falb, D., Briner, T.J., Sunshine, G.H., Bourque, C.R., Luqman, M., Gefter, M.I. and Kamradt, T. (1996). Peripheral tolerance in T cell receptor-transgenic mice: evidence for T cell anergy. *Eur. J. Immunol.* **26**, 130–135.
96. Bianchi, R., Grohmann, U., Belladonna, M.L., Silla, S., Fallarino, F., Ayroldi, E., Fioretti, M.C. and Puccetti, P. (1996). IL-12 is both required and sufficient for initiating T-cell reactivity to a class I-restricted tumor peptide (P815AB) following transfer of P815AB-pulsed dendritic cells. *J. Immunol.* **157**, 1589–1597.
97. Mayordomo, J.I., Zorina, T., Strokus, W.J., Zitvogel, L., Celluzzi, C., Falo, L.D., Melief, C.J., Ildstad, S.T., Kast, W.M., Deleo, A.B. *et al.* (1995). Bone marrow-derived dendritic cells pulsed with synthetic

tumour peptides elicit protective and therapeutic antitumour immunity. *Nature Medicine* **1**, 1297–1302.

98. Bakker, A.B., Marland, G., de Boer, A.J., Huijbens, R.J., Danen, E.H., Adema, G.J. and Figdor, C.G. (1995). Generation of antimelanoma cytotoxic T lymphocytes from healthy donors after presentation of melanoma-associated antigen-derived epitopes by dendritic cells *in vitro*. *Cancer Res.* **55**, 5330–5334.
99. Gong, J., Chen, D., Kashiwaba, M. and Kufe, D. (1997). Induction of antitumor activity by immunization with fusions of dendritic and carcinoma cells. *Nature Medicine* **3**, 558–561.

CHAPTER 17
Langerhans Cell Migration and Cellular Interactions

Ian Kimber[1], Marie Cumberbatch[1], Rebecca J. Dearman[1] and Stella C. Knight[2]
[1]Zeneca Central Toxicology Laboratory, Alderley Park, Macclesfield, Cheshire, UK; [2]Antigen Presentation Research Group, Imperial College School of Medicine at Northwick Park Institute for Medical Research, Harrow, Middlesex, UK

INTRODUCTION: THE BIOLOGY OF LANGERHANS CELLS

Networks of dendritic cells (DC) are found in nonlymphoid tissues, and in particular in those tissues that come into closest contact with the external environment. The best-characterized of these are epidermal Langerhans cells (LC), cells that are uniquely positioned to act as sentinels of the immune system at skin surfaces. The physiological relevance of LC and their contribution to the initiation of cutaneous immune responses are considered below. It should be borne in mind, however, that LC form part of an integrated skin immune system and that other cutaneous DC within the epidermis, the dermis and the afferent lymphatics contribute to this (Silberberg-Sinakin *et al.*, 1980; Knight *et al.*, 1982; Tse and Cooper, 1990; Kimber and Cumberbatch, 1992a; Lenz *et al.*, 1993; Nestle *et al.*, 1993; Steinman *et al.*, 1995; Lappin *et al.*, 1996). While the role of other DC, although poorly understood, is acknowledged, the focus of attention here is on epidermal LC and their migration from the skin to draining lymph nodes.

Langerhans cells display a unique phenotype. They constitutively express major histocompatibility complex (MHC) class II molecules, have a dendritic morphology, the dendrites interdigitate between keratinocytes, and contain an intracytoplasmic organelle, the Birbeck granule (Romani and Schuler, 1992). In addition they express Fc receptors for both IgG and IgE (FcγRII; CD32 and FcεRII; CD23), some cytokine receptors (including those for interleukins 1 and 6, tumour necrosis factor-α and interferon-γ) and a range of adhesion molecules (Romani and Schuler, 1992; Larregina *et al.*, 1996; Lappin *et al.*, 1996). In the skin their main and most important functions appear to be antigen recognition, antigen capture and antigen processing (Streilein and Grammer, 1989; Streilein *et al.*, 1990). LC are able to ingest antigen and this may be facilitated by their expression of Fc receptors and receptors for complement. Following internalization, exogenous antigens are localized in endolysosomal compartments and subsequently expressed at the cell surface in the context of MHC determinants (Girolomoni

Dendritic Cells: Biology and Clinical Applications
ISBN 0-12-455860-7

et al., 1990; Bartosik, 1992; Reis e Sousa *et al.*, 1993; Kleijmeer *et al.*, 1994). Langerhans cells are, however, comparatively ineffective antigen-presenting cells. This property is acquired following functional maturation during the migration of LC from the skin to draining lymph nodes or after culture of freshly isolated LC in the presence of appropriate cytokines (Schuler and Steinman, 1985; Streilein *et al.*, 1990). This development of LC into immunostimulatory DC which are capable of presenting antigen very effectively to naive T-lymphocytes is mediated by cytokines, among the most important being interleukin-1 (IL-1) and granulocyte/macrophage colony-stimulating factor (GM-CSF) (Witmer-Pack *et al.*, 1987; Heufler *et al.*, 1988; Picut *et al.*, 1988; Koch *et al.*, 1990). This maturation of LC is associated with their increased expression of molecules required for interaction with, and presentation of antigen to, responsive T-lymphocytes. Thus, following differentiation *in vitro*, or following movement from the epidermis to draining lymph nodes, there is elevated expression of MHC class II (Ia) molecules, intercellular adhesion molecule-1 (ICAM-1; CD54) and B7 (CD80 and CD86) costimulatory molecules (Schuler and Steinman, 1985; Cumberbatch *et al.*, 1991; Cumberbatch *et al.*, 1992; Larsen *et al.*, 1992; Hart *et al.*, 1993; Razi-Wolf *et al.*, 1994; Inaba *et al.*, 1994). The acquisition by LC of immunostimulatory potential is at the cost of the ability to process antigen, this facility being lost rapidly following differentiation into antigen-presenting DC (Streilein and Grammer, 1989; Streilein *et al.*, 1990). The expression of MHC class II molecules is high on the surface of lymph node DC, but these mature cells show reduced synthesis of these molecules. In such DC the capacity for antigen uptake is reduced and there is a loss of Fc receptor expression and impaired intracellular processing of native antigen and other associated changes (Romani *et al.*, 1989a,b; Stossel *et al.*, 1990; Pure *et al*, 1990; Reis e Sousa *et al.*, 1993; Pierre *et al.*, 1997). Langerhans cells are able, therefore, to display two functionally discrete phenotypes that are dependent upon differentiation status and that match the activity of the cells to their local tissue microenvironment. At the skin surface, where foreign antigen is encountered, LC have the ability to process exogenous antigen. However, following receipt of the signal to migrate from the epidermis, this activity is reduced during differentiation into an antigen-presenting phenotype necessary for activation of T lymphocytes in the peripheral lymphoid tissue. Before considering in detail the nature of the signals required for LC migration it is helpful to consider the immunological context in which they reside in the skin and, in particular, the constitutive and inducible production by epidermal cells of cytokines.

EPIDERMAL CYTOKINES

The skin, and the epidermis in particular, is a rich source of cytokines. Some cytokines are produced exclusively by keratinocytes, some only by LC, and others by both cell types. It is clear that certain cytokines are expressed constitutively by epidermal cells, whereas for others production is dependent upon delivery of an appropriate stimulus. A list of epidermal cytokines and their cellular source or sources is shown in Table 1. There is now firm evidence that several of these are able to effect maturational changes in cultured LC; the implication is that they perform identical, or at least similar, roles *in vivo* during migration of LC to regional lymph nodes. As described above, it is known that IL-1 and GM-CSF play important roles in the functional differentiation of LC (Witmer-Pack *et al.*, 1987; Heufler *et al.*, 1988; Picut *et al.*, 1988; Koch *et al.*, 1990). It is

Table 1. Native and inducible epidermal cytokines

Cytokine	Langerhans cells	Keratinocytes
Interleukins		
IL-1α	−	+
IL-1β	+	−
IL-6	+	+
IL-7	−	+
IL-8	−	+
IL-10	−	+[a]
IL-12	+	+
IL-15	+	+
IL-18	+	+
Granulocyte/macrophage colony-stimulating factor (GM-CSF)	−	+
Tumour necrosis factor-α (TNF-α)	−	+
Macrophage inflammatory protein-1α (MIP-1α)	+	−
Macrophage inflammatory protein-1γ (MIP-1γ)	+	−
Macrophage inflammatory protein-2 (MIP-2)	+	+
Interferon-γ (IFN-γ)	−	+[b]

Summarized from available human and/or mouse data (Schreiber *et al.*, 1992; Heufler *et al.*, 1992; Heufler *et al.*, 1993; Matsue *et al.*, 1992; Enk and Katz, 1992a,b; Aragne *et al.*, 1994; Kimber, 1994; Howie *et al.*, 1997; Kang *et al.*, 1996; Blauvelt *et al.*, 1996; Mohamadzadeh *et al.*, 1996; Cumberbatch *et al.*, 1996a; Teunissen *et al.*, 1997; Stoll *et al.*, 1997a,b).
[a]Possibly in mice only.
[b]Possibly in humans only.

likely that tumour necrosis factor-α (TNF-α) also participates in this process and that certain combinations of cytokines act in synergistic or cooperative fashion to mediate the upregulated expression of costimulatory molecules (Furue *et al.*, 1996; Ozawa *et al.*, 1996b). It has also been shown that addition of interleukin-12 (IL-12) to maturing DC can cause upregulation of CD80 and enhance allostimulatory activity (Kelleher and Knight, 1998). Several cytokines, notably interleukin-10 (IL-10), have the potential to regulate negatively the expression by LC of costimulatory molecules and their antigen-presenting cell activity (Chang *et al.*, 1995; Ozawa *et al.*, 1996a; De Smedt *et al.*, 1997) and may therefore exert a controlling influence on the induced maturation of LC *in vivo*. A similar role may be played by the neuropeptide calcitonin gene-related peptide (CGRP). It has been shown that CGRP-containing nerve fibres are associated intimately with LC in the human epidermis and that this peptide is able to inhibit the antigen-presenting cell activity of LC (Hosoi *et al.*, 1993).

The question addressed here is whether, in addition to influencing the maturation of LC, epidermal cytokines also serve to stimulate and regulate their migration from the skin to draining lymph nodes.

LC MIGRATION

It has been appreciated for some time that topical exposure of mice to skin-sensitizing chemicals causes the accumulation of DC (a proportion of which bear high levels of antigen) in lymph nodes draining the site of application (Silberberg-Sinakin *et al.*, 1980; Knight *et al.*, 1985; Macatonia *et al.*, 1986, 1987; Kinnaird *et al.*, 1989; Kimber *et al.*, 1990; Cumberbatch *et al.*, 1990, Kripke *et al.*, 1990); the interpretation is that these cells derive from epidermal LC. There is both direct and indirect evidence to support this view, although it should be borne in mind that some of the DC which arrive in antigen-activated skin-draining lymph nodes may originate from the dermis rather than epidermis. Skin sensitization of mice results also in increased DC numbers in lymph nodes distant from the site of exposure to allergen, suggesting that systemic cytokine signals for LC migration may be induced (Hill *et al.*, 1990). Topical administration of skin-sensitizing or skin-irritant chemicals results in rapid upregulation of the expression of various epidermal cytokines including, among others, IL-l, TNF-α, GM-CSF, macrophage inflammatory protein-2 (MIP-2) and interleukin-6 (IL-6) (Enk and Katz, 1992a,b; Kimber *et al.*, 1995; Holliday *et al.*, 1996a,b; Holliday *et al.*, 1997). It is therefore reasonable to speculate that some at least of these same cytokines may play important roles in the initiation of LC migration.

Tumour Necrosis Factor-α

Investigations focused initially upon TNF-α, a keratinocyte cytokine. Increased message for TNF-α has been demonstrated in mouse epidermis within 1 h of application of the allergen trinitrochlorobenzene (Enk and Katz, 1992a). Cutaneous TNF-α protein is maximally induced in mice at approximately 2 h after topical exposure to skin allergens (such as oxazolone and dinitrochlorobenzene) and declines rapidly thereafter (Holliday *et al.*, 1997). It was found that the intradermal exposure of mice to homologous recombinant TNF-α (via ear pinnae) induced a time- and dose-dependent loss of a proportion of LC from the local epidermis and that this was associated, some time later, with an accumulation of DC in draining lymph nodes (Cumberbatch and Kimber, 1992; Kimber and Cumberbatch, 1992b; Cumberbatch *et al.*, 1994). A significant decrease in the frequency of epidermal LC was observed within 30 min of exposure to TNF-α and increased numbers of DC within draining nodes were first detectable at 2 h. The inference drawn was that TNF-α could provide one signal for LC migration; a supposition consistent with the rapid induction of this cytokine following skin sensitization. An interesting observation made during the course of these investigations was that the ability of TNF-α to cause LC migration is species specific, or at least species restricted. Thus, intradermal injection of human recombinant TNF-α failed to stimulate in mice either LC migration or DC accumulation, despite the fact that the heterologous cytokine was administered at biologically active concentrations, insofar as treatment resulted in the induced expression by keratinocytes of ICAM-1 (Cumberbatch and Kimber, 1992; Cumberbatch *et al.*, 1994). This species selectivity is almost certainly a function of the expression by LC of TNF-R2 receptors only. There have been described two main types of membrane receptor for TNF-α, designated TNF-R1 and TNF-R2. The former is a 55 kDa transmembrane protein that exhibits considerable interspecies homology in the extracellular ligand-binding domains. In contrast, the 75 kDa TNF-R2 receptor shows homology primarily in the intracellular domains and for this reason is bound by TNF-α in a species-specific fashion (Lewis *et al.*, 1991). There is now good evidence that epidermal LC display only type 2 receptors for TNF (Koch *et al.*, 1990; Ryffel *et al.*, 1991; Larregina *et al.*, 1996, 1997). Consistent with the conclusion that TNF-α induces LC migration via TNF-R2 receptors are results from experiments performed using TNF-R1 gene-targeted mutant mice. In these animals there was a normal accumulation of antigen-bearing DC in draining lymph nodes following skin sensitization with the allergenic fluorochrome fluorescein isothiocyanate (Wang *et al.*,

1996). The importance of TNF-α for the stimulation of LC migration is revealed by the fact that systemic administration to mice (by intraperitoneal injection) of neutralizing anti-TNF-α antibody inhibits very markedly the accumulation of DC within draining lymph nodes induced by topical sensitization. Such treatment served also to compromise the development of contact sensitization (Cumberbatch and Kimber, 1995). Similar results were reported by Wang *et al.* (1996), who found using TNF-R1 gene knockout mice that allergen-induced DC accumulation in draining lymph nodes was similarly inhibited following treatment with neutralizing anti-TNF-α antibody.

The activity of TNF-α raises an important issue regarding the nature of cutaneous insults that cause LC migration. As described above, encounter with antigen in the skin stimulates TNF-α production. It is clear, however, that other forms of cutaneous insult result in increased expression of this cytokine. It has been shown that ultraviolet light (UV) causes the production by keratinocytes of TNF-α (Kock *et al.*, 1990). Similarly, some nonsensitizing skin irritants, such as sodium lauryl sulfate (SLS), are known to stimulate the local production of this cytokine (Enk and Katz, 1992a; Lisby *et al.*, 1994). Both UV irradiation and topical administration of SLS induce in mice DC accumulation in skin-draining lymph nodes, and in both cases this migration can be inhibited with neutralizing anti-TNF-α antibody (Moodycliffe *et al.*, 1992; Moodycliffe *et al.*, 1994; Cumberbatch *et al.*, 1993). The conclusion drawn is that many forms of dermal trauma, those of the type and severity necessary to induce the upregulated expression of TNF-α, will stimulate the migration of LC away from the epidermis, irrespective of an overt antigen challenge. The ability of some skin irritants to induce TNF-α production and LC migration may go some way to explain why local irritation and inflammation is in some instances associated with more effective skin sensitization (Cumberbatch *et al.*, 1993).

Two other interesting questions can be addressed. First, is the ability of TNF-α to provoke the migration of DC from peripheral tissue to regional lymph nodes restricted to the epidermis and LC? Second, does TNF-α perform a similar role in humans? With respect to the first question the assumption is that TNF-α will initiate migration of DC from other sites including the gastrointestinal and respiratory epithelia. There is some limited evidence available to support this view. Endotoxin given intravenously to rats causes the increased release of intestinal DC into lymph, an effect that was found to be almost totally blocked by a neutralizing anti-TNF-α antibody (MacPherson *et al.*, 1995). There are few data available regarding the ability of TNF-α to cause LC migration in humans, although it is assumed that such migration does occur as it has been shown that exposure of volunteers to SLS causes a significant increase in the flow and cellular content of lymph (Brand *et al.*, 1992). The only direct evidence for TNF-α playing a similar role in humans derives from investigations reported by Groves *et al.* (1995), who found that the intradermal injection of human recombinant TNF-α into healthy male volunteers was associated with a dose- and time-dependent decrease in the frequency of CD1a$^+$ LC in the epidermis and an increase in CD1a$^+$ dermal cells.

Despite the information cited above, there still exists some controversy about the role of TNF-α in LC migration and its effects on these cells. This arises from the fact that Streilein and colleagues have proposed that TNF-α serves to immobilize LC in the epidermis and thereby prevent their effective migration to draining lymph nodes (Streilein *et al.*, 1990; Vermeer and Streilein, 1990). Nonetheless, it is relevant that in the studies reported by these investigators there was in response to TNF-α a reduction in the frequency of Ia^+ epidermal LC (Streilein *et al.*, 1990; Vermeer and Streilein, 1990). In an attempt to resolve these apparently conflicting views it has been proposed recently, based on the results of experiments conducted *in vitro*, that TNF-α has variable dose-dependent effects on LC. Specifically, the suggestion is that at lower doses TNF-α induces or increases LC migration, whereas at much higher concentrations TNF-α has the opposite effect and inhibits their movement (Stoitzner *et al.*, 1997). Attractive as this suggestion may appear in the context of reconciling apparently conflicting data, evidence to date indicates that at all concentrations administered *in vivo* homologous recombinant TNF-α causes in mice a rapid and significant loss of LC from the local epidermis. Taken together, the information available indicates that TNF-α provides an important, and probably mandatory, signal for LC migration from the skin.

Before turning to consideration of the signalling roles played by cytokines other than TNF-α, it is relevant to address the question why injection of TNF-α (and topical sensitization) causes the migration from the skin of only a proportion of LC resident in the epidermis (usually about 20–30%). There is no clear answer available and no data which point to a possible explanation. It is, however, tempting to speculate that at any one time only a proportion of epidermal LC is responsive and able to move away from the skin. One possibility might be that only some LC in the epidermis express TNF-R2 receptors at a density sufficient for them to respond productively to the stimulus provided by TNF-α. It must be emphasized, however, that there is no evidence to support this suggestion and that a greater investment in the examination of functional heterogeneity among epidermal LC will be required to provide a definitive answer.

Interleukin-1β

There are several reasons why IL-1β is of interest in the context of skin sensitization and the induction of cutaneous immune responses. In the mouse epidermis IL-1β is a product exclusively of LC (Enk and Katz, 1992a; Matsue *et al.*, 1992; Heufler *et al.*, 1992; Schreiber *et al.*, 1992). Following skin sensitization the expression by LC of this cytokine is upregulated very rapidly, with increased mRNA levels being detectable within 15 min (Enk and Katz 1992a,c). In addition, it has been found that intradermal injection of IL-1β into mice causes many of the changes in cytokine expression associated with skin sensitization and, importantly in the context of LC migration, stimulates the upregulated expression of mRNA for TNF-α (Enk *et al.*, 1993). Finally, IL-1β appears to be essential for the normal development of skin sensitization. It has been shown that intradermal injection of anti-IL-1β antibody inhibits very markedly the development of contact hypersensitivity to trinitrochlorobenzene applied at the same site (Enk *et al.*, 1993). In the same manner, contact sensitization is impaired in IL-1β gene knockout mice (Shornick *et al.*, 1996).

Recent evidence indicates that IL-1β plays an important and probably essential role in LC migration (Cumberbatch *et al.*, 1997a,b). It was shown that homologous recombinant IL-1β injected intradermally into ear pinnae of mice resulted in both a reduction in the frequency of epidermal LC and an increase in the number of DC found in draining lymph nodes (Cumberbatch *et al.*, 1997a). The effects were comparable with those observed following similar treatment with TNF-α, with the exception that the changes induced by IL-1β exhibited somewhat slower kinetics. Thus, with IL-1β a significant decrease in the number of LC was not observed until 2 h following administration of the cytokine, compared with a reduction in LC frequency recorded after only 30 min with TNF-α (Cumberbatch *et al.*, 1997a). Associated with this was a slower tempo of DC accumulation in draining lymph nodes with IL-1β when compared with TNF-α. In the case of TNF-α significant increases in DC numbers were found within 2 h of treatment, whereas with IL-1β comparable increases required 4 h (Cumberbatch *et al.*, 1997a). In subsequent experiments, using a neutralizing anti-IL-1β antibody, it was demonstrated that the stimulation by oxazolone of DC accumulation in draining lymph nodes is dependent upon IL-1β. Thus, intraperitoneal injection into mice of anti-TNF-α or with anti-IL-1β in both instances caused a very substantial inhibition of oxazolone-induced DC accumulation (Cumberbatch *et al.*, 1997b). A representative experiment is illustrated in Fig. 1.

An attractive hypothesis suggested by the data summarized above is that following topical exposure to skin-sensitizing chemicals there is upregulated expression by LC of IL-1β and that this cytokine acts on neighbouring keratinocytes in paracrine fashion to stimulate the production of TNF-α which then acts on LC to trigger migration. Certainly such a hypothesis would be consistent with the relative kinetics of changes induced by IL-1β and TNF-α, the argument being that for migration to be induced following administration of IL-1β this cytokine must first act on keratinocytes to elicit TNF-α production, whereas an exogenous source of TNF-α will interact directly with LC to initiate their migration. In support of this is the fact that the stimulation of LC migration by intradermal injection of IL-1β is inhibited if mice are treated first with a neutralizing anti-TNF-α antibody (see Fig. 2). However, the situation is clearly more complex than this since it is apparent also from the data illustrated in Fig. 2 that the induction of LC migration by intradermal injection of TNF-α is similarly inhibited if mice are pretreated systemically with an anti-IL-1β antibody (Cumberbatch *et al.*, 1997b). Taken together, the results demonstrate that at least two signals are required for LC migration, one being supplied by TNF-α, via TNF-R2 receptors, the other by IL-1β. Such a scheme is certainly compatible with evidence that treatment of mice with neutralizing antibodies specific for either cytokine causes a substantial inhibition of both LC migration and DC accumulation. If two independent signals are required

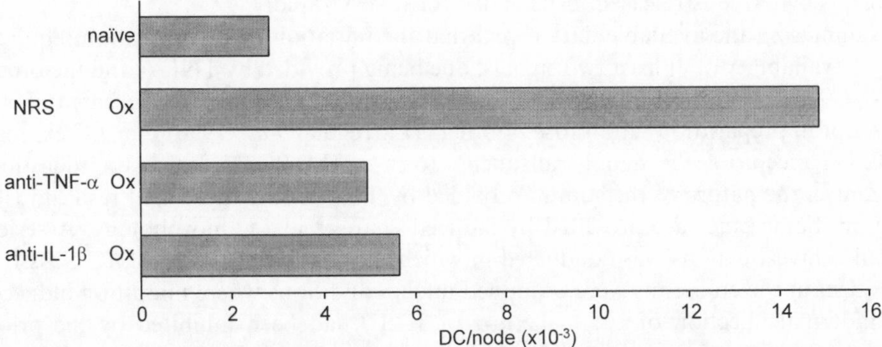

Fig. 1. Migration of DC into lymph nodes is dependent on both IL-1β and TNF-α. Groups of mice ($n = 10$) received a single 100 µl injection (i.p.) of either anti-IL-1β, anti-TNF-α or normal rabbit serum (NRS), each diluted 1:5 in sterile phosphate-buffered saline. Two hours later mice were treated on the dorsum of both ears with 25 µl of 0.5% oxazolone (Ox) in 4:1 acetone:olive oil. Control mice were untreated. Draining auricular lymph nodes were removed 18 h later and the number of DC/node was measured.

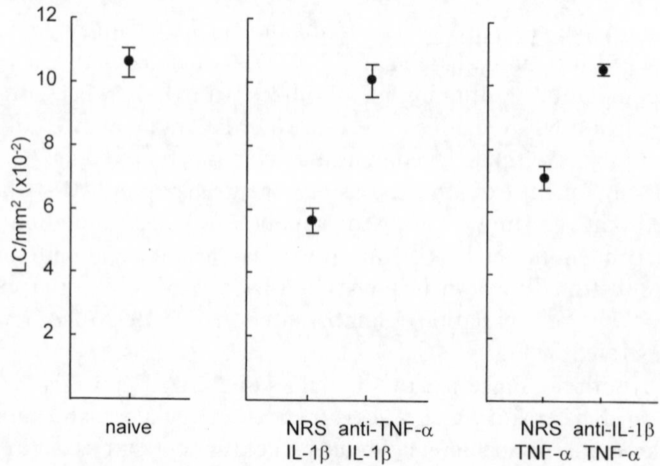

Fig. 2. TNF-β or IL-1β cause migration of Langerhans cells from the epidermis. Groups of mice ($n = 3$) received a single 100 μl injection (i.p.) of either anti-TNF-α, anti-IL-1β or normal rabbit serum (NRS) diluted 1:5 in sterile phosphate-buffered saline. Two hours later mice received 30 μl intradermal injections into both ear pinnae of 50 ng of either murine IL-1β or murine TNF-α. Control mice were untreated. Ears were removed 17 h following administration of IL-1β or 30 min after treatment with TNF-α. Epidermal sheets were prepared following incubation (2 h, 37°C) of dorsal ear halves in 0.02 M ethylenediamine tetraacetic acid and the frequency of MHC class II$^+$ LC was measured by indirect immunofluorescence. Results are expressed as the mean number of cells/mm^2 ($\pm$ SE) derived from examination of 10 fields/sample for each of four samples.

then it is necessary to consider why TNF-α and IL-1β when individually injected intradermally into mice each stimulate LC migration. The assumption is that exogenous IL-1β is effective because it is able to induce the production of TNF-α by keratinocytes. In the case of TNF-α the argument is either that there is sufficient constitutive IL-1β present to provide the second signal, or alternatively that TNF-α in some way induces the increased expression and/or release of IL-1β. The tempo of responses stimulated by exogenous TNF-α would suggest either that there is already sufficient IL-1β available, or that this cytokine is released in its active form very rapidly.

To summarize, the available data reveal that the initiation of LC migration requires the local availability of at least two signals, one being provided by TNF-α and the other by IL-1β. This conclusion is supported by our own observations (Cumberbatch *et al.*, manuscript in preparation) and those of others (Larregina *et al.*, 1996) that LC express type 1 IL-1 receptors, the signal-transducing form of IL-1R. The interesting question is, of course, the nature of the stimuli provided by TNF-α and IL-1β that result in LC migration. Some clues are provided by induced changes in LC morphology. A series of detailed investigations was conducted in which the characteristics of MHC class II$^+$ LC resident in the epidermis were examined under conditions where migration induced by intradermal injection of either TNF-α or IL-1β had been inhibited by the prior systemic administration, respectively, of neutralizing anti-IL-1β or anti-TNF-α antibody (Cumberbatch *et al.*, 1997b). The results of these investigations revealed interesting differences. It was found in mice pretreated with anti-IL-1β that, as expected, TNF-α failed to reduce the frequency of epidermal LC. However, at the site of injection it was clear that a proportion of LC had detached themselves from the surrounding keratinocytes and had adopted a rounded appearance. A different picture emerged when the converse experiment was performed. In mice pretreated with anti-TNF-α and exposed locally to IL-1β, the LC assumed what appeared to be an activated, aggressive morphology with enhanced expression of Ia. However, in this case all LC were apparently attached securely to keratinocytes and retained a highly dendritic morphology. Such changes suggest that TNF-α and IL-1β may have discrete influences on the expression by LC and/or neighbouring cells of adhesion molecules, the enhanced or downregulated expression of which may be necessary for effective migration away from the skin.

ADHESION MOLECULES AND LC MIGRATION

Of particular relevance for effective LC migration may be E-cadherin. It has been demonstrated that this homophilic adhesion molecule is expressed in the epidermis by both LC and keratinocytes (Tang *et al.*, 1993; Blauvelt *et al.*, 1995). It is proposed that E-cadherin represents the 'cement' that, under normal circumstances, maintains cellular contact between keratinocytes and LC and allows the latter to be embedded firmly within the epidermal tissue matrix. If such is the case then the migration of LC away from the skin will demand that this association is broken and that E-cadherin expression is lost, or at least downregulated. It has now been shown that LC migration is associated with the loss by these cells of E-cadherin, the DC which accumulate in draining lymph nodes having little or no detectable E-cadherin (Borkowski *et al.*, 1994; Cumberbatch *et al.*, 1996b). Consistent with these data are results of experiments in which the ability of allergen and epidermal cytokines to influence the expression by LC *in situ* of E-cadherin was investigated. Treatment of mice topically with an allergen was found to cause a substantial reduction in the level of E-cadherin displayed by a proportion of local LC. In parallel investigations it was demonstrated that the injection of TNF-α or of IL-1β, but not of other cytokines, could induce similar changes in E-cadherin expression by LC (Schwarzenberger and Udey, 1996). More recently, the influence of TNF-α and IL-1β on the expression *in vitro* of E-cadherin by LC-like cells expanded from murine fetal skin has been described. Both cytokines were reported to cause a rapid reduction in the expression of mRNA for E-cadherin which preceded lower membrane expression of this molecule (Jakob and Udey, 1997). The conclusion drawn is that pro-inflammatory epidermal cytokines induced or upregulated following exposure to allergen serve to transcriptionally inhibit the expression by LC of E-cadherin. This in turn will permit LC to disassociate from surrounding keratinocytes as a mandatory first step in their mobilization for migration. The data summarized above, where it was reported that intradermal administration of TNF-α to mice pretreated with an anti-IL-1β antibody causes a proportion of LC to detach themselves from surrounding cells and to adopt a rounded appearance, suggest that the more important cytokine in effecting the reduced expression of E-cadherin *in vivo* may be TNF-α.

Another adhesion molecule of importance in LC migration is ICAM-1. As described above, the movement of LC from the skin is associated with a very marked induction of ICAM-1 expression (Cumberbatch *et al.*, 1992). Although this is consistent with the acquisition by LC of antigen-presenting activity, induced ICAM-1 expression may be relevant for the process of migration itself, or at least for the successful accumulation of cells in the draining lymph nodes. Ma *et al.* (1994) investigated in sensitized mice the influence of antibodies specific for ICAM-1 or for its ligand, leukocyte function-associated antigen-1 (LFA-1), on the accumulation within draining lymph nodes of antigen-bearing DC. Treatment with either antibody alone caused a significant reduction in the numbers of DC bearing high levels of antigen within draining lymph nodes. Treatment with these antibodies in combination completely inhibited the development of contact sensitization and the draining lymph nodes of treated mice were devoid of antigen-bearing DC. In similar experiments it was found that treatment of mice prior to allergen exposure with these antibodies caused an inhibition of contact sensitization and that this was associated with the reduced production by draining lymph node cells of interleukin 2 (IL-2) (Murayama *et al.*, 1997). Taken together, these reports suggest that the elevated expression by LC of ICAM-1 may be relevant not only for the development of immunostimulatory activity, but also for the successful accumulation of antigen-bearing cells in draining lymph nodes. It is assumed that TNF-α, and possibly other pro-inflammatory epidermal cytokines, serve to induce ICAM-1 expression by LC.

Of interest also is CD44, an adhesion molecule that has been implicated in the movement of a variety of cell types (Hogg and Landis, 1993). There are some conflicting data relating to the role of CD44, a cellular receptor for hyaluronate, in LC migration. In one series of investigations it was found that both LC and lymph node DC express CD44, but that there are no differences between these cell types with respect to level of expression (Cumberbatch *et al.*, 1996b). There is, however, evidence that epidermal cytokines are able to regulate the expression by LC of CD44. Studies *in vitro* demonstrated that TNF-α and IL-10 exerted reciprocal dose-dependent effects on the level of CD44 displayed by cultured LC; the former caused upregulated expression, while IL-10 lowered expression (Osada *et al.*, 1995). When added to LC cultures in combination, TNF-α and IL-10 were mutually antagonistic, suggesting that altered expression of CD44 is dependent upon the nature of the cytokine microenvironment. Irrespective of changes in CD44 expression and the mechanisms through which this might be regulated, a role for this glycoprotein in LC migration was suggested by the investigations of Gabrilovich *et al.* (1994), who found in mice that impaired DC accumulation in draining lymph nodes and reduced contact sensitization caused by retroviral infection was associated with reduced expression of CD44 (and ICAM-1). However, in virus-infected mice treated with IL-12, contact sensitivity was normalized despite lymph node DC continuing to display a reduced expression of CD44 (Williams *et al.*, 1998). Such data argue against an obligatory role for CD44 in LC migration and function. It may prove that examination of the native CD44 molecule in this context is misleading. It has been found that incubation of cultured DC with TNF-α results in the increased expression of a number of membrane determinants (including ICAM-1) and in the appearance of CD44-v9, a CD44 exon 9 splice variant (Sallusto and Lanzavecchia, 1994). The suggestion is that the stimulation by TNF-α of a CD44 isoform carrying the v9 exon may be involved in the migration of LC from the epidermis; certainly the expression of this molecule has been found to confer metastatic potential on carcinoma cells (Gunthert *et al.*, 1991). Recent studies appear to support this. Antibodies to CD44 epitopes encoded by variant exons were found to inhibit the migration of LC from the epidermis and the localization of DC within the paracortical regions of lymph nodes (Weiss *et al.*, 1997). The exact roles played by CD44 isoforms in LC migration and the signals that regulate their expression have still to be elucidated. Nevertheless, it may be that TNF-α and other epidermal cytokines serve as important determinants of CD44 isoform expression.

Finally, it is pertinent to consider how LC are able to pass across basement membrane during their journey to lymph nodes. Certainly the expression by LC of gelatinase will be of central importance. It has been found in mice that topical administration of contact allergens results in the rapid (within 6 h) induction of type IV collagenase (matrix metalloproteinase 9; MMP-9) expression by LC and that this is associated with development of strong gelatinolytic activity (Kobayashi, 1997). Certainly both TNF-α and IL-1β may be regarded as candidate stimulators for the induction of this activity (Saren *et al.*, 1996). Passage across the basement membrane would be facilitated also by the interaction of LC with laminin. The main cellular determinant that confers laminin-binding activity is very late antigen 6 (VLA-6), which comprises α_6 and β_1 integrins. It has been found recently that the migration of LC *in vitro* and the movement of LC from the epidermis and their accumulation in lymph nodes *in vivo*, are inhibited very effectively with a monoclonal antibody specific for α_6 integrin. In parallel experiments, a control antibody reactive with α_4 integrin was without effect on either LC migration or the arrival of DC in draining lymph nodes (Price *et al.*, 1997). One may speculate that epidermal cytokines are important for the maintained or elevated expression of VLA-6 that permits the interaction of LC with the basement membrane.

In summary, it is likely that those cytokines which are known to be responsible for the mobilization of LC (TNF-α and IL-1β) exert their influence, at least in part, through induced changes in the expression by LC of adhesion molecules. It is proposed that such changes allow LC to free themselves from keratinocytes within the epidermis and also provide them with the cellular receptors necessary for effective migration through the extracellular tissue matrix.

CONCLUDING COMMENTS

An important aspect of Langerhans cell function is their migration from the epidermis to peripheral lymph nodes; a process during which LC assume the characteristics of immunostimulatory dendritic cells to ensure the effective presentation of transported antigen to responsive T lymphocytes. Essential signals for LC migration are provided by epidermal cytokines, both TNF-α and IL-1β being required. It is proposed that these, and possibly other cytokines, stimulate the changes necessary for the mobilization of LC and their directed movement through the skin and afferent lymphatics to draining lymph nodes.

REFERENCES

Aragne, Y., Reimann, H., Bhardwaj, R.S., Schwartz, A., Sawada, Y., Yamada, H., Luger, T.A., Kubin, M., Trinchieri, G. and Schwartz, T. (1994). IL-12 is expressed and released by human keratinocytes and epidermoid carcinoma cell lines. *J. Immunol.* **13**, 5366–5372.

Bartosik, J. (1992). Cytomembrane-derived Birbeck granules transport horseradish peroxidase to the endosomal compartment in the human Langerhans cell. *J. Invest. Dermatol.* **99**, 53–58.

Blauvelt, A., Katz, S.I. and Udey, M.C. (1995). Human Langerhans cells express E-cadherin. *J. Invest. Dermatol.* **104**, 293–296.

Blauvelt, A., Asada, H., Klaus-Kovtun, V., Lacey, D.R. and Katz, S.I. (1996). Interleukin-15 mRNA is expressed by human keratinocytes, Langerhans cells, and blood-derived dendritic cells and is downregulated by ultraviolet B radiation. *J. Invest. Dermatol.* **106**, 1047–1052.

Borkowski, T.A., Van Dyke, B.J., Schwarzenberger, K., McFarland, V.W., Farr, A.G. and Udey, M.C. (1994). Expression of E-cadherin by murine dendritic cells. E-cadherin as a dendritic cell differentiation antigen characteristic of epidermal Langerhans cells and related cells. *Eur. J. Immunol.* **24**, 2767–2774.

Brand, C.U., Hunziker, T. and Braathen, L.R. (1992). Isolation of human skin-derived lymph: flow and output of cells following sodium lauryl sulphate-induced contact dermatitis. *Arch. Dermatol. Res.* **284**, 123–126.

Chang, C-H., Furue, M. and Tamaki, K. (1995). B7-1 expression of Langerhans cells is up-regulated by proinflammatory cytokines and is down-regulated by interferon-γ or by interleukin 10. *Eur. J. Immunol.* **25**, 394–398.

Cumberbatch, M. and Kimber, I. (1990). Phenotypic characteristics of antigen-bearing cells in the draining lymph nodes of contact sensitized mice. *Immunology* **71**, 404–410.

Cumberbatch, M. and Kimber, I. (1992). Dermal tumour necrosis factor-α induces dendritic cell migration to draining lymph nodes, and possibly provides one stimulus for Langerhans cell migration. *Immunology* **75**, 257–263.

Cumberbatch, M. and Kimber, I. (1995) Tumour necrosis factor-α is required for accumulation of dendritic cells in draining lymph nodes and for optimal contact sensitization. *Immunology* **84**, 31–35.

Cumberbatch, M., Gould, S.J., Peters, S.W. and Kimber, I. (1991). MHC class II expression by Langerhans cells and lymph node dendritic cells: possible evidence for the maturation of Langerhans cells following contact sensitization. *Immunology* **74**, 414–419.

Cumberbatch, M., Peters, S.W., Gould, S.J. and Kimber, I. (1992) Intercellular adhesion molecule-1 (ICAM-1) expression by lymph node dendritic cells: comparison with epidermal Langerhans cells. *Immunol. Lett.* **32**, 105–110.

Cumberbatch, M., Scott, R.C., Basketter, D.A., Scholes, E.W., Hilton, J., Dearman, R.J. and Kimber, I. (1993). Influence of sodium lauryl sulphate on 2,4-dinitrochlorobenzene-induced lymph node activation. *Toxicology* **77**, 181–191.

Cumberbatch, M., Fielding, I. and Kimber, I. (1994). Modulation of epidermal Langerhans cell frequency by tumour necrosis factor-α. *Immunology* **81**, 395–401.

Cumberbatch, M., Dearman, R.J. and Kimber, I. (1996a), Constitutive and inducible expression of interleukin-6 by Langerhans cells and lymph node dendritic cells. *Immunology* **87**, 513–518.

Cumberbatch, M., Dearman, R.J. and Kimber, I. (1996b). Adhesion molecule expression by epidermal Langerhans cells and lymph node dendritic cells: a comparison. *Arch. Dermatol. Res.* **288**, 739–744.

Cumberbatch, M., Dearman, R.J. and Kimber, I. (1997a). Interleukin 1β and the stimulation of Langerhans cell migration: comparisons with tumour necrosis factor α. *Arch. Dermatol. Res.* **289**, 277–284.

Cumberbatch, M., Dearman, R.J. and Kimber, I. (1997b). Langerhans cells require signals from both tumour necrosis factor-α and interleukin-1β for migration. *Immunology* **92**, 388–395.

De Smedt, T., Van Mechelen, M., De Becker, G., Urbain, J., Leo, O. and Moser, M. (1997). Effect of interleukin-10 on dendritic cell maturation and function. *Eur. J. Immunol.* **27**, 1229–1235.

Enk, A.H. and Katz, S.I. (1992a). Early molecular events in the induction phase of contact sensitivity. *Proc. Natl Acad. Sci. USA* **89**, 1398–1402.

Enk, A.H. and Katz, S.I. (1992b) Identification and induction of keratinocyte-derived IL-10. *J. Immunol.* **149**, 92–95.

Enk, A.H. and Katz, S.I. (1992c). Early events in the induction phase of contact sensitivity. *J. Invest. Dermatol.* **99**, 39S–41S.

Enk, A.H., Angeloni, V.L., Udey, M.C. and Katz, S.I. (1993). An essential role for Langerhans cell-derived IL-1β in the initiation of primary immune responses in the skin. *J. Immunol.* **150**, 3698–3704.

Furue, M., Chang, C. H. and Tamaki, K (1996) Interleukin-1 but not tumour necrosis factor α synergistically upregulates the granulocyte-macrophage colony-stimulating factor-induced B7-1 expression of murine Langerhans cells. *Br. J. Dermatol.* **135**, 194–198.

Gabrilovich, D.I., Woods, G.M., Patterson, S., Harvey, J.J. and Knight, S.C. (1994). Retrovirus-induced immunosuppression via blocking of dendritic cell migration and down-regulation of adhesion molecules. *Immunology* **82**, 82–87.

Girolomoni, G., Cruz, P.D. Jr. and Bergstresser, P.R. (1990). Internalization and acidification of surface HLA-DR molecules by epidermal Langerhans cells: a paradigm for antigen processing. *J. Invest. Dermatol.* **94**, 753–760.

Groves, R.W., Allen, M.H., Ross, E.L., Barker, J.N.W.N. and Macdonald, D.M. (1995). Tumour necrosis factor alpha is pro-inflammatory in normal human skin and modulates cutaneous adhesion molecule expression. *Br. J. Dermatol.* **132**, 345–352.

Gunthert, U., Hofmann, M., Rudy, W., Reber, S., Zoller, M., Haussmann, I., Matzku, S., Wenzel, A., Ponta, H. and Herrlich, P. (1991). A new variant of glycoprotein CD44 confers metastatic potential to rat carcinoma cells. *Cell* **65**, 13–24.

Hart, D.N.J., Starling, G.C., Calder, V.L. and Fernando, N.S. (1993). B7/BB1 is a leukocyte differentiation antigen on human dendritic cells induced by activation. *Immunology* **79**, 616–620.

Heufler, C., Koch, F. and Schuler, G. (1988). Granulocyte/macrophage colony-stimulating factor and interleukin 1 mediate the maturation of murine epidermal Langerhans cells into potent immunostimulatory dendritic cells. *J. Exp. Med.* **167**, 700–705.

Heufler, C., Topar, G., Koch, F., Trockenbacher, B., Kampgen, E., Romani, N. and Schuler, G. (1992). Cytokine gene expression in murine epidermal cell suspensions: interleukin 1β and macrophage inflammatory protein 1α are selectively expressed in Langerhans cells but are differentially regulated in culture. *J. Exp. Med.* **176**, 1221–1226.

Heufler, C., Topar, G., Grasseger, A., Stanzl, U., Koch, F., Romani, N., Namen, A. E. and Schuler, G. (1993). Interleukin 7 is produced by murine and human keratinocytes. *J. Exp. Med.* **178**, 1109–1114.

Hill, S., Edwards, A.J., Kimber, I. and Knight, S.C. (1990). Systemic migration of dendritic cells during contact sensitization. *Immunology* **71**, 277–281.

Hogg, N. and Landis, R.C. (1993). Adhesion molecules in cell interactions. *Curr. Opin. Immunol.* **5**, 383–390.

Holliday, M.R., Dearman, R.J., Basketter, D.A. and Kimber, I. (1996a). Stimulation by oxazolone of increased IL-6, but not IL-10, in the skin of mice. *Toxicology* **106**, 237–242.

Holliday, M.R., Dearman, R.J., Corsini, E., Basketter, D.A. and Kimber, I. (1996b). Selective stimulation of cutaneous interleukin 6 expression by skin allergens. *J. Appl. Toxicol.* **16**, 65–70.

Holliday, M.R., Corsini, E., Smith, S., Basketter, D.A., Dearman, R.J. and Kimber, I. (1997). Differential induction of TNF-α and IL-6 by topically applied chemicals. *Am. J. Contact Dermatol.* **8**, 158–164.

Hosoi, J., Murphy, G.F., Egan, C.L., Lerner, E.A., Grabbe, S., Asahina, A. and Granstein, R.D. (1993). Regulation of Langerhans cell function by nerves containing calcitonin gene-related peptide. *Nature* **363**, 159–163.

Howie, S.E.M., Aldridge, R.D., McVittie, E., Forsey, R.J., Sands, C. and Hunter, J.A.A. (1997). Epidermal keratinocyte production of interferon-γ immunoreactive protein and mRNA is an early event in allergic contact dermatitis. *J. Invest. Dermatol.* **106**, 1218–1223.

Inaba, K., Witmer-Pack, M., Inaba, M., Hathcock, K.S., Sakuta, H., Azuma, M., Yagita, H., Okumura, K., Linsley, P.S., Ikehara, S., Muramatsu, S., Hodes, R.J. and Steinman, R.M. (1994). The tissue distribution of the B7-2 costimulator in mice: abundant expression on dendritic cells in situ and during maturation in vitro. *J. Exp. Med.* **180**, 1849–1860.

Jakob, T. and Udey, M.C. (1997). E-cadherin-mediated adhesion in Langerhans cell-like dendritic cells is regulated by cytokines that mobilize Langerhans cells in vivo. *J. Invest. Dermatol.* **109**, 257 (Abstract).

Kang, K., Kubin, M., Cooper, K.D., Lessin, S.R., Trinchieri, G. and Rook, A.H. (1996). IL-12 synthesis by human Langerhans cells. *J. Immunol.* **156**, 1402–1407.

Kelleher, P. and Knight, S.C. (1998). Interleukin-12 increases CD80 expression and the stimulatory capacity of bone marrow derived dendritic cells. *Int. Immunol.* **10**, in press.

Kimber, I. (1994). Cytokines and the regulation of allergic sensitization to chemicals. *Toxicology* **93**, 1–11.

Kimber, I. and Cumberbatch, M. (1992a). Dendritic cells and cutaneous immune responses to chemical allergens. *Toxicol. Appl. Pharmacol.* **117**, 137–146.

Kimber, I. and Cumberbatch, M. (1992b). Stimulation of Langerhans cell migration by tumor necrosis factor α (TNF-α). *J. Invest. Dermatol.* **99**, 48S–50S.

Kimber, I., Kinnaird, A., Peters, S.W. and Mitchell, J.A. (1990). Correlation between lymphocyte proliferative responses and dendritic cell migration to regional lymph nodes following skin painting with contact-sensitizing agents. *Int. Arch. Allergy Appl. Immunol.* **93**, 47–53.

Kimber, I., Holliday, M.R. and Dearman, R.J. (1995). Cytokine regulation of chemical sensitization. *Toxicol. Lett.* **82/83**, 491–496.

Kinnaird, A., Peters, S.W., Foster, J.R. and Kimber, I. (1989). Dendritic cell accumulation in draining lymph nodes during the induction phase of contact allergy in mice. *Int. Arch. Allergy Appl. Immunol.* **89**, 202–210.

Kleijmeer, M.J., Oorschot, V.M.J. and Geuze, H.J. (1994). Human resident Langerhans cells display a lysosomal compartment enriched in MHC class II. *J. Invest. Dermatol.* **103**, 516–523.

Knight, S.C., Balfour, B.M., O'Brien, J., Buttefant, L., Sumerska, T. and Clark, J. (1982). Role of veiled cells in lymphocyte activation. *Eur. J. Immunol.* **12**, 1057–1060.

Knight, S. C., Krejci, J., Malkovsky, M., Collizzi, V., Gautam, A. and Asherson, G.L. (1985). The role of dendritic cells in the initiation of immune responses to contact sensitizers. I. In vivo exposure to antigen. *Cell. Immunol.* **94**, 427–434.

Kobayashi, Y. (1997). Langerhans cells produce type IV collagenase (MMP-9) following epicutaneous stimulation with haptens. *Immunology* **90**, 496–501.

Koch, F., Heufler, C., Kampgen, E., Schneeweiss, D., Bock, G. and Schuler, G. (1990). Tumor necrosis factor alpha maintains the viability of murine epidermal Langerhans cells in culture but in contrast to granulocyte/macrophage colony-stimulating factor, does not induce their functional maturation. *J. Exp Med.* **171**, 159–172.

Kock, A., Schwartz, T., Kirnbauer, R., Urbanski, A., Perry, P., Ansel, J.C. and Luger, T.A. (1990). Human keratinocytes are a source for tumor necrosis factor α: evidence for synthesis and release upon stimulation with endotoxin or ultraviolet light. *J. Exp. Med.* **172**, 1609–1614.

Kripke, M.L., Munn, C.G., Jeevan, A., Tang, J.M. and Bucana, C. (1990) Evidence that cutaneous antigen-presenting cells migrate to regional lymph nodes during contact sensitization. *J. Immunol.* **145**, 2833–2838.

Lappin, M.B., Kimber, I. and Norval, M. (1996). The role of dendritic cells in cutaneous immunity. *Arch. Dermatol. Res.* **288**, 109–121.

Larregina, A., Morelli, A., Kolkowski, E. and Fainboim, L. (1996). Flow cytometric analysis of cytokine receptors on human Langerhans cells. Changes observed after short term culture. *Immunology* **87**, 317–325.

Larregina, A.T., Morrelli, A.E., Kolkowski, E., Sanjuan, N., Barboza, M.E. and Fainboim, L. (1997). Pattern of cytokine receptors expressed by human dendritic cells migrated from dermal explants. *Immunology* **91**, 303–313.

Larsen, C.P., Ritchie, S.C., Pearson, T.C., Linsley, P.S. and Lowry, R.P. (1992). Functional expression of the costimulatory molecule, B7/BB1, in murine dendritic cell populations. *J. Exp. Med.* **176**, 1215–1220.

Lenz, A., Heine, M., Schuler, G. and Romani, N. (1993). Human and murine dermis contain dendritic cells. Isolation by means of a novel method and phenotypical and functional characterization. *J. Clin. Invest.* **93**, 2587–2596.

Lewis, M., Tartaglia, L.A., Lee, A., Bennett, G.L., Rice, G.C., Wood, G.H.W., Chen, E.Y. and Goeddel, D.V. (1991). Cloning and expression of cDNAs for two distinct murine tumor necrosis factor receptors demonstrate one receptor is species specific. *Proc. Natl Acad. Sci. USA* **88**, 2830–2834.

Lisby, S., Muller, K.M., Jongeneel, V., Saurat, J-H. and Hauser, C. (1994). Nickel and skin irritants up-regulate tumor necrosis factor-α mRNA in keratinocytes by diferent but potentially synergistic mechanisms. *Int. Immunol.* **7**, 343–352.

Ma, J., Wing, J-H., Guo, Y-J., Sy, M-S. and Bigby, M. (1994) In vivo treatment with anti-ICAM-1 and anti-LFA-1 antibodies inhibits contact sensitization-induced migration of epidermal Langerhans cells to regional lymph nodes. *Cell. Immunol.* **158**, 389–399.

Macatonia, S.E., Edwards, A.J. and Knight, S.C. (1986). Dendritic cells and the initiation of contact sensitivity to fluorescein isothiocyanate. *Immunology* **59**, 509–514.

Macatonia, S.E., Knight, S.C., Edwards, A.J., Griffiths, S. and Fryer, P. (1987). Localization of antigen on lymph node dendritic cells after exposure to the contact sensitizer fluorescein isothiocyanate. Functional and morphological studies. *J. Exp. Med.* **166**, 1654–1667.

MacPherson, G.G., Jenkins, C.D., Stein, M.J. and Edwards, C. (1995). Endotoxin-mediated dendritic cell release from the intestine. Characterization of released dendritic cells and TNF dependence. *J. Immunol.* **154**, 1317–1322.

Matsue, H., Cruz, P.D. Jr., Bergstresser, P.R. and Takashima, A. (1992). Langerhans cells are the major source of mRNA for IL-1β and MIP-1α among unstimulated mouse epidermal cells. *J. Invest. Dermatol.* **99**, 537–541.

Mohamadzadeh, M., Poltorak, A.N., Bergstresser, P.R., Beutler, B. and Takashima, A. (1996). Dendritic cells produce macrophage inflammatory protein-1γ, a new member of the CC chemokine family. *J. Immunol.* **156**, 3102–3106.

Moodycliffe, A.M., Kimber, I. and Norval, M. (1992). The effect of ultraviolet B irradiation and urocanic acid isomers on dendritic cell migration. *Immunology* **77**, 394–399.

Moodycliffe, A.M., Kimber, I. and Norval, M. (1994). Role of tumour necrosis factor-α in ultraviolet B light-induced dendritic cell migration and suppression of contact hypersensitivity. *Immunology* **81**, 79–84.

Murayama, M., Yasuda, H., Nishimura, Y. and Asahi, M. (1997). Suppression of mouse contact hypersensitivity after treatment with antibodies to leukocyte function-associated antigen-1 and intercellular adhesion molecule-1. *Arch. Dermatol. Res.* **289**, 98–103.

Nestle, F.O., Zheng, X-G., Thompson, C.B., Turka, L.A. and Nickoloff, B.J. (1993). Characterization of dermal dendritic cells obtained from normal human skin reveals phenotypically and functionally distinct subsets. *J. Immunol.* **151**, 6535–6545.

Osada, A., Nakashima, H., Furue, M. and Tamaki, K. (1995). Up-regulation of CD44 expression by tumor necrosis factor-α is neutralized by interleukin-10 in Langerhans cells. *J. Invest. Dermatol.* **105**, 124–127.

Ozawa, H., Aiba, S., Nakagawa, S. and Tagami, H. (1996a). Interferon-γ and interleukin-10 inhibit antigen presentation by Langerhans cells for T helper type 1 cells by suppressing their CD80 (B7-1) expression. *Eur. J. Immunol.* **26**, 648–652.

Ozawa, H., Nakagawa, S., Tagami, H. and Aiba, S. (1996b). Interleukin-1β and granulocyte-macrophage colony-stimulating factor mediate Langerhans cell maturation differently. *J. Invest. Dermatol.* **106**, 441–445.

Picut, C.A., Lee, C.S., Dougherty, E.P., Anderson, K.L. and Lewis, R.M. (1988). Immunostimulatory capabilities of highly enriched Langerhans cells in vitro. *J. Invest. Dermatol.* **90**, 201–206.

Pierre, P., Turley, S.J., Gatti, E., Hull, M., Meltzer, J., Mirza, A., Inaba, K., Steinman, R.M. and Mellman, I. (1997). Developmental regulation of MHC class II transport in mouse dendritic cells. *Nature* **388**, 787–792.

Price, A.A., Cumberbatch, M., Kimber, I. and Ager, A. (1997). α6 integrins are required for Langerhans cell migration from the epidermis. *J. Exp. Med.* **186**, 1–11.

Pure, E., Inaba, K., Crowley, M.T., Tandelli, I., Witmer-Pack, M.D., Roberts, G., Fathman, G. and Steinman, R.M. (1990). Antigen processing by epidermal Langerhans cells correlates with the level of biosynthesis of major histocompatability complex class II molecules and expression of invariant chain. *J. Exp. Med.* **172**, 1459–1469.

Razi-Wolf, Z., Falo, L.D. Jr. and Reiser, H. (1994). Expression and function of the costimulatory molecule B7 on murine Langerhans cells: evidence for an alternative CTLA-4 ligand. *Eur. J. Immunol.* **24**, 805–811.

Reis e Sousa, C., Stahl, P.D. and Austyn, J.M. (1993). Phagocytosis of antigens by Langerhans cells in vitro. *J. Exp. Med.* **178**, 509–519.

Romani, N. and Schuler, G. (1992). The immunologic properties of epidermal Langerhans cells as part of the dendritic cell system. *Springer Semin. Immunopathol.* **13**, 265–279.

Romani, N., Koide, S., Crowley, M., Witmer-Pack, M., Livingstone, A.M., Fathman, C.G., Inaba, K. and Steinman, R.M. (1989a). Presentation of exogenous protein antigens by dendritic cells to T cell clones. Intact protein is presented by immature, epidermal Langerhans cells. *J. Exp. Med.* **169**, 1169–1178.

Romani, N., Lenz, A., Glassel, H., Stossel, H., Stanzl, U., Majdic, O., Fritsch, P. and Schuler, G. (1989b). Cultured human Langerhans cells resemble lymphoid dendritic cells in phenotype and function. *J. Invest. Dermatol.* **93**, 600–609.

Ryffel, B., Brockhaus, M., Greiner, B., Mihatsch, M.J. and Gudat, F. (1991). Tumour necrosis factor receptor distribution in human lymphoid tissue. *Immunology* **74**, 446–452.

Sallusto, F. and Lanzavecchia, A. (1994). Efficient presentation of soluble antigen by cultured human dendritic cells is maintained by granulocyte/macrophage colony-stimulating factor plus interleukin 4 and is downregulated by tumor necrosis factor α. *J. Exp. Med.* **179**, 1109–1118.

Saren, P., Welgus, H.G. and Kovanen, P.T. (1996) TNF-α and IL-1β selectively induce expression of 92-kDa gelatinase by human macrophages. *J. Immunol.* **157**, 4159–4165.

Schreiber, S., Kilgus, O., Payer, E., Kutil, R., Elbe, A., Mueller, C. and Stingl, G. (1992). Cytokine pattern of Langerhans cells isolated from murine epidermal cell cultures. *J. Immunol.* **149**, 3525–3534.

Schuler, G. and Steinman, R.M. (1985). Murine epidermal Langerhans cells mature into potent immunostimulatory dendritic cells in vitro. *J. Exp. Med.* **161**, 526–546.

Schwarzenberger, K. and Udey, M.C. (1996). Contact allergens and epidermal proinflammatory cytokines modulate Langerhans cell E-cadherin expression in situ. *J. Invest. Dermatol.* **106**, 553–558.

Shornick, L.P., De Togni, P., Mariathasan, S., Goeliner, J., Strauss-Schoenberger, J., Karr, R.W., Ferguson, T.A. and Chaplin, D.D. (1996). Mice deficient in IL-1β manifest impaired contact hypersensitivity to trinitrochlorobenzene. *J. Exp. Med.* **183**, 1427–1436.

Silberberg-Sinakin, I., Gigli, I., Baer, R.L. and Thorbecke, G.J. (1980). Langerhans cells: role in contact hypersensitivity and relationship to lymphoid dendritic cells and to macrophages. *Immunol. Rev.* **53**, 203–232.

Steinman, R., Hoffman, L. and Pope, M. (1995). Maturation and migration of cutaneous dendritic cells. *J. Invest. Dermatol.* **105**, 2S–7S.

Stoitzner, P., Koch, F., Janke, K. and Romani, N. (1997). Differential effects of TNF-α in the migration of murine Langerhans cells. *J. Invest. Dermatol.* **109**, 265 (Abstract).

Stoll, S., Muller, G., Kurimoto, M., Saloga, J., Tanimoto, T., Yamauchi, H., Knop, J. and Enk, A.H. (1997a). Murine dendritic cells produce IL-18 mRNA and functional protein. *J. Invest. Dermatol.* **109**, 266 (Abstract).

Stoll, S., Muller, G., Kurimoto, M., Saloga, J., Tanimoto, T., Yamauchi, H., Okamura, H., Knop, J. and Enk, A.H. (1997b). Production of IL-18 (IFN-γ-inducing factor) messenger RNA and functional protein by murine keratinocytes. *J. Immunol.* **159**, 298–302.

Stossel, H., Koch, F., Kampgen, E., Stoger, P., Lenz, A., Heufler, C., Romani, N. and Schuler, G. (1990). Disappearance of certain acidic organelles (endosomes and Langerhans cell granules) accompanies loss of antigen processing capacity upon culture of epidermal Langerhans cells. *J. Exp. Med.* **172**, 1471–1482.

Streilein, J.W. and Grammer, S.F. (1989). In vitro evidence that Langerhans cells can adopt two functionally distinct forms capable of antigen presentation to T lymphocytes. *J. Immunol.* **143**, 3925–3933.

Streilein, J.W., Grammer, S.F., Yoshikawa, T., Demidem, A. and Vermeer, M. (1990). Functional dichotomy between Langerhans cells that present antigen to naive and memory/effector T lymphocytes. *Immunol. Rev.* **117**, 159–183.

Tang, A., Amagai, M., Granger, L.G., Stanley, J.R. and Udey, M.C. (1993). Adhesion of epidermal Langerhans cells to keratinocytes mediated by E-cadherin. *Nature* **361**, 82–85.

Teunissen, M.B.M., Koomen, C.W., Jansen, J., de Waal Malefyt, R., Schmitt, E., van den Wijngaard, R.M.J.G.J., Das, P.K. and Bos, J.D. (1997). In contrast to their murine counterparts, normal human keratinocytes and human epidermoid cell lines A431 and HaCaT fail to express IL-10 mRNA and protein. *Clin. Exp. Immunol.* **107**, 213–223.

Tse, Y. and Cooper, K.D. (1990). Cutaneous dermal Ia$^+$ cells are capable of initiating delayed-type hypersensitivity responses. *J. Invest. Dermatol.* **94**, 267–272.

Vermeer, M. and Streilein, J.W. (1990). Ultraviolet B light-induced alterations in epidermal Langerhans cells is mediated in part by tumor necrosis factor-alpha. *Photodermatol. Photoimmunol. Photomed.* **7**, 258–265.

Wang, B., Kondo, S., Shivh, G.M., Fujisawa, H., Mak, T.W. and Sauder, D.N. (1996). Tumour necrosis factor receptor II (p75) signalling is required for the migration of Langerhans cells. *Immunology* **88**, 284–288.

Weiss, J.M., Sleeman, J., Renkl, A.C., Dittmar, H., Termeer, C.C., Taxis, S., Howells, N., Hofmann, M., Kohler, G., Schopf, E., Ponta, H., Herrlich, P. and Simon, J.C. (1997). An essential role for CD44 variant isoforms in epidermal Langerhans cell and blood dendritic cell function. *J. Cell. Biol.* **137**, 1137–1147.

Williams, N.J., Harvey, J.J., Duncan, I., Booth, R. and Knight, S.C. (1998). IL-12 restores dendritic cell function and cell mediated immunity in retrovirus infected mice. *Cell. Immunol.* **183**, 121–130.

Witmer-Pack, M.D., Olivier, W., Valinsky, J., Schuler, G. and Steinman, R.M. (1987). Granulocyte/macrophage colony-stimulating factor is essential for the viability and function of cultured murine epidermal Langerhans cells. *J. Exp. Med.* **166**, 1484–1498.

CHAPTER 18
Dendritic Cells in the Reproductive Tract

Adriana Larregina and Adrian Morelli
Molecular Medicine Unit, Department of Medicine, University of Manchester, Manchester, UK

DENDRITIC CELLS IN THE FEMALE GENITAL TRACT

Anatomical Distribution

The uterine cervix is composed of three different anatomical regions with distinct histology and physiology: (i) the ectocervix; (ii) the endocervix; and (iii) the transformation zone. The ectocervix consists of stratified squamous epithelium overlying a vascular chorion. The ectocervical epithelium is continuous with the simple columnar epithelium of the endocervix. The junction between the stratified squamous and columnar epithelium is termed the transformation zone, and is of particular importance because it is the cervical site with the highest incidence of viral infections and related preneoplastic and neoplastic conditions.

Since 1968, when Langerhans cells (LC) were discovered in the human ectocervix by means of electron microscopy (Younes *et al.*, 1968; Hackemann *et al.*, 1968), several investigators have studied the population of dendritic cells (DC) in the normal cervix uteri (Figueroa and Caorsi, 1980; Morris *et al.*, 1983a; Edwards and Morris, 1985; Caorsi and Figueroa, 1986; Hawthorn and MacLean 1987; Morelli *et al.*, 1992a). The use of different staining techniques for detection of LC, the utilization of distinct methods of sample processing (vertical sections versus epithelial sheets), and the existence of local variations in the LC number in different areas of the cervix gave rise to controversial results for the density and distribution of LC in human cervix uteri. As in other stratified squamous epithelia (i.e. epidermis), ectocervical LC show dendritic morphology; express HLA-DR, CD1a, CD1c, CD32, S-100, CD4, and membrane ATPase; and are located among the basal, parabasal and intermediate layers of keratinocytes. Basal LC have fewer cytoplasmic processes than LC in the mid-zone of the epithelium. Some basal LC extend their processes through the basement membrane, a finding that might represent partially migrated LC, either entering or leaving the epithelium. The mean LC density in human ectocervix is 511 ± 89 cells/mm^2 of epithelial surface (Morelli *et al.*, 1992a). LC are more abundant near the cervical external orifice and in the vicinity of the fornix than in the central area of the ectocervix (Figueroa and Caorsi, 1980; Morelli *et al.*, 1992a). There is no significant difference in the density of

Dendritic Cells: Biology and Clinical Applications
ISBN 0-12-455860-7

ectocervical DC between premenopausal and postmenopausal women. DC are also present in the subepithelial stroma of the ectocervix (Roncalli *et al.*, 1988).

The endocervix consists of a simple layer of columnar mucous secreting cells and subcolumnar reserve cells overlying a submucosa. Epithelial infoldings, from the lumen of the endocervical canal into the underlying submucosa, create false glands or crypts termed endocervical glands. Different groups have reported in humans and monkeys the presence of LC within the columnar epithelium of the endocervical canal, in the endocervical glands, and even in the subepithelial submucosa of endocervix (Puts *et al.*, 1986; Miller *et al.*, 1992; Hussain *et al.*,1992).

Depending on external stimuli, the original columnar epithelium of the transformation zone can be replaced with squamous epithelium by a process known as squamous cell metaplasia. When the metaplasia is complete and the squamous epithelium is fully mature and no columnar cells remain, LC are present at a density and distribution and with a morphology similar to those observed in ectocervical epithelium (DiGirolamo *et al.*, 1985; Roncalli *et al.*, 1988; Morelli *et al.*, 1991). However, during the early stages of metaplasia, the immature squamous epithelium, instead of having typical LC, is populated by round-shaped cells, some of them with short and unbranched dendrites, that are positive for CD1a, CD1c and HLA-DR and with frequent mitotic images. As described in other squamous epithelia (i.e. epidermis), it is likely that this subpopulation represents DC precursors colonizing a just-generated squamous epithelium. However, it remains unknown whether LC precursors (i) arrive from the endocervical columnar epithelium, the underlying chorion, or the neighbouring squamous ectocervical epithelium; or (ii) arrive from bone marrow and, via bloodstream–chorion, reach the metaplastic epithelium.

The inner surface of the uterine body is covered by the endometrium, a mucosa composed of a columnar secreting epithelium with tubular glands overlying a lamina propria. In rodents, endometrial DC are located in the connective tissue between the glands, and in the glandular stroma (Head and Billingham, 1986; Head and Gaede, 1986). Beyond the uterine mucosa, DC can be detected between the two muscle layers of the myometrium and in the serosa, around blood vessels. In humans, cells expressing HLA-DR and with DC morphology were detected in proliferative and secretory endometrium (Bulmer *et al.*, 1988).

The vagina is composed of a stratified squamous epithelium overlying a vascular chorion. LC are located in the basal and parabasal cell layers of vaginal epithelium, as well as in the underlying chorion (Burgos and Roig de Vargas-Linares,1978; Miller *et al.*, 1992; Witkin, 1993). They are more sparsely distributed than in the ectocervix, so the density of LC in vagina is lower than in cervical epithelium (Edwards and Morris, 1985).

Variation During the Hormonal Cycle

In cervix and vagina, LC are surrounded by hormone-dependent and cyclically changing epithelium. In fact, the thickness of cervical and vaginal epithelium changes significantly along the course of the menstrual cycle in humans and monkeys, and during the oestrous cycle in rodents. In mice, there is an inverse relationship between the intraepithelial LC density in vagina and the mitotic activity of the epithelium. Thus, the density of LC is significantly lower in pro-oestrus and oestrus, than in metoestrus and early dioestrus (Young, 1985; Young *et al.*, 1985). During the beginning of the oestrous cycle (pro-oestrus and oestrus), LC decrease as a result of the increase both in thickness and breadth of the basal, parabasal, and intermediate epithelial compartments caused by the epithelial proliferation induced by oestrogens. On the other hand, there is no relationship between LC density and the keratinization stage of the upper epithelial strata (Young and Hosking, 1986). Apoptosis of epithelial cells occurs between late metoestrus and early dioestrus, in response to the decline of oestrogen and progesterone. During that period, LC in vagina are less dendritic, are dispersed throughout the epithelial thickness, and are involved in phagocytosis of epithelial apoptotic cells (Parr and Parr 1990; Parr *et al.*, 1991a).

As in vagina, the density of DC in endometrium is also affected by the circulating levels of oestrogens and progesterone, though in the opposite way. Thus, the highest density of DC in rat endometrium is observed at oestrus, and the lowest at dioestrus. Moreover, in ovariectomized rats, oestradiol causes a significant increase in the number of DC in endometrium, an effect that is blocked by progesterone (Head and Gaede, 1986). During pregnancy in rats, DC become very sparse in the decidua, and they are practically absent in the central decidua, adjacent to the site of implantation (Head and Billingham, 1986). Such a phenomenon might be viewed as a safety mechanism to isolate maternal DC from the conceptus, which can be considered as a semi-allogeneic implant. On the other hand, in nondecidualized areas, distant from the implantation area, DC are abundant. After 10 days of implantation, maternal DC appear at the materno-fetal interface and, by that time, the success of the fetal semi-allograft must depend on other immune-protective mechanisms. In humans, several authors have reported the presence of DC in decidua at 36 weeks and later (Dorman and Searle, 1988).

In human ectocervix, LC density is significantly lower during the oestrogenic phase of the cycle, when the epithelium is in active replication. LC density reaches its maximum by the ovulatory peak and then decreases again during the progestational phase (Morelli *et al.*, 1993b). The LC number is lower in the cervix of pregnant women compared to non-pregnant controls (Poppe *et al.*, 1996a). It is interesting that, in spite of the epithelial changes along the menstrual cycle, LC remain in the basal and parabasal strata of the ectocervical epithelium. That can explain why LC cells are never found in cervical smears, which only contain epithelial cells exfoliated from the ectocervical surface (Figueroa *et al.*, 1989). In contrast, they are detected in cervical smears from patients with cervical squamous carcinoma and cervical intraepithelial neoplasia, where LC are located throughout the thickness of the epithelium.

Function as Antigen Processing and Presenting Cells

LC located in vaginal and cervical epithelium of mice can internalize soluble proteins from the vaginal lumen (Parr and Parr 1990; Parr *et al.*, 1991b). This observation supports the concept that LC in the reproductive tract, as reported in other tissues, have a principal role in the uptake of external antigens. However, the antigen uptake in vaginal mucosa also depends on the hormonal status of the epithelium being much more efficient at dioestrus than at oestrus (Parr and Parr, 1990). Although the LC density in vagina is higher at dioestrus, the increase in antigen uptake and presentation seems to be related to differences in thickness and permeability in the epithelium. When the epithelial permeability increases, antigens can reach the lower half of the epithelium where LC reside. In mice at dioestrus, under the effects of progesterone, the epithelium is more permeable to proteins (40–450 kDa) than at oestrus, when it is under oestrogen control. In agreement with that observation, several reports have demonstrated that vaginal immunization in mice is more effective at dioestrus or after exogenous administration of progesterone (Wira and Rossol, 1995a; Hopkins *et al.*, 1995). The control exerted by oestrogens and progesterone upon the antigen permeability in vaginal epithelium might explain why progesterone enhances the intravaginal transmission of certain viral infections, such as herpes simplex virus type 2 in mice, and simian immunodeficiency virus in monkey (Parr *et al.* 1994; Marx *et al.*, 1996). The physiological role of such differential antigen sampling during the different phases of the hormonal cycle is unknown. It is likely that the block to antigen uptake at oestrus might minimize sensitization to sperm antigens at the time of mating (Parr and Parr, 1990).

Antigen-presenting cells (APC) from lamina propria of rat endometrium exhibit an inverse response to oestrogens in comparison to vaginal epithelium. Thus, the antigen presentation by APC from endometrial lamina propria is highest at oestrus and lowest at dioestrus (Wira and Rossoll, 1995b). The regulation of the antigen-presenting capacity of selected areas of the reproductive tract by oestrogens and progesterone along the sexual cycle might confer a window of immunosuppression during fertilization and implantation (i.e. low antigen-presenting capacity in vagina at oestrus to avoid immunization with sperm antigens during mating; and low antigen-presenting capacity in endometrial stroma at diestrus to allow implantation of conceptus) (Wira and Rossoll, 1995b).

DENDRITIC CELLS AND VIRAL INFECTIONS OF THE FEMALE GENITAL TRACT

Human Papillomavirus (HPV)

The lower female and male genital tracts can be the target of infection by mucotropic types of HPV, such as types 6, 11, 16, 18, 31, 33, and 35. HPV 6 and 11 are associated with genital condylomas (warts) and/or low-degree intraepithelial neoplasias with favourable clinical evolution. By contrast, the genomes of HPV 16, 18, and less frequently HPV 31, 33 and 35, are found in high degree intraepithelial neoplasias and invasive genital carcinomas (Schneider, 1993). Much of the transforming potential of HPV 16 and 18 arises from the biological effects of their E6 and E7 oncoproteins, which have the capacity to bind and affect the function of the regulatory proteins p53 and the retinoblastoma gene product p105-RB which control cell cycle and DNA repair. However, HPV per se is not sufficient to give rise to invasive genital cancer. It has been postulated that the host immune surveillance plays an important role in the control of the persistence, progression, regression, and malignant transformation of condylomas caused by HPV infection. Although the nature of an effective immune response against the HPV infection is not completely understood, studies in skin warts suggest that the cell-mediated immune response is more important than humoral immunity. As in many other tissues, in the genital tract LC are the professional APC in charge of generating T cell responses to viral infections and neoplasms. LC are particularly affected in epithelial lesions caused by HPV.

LC in HPV Infection of the Genital tract

Different authors have demonstrated that cervical condylomas are associated with a significant depletion of intraepithelial LC. The decrease in LC number after HPV infection might be due either to a reduction in the absolute number of LC or to a downregulation of the markers used to detect DC in cervical epithelium. However, the latter hypothesis seems unlikely, because a similar reduction in the number of epithelial LC in cervical condylomas has been reported by several groups by means of different DC markers (i.e. CD1a, HLA-DR, S-100) or different histochemical techniques (i.e. ATPase, zinc–iodide–osmium stain) (Morris *et al.*, 1983b; McArdle and Muller, 1986; Barton *et al.*, 1988; Hachisuga *et al.*, 1989, Morelli *et al.*, 1993a; Al-Saleh *et al.*, 1995).

Although, so far, there is no experimental evidence, it is likely that the reduction in the number of intraepithelial LC in cervical condylomas might weaken the afferent limb of the epithelial immune system. Several authors have postulated the LC decrease as a cofactor that might favour the persistence of HPV infection and, as a consequence, the malignant transformation induced by certain types of HPV in the cervical epithelium (e.g. cervical intraepithelial neoplasia; CIN) (Morris *et al.*, 1983b; McArdle and Muller, 1986).

The mechanism(s) for the partial reduction and morphological alteration of cervical LC during HPV infections remains unknown and may be interpreted in several ways. HPV infection alters keratinocyte maturation, inducing acanthosis and parakeratosis in ectocervical epithelium. Such changes might affect the intraepithelial LC trafficking or differentiation (cervical LC express higher levels of MHC class II molecules during HPV infection; Hughes *et al.*, 1988). Alternatively, LC abnormalities might be the result of a direct cytotoxic effect induced by HPV. However, the restricted cytotropism of HPV, and the lack of evidence demonstrating that LC can be infected by HPV, make this hypothesis unlikely.

The low number of LC in cervical HPV infection appears to be related to a productive HPV infection, and to the presence of koilocytosis and tetraploidy in epithelial cells, rather than the type of HPV (McArdle and Muller, 1986; Lehtinen *et al.*, 1993). In fact, in cervical condylomas and low-degree CIN, those HPV types not associated with malignant transformation (HPV 6 and 11) cause a LC decrease similar to that induced by HPV 16 or 18 (Viac *et al.*, 1990; Morelli *et al*, 1993a; Al-Saleh *et al.*, 1995). These data support the idea that the reduction in the number of LC is not associated with the different clinical progressions observed in distinct types of HPV in cervix uteri. In agreement with this observation, HPV infection in epithelia with low incidence of malignant transformation, such as vulva and penis, also causes a significant decrease of LC number (Morelli *et al.*, 1992b; Morelli *et al.*, 1994).

LC in Cervical Intraepithelial Neoplasia (CIN)

In CIN, LC are detected throughout the entire thickness of the epithelium and their dendrites are much shorter and less numerous. The abnormal DC morphology and distribution have been attributed to a defect in cell maturation or trafficking, or as a result of DC compression by adjacent neoplastic cells, many of which are abnormally orientated in the epithelium. Normal cervical epithelial cells have been shown to produce and secrete in culture IL-1β, GM-CSF and TNF-α, all cytokines involved in LC maturation (Woodworth and Simpson, 1993). Interestingly, when the same cultures are immortalized *in vitro* by HPV 16 or 18 DNA, there is a significant reduction in the levels of IL-1β and GM-CSF released (Woodworth and Simpson, 1993). Another possibility is that IL-10, which is known to be expressed in cervical intraepithelial lesions caused by HPV, plays some role in depleting or inhibiting cervical LC (Al-Saleh *et al.*, 1995).

Several groups have scored the density of LC in different grades of CIN (e.g. CIN 1, CIN 2 and CIN 3) with contradictory results depending on the protocol used to assess epithelial DC (tissue sections vs epithelial sheets; paraffin-embedded vs frozen tissue; DC markers; etc.). In general, most authors agree that the number of LC detected in CIN is higher than in condylomas. Although some early studies suggested an increase in LC in CIN compared to normal epithelium (Morris *et al.*, 1983b; Caorsi and Figueroa, 1986; McArdle and Muller, 1986; Hachisuga *et al.*, 1989), most of the following reports have shown a significant LC depletion compared to unaffected controls (Puts *et al.*, 1986; Tay *et al.*, 1987; Hughes *et al.*, 1988; Barton *et al.*, 1988, Morelli *et al.*, 1993a; Cristoforoni *et al.*, 1995). In CIN, the number of LC seems to be particularly affected by HPV 18 even when its genome is present at low copy number (less than 10 copies per cell) (Hawthorn *et al.*, 1988).

There is an inverse relationship between the density of intraepithelial LC and factor XIII-positive stromal DC in cervical HPV lesions. Al-Saleh *et al.* (1995) found that the number of factor XIII-positive stromal dendrocytes increased in cervical HPV condylomas and in CIN.

LC, Cervical HPV Lesions, and Immunosuppression

It is well known that patients positive for human immunodeficiency virus (HIV) have a high incidence of genital HPV infections and HPV-associated neoplasia (Schneider, 1993). This observation is explained by the alteration of the immune system in the HIV-infected population, which increases the risk of acquisition, reactivation, progression, relapsing after treatment, and malignant transformation of an HPV infection. Spinillo *et al.* (1993) demonstrated that the number of LC in cervix uteri is significantly lower in HIV-infected women than observed in noninfected matched controls. Moreover, the LC depletion observed in samples of CIN obtained from HIV-seropositive patients is more severe in comparison to CIN from HIV negative women (Spinillo *et al.*, 1993). HIV might act on the progression of HPV-related lesions by first infecting and then impairing the function of or killing LC in the genital tract.

LC from cervix uteri are also susceptible to the effects of cigarette smoke constituents present in cervical mucus of women who smoke (Poppe *et al.*, 1996b). Barton *et al.* (1988) demonstrated that there are significantly fewer LC in normal cervical epithelium of smokers in comparison to nonsmokers and ex-smokers. The number of LC in HPV infection and CIN is significantly lower in smokers than in matched controls (Barton *et al.*, 1988).

Cervical LC are also reduced in number in other immune-suppressive states such as chronic renal failure (McKerrow *et al.*, 1989) and in certain autoimmune diseases including Sjögren's syndrome (Oxholm *et al.*, 1986).

Human Immunodeficiency Virus (HIV)

HIV is the aetiological agent of acquired immunodeficiency syndrome (AIDS). The transmission of HIV-1, the main type of the AIDS virus, can occur through vaginal intercourse, through male homosexual activity or through contact with infected blood (i.e. during intravenous drug use or blood transfusions). Whereas heterosexual transmission is the major route of infection in Africa and Southeast Asia, the other models are most common in North America and Europe.

Strong evidence suggests that DC play an important role during the initial spread of HIV; (i) LC and other subpopulations of DC express CD4 glycoprotein, the main cellular receptor for HIV; (ii) HIV particles have been identifed by electron microscopy in LC from AIDS patients; and (iii) purified DC can be infected *in vitro* with HIV.

Semen from AIDS patient bears HIV-free virions and HIV-infected T cells. Different mechanisms were postulated to explain how cell-free or cell-associated HIV virions might cross through the female genital mucosa. HIV may be taken up, via CD4, by vaginal or cervical LC. It is known that LC from vaginal epithelium, ectocervix, transformation zone, endocervical epithelium, and subepithelial stroma express CD4 (Hussain *et al.*, 1992). Alternatively, vaginal and cervical LC, which express FcγRII (CD32) and FcγRIII (CD16) might also take up HIV–antibody complexes via Fc receptors (Hussain *et al.*, 1992). In a second step, HIV-infected LC could leave the genital tract via the submucosal lymphatic vessels and migrate towards the paracortical area of the draining lymph nodes. Once in the satellite lymph node, DC could be able to cluster and infect a high number of CD4 T cells. Infected T cells and free virus could leave the lymph node through the efferent lymphatic vessels and disseminate the infection systemically.

HIV cell-free virions might also cross the epithelial barrier through transepithelial transport of virus carried in intracytoplasmic vesicles by the columnar cells of the endocervix. It is known that HIV-infected T cells, such as those present in the seminal fluid, can adhere to the luminal surface of epithelial surfaces. Such cellular union might facilitate viral uptake by host cells, and might even be the first step during a process of transepithelial migration. However, the relevance of such mechanisms in the human genital tract is unknown (Kraehenbuhl and Wain-Hobson, 1996). Epithelial breaches in the genital mucosa also represent a passage of entry for HIV. CD4-positive T cells and CD4-positive tissue macrophages, mostly located in the submucosa of the female genital tract, can also be the target of HIV infection: directly by HIV virions that after crossing the epithelium reached the subepithelial stroma; indirectly via HIV-infected DC.

Spira *et al.* (1996), using a model in *Macacus rhesus*, studied the earliest events that follow the intravaginal administration of simian immunodeficiency virus (SIV). In this model, the first cellular targets of infection were cells with DC morphology, and lymphocytes, located in the submucosa of vagina, ectocervix and endocervix. Some of the SIV-positive cells were also positive for HLA-DR and S-100, both DC markers, and were negative for CD68, a molecule expressed by macrophages and absent in DC. The authors also demonstrated that the SIV dissemination first takes place in the draining lymph nodes of genital tract (internal iliac), and later systemically to other nonsatellite lymph nodes. An interesting observation is that the SIV-positive cells from the genital tract follow the pattern of migration described for DC (present in the paracortical T cell areas, and absent in germinal centres of lymph nodes).

The existence of subtypes of HIV-1 raised the question whether different viral variants might infect DC and other cell targets with different efficiency. Based on the fact that HIV-1E grows quite well in LC *in vitro*, and that HIV-1B hardly grows at all in

LC but grows well in lymphocytes and monocytes, Soto-Ramirez *et al.* (1996) suggested a putative explanation for the different ways of epidemic spreading of HIV-1. In undeveloped countries (in Africa and Southeast Asia), where HIV-1-C, -E, -D and -A predominate, the first cellular HIV-1 target would be the LC of the genital tract, and DC infection would occur through vaginal intercourse. In developed countries (Europe and the United States), where HIV-1B is the main viral subtype, the primary cell targets would be lymphocytes and monocytes and their infection would take place through blood and homosexual intercourse. However, recent evidence does not support the concept that different subtypes of HIV-1 show a differential cell type-specific tropism for DC (Pope *et al.*, 1997; Dittmar *et al.*, 1997).

DENDRITIC CELLS IN THE MALE GENITAL TRACT

A few reports have demonstrated the presence of intraepithelial LC in the stratified squamous epithelium that lines the foreskin, urethral meatus, and fossa navicularis in mice and humans (Weiss *et al.*, 1993; Quayle, 1994; Pudney and Anderson, 1995). However, macrophages appear to be the primary APC in the stratified columnar epithelium that covers the penile urethra beyond the fossa navicularis. In fact, so far, no DC have been reported in the epithelium of this region (Weiss *et al.*, 1993; Quayle, 1994; Pudney and Anderson, 1995).

The squamous epithelium that covers the penis and the urethral meatus can be the target of HPV infection, and even malignant transformation of HPV-associated lesions (i.e. penile intraepithelial neoplasia; PIN). Penile condylomas caused by HPV show a significant depletion and morphological alterations of intraepithelial LC, similar to those observed in condylomas of the female genital tract (Morelli *et al.*, 1992b).

REFERENCES

Al-Saleh, W., Delvenne, P., Arrese, J., Nikkels, A., Pierard, G. and Boniver, J. (1995). Inverse modulation of intraepithelial Langerhans' cells and stromal macrophage/dendrocyte populations in human papillomavirus-associated squamous intraepithelial lesions of the cervix. *Virchows Arch.* **427**, 41–48.

Barton, S., Maddox, P., Jenkins, D., Edwards, R., Cuzick, J. and Singer, A. (1988). Effect of cigarette smoking on cervical epithelial immunity: mechanism for neoplastic change? *Lancet* **2** (8612), 652–654.

Bulmer, J., Lunny, D. and Hogin, S. (1988). Immunohistochemical characterization of stromal leukocytes in non-pregnant human endometrium. *Am. J. Reprod. Immunol. Microbiol.* **17**, 83–90.

Burgos, M. and Roig de Vargas-Linares, C. (1978). Ultrastructure of the vaginal mucosa. In: *The Human Vagina* (ed. H. Hafez and E. Evans). Elsevier, Amsterdam, p. 63.

Caorsi, I. and Figueroa, C. (1986). Langerhans cell density in the normal exocervical epithelium and in the cervical intraepithelial neoplasia. *Br. J. Obset. Gynaecol.* **93**, 993–998.

Cristoforoni, P., Favre, A., Cennamo, V., Giunta, M., Corte, G. and Grossi, E. (1995). Expression of a novel β_1 integrin in the dysplastic progression of the cervical epithelium. *Gynecol. Oncol.* **58**, 319–326.

DiGirolamo, W., Goni, J. and Laguens, R. (1985). Langerhans' cells in squamous metaplasia of the human uterine cervix. *Gynecol. Obstet. Invest.* **19**, 38–41.

Dittmar, M., Simmons, G., Hibbits, M., O'Hare M., Louisirirotchanakul, S., Beddows, S., Weber, J., Clapham, R. and Weiss, R. (1997). Langerhans cell tropism of human immunodeficiency virus type 1 subtype A through F isolates derived from different transmission groups. *J. Virol.* **71**, 7978–7983.

Dorman, P. and Searle, R. (1988). Alloantigen presenting capacity of human decidual tissue. *J Reprod. Immunol.* **13**, 101–112.

Edwards, J. and Morris, H. (1985). Langerhans cells and lymphocyte subsets in the female genital tract. *Br. J. Obstet. Gynaecol.* **92**, 974–982.

Figueroa, C. and Caorsi, I. (1980). Ultrastructural and morphometric study of the Langerhans' cells in the normal human exocervix. *J. Anat.* **131**, 669–682.

Figueroa, C., Concha, M. and Caorsi, I. (1989). Immunocytochemical demonstration of Langerhans' cells in smears and pellets of exfoliated cells from human exocervices. *Acta Cytol.* **33**, 219–222.

Hackemann, M., Grubb, C. and Hill, K. (1968). The ultrastructure of normal squamous epithelium of the human cervix uteri. *J. Ultrastruct. Res.* **22**, 443–457.

Hachisuga, T., Fukuda, K., Hayashi, Y., Iwasaka, T. and Sugimori, H. (1989), Immunohistochemical demonstration of histiocytes in normal ectocervical epithelium and epithelial lesions of the uterine cervix. *Gynecol. Oncol.* **33**, 273–278.

Hawthorn, R. and MacLean, A. (1987). Langerhans cell density in the normal exocervical epithelium and in the cervical intraepithelial neoplasia. *Br. J. Obstet. Gynaecol.* **94**, 815–816.

Hawthorn, R., Murdoch, J., MacLean, A. and MacKie, R. (1988) Langerhans' cells and subtypes of human papillomavirus in cervical intraepithelial neoplasia. *Br. Med. J.* **297**, 643–646.

Head, J. and Billingham, R. (1986). Concerning the immunology of the uterus. *Am. J. Reprod. Immunol Microbiol.* **10**, 76–81.

Head, J. and Gaede, S. (1986). Ia antigen expression in rat uterus. *J. Reprod. Immunol.* **9**, 137–153.

Hopkins, S., Kraehenbuhl, J., Schodel, F., Potts, A., Petterson, D., deGrandi, P. and Nardelli-Haefriger, D. (1995). A recombinant *Salmonella typhimurium* vaccine induces local immnunity by four different routes of immunization. *Infect. Immun.* **63**, 3279–3286.

Hughes, R., Norval, M. and Howie, S. (1988). Expression of major histocompatibility class II antigens by Langerhans's cells in cervical intraepithelial neoplasia. *J. Clin. Pathol.* **41**, 253–259.

Hussain, L., Kelly, C., Fellowes, R., Hecht, E., Wilson, J. and Chapman, M. (1992). Expression and gene transcript of Fc receptor for IgG, HLA class II antigens and Langerhans cells in human cervico-vaginal epithelium. *Clin. Exp. Immunol.* **90**, 530–538.

Kraehenbuhl, J. and Wain-Hobson, S. (1996). Breaching barriers. SIV vaginal transmission in monkeys may be enhanced by progesterone. *Nature Medicine* **2**, 1080–1082.

Lehtinen, M., Rantala, I., Toivonen, A., Luoto, H., Aine, R., Lauslahti, K., Yla-Outinen, A., Romppanen, U. and Paavonen, J. (1993). Depletion of Langerhans cells in cervical HPV infection is associated with replication of the virus. *APMIS* **101**, 833–837.

Marx, P., Spira, A., Gettie, A., Dailey, P., Veazey, R., Lackner, A., Mahoney, C., Miller, C., Claypool, L., Ho, D. and Alexander, N. (1996). Progesterone implants enhance SIV vaginal transmission and early virus load. *Nature Medicine* **2**, 1084–1089.

McArdle, J. and Muller, K. (1986). Quantitative assessment of Langerhans'cells in human cervical intraepithelial neoplasia and wart virus infection. *Am. J. Obstet. Gynecol.* **154**, 509–515.

McKerrow, K., Hawthorn, R. and Thompson, W. (1989). An investigation of circulating and *in situ* lymphocyte subsets and Langerhans cells in the skin and cervix of patients with chronic renal failure. *Br. J. Dermatol.* **120**, 745–755.

Miller, C., McChesney, M. and Moore, P. (1992) Langerhans cells, macrophages and lymphocyte subsets in the cervix and vagina of rhesus macaques. *Lab. Invest.* **67**, 628–634.

Morelli, A, Larregina, A., DiPaola, G. and Fainboim, L. (1991) Intraepithelial CD1 positive Langerhans cell precursors in transformations zone squamous metaplasia. *The Cervix & Lower Female Genital Tract* **9**, 69–75.

Morelli, A., DiPaola, G. and Fainboim, L. (1992a). Density and distribution of Langerhans cells in the human uterine cervix. *Arch. Gynecol. Obstet.* **252**, 65–71.

Morelli, A., Ronchetti, R., Secchi, A., Cufre, M., Paredes, A. and Fainboim, L. (1992b). Assessment by planimetry of Lagerhans cell density in penile epithelium with human papillomavirus infection: changes observed after topical treatment. *J. Urol.* **147**, 1268–1273.

Morelli, A., Sananes, C., DiPaola, G., Paredes, A. and Fainboim, L. (1993a). Relationship between types of human papillomavirus and Langerhans' cells in cervical condyloma and intraepithelial neoplasia. *Am. J. Clin. Pathol.* **99**, 200–206.

Morelli, A., Tatti, S., DiPaola, G., Paredes, A. and Fainboim, L. (1993b). Langerhans cell variation in the human uterine cervix during the menstrual cycle. *The Cervix & Lower Female Genital Tract* **11**, 99–101.

Morelli, A., Belardi, G., DiPaola, G., Paredes, A. and Fainboim, L. (1994). Cellular subsets and epithelial ICAM-1 and HLA-DR expression in human papillomavirus infection of the vulva. *Acta. Dermatol. Venereol (Stockh)* **74**, 45–50.

Morris, H. Gatter, K., Stein, H. and Mason, D. (1983a). Langerhans cells in human cervical epithelium: an immunohistological study. *Br. J. Obstet. Gynaecol.* **90**, 400–411.

Morris, H., Gatter, K., Sykes, G., Casemore, V. and Mason, D. (1983b) Langerhans' cells in human cervical epithelium: effects of wart virus infection and intraepithelial neoplasia. *Br. J. Obstet. Gynaecol.* **90**, 412–420.

Oxholm, P., Manthorpe, T., Manthorpe, R. and Oxholm, A. (1986) *In vivo* IgG deposits and reduced density of Langerhans cells in the surface epithelium of cervix uteri of patients with primary Sjögren's syndrome. *Scand. J. Rheumatol (Suppl.)* **61**, 177–180.

Parr, M. and Parr, E. (1990). Antigen recognition in the female reprodutive tract: Uptake of intraluminal protein tracers in the mouse vagina. *J. Reprod. Immunol.* **7**, 101–114.

Parr, M., Kepple, L. and Parr, E. (1991a). Langerhans cells phagocytose vaginal epithelial cells undergoing apoptosis during the murine cycle. *Biol. Reprod.* **45**, 252–260.

Parr M., Kepple, L. and Parr, E. (1991b). Antigen recognition in the female reproductive tract. II. Endocytosis of horseradish peroxidase by Langerhans cells in murine vaginal epithelium. *Biol. Reprod.* **45**, 261–265.

Parr, M., Kepple, L., McDermott, M., Drew, M., Bozzola, J. and Parr, E. (1994). A mouse model for studies of mucosal immunity to vaginal infection by herpes simplex virus type 2. *Lab. Invest.* **70**, 369–380.

Pope, M., Frankel, S., Mascola, J., Trkola, A., Isdell, F., Birx, D., Burke, D., Ho, D. and Moore, J. (1997). Human immunodeficiency virus type I strain of subtype B and E replicate in cutaneous dendritic-T-cell mixtures without displaying subtype-specific tropism. *J. Virol.* **71**, 8001–8007.

Poppe, W., Drijkoningen, M., Ide, P., Lauweryns, J. and Van-Assche, F. (1996a). Langerhans' cells and L1 antigen expression in normal and abnormal squamous epithelium of the cervical transformation zone. *Gynecol. Obstet. Invest.* **41**, 207–213.

Poppe, W., Peeters, R., Drijkoningen, M., Ide, P., Daenens, P., Lauweryns, J. and Van-Assche, F. (1996b). Cervical cotinine and macrophage–Langerhans cell density in the normal human uterine cervix. *Gynecol. Obstet. Invest.* **41**, 253–259.

Pudney, J. and Anderson, D. (1995). Immunobiology of the human penile urethra. *Am. J. Pathol.* **147**, 155–165.

Puts, J., Moesker, O., de Wall, R., Kenemans, P., Vooijs, G. and Ramaekers, F. (1986). Immunohistochemical identification of Langerhans cells in normal epithelium and in epithelial lesions of the uterine cervix. *Int. J. Gynecol. Pathol.* **5**, 151–162.

Quayle, A., Pudney, J., Munoz, D. and Anderson, D. (1994). Characterization of T lymphocytes and antigen-presenting cells in the murine male urethra. *Biol. Reprod.* **51**, 809–820.

Roncalli, M., Sideri, M., Gie, P. and Servida, E. (1988). Immunophenotypic analysis of the transformation zone of human cervix. *Lab. Invest.* **58**, 141–149.

Schneider, A. (1993). Pathogenesis of genital HPV infection. *Genitourin. Med.* **69**, 165–173.

Soto-Ramirez, L., Renjifo, B., McLane, M., Marlink, R., O'Hara, C., Sutthent, R., Wasi, C., Vithayasai, P., Vithayasai, V., Apichartpiyacul, C., Auewarakul P., Cruz, V., Chui, D., Osathanondh, R., Mayer, K., Lee, T. and Essex, M. (1996). HIV-1 Langerhans' cell tropism associated with heterosexual transmission of HIV. *Science* **271**, 1291–1293.

Spinillo, A., Tenti, P., Zappatore, R., DeSeta, F., Silini, E. and Guaschino, S. (1993). Langerhans' cell counts and cervical intraepithelial neoplasia in women with human immunodeficiency virus infection. *Gynecol. Oncol.* **48**, 210–213.

Spira, A., Marx, P., Patterson, B., Mahoney, J., Koup, R., Wolinsky, S. and Ho, D. (1996). Cellular targets of infection and route of viral dissemination after intravaginal inoculation of simian immunodeficiency virus into rhesus macaques. *J. Exp. Med.* **183**, 215–225.

Tay, S., Jenkins, D., Maddox, P., Campion, M. and Singer, A. (1987). Subpopulations of Langerhans' cells in cervical neoplasia. *Br. J. Obstet. Gynaecol.* **94**, 10–15.

Viac, J., Guerin-Reverchon, I., Chardonet, Y. and Bremond, A. (1990). Langerhans cells and epithelial cell modifications in cervical intraepithelial neoplasia: correlation with human papillomavirus infection. *Immunobiology* **180**, 328–338.

Weiss, G., Sanders, M. and Westbrook, K. (1993). The distribution and density of Langerhans cells in the human prepuce: site of a diminished immune response? *Isr. J. Med. Sci.* **29**, 42–43.

Wira, C. and Rossoll, R. (1995a). Antigen presenting cells in the female reproductive tract: influence of sex hormones on antigen presentation in the vagina. *Immunology* **84**, 505–508.

Wira, C. and Rossoll, R. (1995b). Antigen-presenting cells in the female reproductive tract: influence of the estrous cycle on antigen presentation by uterine epithelial and stromal cells. *Endocrinology* **136**, 4526–4534.

Witkin, S. (1993). Immunology of the vagina. *Clin. Obstet. Gynecol.* **36**, 122–128.

Woodworth, C. and Simpson, S. (1993). Comparative lymphokine secretion by cultured normal human cervical keratinocytes, papillomavirus-immortalized, and carcinoma cell lines. *Am. J. Pathol.* **142**, 1544–1555.

Younes, M., Robertson, E. and Bencosme, S. (1968). Electron microscope observations on Langerhans' cells in the cervix. *Am. J. Obstet. Gynecol.* **102**, 397–403.

Young, W. (1985). Epithelial kinetics affect Langerhans' cells of mouse vaginal epithelium. *Acta Anat.* **123**, 131–136.

Young, W. and Hosking, A. (1986). Langerhans cells in murine vaginal epithelium affected by oestrogen and topical vitamin A. *Acta Anat.* **125**, 59–64.

Young, W., Newcomb, G. and Hosking, A. (1985). The effect of atrophy, hyperplasia, and keratinization accompaning the estrous cycle on Langerhans' cells in mouse vaginal epithelium. *Am J. Anat.* **174**, 173–186.

IV DENDRITIC CELLS IN DISEASE

CHAPTER 19
Cancer

Michael T. Lotze and Ronald Jaffe
University of Pittsburgh Medical Center, Pittsburgh, Pennsylvania, USA

> There is no royal road to science, and only those who do not dread the fatiguing climb of its steep paths have a chance of gaining its luminous summits
>
> Karl Marx

INTRODUCTION

Following the identification of dendritic cells (DC) as the Langerhans cell in the skin, as the interstitial cell within tissues and lymph nodes, and as the veiled cell in lymph, it was subsequently recognized by clinical pathologists that there was a direct relationship between the presence of DC within various lung tumors, head and neck tumors, breast cancer, cervical cancer, endometrial cancer, esophageal cancer, gastric cancer, Hodgkin disease, lung cancer, mycosis fungoides, prostate cancer, and other tumors (Lotze, 1997) and prognosis (Tables 1 and 2). It appears that the presence of greater numbers of DC is associated with a better prognosis (Zeid and Muller, 1993; Furihata *et al.*, 1992; Tsujitani *et al.*, 1993; Ambe *et al.*, 1989; Inoue *et al.*, 1993, for example). We have recently confirmed these findings in tumors of the oral tongue (Goldman *et al.*, 1998) and in patients with pancreatic (Dallal *et al.*, in press) and colon cancer (Clarke and Sikora, in preparation). The initial notion, that DC are present within tumors to pick up tumor antigen and shuttle it to the lymph node and elicit the adaptive immune response, may be a bit too simplistic to explain this curious set of observations. In fact many individuals have documented the inability of tumor derived DC to express appropriate costimulatory molecules as well as class II MHC molecules and the characteristic DC processes associated with their nominal 'immunosuppressed state' (Gabrilovich *et al.*, 1996a, 1996b; Nestle *et al.*, 1997; Chaux *et al.*, 1997).

An alternative explanation is that they are there to provide costimulation and cytokines to prevent apoptotic death for recruited effector T cells. Perhaps one of the most remarkable findings of recent years has been that a number of tumor types, including melanoma, colorectal cancer, hepatoma, and lung cancer (Hahne *et al.*, 1996; Niehans *et al.*, 1997; O'Connell *et al.*, 1996) all express Fas ligand (FasL), a molecule on the cell surface which is a counterreceptor for the Fas receptor, expressed on virtually all mammalian cells including activated T cells coming into the tumor site. This causes, in susceptible T cells, the induction of apoptosis, and thus we have the seemingly

Dendritic Cells: Biology and Clinical Applications
ISBN 0-12-455860-7

Table 1. Relationship between DC infiltration of head and neck cancers/oral cavity cancers and prognosis

Tumor	Reference	DC infiltration
Larynx	*Otolaryngology* **53**, 349 (1991)	Present in tumors
Nasopharyngeal	*Laryngoscope* **101**, 487 (1991)	Markedly improved prognosis
Larynx	*Chin. J. Otorhinol.* **27**, 297 (1992)	Markedly improved prognosis
Oral	*J. Oral Pathol. Med.* **21**, 100 (1992)	Less with smokeless tobacco
Oral	*J. Cutan. Pathol.* **19**, 398 (1992)	Less in tumors
Head and neck	*Cancer Immunother.* **36**, 108 (1993)	PBMC DC less functional
Larynx	*In vivo* **8**, 229 (1993)	Improved prognosis
Head and neck	*Cancer Immunother.* **38**, 31 (1994)	Present in some tumors
Oropharynx	*In Vivo* **8**, 543 (1994)	Less in tumors
Oral squamous	*J. Oral Pathol. Med.* **24**, 61 (1995)	No relationship with prognosis
Oral tongue	*Laryngoscope* (Goldman *et al.*, in press)	Peritumoral CD1 infiltrate associated with prognosis

This has also been observed in other tumors including bladder, lung, esophageal, and gastric carcinoma.

Table 2. Relationship between DC infiltration and prognosis in malignancy

Tumor	Reference	DC infiltration
Arsenical skin	*Proc. Natl Cl. Ch.* **16**, 127 (1992)	Less compared with normal skin
Basal cell	*Br. J. Dermatol.* **130**, 273 (1994)	Less in tumors*
Basal cell	*Br. J. Dermatol.* **127**, 575 (1992)	?Improved
Breast	*J. Pathol.* **163**, 25 (1991)	?Improved prognosis
Bronchoalveolar	*Eur. J. Cancer* **28A**, 1365 (1992)	No effect
Cervix	*Am. J. Clin. Pathol.* **99**, 200 (1993)	Less in HPV^{+} tumors
Cervix	*Cancer* **70**, 2839 (1992)	Improved*
Cervix, stage III	*In Vivo* **7**, 257 (1993)	Marked improved prognosis*
Cervix/penile	*J. Urol* **147**, 1268 (1992)	Less with HPV infection
Cervix/HIV	*Gynecol. Oncol.* **48**, 210 (1993)	Less in AIDS
Endometrial	*Hum. Pathol.* **29**, 455 (1988)	Langerhans infiltration favorable
Esophageal	*Virchows Arch.* **61**, 409 (1992)	Marked improved prognosis
Esophageal	*In Vivo* **7**, 239 (1993)	Direct relationship to grade
Gastric	*Int. Surg.* **77**, 238 (1992)	Marked improved prognosis*
Gastric	*Cancer* **75**, 1478 (1995)	More in tumor draining lymph nodes
Gastric, stage III	*In Vivo* **7**, 233 (1993)	Marked improved prognosis*
Hodgkin disease	*Am. J. Clin. Pathol.* **101**, 761 (1994)	FDC improve prognosis*
Lung	*Pathology* **25**, 338 (1993)	Marked improved prognosis*
Lung	*J. Clin. Invest.* **91**, 566 (1993)	Related GM-CSF production
Melanoma	*J. Invest. Dermatol.* **100**, 269 (1993)	Inverse with tumor thickness
Mycosis fungoides/SS	*In Vivo* **7**, 277 (1993)	Marked improved prognosis*
Prostate	*Prostate* **19**, 73 (1991)	Improved prognosis
Skin tumors	*Arch. Dermatol.* **131**, 187 (1995)	Less in tumors
Thyroid (papillary)	*Z. f. Chir.* **117**, 603 (1992).	No effect

*Indicates statistically significant difference when compared to either normal or fewer DC.

paradoxical situation of tumors killing T cells instead of T cells killing tumors. For that reason, means of preventing premature T cell apoptotic death and the engagement of so-called 'T cell futile cycles' is another goal of the immunologist. DC, by virtue of their expression of so-called costimulatory molecules such as CD80 (B7.1) and CD86 (B7.2) and several 'dendrikines' including interferon-α and IL-12, may be uniquely capable of preventing premature T cell death and thus becoming the mediators of T cell survival.

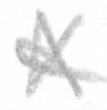

The recognition of several distinct pathologic entities now known collectively as Langerhans cell disorders or tumors allows some insight into the pathologic manifestations of these cells themselves. A fascinating array of histologic appearances and clinical presentations from the banal to the rapidly lethal have been identified. These are dealt with in some detail below.

THE IDENTIFICATION OF HUMAN DC *IN SITU*

Dendritic cells, or cells with a dendritic appearance in extraneural tissues, have long been recognized by their shape and their ability to bind silver metals (Marshall, 1956). It is likely that some of the curious cells described by Marshall are the same cells that we recognize today as the 'dendritic' antigen-presenting cells, but using a completely different set of criteria. Dendritic, professional antigen-processing cells are best characterized by a combination of attributes; their shape, motility, phenotype, and their striking ability to induce primary T cell responses. No single feature or phenotypic marker will identify all DC in all tissues.

The identification of DC in tissues has been problematical for two main reasons. First, the specificity of the markers used to date has been low. DC share many of their surface and cytoplasmic proteins and enzymes with macrophages, with which they share a close affiliation, and with other activated cells, lymphoid or endothelial. Second, the sensitivity of putative DC staining has been an issue. Markers in use to date have highlighted only subpopulations of DC, not all DC, and only recently have markers come into use that have the potential to be more broadly applicable to a wider spectrum of DC. There are also various types of DC that have phenotypic and functional heterogeneity, and no single marker is generally applicable across the board. Most of the information available in humans at present pertains to the so-called myeloid DC. Little information on the human putative lymphoid DC exists other than a suggestion that the plasmacytoid T cells can be induced to display DC characteristics when incubated with IL-3 but not GM-CSF (Grouard *et al.*, 1997). Importantly, too, even the best-characterized subtypes of DC, such as Langerhans' cells, undergo a life-cycle that involves differentiation, maturation, and functional activation that may be accompanied by changes in enzyme activity and phenotype at each stage.

The search has been for markers that will be informative in fixed and embedded tissues so that the vast repositories of the pathology departments can be tapped. Markers applicable only on fresh cells or frozen tissues are important, but of limited potential. Markers that promise to be applicable to the tissue demonstration of subsets of DC include CD83 (Zhou *et al.*, 1992, 1995), CMRF-44 (Hock *et al.*, 1994) and CMRF-56, activation and differentiation associated DC antigens (Hart, 1997), fascin (p55) (Mosialos *et al.*, 1996), and high expression of the IL-3α receptor (Olweus *et al.*, 1997).

The most commonly applied markers for DC in human tissues identify the HLA-II molecules and the associated invariant chain, expressed in high density on the cell surface (Steinman, 1991). Many anti-HLA class II antibodies will react with DC in frozen tissues, less well in fixed, embedded tissue, but are not specific for the DC, being expressed also on macrophages, B cells, endothelial cells, and assorted other activated cells, including T cells and epithelia. The high concentration of class II MHC molecules on the DC, both constitutive and following inflammatory induction (Cella, 1997a), has been used to identify them by resorting to high dilutions of anti-HLA-II antibodies, effectively diluting out the staining of competing cells. A number of antibodies have been specifically produced to demonstrate class II MHC in formalin-fixed tissues; the most widely used is LN3, which recognizes the DR subregion (Mardee *et al.*, 1985). Other antibodies produced specifically to react with human DC also bind the class II MHC molecule, such as RFD-1, which reacts with an HLA-DQ associated antigen, and RFDR1, reacting with HLA-DR, DQ, and DP (Poulter *et al.*, 1986). The use of anti-class II MHC antibodies as DC markers in fixed tissues suffers from the limitations of low specificity, and it is not possible to know that any stained cell is, in fact, a DC.

The S100 family of intracytoplasmic calcium-binding proteins is implicated in a wide range of cellular functions, and has traditionally been used to demonstrate dendritic populations such as Langerhans cells and the lymph node interdigitating DC (Takahashi *et al.*, 1982; Uccini *et al.*, 1986). Specificity of staining when polyclonal antibodies are used is low since there are many other cell types, including S100-reactive lymphoid cells, nerve, fat, chondrocytes, and melanocytes that also express S100 proteins, but in the context of tissue reactions, these other cells can be visually discriminated. As other DC markers become available, it is also becoming evident that the use of polyclonal anti-S100 protein antibodies reveals only subpopulations of DC. DC contain largely S100β with two β chains, and there are monoclonal antibodies to the S100β. Neural tissues contain mostly S100α, but S100α itself has an α and a β chain, so that cross-reaction is still possible. The available S100β monoclonal antibodies are poorly reactive in fixed tissues.

CD68 is a lysosome-associated molecule, the human homologue of mouse macrosialin, a member of the LAMP family with a macrophage-specific mucin-like domain. Antibodies to CD68 stain tissue macrophages in a vacuolar cytoplasmic pattern (Weiss and Keller, 1993). Even though there are CD68 antibodies that recognize the presence of a paranuclear dot of CD68 in DC (Betjes *et al.*, 1991), CD68 can not be considered a marker for DC because macrophages, developing myeloid cells, and other tumor cells express the antigen (Gloghini *et al.*, 1995). Some of the immune accessory molecules, such as CD40, CD80, CD86, and the adhesion molecules CD11c, ICAM-1, and ICAM-3 (CD54 and CD102), may be present in high concentration on DC at various times, but the sensitivity and specificity of their detection in tissues are too low to allow these to be used as unique markers of DC.

There are markers that are expressed normally only on certain DC subsets. CD1a outside of the thymus serves as a good marker of the Langerhans cell in tissue (Murphy *et al.*, 1981), though it should be borne in mind that CD1a will be expressed on the surface of monocytes stimulated with GM-CSF (Kasinrerk *et al.*, 1993) and on some monocytic and myelomonocytic leukemias (Misery *et al.*, 1992). The Lag antibody demonstrates an antigen associated with the Langerhans cell Birbeck granule (Kashihara *et al.*, 1986), an organelle considered to be the hallmark of the Langerhans cell.

Follicular DC (FDC) are marked by their expression of CD21, CD35, and other FDC-related antibodies, such as Ki-M4. S100 and fascin are variably demonstrable on follicular DC (Said *et al.*, 1997). Dermal and interstitial DC express a tissue transglutaminase, factor XIIIa (Cerio *et al.*, 1989a). An antibody, Ki-M9, that identifies a putative lymph node sinus DC has been described (Wacker *et al.*, 1997) and these same cells express factor XIIIa and fascin.

Newer molecules of interest for the study of DC *in situ* include p55 (fascin), CD83, DEC-205, and CMRF-44 (Plate 19.1). DEC-205, a multilectin receptor for antigen presentation, is recognized by a rat monoclonal, NLDC-145. Although the human homologue has been identified, topographic information is currently limited to the mouse, in which a number of other cell types are also noted to express the glycoprotein (Witmer-Pack, 1995). CD83 appears to be unique in the blood to DC (Zhou *et al.*, 1995). Tissue application in frozen tissue reveals strong staining of lymph node paracortical interdigitating cells (Zhou *et al.*, 1992) and freshly isolated Langerhans cells (McLellan, 1996). A population of smaller lymphoid cells also stains, and Hodgkin cells stain using both frozen and fixed tissues (Sorg *et al.*, 1997).

Fascin, a 55 kDa actin-bundling protein, has widespread reactivity on tissue DC, interdigitating, follicular, thymic, splenic and dermal, but is not detected on Langerhans cells *in situ* (Said *et al.*, 1997). The usefulness of fascin as a tissue marker is, however, limited by the low specificity, since other cell types, most notably capillary endothelial cells, also express the antigen. Interestingly, Hodgkin cells have been shown to express both fascin (Said *et al.*, 1997) and CD83 (Sorg *et al.*, 1997). Its application to the differential diagnosis of histiocytic disorders in children reveals that Langerhans cell lesions can be distinguished from so-called indeterminate cell histiocytomas because the first have Birbeck granules, are Lag$^+$, CD1a$^+$, and are fascin$^-$, and the second are CD1a$^+$, fascin$^+$, but lack Birbeck granules (Jaffe *et al.*, 1998). Pincus and colleagues (1997) have reported, in contrast, that Langerhans cell lesions can be shown to express fascin after heat retrieval. Juvenile xanthogranuloma cells, which are presumably dermal or interstitial DC, and also those DC expressing factor XIIIa, also mark with fascin.

CMRF-44, a monoclonal antibody to a DC surface membrane, identifies activated blood-derived DC after a brief period in culture (Fearnley *et al.*, 1997). Tissue exploration with this antibody and the rat antibody to OX40 ligand in humans (Ohshima *et al.*, 1997) remains to be described. Mannose receptors are important for internalization of glycosylated ligands, a property of both macrophages and DC in their phase of antigen uptake. Mannose receptors can be demonstrated on immunosupressed macrophages but not on monocytes or activated macrophages, and in tissues, on thymic cortical DC, lymph node paracortical DC, and on bone marrow macrophages (Noorman *et al.*, 1997). Consequently mannose receptor demonstration will demonstrate DC in tissue but will not distinguish them from macrophages.

Identification of Dendritic Cells within Human Tumors

Many of the studies designed to evaluate DC infiltration into tumors were done 5–10 years ago, before the explosion of interest in DC biology. What had become apparent in many murine experimental studies was that DC were either decreased in number or dysfunctional, associated with decreased expression of a number of costimulatory molecules. It has also been envisioned that DC could be dysfunctional based on failure to generate them in the bone marrow (Gabrilovich, 1996a, b, c), failure to migrate across endothelial barriers that did not permit their emigration (Piali *et al.*, 1995), rapid destruction of such cells as demonstrated recently by Michael Shurin in our group

(Shurin, 1997b), or enhanced migration out of the tumor site related to increased expression of molecules promoting DC maturation and migration such as TNF-α. Some investigators (Halliday *et al.*, 1991, 1992) have also suggested that the tumor represents a 'black hole' for DC and that they succumb to apoptotic death at those sites, explaining the paucity of DC in poor-prognosis tumors. Interestingly, they observed an enhanced number of DC in nonimmunogenic tumors and attributed this to a cytokine which recruited DC into a site but prevented their emigration.

Most of the observations in human tumors have been descriptive and allowed pathologists the opportunity to suggest that the increased number of DC being associated with good prognosis might be attributable to direct lysis of tumors by DC. This seemed implausible initially, but we now have some data from experimental models in the mouse (Shimamura and Baar, unpublished) that suggest that DC may indeed cause limited apoptotic death in some tumors. This may be related to their ability to rapidly take up both particulate antigen as well as free, unattached cells (to each other and to the stroma and basement membrane). Furthermore, Fas mediated pathways wherein either lymphoid or myeloid DC expressing FasL could be envisioned to mediate Fas cross-linking and induction of apoptotic death. This is being actively tested at this time.

Other Findings Related to Tumors

In patients with lung cancer (Nakajima *et al.*, 1985; Zeid *et al.*, 1993) S100-positive Langerhans-like cells have been identified and shown to be at highest density in bronchoalveolar (alveolar II) and well and moderately differentiated squamous cell carcinoma. There are fewer cells observed in small-cell lung cancer and poorly differentiated squamous cell carcinoma. Similar findings have been observed in esophageal squamous cell carcinoma in which a dense infiltration of class II-positive DC is associated with an improvement in survival rate ($p < 0.01$) (Furihata *et al.*, 1992; Imai and Yamakawa, 1993). In patients with gastric cancer, improvements in survival were limited to patients with stage III disease (Tsujitani *et al.*, 1993), with marked infiltration associated with greater survival time ($p < 0.001$). In colorectal cancer (Ambe *et al.*, 1989), the grade of S100-positive DC infiltration was related to the density of lymphocytic infiltration in the tumor ($p < 0.05$). Patients survived longer when they had more than 30 cells per 10 high-power fields (HPF) than those with fewer cells (less than 30 cells/HPF) ($p < 0.001$). In bladder carcinoma (Inoue *et al.*, 1993) it appears that the most important factor affecting prognosis was distant organ and/or lymph node metastasis ($p < 0.01$ as well as number of S100$^+$ DC, with a hazard ratio of 0.26 ($p < 0.01$). Interestingly, class II expression of the tumor was also a prognostically important factor ($p < 0.05$). This probably relates to the presence of interferon-γ expressed locally. A recent evaluation of malignant ascites revealed that DC identified as lineage-negative, class II-positive cells were present in up to 3% of the mononuclear cells (Melichar *et al.*, 1998) but expressed less class II and low levels of CD80, again consistent with a nonstimulatory or immunosuppressed phenotype. The concentration of neopterin, reflecting macrophage activation, in ascitic fluid correlated inversely with the number of lineage-negative HLA-DR$^+$ cells found in ascites (Spearman correlation coefficient -0.44; $p = 0.05$) and directly with the concentration of interleukin-10 in ascitic fluid (Spearman correlation coefficient -0.40; $p = 0.05$). Thus factors associated with the tumor microenvironment appear to influence both the number of DC and their expression of costimulatory molecules. Recently it has become clear that the killer inhibitory receptor family of molecules, which had previously been identified in T cells and NK cells, also exists as closely related family members, so-called LIRS or ILT-3 (Cella *et al.*, 1997b). These molecules may be critically important for class I detection by infiltrating DC, which may lead to unique DC effector functions and which we are now exploring in the laboratory.

Savary and colleagues investigated flow cytometry as a means of evaluating the number and maturation/activation status of DC in peripheral blood mononuclear cells (PBMC) of both normal donors and cancer patients (Savory *et al.*, 1998). DC were identified as HLA-DR$^+$ lineage$^-$ cells (less than 1% mononuclear cells). They had high forward light-scatter characteristics and coexpressed CD4, CD86, and CD54 surface antigens, but lacked the lineage-associated surface markers of T cells, B cells, monocytes, granulocytes or NK cells. Interestingly, the frequency of DC-like cells in PBMC of chemotherapy-treated cancer patients was lower than that of normal individuals (mean $\pm$ SE 0.36 $\pm$ 0.05%, 0.14 $\pm$ 0.06%, and 0.75 $\pm$ 0.04%, respectively). There are other novel markers that could be used to distinguish DC from other cells. These include CD1, S100 staining, high expression of the MHC class II molecules, and, most recently, expression of the p55 actin-bundling protein, a cytosolic marker that was found within EBV-transformed B cells (Sonderbye *et al.*, 1997), within both follicular and nonfollicular DC, but more recently also within the Reed–Sternberg cells in all but the lymphocyte-predominant forms of Hodgkin disease (Pincus *et al.*, 1997).

DC AND THEIR DISORDERS

The various subtypes of DC in the human can be characterized *in situ* by a combination of topography and phenotype. Table 3 lists the major forms and the lesions that can now be ascribed to the DC types.

DC-related Disorders: Proliferation(s)

Langerhans Cell Histiocytosis

Many aspects of Langerhans disease have been summarized in a publication stemming from the Nikolas symposium, an annual 'think-tank' dedicated to the histiocytos (Pritchard *et al.*, 1994; Egeler and D'Angio 1998). Basically, Langerhans cell histiocytosis (LCH), is a clonal disorder in which abnormal Langerhans cells accumulate at

Table 3. DC and their disorders

DC	Phenotype	Disorder
Langerhans cell	CD1a, S100, LCG, Lag[a]	Langerhans cell histiocytosis
Indeterminate cell	CD1a, S100, fascin	DC histiocytoma, indeterminate
Interdigitating DC	S100, fascin, IL-3Rα^{hi}	DC histiocytoma, IDC type
Dermal dendrocytes (and subtypes)	Factor XIIIa, fascin, CD68	Xanthogranuloma family, dermal dendrocytomas
Follicular DC	CD21, CD35, Ki-M4, S100$^+$/$^-$, fascin	DC histiocytoma, FDC type
Sinus DC	Ki-M9, fascin, CD68, S100	?Rosai–Dorfman disease

[a]Lag, Lag antigen.

various body sites not usually known to harbor them (Willman *et al.*, 1994; Yu *et al.*, 1994). Diagnosis in all of the varied clinical forms, localized, multifocal and visceral, rests on identifying the Langerhans cell in the tissue lesions, which has, until recently, required the demonstration, within the cells, of the characteristic Langerhans granule or Birbeck granule. Now the demonstration of the CD1a molecule at the cell surface, in a lesion that has the morphologic hallmarks of Langerhans cell disease, is sufficient to confirm the diagnosis (Favara *et al.*, 1997) The 010 antibody has the required sensitivity and specificity to demonstrate CD1a in paraffin-embedded tissues, and will mark LCH cells (Emile *et al.*, 1994, 1995) (Plate 19.2). The cells of LCH have the phenotype of activated rather than newly isolated Langerhans' cells because CD11b, CD24, and CD80/86 were demonstrable on the LCH cells but not the Langerhans cells (Emile *et al.*, 1994, 1995). Paradoxically, though, LCH cells retain their Birbeck granules, while activated Langerhans cells tend to lose theirs. In addition to CD1a, LCH cells, which, despite their affiliation, are oval and not dendritic in shape, will express HLA-II, S100 protein, and CD4, but not fascin or CD83 (Jaffe *et al.*, 1998) (Plate 19.3). The Lag antigen identifies the intracytoplasmic Birbeck granule and antibody detection is possible (Kashihara *et al.*, 1986).

Secondary DC Reactions

Clusters of Langerhans cells have been described in the tissues in a number of conditions, usually designated as Langerhans cell histiocytosis and arising in association with the underlying disorder. Such collections are described in malignant lymphomas (Willman *et al.*, 1994), in the thymus in myasthenia gravis, and in association with other tumors (Egeler *et al.*, 1993; Burns *et al.*, 1983). There is no information on the clonality of the process, but it is best thought of as a reactive hyperplasia of Langerhans cells, possibly an immune reaction to the tumor, and not an independent disease process (Favara *et al.*, 1997).

Juvenile Xanthogranuloma and Related Disorders

The cutaneous lesion juvenile xanthogranuloma (Hernando-Martin *et al.*, 1997), and its systemic counterpart which can involve deep soft tissues, brain, and meninges as well as other organs (Freyer *et al.*, 1996) appear to be lesions of the dermal and interstitial DC (Sangueza *et al.* 1995; Nascimento, 1997; De Graaf *et al.*, 1992) (Plate 19.4). The histology encompasses a mixture of angular histiocytes, lipid-filled xanthomatous forms, and multinucleated Touton-type giant cells. The *in situ* phenotype is generally fascin^{+}, factor XIIIa^{+}, CD68^{+} (especially when using the PG-M1 antibody), S100^{-} and CD1a^{-}, though some deep lesions are said to be CD1a^{+} (De Graaf *et al.*, 1992). It is likely that their phenotype changes over time as the dendritic histiocytes become lipidized and take on more fibrous or macrophage-like characteristics while losing their dermal dendritic features. Healing lesions are fibrotic and lose the macrophage population, and are generally referred to as dermatofibromas. The same dermal DC type is involved in a number of other dermal and soft-tissue masses and some systemic disorders that have been given a variety of names over the years. It is likely that cellular xanthogranulomas, benign cephalic histiocytosis, papular xanthoma, progressive nodular histiocytosis, spindle cell xanthogranuloma, xanthoma disseminatum, and

Erdheim–Chester disease are the same lesion with varying site or clinical presentation (Zelger *et al.*, 1995). An important feature that they share is their biological behavior, which tends to be self-limiting, albeit slowly, with regression over months to years, so that aggressive chemotherapy should be averted by correct diagnosis.

Xanthogranuloma can behave much like Langerhans' cell disease in its systemic manifestations, but xanthogranulomas may also be noted in patients with LCH and myelomonocytic leukemias, accentuating the close relationship between the disorders.

Xanthoma disseminatum is a normolipemic mucocutaneous variant of the juvenile xanthogranuloma family that affects young adults with many dermal lesions and involvement of mucosa, often that of the upper airways (Weiss and Keller, 1993). Brain involvement occurs and diabetes insipidus, a hallmark of Langerhans cell disease, is seen transiently in up to 40% of patients. The histopathology and phenotype are that of juvenile xanthogranuloma, (factor XIIIa$^+$, CD68$^+$, S100$^-$, CD1a$^+$). Erdheim–Chester disease has histopathologic features very much like those of the xanthogranulomas and is distinguished by the symmetrical metaphyseal and diaphyseal osteosclerosis demonstrable on radiography.

Non-Langerhans DC Histiocytomas

There are a number of descriptions of dermal or soft-tissue lesions that have an appearance and phenotype very similar to the Langerhans cell lesions but differ in that Birbeck granules are not demonstrable, so-called indeterminate cell lesions (Wood *et al.*, 1985; Manente *et al.*, 1997; Sidoroff *et al.*, 1996). Since Birbeck granules can only be demonstrated in 2–69% of Langerhans cells in LCH (Mierau *et al.*, 1986), this distinction alone seems tenuous, but the demonstration of fascin in these lesions but not in Langerhans cell disease adds another distinguishing feature (Jaffe *et al.*, 1998) The biological behavior of the dermal and soft-tissue lesions appears to be benign, but intracranial lesions and a neck lesion have recurred with more aggressive growth. The phenotype is generally CD1a$^+$, Birbeck granule$^-$, fascin$^+$, factor XIIIa$^+$ CD86$^+$, and S100 variable. Lesions of this kind have been referred to as dermal dendrocytomas (Cerio *et al.*, 1989a, 1989b; Nickoloff *et al.*, 1990), though they are not limited to the skin and may even be intracranial.

Monocytic and Myelomonocytic Leukemias with Dermal Lesions of Dendritic Phenotype

Adults are described who have myelomonocytic or monocytic leukemias that have pre-DC phenotype or develop one in culture (Misery *et al.*, 1992; Srivastava *et al.*, 1994). In some of these patients there are dermal (Lauritzen *et al.*, 1994) or disseminated DC lesions that have the features of Langerhans cell disease (Claudy, 1989). In one of these (Takahashi *et al.*, 1992) a serum factor was isolated that caused a human monocytic cell line to mature to interdigitating-type DC.

DC Sarcomas

Soft-tissue and lymph node-based lesions have been described, some of which have the biological potential for recurrence, metastasis, and resistance to chemotherapy sufficient for them to be deemed malignant. The lesions are generally composed of spindled cells without other distinguishing morphological features, but on phenotyping have been assigned to one or other of the DC forms, so that follicular DC sarcomas Ki-M4$^+$, CD21$^+$, CD35$^+$ (Chan *et al.*, 1997; Masunaga *et al.*, 1997), interdigitating DC sarcomas HLA-DR$^+$, CD68$^+$, S100$^+$ (Nakamura *et al.*, 1994; Rousselet *et al.*, 1994; Meittinen *et al.*, 1993), and Langerhans cell sarcomas CD1a$^+$ (Lauritzen *et al.*, 1994) are described.

SUMMARY

Much has been learned about the various manifestations of DC in human tissues and in particular in the setting of cancer over the last 25 years since the DC was first defined as an identifiable cell type. Future challenges will be to understand the natural biology of these cells as they traverse tissues, the manifestations of arrested biology revealed by neoplastic DC, and the errant findings of DC within tumor and how their recruitment, maturation, or emigration is modified. Of particular interest will be the determination of the role of the more recently identified lymphoid dendritic cell and how it migrates through various tissues and, in particular, whether a nominal tumor-pathologic variant might be identified. Tissue markers for DC of varying kind are needed for a number of reasons. Clearly, in order to understand the role of the DC in the immune regulation of cancer it is important to know which are antigen-acquiring and which the effector DC. To gain insight into the nature and biology of lesions made up of DC it requires that there be standardized ways of looking at these cells and categorizing them. This is an area of evolution, and dendritic cell phenotyping *in situ* lags behind the functional understanding of DC capabilities.

REFERENCES

Ambe, K., Mori, M. and Enjoji, M.S. (1989). S-100 protein-positive dendritic cells in colorectal adenocarcinomas. Distribution and relation to the clinical prognosis. *Cancer* **63**(3), 496–503.

Betjes, M.G.H., Haks, M.C., Tuk, C.W. and Beelan, H.J. (1991). Monoclonal antibody EBM11 (anti-CD68) discriminates between dendritic cells and macrophages after short-term culture. *Immunobiology* **183**, 79–87.

Burns, B.F. Colby, T.F. and Dorfman, R.F. (1983). Langerhans cell granulomatosis (histiocytosis X) associated with malignant lymphomas. *Am. J. Surg. Pathol.* **7**, 529–533.

Cella, M., Engering, A., Pinet, V., Pieters, J. and Lanzavecchia, A. (1997a). Inflammatory stimuli induce accumulation of MHC class II complexes on dendritic cells. *Nature* **388**, 782–787.

Cella, M., Dohring, C., Samaridis, J., Dessing, M., Brockhaus, M., Lanzavecchia, A. and Colonna, M.A. (1997b). A novel inhibitory receptor (ILT3) expressed on monocytes, macrophages and dendritic cells involved in antigen processing. *J. Exp. Med.* **185**(10), 1743–1751.

Cerio, R., Spaull, J. and Wilson-Jones, E. (1989a). Histiocytoma cutis; a tumor of dermal dendrocytes (dermal dendrocytoma). *Br. J. Dermatol.* **120**, 197–206.

Cerio, R., Griffiths, C.E.M, Cooper, K.D., Nickoloff, B.J. and Headington, J.T. (1989b). Characterization of factor XIIIa positive dermal dendritic cells in normal and inflamed skin. *Br. J. Dermatol.* **121**, 421–431.

Chan, J.K., Fletcher, C.D., Nayler, S.J. and Cooper, K. (1997). Follicular dendritic cell sarcoma. Clinicopathologic analysis of 17 cases suggesting a malignant potential higher than currently recognized. *Cancer* **79**, 294–313.

Chaux, P., Favre, N., Bonnotte, B., Moutet, M., Martin, M., Martin, F., Claudy, A.L., Larbre, B., Colomb, M., Levigne, V. and Deville, V. (1989). Letter–Siwe disease and subacute monocytic leukemia. *J. Am. Acad. Dermatol.* **21**, 1105–1106.

Chaux, P., Favre, N., Martin, M. and Martin, F. (1997). Tumor-infiltrating dendritic cells are defective in their antigen-presenting function and inducible B7 expression in rats. *Int. J. Cancer* **72**(4), 619–624.

Claudy, A.L., Larbre, B., Colomb, M., Levigne, V. and Deville, V. (1989). Letterer–Siwe disease and subacute monocytic leukemia. *J. Am. Acad. Dermatol.* **21**(5 Pt 2), 1105–1106.

Coppola, D., Fu, L., Cicosia, S.V., Kounelis, S. and Jones, M. (1998). Prognostic significance of p53, bdl-2, vimentin and S100 protein-positive Langerhans cells in endometrial carcinoma. *Hum. Pathol.* **29**, 455–462.

Dallal, R.M., Christakos, P. and Lotze, M.T. Paucity of dendritic cell (DC) infiltrate in pancreatic carcinoma (PCa) predicts poor prognosis. *Surg. Res.*, in press.

De Graaf, J., Timens, W., Tamminiga, R.Y.J. and Molenaar, W.M. (1992). Deep juvenile xanthogranuloma: a lesion related to dermal indeterminate cells. *Hum. Pathol.* **23**, 905–910.

Egeler, R.M., Neglia, J. and Puccetti, D.M, *et al.* (1993). The association of Langerhans cell histiocytosis with malignant neoplasms. *Cancer* **71**, 865–873.

Egeler, R.M. and D'Angio, A. J. (1988). Langerhans cell histiocytosis. *Hematol. Oncol. Clin. N. Am.* **12**(2), 1998.

Emile, J.F., Fraitag, S., Leborgne, M., de Prost, Y. and Brousse, N. (1994). Langerhans' cell histiocytosis cells are activated Langerhan's cells. *J. Pathol* **174**, 71–76.

Emile, J.F., Wechsler, J. and Brousse, N., *et al.* (1995). Langerhans' cell histiocytosis. Definitive diagnosis with the use of the monoclonal antibody 010 on routinely paraffin-embedded samples. *Am. J. Surg. Pathol.* **19**, 636–641.

Enk, A.H., Jonuleit, H., Saloga, J. and Knop, J. (1997). Dendritic cells as mediators of tumor-induced tolerance in metastatic melanoma. *Int. J. Cancer* **73**(3), 309–316.

Favara, B.E. and Feller, A.C. *et al.* (1997). Contemporary classification of histiocytic disorders. *Med. Ped. Oncol.* **29**, 157–166.

Fearnley, D.B., McLellan, A.D., Mannering, S.I., Hock, B.D. and Hart, D.N.J. (1997). Isolation of human blood dendritic cells using the CMRF-44 monoclonal antibody—implications for studies on antigen-presenting cell function and immunotherapy. *Blood* **89**, 3708–3716.

Freyer, D.R., Kennedy, R., Bostrom, B.C., Kohut, G. and Dehner, L.P. (1997). Juvenile xanthogranuloma; forms of systemic disease and their clinical implications. *J. Pediatr.* **129**, 227–237.

Furihata, M., Ohtsuki, Y., Ido, E., Iwata, J., Sonobe, H., Araki, K., Ogoshi, S. and Ohmori, K. (1992). HLA-DR antigen- and S-100 protein-positive dendritic cells in esophageal squamous cell carcinoma—their distribution in relation to prognosis. *Virchows Arch. B. Cell. Pathol. Incl. Mol. Pathol.* **61**(6), 409–414.

Gabrilovich, D.I., Nadaf, S., Corak, J., Berzofsky, J.A. and Carbone, D.P. (1996a). Dendritic cells in antitumor immune responses. II. Dendritic cells grown from bone marrow precursors, but not mature DC from tumor-bearing mice, are effective antigen carriers in the therapy of established tumors. *Cell. Immunol.* **171**(1), 111–119.

Gabrilovich, D.I., Ciernik, I.F. and Carbone, D.P. (1996b). Dendritic cells in antitumor immune responses. I. Defective antigen presentation in tumor-bearing hosts. *Cell. Immunol.* **170**(1), 101–110.

Gabrilovich, D.I., Chen, H.L., Girgis, K.R., Cunningham, H.T., Meny, G.M., Madaf, S., Kavanaugh, D. and Carbone, D.P. (1996c). Production of vascular endothelial growth factor by human tumors inhibits the functional maturation of dendritic cells. *Native Medicine* **2**, 1096–1103.

Gloghini, A., Rizzo, A., Zanette, I., Canal, B., Rupolo, G., Bassi, P. and Carbone, A. (1995). KPI/CD68 expression in malignant neoplasms including lymphomas, sarcomas, and carcinomas. *Am. J. Clin. Pathol.* **103**, 425–431.

Goldman, S.A., Baker, E., Weyent, R.J., Clarke, M.R., Myers, J. and Lotze, M.T. Peritumoral CD1a-positive dendritic cells are associated with survival, recurrence and tumor stage in oral tongue squamous cell carcinoma. *Head Neck Surg.*, in press.

Grouard, G., Rissoan, M.C., Filgueira, L., Durand, I., Banchereau, J. and Liu, Y.-J. (1997). The enigmatic plasmacytoid T cells develop into dendritic cells with interleukin (IL)-3 and CD40-ligand. *J. Exp. Med.* **185**(6), 1101–1111.

Hahne, M., Rimoldi, D., Schröter, Romero, M., Schreier, M., French, L.E., Schneider, P., Bornand, T., Fontana, A., Lienard, D., Cerottini, J.-C. and Tschopp, J. (1996). Melanoma cell expression of Fas(Apo-1/CD9S) ligand: implications for tumor immune escape. *Science* **274**, 1363–1366.

Halliday, G.M., Reeve, V.E. and Barnetson, R.S. (1991). Langerhans cell migration into ultraviolet light-induced squamous skin tumors is unrelated to anti-tumor immunity. *J. Invest. Dermatol.* **97**(5), 830–834.

Halliday, G.M., Lucas, A.D. and Barnetson, R.S. (1992). Control of Langerhans' cell density by a skin tumour-derived cytokine. *Immunology* **77**(1), 13–18.

Hart, D.N.J. (1997). Dendritic cells: unique leukocyte populations which control the primary immune response. *Blood* **90**, 3245–3278.

Hernando-Martin, A., Baselga, E., Drolet, B.A. and Esterley, N.B. (1997). Juvenile xanthogranuloma. *J. Am. Acad. Dermatol.* **36**, 355–367.

Hock, B.D., Starling, G,C., Daniel, P.B. and Hart, D.N.J. (1994). Characterization of CMRF-44, a novel monoclonal antibody to an activation antigen expressed by allostimulatory cells within peripheral blood, including dendritic cells. *Immunology* **83**, 573–581.

Imai, Y. and Yamakawa, M. (1993). Dendritic cells in esophageal cancer and lymph node tissues. *In Vivo* **7**(3), 239–248.

Inoue, K., Furihata, M., Ohtsuki, Y. and Fujita, Y. (1993). Distribution of S-100 protein-positive dendritic cells and expression of HLA-DR antigen in transitional cell carcinoma of the urinary bladder in relation to tumour progression and prognosis. *Virchows Arch. A. Pathol. Anat. Histopathol.* **422**(5), 351–355.

Jaffe, R., DeVaughn, D. and Langhoff, E. (1998). Fascin and the differential diagnosis of childhood histiocytic lesions. *Pediatr. Dev. Pathol.* **1**, 216–221.

Kakeji, Y., Maehara, Y., Korenaga, D., Tsujitani, S., Haraguchi, M., Watanabe, A., Orita, H. and Sugimachi, K. (1993). Prognostic significance of tumor–host interaction in clinical gastric cancer: relations between DNA ploidy and dendritic cell infiltration. *J. Surg. Oncol.* **52**(4), 207–212.

Kashihara, M., Ueda, M., Horiguchi, Y., Furukawa, F., Hanaoka, M. and Imamura, S.A. (1986). A monoclonal antibody specifically reactive to human Langerhans cells. *J. Invest. Dermatol.* **87**, 602–607.

Kasinrerk, W., Baumruker, T., Madjic, O., Lnapp, W. and Stockinger, H. (1993). CD1 molecule expression on human monocytes induced by GM-CSF. *J. Immunol.* **150**, 579.

Lauritzen, A.F., Delsol, G., Hansen, N.E., Horn, T., Ersboll, J., Hou-Jensen, K. and Ralfkiaer, E. (1994). Histiocytic sarcomas and monoblastic leukemias. A clinical, histologic, and immunophenotypical study. *Am. J. Clin. Pathol.* **102**, 45–54.

Lotze, M.T. (1997). Getting to the source: dendritic cells as therapeutic reagents for the treatment of cancer patients (Editorial). *Ann. Surg.* **226**, 1–5.

Manente, L., Contellessa, C., Schmitt, I., Peris, K., Torlone, G., Muda, A.O., Romano, M.C. and Chementi, S. (1997). Indeterminate cell histiocytosis; a rare histiocytic disorder. *Am. J. Dermatopathol.* **19**, 276–283.

Marder, R.J., Variakojis, D., Silver, J. and Epstein, A.L. (1985). Immunohistochemical analysis of human lymphomas with monoclonal antibodies to B cell and Ia antigens reactive in paraffin sections. *Lab. Invest.* **52**, 497–504.

Marshall, A.H.E. (1956). *An Outline of the Cytology and Pathology of Reticular Tissue.* London.

Masunaga, A., Nakamura, H., Katata, T., Furubayashi, T., Kanayama, Y., Yamada, A., Shiroko, Y. and Itoyama, S. (1997). Follicular DC tumor with histiocytic characteristics and fibroblastic antigen. *Pathol. Int.* **47**, 707–712.

McLellan, A.D., Sorg, R.V., Fearnley, D.B. and Hart, D.N.J. Fresh human Langerhans cells express the CD83 and CMRF-44 differentiation/activation antigens and costimulate T lymphocytes via CD86 (submitted).

Meittinen, M., Fletcher, C.D.M. and Lasota, J. (1993). True histiocytic lymphoma of small intestine. Analysis of two S100 protein-positive cases with features of interdigitating reticulum cell sarcoma. *Am. J. Clin. Pathol.* **100**, 285–292.

Melichar, B., Savary, C., Kudelka, A.P., Verschraegen, C., Kavanagh, J.J., Edwards, C.L., Platsoucas, C.D. and Freedman, R.S. (1998). Lineage-negative human leukocyte antigen-DR$^+$ cells with the phenotype of undifferentiated dendritic cells in patients with carcinoma of the abdomen and pelvis. *Clin. Cancer Res.* **4**(3), 799–809.

Mierau, G.W., Favara, B.E. and Brenman, J.M. (1986). Electron microscopy in histiocytosis X. *Ultrastruct. Pathol.* **3**, 137–142.

Misery, L., Campos, L., Dezutter-Dambuyant, C., Guyotat, D., Trielle, D., Schmitt, D. and Thivolet, J. (1992). CD1a-reactive leukemic cells in bone marrow: presence of Langerhans cell marker on leukemic monocytic cells. *Eur. J. Haematol.* **48**, 27–32.

Mosialos, G., Birkenbach, M., Ayehunie, S., Matsumara, F., Pincus, G.S., Kieff, E. and Langhoff, E. (1996). Circulating human dendritic cells differentially express high levels of a 55-Kd actin-binding protein. *Am. J. Pathol.* **148**, 593–600.

Murphy, G.F., Bhan, A.K., Sato, S., Harrist, T.J. and Mihm, M.C. Jr. (1981). Characterization of Langerhans cells by the use of monoclonal antibodies. *Lab. Invest.* **45**, 465–468.

Nakajima, T., Kodama, T., Tsumuraya, M., Shimosato, Y. and Kameya, T.S. (1985). S-100 protein-positive Langerhans cells in various human lung cancers, especially in peripheral adenocarcmomas. *Virchows Arch. A. Pathol. Anat. Histopathol.* **407**(2), 177–189.

Nakamura, S., Koshikawa, T., Kitoh, K., Nakayama, M., Imai, Y., Ishii, K., Fujita, M. and Suchi, T. (1994). Interdigitating cell sarcoma: a morphologic and immunologic study of lymphnode lesions in four cases. *Pathol. Int.* **44**, 374–386.

Nascimento, A.G. (1997). A clinicopathologic and immunohistochemical comparative study of cutaneous and intramuscular forms of juvenile xanthogranuloma. *Am. J. Surg. Pathol.* **21**, 645–652.

Nestle, F.O., Burg, G., Fah, J., Wrone-Smith, T. and Nickoloff, B.J. (1997). Human sunlight-induced basal-cell-carcinoma-associated dendritic cells are deficient in T cell co-stimulatory molecules and are impaired as antigen-presenting cells. *Am. J. Pathol.* **150**(2), 641–651.

Nickoloff, B.J., Weed, G.S. and Chu, M., *et al.* (1990). Disseminated dermal dendrocytoma: a new cutaneous fibrohistiocytic proliferation? *Am. J. Surg. Pathol.* **14**, 867–871.

Niehans, G.A., Brunner, T., Frizelle, S.P., Liston, J.C., Salerno, C.T., Knapp, D.J., Green, D.R. and Kratzke, R.A. (1997). Human lung carcinomas express Fas ligand. *Cancer Res.* **57**, 1007–1012.

Noorman, F., Braat, E.A., Barrett-Bergshoeff, M., Barbe, E., van Leeuwen, A., Lindeman, J. and Rijken, D.C. (1997). Monoclonal antibodies against the human mannose receptor as a specific marker in flow cytometry and immunohistochemistry for macrophages. *J. Leukocyte Biol.* **61**, 63–72.

O'Connell, J., O'Sullivan, G.C., Collins, J.K. and Shanahan. F. (1996). The Fas counterattack: Fas-mediated T cell killing by colon cancer cells expressing Fas ligand. *J. Exp. Med.* **184**, 1075–1082.

Ohshima, Y., Tanaka, Y., Tozawa, H., Takahashi, Y., Maliszewski, C. and Delespesse, G. (1997). Expression and function of OX40 ligand on human dendritic cells. *J. Immunol.* **159**, 3838–3848.

Olweus, J., BitMansour, A., Warnke, R., Thompson, P.A., Carballido, J., Picker, L.J. and Lund-Johansen, F. (1994). Dendritic cell ontogeny: a human dendritic cell lineage of myeloid origin. *Proc. Natl Acad. Sci. USA* **94**(23), 12551–12556.

Piali, L., Fichtel, A., Terpe, H.J., Imhof, B.A. and Gisler, R.H. (1995). Endothelial vascular cell adhesion molecule 1 expression is suppressed by melanoma and carcinoma. *J. Exp. Med.* **181**(2), 811–816.

Pinkus, G.S., Pinkus, J.L., Langhoff, E., Matsumura, F., Yamashiro, S., Mosialos, G. and Said, J.W. (1997). Fascin, a sensitive new marker for Reed–Sternberg cells of Hodgkin's disease. Evidence for a dendritic or B cell derivation? *Am. J. Pathol.* **150**(2), 543–562.

Pinkus, G.S., Pinkus, J.L., Lones, M.A., Matsumata, F., Yamashiro, S. and Said, J.W. (1998). Fascin: a marker for Langerhans cell histiocytosis (abstract) *Lab. Invest.* **78**, 138A.

Poulter, L.W., Campbell, D.A., Munroe, C. and Janossy, G. (1986). Discrimination of human macrophages and dendritic cells by means of monoclonal antibodies. *Scand. J. Immunol.* **24**, 351–357.

Pritchard, J., Beverley, P.C.L., Chu, A.C., D'Angio, G.J., Davis, I.C. and Malpas, J.S. (1994). The proceedings of the Nikolas symposia on the histiocytoses 1989–1993. *Br. J. Cancer* **70** (Supplement XXIII).

Qin, Z., Noffz, G., Mohaupt, M. and Blankenstein, T. (1997). Interleukin-10 prevents dendritic cell accumulation and vaccination with granulocyte-macrophage colony-stimulating factor gene-modified tumor cells. *J. Immunol.* **159**(2), 770–776.

Rousselet, M.C., Croue, F.S., Maigre, M., Saint-Andre, J.P. and Ifrah, N. (1994). A lymphnode interdigitating reticulum cell sarcoma. *Arch. Pathol. Lab. Med.* **118**, 183–188.

Said, J.W., Pinkus, J.L., Yamashita, J., Mishalani, S., Matsumura, F., Yamashiro, S., *et al.* (1997). The role of follicular and interdigitating dendritic cells in HIV-related lymphoid hyperplasia: localization of fascin. *Mod. Pathol.* **10**, 421–427.

Sangueza, O.P., Salmon, J.K., White, C.R. and Beckstead, J.H. (1995). Juvenile xanthogranuloma; a clinical, histopathologic and immunohistochemical study. *J. Cutan. Pathol.* **22**, 327–335.

Savary, C.A., Grazziutti, M.L., Melichar, B., Przepiorka, D., Freedman, R.S., Cowart, R.E., Cohen, D.M., Anaissie, E.J., Woodside, D.G., McIntyre, B.W., Pierson, D.L., Pellis, N.R. and Rex, J.H. (1998). Multidimensional flow-cytometric analysis of dendritic cells in peripheral blood of normal donors and cancer patients. *Cancer Immunol. Immunother.* **45**(5), 234–240.

Shurin, M.R., Pandharipande, P.P., Zorina, T.D., Haluszczak, C., Subbotin, V.M., Hunter, O., Brumfield, A., Storkus, W.J., Maraskovsky, E. and Lotze, M.T. (1997a). FLT3 ligand induces the generation of functionally active dendritic cells in mice. *Cell. Immunol.* **179**(2), 174–184.

Shurin, M.R., Esche, C., Lokshin, A. and Lotze, M.T. (1997b). Tumors induce apoptosis of dendritic cells *in vitro*. *J. Immunother.* **20**, 403.

Sidoroff, A., Zelger, B., Steiner, H. and Smith, N. (1996). Indeterminate cell histiocytosis—a clinico-pathological entity with features of both X and non-X histiocytosis. *Br. J. Dermatol.* **134**, 525–532.

Sonderbye, L., Magerstadt, R., Blatman, R.N., Preffer, F.I. and Langhoff, E. (1997). Selective expression of human fascin (p55) by dendritic leukocytes. *Adv. Exp. Med. Biol.* **417**, 41–46.

Sorg, U.R., Morse, T.M., Patton, W.N., Hock, B.D., Angus, H.B., Robinson, B.A., Colls, B.M. and Hart, D.N. (1997). Hodgkin's cells' express CD83, a dendritic cell lineage associated antigen. *Pathology* **29**, 294–299.

Srivastava, B.I.S., Srivastava, A. and Srivastava, M.D. (1994). Phenotype, genotype and cytokine production in acute leukemia involving progenitors of dendritic Langerhans' cells. *Leukemia Res.* **18**, 499–511.

Steinman, R.M. (1991). The dendritic cell system and its role in immunogenicity. *Annu. Rev. Immunol.* **9**, 271–289.

Takahashi, Y., Yamaguchi, H., Ishizeki, J., Nakajima, T. and Nakazota, Y. (1982). Immunohistochemical and immunoelectron microscopic localization of S100 protein in the interdigitating reticulum cells of the human lymphnode. *Virchows Arch. (Cell. Pathol.)* **37**, 125–132.

Takahashi, K., Miyatani, K., Yanai, H., Jeon, H.J., Fujiwara, K., Yoshino, T., Hayashi, K., Akagi, T., Tsutsui, K. and Mizobuchi, K. (1992). Induction of interdigitating reticulum cell-like differentiation in human monocytic leukemia cells by conditioned medium from IL-2-stimulated helper T-cells. *Virchows Arch. B. Cell. Pathol. Incl. Mol. Pathol.* **62**(2), 105–113.

Thurnher, M., Radmayr, C., Ramoner, R., Ebner, S., Bock, G., Klocker, H., Romani, N. and Bartsch, G. (1996). Human renal-cell carcinoma tissue contains dendritic cells. *Int. J. Cancer.* **68**(1), 1–7.

Tsujitani, S., Kakeji, Y., Maehara, Y., Sugimachi, K. and Kaibara, N. (1993). Dendritic cells prevent lymph node metastasis in patients with gastric cancer. *In Vivo* **7**(3), 233–237.

Uccini, S., Vitolo, D., Stoppacciaro, A., Paliotta, D., Cassano, A.M., Barsotti, P., Ruco, L.P. and Baroni, C.D. (1986). Immunoreactivity for S100 protein in dendritic and in lymphocyte-like cells in human lymphoid tissues. *Virchows Arch. B. Cell. Pathol.* **52**, 129–141.

Wacker, H.H., Frahm, S.O., Heidebrecht, H.J. and Parwaresch, R. (1997). Sinus-lining cells of the lymphnodes recognized as a dendritic cell by the new monoclonal antibody Ki-M9. *Am. J. Pathol.* **151**, 423–434.

Weiss, N. and Keller, C. (1993). Xanthoma disseminatum; a rare normolipemic xanthomatosis. *Clin. Invest.* **71**, 233-238.

Weiss, L.M., Arber, D.A. and Chang, K.L. (1994). CD68. A review. *Appl. Immunohistochem.* **2**, 2–8.

Willman, C.L., Busque, L., Griffith, B.B., Favara, B.E., McClain, K.L., Gresik, V.M., Duncan, M.H., Isaacson, P.G. and Gilliland, D.G. (1994). Langerhans cell histiocytosis (histiocytosis X): a clonal proliferative disease. *N. Engl. J. Med.* **331**, 154–160.

Witmer-Pack, M.D., Swiggard, W.J., Mirza, A., Inaba, K. and Steinman, R.M. (1995). Tissue distribution of the DEC-205 protein that is detected by the monoclonal antibody NLDC-145. Expression *in situ* in lymphoid and non-lymphoid tissues. *Cell. Immunol.* **163**, 157–162.

Wood, G.S., Chung-Hong, H., Beckstead, J.H., Turner, R.R. and Winkelmann, R.K. (1985). The indeterminate cell proliferative disorder; report of a case manifesting as an unusual cutaneous histiocytosis. *J. Dermtol. Surg. Oncol.* **11**, 1111–1119.

Yu, R.C., Chu, C., Buluwela, L. and Chu, A.C. (1994). Clonal proliferations of Langerhans cells in Langerhans cell histiocytosis. *Lancet* **343**, 767–768.

Zeid, N.A. and Muller, H.K. (1993). S100 positive dendritic cells in human lung tumors associated with cell differentiation and enhanced survival. *Pathology* **25**(4), 338–343.

Zelger, B.G., Zelger, B., Steiner, H. and Mikuz, G. (1995). Solitary giant xanthogranuloma and benign cephalic histiocytosis—variants of juvenile xanthogranuloma. *Arch. Dermatol.* **131**, 904–908.

Zhou, L. and Tedder, T.F. (1995). Human blood dendritic cells selectively express CD83, a member of the immunoglobulin superfamily. *J. Immunol.* **154**, 3821-3835.

Zhou, L., Schwarting, R., Smith, H.M. and Tedder, T.F. (1992). A novel cell-surface molecule expressed by human interdigitating reticulum cells, Langerhans cells, and activated lymphocytes is a new member of the Ig superfamily. *J. Immunol.* **149**, 735–742.

CHAPTER 20
Dendritic Cells in Rejection and Acceptance of Solid Organ Allografts

A.J. Demetris[1], N. Murase[2], J.J. Fung[2] and T.E. Starzl[2]
Thomas E. Starzl Transplantation Institute, Departments of [1]Pathology and [2]Surgery, Divisions of Transplantation, University of Pittsburgh Medical Center, Pittsburgh, Pennsylvania, USA

INTRODUCTION

The field of solid organ transplantation is based largely on the concept that replacement of irreversibly damaged organ in an otherwise 'healthy' recipient can significantly prolong survival or even cure some diseases. Although the hope for clinical success is based on this premise, many allograft recipients suffer from recurrence of the original disease. For example, chronic viral hepatitis types B and C almost invariably attack the new liver after hepatic replacement [1, 2]. This unfortunate reality illustrates the importance of a systemic, or nonlocal, perspective in transplantation biology: a specific disease may primarily manifest in a single organ, but for many disorders this simply represents a local manifestation of a more pervasive problem. An exception to this generalization is organ-specific toxic injury or organ-based metabolic diseases where replacement of the defective organ corrects a systemic problem and brings about a true cure.

A systemic perspective is also of importance in the study of transplantation physiology, including allograft immunobiology. For example, insulin secreted by islet allografts can regulate the recipient blood sugar; and a new liver will receive blood and nutrients from the recipient intestines, from which it will synthesize cholesterol used to construct new 'recipient' cells. Fortunately, clinical physicians rarely have to be concerned about physiological compatibility between the donor and recipient. Most of the complex systems involved have 'nonlocal' properties that enable a donor organ to spontaneously adjust to its new environment. The integration occurs so naturally that one rarely even thinks about the interface between donor and recipient, unless something goes wrong.

The most important exception to the above generalization is the immune system: its 'local' properties result in an inability to spontaneously integrate the donor with the recipient, and vice versa, which in turn leads to significant problems for the transplant surgeon. Unless the patient is heavily immunosuppressed, the allograft is eventually rejected. There are, however, situations in experimental animals where allografts are accepted without immunosuppression, and in humans where immunosuppression can

Dendritic Cells: Biology and Clinical Applications
ISBN 0-12-455860-7

be completely withdrawn and the allografts function for the lifetime of the recipient. Thus, the local properties of the immune system were not designed to frustrate transplant clinicians, instead, they can be predictably redesigned under certain circumstances.

Consequently, the entire field of clinical transplantation could be thought of as an experiment conducted to investigate the local properties of the immune system, among others, including the role of MHC antigens and the consequences of MHC antigen expression on different cell types. Since these antigens, as well as sex chromosomes, can be used to mark the genetic fidelity of an individual cell, double labeling techniques can be used to trace specific donor and recipient cell types after solid organ transplantation to assess problems with integration. Discoveries made using this technology have brought together two previously unlinked research fields in transplantation immunology: the deleterious and the beneficial functions of donor hematolymphoid cells. The sections below overview both lines of investigation and highlight the role of dendritic cells (DC) in allograft rejection and acceptance.

ORGAN-BASED IMMUNE NETWORKS

Before proceeding directly to a discussion of the role of DC in transplantation, it is important first to briefly overview organ-based immune physiology. This refers to a dynamic network of hematolymphoid cells that travel into and out of, and transiently occupy, the interstitium of all solid organs. These cells monitor the microenvironment and communicate with central lymphoid organs, and regional lymph nodes via the circulatory system and lymphatics [3]. An understanding of this system is of particular importance in organ transplantation, since problems with assimilation of the donor immune system affect many aspects of transplantation biology, as well as patient management. Examples include the susceptibility to rejection, the clinical and histopathological manifestations of both acute and chronic rejection, infections, and the interface between infection and rejection.

Organ-based immune cells are primarily derived from progenitors that migrate from the bone marrow, although maturation from local precursors, including intraorgan hematopoietic stem cells, can also contribute to this pool. Even in an adult, the liver has enough hematopoietic stem cells to fully reconstitute, for the long term, a lethally irradiated recipient [4, 5]. The important point is that intraorgan immune cells are a dynamic population: they continuously mature and migrate and therefore must ultimately be maintained by a stem cell population.

Normal physiology accounts for the considerable variation among different organs in the quantity and quality of organ-based immune cells [6, 7]. Organs in direct contact with the external environment, such as the lungs and intestines, have an exaggerated complement of organ-associated lymphoid tissue, generally termed 'mucosal-associated lymphoid tissue'. After contact with commensal bacteria in neonatal life, the immune cells spontaneously arrange into an organized complex structure, which is identical to that seen in lymph nodes, replete with B cell follicles and T cell-rich interfollicular zones rich in DC [8–10]. Thereafter, a delicate balance is maintained between reaction to antigens from the environment and local tissue damage. The liver, on the other hand, is indirectly exposed to the external environment, since it drains blood from the intestines. It is richly endowed with a large component of cells from the monocyte/macrophage lineage, consistent with its role as a filter of various opsonized materials, including microorganisms, activated platelet aggregates, and coagulated proteins [11]. Heart [6, 7, 12, 13] and kidneys [6, 14, 15] also have considerable, but less well developed immune networks in comparison to the above organs.

Common to vascularized organs is a population of DC precursors at various stages of maturation located in the interstitial connective tissue [14–19]. The 'immature' state of many intraorgan DC [18, 20–22], except for those in the lymphoid tissue of the lung and intestines [18, 19], is characterized by phagocytic capacity, which is absent in mature DC [18, 21, 22]; relatively inefficient stimulatory capacity in a mixed leukocyte reaction (MLR) [22]; and low density of MHC class II [21] or costimulatory molecule expression [19]. Organ-based DC precursors can also be identified with a series of monoclonal antibodies directed at certain differentiation markers, covered elsewhere in this book.

Dendritic cells and their precursors reside near terminal lymphatics throughout the interstitium of organs, and are concentrated near draining efferent lymphatic vessels in the adventitia of arteries; epithelial-lined conduits that are in contact with the external environment, such as the mucosal-associated lymphoid tissue of the lungs [23] and intestines [18, 19]; and portal tracts of the liver [17, 21, 24]. At these sites, they monitor the microenvironment for foreign, or dangerous antigens [25], exposure to which stimulates DC maturation and migration via efferent lymphatics to the paracortex of regional lymph nodes where they stimulate a T cell response [18, 22, 26–30]. The factors involved in DC activation, maturation, and migration are covered in more detail in Chapter 11. Thus, the vasculature and lymphatics represent important lines of communication between the intraorgan immune network, the regional lymph nodes, and eventually the thymus and spleen.

HEMATOLYMPHOID AND DENDRITIC CELLS AS POTENTIATORS AND FACILITATORS OF REJECTION

Acute 'Cellular' Rejection

When an organ becomes an allograft, the nascent hematolymphoid cells become known as 'passenger leukocytes'. The idea that these particular donor cells are especially immunogenic was first proposed by Snell [31]. Steinmuller [32] provided experimental evidence for this concept by showing that chimeric donor skin allografts in which the passenger leukocytes were allogeneic, but the epidermal cells were syngeneic to the recipient, resulted in permanent graft acceptance. However, the recipients became sensitized to the alloantigens on the hematopoietic cells.

The relative importance of passenger leukocytes in precipitating rejection was further addressed by Guttmann *et al.* [33], who constructed chimeric donor organs by lethally irradiating rats and reconstituting them with allogeneic bone marrow. He showed that the 'immunogenicity' of the organs could be greatly reduced when the passenger leukocytes were syngeneic to the recipient. Several other experimental manipulations also showed conclusively that the passenger leukocytes were more immunogenic than the parenchyma. These included pretransplant *in vitro* culturing to eliminate or reduce the complement of passenger leukocytes [34–36], and so-called 'parking' experiments [37–40]. In the latter, allografts are transplanted into intermediate hosts that are kept immunosuppressed or are naturally immuno-incompetent for one reason or another. Once the original passenger leukocytes have been replaced, the composite grafts are then retransplanted into a second recipient, that is syngeneic with either the parenchymal and stroma or the passenger leukocyte population. Regardless of the technique used, the important concept was that depletion of allogeneic passenger leukocytes led to prolonged allograft survival.

Lechler and Batchelor [40] provided a key piece of evidence bringing DC to the forefront as the passenger leukocyte prototype. They showed that the immunogenicity of long-surviving enhanced (AS X AUG)F1 renal allografts retransplanted into secondary AS recipients could be restored by the injection of as few as 1×10^4 to 5×10^4 DC of donor strain derived from afferent lymph [40]. In contrast, neither the passenger volume of donor strain blood, nor 5×10^6 T- or B-lymphocytes were able to do so, thereby demonstrating more than a 100-fold difference in immunogenic potency. These findings were consistent with observations about the functional activities of DC originally made by Steinman and colleagues [41–43] and later confirmed by many others.

Disrupted Local Lymphatics

It should be remembered that donor organ harvesting and reimplantation disrupts the efferent lymphatic channels. This blocks an important migratory circuit for immune cells that are either already present in or enter the allograft interstitium, until connections with regional lymph nodes are reestablished within 2–3 weeks [44–48]. In fact, efferent lymphatic disruption, along with ischemic injury contributes to a 'reimplantation' response, which by itself can precipitate activation of the intraorgan immune network [46–51]. Thus, this purely mechanical problem can, in some respects, simulate an antigen-driven immune response [51] and is one of the first difficulties, but by no means the only one, encountered when the immune system of the donor attempts assimilation with that of the recipient.

The presence of MHC, adhesion and costimulating molecules on DC causes them to spontaneously form clusters with and directly activate allogeneic lymphocytes [24, 52]. In an allograft, activated recipient T cells in such clusters proliferate [24] and produce cytokines that recruit other immune cells that have the potential to damage the organ. In fact, the distribution of mononuclear cells at the initiation of acute rejection reflects the intraorgan distribution of DC [24, 52]: in kidney allografts it preferentially localizes to the cortex and outer medulla [14, 15], whereas, in the liver, portal tracts and perivenular regions are preferentially targeted [17, 24, 53]. Conversely, the absence of renal cortex or portal tracts in an allograft kidney or liver biopsy, respectively, renders such samples inadequate for the evaluation of rejection. Altogether, this process is referred to as 'peripheral sensitization', or recognition of the allograft in the periphery via direct alloantigenic stimulation. Subsequently, upregulation of adhesion molecules on the surrounding vasculature and recruitment of lymphoid and nonlymphoid effector cells and local tissue damage signal the development of acute 'cellular' rejection.

In organs with mucosal-associated lymphoid tissue, such as the lung and intestines, recipient lymphocytes trafficking into the allograft following the same migratory routes as they normally would: they enter the T cell-dependent areas of the bronchial (BALT) and mucosal (MALT) associated lymphoid tissue, respectively [12, 54–58]. Here they encounter donor DC and participate in a bidirectional '*in vivo* mixed leukocyte response' [12, 54–59], which is the same type of response as described above for the interstitium of organs except that the surrounding microenvironment contains immunologically active donor T- and B-lymphocytes.

Passenger Leukocytes

Passenger leukocytes from the donor immune network, including DC, leave the allograft, either hematogenously or via intact regional efferent lymphatics that drain to *donor* regional lymph nodes transplanted *en bloc* with the allograft [56, 57, 59]. Larsen and colleagues [60, 61] were the first to show that donor DC from a heart allograft migrate hematogenously to the recipient spleen. The same thing occurs after transplantation of a liver allo- or xenograft [24, 62]. Donor DC leaving these allografts migrate to the periarterial lymphatic sheath and marginal zone of the spleen, where their appearance is associated with a proliferative response in the recipient lymphoid cells (Plate 20.1) [24, 63]. Altogether, this process is referred to as 'central sensitization' [24, 60, 61, 63], or central recognition of the allograft, again via direct alloantigenic stimulation. The passenger leukocyte population also contains hematopoietic stem cells, as well as T and B cells, macrophages, and mature and progenitor DC (Plate 20.2). This is evidenced by their ability to reconstitute lethally irradiated experimental animal recipients [4, 5] and to convert the blood type of human recipients [64]. Thus, at the progenitor level, donor cells will have access to the recipient bone marrow, to regional and distant lymph nodes, and even to the thymic medulla [3, 63, 65–68].

Once recipient T cells are activated within the allograft and rejection effector mechanisms begin to damage the organ, there is an increased production of lymph and disruption of the lymphatic and capillary microvascular endothelial junctions. This retards immune cell traffic and lymph flow [45–48, 69–71] and contributes to the reappearance of graft edema and swelling typically seen during acute rejection [45, 69–72]. The result is an endless cycle of immune activation and damage, graft edema, retarded immune cell trafficking and diminished blood flow. Unless interrupted by increased immunosuppression, the process usually leads to allograft failure.

Considering the completeness of the data outlined above, it was reasonable to conclude that the passenger leukocyte population should be removed from the allograft before transplantation. Thus, various types of irradiation [73] and monoclonal antibodies directed at common leukocyte [74–76] or MHC class II [77–79] antigens were used in an effort to deplete these cells. In general, all of these pretreatment regimens prolonged allograft survival, but the long-term beneficial effects were less than expected.

Targeting Donor DC

Blocking costimulatory molecules such as the B7 family [80–85] and CD40 [81, 86] interrupts cell signaling mediated by interactions of these molecules with their ligands and significantly diminishes acute rejection, resulting in prolongation of graft survival [81–88]. In some models, there is even an absence [81] or amelioration of chronic rejection (CR) [82–86]. However, in some of the models used, CR develops directly from acute rejection, which is nonlethal because of genetic compatibility between the donor and recipient [83–85], and may not reflect the clinical scenario in most cases of CR [89]. In addition, the presence of infiltrates within the treated allografts [82, 84] or actual allograft vasculopathy [82–85] suggests that tolerance without a susceptibility to CR has not been achieved. Nevertheless, this line of research represents an important advance in our understanding of how acute rejection damages an allograft.

It is interesting to note that the beneficial effect of costimulatory molecule blockade was *diminished* by immunosuppression and was *augmented* by the addition of donor antigen in the form of donor splenocytes [85]. In addition, the B7-CD28 blockade does not completely stop cytokine mRNA production within the allograft. Instead it is shifted toward a T_H2-type 'tolerogenic' pathway [87]. Paradoxically, the beneficial effect is still observed in IL-4 deficient mice [88]. These observations suggest, but do not prove, that tolerance requires T cell activation, and that stimulation is best provided by the passenger leukocyte population [36, 90, 91].

Nonetheless, the logical conclusion of this line of reasoning is to construct allografts completely devoid of passenger leukocytes. The idea is that the stimulatory DC are removed and forms of donor antigen other than hematopoietic cells, such as the allograft parenchyma and stroma [25, 92, 93] and soluble MHC antigens [94, 95] or peptides [94–97], may actually be tolerogenic [90]. Although this line of reasoning has several important conceptual flaws, it is based on the concept that more than one signal is needed to trigger T cell activation and proliferation [25].

In vitro, presentation of antigen without proper costimulation can result in anergy [25]. When this concept is tested *in vivo* using transgenic mice, the results are not clear cut. For example, the immune system of mice carrying allogeneic MHC transgenes on nonimmune cells, such as islets of Langerhans, simply 'ignores' alloantigen expression until it is presented to the immune system in the proper context by DC and other antigen-presenting cells. This most often occurs during tissue damage from viral infection or other insults that cause local immune stimulation [98–100].

In a vascularized allograft, immune activation, and thus immunological cognition of the allograft, is extremely difficult, if not impossible to avoid. Organ harvesting and reimplantation, ischemia, preexisting donor diseases and efferent lymphatic disruption can all potentially contribute to intragraft immune activation, which in turn creates an immune environment conducive to allorecognition, even if donor DC are not present. Migration of potently allostimulatory cells from the allograft assures central allorecognition. Thus, from a practical perspective in clinical transplantation, it is our opinion that, initially, very few allografts are 'ignored', which is evidenced by the fact that all allograft recipients require immune suppression to prevent acute rejection.

Nevertheless, certain tissue allografts, such as pure epithelial [35, 101, 102], fibroblast [103], and corneal [104] allografts, can be completely depleted of donor hematopoietic cells. Unfortunately, these allografts are still often rejected [35, 101, 102], particularly if they are placed into an immunologically active environment [105], similar to the observations described above for the transgenic mice. Thus, despite an absence of passenger leukocytes or DC, rejection still occurs, albeit more slowly, and probably via the indirect pathway of alloantigen presentation [35, 104, 106–109].

Transitional Phase

Since passenger leukocytes are bone marrow-derived or stem cell-dependent, they exist for a relatively short period in the periphery. Thus, replacement of the donor intraorgan immune network (including DC) after transplantation with similar recipient cells is an expected finding [57, 110–118]. Indeed, this occurs to some extent in all allografts, since trafficking of immune cells is part of the normal 'nonlocal' immune physiology. However, as discussed above, when recipient T cells encounter donor DC (and vice versa), the transitional process has to be chaperoned by immunosuppressive drugs because it usually precipitates acute rejection. For DC, the replacement phenomenon likely occurs at a precursor cell stage, since mature recipient DC do not appear to home to allograft tissues [119].

It is likely that the same factors that control activation, maturation, and migration of DC precursors in nonallograft organs contribute to donor and recipient DC trafficking in allografts. For example, it is known that the intraorgan cytokine milieu contributes to activation, recruitment, and migration of both macrophages and DC. In allografts, the cytokine-rich milieu of rejection [120] quickens the rate and extent of donor macrophage replacement [111, 121]. Infiltrates associated with T_H1-type cytokines, such IFN-γ and macrophage-activating chemokines like IL-12, mobilize donor macrophages and foster the influx of activated recipient cells (unpublished observation).

An orderly transition from donor to recipient cells in the intraorgan immune network, however, is dependent on preventing architectural damage during the transition [57]. If this can be accomplished, recipient cells can function alongside donor ones, as a chimeric intraorgan immune network. If not, irreversible structural damage may prevent reestablishment of a normally functioning intraorgan immune network, with lines of communication to regional lymph nodes. The architectural damage can occur at the level of the BALT [116, 122, 123] or GALT [57, 118, 124], lymphatic drainage from the organ, and/or the regional donor lymph nodes [57]. Subsequently, any cause of allograft inflammation, such as environmental irritants or infection, may result in an ineffectual local immune response and persistence of the insult(s). This, in turn, can cause cytokine release that facilitates alloimmune injury, and the allograft then becomes trapped in a relentless downward spiral of declining organ function that eventually ends in allograft failure (see below).

Chronic Rejection

Chronic rejection (CR), in any organ, can be broadly defined as a largely indolent but progressive form of allograft injury, characterized primarily by persistent but patchy inflammation of the allograft, interstitial fibrosis, fibrointimal hyperplasia of arteries, and destruction and atrophy of parenchymal elements and organ-associated lymphoid tissue [89, 120, 125]. The term chronic implies a temporally prolonged course and, in general, CR more indolently compromises organ function than acute rejection. However, it clearly develops in many cases from inadequately controlled acute rejection and in patients not compliant with immunosuppressive therapy. In others, CR more indolently compromises allograft function over a period of months to years, without an apparent precipitating event [89]. Our emphasis here will be on DC. The reader interested in a broader perspective of CR is referred to several recent reviews [89, 126–128].

The intragraft inflammatory infiltrates associated with CR are often arranged into nodular aggregates, some of which contain germinal centers [89] reminiscent of the development of mucosal-associated lymphoid tissue, discussed above. Immunophenotypic analysis reveals a predominance of $CD4^+$ and $CD8^+$ T cells and macrophages with fewer B cells, although those present can form small primary and secondary follicles. This is in contrast to the infiltrates associated with acute rejection, which have fewer B cells and no follicles and tend to be more diffusely distributed throughout the interstitium, lacking an organized structure.

Few studies have specifically investigated DC in chronically rejecting organs. Oguma *et al.* (129) suggested that DC of *recipient* origin participated in the CR process by coordinating antigenic presentation in arteries affected by obliterative arteriopathy and in the interstitium. Subsequent studies have verified these findings and found that the number of recipient DC in chronically rejecting organs correlates directly with the overall severity of inflammation [116, 120, 130]. Moreover, the *recipient* DC are concentrated amidst the lymphoid aggregates [116, 120, 122, 129], suggesting that they are coordinating antigen presentation, an assumption based on the spatial relationship between the DC and the lymphoid infiltrates. These morphological and immunohistochemical observations are consistent with the concept that indirect (rather than direct), MHC-restricted alloantigen presentation importantly contributes to CR [106–108], and that chronic antigenic stimulation occurring outside the lymph nodes can result in the development of intraorgan lymphoid tissue [131, 132], similarly to autoimmune disorders such as Hashimoto's thyroiditis, primary biliary cirrhosis, and Crohn's disease [131].

As alluded to above, chronically rejecting allografts also develop another significant problem: the persistent or severe injury during the transitional phase selectively damages mucosal-associated lymphoid tissue normally present in the lung [72, 133] and intestines [56, 58] and focally disrupts intraorgan lymphatics in other organs [46, 89, 120]. Eventually these structures can be completely destroyed and replaced by fibrosis [56, 58, 133, 134]. Consequently, the organizational structure of the immune network and migratory routes of DC are disrupted. This undoubtedly contributes to the inability of the intraorgan immune network to adequately process infectious and other antigens. Thus, it is tempting to speculate that this accounts for the frequent association between infection and CR [123, 133, 135–139]: chronically rejecting organs may simply be unable to adequately handle infections or other antigenic insults.

HEMATOLYMPHOID AND DENDRITIC CELLS AS FACILITATORS OF TOLERANCE INDUCTION

There are two lines of transplantation research in which studies show how donor hematopoietic cells in general, and DC specifically, might induce tolerance to solid organ allografts. The first of these is activation-induced clonal deletion and the second is induction of hematopoietic chimerism.

Donor Dendritic Cells as Mediators of Peripheral Clonal Deletion

Implantation of any solid organ allograft results in a characteristic cycle of heightened immune activation, followed by evolution toward a more stable relationship between the allograft and the recipient when immunosuppression can be considerably lowered or even withdrawn [140, 141]. With the understanding brought about by the appreciation of donor hematopoietic cell migration after transplantation [24, 63, 113, 142], this prototypic series of events can likely be attributed, in large part, to the initial engagement of donor and recipient immune cells in the allograft and recipient lymphoid tissues.

During this time, it is possible that the intense immune activation results in a form of clonal deletion called clonal stripping [143], deletion or purging through apoptosis [144–146]. It might be crudely thought of as the peripheral equivalent of negative selection in the thymus, which is a very efficient means of controlling reactivity in a lymphocyte population. Current research suggests that DC may be involved in this process: blocking of costimulation on mature DC allows exhibition of their apoptosis-inducing potential and they thus may be particularly adept at mediating such a process [27, 147, 148]. In fact, it is tempting to speculate that the combination of clonal deletion via apoptosis after a strong rejection reaction, followed by replacement of the intra-graft immune network (graft adaptation), ultimately causes the immune system to ignore the allograft.

Unfortunately, on a practical level, the harsh reality is that, even in combination, the above mechanisms are unable to prevent rejection in the majority of long-term survivors without the aid of exogenous immunosuppression [89]. At best, there exists an uneasy truce between an adapted allograft and a recipient that can be triggered into a rejection reaction at the slightest provocation. In the worst case, most long-term recipients are slowly rejecting their organs. This also holds true for liver allograft recipients, who are resistant to CR compared to recipients of other vascularized allografts [89, 149]: even this 'favorable' recipient population requires chronic immunosuppression in over 80% of long-term survivors [141]. Thus, while clonal deletion or stripping, veto or regulatory cells, or other mechanisms may contribute to graft acceptance in immunosuppressed recipients, they are insufficient in the majority of patients to allow cessation of immunosuppressive therapy.

Dendritic Cells as Mediators of the Effects of Hematopoietic Chimerism

Owen [150] was the first to show that twin cattle sharing a placental circulation develop chimeric immune systems, each composed of immune cells from both individuals [150]. He found that this condition enabled them to exchange other tissues without the fear of rejection, or a need for immunosuppression. When attempts were made to create chimeric immune systems in adult animals, it was quickly realized that lethal or sublethal irradiation and other harsh conditioning regimens were required to ablate the recipient immune system and to make 'physiological space' for the engraftment of infused donor bone marrow [151–159]. Unfortunately, this limits clinical implementation of the concept. Two major problems exist: graft-versus-host disease [160, 161] and the morbidity associated with the conditioning regimens [158, 162]. Current approaches to decreasing morbidity without compromising donor stem cell engraftment include lower doses of irradiation, facilitator cells [163, 164], and/or higher doses or repeated infusions of donor bone marrow [159, 162, 165].

Nevertheless, when donor stem cell engraftment results in long-term mixed hematopoietic chimerism, there is complete assimilation of the donor immune system in some cases, and an undeniable association with tolerance. In the mixed chimeric animals, intraorgan immune networks are composed of cells from both individuals [154, 166], and tolerance is strictly dependent on the persistence of hematopoietic chimerism: loss of chimerism and loss of tolerance go together [167, 168]. This has been observed in humans given fetal liver cell allografts [169–171], and in a number of small experimental animal models [151–155, 157–159].

The experimental models have been useful in determining the role of DC in tolerance induction. For example, mixed chimeric animals specifically lack donor responsiveness in a MLR, accept allografts without immunosuppression, and are resistant to CR [172, 173]. Central deletional tolerance is primarily responsible for these observations [154, 155, 158], although peripheral mechanisms also likely contribute to the process [174, 175]. Thus, the situation is similar to the nontransplantation setting, where both central and peripheral mechanisms contribute to 'self' tolerance, which is a 'local' property of the immune system.

In the nontransplantation setting, central or thymic tolerance involves a complex set of thymic epithelial and stromal interactions with immature T cells that first mediate positive selection of developing thymocytes, based on 'self' reactivity [176–179]. Subsequently, thymic medullary DC play a predominant role in negative selection [176, 178, 180–186], where cells that react too strongly with the DC are deleted. Similar observations have been made in the mixed allogeneic chimeras: thymic stromal and epithelial elements appear to mediate positive selection, even if there is MHC mismatching between the lymphoid and nonlymphoid populations [169, 171, 187], whereas donor thymic hematopoietic cells appear to mediate negative selection [158, 166, 168, 169, 171, 174, 187]. Although more studies are needed to identify the population of donor cells that mediate negative selection in chimeras, the characteristics identified to date make donor DC a likely candidate [3, 63, 65–68].

FINDINGS THAT BRIDGE THE GAP BETWEEN IMMUNOGENIC AND TOLEROGENIC DC

In the late 1980s, a series of experiments were carried out to examine the sequence of histopathological changes associated with acute intestinal allograft rejection [56, 57]. During these studies, it was necessary to distinguish between donor and recipient lymphoid cells, so that one could unravel the underlying immune pathophysiology. This was achieved with the development of a monoclonal antibody that reacted with the class II major histocompatibility antigens of most rat strains, except the Brown Norway (BN) [188]. Subsequently, it was possible to show that Lewis cells emigrated into the BN GALT and mesenteric lymph node of intestinal allografts, where they replaced cells of donor origin in the organ-based immune network. This occurred within the first several weeks after transplantation [57]. Similar findings were observed in human small-intestinal allograft recipients [112].

The above studies prompted an investigation of the fate of donor cells that had emigrated from the allograft. Up to that time, very few such studies had appeared in the literature [24, 60, 65, 189, 190], and all came to the same conclusion discussed above—donor passenger leukocytes, especially DC, were essentially deleterious to allograft survival because they served only to precipitate and/or amplify a rejection reaction. However, all of these studies were conducted in nonimmunosuppressed recipients, which resulted in rapid rejection of the allografts, as expected. Had similar studies been carried out on the fate of passenger leukocytes in either transiently or continuously immunosuppressed recipients, the conclusion about the role of DC in organ transplantation might have been different. In essence, that is what was done in the early 1990s.

A quick survey of available long-term experimental animal and several humans organ allograft recipients revealed a surprising finding—the donor hematolymphoid cells persisted in long-term survivors (Plate 20.3), some of whom were chronically free of immunosuppressive therapy [65, 113, 166]. Moreover, the donor cells were ubiquitously distributed throughout the lymphoid and nonlymphoid tissues, and some had the characteristics of DC [65, 166]. This included a strong surface expression of MHC class II antigens, a dendritic shape, and a location in the interstitium of organs, the paracortex of lymph nodes, the thymic medulla [63, 65–68], and the periarterial lymphatic sheath of the spleen. These are all sites where DC normally reside. Further studies by Lu and Thomson [21, 66, 191, 192] showed conclusively that DC and their precursors were included among the passenger leukocytes persisting in organ allograft recipients.

These observations led to the suggestion that 'microchimerism' or the persistence of donor hematopoietic cells was necessary, but alone not sufficient, for the induction of tolerance [113–115, 193]. Since the donor cells persisted for decades in some patients, it was assumed that they are sustained by 'engrafted' donor stem cells transplanted with the organ (Plate 20.2). The important conceptual point is that donor hematolymphoid cells appear to have integrated successfully into the recipient immune system, similarly to the chimeras made by irradiation. However, the number of donor cells present is much smaller in microchimeras than in macrochimeras made by irradiation, and this likely affects the relative contribution of various mechanisms to the tolerant phenotype. For example, it is unlikely that only a few donor DC that make their way to the recipient thymus would be able to completely delete donor reactive T cells (Plate 20.3), but there may be enough to activate autoregulatory circuits. In the meanwhile, other studies confirmed that passenger leukocytes persisted in experimental animals and in humans, but the authors did not necessarily agree with our interpretation [92, 93, 194–201].

Initially this discovery did not fit easily into the current understanding of donor DC in transplantation immunobiology. It was not immediately clear how the most potentially potent allogeneic simulator could survive long term in a recipient who no longer required immunosuppression. This was especially true for DC in the periphery, even though freshly isolated DC from nonlymphoid tissues are relatively inefficient antigen-presenting cells. It was clear, however, that long-term persistence of donor DC in the allograft was associated with freedom from chronic rejection [120] and, therefore, they might mediate tolerogenic reactions. In addition, trafficking of donor hematopoietic stem and progenitor cells from the allograft to the recipient bone marrow and thymus was not widely appreciated. However, analogies were drawn between this situation and that of mixed allogeneic chimeras achieved with irradiation. In the periphery, only a few studies had suggested that DC might mediate tolerogenic reactions [202, 203]. More recently, however, there is an increasing awareness that DC can and do mediate eventual 'nonresponsiveness' [27, 204–207]. How this is achieved is covered in greater detail in Chapter 26.

In the nontransplantation setting, there is now convincing evidence that DC can mediate both stimulatory and tolerogenic immune reactions. The context of presentation is certainly of great importance in determining which pathway is chosen. This is also true for transplantation. Without transient immunosuppression, mature DC invariably precipitate rejection that causes graft failure. With immunosuppression, acute rejection is avoided and the persistence of donor DC is associated with allograft protection from CR [120]. These probably arise from engrafted stem cells and/or other precursors. Emerging details about the mechanism(s) in stimulatory and tolerogenic reactions involved are covered in Chapter 26.

What, then, has been learned about the immune system, MHC antigens and the role of DC in the experiment of transplantation? First, it is clear that an immune system has 'local' properties, which greatly complicate the ability to take an organ from one person and implant it into another one. We have also learned that MHC antigens and DC both play important roles in defining these local properties, and successful long-term freedom from rejection probably requires transfer of the donor immune system. DC appear to exert this effect via their ability to stimulate immune reactions that either prevent or facilitate assimilation of the donor immune system and its accompanying organ into the recipient, which in turn depends on their phenotype and maturational stage. Thus, in a generic sense, at least part of the 'local' properties of the immune system are self-defined by DC, and the other immune cells with which they interact, both in the thymus and in the periphery. However, this occurs in the context of the environment and is dependent on, but not strictly limited by, the recipient MHC genes/antigens. Consequently, it appears that the local properties of the immune system and MHC antigens were not designed for the purpose of preventing allogeneic transplantation but to enable species adaptability [208–210]. The key to understanding, and thus controlling, the immune system for the purpose of transplantation will come from a knowledge of its local and nonlocal properties so that the latter can be exploited [90, 211].

ACKNOWLEDGMENT

Supported by NIH 1 RO1 DK49615-01 and NIH RO1 AI40329-02.

REFERENCES

1. Demetris, A.J., Jaffe, R., Sheahan, D.D. *et al.* (1986). Recurrent hepatitis B in liver allograft recipients. Differentiation between viral hepatitis B and rejection. *Am. J. Pathol.* **125** (1), 161–172.
2. Randhawa, P.S. and Demetris, A.J. (1995). Hepatitis C virus infection in liver allografts. [Review]. *Pathol. Annu.* **2**, 203–226.
3. Beschorner, W.E., Yao, X. and Divic, J. (1995). Recruitment of semiallogeneic dendritic cells to the thymus during post-cyclosporine thymic regeneration. *Transplantation* **60** (11), 1326–1330.
4. Murase, N., Starzl, T.E., Ye, O. *et al.* (1996). Multilineage hematopoietic reconstitution of supralethally irradiated rats by syngeneic whole organ transplanation: with particular reference to the liver. *Transplantation* **61**, 1–4.
5. Taniguchi, H., Toyoshima, T., Fukao, K. and Nakauchi, H. (1996). Presence of hematopoietic stem cells in the adult liver. *Nature Medicine* **2**, 198–203.
6. Murase, N., Starzl, T.E., Tanabe, M. *et al.* (1995). Variable chimerism, graft-versus-host disease, and tolerance after different kinds of cell and whole organ transplantation from Lewis to brown Norway rats. *Transplantation* **60** (2), 158–171.
7. Holzinger, C., Zuckermann, A., Reinwald, C. *et al.* (1996). Are T cells from healthy heart really only passengers? Characterization of cardiac tissue T cells. *Immunol. Lett.* **53** (2–3), 63–67.
8. Anderson, J.C. (1977). The response of gut-associated lymphoid tissue in gnotobiotic piglets to the presence of bacterial antigen in the alimentary tract. *J. Anat.* **124** (3), 555–562.
9. Gordon, J.I., Hooper, L.V., McNevin, M.S., Wong, M. and Bry, L. (1997). Epithelial cell growth and differentiation. III. Promoting diversity in the intestine: conversations between the microflora, epithelium, and diffuse GALT. *Am. J. Physiol.* **273** (3 Pt 1), G565–570.

10. Woolverton, C.J., Holt, L.C., Mitchell, D. and Sartor, R.B. (1992). Identification and characterization of rat intestinal lamina propria cells: consequences of microbial colonization. *Vet. Immunol. Immunopathol.* **34** (1–2), 127–138.
11. Wardle, E.N. (1987). Kupffer cells and their function. *Liver* **7**, 63–75.
12. Prop, J., Kuijpers, K., Petersen, A.H., Bartels, H.L., Nieuwenhuis, P. and Wildevuur, C.R. (1985). Why are lung allografts more vigorously rejected than hearts? *J. Heart Transplant.* **4** (4), 433–436.
13. Eiref, S.D., Zhang, W., Popma, S.H., Shah, L.J., Moore, J.S. and Rosengard, B.R. (1997). Creation of chimeric hearts: a tool for testing the 'passenger leukocyte' hypothesis. *Ann. Thorac. Surg.* **4** (3), 628–633.
14. Kaissling, B. and Le Hir, M. (1994). Characterization and distribution of interstitial cell types in the renal cortex of rats. *Kidney Int.* **45** (3), 709–720.
15. Kaissling, B., Hegyi, I., Loffing, J. and Le Hir, M. (1996). Morphology of interstitial cells in the healthy kidney. *Anat Embryol. (Berl)* **193** (4), 303–318.
16. Hart, D.N.J. and McKenzie, J.L. (1990). Interstitial dendritic cells. *Int. Rev. Immunol.* **6**, 128–149.
17. Prickett, T.C.R., McKenzie, J.L. and Hart, D.N.J. (1988). Characterization of interstitial dendritic cells in human liver. *Transplantation* **46**, 754–761.
18. Rao, A.S., Roake, J.A., Larsen, C.P., Hankins, D.F., Morris, P.J. and Austyn, J.M. (1993). Isolation of dendritic leukocytes from non-lymphoid organs. *Adv. Exp. Med. Biol.* **329**, 507–512.
19. Inaba, K., Witmer-Pack, M., Inaba, M. *et al.* (1994). The tissue distribution of the B7-2 costimulator in mice: abundant expression on dendritic cells in situ and during maturation in vitro. *J. Exp. Med.* **180** (5), 1849–1860.
20. Roake, J.A. and Austyn, J.M. (1993). The role of dendritic cells and T cell activation in allograft rejection. *Exp. Nephrol.* **1** (2), 90–101.
21. Lu, L, Woo, J., Rao, A.S. *et al.* (1994). Propagation of dendritic cell progenitors from normal mouse liver using granulocyte/macrophage colony-stimulating factor and their maturational development in the presence of type-1 collagen. *J. Exp. Med.* **179** (6), 1823–1834.
22. Austyn, J.M., Hankins, D.F., Larsen, C.P., Morris, P.J., Rao, A.S. and Roake, J.A. (1994). Isolation and characterization of dendritic cells from mouse heart and kidney. *J. Immunol.* **152** (5), 2401–2410.
23. Gong, J.L., McCarthy, K.M., Telford, J., Tamatani, T., Miyasaka, M. and Schneeberger, E.E. (1992). Intraepithelial airway dendritic cells: a distinct subset of pulmonary dendritic cells obtained by microdissection. *J. Exp. Med.* **175** (3), 797–807.
24. Demetris, A., Qian, S., Sun, H. *et al.* (1991). Early events in liver allograft rejection: delineation of sites of simultaneous intragraft and recipient lymphoid tissue sensitization. *Am. J. Pathol.* **138**, 609.
25. Matzinger, P. (1994). Tolerance, danger, and the extended family. *Annu. Rev. Immunol.* **12**, 991–1045.
26. Steinman, R.M. (1991). The dendritic cell system and its role in immunogenicity. [Review]. *Annu. Rev. Immunol.* **9**, 271–296.
27. Steinman, R.M., Pack, M. and Inaba, K. (1997). Dendritic cells in the T-cell areas of lymphoid organs. *Immunol. Rev.* **156**, 25–37.
28. Wright-Browne, V., McClain, K.L., Talpaz, M., Ordonez, N. and Estrov, Z. (1997). Physiology and pathophysiology of dendritic cells. *Hum. Pathol.* **28** (5), 563–579.
29. Ni, K. and O'Neill, H.C. (1997). The role of dendritic cells in T cell activation. *Immunol. Cell. Biol.* **75** (3), 223–230.
30. Cella, M., Sallusto, F. and Lanzavecchia, A. (1997). Origin, maturation and antigen presenting function of dendritic cells. *Curr. Opin. Immunol.* **9** (1), 10–16.
31. Snell, G.D. (1957). The homograft reaction. *Annu. Rev. Microbiol.* **11**, 439–458.
32. Steinmuller, D. (1967). Immunization with skin isografts taken from tolerant mice. *Science* **158**, 127–129.
33. Guttmann, R.D., Lindquist, R.R. and Ockner, S.A. (1969). Renal transplantation in the inbred rat. IX. Hematopoietic origin of an immunogenic stimulus of rejection. *Transplantation* **8** (4), 472–484.
34. Lafferty, K.J., Cooley, M.A., Woolnough, J. and Walker, K.Z. (1975). Thyroid allograft immunogenicity is reduced after a period in organ culture. *Science* **188** (4185), 259–261.
35. Rouabhia, M., Germain, L., Belanger, F. and Auger, F.A. (1993). Cultured epithelium allografts: Langerhans cell and Thy-1^+ dendritic epidermal cell depletion effects on allograft rejection. *Transplantation* **56** (2), 259–264.

36. Coulombe, M., Yang, H., Guerder, S., Flavell, R.A., Lafferty, K.J. and Gill, R.G. (1996). Tissue immunogenicity: the role of MHC antigen and the lymphocyte costimulator B7-1. *J. Immunol.* **157** (11), 4790–4795.
37. Stuart, F.P., Bastien, E., Holter, A., Fitch, F.W. and Elkins, W.L. (1971). Role of passenger leukocytes in the rejection of renal allografts. *Transplant. Proc.* **3** (1), 461–464.
38. Hart, D.N., Winearls, C.G. and Fabre, J.W. (1980). Graft adaptation: studies on possible mechanisms in long-term surviving rat renal allografts. *Transplantation* **30** (1), 73–80.
39. Lechler, R.I. and Batchelor, J.R. (1982). Immunogenicity of retransplanted rat kidney allografts. Effect of inducing chimerism in the frst recipient and quantitative studies on immunosuppression of the second recipient. *J. Exp. Med.* **156** (6), 1835–1841.
40. Lechler, R.I. and Batchelor, J.R. (1982). Restoration of immunogenicity to passenger cell-depleted kidney allografts by the addition of donor strain dendritic cells. *J. Exp. Med.* **155** (1), 31–41.
41. Steinman, R.M. and Cohn, Z.A. (1973). Identification of a novel cell type in peripheral lymphoid organs of mice. I. Morphology. *J. Exp. Med.* **137**, 1142–1162.
42. Steinman, R.M. and Cohn, Z.A. (1974). Identification of a novel cell type in peripheral lymphoid organs of mice. II. Functional properties in vitro. *J. Exp. Med.* **139**, 380–397.
43. Steinman, R.M., Lustig, D.S. and Cohn, Z.A. (1974). Identification of a novel cell in peripheral lymphoid organs in mice. III. Functional properties in vivo. *J. Exp. Med.* **139**, 1431–1445.
44. Kocandrle, V., Houttuin, E. and Prohaska, J.V. (1966). Regeneration of the lymphatics after autotransplantation and homotransplantation of the entire small intestine. *Surg. Gynecol. Obstet.* **122** (3), 587–592.
45. Malek, P., Vrubel, J. and Kolc, J. (1969). Lymphatic aspects of experimental and clinical renal transplantation. *Bull. Soc. Int. Chirurg.* **28** (1), 110–114.
46. Kline, I.K. and Thomas, P.A. (1976). Canine lung allograft lymphatic alterations. *Ann. Thorac. Surg.* **21** (6), 532–535.
47. Cuttino, J.T., Jr, Clark, R.L., Mandel, S.R., Webster, W.P. and Jaques, P.F. (1978). Lymphatic visualization during renal transplant rejection. *Invest. Radiol.* **13** (4), 328–333.
48. Rabin, A.M., Abramson, A.F., Manzarbeitia, C. *et al.* (1991). Dilated periportal lymphatics mimicking an anastomotic bile leak after liver transplantation. *Gastrointest. Radiol.* **16** (4), 337–338.
49. Shibuya, H., Ohkohchi, N., Tsukamoto, S. and Satomi, S. (1997). Tumor necrosis factor-induced, superoxide-mediated neutrophil accumulation in cold ischemic/reperfused rat liver. *Hepatology* **26** (1), 113–120.
50. Rao, P.N., Liu, T., Synder, J.T., Platt, J.L. and Starzl, T.E. (1991). Reperfusion injury following cold ischemia activates rat liver Kupffer cells. *Transplant. Proc* **23** (1 Pt 1), 666–669.
51. Galkowska, H. and Olszewski, W.L. (1992). Spontaneous cluster formation of dendritic (veiled) cells and lymphocytes from skin lymph obtained from dogs with chronic lymphedema. *Lymphology* **25** (3), 106–113.
52. Forbes, R.D., Parfrey, N.A., Gomersail, M., Darden, A.G. and Guttmann, R.D. (1986). Dendritic cell-lymphoid aggregation and major histocompatibility antigen expression during rat cardiac allograft rejection. *J. Exp. Med.* **164**, 1239–1258.
53. van den Oord, J.J., Volpes, R. and Desmet, V.J. Dendritic cells and the liver. [Review]. *Apmis* (Supplement) **23**, 68–76.
54. Prop, J., Nieuwenhuis, P. and Wildevuur, C.R. (1985). Lung allograft rejection in the rat. I. Accelerated rejection caused by graft lymphocytes. *Transplantation* **40** (1), 25–30.
55. Prop, J., Wildevuur, C.R. and Nieuwenhuis, P. (1985). Lung allograft rejection in the rat. II. Specific immunological properties of lung grafts. *Transplantation* **40** (2), 126–131.
56. Murase, N., Demetris, A.J., Kim, D.G., Todo, S., Fung, J.J. and Starzl, T.E. (1990). Rejection of multivisceral allografts in rats: a sequential analysis with comparison to isolated orthotopic small-bowel and liver grafts. *Surgery* **108** (5), 880–889.
57. Murase, N., Demetris, A.J., Matsuzaki, T. *et al.* (1991). Long survival in rats after multivisceral versus isolated small-bowel allotransplantation under FK 506. *Surgery* **110** (1), 87–98.
58. Lee, R.G., Nakamura, K., Tsamandas, A.C. *et al.* (1996). Pathology of human intestinal transplantation [see comments]. *Gastroenterology* **110** (6), 1820–1834.
59. Fung, J., Zeevi, A., Demetris, A.J. *et al.* (1989). Origin of lymph node derived lymphocytes in human hepatic allografts. *Clin. Transplant.* **3**, 316–324.

60. Larsen, C.P., Morris, P.J. and Austyn, J.M. (1990). Migration of dendritic leukocytes from cardiac allografts into host spleens. A novel route for initiation of rejection. *J. Exp. Med.* **171**, 307–314.
61. Larsen, C.P., Austyn, J.M. and Morris, P.J. (1990). The role of graft-derived dendritic leukocytes in the rejection of vascularized organ allografts. Recent findings on the migration and function of dendritic leukocytes after transplantation. [Review]. *Ann. Surg.* **212** (3), 308–315.
62. Langer, A., Valdivia, L.A., Murase, N. *et al.* (1993). Humoral and cellular immunopathology of hepatic and cardiac hamster-into-rat xenograft rejection. Marked stimulation of IgM^{++}/bright/IgD^{+}dull splenic B cells. *Am. J. Pathol.* **143** (1), 85–98.
63. Demetris, A.J., Murase, N., Fujisaki, S., Fung, J.J., Rao, A.S. and Starzl, T.E. (1993). Hematolymphoid cell trafficking, microchimerism, and GVH reactions after liver, bone marrow, and heart transplantation. *Transplant. Proc.* **25** (6), 3337–3344.
64. Collins, R.H., Anastasi, J., Terstappen, L.W.W.M. *et al.* (1993). Brief report: Donor-derived long-term multilineage hematopoiesis in a liver-transplant recipient. *N. Engl. J. Med.* **328**, 762–765.
65. Demetris, A.J., Murase, N. and Starzl, T.E. (1992). Donor dendritic cells after liver and heart allotransplantation under short-term immunosuppression [letter]. *Lancet* **339** (8809), 1610.
66. Lu, L., Rudert, W.A., Qian, S. *et al.* (1995). Growth of donor-derived dendritic cells from the bone marrow of murine liver allograft recipients in response to granulocyte/macrophage colony-stimulating factor. *J. Exp. Med.* **182** (2), 379–387.
67. Kobayashi, E., Kamada, N., Delriviere, L. *et al.* (1995). Migration of donor cells into the thymus is not essential for induction and maintenance of systemic tolerance after liver transplantation in the rat. *Immunology* **84** (2), 333–336.
68. Lord, R., Goto, S., Vari, F. *et al.* (1997). Differences in the rate of donor leucocyte migration between natural and drug-assisted tolerance following rat liver transplantation. *Clin. Exp. Immunol.* **108** (2), 358-365.
69. Malek, P. and Vrubel, J. (1968). Lymphatic system and organ transplantation. [Review]. *Lymphology* **1** (1), 4–22.
70. Cockett, A.T., Sakai, A. and Netto, I.C. (1973). Kidney lymphatics: an important network in transplantation. *Trans. Am. Ass. Genito Urinary, Surg.* **65**, 73–76.
71. Eliska, O., Eliskova, M. and Mirejovsky, P. (1986). Lymph vessels of the transplanted kidney. *Nephron* **44** (2), 136–141.
72. Ruggiero, R., Fietsam, R., Jr, Thomas, G.A. *et al.* (1994). Detection of canine allograft lung rejection by pulmonary lymphoscintigraphy. *J. Thorac. Cardiovasc. Surg.* **108** (2), 253–258.
73. von Gaudecker, B., Petersen, R., Epstein, M., Kaden, J. and Oesterwitz, H. (1993). Down-regulation of MHC-expression on dendritic cells in rat kidney grafts by PUVA pretreatment. *Adv. Exp. Med. Biol.* **329**, 495–499.
74. Brewer, Y., Palmer, A., Taube, D. *et al.* (1989). Effect of graft perfusion with two CD45 monoclonal antibodies on incidence of kidney allograft rejection. *Lancet* **2** (8669), 935–937.
75. Goldberg, L.C., Bradley, J.A., Connolly, J. *et al.* (1995). Anti-CD45 monoclonal antibody perfusion of human renal allografts prior to transplantation. A safety and immunohistological study. CD45 Study Group. *Transplantation* **59** (9), 1285–1293.
76. Goldberg, L.C., Cook, T. and Taube, D. (1994). Pretreatment of renal transplants with anti-CD45 antibodies: optimization of perfusion technique. *Transplant. Immunol.* **2** (1), 27–34.
77. Lloyd, D.M., Cotler, S.J., Letai, A.G., Stuart, F.P. and Thistlethwaite, J.R. Jr. (1989). Pancreas-graft immunogenicity and pretreatment with anti-class II monoclonal antibodies. *Diabetes* **38** (Suppl. 1), 104–108.
78. Krzymanski, M., Waaga, A.M., Ulrichs, K. *et al.* (1991). The influence of MHC class II antigen blockade by perfusion with a monoclonal antibody on rat renal graft survival. *Transplant. Int.* **4** (3), 180–185.
79. Krzymanski, M. and Muller-Ruchholtz, W. (1992). Tissue distribution of MHC class II-positive cells, their down-manipulation by monoclonal antibodies and potential role in organ allograft immunogenicity. *Arch. Immunol. Ther. Exp.* (*Warsz*) **40** (3–4), 177–181.
80. Larsen, C.P., Ritchie, S.C., Pearson, T.C., Linsley, P.S. and Lowry, R.P. (1992). Functional expression of the costimulatory molecule, B7/BB1, on murine dendritic cell populations. *J. Exp. Med.* **176** (4), 1215–1220.
81. Larsen, C.P., Elwood, E.T., Alexander, D.Z. *et al.* (1996). Long-term acceptance of skin and cardiac allografts after blocking CD40 and CD28 pathways. *Nature* **381** (6581), 434–438.

82. Steurer, W., Nickerson, P.W., Steele, A.W., Steiger, J., Zheng, X.X. and Strom, T.B. (1995). Ex vivo coating of islet cell allografts with murine CTLA4/Fc promotes graft tolerance. *J. Immunol.* **155** (3), 1165–1174.
83. Russell, M.E., Hancock, W.W., Akalin, E. *et al.* (1996). Chronic cardiac rejection in the LEW to F344 rat model. Blockade of CD2B-B7 costimulation by CTLA4Ig modulates T cell and macrophage activation and attenuates arteriosclerosis. *J. Clin. Invest.* **97** (3), 833–838.
84. Azuma, H., Chandraker, A., Nadeau, K. *et al.* (1996). Blockade of T-cell costimulation prevents development of experimental chronic renal allograft rejection [see comments]. *Proc. Natl Acad. Sci. USA* **93** (22), 12439–12444.
85. Chandraker, A., Russell, M.E., Glysing-Jensen, T., Willett, T.A. and Sayegh, M.H. (1997). T-cell costimulatory blockade in experimental chronic cardiac allograft rejection: effects of cyclosporine and donor antigen. *Transplantation* **63** (8), 1053–1058.
86. Larsen, C.P., Alexander, D.Z., Hollenbaugh, D. *et al.* (1996). CD40-gp39 interactions play a critical role during allograft rejection. Suppression of allograft rejection by blockade of the CD40-gp39 pathway. *Transplantation* **61** (1), 4–9.
87. Lin, H., Wei, R.Q., Goodman, R.E. and Bolling, S.F. (1997). CD28 blockade alters cytokine mRNA profiles in cardiac transplantation. *Surgery* **122** (2), 129–137.
88. Lakkis, F.G., Konieczny, B.T., Saleem, S. *et al.* (1997). Blocking the CD28-B7 T cell costimulation pathway induces long term cardiac allograft acceptance in the absence of IL-4. *J. Immunol.* **158** (5), 2443–2448.
89. Demetris, A.J., Murase, N., Lee, R.G. *et al.* (1997). Chronic rejection. A general overview of histopathology and pathophysiology with emphasis on liver heart and intestinal allografts. *Transplant. Ann.* **2**, 27–44.
90. Demetris, A.J., Murase, N., Rao, A.S. and Starzl, T.E. (1994). The role of passenger leukocytes in rejection and 'tolerance' after solld organ transplantation: a potential explanation of a paradox. In: *Rejection and tolerance* (eds. J.L. Touraine *et al.*) Kluwer Academic, Dordrecht, pp. 325–392.
91. Gill, R.G., Coulombe, M. and Lafferty, K.J. (1996). Pancreatic islet allograft immunity and tolerance: the two-signal hypothesis revisited. *Immunol. Rev.* **149**, 75–96.
92. Bushell, A., Pearson, T.C., Morris, P.J. and Wood, K.J. (1995). Donor–recipient microchimerism is not required for tolerance induction following recipient pretreatment with donor-specific transfusion and anti-CD4 antibody. Evidence of a clear role for short-term antigen persistence [see comments]. *Transplantation* **59** (10), 1367–1371.
93. Shirwan, H., Wang, H.K., Barwari, L., Makowka, L. and Cramer, D.V. (1996). Pretransplant injection of allograft recipients with donor blood or lymphocytes permits allograft tolerance without the presence of persistent donor microchimerism. *Transplantation* **61** (9), 1382–1386.
94. Oluwole, S.F., Jin, M.X., Chowdhury, N.C., Engelstad, K., Ohajekwe, O.A. and James, T. (1995). Induction of peripheral tolerance by intrathymic inoculation of soluble alloantigens: evidence for the role of host antigen-presenting cells and suppressor cell mechanism. *Cell. Immunol.* **162** (1), 33–41.
95. Oluwole, S.F., Chowdhury, N.C., Jin, M.X. and Hardy, M.A. (1993). Induction of transplantation tolerance to rat cardiac allografts by intrathymic inoculation of allogeneic soluble peptides. *Transplantation* **56** (6), 1523–1527.
96. Sayegh, M.H., Perico, N., Imberti, O., Hancock, W.W., Carpenter, C.B. and Remuzzi, G. (1993). Thymic recognition of class II major histocompatibility complex allopeptides induces donor-specific unresponsiveness to renal allografts. *Transplantation* **56** (2), 461–465.
97. Sayegh, M.H., Khoury, S.J., Hancock, W.W., Weiner, H.L. and Carpenter, C.B. (1996). Mechanisms of oral tolerance by MHC peptides. *Ann. NY Acad. Sci.* **778**, 338–345.
98. Heath, W.R., Karamalis, F., Donoghue, J. and Miller, J.F. (1995). Autoimmunity caused by ignorant $CD8^+$ T cells is transient and depends on avidity. *J. Immunol.* **155** (5), 2339–2349.
99. Miller, J.F. and Heath, W.R. (1993). Self-ignorance in the peripheral T-cell pool. [Review]. *Immunol. Rev.* **133**, 131–150.
100. Nossal, G.J., Herold, K.C. and Goodnow, C.C. (1992). Autoimmune tolerance and type 1 (insulin-dependent) diabetes mellitus. *Diabetologia* **35** (Suppl. 2), S49–59.
101. Hoffman, D.K., Sibley, R.K., Korman, J.M. and Press, B.H. (1994). Light microscopic and immunohistochemical features in serial biopsies of epidermal versus dermal allografts. *Ann. Plast. Surg.* **33** (3), 295–299.

102. Kawai, K., Ikarashi, Y., Tomiyama, K., Matsumoto, Y. and Fujiwara, M. (1993). Rejection of cultured keratinocyte allografts in presensitized mice. *Transplantation* **56** (2), 265–269.
103. Hultman, C.S., Brinson, G.M., Siltharm, S. *et al.* (1996). Allogeneic fibroblasts used to grow cultured epidermal autografts persist in vivo and sensitize the graft recipient for accelerated second-set rejection. *J. Trauma* **41** (1), 51–58; discussion, 58–60.
104. Sano, Y., Ksander, B.R. and Streilein, J.W. (1996). Minor H, rather than MHC, alloantigens offer the greater barrier to successful orthotopic corneal transplantation in mice. *Transplant. Immunol.* **4** (1), 53–56.
105. Sano, Y., Ksander, B.R. and Streilein, J.W. (1997). Murine orthotopic corneal transplantation in high-risk eyes. Rejection is dictated primarily by weak rather than strong alloantigens. *Invest. Ophthalmol. Vis. Sci.* **38** (6), 1130–1138.
106. Braun, M.Y., McCormack, A., Webb, G. and Batchelor, J.R. (1993). Mediation of acute but not chronic rejection of MHC-incompatible rat kidney grafts by alloreactive CD4 T cells activated by the direct pathway of sensitization. *Transplantation* **55** (1), 177–182.
107. Batchelor, J.R. and Braun, M.Y. (1994). Distinct T cells mediating acute and chronic rejection. In: *Rejection and Tolerance* (ed. Touraine, J.J., *et al.*), vol. 25. Kluwer Academic, Dordrecht, pp. 103–110.
108. Bradley, J.A. (1996). Indirect T cell recognition in allograft rejection. *Int. Rev. Immunol.* **13** (3), 245–255.
109. Sayegh, M.H. and Carpenter, C.B. (1996). Role of indirect allorecognition in allograft rejection. *Int. Rev. Immunol.* **13** (3), 221–229.
110. Porter, K.A. (1969). Pathology of the orthotopic homograft and heterograft. *Experience in Hepatic Transplantation* (ed. Starzl, T.E.) W.B. Saunders, pp. 422–471.
111. Gouw, A.S., Houthoff, H.J., Huitema, S., Beelen, J.M., Gips, C.H. and Poppema, S. (1987). Expression of major histocompatibility complex antigens and replacement of donor cells by recipient ones in human liver grafts. *Transplantation* **43** (2), 291–296.
112. Iwaki, Y., Starzl, T.E., Yagihashi, A. *et al.* (1991). Replacement of donor lymphoid tissue in small-bowel transplants. *Lancet* **337** (8745), 818–819.
113. Starzl, T.E., Demetris, A.J., Murase, N., Ildstad, S., Ricordi, C. and Trucco, M. (1992). Cell migration, chimerism, and graft acceptance [see comments]. [Review]. *Lancet* **339** (8809), 1579–1582.
114. Starzl, T.E., Demetris, A.J., Trucco, M. *et al.* (1993). Chimerism after liver transplantation for type IV glycogen storage disease and type 1 Gaucher's disease [see comments]. *N. Engl. J. Med.* **328** (11), 745–749.
115. Starzl, T.E., Demetris, A.J., Trucco, M. *et al.* (1993). Cell migration and chimerism after whole-organ transplantation: the basis of graft acceptance [see comments]. [Review]. *Hepatology* **17** (6), 1127–1152.
116. Uyama, T., Winter, J.B., Sakiyama, S., Monden, Y., Groen, G. and Prop, J. (1993). Replacement of dendritic cells in the airways of rat lung allografts. *Am. Rev. Respir. Dis.* **148** (3), 760–767.
117. Valdivia, L.A., Demetris, A.J., Langer, A.M., Celli, S., Fung, J.J. and Starzl, T.E. (1993). Dendritic cell replacement in long-surviving liver and cardiac xenografts. *Transplantation* **56** (2), 482–484.
118. Langrehr, J.M., Demetris, A.J., Banner, B. *et al.* (1994). Mucosal recipient-type mononuclear repopulation and low-grade chronic rejection occur simultaneously in indefinitely surviving recipients of small bowel allografts. *Transplant. Int.* **7** (2), 71–78.
119. Larsen, C.P., Barker, H., Morris, P.J. and Austyn, J.M. (1990). Failure of mature dendritic cells of the host to migrate from the blood into cardiac or skin allografts. *Transplantation* **50** (2), 294–301.
120. Demetris, A.J., Murase, N., Ye, Q. *et al.* (1997). Analysis of chronic rejection and obliterative arteriopathy. Possible contributions of donor antigen-presenting cells and lymphatic disruption. *Am. J. Pathol.* **150** (2), 563–578.
121. Steinhoff, G., Wonigeit, K., Sorg, C. *et al.* (1989). Patterns of macrophage immigration and differentiation in human liver grafts. *Transplant. Proc.* **21**, 398–400.
122. Uyama, T., Winter, J.B., Groen, G., Wildevuur, C.R., Monden, Y. and Prop, J. (1992). Late airway changes caused by chronic rejection in rat lung allografts. *Transplantation* **54** (5), 809–812.
123. Siddiqui, M.T., Garrity, E.R. and Husain, A.N. (1996). Bronchiolitis obliterans organizing pneumonia-like reactions: a nonspecific response or an atypical form of rejection or infection in lung allograft recipients? *Hum. Pathol.* **27** (7), 714–719.

124. Li, X.C., Tucker, J., Zhong, R., Jevnikar, A. and Grant, D. (1993). The role of gut-associated lymphoid tissue in intestinal rejection. Allogeneic response to rat intestinal lymphocytes. *Transplantation* **56** (1), 244–247.
125. Hayry, P., Isoniemi, H., Yilmaz, S. *et al.* (1993). Chronic allograft rejection. *Immunol. Rev.* **134**, 33–81.
126. Azuma, H. and Tilney, N.L. (1994). Chronic graft rejection. [Review]. *Curr. Opin. Immunol.* **6** (5), 770–776.
127. Hayry, P., Mennander, A., Yilmaz, S. *et al.* (1992). Towards understanding the pathophysiology of chronic rejection. [Review]. *Clin. Invest.* **70** (9), 780–790.
128. Paul, L.C. (1995). Immunobiology of chronic renal transplant rejection. [Review]. *Blood Purif.* **13** (3–4), 206–218.
129. Oguma, S., Banner, B., Zerbe, T., Starzl, T. and Demetris, A.J. (1988). Participation of dendritic cells in vascular lesions of chronic rejection of human allografts. *Lancet* **2** (8617), 933–936.
130. Wakabayashi, T. and Onoda, H. (1991). Interdigitating reticulum cells in human renal grafts. *Virchows Arch. A: Pathol. Anat. Histopathol.* **418** (2), 105–110.
131. Zinkernagel, R.M., Ehl, S., Aichele, P., Oehen, S., Kundig, T. and Hengartner, H. (1997). Antigen localisation regulates immune responses in a dose- and time-dependent fashion: a geographical view of immune reactivity. *Immunol. Rev.* **156**, 199–209.
132. Zinkernagel, R.M. (1997). Immunology and immunity studied with viruses. *Ciba Found. Symp.* **204**, 105–125; discussion, 125–129.
133. Hruban, R.H., Beschorner, W.E., Baumgartner, W.A. *et al.* (1988). Depletion of bronchus-associated lymphoid tissue associated with lung allograft rejection. *Am. J. Pathol.* **132** (1), 6–11.
134. MacPherson, G.G., Murphy, M.J. Jr, and Morris, B. (1977). The traffic of mononuclear phagocytes through renal allografts in sheep. *Transplantation* **24** (1), 16–28.
135. Durham, J.R., Nakhleh, R.E., Levine, A. and Levine, T.B. (1995). Persistence of interstitial inflammation after episodes of cardiac rejection associated with systemic infection. *J. Heart Lung Transplant.* **14** (4), 774–780.
136. Heemann, U.W., Tullius, S.G., Schmid, C., Philipp, T. and Tilney, N.L. (1996). Infection-associated cellular activation accelerates chronic renal allograft rejection in rats. *Transplant. Int.* **9** (2), 137–140.
137. Manez, R., White, L.T., Linden, P. *et al.* The influence of HLA matching on cytomegalovirus hepatitis and chronic rejection after liver transplantation. *Transplantation* **55** (5), 1067–1071.
138. Wallwork, J. (1994). Risk factors for chronic rejection in heart and lungs—why do hearts and lungs rot? *Clin. Transplant.* **8** (3 Pt 2), 341–344.
139. Whitehead, B., Rees, P., Sorensen, K. *et al.* Incidence of obliterative bronchiolitis after heart-lung transplantation in children. *J. Heart Lung Transplant.* **12** (6 Pt 1), 903–908.
140. Starzl, T.E., Marchioro, T.L. and Waddell, W.R. (1963). The reversal of rejection in human renal homografts with subsequent development of homograft tolerance. *Surg. Gynecol. Obstet.* **117**, 385–395.
141. Mazariegos, G.V., Reyes, J., Marino, I.R. *et al.* (1997). Weaning of immunosuppression in liver transplant recipients. *Transplantation* **63** (2), 243–249.
142. Larsen, C.P., Morris, P.J. and Austyn, J.M. (1990). Migration of dendritic leukocytes from cardiac allografts into host spleens. A novel pathway for initiation of rejection. *J. Exp. Med.* **171** (1), 307–314.
143. Starzl, TE. (1964). *Host-Graft Adaptation. Experience in Renal Transplantation.* W.B. Saunders, Philadelphia PA, pp. 164–170.
144. Webb, S., Morris, C. and Sprent, J. (1990). Extrathymic tolerance of mature T cells: clonal elimination as a consequence of immunity. *Cell* **63** (6), 1249–1256.
145. Sprent, J., Gao, E.K. and Webb, S.R. (1990). T cell reactivity to MHC molecules: immunity versus tolerance. *Science* 1990, **248** (4961), 1357–1363.
146. Webb, S.R., Hutchinson, J., Hayden, K. and Sprent, J. (1994). Expansion/deletion of mature T cells exposed to endogenous superantigens in vivo. *J. Immunol.* **152** (2), 586–597.
147. Lu, L., Qian, S., Starzl, T.E., Lynch, D.H. and Thomson, A.W. (1997). Blocking of the B7-CD28 pathway increases the capacity of $FasL^+$ ($CD95L^+$) dendritic cells to kill alloactivated T cells. *Adv. Exp. Med. Biol.* **417**, 275–282.
148. Lu, L., Qian, S., Hershberger, P.A., Rudert, W.A., Lynch, D.H. and Thomson, A.W. (1997). Fas ligand (CD95L) and B7 expression on dendritic cells provide counter-regulatory signals for T cell survival and proliferation. *J. Immunol.* **158** (12), 5676–5684.

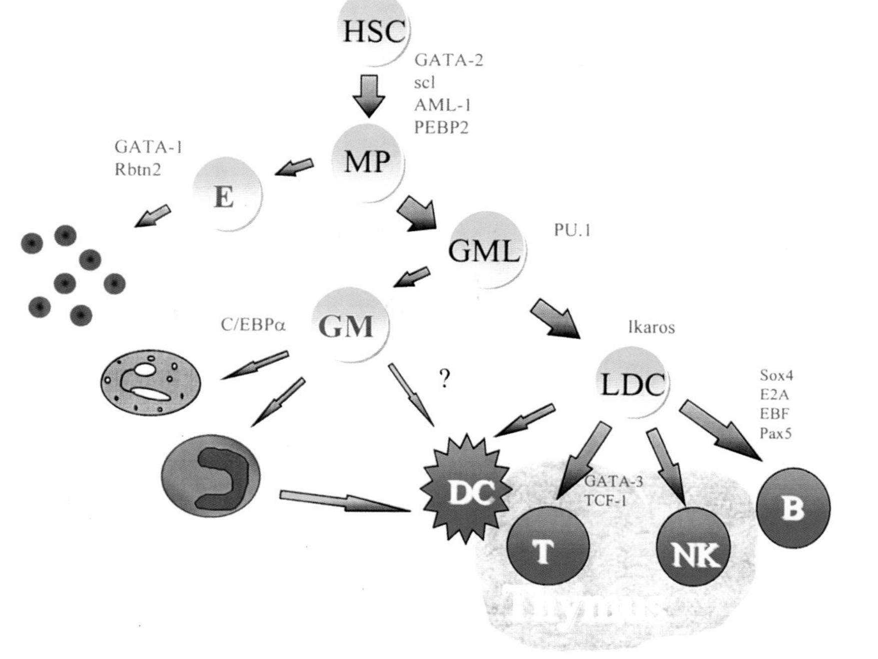

Plate 1.1. Hypothetical pathway for the production of lymphocytes and DC and essential transcriptional regulators. Hematopoietic stem cells (HSC) differentiate sequentially into multipotent progenitors (MP) that have lost the ability to repopulate marrow for long periods of time, then into progenitors of restricted hematopoietic differentiation potential (G = granulocyte, M = monocyte, L = lymphocyte). A common lymphoid-DC-restricted progenitor (L/DC) gives rise to all classes of lymphocytes and to lymphoid-related DC. Presumably this cell could seed the thymus to give rise to intrathymic T, B,NK, and DC but may also develop in a thymic-independent fashion since neither B, NK, or DC are thymic-dependent. DCs can arise from lymphoid-related progenitors or from monocytes. It is not clear whether a myeloid-restricted pathway not involving lymphocytes contributes to the production of DC before they become monocytes. Transcription factors that control hematopoietic cell fate are indicated at the presumed developmental checkpoints that they critically control.

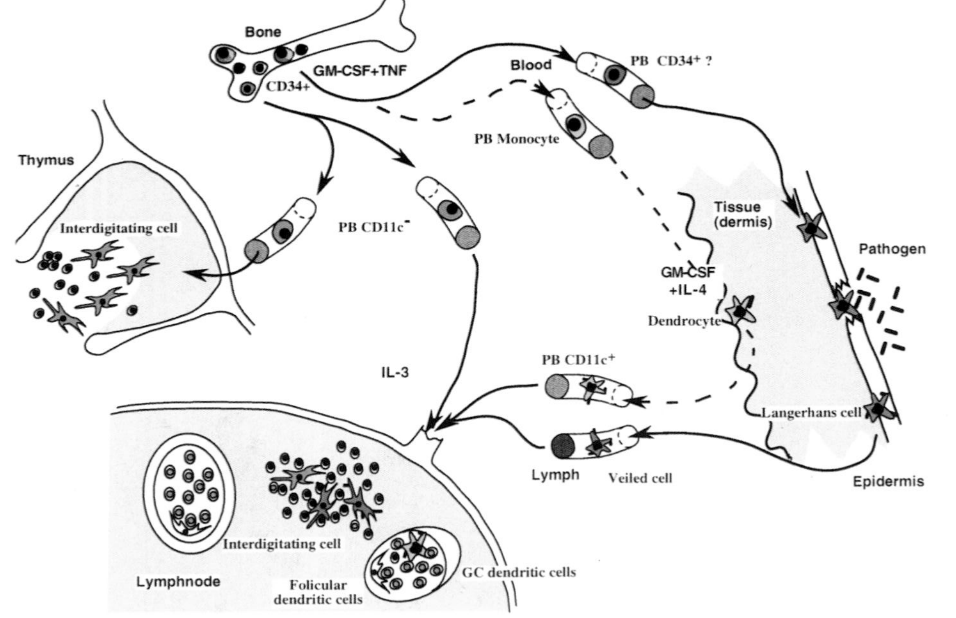

Plate 5.5. Different pathways of DC development: potential relationship with *in vivo* DC populations. *In vitro* and *in vivo* studies in mice and humans suggest that several DC subsets may originate from at least three different progenitors. A progenitor cell common for granulocytes, monocytes, and DCs (myeloid progenitor, $CD33^+$), identified in semisolid medium, further differentiates into several lineage-specific precursors. DC specific precursors (CL^+CD1a^+) lead to Langerhans cell type DC. Langerhans cells further differentiate into interdigitating cells and might be more specifically involved in cellular immune responses. Monocytes might differentiate into DC during migration from blood to lymph tissues. Monocyte-derived DC are more related to interstitial DC, $CD11c^+$ blood DC, and germinal center DC. Those cells, in view of their localization in lymphoid organs and activity on B cells, might be more specifically involved in humoral immune responses. Finally, the existence of a third progenitor for thymic DC has also been demonstrated in mice. This progenitor displays T and B lymphoid, but no myeloid, differentiation potential. In humans, this progenitor ($CD10^+$?) might lead to $CD11c^-$ DC precursor identified in blood and tonsils, which would further differentiate into a subset of IDC (interdigitating DC). The function of this subset is unknown but this population has been proposed to be involved in maintenance of peripheral tolerance.

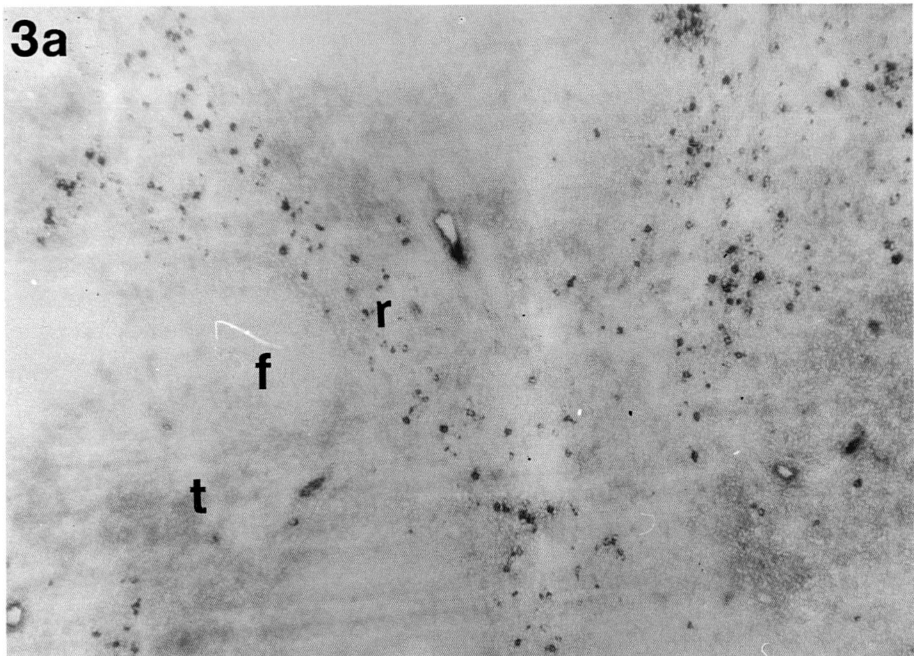

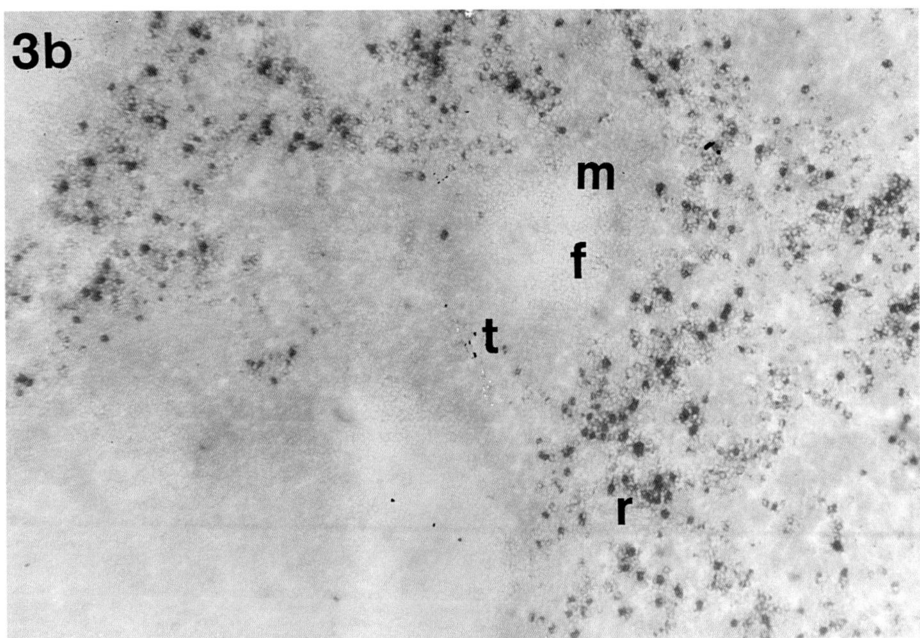

Plate 6.3. Immunohistochemical analysis of DC subsets in spleens of FL-treated and control mice. CD11c (brown), CD11b (blue) co-staining of splenic sections from control (a) and FL-treated (b) mice. Magnifications ×40. CD11c staining is predominantly found in the T cell areas and the marginal zones. CD11b$^+$ cells are apparent in the red-pulp and marginal zones of control and FL-treated mice, but not in the white-pulp. FL-treated mice have increased numbers of CD11b$^+$ cells in these areas.

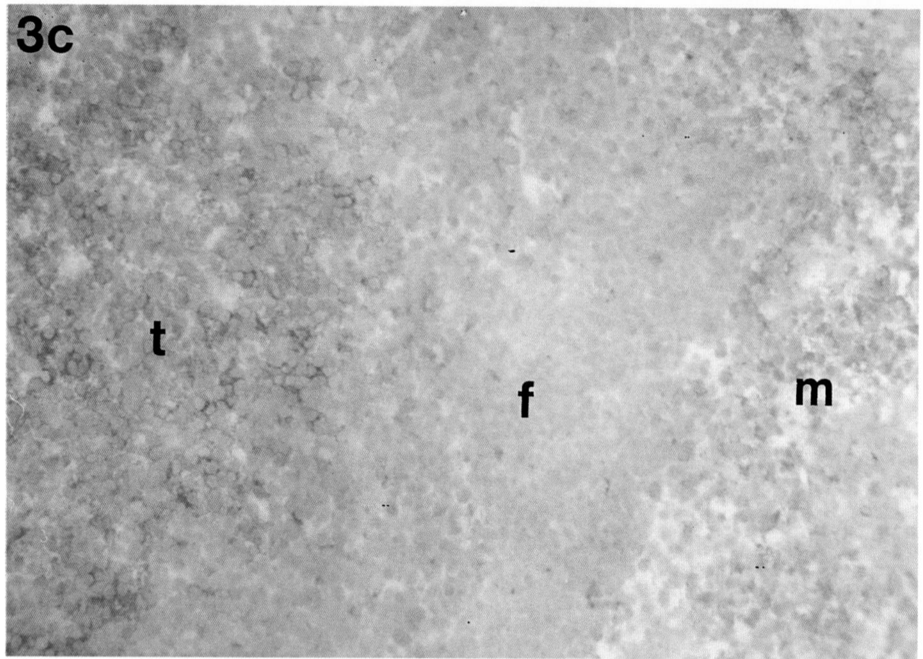

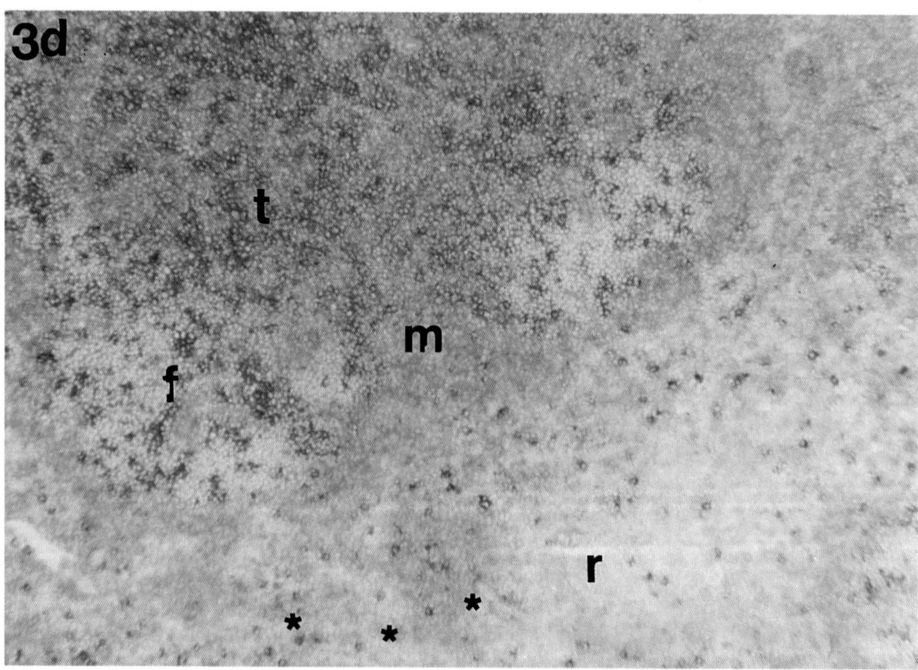

Plate 6.3. (Continued) (c) CD8α staining (red) is observed mainly in the T cell zones. CD11c staining (brown) is observed in both the T cell zones and in the marginal zones. Magnification × 80. (d) CD11c (brown) versus CD4 (blue) staining of splenic section from FL-treated mice. Note the CD11c^{bright} cells in the T cell areas, and in the marginal zones. Cells staining weakly for CD11c are highlighted with asterisks, and can be observed in the red-pulp and the red-pulp/marginal zone border in FL-treated spleens. Magnification × 60. f = follicle; m = marginal zones; r = red-pulp; t = T cell areas. (Asterisk represents CD11c^{dull} cells in marginal zones/red-pulp border). Reproduced with kind permission from J*ournal of Immunology* **159**, 2222–2231. Copyright © 1997 The American Association of Immunologists.

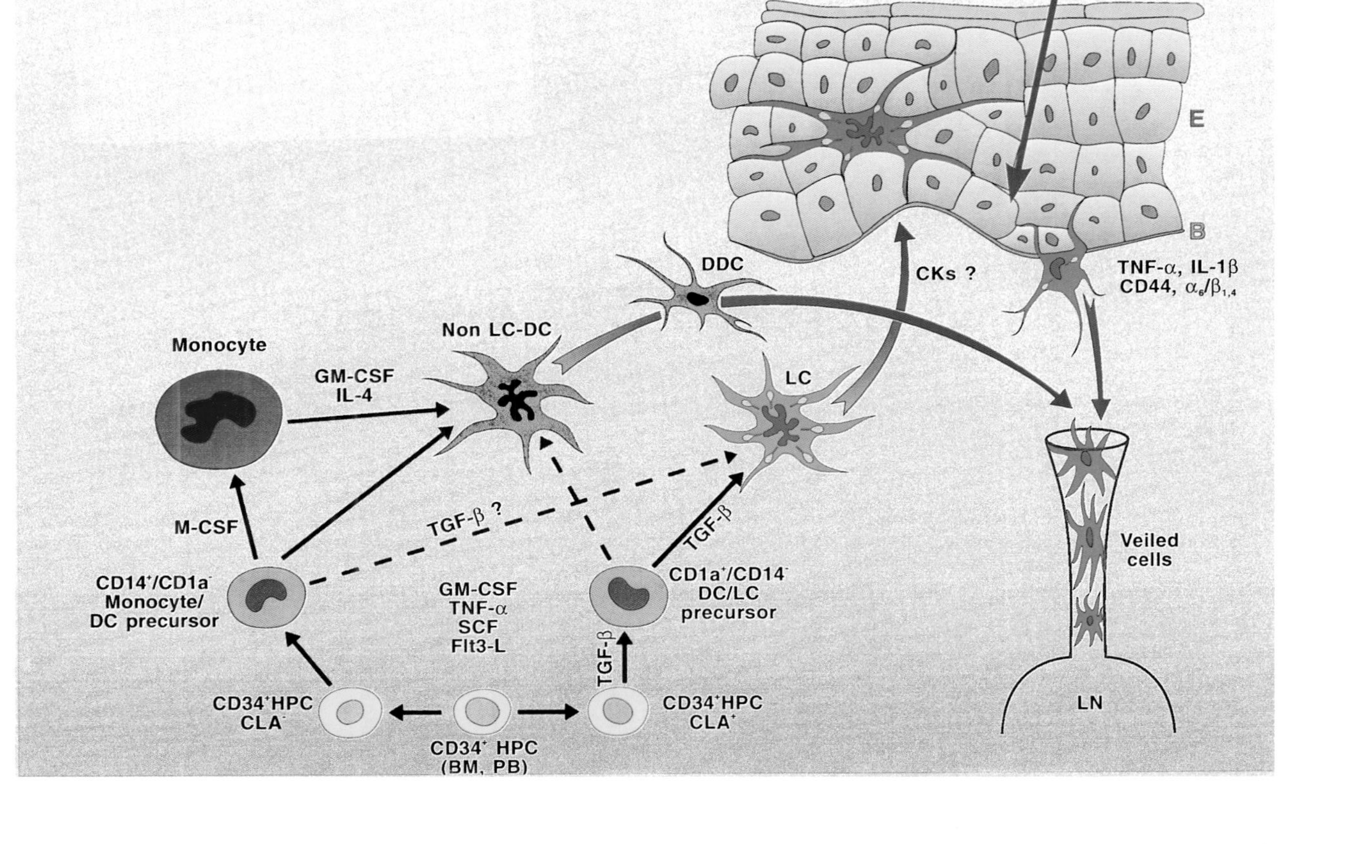

Plate 7.2. Schematic representation of ontogenetic, migration and maturation pathways of cutaneous dendritic leukocytes. E, epidermis; B, basement membrane; HPC, hemopoietic cell; DC, dendritic cell; LC, Langerhans cell; DDC, dermal dendritic cell; BM, bone marrow; PB, peripheral blood; LN, lymph node; IL-1β, interleukin-1β; IL-4, interleukin-4; SCF, stem cell factor; GM-CSF, granulocyte/macrophage colony-stimulating factor; M-CSF, macrophage colony-stimulating factor; TNF-α, tumor necrosis factor-α; CKs, chemokines; TGF-β, transforming growth factor-β; CLA, cutaneous leukocyte antigen; Flt-3-L, Flt-3 ligand; $\alpha_6/\beta_{1,4}$, $\alpha_6/\beta_{1,4}$ integrins interloukin-1β.

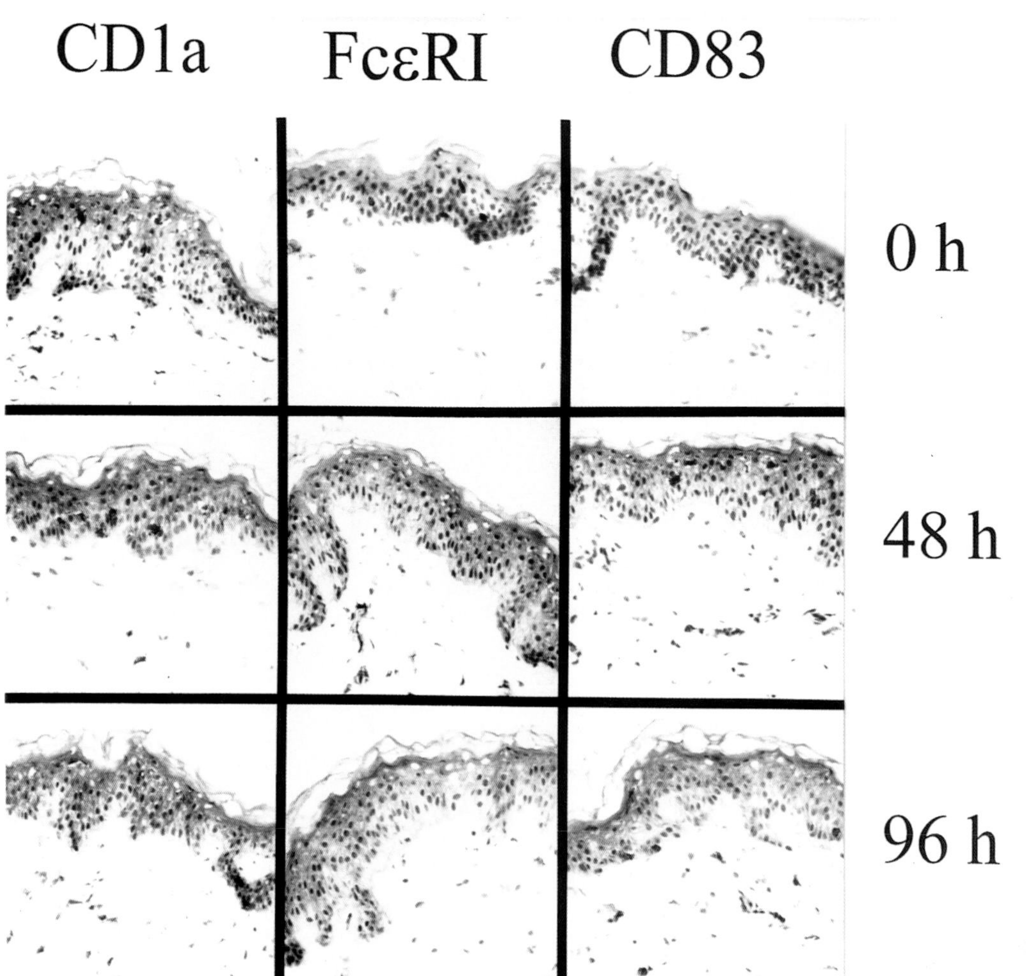

Plate 7.3. Phenotypic changes and emigration of epidermal Langerhans cells (LC) after perturbation of the cutaneous microenvironment. Cryostat sections of freshly excised or *ex vivo* cultured (48 h, 96 h) human split-thickness skin were reacted with antibodies against CD1a, FcεRI, or CD83 and then processed for peroxidase immunolabeling. Before culture, LC are $CD1a^+$, $Fc\varepsilon RI^+$, $CD83^-$ and reside mainly at a suprabasal position within the epidermis. In skin organ culture, LC progressively lose surface-bound CD1a and FcεRI, begin to express CD83, and move downward. (Original magnification × 40.)

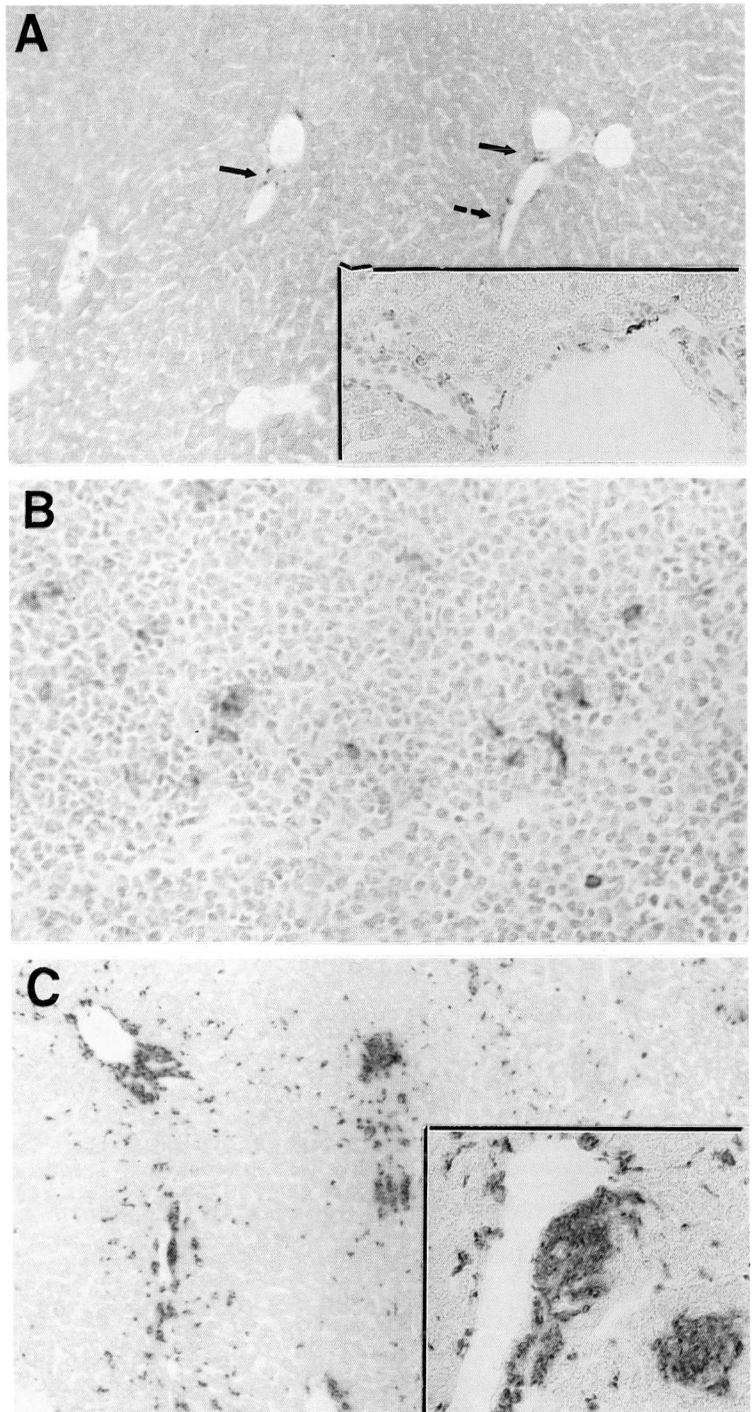

Plate 10.1. DC within the liver. (A) Photomicrograph of normal mouse liver (C576BL/10) stained with anti-MHC class II (I-A^b). Note the restricted localization of immunopositive cells to portal areas (arrows). Inset: High-power view of portal area demonstrating dendriform morphology of I-A^{b+} cells. (B) Donor (C57BL/10)-derived MHC class II^+ (I-A^{b+}) cells in recipient (C3H) spleen 24h following orthotopic liver transplantation. (C) Anti-MHC class II (I-A^b) immunostaining of liver from a C57BL/10 mouse treated with Flt3 ligand (10μg/day × 10 days). Note the presence of large infiltrates of MHC class II^+ cells in periportal areas and also throughout the parenchyma. Single MHC class II^+ cells are also present distributed throughout the parenchyma. Inset: high-power view of cellular infiltrates (anti-I-A^b)

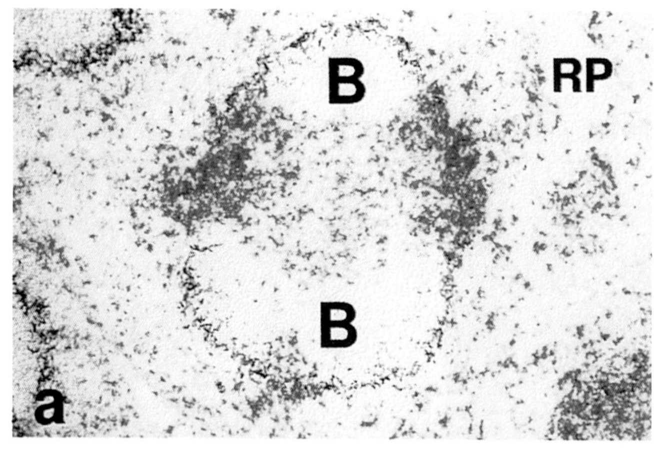

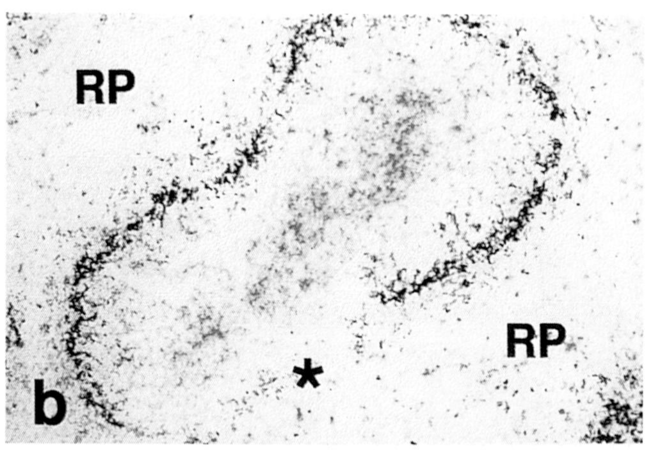

Plate 11.1. CD11c and DEC-205 expression in mouse spleen (from Steinman *et al.*, 1997). Double label immunocytochemistry of mouse spleen. (a) CD11c-positive DC are in blue and sialoadhesin-positive marginal zone macrophages are in brown. 'Nests' of CD11c-positive DC interrupt the marginal zone macrophages, and the DC extend into T cell areas (centre) but not B cell follicles (above and below centre, labelled B). (b) DEC-205-positive DC are in blue and sialoadhesin-positive marginal zone macrophages are in brown; note the interrupted area (*). DEC-205-positive DC ('interdigitating cells') occupy the central white pulp (T cell areas) and do not extend to the periphery (compare with (a)). RP, red pulp. (Copyright with permission. Copyright of Munksgaard International Publishers Ltd, Demark 1997).

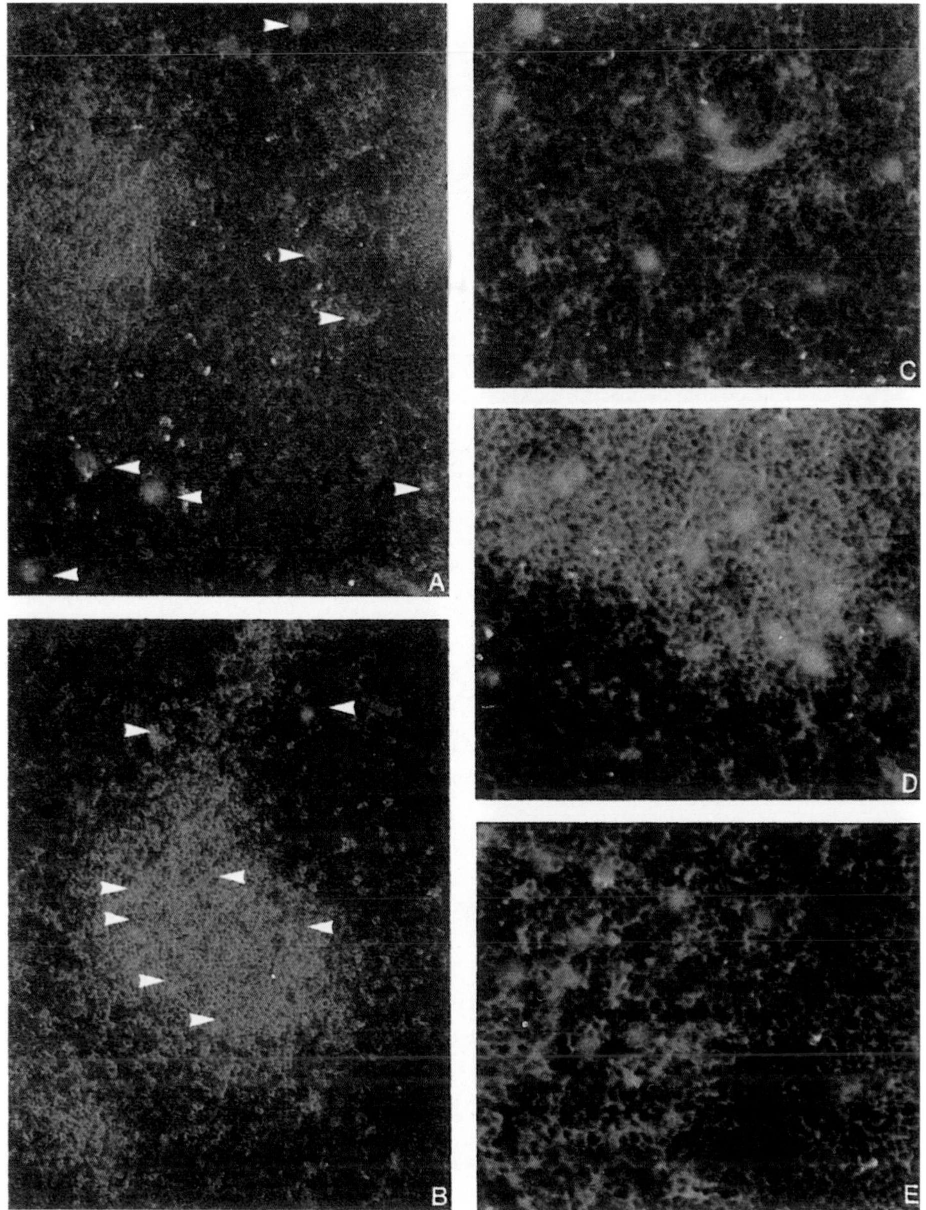

Plate 11.2. Migration of DC from blood to spleen in mouse (from Austyn *et al.*, 1988). Double label fluorescence and immunofluorescence of mouse spleen. DC purified from mouse spleen were labelled with H33342 (blue) and injected intravenously into syngeneic recipients. At 3 h (A, C) or at 24 h (B, D, E) after injection, spleens were removed and frozen sections were FITC-labelled (green) for T cells (A–D) or MHC class II (E). Low power (A, B; arrows indicate positions of blue fluorescence) and high power(C–E) fields were viewed by ultraviolet microscopy and photographed. DC are found predominantly in red pulp at 3 h (A, C), and in T cell areas at 24 h (B, D, E). In (E), the large and bright MHC class II-positive cells (to the left) are interdigitating cells in T cell areas; the smaller and less strongly labelled cells (to the right) are B cells in a follicle. (Reprinted with permission. Copyright of Rockerfeller University Press, New York, 1998).

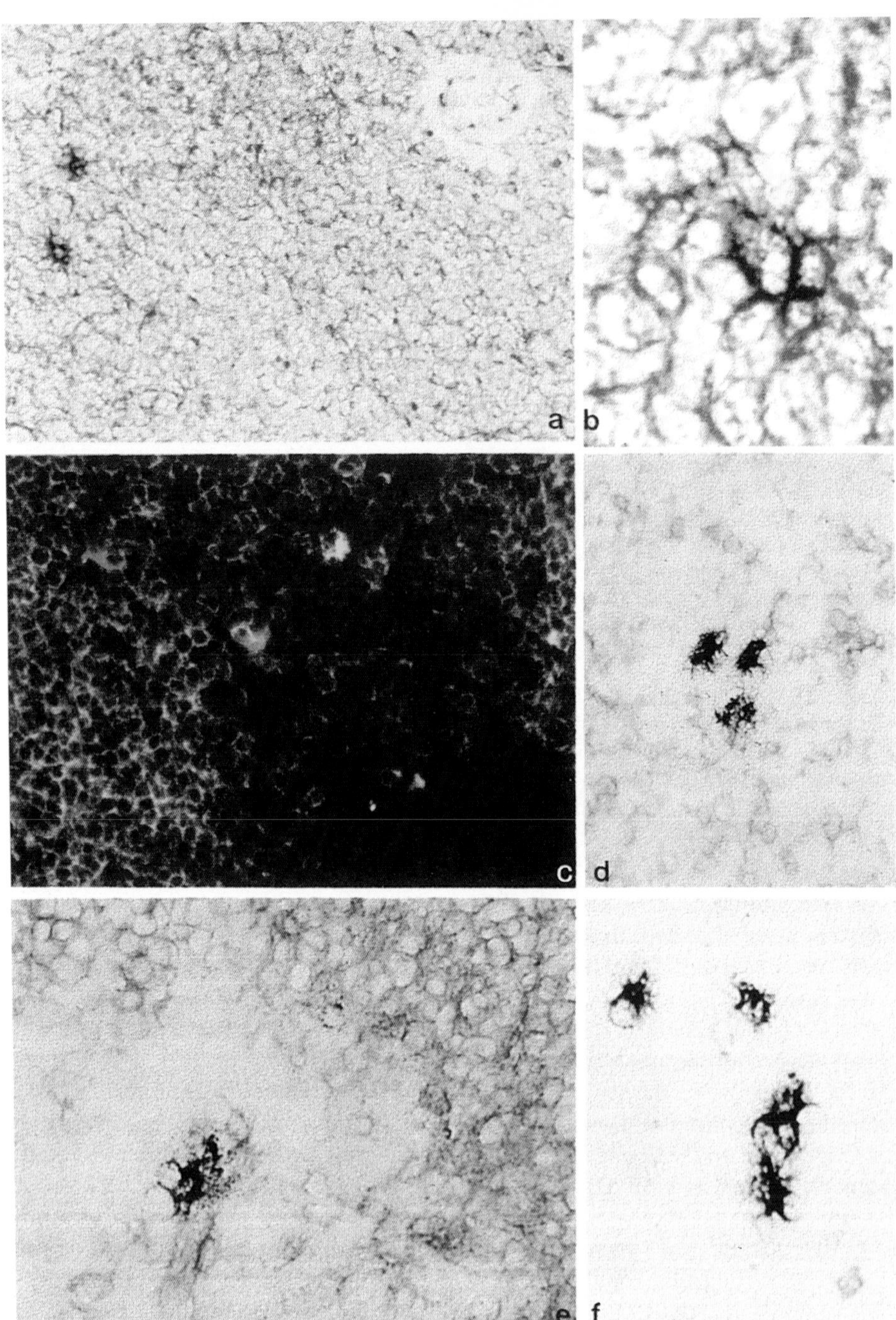

Plate 11.3. Migration of DC from cardiac allografts to spleen in mouse (from Larsen *et al.*, 1990a). Single and double label immunocytochemistry of mouse spleen. Hearts were transplanted as fully vascularized heterotopic allografts to allogeneic recipients. Two days later, recipient spleens were removed and frozen sections were labelled for donor MHC class II, either alone (a, b) or in combination with other markers (c–f). (a, b) At 2 days, donor DC in recipient spleens are distant from the central arteriole (a, top right, low power), but have dendritic morphology (b, high power). (c) Double labelling for donor MHC class II (green) and recipient MHC class II (red) reveals donor DC within B cell areas or at the border of B cell and T cell areas, but not in central white pulp (c, low power view). (d–f) Within peripheral white pulp, DC (black) preferentially associate with CD4-positive T cells (brown: d, low power; e, intermediate power) but not CD8-positive T cells (e, intermediate power). Subsequent studies (Roake *et al.*, 1995b) demonstrated that allogeneic DC move into central white pulp at later time points. Reprinted with permission.

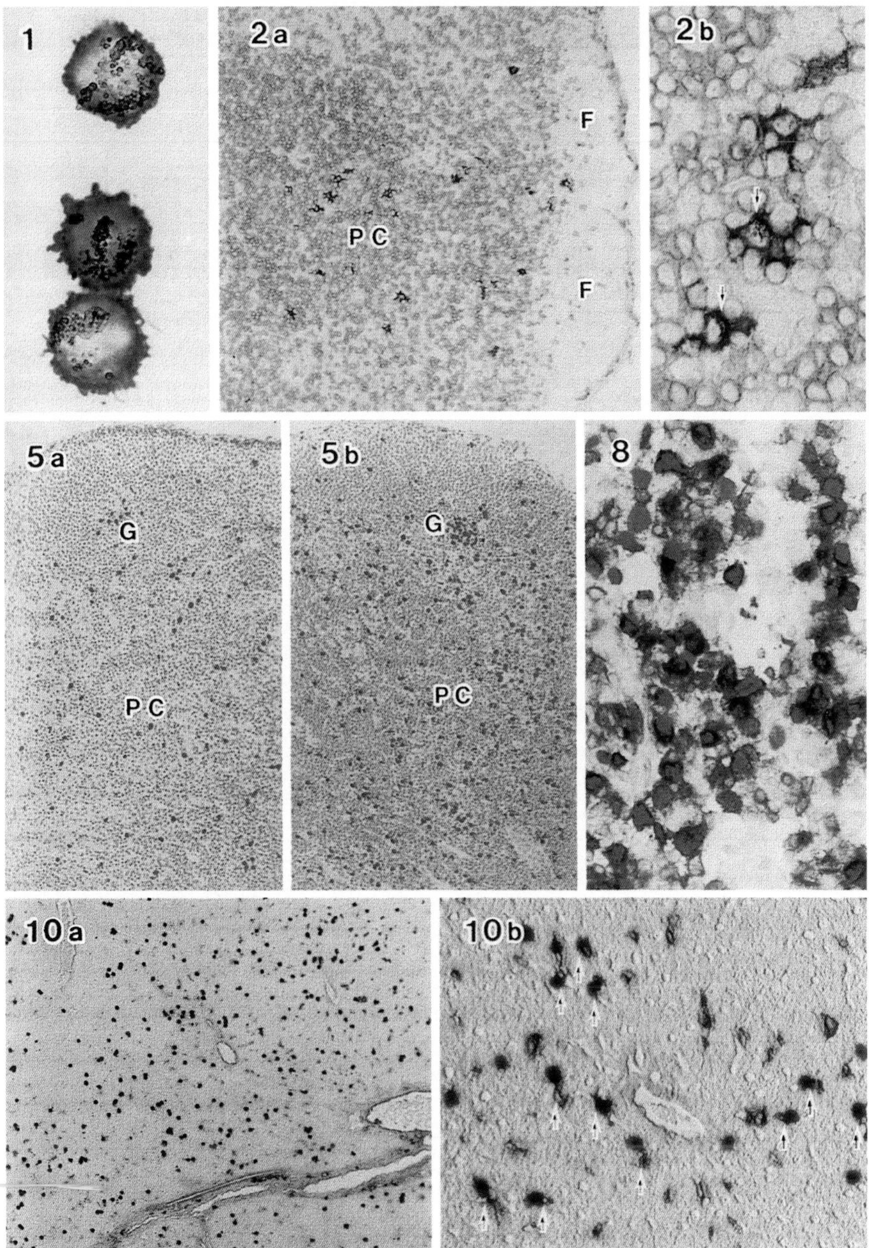

Plate 11.4. Migration of dendritic cells from blood to celiac lymph nodes in rat (from Kudo *et al.*, 1997). Single and double label immunocytochemistry of rat cells and tissues. Panel 1: Rats were injected intravenously with paramagnetic latex particles. DC isolated from hepatic lymph (see text) expressed MHC class II molecules (blue) and contained phagocytosed latex particles. Panel 2a (low power): One day after injection of latex-laden DC (see panel 1) into the bloodstream of allogeneic rats, the DC (blue) could be detected in the paracortex (PC) of celiac lymph nodes, where host T cells (brown) are localized, but not within the follicles (F). Panel 2b (a high power view of part of the field in panel 2a): Many of the cells (blue) had a dendritic morphology and contained particles in the cytoplasm (arrows). Panels 5a, 5b (low power) and 8 (high power): Three days after transfer of latex-laden DC to allogeneic rats, significant cell proliferation was evident in the celiac lymph nodes by bromodeoxyuridine labelling (red) (panel 5b), over and above that within control nodes (panel 5a). Many of the proliferating cells (red) were T cells (blue) (panel 8). G, germinal centre; PC, paracortex. Panels 10a (low power) and 10b (high power): DC isolated from hepatic lymph (blue-black) can adhere to frozen sections of liver, with a similar distribution to that of Kupffer cells (brown); the two cell types are often closely associated (panel 10b, arrows). (Reprinted with permission. Copyright of Rockfeller University Press, New York, 1997)

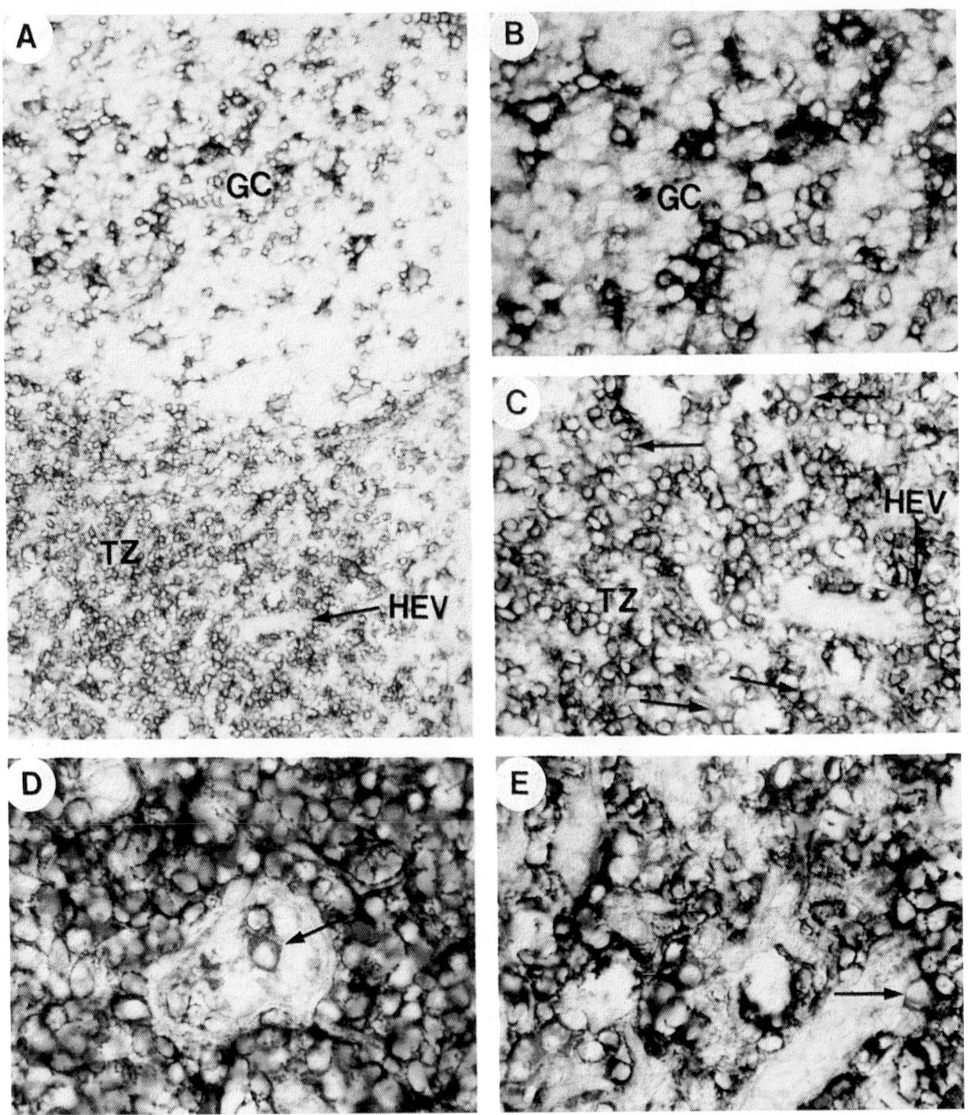

Plate 11.5. Plasmacytoid T cells, a possible lymphoid DC precursor, in human tonsils (from Grouard *et al.*, 1997). Double label immunocytochemistry of human tonsil. (A) Low power view of tonsil showing a germinal centre (GC), a portion of the T cell area (TZ) and a high endothelial venule (HEV). (B) At higher power, the same germinal centre (GC) as in (A) contains $CD4^{+}CD11c^{+}$ germinal centre DC (black). (C) In contrast, the same T cell area (TZ) as in (A) contains $CD4^{+}CD11c^{-}$ plasmacytoid T cells (red, arrows) located close to the high endothelial venule (HEV), together with T cells (black). (D, E) At high power, $CD4^{+}CD11c^{-}$ plasmacytoid T cells (red, arrows) can also be detected within the lumen (D) and the wall (E) of high endothelial venules. (Reprinted with permission. Copyright Rockfeller University Press, New York, 1997).

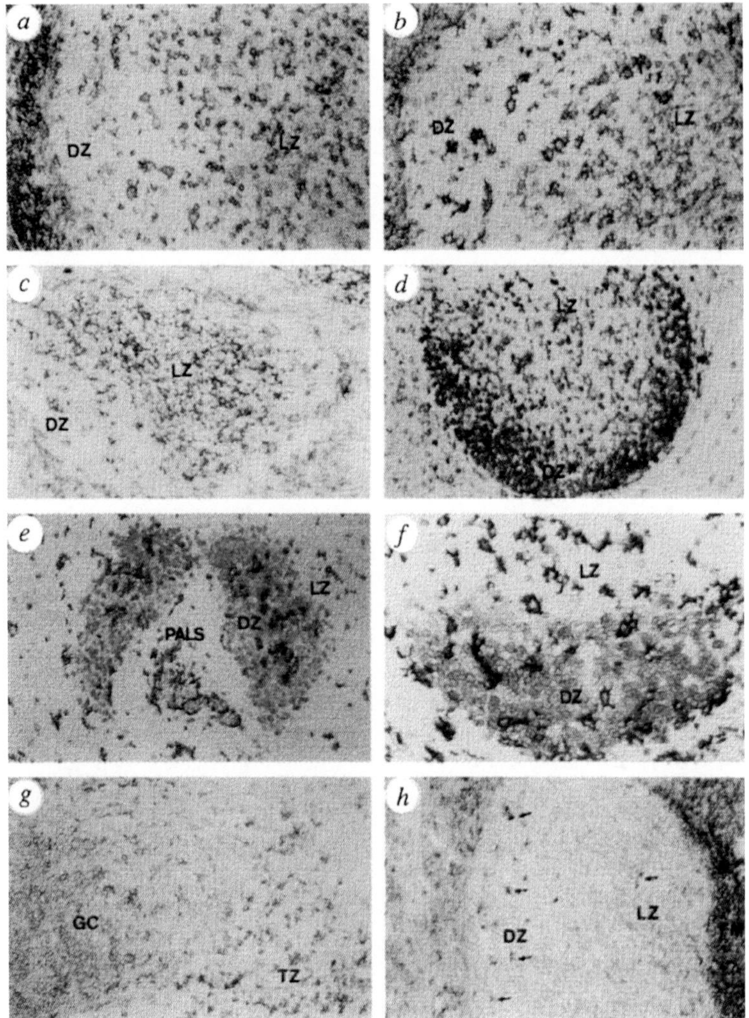

Plate 11.6. Germinal centre dendritic cells in human tonsil, spleen and lymph nodes (from Grouard *et al.*, 1996). Double label immunocytochemistry of human tissues. (a) Large $CD4^{+}CD3^{-}$ germinal centre dendritic cells (GCDC, red) and small $CD4^{+}CD3^{+}$ T cells (black) in a germinal centre. DZ, dark zone; LZ, light zone. (b) All large $CD4^{+}$GCDC (purple) but not small T cells (red) express CD11c. (c) $CD4^{+}CD11c^{+}$ GCDC (red) do not express follicular dendritic cell (FDC) antigens (blue), and FDC do not express CD11c (red). (d) $CD4^{+}CD11c^{+}$ GCDC (red) are distributed both in the dark zone (DZ), containing proliferating centroblasts (blue), and the light zone (LZ) of tonsillar germinal centres. (e) Similar staining as in (d) for GCDC in a germinal centre of spleen. DC in the periarteriolar lymphoid sheath (PALS, T cell areas) represent interdigitating cells. (f) Similar staining as in (d) for GCDC in a germinal centre of lymph node. (g) GCDC in germinal centres (GC) express low levels of CD40 (red), whereas interdigitating cells in T cells areas (TZ) express high levels of CD40 (dark blue). (h) Whereas GCDC are distributed throughout germinal centres (see (a)–(g)), tingible body macrophages (arrows) are mainly located in the dark zone in low numbers; the follicular mantle is in blue. (Reprinted with permission.)

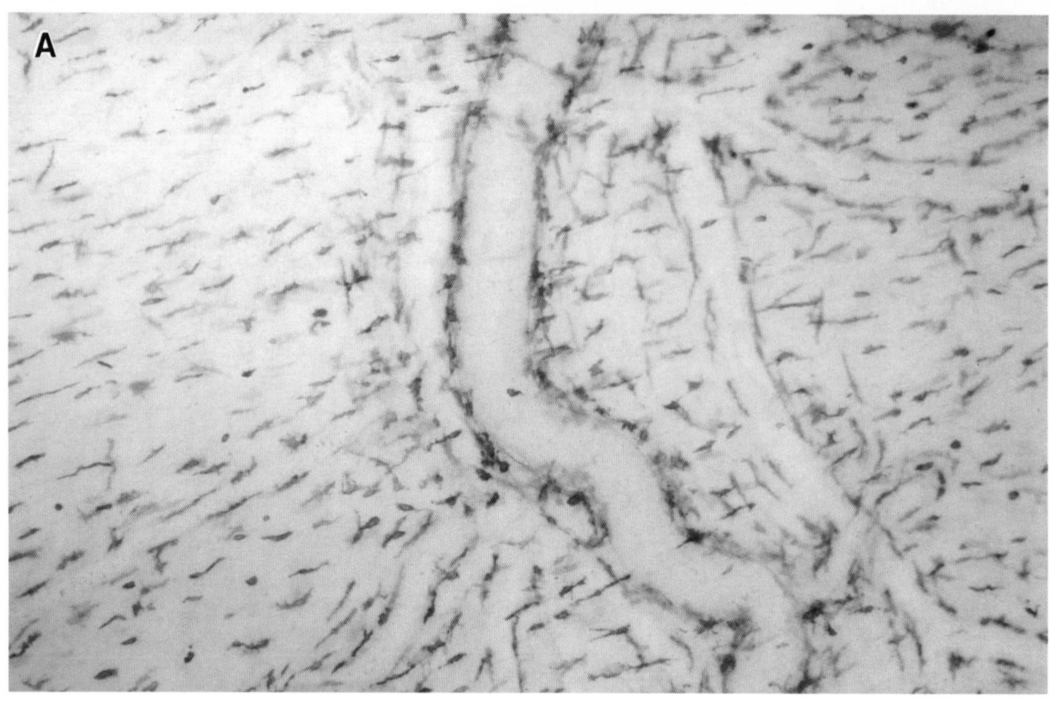

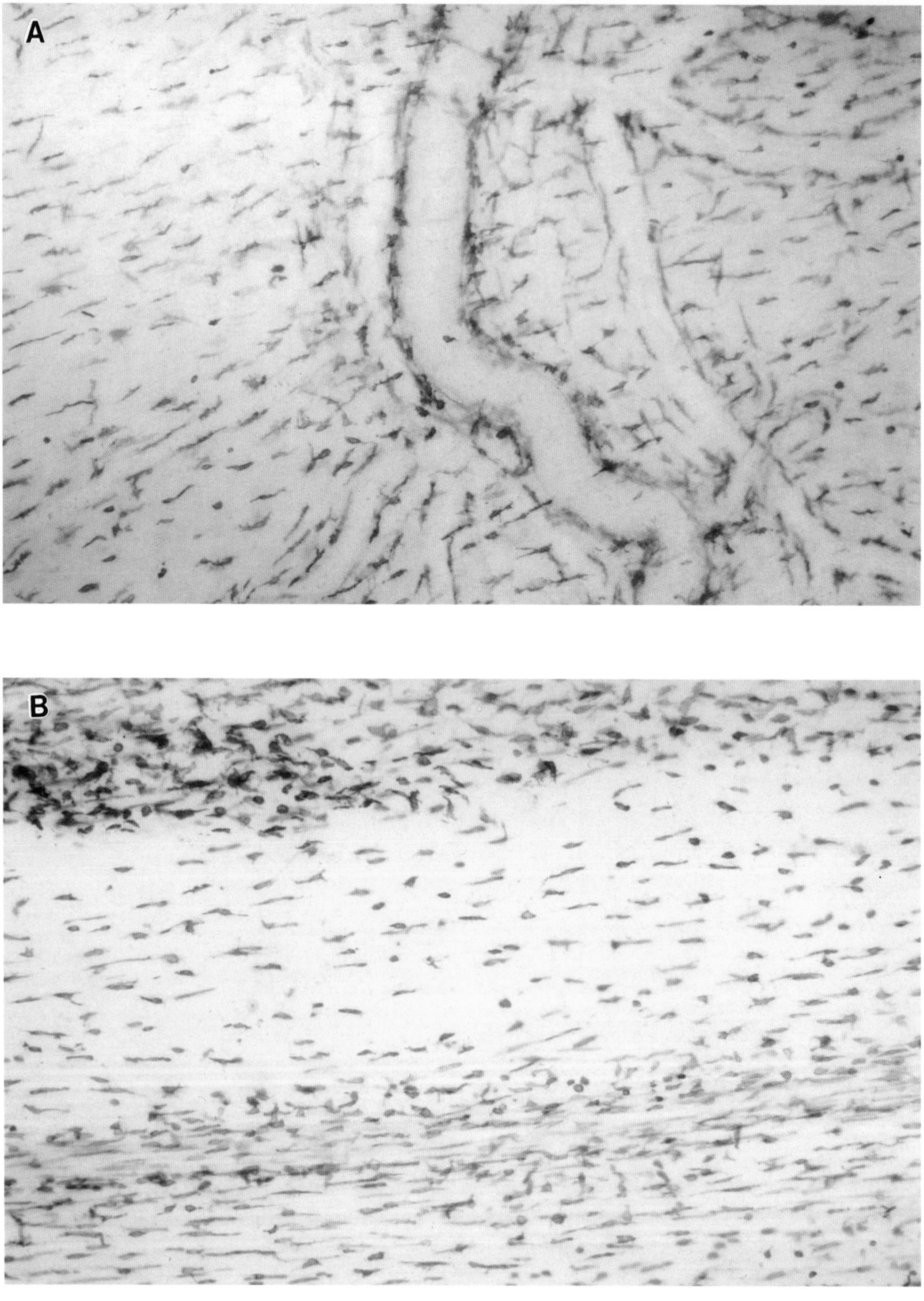

Plate 12.9. Rat dural wholemounts stained with the mAb ED2 specific for resident tissue macrophages. (A) Meningeal vessels, note predominant perivascular distribution. (B) Region in which vessels are less evident and macrophages are orientated parallel to the connective-tissue fibres in the dura (× 150).

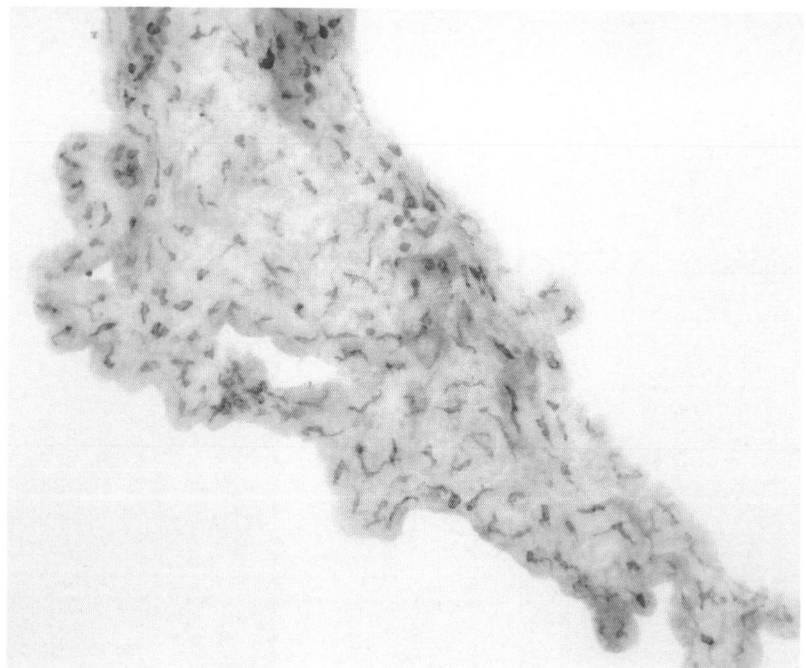

Plate 12.13. Rat choroid plexus wholemount stained with mAb Ox62 (anti-DC marker) (× 220).

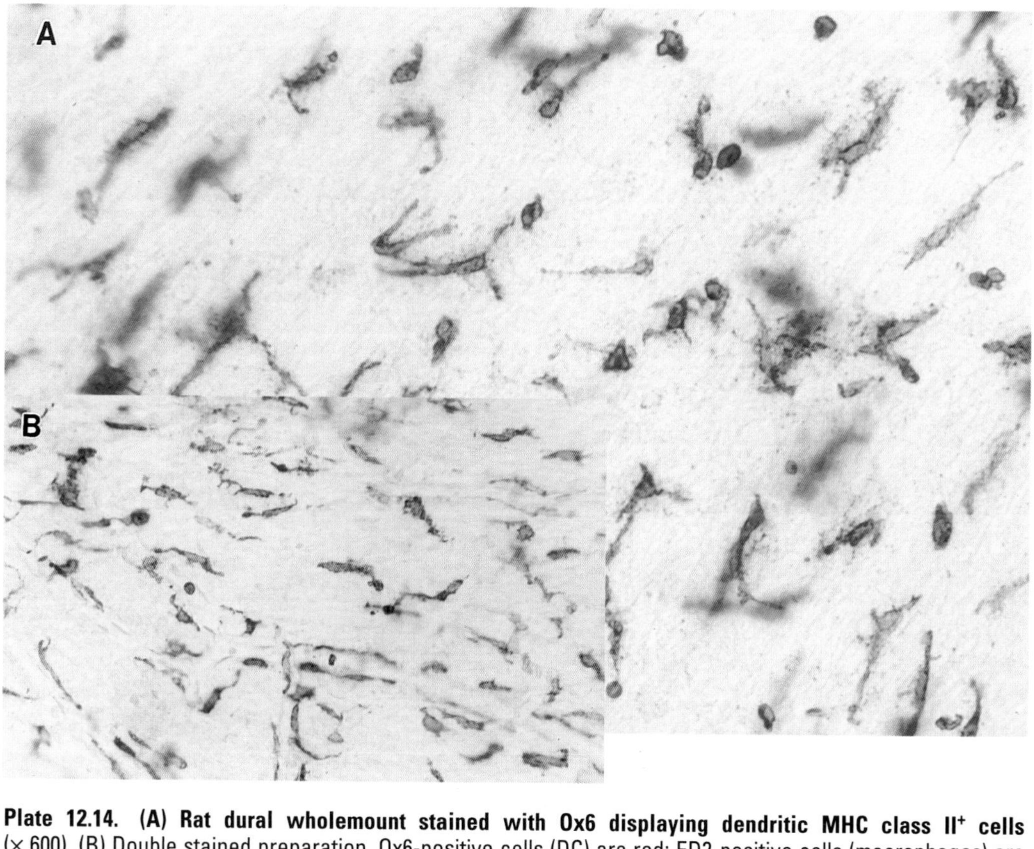

Plate 12.14. (A) Rat dural wholemount stained with Ox6 displaying dendritic MHC class II$^+$ cells (× 600). (B) Double stained preparation. Ox6-positive cells (DC) are red; ED2-positive cells (macrophages) are blue (× 220).

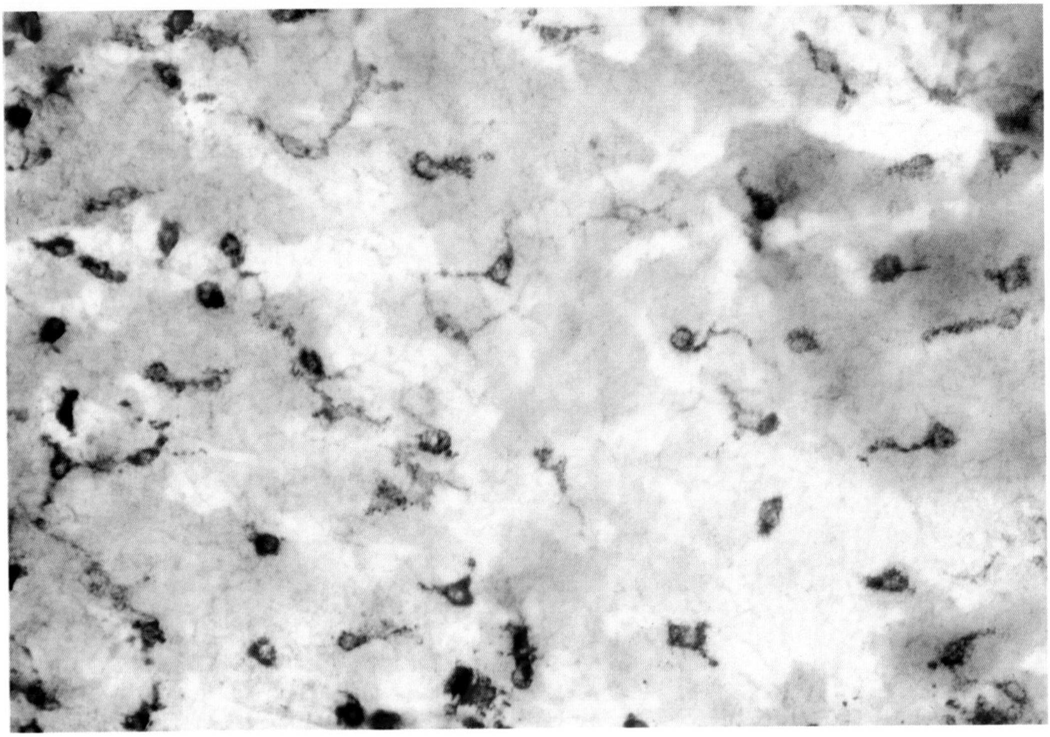

Plate 12.15. Pia mater wholemount double stained as in Plate 12.14 (DC, red; macrophages, blue) (× 600).

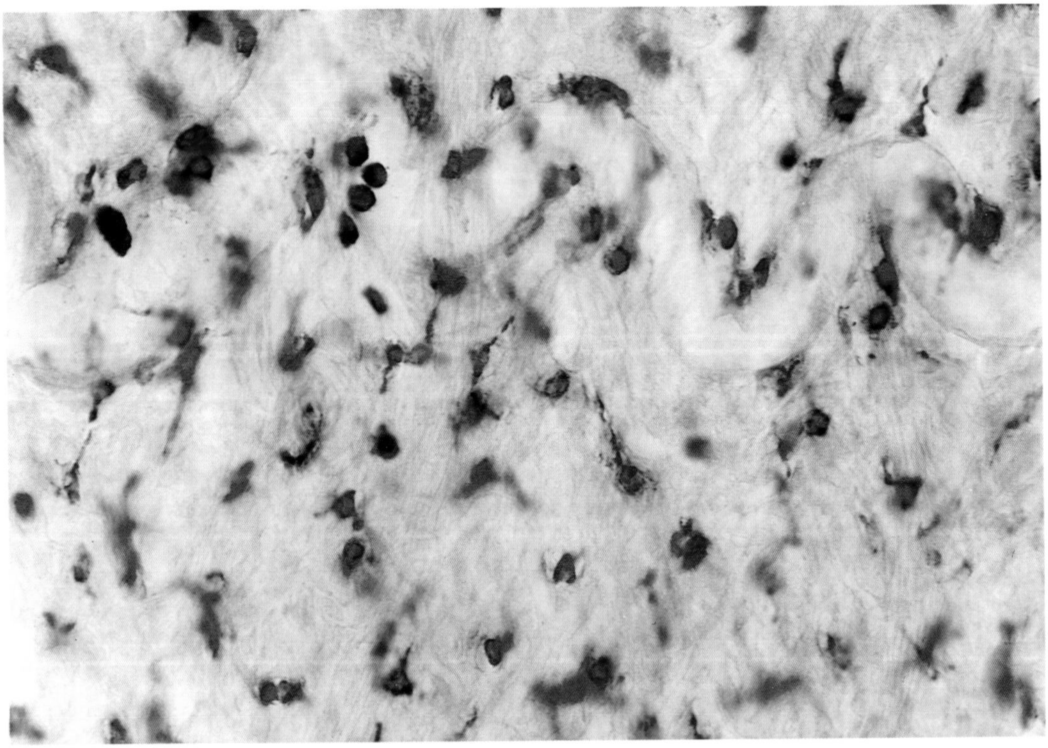

Plate 12.17. Double colour immunostaining of rat iris wholemount. Red, DC (Ox6); blue, macrophages (ED2) (× 600).

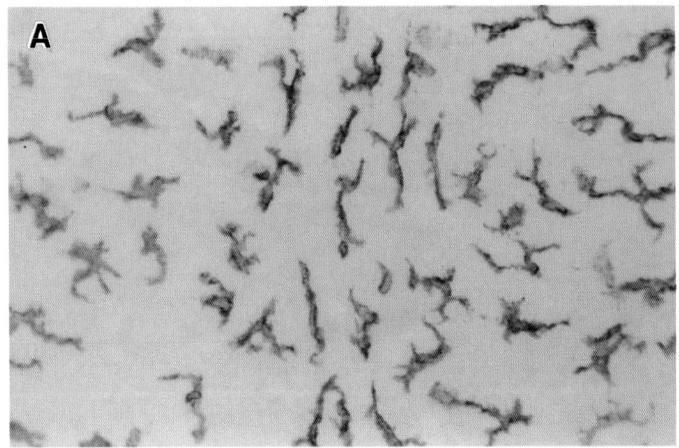

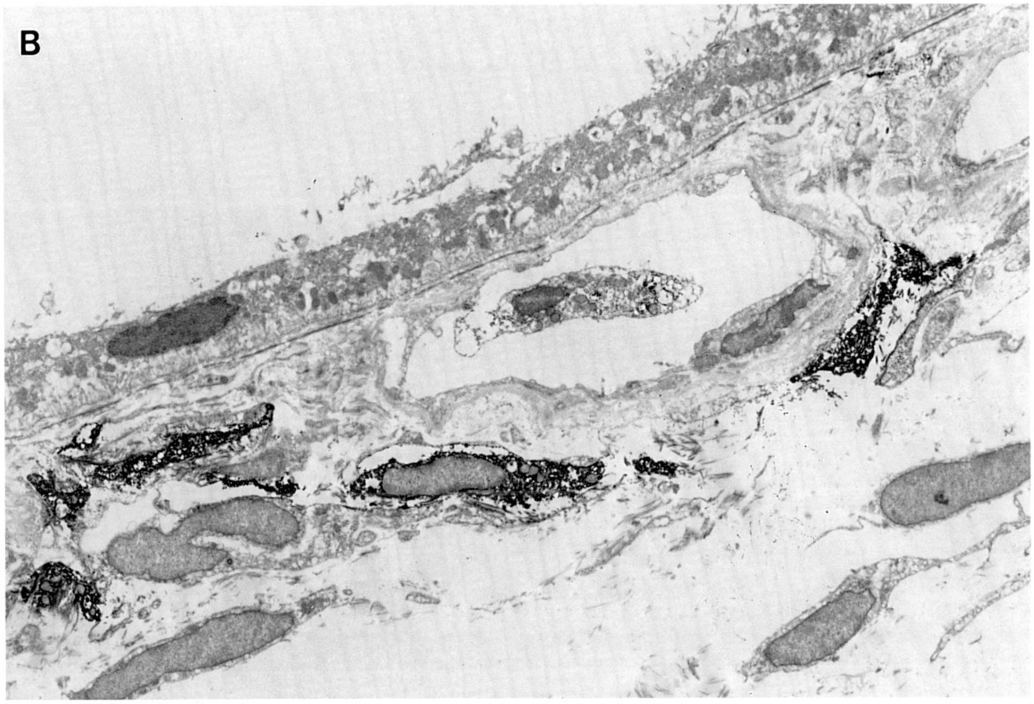

Plate 12.20. (A) DCs in mouse choroid wholemount stained with anti-MHC class II (M5/114) (× 200). (B) Transmission electron micrograph of rat choroid stained with anti-MHC class II mAb (Ox6). Note the monolayer of RPE cells resting on Bruch's membrane. Immunopositive cells are distributed throughout the choroid including directly beneath the 'pigment' epithelium (albino Lewis rat) (× 2200).

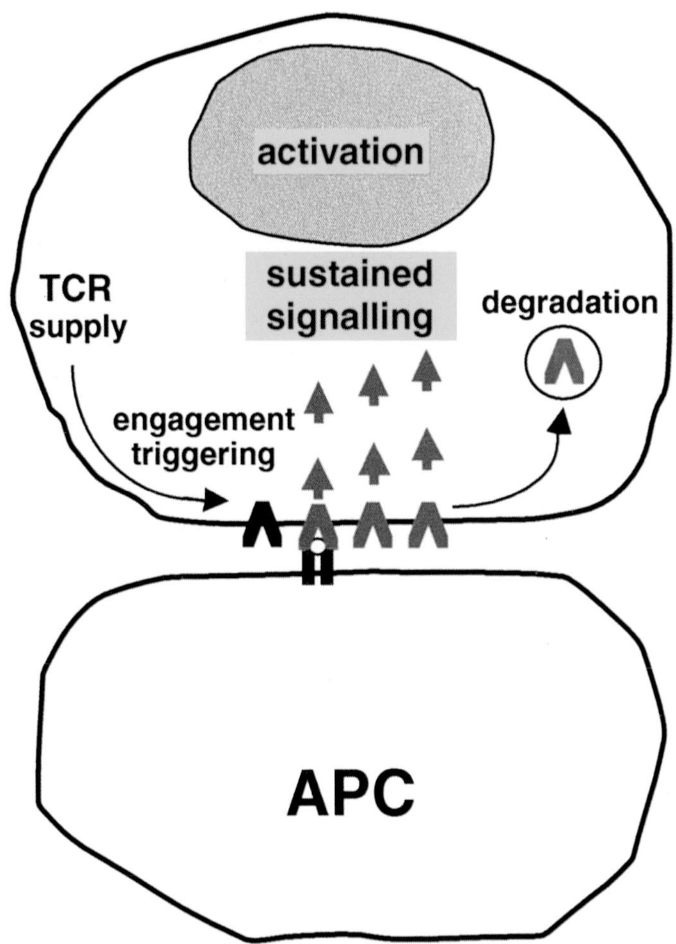

Plate 13.1. The sustained signalling that eventually leads to T cell activation is maintained by a dynamic process of TCR serial triggering. During the prolonged interaction between T and APC every peptide–MHC complex triggers and downregulates many TCRs (typically 100 complexes trigger up to 20000 TCRs). This process of serial triggering depends on an appropriate kinetics of TCR–ligand interaction that can be adjusted by CD4/CD8 coreceptors. CD28 increases the signal transduced by triggered TCRs, allowing T cells to become committed more rapidly and at lower thresholds of TCR triggering. Adhesion molecules stabilize T–APC conjugates and thus allow the signal to be sustained for hours. The duration of signalling is the major factor determining T cell fate: naive T cells require >20 h while effector T cells require about 1 h.

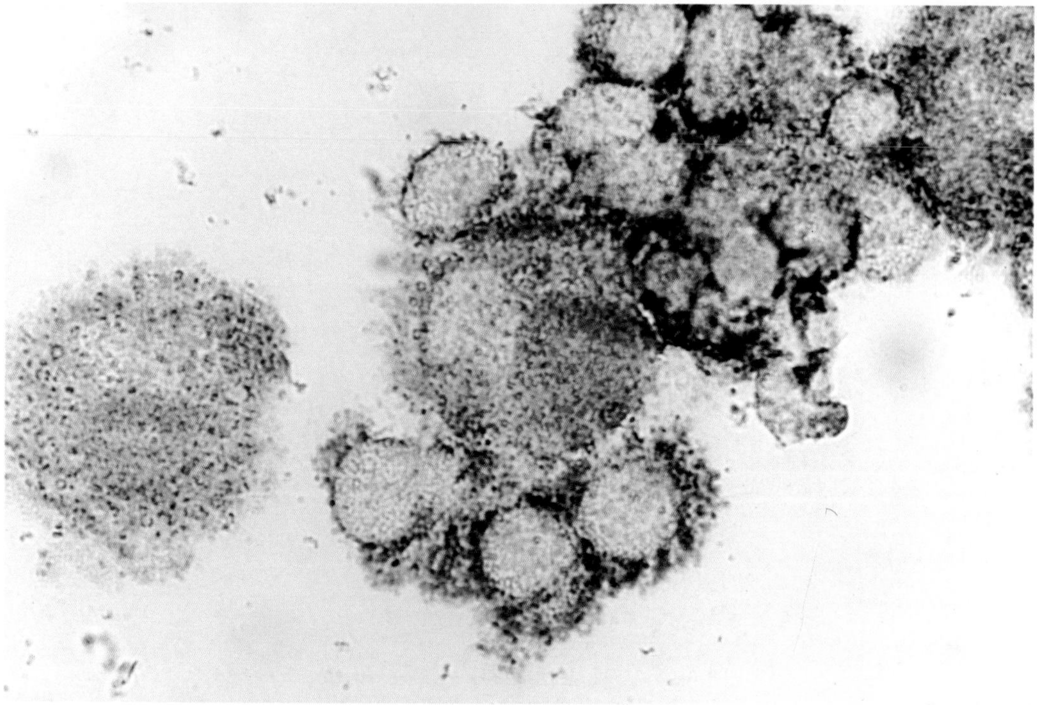

Plate 15.1. Clusters of DC and B lymphocytes. Purified B cells (10^5 cells) were cultured in 24-well plates over 2.5×10^4 irradiated CD40 ligand-transfected B cells and 5×10^4 DC. After 8 days of coculture, cells were harvested, cytocentrifuged and used for double anti-HLA-DR (red) and anti-CD20 (blue) staining. Magnification $\times$ 1000.

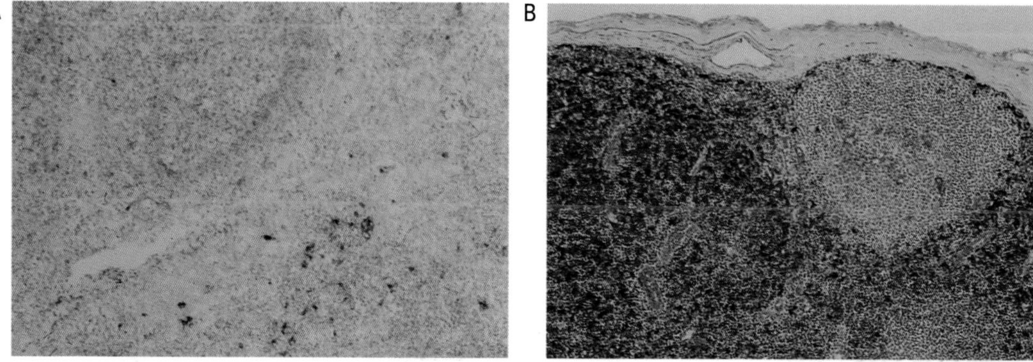

Plate 19.1. Identification of DC in normal and abnormal lymph nodes. (A) Frozen lymph node immunostained to reveal the presence of CD83. In the normal node there is a scattering of paracortical cells (HB 15A antibody, DAB). The fixed embedded counterpart revealed identical staining. (B) A lymph node with an exuberant example of a dermatopathic reaction reveals the vast numbers of interdigitating paracortical cells when stained for fascin (p55 antibody, DAB)

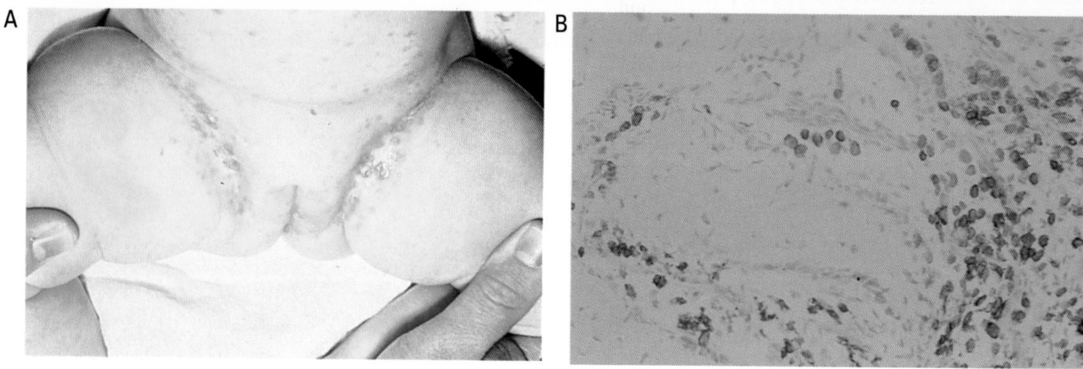

Plate 19.2. Langerhans cell disease. (A) Five-month-old girl with the petechial eczematous rash of the skin folds seen in Langerhans' cell disease. (B) Langerhans cell disease is confirmed by demonstrating the presence of CD1a on the histiocytes by immunohistochemistry in the bone section (010 antibody, DAB).

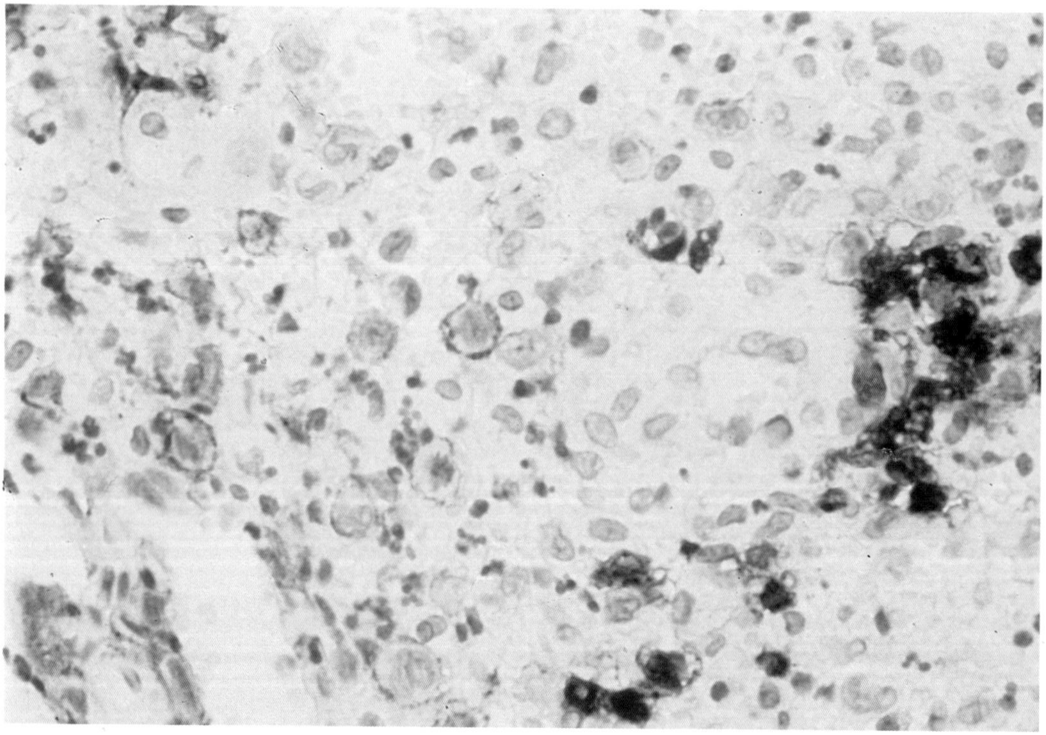

Plate 19.3. Langerhans cell disease. The LCH cells are immunostained for CD1a, in red. A population of perivascular dendritic cells stains intensely for the presence of fascin, but the LCH cells are unstained.

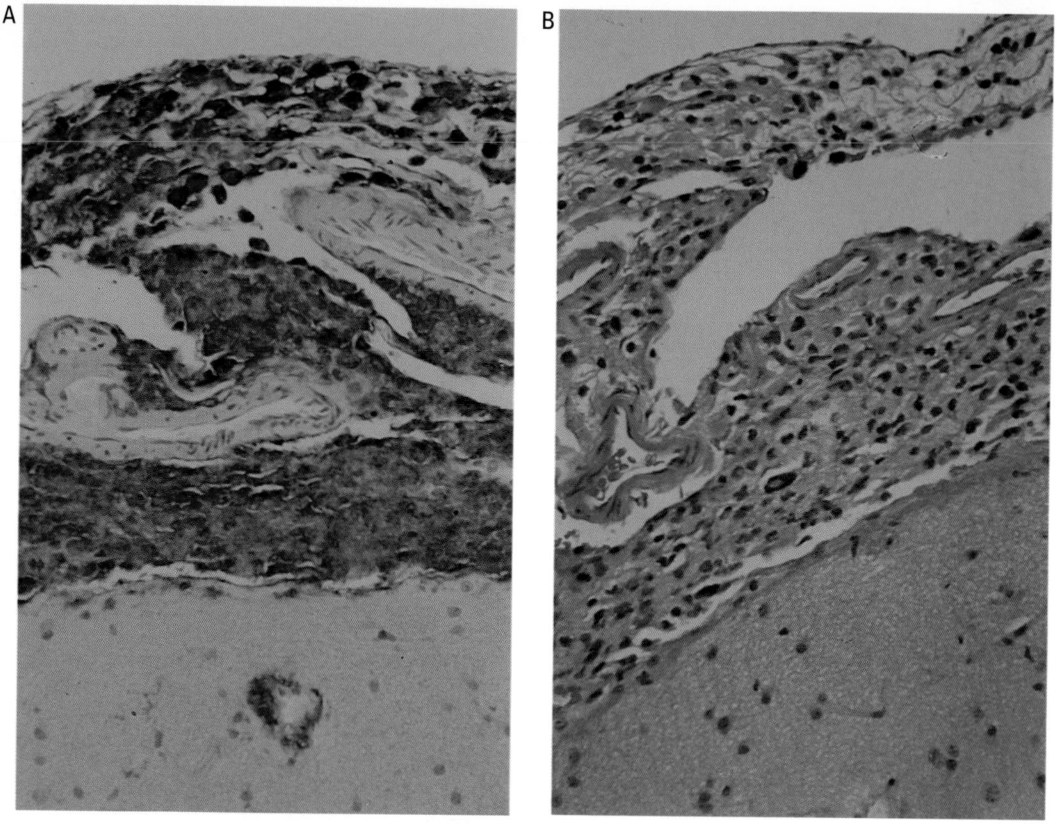

Plate 19.4. Juvenile xanthogranuloma family. (A) 12-year-old girl had meningitic involvement. (B) Fascin immunostain is strongly positive on JXG cells.

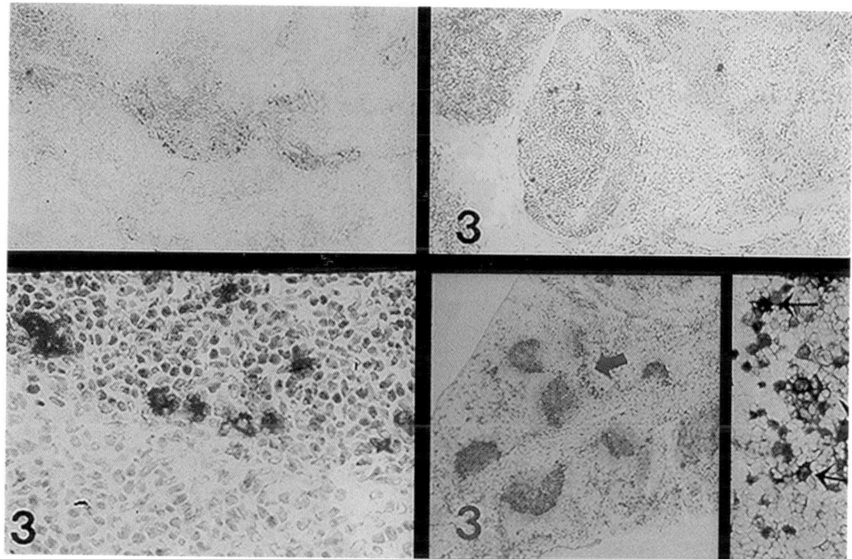

Plate 20.1. Identification of donor cells in the recipient spleen and thymus. Series of photomicrographs taken from sections of the recipient spleen (all except upper right frame) and thymus (upper right frame), 3 days after transplantation of a rat liver allograft. The recipients were treated with immunosuppression and all of the tissues are stained with a monoclonal antibody that reacts with MHC class II antigens of the donor, but not that of the recipient [188]. Note the presence of donor cells in the marginal zone and B cell follicles in the spleen in the upper left, lower left and lower right frames. Donor MHC class II$^+$ cells are also detected in the thymic medulla (upper right). In the lower right frames, the tissue is also stained for BrdU, which labels cells synthesizing DNA. Note that the presence of donor cells in the recipient spleen is associated with proliferation of both cell populations [63].

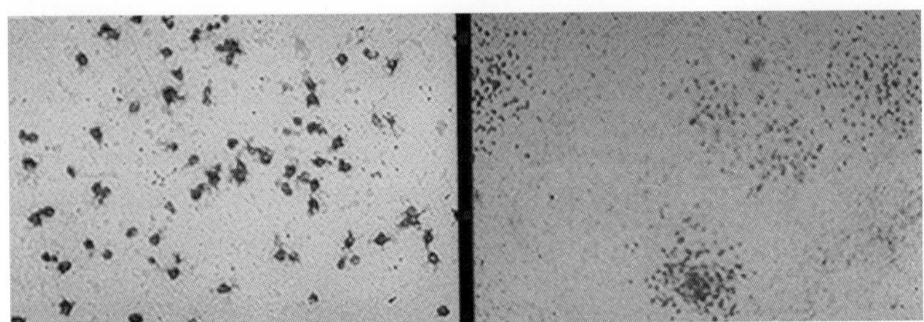

Plate 20.2. Donor CFU-C in recipient bone marrow. Photomicrographs of a colony-forming unit-culture (CFU-C) assay using a fibrin clot system. The cultured cells were obtained from the bone marrow of a recipient rat, 10 days after liver transplantation, and stained for donor MHC class II antigens. Note the presence of donor hematopoietic colonies on the right. On the left, note the presence of myelomono-cytic cells, some of which have a characteristic dendritic morphology, typical of rat dendritic cells [212, 213].

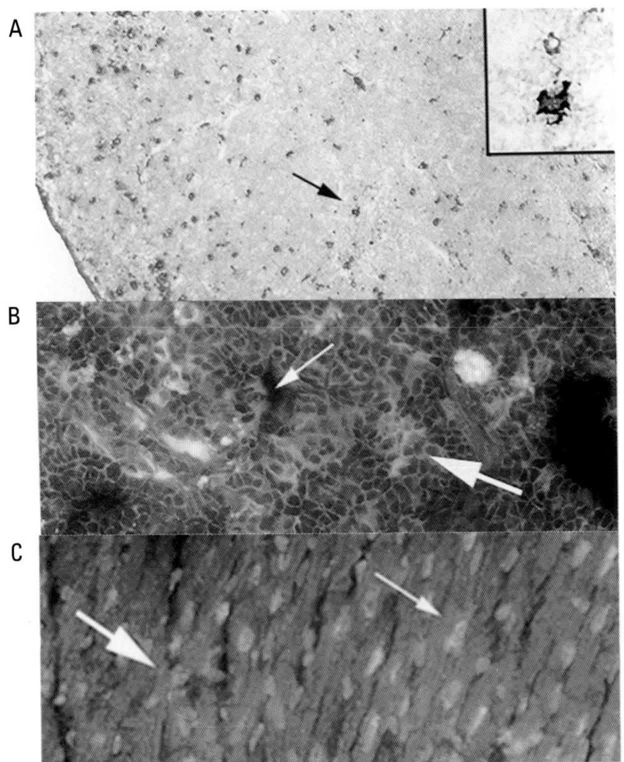

Plate 20.3. Donor dendritic cells within recipient thymus. Thymus of a rat liver allograft recipient, 30 days after transplantation. The tissue is double stained for donor MHC class II-positive cells (rust color) and ED2 (blue), which highlights tissue macrophages. Note the presence of the donor dendritic-shaped cell in the recipient thymus (arrow and inset). The 'shrunken' medulla in this recipient can be attributed to the transient 2-week course of FK506, which is known to cause damage to the thymic medulla [214]. It may also create a milieu conducive to the recruitment of donor DC progenitors [3, 214]. (B) Donor DC can also be detected in the spleen. This is a section of recipient spleen, obtained 30 days after liver transplantation and double stained for donor MHC class II (red) and OX62, an integrin, known to be expressed by rat DC [213]. Note the presence of the yellow, doubly labeled donor DC. (C) Challenge donor heart allograft 100 days after transplantation in a recipient rendered tolerant to the donor by a previous liver allograft. This section is double stained for donor MHC class II (red) and OX62. Note the red, single positive MHC class II^+ donor interstitial cell (large arrow) and yellow, double positive donor DC. Even though this recipient received no immunosuppression, donor DC persisted in the challenge allograft and it was resistant to chronic rejection [120].

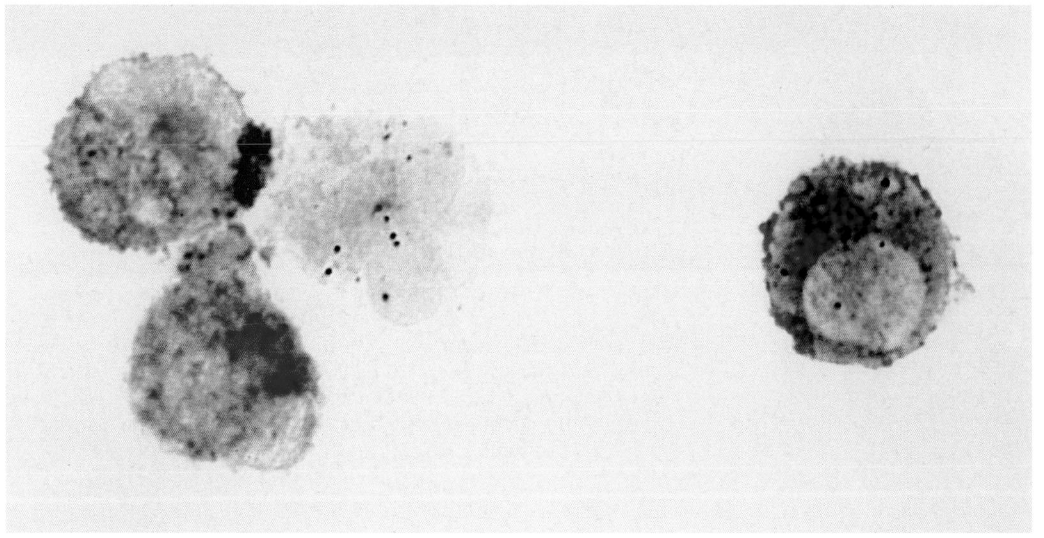

	Fresh	3 days	6 days
CD1a	++	80% ++	20% +
CD14	–/±	10% ++	70% ++
CD68	+	++	++
RFD7	–	–	–
RFD9	–	+	++
APh	–/±	–/±	90% ++

Plate 21.1. DC from bronchoalveolar lavage. The table shows the immunophenotype of freshly isolated CD1a$^+$ DC from the bronchoalveolar lavage of healthy individuals, exposed to lipopolysaccharide in culture for 3 and 6 days (for isolation techniques see van Haarst *et al.*, 1994). Data show the staining intensity: – = negative; ± = weakly positive; + = positive; ++ = strongly positive. Staining intensity applies to all cells unless indicated otherwise by percentage positive cells. Note that a prototype of the DCs, viz. a CD1a$^+$, CD14$^-$, acid phosphatase$^-$ stellate-shaped cell gradually turns into a macrophage-like cell (CD14$^+$, CD68$^+$, RFD9$^+$, acid phsophatase$^+$ round cell). The photomicrographs show transitional forms during culture, viz. a round cell both positive for CD1a (blue) and acid phosphatase (red).

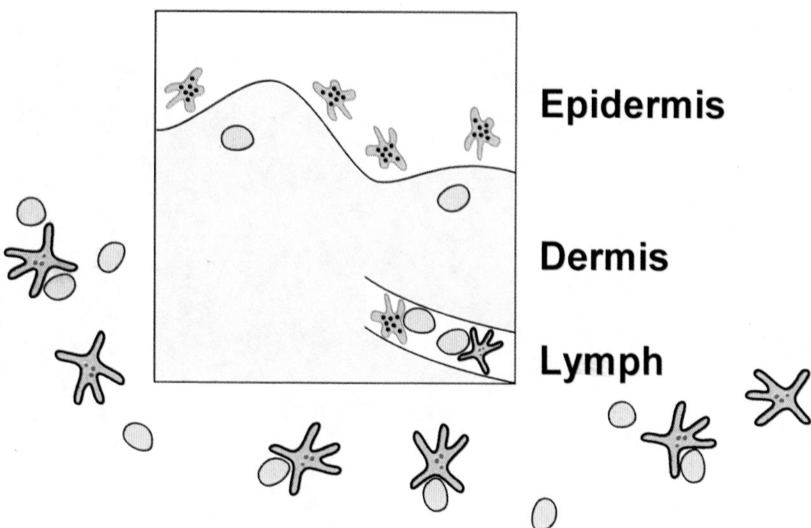

Plate 23.1. Maturation and migration of DC from a body surface like skin. *In situ*, the DC have large stores of intracellular MHC class II products within specialized vacuoles (dark granules) that contain lysosomal membrane glycoproteins. As the DC migrate, the MHC II is sorted as MHC II–peptide complexes to the cell surface (thick line) for presentation to T cells. Not shown is the fact that during maturation and migration, several new molecules are expressed such as CD86, CD83, and p55.

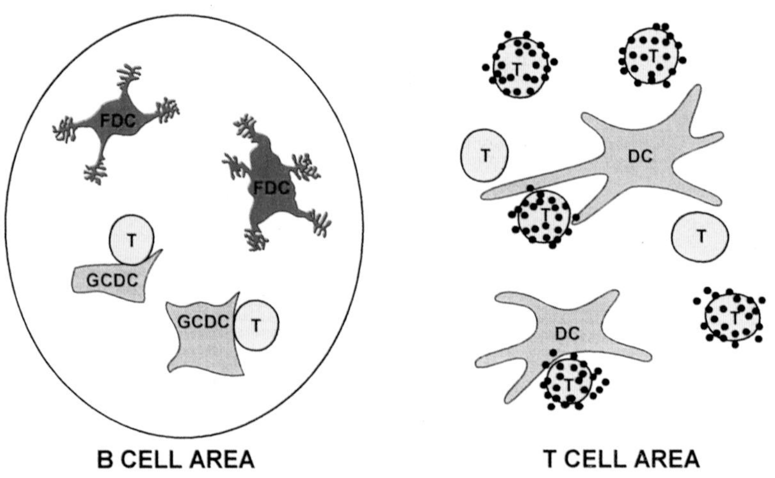

Immune status: HIV-1 reactive CD4$^+$ T cells present; CD8$^+$ T cells absent

No HIV-1 antibody to bring virus to FDC and GCDC

Plate 23.2. Viral RNA (*in-situ* hybridization with radiolabeled antisense probes) localized in an acutely infected lymph node. Most of the silver grains from the antisense probe (black dots) are localized over CD4$^+$ T cells, but tissue culture experiments suggest that this virus can originate from DC that have captured virus beforehand, e.g., at a body surface.

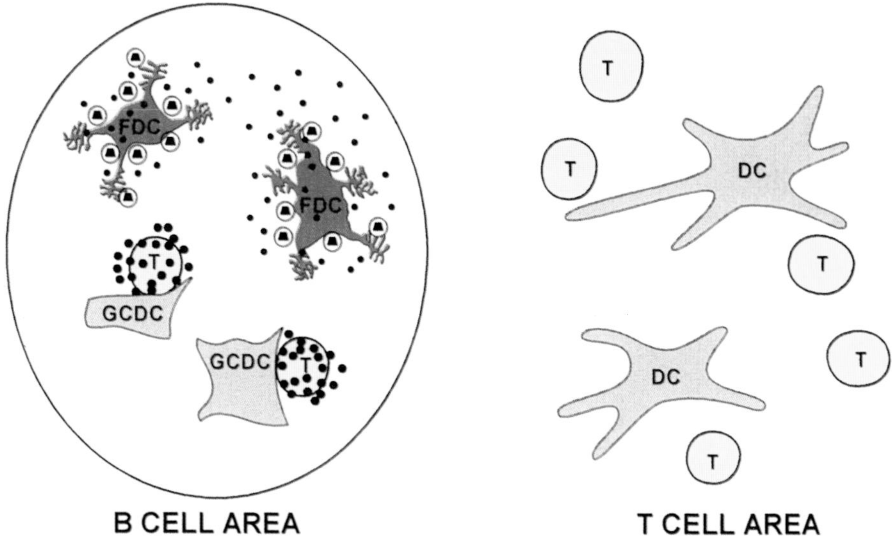

Immune status: HIV-1 reactive CD4$^+$ T cells absent; CD8$^+$ T cells present

HIV-1 antibodies to bring virus to FDC and GCDC

Plate 23.3. Viral RNA (*in-situ* hybridization with radiolabeled antisense probes) localized in a chronically infected lymph node. Most of the silver grains (black dots) are found in the germinal center, either as diffuse labeling of immune-complexed virions on FDC, or as much 'hotter' CD4$^+$ T cells. The latter may receive virus from germinal center DC (GCDC) or from the FDC network.

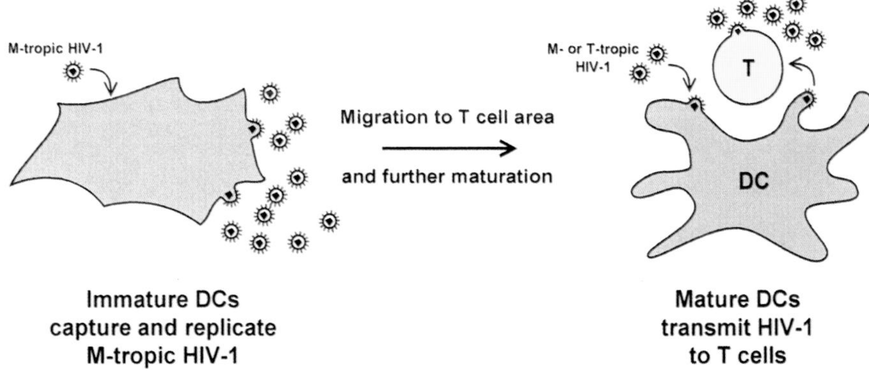

Plate 23.4. Contrasting roles of immature and mature DC in promoting viral replication. Purified, immature cells replicate M-tropic strains of HIV-1 directly, but not T-tropic virus. Mature cells do not replicate virus but capture and transmit both M-tropic and T-tropic strains T cells. One suggested mechanism is diagrammed, i.e., the virus persists as RNA beneath the DC surface until the appropriate T cell is bound.

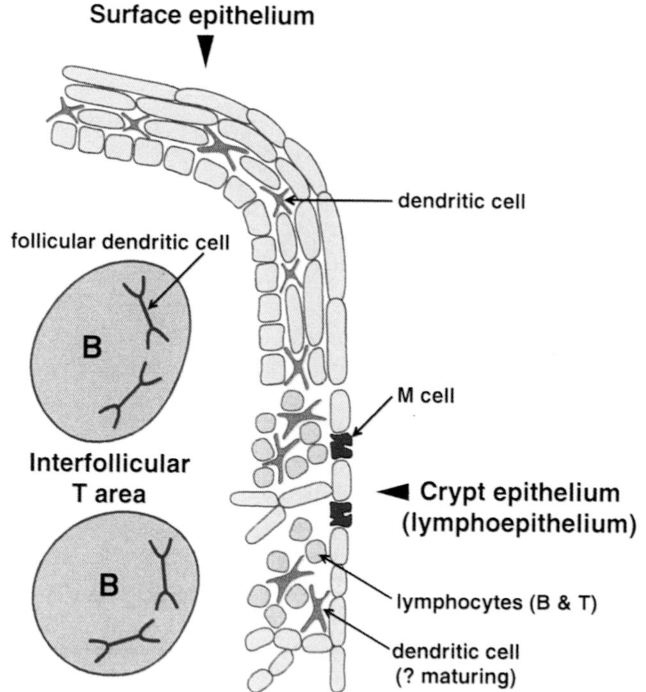

Plate 23.5. The lymphoepithelial surfaces of mucosal-associated, oropharyngeal, lymphoid tissue, or tonsils. M-cells transport antigens into the lymphoepithelium, a region that contains both DC and memory lymphocytes. Beneath the lymphoepithelium lie typical B and T cell areas with FDC and DC, respectively.

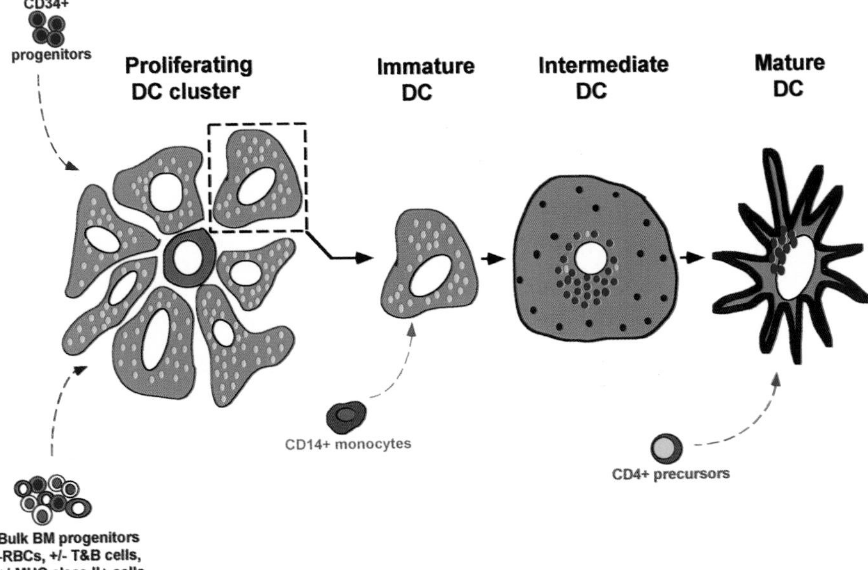

Plate 28.1. Stages of maturation during DC development. Clusters of newly forming DC can be generated by bone marrow- and/or blood-derived proliferating progenitors. DC formed in proliferating clusters pass through three distinct stages of maturation, mimicking the developmental pathway of DC *in vivo*. DC can also be formed from nonproliferating progenitors such as the $CD14^+$ blood monocyte and the $CD4^+$ lymphoid precursor. Growth requirements differ for each pathway (see text).

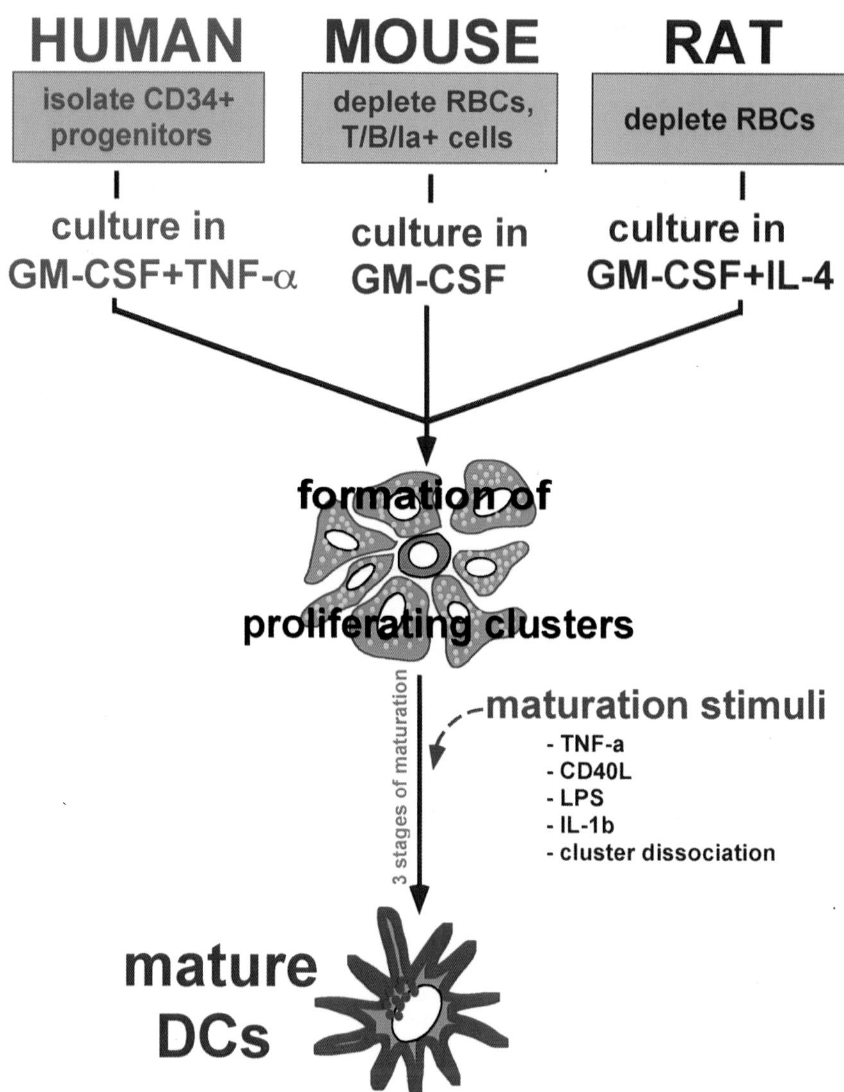

Plate 28.2. Methods for obtaining cultures of developing DC from proliferating progenitors. Growth requirements and starting populations are different for each species. For human, $CD34^+$ progenitors can be obtained from blood and/or bone marrow. For mouse and rat, proliferating progenitors are obtained from bone marrow.

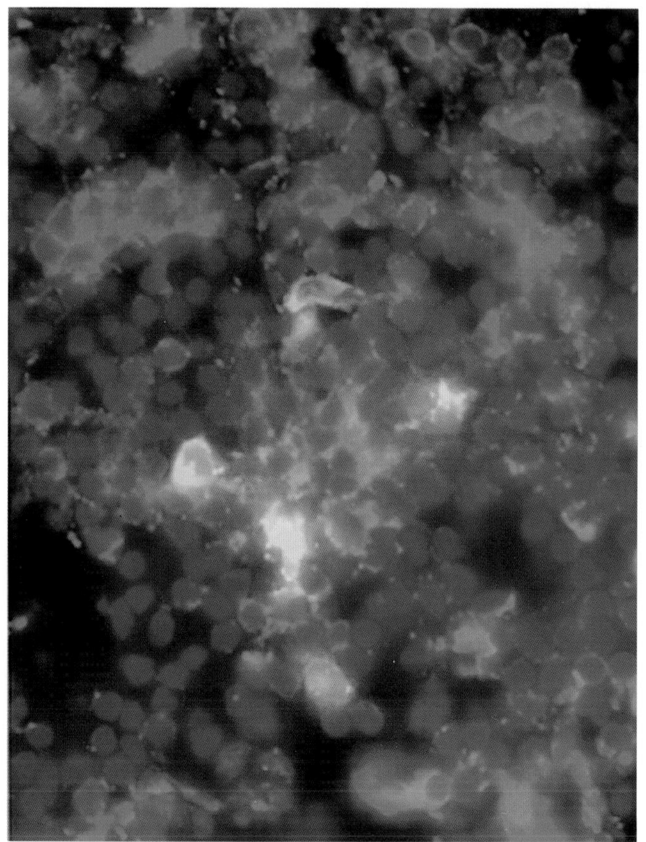

Plate 31.1. Dendritic cells which localize in the draining lymph node after subcutaneous injection maintain high-level expression of MHC class II molecules. Chimpanzee dendritic cells were cultured from peripheral blood mononuclear cells using recombinant cytokines (Barratt-Boyes *et al.*, 1996) and labelled with a lipophilic carbocyanine dye, DiIC^{18}(5), which flouresces red. Labelled cells were injected subcutaneously in the thigh of the donor chimpanzee and the draining inguinal lymph node harvested 48h later. Cryosectioned tissues were labelled with antibody to HLA-DR (green) and Hoescht 33322 (blue) and examined by fluorescence microscopy (Barratt-Boyes *et al.*, 1997). The injected dendritic cells in the center of the field (double labelled; orange) and the surrounding endogenous interdigitating dendritic cells (green) are strongly class II-positive. (Image by Center for Biologic Imaging, University of Pittsburgh.)

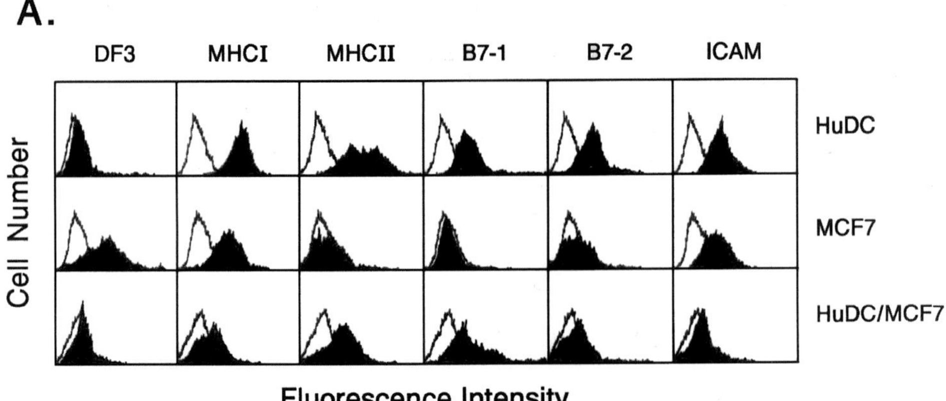

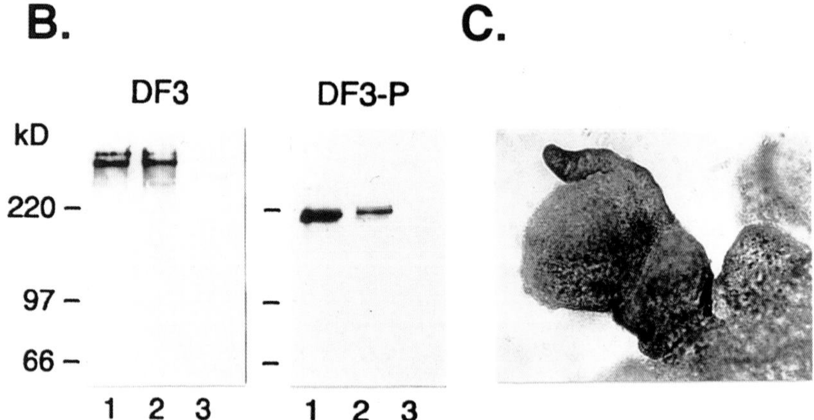

Plate 33.6 Expression of MHC molecules and tumor antigens on DC/tumor fusion cells. (A) Expression of MHC class I, class II and costimulatory ligands on HuDC/MCF-7 fusion cells compared with autologous DC and unfused MCF-7 cells. Solid areas are cells stained with indicated mAbs. Open areas are cells stained with control antibodies. (B) Lysates from HuDC/MCF-7 fusion cells (lane 1), MCF-7 cells (lane 2) and HuDC (lane 3) were analyzed by immunoblotting with mAbs DF3 and DF3-P. (C) Cytocentrifuge preparations of HuDC/MCF-7 were double stained with mAb HLA-DR (anti-MHC II, blue) and mAb DF3 (anti-MUC1, red).

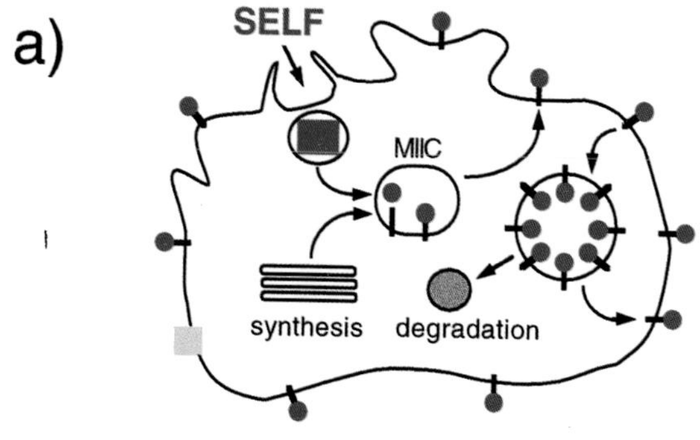

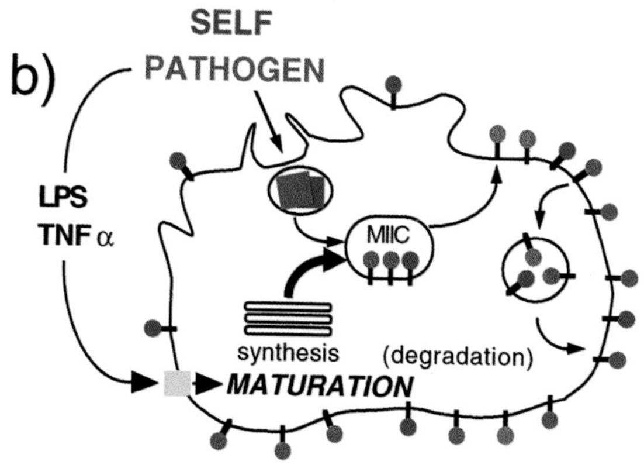

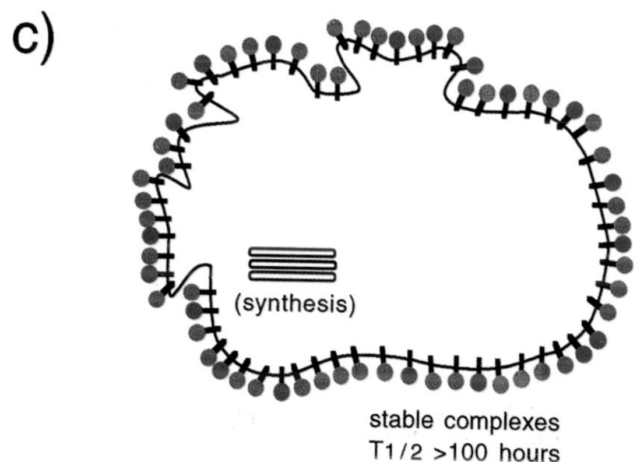

Plate 34.3 DC optimize presentation of infectious antigens by modulating class II synthesis and stability. (a) Immature DC efficiently capture self-antigens (green). The processed peptides are loaded onto newly synthesized as well as recycling class II molecules. Because of the high endocytic activity the mature molecules are degraded at a high rate with half-lives of about 10h. (b) An infectious antigen (red) induces DC maturation either directly via LPS or indirectly via stimulation of an inflammatory response. Increased levels of class II biosynthesis allow formation of peptide–MHC complexes at a higher rate. Many of these complexes contain peptides derived from infectious antigens (red dots). Together with a decrease in the endocytic activity, degradation of class II molecules also progressively decreases until finally the class II molecules acquire a half-life of more than 100h. (c) At later times (2 days), synthesis of class II molecules is shut off, DC retain the complexes formed during maturation. This figure has been adapted from Watts (1997).

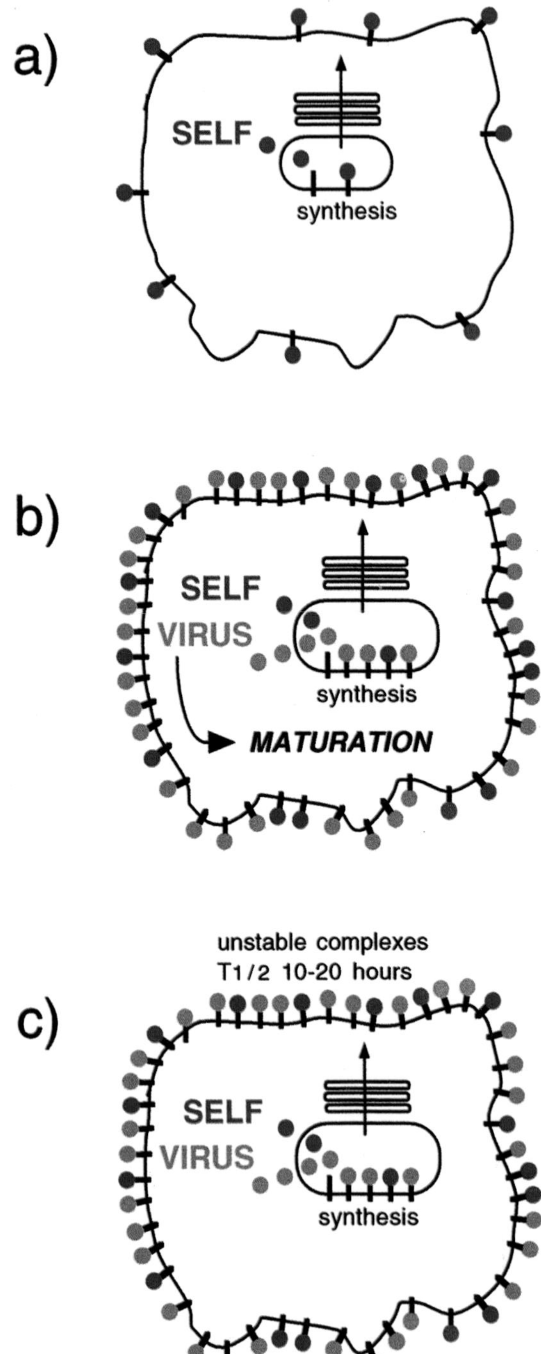

Plate 34.4 Sustained upregulation of class I synthesis by maturation. (a) Immature DC synthesize class I molecules at low rates. These are loaded with self-peptides (blue). (b) Maturation induced by exogenous stimuli or by viral infection upregulates class I synthesis. More complexes are formed, many of which contain viral peptides (red). (c) In mature DC, class I synthesis is sustained at high levels, allowing continuous loading of viral peptides while the surface complexes have relatively short half- lives (10–20h).

149. Demetris, A.J., Murase, N., Delaney, C.P., Woan, M., Fung, J.J. and Starzl, T.E. (1995). The liver allograft, chronic (ductopenic) rejection, and microchimerism: what can they teach us? *Transplant. Proc.* **27** (1), 67–70.
150. Owen, R.D. (1945). Immunogenetic consequences of vascular anastomoses between bovine twins. *Science* **102**, 400–401.
151. Main, J.M. and Prehn, R.T. (1955). Successful skin homografts after the administration of high dosage X radiation and homologous bone marrow. *J. Natl Cancer Inst.* **15**, 1023–1029.
152. Monaco, A.E., Wood, M.L. and Russell, P.S. (1966). Studies of heterologous anti-lymphocyte serum in mice. III. Immunologic tolerance and chimerism produced across the H-2 locus with adult thymectomy and anti-lymphocyte serum. *Ann. NY Acad. Sci.* **129**, 190–209.
153. Slavin, S., Fuks, Z., Weiss, L. and Morecki, S. (1989). Mechanisms of tolerance in chimeric mice prepared with total lymphoid irradiation. *ICN-UCLA Symp. Mol. Cell. Biol.* **17**, 383.
154. Ildstad, S.T. and Sachs, D.H. (1984). Reconstitution with syngeneic plus allogeneic or xenogeneic bone marrow leads to specific acceptance of allografts or xenografts. *Nature*, **307** (5947), 168–170.
155. Ildstad, S.T., Wren, S.M., Bluestone, J.A., Barbieri, S.A. and Sachs, D.H. (1985). Characterization of mixed allogeneic chimeras. Immunocompetence, in vitro reactivity, and genetic specificity of tolerance. *J. Exp. Med.* **162** (1), 231–244.
156. Alard, P., Matriano, J.A., Socarras, S., Ortega, M.A. and Streilein, J.W. (1995). Detection of donor-derived cells by polymerase chain reaction in neonatally tolerant mice. Microchimerism fails to predict tolerance. *Transplantation* **60** (10), 1125–1130.
157. Hayashi, H., LeGuern, C., Sachs, D.H. and Sykes, M. (1996). Long-term engraftment of preculture post-5-fluorouracil allogeneic marrow in mice conditioned with a nonmyeloablative regimen: relevance for a gene therapy approach to tolerance induction. *Transplant. Immunol.* **4** (1), 86–90.
158. Sykes, M. (1996). Chimerism and central tolerance. *Curr. Opin. Immunol.* **8** (5), 694–703.
159. Sykes, M., Szot, G.L., Swenson, K.A. and Pearson, D.A. (1997). Induction of high levels of allogeneic hematopoietic reconstitution and donor-specific tolerance without myelosuppressive conditioning. *Nature Medicine* **3** (7), 783–787.
160. Billingham, R. and Brent, L. (1956). Quantitative studies on transplantation immunity. IV. Induction of tolerance in newborn mice and studies on the phenomenon of runt disease. *Phil. Trans. R. Soc. Lond. (Biol.)* **242**, 439–477.
161. Russell, P.S. (1962). Modification of runt disease in mice by various means. *Transplantation: Ciba Foundation Symposium* (eds. Wolstenholme, C.E.W., Cameron, M.P., London, J., Churchill, A). Little Brown, Boston.
162. Jankowski, R.A. and Ildstad, S.T. (1997). Chimerism and tolerance: from freemartin cattle and neonatal mice to humans. *Hum. Immunol.* **52** (2), 155–161.
163. Kaufman, C.L., Colson, Y.L., Wren, S.M., Watkins, S., Simmons, R.L. and Ildstad, S.T. (1994). Phenotypic characterization of a novel bone marrow-derived cell that facilitates engraftment of allogeneic bone marrow stem cells. *Blood* **84** (8), 2436–2446.
164. Gaines, B.A., Colson, Y.L., Kaufman, C.L. and Ildstad, S. (1996). Facilitating cells enable engraftment of purified fetal liver stem cells in allogeneic recipients. *Exp. Hematol.* **24** (8), 902–913.
165. Ricordi, C., Karatzas, T., Selvaggi, G. *et al.* (1995). Multiple bone marrow infusions to enhance acceptance of allografts from the same donor. *Ann. NY Acad Sci.* **770**, 345–350.
166. Ricordi, C., Ildstad, S.T., Demetris, A.J., Abou el-Ezz, A.Y., Murase, N. and Starzl, T.E. (1992). Donor dendritic cell repopulation in recipients after rat-to-mouse bone-marrow transplantation [letter]. *Lancet* **339** (8809), 1610–1611.
167. Sharabi, Y., Abraham, V.S., Sykes, M. and Sachs, D.H. (1992). Mixed allogeneic chimeras prepared by a non-myeloablative regimen: requirement for chimerism to maintain tolerance. *Bone Marrow Transplant.* **9** (3), 191–197.
168. Khan, A., Tomita, Y. and Sykes, M. (1996). Thymic dependence of loss of tolerance in mixed allogeneic bone marrow chimeras after depletion of donor antigen. Peripheral mechanisms do not contribute to maintenance of tolerance. *Transplantation* **62** (3), 380–387.
169. Touraine, J.L., Roncarolo, M.G., Plotnicky, H., Bachetta, R. and Spits, H. (1993). T lymphocytes from human chimeras do recognize antigen in the context of allogeneic determinants of the major histocompatibility complex. *Immunol. Lett.* **39** (1), 9–12.

170. Roncarolo, M.G., Bacchetta, R., Bigler, M., Touraine, J.L., de Vries, J.E. and Spits, H. (1991). A SCID patient reconstituted with HLA-incompatible fetal stem cells as a model for studying transplantation tolerance. *Blood Cells* **17** (2), 391–402.
171. Roncarolo, M.G., Yssel, H., Touraine, J.L. *et al.* (1988). Antigen recognition by MHC-incompatible cells of a human mismatched chimera. *J. Exp. Med.* **168** (6), 2139–2152.
172. Orloff, M.S., DeMara, E.M., Coppage, M.L. *et al.* (1995). Prevention of chronic rejection and graft arteriosclerosis by tolerance induction. *Transplantation* **59** (2), 282–288.
173. Colson, Y.L., Zadach, K., Nalesnik, M. and Ildstad, S.T. (1995). Mixed allogeneic chimerism in the rat. Donor-specific transplantation tolerance without chronic rejection for primarily vascularized cardiac allografts. *Transplantation* **60** (9), 971–980.
174. Tomita, Y., Khan, A. and Sykes, M. (1994). Role of intrathymic clonal deletion and peripheral anergy in transplantation tolerance induced by bone marrow transplantation in mice conditioned with a nonmyeloablative regimen. *J. Immunol.* **153** (3), 1087–1098.
175. Thomas, J., Carver, M., Cunningham, P., Park, K., Gonder, J. and Thomas, F. (1987). Promotion of incompatible allograft acceptance in rhesus monkeys given posttransplant antithymocyte globulin and donor bone marrow. I. In vivo parameters and immunohistologic evidence suggesting microchimerism. *Transplantation* **43** (3), 332–338.
176. Anderson, G., Moore, N.C., Owen, J.J. and Jenkinson, E.J. (1996). Cellular interactions in thymocyte development. *Annu. Rev. Immunol.* **14**, 73–99.
177. DeKoning, J, DiMolfetto, L, Reilly, C., Wei, Q., Havran, W.L. and Lo, D. (1997). Thymic cortical epithelium is sufficient for the development of mature T cells in relB-deficient mice. *J. Immunol.* **158** (6), 2558–2566.
178. Lo, D., Reilly, C.R., Burkly, L.C., DeKoning, J., Laufer, T.M. and Glimcher, L.H. (1997). Thymic stromal cell specialization and the T-cell receptor repertoire. *Immunol. Res.* **16** (1), 3–14.
179. Markowitz, J.S., Auchincloss, H. Jr., Grusby, M.J. and Glimcher, L.H. (1993). Class II-positive hematopoietic cells cannot mediate positive selection of $CD4^+$ T lymphocytes in class II-deficient mice. *Proc. Natl Acad. Sci. USA* **90** (7), 2779–2783.
180. Kappler, J.W., Roehm, N. and Marrack. P. (1987). T cell tolerance by clonal elimination in the thymus. *Cell* **49** (2), 273–280.
181. Zepp, F., Cussler, K., Mannhardt, W., Schofer, O. and Schulte-Wissermann, H. (1987). Intrathymic tolerance induction: determination of tolerance to class II major histocompatibility complex antigens in maturing T lymphocytes by a bone marrow-derived non-lymphoid thymus cell. *Scand. J. Immunol.* **26** (6), 589–601.
182. Hengartner, H., Odermatt, B., Schneider, R. *et al.* (1988). Deletion of self-reactive T cells before entry into the thymus medulla. *Nature* **336** (6197), 388–390.
183. Speiser, D.E., Lees, R.K., Hengartner, H., Zinkernagel, R. MacDonald, H.R. (1989). Positive and negative selection of T cell receptor V beta domains controlled by distinct cell populations in the thymus. *J. Exp. Med.* **170** (6), 2165–2170.
184. Tanaka, Y., Mamalaki, C., Stockinger, B. and Kioussis, D. (1993). In vitro negative selection of alpha beta T cell receptor transgenic thymocytes by conditionally immortalized thymic cortical epithelial cell lines and dendritic cells. *Eur. J. Immunol.* **23** (10), 2614–2621.
185. Ferrero, I., Anjuere, F., MacDonald, H.R. and Ardavin, C. (1997). In vitro negative selection of viral superantigen-reactive thymocytes by thymic dendritic cells. *Blood* **90** (5), 1943–1951.
186. Naspetti, M., Aurrand-Lions, M., DeKoning, J. *et al.* (1997). Thymocytes and RelB-dependent medullary epithelial cells provide growth-promoting and organization signals, respectively, to thymic medullary stromal cells. *Eur. J. Immunol.* **27** (6), 1392–1397.
187. Roncarolo, M.G., Yssel, H., Touraine, J.L., Betuel, H., De Vries, J.E. and Spits, H. (1988). Autoreactive T cell clones specific for class I and class II HLA antigens isolated from a human chimera. *J. Exp. Med.* **167** (5), 1523–1534.
188. Yagihashi, A., Takahashi, S., Murase, N., Starzl, T.E. and Iwaki, Y. (1995). A monoclonal anti-body (L21-6) recognizing an invariant chain expressed on the cell surface in rats with the exception of the BN ($RT1^n$): a study of tissue and strain distribution. *Transplant. Proc.* **27**, 1519–1521.
189. van Schilfgaarde, R., Hermans, P., Terpstra, J.L. and van Breda Vriesman, P.J. (1980). Role of mobile passenger lymphocytes in the rejection of renal and cardiac allografts in the rat. A passenger lymphocyte-mediated graft-versus-host reaction amplifies the host response. *Transplantation* **29** (3), 209–213.

190. Nemlander, A., Soots, A., von Willebrand, E., Husberg, B. and Hayry, P. (1982). Redistribution of renal allograft-responding leukocytes during rejection. II. Kinetics and specificity. *J. Exp. Med.* **156** (4), 1087–1100.
191. Thomson, A.W., Lu, L., Wan, Y., Qian, S., Larsen, C.P. and Starzl, T.E. (1995). Identification of donor-derived dendritic cell progenitors in bone marrow of spontaneously tolerant liver allograft recipients. *Transplantation* **60** (12), 1555–1559.
192. Thomson, A.W., Lu, L., Murase, N., Demetris, A.J., Rao, A.S. and Starzl, T.E. (1995). Microchimerism, dendritic cell progenitors and transplantation tolerance. *Stem Cells* **13** (6), 622–639.
193. Starzl, T.E., Demetris, A.J., Murase, N., Thomson, A.W., Trucco, M. and Ricordi, C. (1993). Donor cell chimerism permitted by immunosuppressive drugs: a new view of organ transplantation. *Immunol. Today* **14** (6), 326–332.
194. Adams, D.H. and Hutchinson, I.V. (1997). Microchimerism and graft tolerance: cause or effect? [comment]. *Lancet* **349** (9062), 1336–1337.
195. Burlingham, W.J., Grailer, A.P., Fechner, J.H. Jr., *et al.* (1995). Microchimerism linked to cytotoxic T lymphocyte functional unresponsiveness (clonal anergy) in a tolerant renal transplant recipient. *Transplantation* **59** (8), 1147–1155.
196. Caillat-Zucman, S., Legendre, C., Suberbielle, C. *et al.* (1994). Microchimerism frequency two to thirty years after cadaveric kidney transplantation. *Hum. Immunol.* **41** (1), 91–95.
197. Reinsmoen, N.L., McSherry, C., Chavers, B., Hertz, M.I. and Matas, A.J. (1995). Correlation of donor antigen-specific hyporeactivity with allogeneic microchimerism in kidney and lung recipients. *Pediatr. Nephrol.* **9** (Suppl.), S35–39.
198. Schlitt, H.J., Hundrieser, J., Hisanaga, M. *et al.* (1994). Patterns of donor-type microchimerism after heart transplantation. *Lancet* **343** (8911), 1469–1471.
199. Schlitt, H.J., Hundrieser, J., Ringe, B. and Pichlmayr, R. (1994). Donor-type microchimerism associated with graft rejection eight years after liver transplantation [letter]. *N. Engl. J. Med.* **330** (9), 646–647.
200. Sivasai, K.S., Alevy, Y.G., Duffy, B.F. *et al.* (1997). Peripheral blood microchimerism in human liver and renal transplant recipients: rejection despite donor-specific chimerism. *Transplantation* **64** (3), 427–432.
201. Suberbielle, C., Caillat-Zucman, S., Legendre, C. *et al.* (1994). Peripheral microchimerism in long-term cadaveric-kidney allograft recipients. *Lancet* **343** (8911), 1468–1469.
202. Matzinger, P. and Guerder, S. (1989). Does T-cell tolerance require a dedicated antigen-presenting cell? *Nature* **338** (6210), 74–76.
203. Zhang, L.I., Martin, D.R., Fung-Leung, W.P., Teh, H.S. and Miller, R.G. (1992). Peripheral deletion of mature $CD8^+$ antigen-specific T cells after in vivo exposure to male antigen. *J. Immunol.* **148** (12), 3740–3745.
204. Fu, F., Li, Y., Qian, S. *et al.* (1996). Costimulatory molecule-deficient dendritic cell progenitors (MHC class II^+, $CD80^{dim}$, $CD86^-$) prolong cardiac allograft survival in nonimmunosuppressed recipients. *Transplantation* **62** (5), 659–665.
205. Finkelman, F.D., Lees, A., Birnbaum, R., Gause, W.C. and Morris, S.C. (1996). Dendritic cells can present antigen in vivo in a tolerogenic or immunogenic fashion. *J. Immunol.* **157** (4), 1406–1414.
206. Inaba, K., Pack, M., Inaba, M., Sakuta, H., Isdell, F. and Steinman, R.M. (1997). High levels of a major histocompatibility complex II-self peptide complex on dendritic cells from the T cell areas of lymph nodes. *J. Exp. Med.* **186** (5), 665–672.
207. Saleem, M., Sawyer, G.J., Schofield, R.A., Seymour, N.D., Gustafsson, K. and Fabre, J.W. (1997). Discordant expression of major histocompatibility complex class II antigens invariant chain in interstitial dendritic cells. Implications for self-tolerance and immunity. *Transplantation* **63** (8), 1134–1138.
208. Kauffman, S.A. (1993). *The Origins of Order: Self-Organization and Selection in Evolution.* Oxford University Press, Oxford.
209. Hill, A.V., Yates, S.N., Allsopp, C.E. *et al.* (1994). Human leukocyte antigens and natural selection by malaria. *Phil. Trans. R. Soc. Lond. B. Biol. Sci.* **346** (1317), 379–385.
210. Klein, J. and O'Huigin, C. (1994). MHC polymorphism and parasites. *Phil. Trans. R. Soc. Lond. B. Biol. Sci.* **346** (1317), 351–357; discussion, 357–358.
211. Coutinho, A. (1989). Beyond clonal selection and network. *Immunol. Rev.* **110**, 63–87.

212. Chen-Woan, M., Delaney, C.P., Fournier, V. *et al.* (1995). A new protocol for the propagation of dendritic cells from rat bone marrow using recombinant GM-CSF, and their quantification using the mAb OX-62. *J. Immunol. Methods* **178** (2), 157–171.
213. Chen-Woan, M., Delaney, C.P., Fournier, V. *et al.* (1996). In vitro characterization of rat bone marrow-derived dendritic cells and their precursors. *J. Leukocyte Biol.* **59** (2), 196–207.
214. Beschorner, W.E. and Armas, O.A. (1991). Loss of medullary dendritic cells in the thymus after cyclosporine and irradiation. *Cell Immunol.* **132** (2), 505–514.

CHAPTER 21
Dendritic Cells in Autoimmunity

H.A. Drexhage, F.G.A. Delemarre, K. Radosevic and P.J.M. Leenen
Department of Immunology, Faculty of Medicine, Erasmus University Rotterdam, The Netherlands

INTRODUCTION

One of the important functions of the immune system is the discrimination between 'self' and 'nonself'. The self needs to be protected, whereas the nonself must be eliminated or ignored. Currently, the distinction between self and nonself is considered to involve a series of complicated and multistep interactions between various cells of the immune system, most notably interactions between dendritic cells (DC), macrophages, B cells and T cells.

Under certain circumstances the cells of the immune system build an immune reaction toward self, in other words 'immune tolerance is broken' and 'autoimmunity' is the result. Autoimmunity per se is not always harmful and sometimes is even desirable (see below). However, in conditions in which the immune reaction is so aberrantly and vigorously self-directed that pathological damage is inflicted on tissues, so-called 'autoimmune diseases' are the result.

The major criteria in the definition of an 'autoimmune disease' are:

1. The presence of IgG autoantibodies and/or autoreactive T lymphocytes specific for antigens of the affected organ or organ systems; this presence correlates to functional and/or morphological lesions of the affected organ or organ systems.
2. The ability to induce these functional and/or morphological lesions in the organs or organ systems by the transfer of disease-related IgG autoantibodies and/or autoreactive T lymphocytes.

There are many pathological conditions fullfilling these criteria and they are generally divided into two main categories: the 'organ-specific' and the 'systemic' autoimmune diseases.

In organ-specific autoimmune diseases, target antigens are generally confined to one organ or organ system. Peculiarly in the majority of organ-specific autoimmune diseases, target antigens are of neuroendocrine character, and hence involve organs or organ systems such as the thyroid; the islets of Langerhans; the intrinsic-factor producing gastric parietal cells; the steroid-producing cells of the adrenal, ovary, and testis;

Dendritic Cells: Biology and Clinical Applications
ISBN 0-12-455860-7

the pituitary; the neuromuscular junction; and the myelin-sheets in the central nervous system. The most extensively studied and best-characterized organ-specific autoimmune diseases are listed in Table 1 and include disorders such as Hashimoto's autoimmune thyroiditis, primary thyroid atrophy, Graves' disease, pernicious anemia, Addison's disease and type 1 diabetes mellitus (autoimmune insulitis).

In the systemic autoimmune diseases, target antigens are, in general, widely distributed in the body, such as nuclear components, collagen components, and IgG itself. Hallmarks of the systemic autoimmune diseases are vasculitis and arthritis. Prototypes are systemic lupus erythematosus (SLE) and rheumatoid arthritis (RA) (Table 1).

Studies on the etiology and pathogenesis of the various autoimmune diseases is restricted in humans, predominantly owing to limited availability of study material. Moreover, autoimmune diseases often show long nonclinical prodromal phases, which can hardly be studied in the human since clinical signs and symptoms are still absent. Over the past 30 years, various inbred animal models of spontaneously occurring variants of the human autoimmune diseases have become available (Table 1). These models have greatly contributed to the knowledge on the etiopathogenesis of the various autoimmune diseases, most notably on the very early prodromal phases. Of note is the fact that the spontaneously occurring animal models of organ-specific autoimmune disease never show systemic autoimmunity, but often have more than one organ-specific autoimmune disease. Conversely, models of systemic autoimmunity never show organ-specific autoimmune disease. This strongly suggests a different etiopathogenetic mechanism for organ-specific versus systemic autoimmune diseases. Of note also is that a spontaneously occurring inbred animal model of RA is lacking, and that the two spontaneously occurring inbred animal models for SLE never show the severe form of destructive arthritis which is characteristic of RA. This suggests that the etiopathogenesis of SLE and RA are different too, and that environmental factors play a prominent role in the development of RA. Indeed, animal models of RA often involve the experimental induction of the disease via immunizations with mycobacteria, anaerobic bacteria, or derived antigens, albeit in animals with a genetic susceptibility for the disease, such as the Lewis rat and the SJL mouse (Table 1).

Apart from the inbred animal models of spontaneously occurring autoimmune diseases there are animal models in which the autoimmune damage to the target tissue is induced by an artificial immunization with the target antigen in adjuvants. This results in a so-called experimental allergic (EA) autoimmune disease, such as EA thyroiditis, EA encephalitis, EA myocarditis, and EA arthritis. Although often self-limiting diseases, the EA models have proved to be useful in studies on the mechanisms of immune destruction (effector phases) of the autoimmune diseases. Experimental models in which autoreactive T cells and/or autoantibodies are transferred to animal recipients have also greatly expanded our knowledge on the effector phases of the diseases.

Taken together, studies over the past 20 years both in patients and various animal models have culminated in the awareness that autoimmune diseases must be regarded as largely autoantigen-driven, excessive immune responses toward self. Regarding their etiopathogenesis, autoimmune diseases are based on unfortunate combinations of various genetic and environmental factors. Multiple genes (at least more than 10) are involved in the aberrant immune response toward self; first of all the genes of the MHC region, but also genes involved in the regulation of the metabolism of the target tissue, e.g. the insulin gene in type 1 diabetes, and genes involved in a general regulation

Table 1. Characteristic autoimmune diseases and animal models

Disease	Autoantigens	Result autoantibodies/T cells	Symptoms	Animal models		
					Experimental (allergic)	
				Spontaneous	Antigen	Animal
Hashimoto's thyroiditis	Thyroperoxidase (TPO) Thyroglobulin (Tg)	ADCC and T_H1-mediated thyrocyte destruction	Goiter, followed by thyroid failure	BB rat NOD mouse OS chicken	Tg in FCA	Normal rats and rabbits
Primary hypothyroidism	TSH receptor (TSH-R)	Antibodies blocking the TSH-R	Hypothyroidism and thyroid atrophy	None	TSH-R	Balb-c mouse
Graves' disease	TSH-R	Antibodies stimulating the TSH-R	Goiter and hyperthyroidism	None	TSH-R$^+$, MHC class II$^+$ fibroblasts	AKR/N mouse
Type 1 diabetes	Insulin GAD IA-2	T_H1-mediated destruction of the β cells	Hyperglycemia	BB rat NOD mouse	Streptozotocin	Normal rats and mice
Pernicious anemia	Na^+/H^+ ATPase Intrinsic factor	T_H1-mediated destruction of gastric parietal cells and neutralization of intrinsic factor by antibodies	Atrophic gastritis Anemia		Tx (3 day)	Balb/c mouse A/J mouse
Addison's disease	21-Hydroxylase 17α-Hydroxylase	T_H1-mediated destruction of steroid-producing cells	Adrenalitis and oöphoritis		Tx (3 day)	Balb/c mouse A/J mouse
SLE	dsDNA other nucleoproteins	Antigen–antibody reaction	Skin Mild arthritis Vasculitis Glomerulonephritis	MRL/lpr mouse NZW/NZB mouse		
RA	IgG Collagen type II	1. Excessive lymphoid tissue development in synovium (pannus formation) 2. Excessive cytokine and rheumatoid factor production in pannus 3. Destruction of cartilage/bone	Severe arthritis with deformations	None	Mycobacteria Anaerobic bacteria	Lewis rat SJL mouse

GAD, glutamic acid decarboxylase; IA-2, tyrosine phosphatase; Tx, 3-day thymectomy model (see text); FCA, Freund's complete adjuvant; ADCC, antibody-dependent cell-mediated cytotoxicity.

of the immune system, e.g. the CTLA-4 gene (Todd and Farrall, 1996). However, genetic polymorphisms are not the whole story; for example, monozygotic twin studies in type 1 diabetes have shown a concordance rate of, at best, 40–50% between twins. This shows the additional importance of environmental eliciting factors. In particular, microbial agents of the gut or lung environment (e.g. anaerobic bacteria, *Yersinia enterocolitica*, Cocksackie virus) and environmental substances damaging to the target tissue (e.g. iodine for thyrocytes, streptozotocin for β cells, and UV light for skin epithelial cells) and/or the immune system are involved.

Although detailed mechanisms are far from clear for the individual autoimmune diseases, some generalizations can be made. The odds are in favor of the following scenarios.

1. The organ-specific autoimmune diseases characterized by organ failure are mainly due to T_H1-mediated target cell destruction. Abnormalities in the growth and metabolism of the organ or organ system prior to autosensitization are the driving force for T cell autosensitization to the various organ-specific antigens. For a full-blown autoimmune disease to develop, additional immunodysregulations are a prerequisite.
2. The SLE-like diseases are mainly due to antigen–antibody complex reactions, in which the antigens are nuclear components and the autoantibodies the result of an abnormal B cell hyperplasia in an immunodysregulated individual.
3. RA is an excessive T and B cell-mediated reaction toward environmental microbial antigens of the gut and/or lung environment. These antigens are spread to and trapped in the joints, where hypersensitization is continued in a locally formed lymphoid tissue. In this hypersensitization the immune reaction is amplified and spread to autoantigens of the joint, such as collagen type II and IgG itself.

Recent research indicates a prime role for dendritic cells in the pathogenesis of the various autoimmune diseases.

PATHOGENESIS AND IMMUNODYSREGULATION IN AUTOIMMUNITY

Autorecognition is the Normal Rule. To Ignore It or Not to Ignore It, That is the Question

The problem of how the immune system copes with its inherent potential for autosensitization was first perceived by Paul Ehrlich almost 100 years ago, but it lay dormant for decades because the scientific community was unable to accept Ehrlich's idea, now universally embraced, that the formation of immune receptors precedes any contact with their corresponding antigens. It was Burnet's idea that the thymus has a key role in eliminating anti-self T cells; however, his view that such autoreactive T cells were abnormal mutants (forbidden clones) has been disproved.

T cells mature in the thymus from prothymocytes to naive T cells with high-affinity receptors to foreign antigens. Since T cell receptor (TCR) rearrangement is random, self-reactive T cells are generated in this process. For these T cells to avoid apoptosis (the normal death program), the binding affinity of the TCR for peptide–MHC complexes displayed on the thymic epithelial cortical cells must be sufficient to transduce intracellular signals that terminate the normal operating cell death program. This process is called positive selection. It is of note that the peptides used for positive selection are thus 'self', at least for the thymus environment, and that in positive selection autoreactive T cells are selected with sufficient but not too high affinity for a MHC–autopeptide complex (Ignatowicz *et al.*, 1996). After generation, the vast majority of T cells which still express TCR with a relatively too high affinity for self-peptide–MHC complexes are deleted via an active induction of apoptosis during further maturation in the thymus. This process is called 'clonal deletion' or 'negative selection'. Dendritic cells (DC) which occur in large numbers in the medulla and at the cortico-medullary junction of the thymus are major players in clonal deletion and curiously express certain self-antigens (e.g. insulin; Vafiadis *et al.*, 1997). Interestingly in view of the different roles of thymus epithelial cells (positive selection) and thymus DC (negative selection), autoantigen handling is also different between thymic DC and cortical thymus epithelial cells (Hadzija *et al.*, 1991).

What finally emerges from the thymus is a population of naive $CD4^+$ and $CD8^+$ T cells that have been selected by virtue of the ability of their receptors to bind to self with an affinity between two extremes. These T cells are polyreactive, i.e. they bind not only to self-peptide–MHC complexes but also to foreign peptide–MHC complexes, among which there are configurations with a higher affinity for the T cell receptor than self-peptide–MHC complexes. The protective function of the T cell limb of the immune system thus depends on deviations from self in the short foreign peptide contained within the groove of the MHC molecule (Schwartz, 1996).

A similar mechanism of selection probably exists for self-reactive B cells in the bone marrow. However, this mechanism is not as well studied as clonal T cell selection in the thymus; nevertheless, it is highly likely that, like T cells, B cells are inherently anti-self. In normal mice the frequency of naive B cells with the potential to secrete IgM anti-DNA antibodies is 10^{-3} to 10^{-2}, and the frequency of those with the capacity to produce autoantibodies against a pool of other intracellular antigens is about 10^{-1}. This very high frequency suggests that a significant fraction of preimmune B cells is anti-self (Schwartz, 1996). A large fraction of circulating B cells from normal humans can also produce autoantibodies when captured as hybridomas, immortalized *in vitro* by Epstein–Barr virus, or cultured in the presence of supernatants from activated T cells. These B cells are most likely the source of so-called natural autoantibodies, which are IgM low-affinity antibodies with the capacity to bind to several different antigens, including nuclear and cytoplasmic constituents, insulin and IgG (rheumatoid factor). All these results suggest that B cells, like their T cell counterparts, may undergo an initial round of selection in which their ability to bind to self-antigens rescues them from apoptosis. The fact that unmutated V genes encode human natural autoantibodies supports the concept that the potential for self-reactivity in immunoglobulins is a property of the germline (Schwartz, 1996).

Instead of viewing naturally occurring autoreactive T cells and autoantibodies as an unwanted stage in the development of our immune repertoire from which we later may recruit forces for our defense system, it is also possible that these autoreactive T cells and autoantibodies play a natural role in homeostasis (e.g. via a neuroendocrine idiotype–anti-idiotype network), in morphogenesis, and in the disposal and removal of effete body components (Mooij and Drexhage, 1993). In this context it is also worthy of note that clonal deletion of T and B cells with high-affinity receptors for endocrine autoantigenic targets is incomplete, as T and B cells with a specificity for thyroglobulin and insulin can easily be found in the circulation (Mooij and Drexhage, 1993). This is partly explained by the fact that not all self-antigens are expressed at sufficient level in the thymus and bone marrow. Some self-antigens, such as ocular lens antigens, only are present in immune-privileged sites and are thus sequestered from the immune system. Other self-antigens, such as sperm antigens, are only expressed during late fetal life or in adult life. Some autoantigens probably never reach the thymus or bone marrow and are never expressed there. This particularly applies to cryptic epitopes. Cryptic epitopes are *de novo* expressed epitopes on self-antigens that are caused by changes in the antigen due to, for instance, an inflammatory process.

What mechanism holds the circulating and thymus-escaped potentially autoreactive T cells in abeyance? A key element for this has turned out to be the silencing of these cells by lack of costimulatory signals. Transgenic animal studies (von Herrath and Holz, 1997) have shown that, even when such potentially autoreactive naive T cells meet their corresponding autoantigen, either as peptides in the context of appropriate MHC molecules on target cells or as soluble molecules, they remain dormant ('ignorant') and do not show clonal expansion, differentiation, and/or receptor affinity maturation. To break this stage of ignorance, costimulatory signals such as are provided by CD80, CD86, and CD40 are essential.

DC Break the State of Ignorance and Trigger the Autoimmune Response by Providing Costimulatory Signals for Autoreactive Naive T Cells

In the early 1980s it was found that target cells in organ-specific autoimmune diseases such as Hashimoto's thyroiditis and Graves' disease aberrantly express MHC class II molecules, and the concept was developed that such aberrant expression represented an initial event for the development of disease and the initial trigger for autoreactive naive T cell clones to expand and mature (Bottazzo *et al.*, 1985). Indeed, MHC class II-positive thyrocytes and β cells are capable of presenting autoantigens to T cells and inducing clonal expansion of autoreactive T cells, but the proviso for this turned out to be that the T cells were no longer in their naive state. In keeping with such a view were experiments using the BB rat and NOD mouse models, which showed that MHC class II expression by thyrocytes and β cells (if occurring at all) is a rather late phenomenon in the autoimmune process, occurring in time after T cell autosensitization and local T cell infiltration (Kabel *et al.*, 1987; Weringer and Like, 1988; Voorbij *et al.*, 1990b; Lo *et al.*, 1993). In particular, cytokines produced by autosensitized memory T cells, such as IFN-γ and TNF-α trigger the endocrine cells to express MHC class II molecules. Hence MHC class II expression by target cells is a late phenomenon and the consequence rather than the cause of the autoimmune process. Importantly, costimulatory molecules are hardly expressed by endocrine cells in endocrine autoimmune disease (Tandon *et al.*, 1994), lending further support to a view that target cells do not act as antigen-presenting cells (APC) early in the autoimmune process. At present the generally held view is that the aberrant expression of MHC class II provides anergic signals to the already begun and excessive autoimmune response. In conditions where sufficient costimulation is provided by the MHC class II-positive endocrine cells, the autoimmune response may be perpetuated and aggravated. Of note is here the experiment of Shimojo *et al.* (1996), showing that injection with fibroblasts transgenically expressing

MHC class II and TSH-R may drive an autoimmune response in mice resulting in the production of TSH-R antibodies and experimental Graves' disease (see also Table 1).

However, the best candidate to break the state of ignorance for the naturally occurring repertoire of autoreactive naive T cells is the DC. The cell is known for its naturally high expression of costimulatory molecules and its superb ability to trigger naive T cells, such as those specific for thyroid antigens which clonally expand and mature upon stimulation by DC (Iwai *et al.*, 1989). Experimental data suggesting that DC may trigger naive autoreactive T cells was first obtained in immunohistological studies on early autoimmune lesions: in the thyroid and pancreas of the BB rat, DC accumulate in the target tissue before autosensitization, i.e. before the swelling of the draining lymph nodes, the T cell proliferation and plasma cell development in these nodes, and the appearance of autoantibodies in the circulation (Kabel *et al.* 1987; Voorbij *et al.*, 1990b). These immunohistological observations have been confirmed amply for the insulitis and thyroiditis processes in the NOD mouse (Lo *et al.*, 1993; Jansen *et al.*, 1994; Many *et al.*, 1995) and the thyroiditis of the OS chicken (Hala *et al.*, 1996). Moreover, it has been shown that such DC contain relevant autoantigens, and also appear in the central lymphoid system (Shimizu *et al.*, 1995). The important role of DC in the development of autoimmune diseases was further suggested by the observation that GM-CSF treatment (a potent activator of DC) of breast cancer patients already positive for TPO-Abs elicits or aggravates the autoimmune thyroiditis in these patients (Hoekman *et al.*, 1991). Mercuric chloride ($HgCl_2$) treatment of BN rats—known to induce autoimmunity in these animals—results in accumulation of $HgCl_2$ in DC (Warfvinghe *et al.*, 1994). More importantly, it has also been shown that transfer of autoantigen-pulsed DC rather than autoantigen-pulsed Mϕ induces autoimmunity in experimental animals (Knight *et al.*, 1988; Gautam and Glynn, 1989). Furthermore the prevention of the infiltration of monocyte-derived cells blocks the development of autoimmunity (Hutchings *et al.*, 1990).

Although there is circumstantial evidence that it is the APC, in particular the DC, that initially breaks the state of ignorance of the autoreactive naive T cells (Nossal *et al.*, 1992), it does not mean that such a process is pathological per se and that the later developing autoimmune response is out of control. For an uncontrolled, excessive immune reaction toward self, additional defects in the immunoregulatory machinery such as defects in T cell deletion or deficiencies in regulator or suppressor T cells are required (see below). Recent data indicate that such immunoregulatory defects may also be induced by abnormal DC or macrophage (Mϕ) function, placing the cells not only at the triggering point of the autoimmune reaction but also in the center of the subsequent faulty immunoregulation leading to the generation of excessive numbers of autoreactive effector T cells and IgG autoantibodies (see below). After such a stage of excessive generation of autoreactive effector T cells and IgG autoantibodies, yet other factors—at least in the thyroid disease of the OS chicken—determine whether or not a full-blown autoimmune disease will develop. A prerequisite for overt thyroid failure in this bird is a susceptibility of the target, the thyrocyte, for an autoimmune attack by the generated autoreactive T cells and IgG autoantibodies. Experiments have shown that this susceptibility factor is genetically determined, and it has been speculated that this factor might be an abnormal (virally-induced?) susceptibility of the thyrocytes for the cytokines produced by the autoreactive immune cells after infiltration in the target tissue (Wick *et al.*, 1993). The EA and transfer models of the various autoimmune diseases indicate that local DC are likely to be involved in such effector phases prior to overt disease and the susceptibility of the target cells for cytokines. Besides the direct cytotoxic effects of immune cells ($CD8^+$ cytotoxic T cells, NK cells, Mϕ) and of autoantibodies on target cells in effector phases, activated autoreactive T cells are seen to communicate with autoantigen-laden local DC at the center of the lesion (see below). These latter interactions between DC and T cells are thought to result in enhanced local cytokine production, which is often by itself sufficient for target cell lysis. The milieu of local DC–T cell interactions also fosters epitope spreading and a further aggravation of the disease.

In sum, the multifactorial character of the pathogenesis of autoimmune diseases involving both environmental and genetic factors is reflected in a multistep process of disease development: first a triggering of the autoimmune response takes place in an immune system with a genetic and/or acquired defect in handling 'self'. This leads in a second phase to an uncontrolled and excessive production of autoreactive effector T cells and autoantibodies. Finally this culminates in a last phase of target or bystander cell destruction. DC are critically involved in all three phases (see below).

HETEROGENEITY OF DC IN VIEW OF THEIR ROLE IN IMMUNIZATION AND TOLERANCE INDUCTION

Heterogeneity of the DC Population

It took until the late 1970s (van Furth, 1980) before it was realized that the Langerhans cells of the skin, the interdigitating cells (IDC) in the thymus and secondary lymphoid organs, the veiled cells (VC) in the lymph, and the splenic DC formed one—though morphologically heterogeneous—cell system of superb antigen-presenting accessory cells (APC). The term 'dendritic' was introduced to refer to the cells of this cellular system (although they are often 'veiled'), and the cells shared a strong expression of MHC class I and II molecules, an active motile/migratory capacity, and an active cluster behavior with T and B cells.

With regard to the origin of the cells, the cytology, the light-microscopic and ultrastructural morphology, and the enzyme histochemistry of DC/VC in skin lymph (Drexhage *et al.*, 1979a,b) and gut mucosa (Wilders *et al.*, 1983; Wilders *et al.*, 1984) showed many transitional forms between monocytes, DC/VC and macrophages. This strongly suggested a place for the cell in the spectrum of the so-called mononuclear phagocyte system, a heterogeneous cell system including cells as distinct as the osteoclast and the Kupffer cell but sharing the blood monocyte as their precursor. Undisputable proof of the monocytic origin of at least part of the DC/VC was given in the mid-1980s (Peters *et al.*, 1987; Kabel *et al.*, 1989b). Other groups of investigators, however, regarded yet unidentified bone marrow-derived precursors as lineage-specific precursors for their splenic DCs. The term dendrocytes or D cells was used to refer to the presumed specific lineage commitment of DC (Austyn, 1987). Later experiments clarified this issue, showing a heterogeneity in the DC/VC population; bone marrow cultures showed on the one hand that Birbeck granule-containing DC/VC may have a separate $CD34^+$ $CD14^-$ blood-borne precursor, but on the other hand that $CD14^+$ monocytes do give rise to $CD1a^+$ but Birbeck granule-negative DC (Caux *et al.*, 1995). The DC/VC stage may not be the end stage of development. We earlier showed that prototypic $CD1a^+$ DC isolated from human bronchoalveolar lavages (Plate 21.1) and monocyte-derived DC (Delemarre *et al.*, 1995a) are able to convert into ruffled, acid phosphatase-positive macrophage-like cells after 1 week of coculture with lipopolysaccharide (LPS). This further underlines the mononuclear phagocyte character of at least some of the DC/VC. Such mononuclear phagocyte character also explains the recently described positivity for macrophage markers of malignant DC in histiocytosis (Kitahama *et al.*, 1996) and of diseased DCs in pemphigus foliaceus (Petzelbauer *et al.*, 1993). A further heterogeneity of the DC system became apparent recently in experiments identifying not a myeloid cell but an early thymic lymphocyte as the precursor of the $CD8\alpha^+$ mouse dendritic cells in the thymus and periphery, the so-called lymphoid DC (Wu and Shortman, 1996).

In view of the heterogeneity of the DC population and the overlap with monocytes/macrophages, it is not surprising that a single separate marker for the DC could not be found despite extensive research. In our hands, combinations of markers have been useful for immunohistochemical identification of DC in human and animal autoimmune diseases, such as the combination of weak to absent positivity for acid phosphatase (if present in a juxtanuclear spot), MHC class II expression, veils/dendritic protrusions, and/or positivity for CD1a, RFD1, L25, S100 in the human, the marker CD11c (N418) and DEC205 (NLDC-145) in the mouse, and the marker Ox-62 in the rat.

Regardless of the heterogeneity of the DC-system, some cells require the same cytokines for their generation, i.e. IL-4, TNF-α and Flt-3 ligand. It is also noteworthy that various hormones such as triiodothyronine (T3) (Mooij *et al.*, 1994), 1,25-dihydroxyvitamin D3 (Canning *et al.*, 1997), follicle-stimulating hormone (FSH), estrogens, and thymic hormones (Hoek *et al.*, 1997), act as regulatory cofactors in such differentiation. Whereas monocytes and macrophages are established sources of cytokines such as interleukin-1 (IL-1), IL-6, and TNF-α, mature human DC have been shown to produce the mRNAs for these cytokines with only a limited production of the peptides (Witmer and Steinman, 1984; Vakkila *et al.*, 1990; Kamperdijk *et al.*, 1994). In general, human DCs are regarded as poor producers of cytokines, and their excellent APC function probably lies in their migratory capacity, their ability to form clusters with T cells via adhesion molecules, and their high constitutive expression of costimulatory molecules such as CD80 and CD86. It is as yet unresolved whether the human DC need other cytokine-producing accessory cells to guide the clonal expansion of naive T cells in a certain direction of development. IL-12 is known to be produced by monocytes and macrophages, and this cytokine is able to push the development of T cells into T_H1 cells that predominantly produce IFN-γ (Trinchieri, 1997); IL-10 (also produced by monocytes and macrophages) downregulates such development, but stimulates T_H2 development (Belardelli, 1995). Although there are reports that human DC can produce IL-12 (Macatonia *et al.*, 1995) and IL-10 (Kalinsky *et al.*, 1997), we (to be published) and others (Granucci *et al.*, 1994) have found that IL-12 production from immature and mature human DC is limited in comparison to that of monocytes. It has, however, become clear recently that CD40 ligation of immature and mature DC (hence contact with other cells) induces further activation of the cell, resulting in enhanced cytokine production, particularly of IL-12, and improved T cell stimulation (Sallusto *et al.*, 1995).

DC in Tolerance Induction

Although the emphasis over the past 10–20 years has been on the immunostimulatory capacity of the DC, one is now realizing that the cell is rather a regulator and conductor of the T cell orchestra than a simple stimulator. Kalinski *et al.* (1997) showed that the addition of prostaglandin E_2 (PGE_2) to GM-CSF and IL-4 in order to induce maturation of monocytes into DC resulted in a population of DC largely devoid of the CD1a marker. This population was superb in stimulating naive T cells, and it appeared that such DC were also strong producers of IL-10, inducing proliferation of T cells with a T_H2 cytokine profile. In contrast, DC in the absence of PGE_2 produced IL-12, inducing proliferation of T cells with a T_H1 cytokine profile. Marth *et al.* (1997) showed that TGF-β-producing ovalbumin-specific T cells (T_H3 cells or 'regulator cells') are generated by ovalbumin-pulsed DC in the presence of anti-IL-12 or anti-IFN-γ. The cytokines involved in stimulation of T_H3 cells could not be identified in their system, but appeared not to be IL-4. IL-10 might be involved (O'Garra *et al.*, 1997).

Tolerogenic signals can also be given by DC *in vivo*: immunization of mice with the rat monoclonal IgG2b antibody 33D1 specific for DC results in a T and B cell tolerance for rat IgG2b (Finkelman *et al.*, 1996). Such tolerance induction is avoided when 33D1 is given not in a soluble but in an aggregated form, or together with IL-1. These observations indicate that DC can present antigens in either a tolerogenic or stimulatory manner, and suggest that pro-inflammatory stimuli can convert an otherwise tolerogenic signal to a stimulatory signal. Also, the concentration of the antigen is important in the dichotomy between stimulation and suppression (Knight *et al.*, 1985). Another example of the *in vivo* tolerogenic potential of DC is the systemic immune deviation, i.e. a deficit in delayed-type hypersensitivity (DTH) reactivity, after injection of antigens into the anterior chamber of the eye. The cells that carry the deviation signal from the eye via the blood to the spleen are most likely DC from the stroma of the iris and ciliary body (Hara *et al.*, 1992).

It is of note that even in overt autoimmune diseases tolerogenic DC are around: DC isolated from the pancreas-draining lymph nodes of NOD mice with an autoimmune insulitis were able to prevent the development of diabetes upon transfer to very young (4-week-old) mice. This protection occurred via the induction of regulatory T cells (Clare-Salzler *et al.*, 1992).

An important and novel approach in the study of DC as conductors of the T cell orchestra has come from recent observations from the groups of Galy and Shortman. Galy *et al.* (1995) found that DC share with T, B, and NK cells a common lymphoid progenitor cell. Shortman and colleagues also found a heterogeneity in the DC system by identifying an early $CD4^-8^-3^-44^+25^+$ lymphocyte in the mouse thymus as the precursor of $CD8\alpha^+$ DC (the presently so-called 'lymphoid' DC as opposed to the 'myeloid' DC; Wu and Shortman, 1996). Such thymic $CD8\alpha^+$ DC—also seeding to the periphery—initially stimulate clonal T cell expansion, but upon further interaction restrict $CD4^+$ T cell responsiveness by initiating apoptosis, which is probably Fas-mediated (Suss and Shortman, 1996). Lymphoid DC restrict $CD8^+$ T cell expansion by limiting their IL-2 production (Kronin *et al.*, 1996) . Such tolerogenic thymic DC may be the explanation for the observation that cell suspensions enriched for thymic DC induce a specific peripheral T cell unresponsiveness toward myelin basic protein (MBP) and its encephalitogenic peptides in EAE (Khoury *et al.*, 1995). It is possible that for such deletional signals autoreactive T cells must re-enter the thymus. However, the homing of $CD8\alpha^+$ lymphoid DC to the periphery suggests that their tolerogenic effect can also be exerted in the secondary lymphoid organs.

In sum, DC constitute a heterogeneous group of cells, sharing a characteristic morphology (veils rather than dendrites), a strong expression of MHC and costimulatory molecules, and a capability to interact and to form clusters with T and B lymphocytes owing to their active migratory behavior. The cells, however, have various origins, i.e. a lymphoid origin (viz. an early thymus lymphocytic precursor) and a myeloid origin (viz. the $CD14^+$ monocyte and an as yet unidentified $CD34^+$ bone marrow-derived cell). Within the group of DC the Langerhans cells may form a separate lineage (Caux *et al.*, 1996; Strunk *et al.*, 1997). With regard to the monocyte-derived DC, transitional forms between the monocyte and the DC and the DC and the macrophage exist. DC are the accessory cells *par excellence*, and *the* conductors of the T-lymphocyte orchestra for both crescendos and diminuendos. The mechanisms via which the orchestra is conducted are not (fully) understood: the various types (lymphoid versus myeloid), maturation stages (monocyte–DC–macrophage), and the endocrine milieu in which the conductor has matured play a role, probably via the differing abilities of such cells to deliver apoptotic signals, cytokine signals (IL-12, IL-10), and other molecular signals (PGE_2).

DC AND THE INITIAL TRIGGERING OF THE AUTOIMMUNE RESPONSE

DC Are Recruited to Endocrine Glands Prior to Endocrine Autoimmune Sensitization

Immunohistological observations on all animal models of spontaneously occurring organ-specific autoimmune diseases have clearly shown the very early infiltration of DC—among other accessory types of macrophages—in the glands to be the eventual target. In the thyroid of the BB rat, acid phosphatase-negative, MHC class II^+ (Ox-6^+) and $Ox62^+$ dendritic-shaped cells rise in number in the gland from 8 weeks of age onward in animals on a normal iodine diet (Voorbij *et al.*, 1990b; Li *et al.*, 1993). The cells form small homotypic clusters in the interfollicular area. A reaction of the draining lymph node and the generation of anti-thyroglobulin antibody-producing plasma cells in these lymph nodes occurs shortly after the intrathyroidal DC accumulation. A high-iodine diet accelerates the early DC accumulation and the subsequent development of autoimmune thyroiditis (Mooij *et al.*, 1993a).

In the majority of NOD strains, autoimmune thyroiditis does not develop spontaneously. However, when thyrocyte necrosis is induced by radical formation a thyroid inflammatory infiltrate composed of various macrophages and DC is formed (Many *et al.*, 1995). This macrophage infiltration is followed in time by a reaction of the thyroid-draining lymph nodes, i.e. a swelling of the T cell area and the development of B lymphoid follicles, and an appearance of anti-colloid antibodies in the circulation. The ultimate result is an autoimmune thyroiditis with a strong accumulation of T and B lymphocytes in the thyroid of the NOD mouse. Also, the autoimmune thyroiditis of the OS chicken begins with an accumulation of macrophages and MHC class II^+ dendritic-shaped cells in the thyroid (Hala *et al.*, 1996).

With regard to animal models of organ-specific autoimmune diseases, other than thyroiditis, the insulitis of the BB rat also starts with an accumulation of MHC class II^+, acid phosphatase-negative dendritic-shaped cells around the islets, followed within a relatively short time by an insular infiltration with lymphocytes and $ED1^+$ and $ED3^+$ macrophages (Voorbij *et al.*, 1989; Ziegler *et al.*, 1992). The very early phases of the NOD insulitis are characterized by an infiltration with $N418^+$ ($CD11c^+$) DC, ER-$MP23^+$ histiocyte-type macrophages, and MOMA-1^+ macrophages around the islets (Jansen *et al.*, 1994; Jansen *et al.*, 1996). Shortly thereafter, peri-insular lymphocytic cuffs are formed, lymphocytes being intermingled with $N418^+$ DC and NLDC-145^+ (DEC-205^+) DC and $BM8^+$ macrophages. Particularly in the female NOD mouse, $BM8^+$ macrophages are found in the islet mass itself. It is of note that virtually all NOD females develop diabetes with significantly higher incidence than males. The macrophages and DC accumulating around the islets in NOD mice were shown to take up relevant autoantigens (Shimizu *et al.*, 1995). Pancreas-draining lymph nodes become swollen, while the DC from these lymph nodes show an enhanced cluster capability with T cells (Clare-Salzler and Mullen, 1992). When I-E molecules are transgenically expressed on primary antigen-presenting cells of the NOD (normally they lack these molecules but express a particular I-A complex consisting of $\alpha^{d}\beta^{g7}$) there is alleviation of insulitis and decrease of subsequent diabetes incidence (Pilstrom and Bohme, 1997). It is also of interest to note that fish oil-enriched diets result in the decrease of insulitis in the low-dose streptozotocin model (Linn *et al.*, 1989) by interfering with the influx of dendritic cells in the islets.

All in all, the mode of histological events in all animal models of spontaneously occurring endocrine autoimmune diseases points in the direction of an abnormal accumulation of APC, including many DC in the target-glands-to-be before any involvement of T or B cells. Also, in human organ-specific autoimmune diseases numerous DC can be found in the diseased glands. However, since we are dealing in human pathology specimens with end stages of the disease, nothing can be concluded about the initial phases of disease, prior to autoantibody production and T cell infiltration. In the diseased human endocrine tissues of Graves' disease, Hashimoto's thyroiditis (Kabel *et al.*, 1988), and type 1 diabetes (Jansen *et al.*, 1993), DC are found with progression of disease first as single, isolated cells between the parenchymal cells, then as cells in small clusters with T and B lymphocytes, and finally as IDC between T cells in the T cell areas of a locally formed lymphoid tissue (see also Chapter 6). Wherever this lymphoid tissue has developed, high endothelial venules (HEVs) are present and positive for various adhesion molecules that are characteristic for HEVs (Kabel *et al.*, 1989a; Faveeuw *et al.*, 1994). These HEVs function in the homing of lymphocytes and monocytes to the diseased endocrine glands (Kabel *et al.*, 1990). The adhesion molecules present on the HEVs can often also be found on the DC and IDC in the glands (Marazuela *et al.*, 1994), underlining the function of the cells as interactors with T and B lymphocytes.

Why Do DC Accumulate in Endocrine Glands prior to Autosensitization?

There are several explanations for the early accumulation of DC in the thyroid and around the islets in the animal models of spontaneously occurring endocrine autoimmune diseases, viz. early vascular abnormalities, an early necrosis of target-cells-to-be, and metabolic or growth disturbances of target-cells-to-be (Fig. 2).

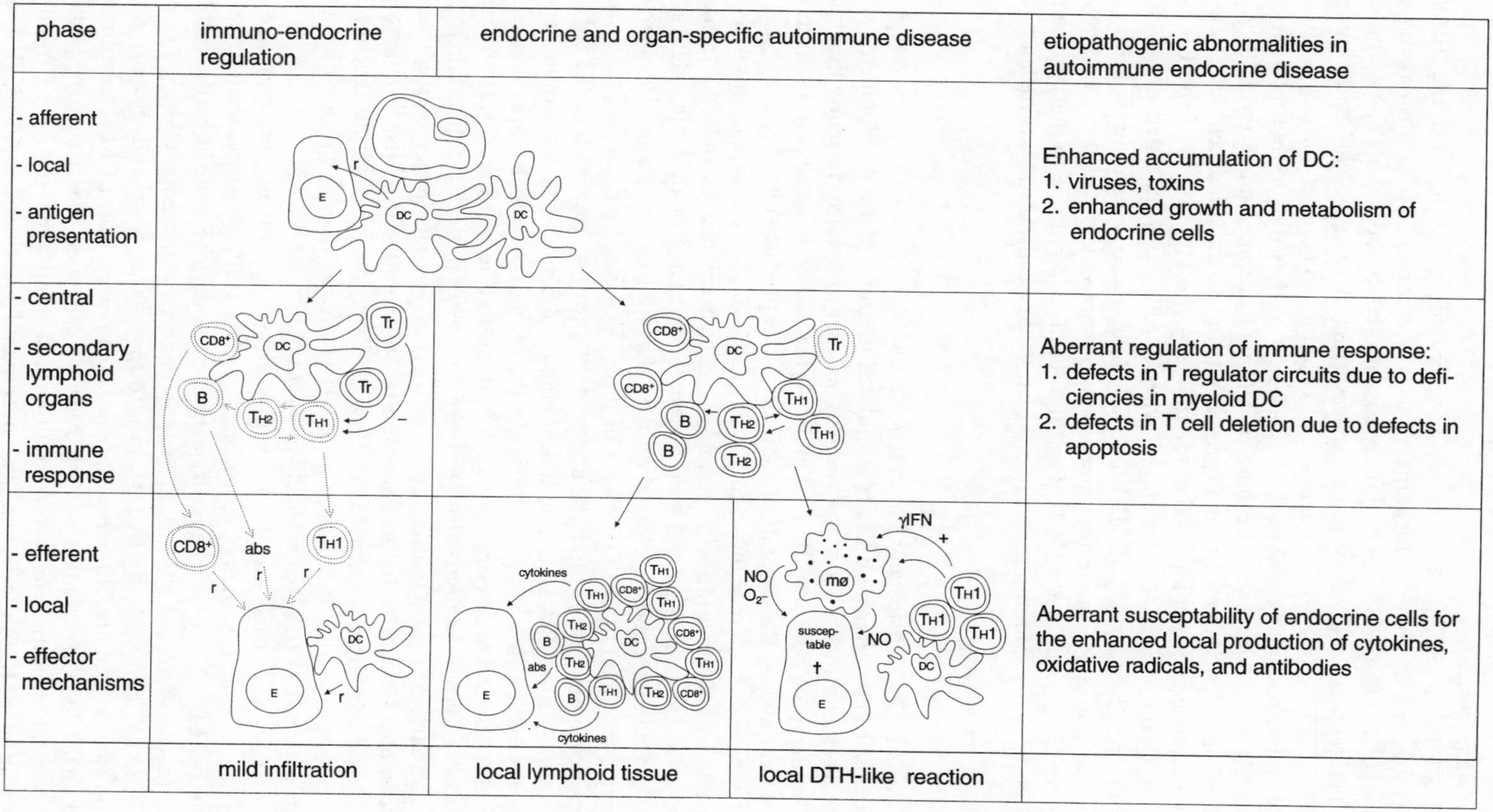

phase	immuno-endocrine regulation	endocrine and organ-specific autoimmune disease		etiopathogenic abnormalities in autoimmune endocrine disease
- afferent - local - antigen presentation	E, DC, r, DC			Enhanced accumulation of DC: 1. viruses, toxins 2. enhanced growth and metabolism of endocrine cells
- central - secondary lymphoid organs - immune response	CD8+, DC, Tr, Tr, B, TH2, TH1, –	CD8+, CD8+, DC, Tr, TH1, B, TH2, TH1, B, TH2		Aberrant regulation of immune response: 1. defects in T regulator circuits due to deficiencies in myeloid DC 2. defects in T cell deletion due to defects in apoptosis
- efferent - local - effector mechanisms	CD8+, abs, TH1, r, r, r, E, DC, r	cytokines, TH1, CD8+, TH1, TH1, TH2, DC, CD8+, B, TH2, TH1, abs, E, B, TH1, TH2, CD8+, cytokines	γIFN, +, NO, O_2^-, mø, suscep-table, †, E, NO, TH1, TH1, TH1, DC	Aberrant susceptability of endocrine cells for the enhanced local production of cytokines, oxidative radicals, and antibodies
	mild infiltration	local lymphoid tissue	local DTH-like reaction	

Fig. 2. The different phases of an immunoendocrine regulatory reaction and of an endocrine (or organ-specific) autoimmune disease. The various etiopathogenic mechanisms leading to disease are also listed. E = endocrine cell; DC = dendritic cell; r = regulation; Tr = T regulator cell; B = B cell; abs = autoantibodies; Mϕ = macrophage; – = downregulation; + = stimulation. For further explanation see text.

Early Vascular Abnormalities

Abnormalities of the pancreatic blood vessels have been described for both the BB rat and the NOD mouse. An abnormal leakiness was found for the BB rat insular blood vessels (Manjo *et al.*, 1987), whereas NOD mouse insular blood vessels show abnormally large periductular and perivascular spaces (Jansen *et al.*, 1994) with higher amounts of connective-tissue components such as laminin (Savino *et al.*, 1993). However, we were unable to detect an abnormal expression of ICAM-1 on thyroidal blood vessels in the BB rat before or at the time of DC infiltration (Simons *et al.*, 1998). Similar studies on adhesion molecule expression prior to immune cell infiltration have not been reported to our knowledge for the early insular process of the BB rat and that of the NOD mouse. At later stages, when T cells have infiltrated or when a local lymphoid tissue has developed, HEV-like blood vessels are present in both BB rat and NOD mouse and are positive for these adhesion molecules (Kabel *et al.*, 1989a; Hanninen *et al.*, 1993; Linn *et al.*, 1994). This situation is comparable to that normally encountered in human autoimmune specimens of full-blown disease (Marazuela *et al.*, 1994).

An Early Necrosis of the Autoimmune Target-Cells-to-Be

During iodine deficiency, thyroid cells are stimulated to grow (goiter development) and to produce higher quantities of oxidative radicals in order to oxidize efficiently the trace amounts of iodine to be built into thyroglobulin. When iodine is subsequently given in large amounts in the diet, the amount of iodine radicals produced by the thyrocytes is so high that the cells die (Toussaint-Demylle *et al.*, 1990). Such thyrocyte necrosis is followed by a local inflammation with various types of macrophages and DC. In fact, this process of thyrocyte necrosis leads to a desired shrinkage of the iodine-deficient goiter, while the cellular debris is cleared by the infiltrating macrophages. In normal, nonautoimmune-prone animals this process of goiter shrinkage has no further consequences. In autoimmune-prone animals, however, the necrosis process and the subsequent infiltration with APC is the initiating factor for the later development of autoimmune thyroiditis (Many *et al.*, 1995). In the human and in the BB rat, iodine intoxication has also been described as an initiating and accelerating factor for the development of autoimmune thyroiditis (Braverman, 1990): in the BB rat, iodine overload leads to an early enhanced infiltration of the thyroid with DC (Mooij *et al.*, 1993b).

Parallels can also be drawn for the initiation of autoimmune insulitis. Streptozotocin—a β cell toxic substance—is able to initiate a β cell-specific autoimmune reaction in autoimmune-prone animals (Cockfield *et al.*, 1989). However, whether an enhanced DC infiltration is involved in this toxic model is as yet unknown.

Not only toxins lead to early target cell necrosis; viruses or viral antigens may also be involved. When the nucleoprotein (NP) or glycoprotein (GP) of lymphocytic choriomeningitis virus (LCMV) is transgenically expressed under the control of the insulin promoter in mouse β cells, they start to express these viral proteins (Oldstone *et al.*, 1991; Ohashi *et al.*, 1991). However, tolerance to these viral proteins does exist since they are expressed in fetal life. But when the mice are infected with LCMV, tolerance is broken and $CD8^+$ LCMV-specific cytotoxic cells are generated that attack the β cells. The relatively small necrotic effect—not resulting in a total β cell loss—is followed in time by a peri-insular DC infiltration in these mice (von Herrath and Holz, 1997). These

DC initiate a β cell-specific autoimmune cascade with an appearance similar to the wild-type autoimmune insulitis of the NOD mouse (von Herrath *et al.*, 1997). This model makes it possible to envisage that any β cell-tropic virus could initiate an insulitis particularly in autoimmune-prone individuals, even when such a virus is hardly β cell-cytotoxic on its own. Interestingly, very early treatment with CD8 antibodies (at 4–6 weeks of age) has been shown to prevent the development of type 1 diabetes in both the BB rat and the NOD mouse (Groen, 1996; Wang *et al.*, 1996). On histology, only a few $CD8^+$ lymphocytes can be seen in the islets of these very young animals.

Metabolic and Growth Disturbances of the Target-Gland-to-Be

It is important to realize that histiocytes and DCs are in fact a normal component of various tissues, including the endocrine glands (Hoek *et al.*, 1997). The cells are present in relatively low numbers in the thyroid and in the islets (Kabel *et al.*, 1988; Voorbij *et al.*, 1989; Lo *et al.*, 1993; Maile and Merker, 1995), and even in relatively high numbers in the normal anterior pituitary (called folliculo-stellate cells) (Allaerts *et al.*, 1996) and in the ovary and testis (Hoek *et al.*, 1997). Upon isolation, pituitary DC and also splenic DC are able to downregulate the growth and hormone production of pituitary and thyroid endocrine cells *in vitro* (Allaerts *et al.*, 1996; Simons *et al.*, 1997). They exert such endocrine regulatory function via short clustering interactions with the endocrine cells while delivering cytokine signals such as IL-1β and IL-6 signals (to be published). Also *in vivo* there is indication of the endocrine regulatory role of monocyte-derived cells in, for example, the islets of Langerhans. Prevention of monocyte infiltration into islets by depletion experiments in a transgenic mouse model of diabetes resulted in a slight but consistent rise in the proliferation of ductal and islet cells (Gu *et al.*, 1995). It is thus possible that the very early accumulation of DC in endocrine tissues that are the later targets of an autoimmune response could be the consequence of an early metabolic or growth disturbance of the endocrine cells. Indeed, numerous reports show that BB rat thyroids (Simons *et al.*, 1998), OS chicken thyroids (Sundick, 1989), BB rat islets (Bone *et al.*, 1997), NOD mouse islets (Homo-Delarche and Boitard, 1996), and NOD mouse salivary glands (Robinson *et al.*, 1996) are inherently abnormal in their proliferation potential as well as in their hormone or oxidative radical production at the time of early DC accumulation. Such metabolic and growth abnormalities are also present in the islets and salivary glands of NOD-SCID mice showing that T and B lymphocytes can be ruled out as initiators of such early glandular abnormalities. It is likely that the growth and metabolic abnormalities of the endocrine glands at the time of or prior to DC influx also have their repercussions for *de novo* autoantigen expression (Ihm *et al.*, 1991).

This mechanism of early DC infiltration for purposes of endocrine regulation also explains the mild thyroid autoimmune response occurring in iodine-deficient humans and rats (Wilders *et al.*, 1990; Bretzel *et al.*, 1990; Mooij *et al.*, 1993b). When iodine-deficient goiter develops in both humans and rats, DC start to infiltrate the goitrous gland (Wilders-Truschnig, 1989; Mooij *et al.*, 1993b) presumably to downregulate the enhanced growth and oxidative radical metabolism of the iodine-deficient thyrocytes. Such infiltration (Fig. 3) results in rats in a relatively mild production of anti-colloid antibodies (Fig. 4) and a relatively mild infiltration with single, isolated lymphocytes as compared to the severe infiltration of autoimmune-prone individuals and animals

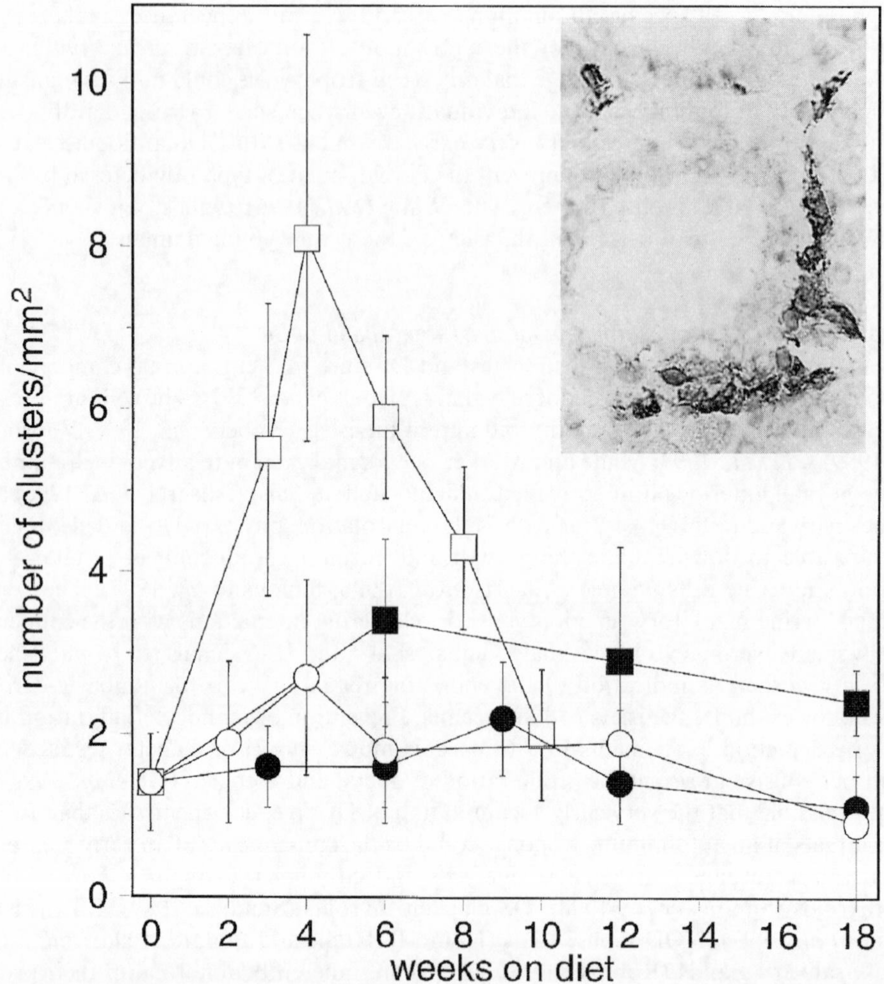

Fig. 3. The photomicrograph shows an enhanced infiltration of MHC class II⁺ dendritic cells (black) around a thyroid follicle of a Wistar rat kept on an iodine-deficient diet. The infiltrated dendritic cells locally form homotypic clusters. The figure represents the number of dendritic cell clusters/mm² surface section of thyroids of Wistar rats kept for up to 18 weeks (commencing at 3 weeks of age; horizontal axis) on various diets (□, severely iodine-deficient diet; ■, mildly iodine-deficient diet; ○, normal diet; ●, diet with excess iodine; for details see Mooij *et al.*, 1993b). Means ± standard deviations are given. Note that in iodine deficiency homotypic clustering as well as infiltration of DC (not shown) are enhanced in the Wistar thyroid, particularly 4 weeks after the introduction of the severely iodine-deficient diet.

(Mooij *et al.*, 1993b). Apparently other abnormalities in immunoregulation are required for an excessive anti-colloid antibody production (see below) to follow such initial DC infiltration. Indeed, an iodine deficiency state in the autoimmune-prone BB rat leads to an acceleration and aggravation of the autoimmune thyroiditis process as compared to the process in the the iodine-sufficient BB rat (unpublished observations).

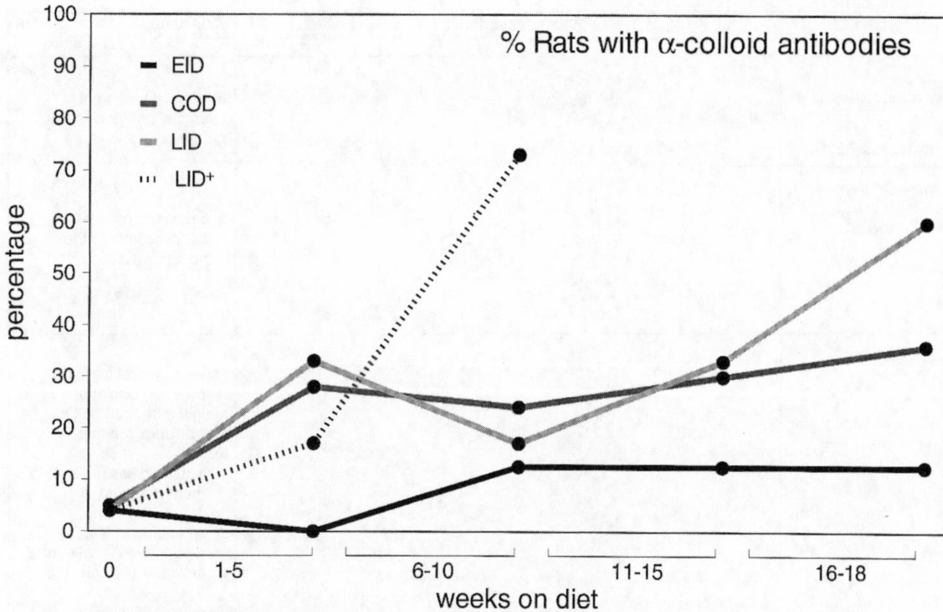

Fig. 4. Deveopment of anti-colloid antibodies. The percentage of Wistar rats developing anti-colloid autoantibodies in the circulation after introduction of a severely iodine-deficient diet (LID$^+$), a mildly iodine-deficient diet (LID), a normal diet (COD), and a diet with excess iodine (EID). For further technical details see Mooij *et al.* (1993b). Note that 70% of Wistar rats on a severely iodine-deficient diet develop anti-colloid antibodies, particularly 6–10 weeks after introduction of the diet (see also Fig. 3).

The Early Phases of SLE and RA prior to Autosensitization

Nothing is known about a possible involvement of DC in the triggering phases of SLE and RA leading to the initial production of antibodies to dsDNA and nuclear proteins and to the production of arthritogenic T cells and/or antibodies, respectively. It has been speculated that—owing to the apoptotic disturbances which presumably underlie SLE (see later)—cellular blebs containing DNA material become available to the immune system. It is unknown at which site this comes available; both the skin and the immune system may be spots of such release. Consequently, the involvement of local DC, viz. skin Langerhans cells or thymic and splenic DC, in the uptake and presentation of such cellular DNA-containing blebs is also speculative. Of note is the high turnover of skin Langerhans cells in discoid LE (Lee *et al.*, 1996).

With regard to the very early phases of RA, a possible sensitization to microbes in the gut or lung environment is involved (Fig. 5) (Klasen *et al.*, 1992; Hayakawa *et al.*, 1996). There is ample evidence of the presence of DC in both the gut (Wilders *et al.*, 1983) and bronchial mucosa (van Haarst *et al.*, 1994), and their involvement in the handling of microbial antigens. Moreover, the bronchus-associated lymphoid tissue (BALT) of RA patients shows a histology reminiscent of a diffuse panbronchiolitis with activated DC and other immune cells, indicating that extrinsic stimulation as well as alterations of the immune response are involved in the more excessive development of BALT in RA patients (Sato *et al.*, 1996; Scherak *et al.*, 1993). Of note is also the

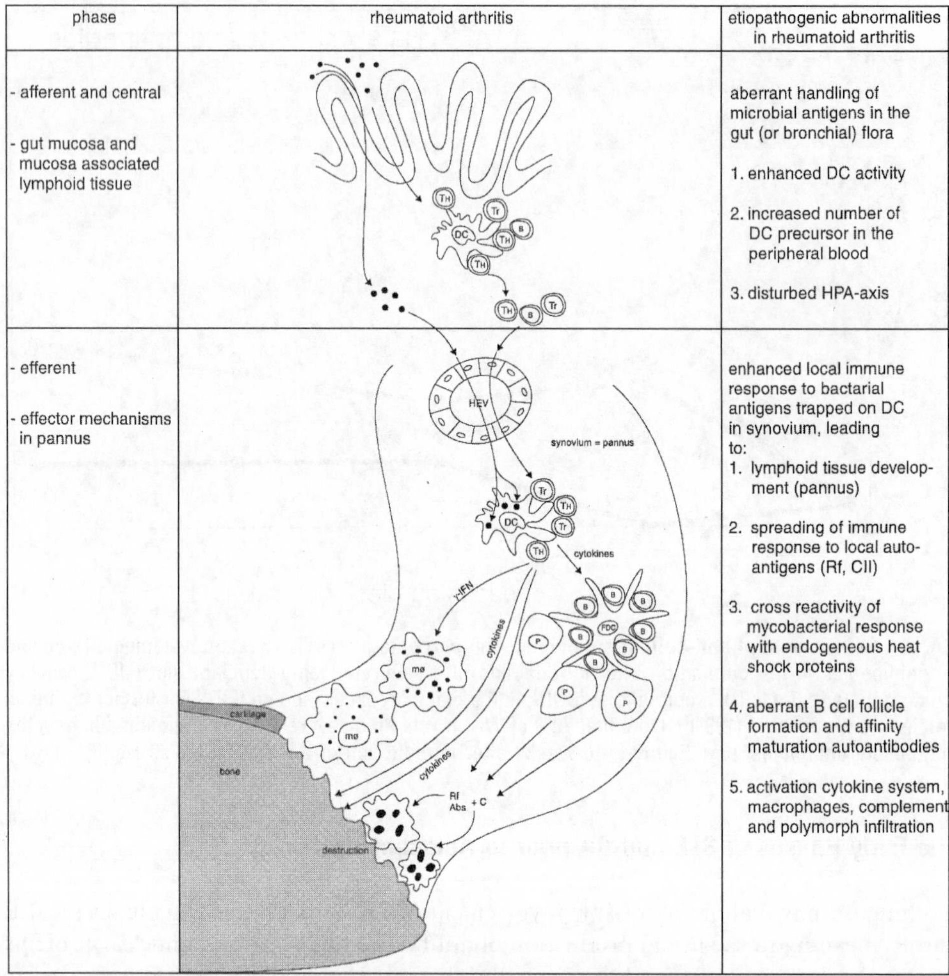

phase
rheumatoid arthritis
etiopathogenic abnormalities in rheumatoid arthritis
- afferent and central
- gut mucosa and mucosa associated lymphoid tissue
aberrant handling of microbial antigens in the gut (or bronchial) flora
1. enhanced DC activity
2. increased number of DC precursor in the peripheral blood
3. disturbed HPA-axis
- efferent
- effector mechanisms in pannus
enhanced local immune response to bactarial antigens trapped on DC in synovium, leading to:
1. lymphoid tissue development (pannus)
2. spreading of immune response to local autoantigens (Rf, CII)
3. cross reactivity of mycobacterial response with endogeneous heat shock proteins
4. aberrant B cell follicle formation and affinity maturation autoantibodies
5. activation cytokine system, macrophages, complement and polymorph infiltration
HEV
synovium = pannus
cytokines
γ-IFN
FDC
cartilage
bone
Rf Abs
+C
destruction

Fig. 5. A hypothetical scheme of the different phases of rheumatoid arthritis. For explanation of abbreviations see also Fig. 2; ●, microbial antigen; HEV, high endothelial venule; FDC, follicular dendritic cell; P, plasma cell; Rf, rheumatoid factor; C, complement; Mϕ = macrophages (surrounded by polymorphonuclear leukocytes). For further explanation see text.

presence of potentially arthritogenic peptidoglycans of the anaerobic microbial flora in both normal gut mucosa and spleen (Klasen *et al.*, 1994; Kool *et al.*, 1994; Hoijer *et al.*, 1995).

It goes without saying that in the artificial EA models of RA, DC located at the injection site take up, process, transport, and present the injected antigens to the immune system.

In sum, DC play a prime role in the initial triggering of the autoimmune response toward the target cells in organ-specific autoimmune diseases (Fig. 2). Various mechanisms are probably involved in their enhanced early attraction to the target tissue prior to autosensitization. Among these are vascular abnormalities, an early limited necrosis of the target cells in response to toxins or viral influences, and innate or acquired metabolic and growth disturbances of the target cells. Whether this leads to enhanced chemokine expression in early phases is as yet unknown. Regardless of the mechanism of the enhanced local accumulation, after arrival in the draining lymph nodes the DC will start to present autoantigens to T cells. This presentation is followed in time by a 'mild' (regulatory?) autoimmune reaction to the various presented autoantigens. Such autoimmune reaction will only get out of hand in individuals with a concomitant immunodysregulation ('autoimmune-prone' individuals, see next section).

DC AND DYSREGULATIONS OF THE CENTRAL IMMUNE RESPONSE IN AUTOIMMUNE DISEASE

In humans there is little information on a possible role of DC in the immunodysregulations linked to autoimmune diseases. However, there is more and intriguing new information about such role of DC in the animal models of spontaneously occurring autoimmune diseases, viz. the neonatal thymectomy model, the BB rat, the NOD mouse, and the MRL/lpr mouse, and in the EA model of RA, the Lewis rat.

DC in Experimental Models of Organ-specific Autoimmune Diseases

Neonatal Thymectomy Model

Neonatal thymectomy in BALB/c mice and A/J mice (but not in C57BL/6 and DBA-2 mice) at day 3 after birth results in thyroiditis, oöphoritis, parotitis, and gastritis (Tung *et al.*, 1987). The inflammation is characterized by the presence of T cell infiltrates in the affected organs and the development of organ-specific antibodies in serum. There is a strict temporal relationship between the development of the autoimmune syndrome and the day of thymectomy, which has to occur between the second and the fifth days after birth (Taguchi and Nishizuka, 1980; Tung *et al.*, 1987). An explanation for this phenomenon is based on the premise that self-reactive $CD4^+$ T cells are generated in the thymus throughout life and exported to the periphery. In euthymic animals, autoimmune disease is not observed because these autoreactive $CD4^+$ T cells are controlled by $CD4^+$ T cells with regulatory or suppressor activity. These cells are also generated in the thymus, but only after the first week of life. Hence thymectomy at day 3, restricting the T cell repertoire to only effector autoimmune $CD4^+$ T cells, explains the spontaneously occurring autoimmune diseases, because the balance between self-reactive T cells and regulatory T cells tips over to the former. The organ-specific autoimmune diseases in this model are directly due to autoimmune T cells, since transfer experiments of $CD4^+$ T cells of thymectomized donors cause disease in young recipients (Sakaguchi *et al.*, 1982; Smith *et al.*, 1991). This transfer of disease can be prevented by infusion of $CD4^+$ $CD5^+$ T cells from normal adult mice in an early stage after the transfer of the $CD4^+$ cells of the thymectomized donors.

With regard to the role of DC in this model, Bonomo *et al.* (1995) demonstrated that lymph node T cells from 3-day thymectomized mice had an enhanced response in the syngeneic MLR (an MLR generally considered to be driven by autoantigenic peptides), and that these T cells appeared to respond preferentially to syngeneic DC. They also showed that intrathymic APC (among which are the intrathymic DC) played a role in the 3-day thymectomy model, most likely by inducing the regulatory T cell population in the thymus.

BB Rat Model

The immunoregulatory defects of the BB diabetes-prone (DP) rat are linked to the severe lymphopenia which the animal gradually develops from birth onward. This lymphopenia is under control of the *lyp* gene, and predominantly affects the $CD8^+$ $RT6^+$ T cell population (Greiner *et al.*, 1986; Markholst, 1997). It is precisely this population that regulates autoimmune responsiveness in the BB-DP rat. A subline of BB rats, i.e. the BB diabetic-resistant (DR) rat lacks the *lyp* gene in an otherwise similar genetic background as the BB-DP rat; this BB-DR rat has normal numbers of $CD4^+$ and $CD8^+$ $RT6^+$ T cells and does not develop autoimmune insulitis and autoimmune thyroiditis (Jiang *et al.*, 1990). Moreover, transfer of $RT6^+$ T cells from the BB-DR rat to the BB-DP rat at young age prevents the development of autoimmune insulitis and thyroiditis (Greiner *et al.*, 1987; McKeever *et al.*, 1990).

With regard to the origin of the lack of T cells, and predominantly of regulatory $RT6^+$ T cells, there are reports that BB-DP bone marrow-derived cells, which are not T cell precursors, influence the maturation environment in the thymus of otherwise normal T cell precursors in such a way that the faulty T cell development characteristic of the BB-DP rat results (Georgiou *et al.*, 1988). These observations suggest the involvement of an abnormal function of intrathymic macrophages and/or IDC. In subsequent experiments it was reported, however, that splenic DC of young BB-DP rats were not abnormal in function (Tafuri *et al.*, 1993), that is they showed a superb APC function in allogeneic MLR (all-MLR). After interaction with macrophages, such splenic DC were capable of even greater stimulatory activity in allo-MLR as compared to DC of control rats, and this phenomenon was ascribed to a higher sensitivity for IL-1 and GM-CSF of the splenic DC of BB-DP rats. We have recently extended these experiments and have shown that splenic DC of young BB-DP rats (3–8 weeks of age) are indeed good stimulators in allo-MLR. However, an important new finding was that the accessory capability of splenic DC of young BB-DP rats was very poor in syngeneic (syn)-MLR (Delemarre *et al.*, 1995b; Delemarre *et al.*, 1996). Of note is that the syn-MLR most likely represents proliferative responses toward self-antigens. Particularly relevant is the observation in our series of experiments that the splenic DC of young BB-DP rats were faulty in the generation of predominantly $CD8^+$ and $RT6^+$ T cells in syn-MLR (Delemarre and Drexhage, 1997).

Collectively these observations lead to a view that the cross-talk between autoantigen-loaded BB-DP DC and T cells is intrinsically disturbed both in the periphery and in the thymus. This leads to an imbalance between regulator and effector T cells, the basis for a tendency to autoimmunity. A concomitant intrinsic defect in the generation of $RT6^+$ T cells (Markholst, 1997) may further complicate the cross-talk between DC and T cells in the BB-DP rat.

Interestingly, the defects of DC characteristic of the BB-DP rat, i.e. a low accessory capability in syn-MLR, have also been reported in autologous MLR in 60–70% of patients with type 1 diabetes (Jansen *et al.*, 1995). These DC defects were present irrespective of the duration of the disease, and were found even before clinical signs and symptoms in islet cell antibody-positive first-degree relatives of index type 1 diabetes cases (Takahashi *et al.*, 1997). This shows the fundamental character of this DC defect for disease development. Similar DC defects are also present in patients with thyroid autoimmune disease (Tas *et al.*, 1991) or autoimmune oöphoritis (Hoek *et al.*, 1995).

NOD Mouse Model

The autoimmune insulitis of the NOD mouse is presently regarded as predominantly a T_H1 cell-mediated phenomenon. CD40 signaling probably plays a prominent role in IL-12 production by DC in stimulating T_H1 patterns of reaction (Kelsall *et al.*, 1996), and the RelB knockout (KO) mouse that lacks functional DC does not develop T_H1 but does T_H2 responses (Lo *et al.*, 1995). Thus, DC are likely involved in the induction of the autoimmune insulitis of the NOD mouse; the immunohistology of early lesions supports such a view (see earlier).

In view of the above-described faulty APC functions of splenic DC of the BB-DP rat in syn-MLR, and in view of the recently found defects of splenic APC of the NOD mouse in HEL-specific memory T cell responses (Piganelli and Haskins, personal communication), we recently studied the capability of splenic and lymph node DC of the young NOD mouse (10 weeks of age, prior to autosensitization) to induce T cell proliferation in syn-MLR. It appeared that such DC were not defective but were very active in T cell stimulation: proliferative responses were in fact prolonged and continued for over 6 days generating more $CD4^+$ CD45 RB low to negative T cells (memory-like) as compared to DC-driven syn-MLRs of various other control mouse strains (Radosevic *et al.*, 1997). More detailed examination of these prolonged and excessive syngeneic T cell responses driven by NOD splenic DC showed a lowered rate of apoptosis. It is tempting to speculate that this is due to a lower function of $CD8\alpha^+$ lymphoid DCs in the splenic NOD DC populations. If such a speculation could be confirmed, it would further support a hypothesis of an intra- and extrathymic defect in the NOD mouse with failure to properly delete the appropriate, i.e. the self T cell, cell repertoire (Thomas-Vaslin *et al.*, 1997). As well as lymphoid DC, thymic and other macrophages are also capable of downregulating DC-driven autologous T cell responses (Georgiou *et al.*, 1995), probably by virtue of their PGE_2, NO and/or IL-10 production (M. Clare-Salzler, personal communication). Peritoneal macrophages of the NOD indeed produce more prostaglandins than control mice (Lety *et al.*, 1992), and studies carried out by Serreze and colleagues (1993a,b) have shown an inappropriate maturation of the precursors of NOD-APC, including DCs and macrophages in the bone marrow.

It is thus not too daring a concept that in the NOD mouse (but also in the BB rat and the human) disturbances in the conductance of the T cell orchestra due to maturation abnormalities of macrophages, myeloid DC, and lymphoid DC result in its off-key tuning: i.e. an overrepresentation of autoreactive T cells, with excessive dominance of effector T cells over regulator T cells and of T_H1 cells over T_H2 cells (Jaramillo *et al.*, 1994).

DC in Experimental Allergic Models of Arthritis

The experimental animal models of autoimmune arthritis resembling human RA require artificial sensitization. As sensitizing antigens, microbial antigens (particularly mycobacteria and peptidoglycans of anaerobic bacteria) or other arthritogenic antigens (collagen type II) are used in strains of rats and mice with a genetic tendency to the disease, most notably the Lewis rat and the SJL mouse. The tendency to the chronic arthritic autoimmune reaction in the Lewis rat has—among other mechanisms—been attributed to a subnormal activity of the hypothalamus–pituitary–adrenal axis (HPA axis), i.e. a low ACTH output upon IL-1 stimulation of the hypothalamus (Wilder, 1996).

Although there are no data on disturbed DC function in the animal models used for induction of experimental allergic arthritis (EAA), it is the presence of DC and their interactions with lymphocytes in the inflamed synovial tissues of the animals that suggest at least a local activation of the cells (Thomas and Lipsky, 1996). The most eye-catching histological finding in human RA-synovitis is, however, the development of secondary lymphoid follicles in the inflamed tissues and the presence of a strong local germinal center reaction (Kavanaugh and Lipsky, 1996). This local B cell reaction likely contributes to a higher affinity maturation of the disease-inducing or disease-accelerating autoantibodies, such as the rheumatoid factors (Rf) and autoantibodies to collagen type II. Interestingly the OS chicken, a model of severe autoimmune thyroiditis, also has HPA axis disturbances and also develops secondary lymphoid follicles in the thyroiditis process (Wick *et al.*, 1993). Also, in this bird the affinity maturation of the thyroid-reactive IgGs contributes to the ultimate thyroid failure. The accessory cells of the secondary follicle playing a role in memory B cell formation and affinity maturation are the follicular dendritic cells (FDC), but also the DC (Grouard *et al.*, 1996). It is generally assumed that fibroblasts are the precursors of FDC (Gadher and Woolley, 1987; Edwards *et al.*, 1993). However, there are reports that the FDC population is heterogeneous, and that DRC-1$^+$ blood-borne precursors do exist for the FDC. The number of such precursors is said to be increased in RA patients (Terashma *et al.*, 1988). In the synovial arthritis of RA, FDC are in a hyperreactive state (Imai and Yamakawa, 1996), and particularly T cell cytokines, IL-1, prostaglandins, mast cell products, and Rf themselves play a role in intrasynovial FDC development and activation (Gadher and Wooley, 1987; Mageed *et al.*, 1991; Edwards *et al.*, 1993). For such development and activation, a previous locally excessive DC–T cell interaction is likely to be essential to provide the high local levels of T cell cytokines and other immune products. In patients suffering from RA there are indeed signs of a hyperactivity of DC progenitors in the peripheral blood: (a) there is increased monocyte adhesiveness, integrin expression, and cytokine release in RA patients (Lioté *et al.*, 1996); (b) GM-CSF, TNF, and stem cell factor produce increased DC progeny in RA patients (Santiago-Schwartz, 1996); and (c) IL-1α-containing dendritic-like cells can be found in the peripheral blood of RA patients to extents as high as $7\frac{1}{2}\%$ (Barkley *et al.*, 1990).

In sum, there is evidence for an enhanced general activity of DC and their blood-borne precursors in RA leading to an excessive response to microbial antigens of the gut (and probably lung) environment (Fig. 5).

DC in Experimental Models of Spontaneously Occurring SLE

The experimental animal model most closely resembling human SLE is the MRL/lpr mouse (Singh, 1995). This mouse has a defect in the expression of the apoptosis-inducing Fas gene resulting in a progressive SLE-like autoimmune syndrome. With few exceptions—such as the presence of massive lymphadenopathy and the inappropriate expansion of very early CD4$^-$ CD8$^-$ thymocytes—the SLE-like autoimmune syndrome in the MRL/lpr mouse has several similarities with human SLE, particularly the autoantibody profile, the immune complex vasculitis and the multiorgan involvement including that of the skin. Interestingly, 60% of human subjects with SLE have elevated levels of the soluble Fas receptor in their serum, suggesting that disturbances in apoptosis may underlie disease development in the human disease also (Rose *et al.*, 1997). The immunopathogenic hallmarks of both murine and human SLE-like syndromes are a polyclonal B cell stimulation and a raised IgG production; in particular, anti-dsDNA antibodies arising in this polyclonal B cell response are pathological and give rise to immune complex vasculitis, particularly at the level of the kidney (Petri, 1996). Whether bacterial DNA and/or abnormal endogeneous DNA drive such excessive B cell responsiveness is unknown (Krieg, 1995), and hence so is a potential role of DCs in such stimulation. *In vitro* antigen-presenting activity of splenic DC obtained from MRL/lpr mice is impaired (Ito *et al.*, 1988); disturbances have been found in Mϕ-differentiation in lupus-prone male BXSB mice (Vieten *et al.*, 1996); and there is also one report (Katagiri, 1992) of a reduced accessory activity of DC in the blood of patients with active SLE.

DC AND THE EFFECTOR PHASES OF AUTOIMMUNE DISEASES

The EA models, the transfer models of T cells and of autoantibodies, as well as some transgenic animal models have proved useful for obtaining a better insight into the effector phase of the autoimmune responses leading to target or bystander cell destruction. From these experimental models it has become clear that, even in stages beyond the generation of autoreactive T cells, DC act as important local APC for already sensitized T cells.

In essence three major patterns of autoimmune effector reactivity can be discerned: (a) a T_H1 pattern of reaction (synonyms: delayed type hypersensitivity (DTH) reaction or type IV reaction); (b) a development of a local lymphoid tissue; and (c) various antigen–antibody-mediated reactions (synonyms: type II (cytotoxic antibody-mediated) and type III (immune complex-mediated) reactions).

DC and T_H1 Reaction Patterns

The effector phases of autoimmune insulitis and other autoimmune endocrinopathies are now generally considered as being largely T_H1-mediated. Destruction of target cells is predominantly reached via the production of γ-IFN by autoreactive $CD4^+$ and $CD8^+$ T cells. This cytokine activates cells of the mononuclear phagocyte series to exert their damaging function on the target tissue (Fig. 2). The prototype of the T_H1-mediated reactions is the DTH skin reaction. The histology of this reaction shows the presence of the players in such reactivity, viz. a local, mostly perivascular accumulation of $CD4^+$ T cells, a few $CD8^+$ T cells, and scavenger (acid phosphatase-positive) macrophages. However, early perivascular infiltration of DC into DTH reactions has also been reported (van de Plassche-Boers *et al.*, 1985; Voorbij *et al.*, 1990a). These DC are often found in apposition to the accumulated $CD4^+$ T cells. Similar histological DTH-like pictures are obtained in the later phases of the autoimmune insulitis of the BB rat (Voorbij and Schumacker, 1989), the autoimmune insulitis of the NOD mouse (Jansen *et al.*, 1993), and the autoimmune oöphoritis of the 3-day thymectomy mouse, showing a peritarget accumulation of $CD4^+$ T cells in close apposition to locally accumulated DCs and an infiltration of the target by scavenger-type macrophages ($ED1^+$ and $ED3^+$ in the rat; $BM8^+$ in the mouse). However, DTH-like infiltration patterns can be seen best in the T cell transfer models of the organ-specific autoimmune diseases. Here, autoreactive T cells are transferred to susceptible recipients to induce diseases: for example, the transfer of islet-specific diabetogenic clonal T cells to young NOD mice leads to diabetes (Bergman and Haskins, 1997); the transfer of TSH-receptor-specific T cells to BALB/c mice leads to thyroiditis (Costagliola *et al.*, 1996); and the transfer of concanavalin-A-stimulated splenic BB T cells to young cyclophosphamide-treated BB rats results in destructive insulitis (Issa-Chergui *et al.*, 1988). The induced lesions are characterized by a simultaneous infiltration in or around the target of T cells, DC, and various types of accessory and scavenger macrophages (Rosmalen *et al.*, 1998). The latter are found close to destroyed target cells.

In the EA models of organ-specific autoimmune diseases, initial autosensitization is artificial and does not take place in the target and target-draining lymph nodes but at a chosen peripheral site, such as the tail and tail-draining lymph nodes. Since this type of active immunization with the autoantigen—often in combination with an adjuvant—is not different from any other form of immunization, it is not surprising that DC locally infiltrated at these remote sites are involved in the handling of the injected autoantigen (Gautam and Glynn, 1991). More peculiar is the finding that in EA models—as in the T cell transfer models—DC are involved in the effector phases, which histologically are reminiscent of DTH reactions:

(a) In EA uveoretinitis, DC infiltrate the ciliary body and iris simultaneously with the T cells (Butler and McMenamin, 1996).
(b) In EA thyroiditis, the first sign of thyroidal involvement is positivity of the vascular endothelium for MHC class II molecules and early infiltration with DC, which is later followed by focal infiltrates of T and B cells (Hassman *et al.*, 1988).
(c) In EA myocarditis, DC are abundantly present around the foci of cardiac muscle cell damage (Suzuki, 1995; Neu *et al.*, 1993). Their close apposition to the destroyed cardiac muscle cells and their ultrastructural intimate contacts with these muscle cells have even led to the view that these DC rather than the locally accumulated lymphocytes are the damaging cells for the cardiac muscle cells (McCombe *et al.*, 1994; Izumi *et al.*, 1995; Matyszak and Perry, 1996). The scavenger macrophages, which also infiltrate the myocardium, would serve for the removal of cellular debris in this model.
(d) In EA encephalomyelitis, MHC class II^+, $Ox62^+$ DC-like cells accumulate perivascularly together with T cells and macrophages in the demyelinating lesions. However, since microglial cells, the putative 'immune cells' of the CNS, share markers and morphology with bone marrow-derived APC, it is almost impossible to distinguish between a neuropil infiltration with DC and an accumulation in the neuropil of microglial cells in EA encephalomyelitis (Bauer *et al.*, 1994).

Collectively, the data described above show that DC–T cell interactions also take place in the target tissue during the effector or destructive phases of organ-specific autoimmune reactions in an immunohistochemical pattern reminiscent of dth (T_H1-like)-reactions (Fig. 2). Interestingly, it has been shown that the target cells themselves need not be recognized by the infiltrating T cells in such reactions for their destruction to take place (Lo *et al.*, 1995). The recognition of the autoantigen by the T cell in the context of the MHC class II molecules on the APC suffices. The excessive local production of cytokines such as IL-1 will create a milieu in which, for example, insular β cells are unable to survive (Mandrup-Poulsen *et al.*, 1987) and they will undergo apoptosis owing to excessive NO radical production (Corbett *et al.*, 1992; Eizirik and Leijerstam, 1994). Thyrocytes are thought to start to express the Fas molecule under such circumstances of enhanced local cytokine production (Berg, 1997) and the expression of this apoptosis-inducing molecule will contribute to their disappearance in the final stages of autoimmune thyroiditis.

DC and the Development of Local Lymphoid Tissue

In organ-specific autoimmune diseases a special type of focal infiltrates of lymphoid cells can be found that are often erroneously described as 'inflammatory' infiltrates. However, these infiltrates are histologically clearly distinct from the destructive DTH reactions described above. Such focal accumulations of lymphoid cells have an architecture similar to the mucosa- and bronchus-associated lymphoid tissues and are composed of a T cell zone with intermingled DC (in this position called IDCs) and HEVs at the periphery of the T cell zone (Fig. 2, Fig. 6) (Kabel *et al.*, 1989a). A smaller B cell area (often without a germinal center) may be part of the lymphoid structure, while plasma cells radiate from the lymphoid tissue between the surrounding parenchymal cells (Voorbij *et al.*, 1990b). Such focal infiltrates of lymphoid cells which do not damage or hardly damage the surrounding parenchymal cells can easily be found in BB rat thyroids, in Graves' goiters, and in TPO-Ab$^+$ human sporadic goiters (Kabel *et al.*, 1989a). The most explicit histological prototype of such lymphoid tissue can, however, be found in a transgenic NOD mouse diabetic model, in which virtually all CD4$^+$ T cells carry a diabetogenic TCR (Rosmalen *et al.*, manuscript submitted). This mouse develops extensive peri-insular lymphoid tissue from the age of 2–3 weeks onward, but in the absence of overt diabetes (Fig. 6). Similar but smaller areas of peri-insular lymphoid tissue can sometimes be observed in wild-type NOD mice. That overt diabetes does not develop might be related to the fact that in the TCR-transgenic NOD mouse, BM8$^+$ scavenger macrophages are totally absent from the peri-insular lymphoid tissue (unlike the DTH reaction described above). It is tempting to speculate that the oxidative and cytokine milieu created by the infiltrating BM8$^+$ scavenger macrophages, and involving IL-1 and NO, is not compatible with β cell survival.

At the edges of the smaller foci of lymphoid tissue occurring in the BB rat thyroid and in human Graves' and sporadic goiters often a few acid phosphatase-positive scavenger macrophages are present in the colloidal spaces of thyroid follicles adjacent to the lymphoid tissue (Mooij *et al.*, 1993a). This suggests that such infiltration is either a sign of colloidophagy and mild thyrocyte destruction via macrophage cytotoxic mechanisms, or alternatively, a sign of removal of debris of some dead thyrocytes.

In Hashimoto's goiter and in the thyroiditis of the OS chicken, focal intrathyroidal lymphoid tissue becomes very prominent and also involves the development of secondary B cell follicles with germinal center reactions (Wick *et al.*, 1993; Postigo *et al.*, 1994). Thyroid follicles adjacent to the local lymphoid tissue are often in an advanced stage of decay. The development of B cell follicles in the intrathyroidal lymphoid tissue suggests an ongoing affinity maturation of the thyroid-reactive autoantibodies. Indeed, thyroglobulin has been found trapped on the FDC in the secondary B lymphoid follicles (Kasajima *et al.*, 1987). It is tempting to speculate that the combination of the local cytokine milieu with the local production of high-affinity anti-thyroid antibodies (also

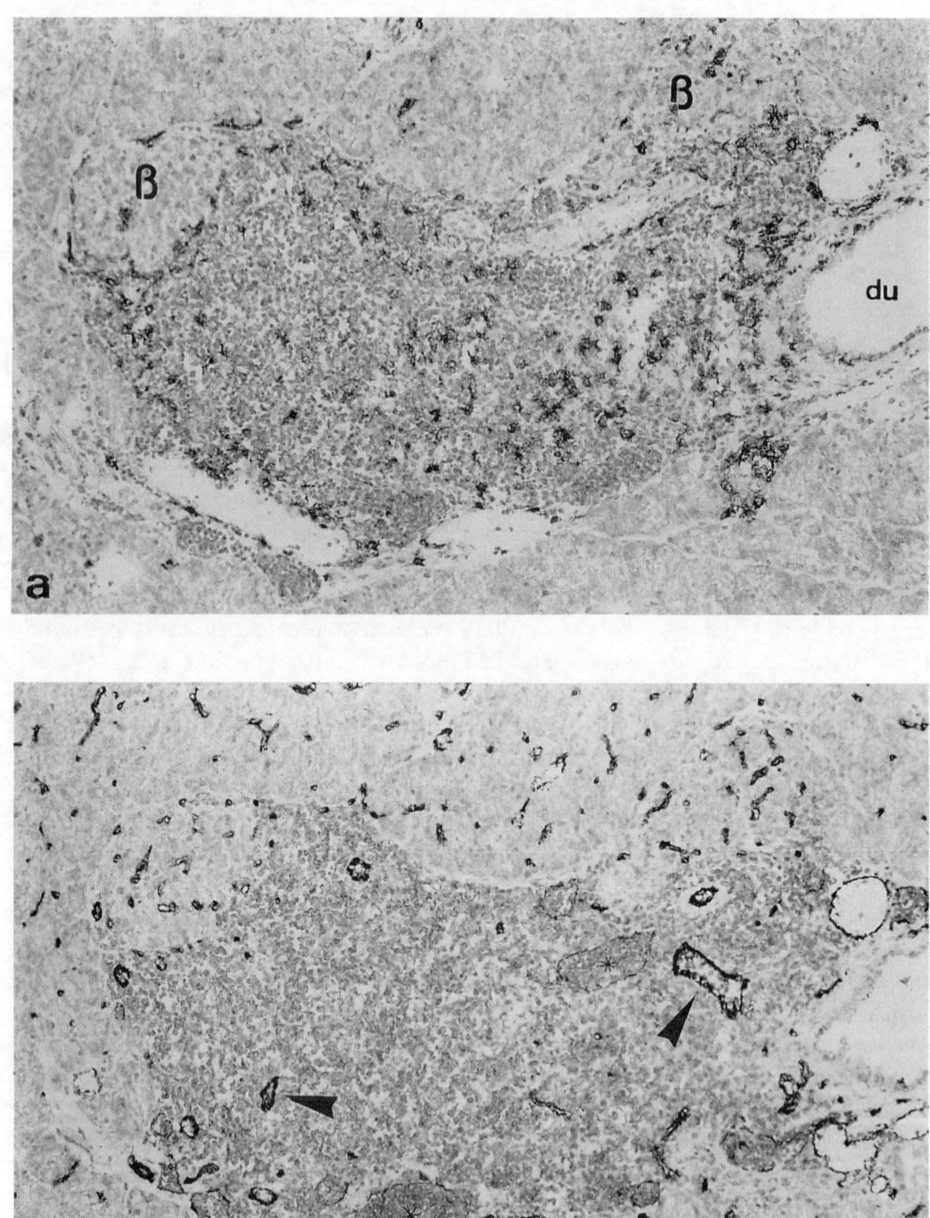

Fig. 6. Immunohistological pictures of a representative peri-islet lymphoid tissue development in a 4-week-old NOD mouse transgenic for a diabetogenic T cell receptor. Original magnification ×90. For details see Rosmalen *et al.* (1998). (a) CD11c (N418) staining, showing the accumulation of DC at the islet-edge (β = islet) and between the lymphocytes (du = ductus). (b) ER-MP23 staining, showing endothelial cells, particularly HEVs (arrow) and lymphatics (asterisk), characteristic of the secondary lymphoid tissue nature of the peri-islet lymphoid cell accumulations in this model.

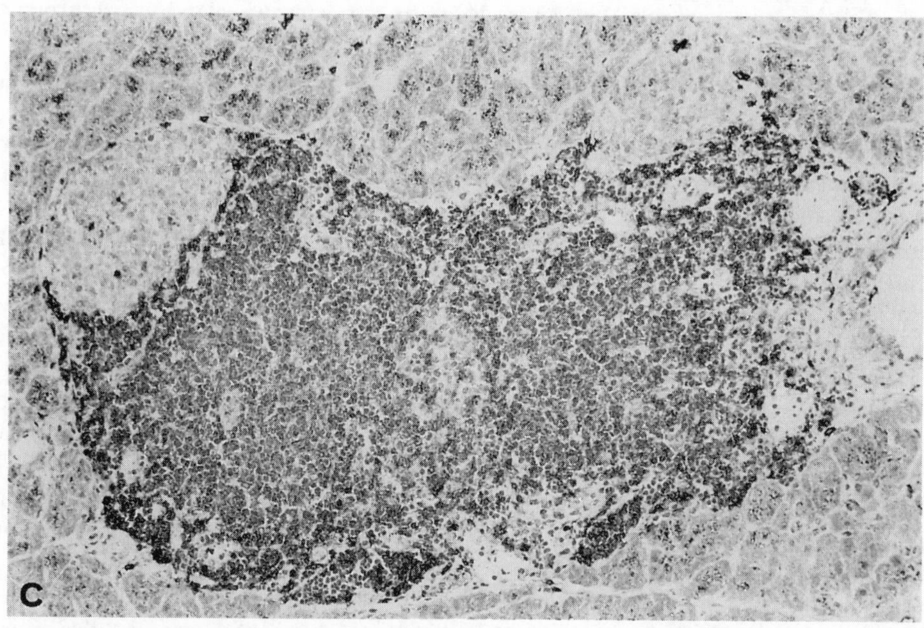

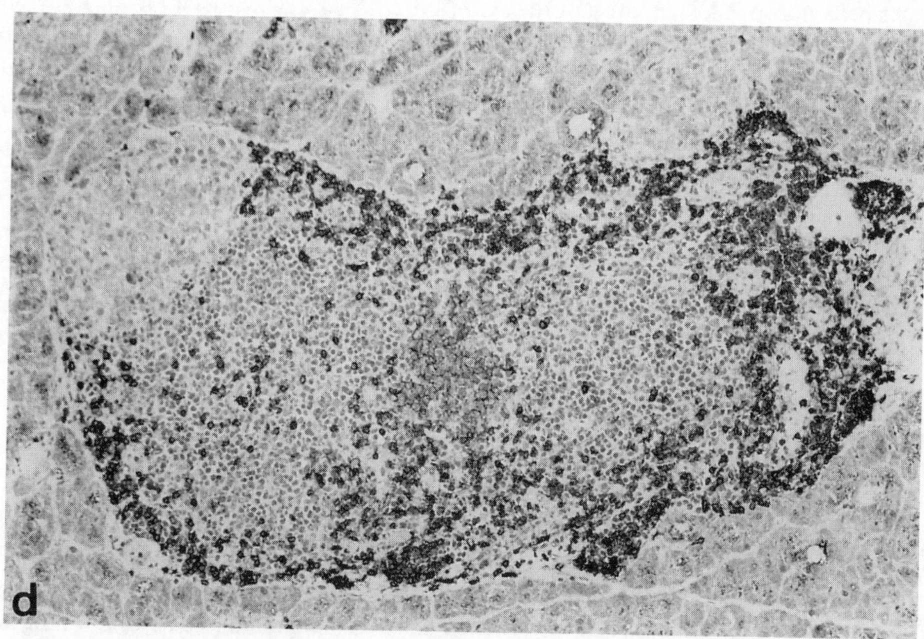

Fig. 6 (*contd.*). (c) and (d) CD3 (T cells) and B220 (B cells) respectively, showing the high grade of organization of the accumulated peri-islet lymphocytes in separate T and B cell areas reminiscent of secondary lymphoid tissue.

leading to immune complex formation) leads to the extensive glandular destruction characteristic of Hashimoto goiter and OS thyroiditis (Wick *et al.*, 1993).

Extensive focal lymphoid infiltrates with germinal center reactions are also the prime hallmark of the synovitis of RA (Fig. 5). In contrast, the arthritis of SLE shows only a very mild synovial infiltration (Holmdahl *et al.*, 1991). DC are a conspicuous part of the T cell zones of the infiltrates in the RA synovium (March, 1987; Waalen *et al.*, 1987a). They have the characteristics of IDC, and are located at strategic positions to interact with the local T cells (Wilkinson *et al.*, 1990; van Dinther-Jansen *et al.*, 1990; Demaziere *et al.*, 1992; Thomas and Quinn, 1996). HEVs are also components of the synovium-associated lymphoid tissue. Regarding the histological picture, it is not surprising that increased numbers of activated DC can be isolated from RA synovial tissue, and that DC-like cell clones have been generated from RA synovial tissue (Goto *et al.*, 1991). The DC are likely to handle and present various trapped microbial antigens to the locally accumulated sensitized T cells (Melief *et al.*, 1995). Peptidoglycans of the anaerobic gut flora, heat shock proteins like antigens of mycobacteria (van Eden *et al.*, 1996), and microbial superantigens (Bhardwaj *et al.*, 1994) may all play a role in this intrasynovial expansion of memory T cells (Travaglio-Encinoza *et al.*, 1995). There are indications that the locally accumulated DC in the RA synovium may be abnormal or in another state of maturation as compared to blood-borne DC populations: their cluster behavior with T cells is lower (Tsai and Zvaifler, 1988) and the DC–T cell clusters easily fall apart (Burns *et al.*, 1992). It has been proposed that anergic and/or $CD8^+$ T cells accumulated in the synovium play a role in this 'abnormal' DC–T cell cluster behavior in RA synovitis (Burns *et al.*, 1992). Also, the synovial DC in RA seem to have a peculiar pattern of expression of costimulatory molecules; CD80 is hardly expressed, but there are conflicting data regarding CD86 expression, varying from high to low levels (Summers *et al.*, 1995; Summers *et al.*, 1996; Thomas and Quinn, 1996). Undisputedly, DCs present in the RA synovial tissue as well as blood-derived DC of RA patients are excellent accessory cells in T cell proliferative reactions, showing a higher stimulatory potential than DC of healthy individuals (Waalen *et al.*, 1987b; Bergroth *et al.*, 1989; Stagg *et al.*, 1991). This functionally strong local DC–T cell interaction in the synovium of RA patients has its consequences, however: it is supposed to create a milieu with excessive local cytokine production. This cytokine milieu attracts monocytes and macrophages, particularly at the periphery of the lymphoid cell accumulations, viz. at the synovium–cartilage junction (Salisbury *et al.*, 1987). The cytokines will not only attract but also activate these macrophages close to the cartilage and bone to produce IL-1, PGE_2 and other products detrimental to these tissues (Bhardwaj *et al.*, 1988, Bhardwaj *et al.*, 1989; Sasano *et al.*, 1990; Ridderstad *et al.*, 1991). Moreover, many B cells will also infiltrate the synovial lymphoid tissue via the newly formed HEVs (Edwards *et al.*, 1993) and will be activated to become plasma cells (Shimuzu *et al.*, 1988). The excessive cytokine milieu will contribute to the FDC development from synovial fibroblasts (Heino *et al.*, 1987). That DC and FDC development are intrinsically abnormal in patients with RA has been suggested (see before) but needs further investigation (Krenn *et al.*, 1996). What is known is that production of autoantibodies does take place in the synovial lymphoid tissue of RA patients (Imai *et al.*, 1989), particularly of autoantibodies specific for type II collagen as well as of rheumatoid factors, both serological hallmarks of RA. Epitope spreading from trapped microbial antigens toward such local autoantigens may be the cornerstone for this autoreactivity (Fig. 5).

Antibodies to type II collagen, when passively transferred to recipients, will induce the development of a synovitis in which the early stages are characterized by complement activation and neutrophil infiltration (Holmdahl *et al.*, 1991). In the later stages activated macrophages, T cells and DC infiltrate the synovia. These transfer data show the disease-promoting activity of antibodies to type II collagen, and the vicious circle that is created via the local production of such autoantibodies. Rheumatoid factors will likewise significantly enhance and perpetuate the arthritis by local complement-mediated reactions and further attraction of inflammatory and immune cells.

In sum, in the RA synovium a local lymphoid tissue (pannus) will develop with strong germinal center reactions and macrophage activation. Enhanced local DC–T cell interactions involving locally trapped microbial antigens of the gut environment are likely cornerstones for such pannus formation. Intrinsic DC and FDC abnormalities may contribute to the local excessive immune reactions in the synovium. The excessive cytokine, autoantibody, and rheumatoid factor production in the pannus are probably the factors leading to cartilage and bone destruction due to local macrophage activation, complement activation, and polymorphonuclear cell infiltration.

DC and Antigen–Antibody Reactions

Immune complex-induced vasculitis is a hallmark of SLE. It is not known whether DC are part of the inflammatory infiltrate of such immune-complex vasculitis. This, however, deserves investigation, since such DC infiltration may contribute to epitope spreading, leading, for example, to involvement of autoantigens of the blood coagulation cascade (anti-phospholipid antibodies). DC have been identified in mild synovitis—another clinical hallmark of SLE—but local antigens are unknown (Holmdahl *et al.*, 1991; Vivino and Schumacker, 1989). DC can also be found in lupus conjunctivitis (Heiligenhaus *et al.*, 1996) and lupus myositis (Pallis *et al.*, 1993).

The skin lesions of SLE—characteristic of the lupus disease process—sometimes occur in an isolated form without multiorgan SLE involvement (the so-called discoid LE). Classically, the skin lesion is an erythematous or maculopapular eruption over the malar eminences and bridge of the nose, creating a butterfly pattern. It is usually exacerbated by exposure to sunlight or to ultraviolet light. Microscopically, the areas of involvement show liquifactive degeneration of the basal epithelial layer of the epidermis, edema at the dermo-epidermal junction, and swelling and fusion of collagen fibers. Deposits of immunoglobulin and complement (most likely interactions of nuclear proteins, autoantibodies to nuclear proteins, and complement) can be seen along the dermo-epidermal junction in both the involved and the uninvolved skin (Petri, 1996). The antigen–antibody interactions at the dermo-epidermal junction may also involve autoantibodies to other skin elements such as the epidermal basement membrane and to the keratinocytes (Aiba *et al.*, 1989). Sun exposure and ultraviolet light may lead to enhanced skin epithelial cell death and apoptosis, in particular in an SLE background where apoptotic defects are suspected anyway (Casciola-Rosen and Rosen, 1997). DNA-containing apoptotic blebs may consequently be released in the skin and might act as an autoantigen package of nuclear proteins. The Langerhans cells of the skin are the most likely candidates to handle these packages. Indeed, increased numbers of Langerhans cells in the central portions of early SLE skin lesions followed by decreases suggest a high turnover of these cells (Kanauchi *et al.*, 1991; Stephansson and Ross, 1993). A report on morphological observations suggests that defects in the cytological differentiation and expression of marker molecules on Langerhans cells are indicative of an impairment of their function in cutaneous SLE (Mori *et al.*, 1994). If so, this may contribute to a local immunodysregulation actually leading to or aggrevating the skin involvement in this disease.

SUMMARY AND CONCLUSIONS

Autoimmune diseases have been defined as diseases which can be experimentally transferred by self-reactive antibodies and/or self-reactive T cells. Autoimmune diseases are generally divided into two polar subgroups: the organ-specific and the systemic autoimmune diseases. In the organ-specific autoimmune diseases the autoimmune reaction is largely restricted to a number of autoantigens in one organ or organ system, such as thyroglobulin, thyroperoxidase, and the TSH receptor in thyroid autoimmune diseases. Many of the organ-specific autoimmune diseases are endocrine diseases, frequently characterized by a final destruction of the endocrine tissues. Prototypes are autoimmune thyroiditis, autoimmune insulitis, and autoimmune adrenalitis/oöphoritis. In the systemic autoimmune diseases the autoimmune reaction is directed against a number of autoantigens not restricted to one organ or organ system, for example against dsDNA and nuclear proteins. Many of these systemic autoimmune diseases are characterized by vasculitis and arthritis. Prototypes of systemic autoimmune disease are SLE and RA. Since studies in patients on the pathogenesis of these diseases have their obvious limitations, various animal models of these diseases have been developed. These include animal models of spontaneously occurring autoimmune diseases and models in which the disease is induced by active immunization with autoantigens in susceptible animals, by passive immunization with autoantibodies or autoreactive T cells, or by the transgenic introduction of an overexpression of autoantigens or of autoreactive TCR. Studies on animal models and patients have led to the view that the etiology and pathogenesis of organ-specific autoimmune diseases, RA, and SLE differ but share the complexity of causal factors leading to the various autoimmune diseases. At present one realizes that the autoimmune diseases are the outcome of unfortunate combinations of various genetic as well as environmental influences.

Three phases can be discerned in the development of the various autoimmune diseases. In these phases, DC are critically involved.

I. In the organ-specific or endocrine autoimmune diseases there is initially—prior to autosensitization—a phase of an enhanced accumulation of APC, among which are many DC in the target-gland-to-be. Experimental data show that this enhanced accumulation of DC can be caused by a variety of genetic and environmental factors. An early mild necrosis of the target cells by viruses or toxins may lead to such DC accumulations, but innate or acquired growth and metabolic abnormalities of the target gland may also result in an enhanced DC infiltration. Regarding the latter mechanism, DC not only act as superb accessory cells in immune responses, but act also as regulator cells in the growth and metabolism of various endocrine cells. The increased early local accumulation of DC in the target-gland-to-be may lead to an enhanced trafficking of the cells to the draining lymph nodes and an enhanced presentation of various organ-specific autoantigens to the lymph nodal lymphocytes.

Although practically nothing is known about this initial afferent phase in SLE and RA, there are some indications that in RA an excessive sensitization toward the microbial flora in the gut and lung environment may play a role in disease initiation. If so, it is clear that the DC in the gut and bronchial mucosa of RA patients must play a prominent role in disease initiation.

II. In the second phase the DC present the organ-specific autoantigens or the microbial gut antigens to an immune system that has inborn or acquired defects in balancing the immune reponse toward an appropriate, i.e. non-self and non-destructive immune response. Data show that DC are likely critically involved in such immunodysregulations:

(a) In endocrine autoimmune patients and the animal models of spontaneously occurring organ-specific autoimmune diseases (the BB rat and NOD mouse), defects in the maturation of myeloid DC from their precursors have been found recently (leading to defects in regulator T cells).
(b) In human RA the blood-borne DC precursors have an intrinsically high T cell stimulatory activity, probably leading to hyperreactivity toward microbial antigens in the gut and lung environment.

In SLE, lack of lymphocytic apoptosis may play a role in repertoire selection and the polyclonal B cell response. The role of DC in this type of immunodysregulation is presently not known.

III. In a last phase, excessively produced autoreactive and/or microbial reactive antibodies and/or autoreactive T cells hit their target. Even in this last phase, DC seem to play a crucial role. Although antibodies (via complement activation) and $CD8^+$ T cells may destroy their targets by direct contact, experiments also show that it suffices that autoreactive T_H1 cells recognize their autoantigen/microbial antigen presented on DC in the vicinity of the 'target' tissue (in fact 'bystander' tissue) to exert a detrimental effect. This target tissue may well show an enhanced sensitivity for destruction by products generated during a localized immune response and concomitant macrophage activation, such as IL-1, TNF, and NO. The initiating DC–T cell interactions lead to local DTH reactions in the target tissue or to the development of local lymphoid tissue with or without germinal centers leading to excessively high local level of cytokines and/or autoantibodies. Particularly in the synovium of RA patients, such excessive generation of local lymphoid tissue (pannus) around DC that have unfortunately trapped gut microbial antigens, and the resulting high local levels of cytokines and autoantibodies (rheumatoid factors and anticollagen type II antibodies), is considered deleterious for the bone and cartilage of the affected joints.

It is the hope that new approaches will further elucidate the role of DC in the various stages of the different autoimmune diseases, and will provide new targets for immunotherapy modulating DC function in early autoimmune disease.

ACKNOWLEDGMENT

The work on dendritic cells and autoimmunity is supported by several grants from NWO-Medical Sciences, NWO-INSERM, and the Dutch Diabetes Fund.

REFERENCES

Aiba, S., Yoshie, O., Tomita, Y. and Tagami, H. (1989). Cross-reactivity of murine monoclonal anti-DNA antibodies with human and murine skin: a possible pathogenetic role in skin lesions of lupus erythematosus. *J. Invest. Dermatol.* **93**, 739–745.

Allaerts, W., Fluitsma, D.M., Hoefsmit, E.C.M., Jeucken, P.H.M., Morreau, H., Bosma, F.T. and Drexhage, H.A. (1996). Immunohistochemical morphological and ultrastructural resemblance between dendritic cells and folliculo-stellate cells in normal human and rat anterior pituitaries. *J. Neuroendocrinol.* **8**, 17–29.

Austyn, J.M. (1987). Lymphoid dendritic cells. *Immunology* **62**, 161–170.

Barkley, D.W., Feldmann, M. and Maini, R.N. (1990). Cells with dendritic morphology and bright interleukin-1 alpha staining circulate in the blood of patients with rheumatoid arthritis. *Clin. Exp. Immunol.* **80**, 25–31.

Bauer, J., Sminia, T., Wouterlood, F.G. and Dijkstra, C.D. (1994). Phagocytic activity of macrophages and microglial cells during the course of acute and chronic relapsing experimental autoimmune encephalomyelitis. *J. Neurosci.* **38**, 365–375.

Belardelli, F. (1995). Role of interferons and other cytokines in the regulation of the immune responses. *APMIS* **103**, 161–179.

Berg, J.P. (1997). Autocrine/paracrine cell death in Hashimoto's thyroiditis. *Eur. J. Endocrinol.* **137**, 122–123.

Bergman, B. and Haskins, K. (1997). Autoreactive T cell clones from the nonobese diabetic mouse. *Proc. Soc. Exp. Biol. Med.* **214**, 41–48.

Bergroth, V., Tsai, V. and Zvaifler, N.J. (1989). Differences in responses of normal and rheumatoid arthritis peripheral blood T cells to synovial fluid and peripheral blood dendritic cells in allogeneic mixed leukocyte reactions. *Arthritis Rheum.* **32**, 1381–1389.

Bhardwaj, N., Lau, L.L., Rivelis, M. and Steinman, R.M. (1988). Interleukin-1 production by mononuclear cells from rheumatoid synovial effusions. *Cell. Immunol.* **114**, 405–423.

Bhardwaj, N., Santhanam, U., Lau, L.L., Tatter, S.B., Ghrayeb, J., Rivelis, M., Steinman, R.M., Sehgal, P.B. and May, L.T. (1989). IL-6/IFN-beta 2 in synovial effusions of patients with rheumatoid arthritis and other arthritides. Identification of several isoforms and studies of cellular sources. *J. Immunol.* **143**, 2153–2159.

Bhardwaj, N., Hodtsev, A.S., Nisanian, A., Kabak, S., Friedman, S.M., Cole, B.C. and Posnett, D.N. (1994). Human T cell responses to *Mycoplasma arthritidis*-derived superantigen. *Infect. Immun.* **62**, 135–144.

Bone, A.J., Hitchcock, P.R. and Dunger, A. (1997). Islet cell cytotoxicity and disease progression in the BB rat. *Diabetologia* **40**, A86 (abstract).

Bonomo, A., Kehn, P.J., Payer, E., Rizzo, L., Cheever, A.W. and Shevach, E.M. (1995). Pathogenesis of post-thymectomy autoimmunity. Role of syngeneic MLR-reactive T cells. *J. Immunol.* **154**, 6602–6611.

Bottazzo, G.F., Dean, M.R.C., McNally, J.M., McKay, E.H., Swift, P.G.F. and Gamble, D.R. (1985). In situ characterization of autoimmune phenomena and expression of HLA molecules in the pancreas in diabetic insulitis. *N. Engl. J. Med.* **313**, 353–360.

Braverman, L.E. (1990). The role of iodine in the pathogenesis of lymphocytic thyroiditis in animal models. In: *The Thyroid Gland, Iodine and Autoimmunity* (eds. H.A. Drexhage *et al.*), Elsevier, Amsterdam, pp. 279–288.

Bretzel, R.G., Platzer, A. and Schaeffer, R. (1990). Immunopathological findings and thyroid autoantibodies in thyroid autonomy. *Acta Med. Austriaca* **17**, 20–24.

Burns, C.M., Tsai, V. and Zvaifler, N.J. (1992). High percentage of $CD8^+$, Leu-7^+ cells in rheumatoid arthritis synovial fluid. *Arthritis Rheum.* **35**, 865–873.

Butler, T.L. and McMenamin, P.G. (1996). Resident and infiltrating immune cells in the uveal tract in the early and late stages of experimental autoimmune uveoretinitis. *Invest. Ophthalmol. Vis. Sci.* **37**, 2195–2210.

Canning, M.O., Haan-Meulman de, M. and Drexhage, H.A. (1997). The immunosuppressive effects of 1,25-dihydroxyvitamin D_3 are partly mediated via negative effects on the differentiation of monocytes into veiled cells. *J. Invest. Dermatol.* **109**, 255 (abstract).

Casciola-Rosen, L. and Rosen, A. (1997). Ultraviolet light-induced keratinocyte apoptosis: a potential mechanism for the induction of skin lesions and autoantibody production in LE. *Lupus* **6**, 175–180.

Caux, C., Liu, Y.J. and Banchereau, J. (1995). Recent advances in the study of dendritic cells and follicular dendritic cells. *Immunol. Today* **16**, 2–4.

Caux, C., Vandervliet, B., Massacrier, C., Dezutter-Dambuyant, C., de Saint-Vis, B., Jacquet, C., Yoneda, K., Imamura, S., Schmitt, D. and Banchereau, J. (1996). $CD34^+$ hematopoietic progenitors from human cord blood differentiate along two independent dendritic cell pathways in response to GM-CSF plus TNF alpha. *J. Exp. Med.* **184**, 695–706.

Clare-Salzler, M. and Mullen, Y. (1992). Marked dendritic cell–T cell cluster formation in the pancreatic lymph node of the non-obese diabetic mouse. *Immunology* **76**, 478–484.

Clare-Salzler, M.J., Brooks, J., Chai, A., van Herle, K. and Anderson, C. (1992). Prevention of diabetes in nonobese diabetic mice by dendritic cell transfer. *J. Clin. Invest.* **90**, 741–748.

Cockfield, S.M., Ramassar, V., Urmson, J. and Halloran, P.F. (1989). Multiple low dose streptozotocin induces systemic MHC expression in mice by triggering T cells to release IFN-gamma. *J. Immunol.* **142**, 1120–1128.

Corbett, J.A., Want, J.L., Sweetland, M.A., Lancaster, J.R. and McDaniel, M.L. (1992). Interleukin-1 beta induces the formation of nitric oxide by beta-cells purified from rodent islets of Langerhans. Evidence for the beta-cell as a source and site of action of nitric oxide. *J. Clin. Invest.* **90**, 2384–2391.

Costagliola, S., Many, M.C., Stalmans-Falys, M., Vassart, G. and Ludgate, M. (1996). Transfer of thyroiditis, with syngeneic spleen cells sensitized with the human thyrotropin receptor, to naive BALB/c and NOD mice. *Endocrinology* **137**, 4637–4643.

Delemarre, F.G.A. and Drexhage, H.A. (1997). Dendritic cells of the BB-DP rat are deficient accessory cells, particularly for $CD8^+$ and $RT6^+$ T cells ('suppressor cells'). *Exp. Clin. Endocrinol. Diabetes* **105**, 5–7.

Delemarre, F.G.A., Mooij, P., de Haan-Meulman, M., Simons, P.J., de Wit, H.J. and Drexhage, H.A. (1995a). Transition of T_3-induced monocyte-derived veiled/dendritic cells into macrophage-like cells by lipopolysaccharide. *Adv. Exp. Med. Biol.* **378**, 57–59.

Delemarre, F.G.A., Simons, P.J. and Drexhage, H.A. (1995b). Reduced function of dendritic cells from spleen and lymph nodes of the BB rat. *Immunol. Suppl.* **1**, 14 (abstract).

Delemarre, F.G.A., de Heer, H.J. and Simons, P.J. (1996). What triggers thyroid autoimmunity? II. Reduced accessory cell function of dendritic cells from the BB rat. *J. Endocrinol. Invest. Suppl.* **6**, 81 (abstract).

Demaziere, A., Leek, R. and Athanasou, N.A. (1992). Histological distribution of the interleukin-4 receptor (IL4R) within the normal and pathological synovium. *Rev. Rheum. Mal. Osteoartic.* **59**, 219–224.

Drexhage, H.A., Mullink, H, de Groot, J., *et al.* (1979a). A study of cells present in peripheral lymph of pigs with special reference to a type of cell resembling the Langerhans cell. *Cell Tiss. Res.* **202**, 407–430.

Drexhage, H.A., Mullink, H. and Balfour, B.M. (1979b). Morphology of cells present in skin lymph of pigs and rats. In: *Proc. VIth International Congress of Lymphology* (eds P. Malek, V. Bartos, H. Weisslader and M.H. White). Thieme Verlag, Stuttgart, pp. 246–249.

Edwards, J.C., Wilkinson, L.S., Speight, P. and Isenberg, D.A. (1993). Vascular cell adhesion molecule 1 and alpha 4 and beta 1 integrins in lymphocyte aggregates in Sjögren's syndrome and rheumatoid arthritis. *Ann. Rheum. Dis.* **52**, 806–811.

Eizirik, D.L. and Leijerstam, F. (1994). The inducible form of nitric oxide synthase (iNOS) in insulin-producing cells (Review). *Diabetes Metab.* **20**, 116–22.

Faveeuw, C., Gagnerault, M.C. and Lepault, F. (1994). Expression of homing and adhesion molecules in infiltrated islets of Langerhans and salivary glands of nonobese diabetic mice. *J. Immunol.* **152**, 5969–5978.

Finkelman, F.D., Lees, A., Birnbaum, R., Gause, W.C. and Morris, S.C. (1996). Dendritic cells can present antigen in vivo in a tolerogenic or immunogenic fashion. *J. Immunol.* **157**, 1406–1414.

Gadher, S.J. and Woolley, D.E. (1987). Comparative studies of adherent rheumatoid synovial cells in primary culture: characterisation of the dendritic (stellate) cell. *Rheumatol. Int.* **7**, 13–22.

Galy, A., Travis, M., Cen, D. and Chen, B. (1995). Human T, B, natural killer, and dendritic cells arise from a common bone marrow progenitor cell subset. *Immunity* **3**, 459–473.

Gautam, A.M. and Glynn, P. (1989). Lewis rat lymphoid dendritic cells can efficiently present homologous myelin basic protein to encephalitogenic lymphocytes. *J. Neuroimmunol.* **22**, 113–121.

Gautam, A.M. and Glynn, P. (1991). Competitive dissociation of encephalitogenic complexes between antigen presenting cells and myelin basic protein. *J. Neuroimmunol.* **34**, 25–31.

Georgiou, H.M., Lagarde, A.C. and Bellgrau, D. (1988). T cell dysfunction in the diabetes-prone BB rat. A role for thymic migrants that are not T cell precursors. *J. Exp. Med.* **167**, 132–148.

Georgiou, H.M., Constantinou, D. and Mandel, T.E. (1995). Prevention of autoimmunity in nonobese diabetic (NOD) mice by neonatal transfer of allogeneic thymic macrophages. *Autoimmunity* **21**, 89–97.

Goto, M., Okamoto, M., Sasano, M., Nishizawa, K., Aotsuka, S., Yamaguchi, N., Obinata, M. and Ikeda, K. (1991). Functional characterization of SV40-transformed adherent synovial cells from rheumatoid arthritis. *Clin. Exp. Immunol.* **86**, 387–392.

Granucci, F., Girolomoni, G., Lutz, M.B., Foti, M., Marconi, G., Gnocchi, P., Nolli, L. and Ricciardi-Castagnoli, P. (1994). Modulation of cytokine expression in mouse dendritic cell clones. *Eur. J. Immunol.* **24**, 2522–2526.

Greiner, D.L., Handler, E.S., Nakano, K., Mordes, J.P. and Rossini, A.A. (1986). Absence of the RT6 T cell subset in diabetes-prone BB/W rats. *J. Immunol.* **136**, 148–151.

Greiner, D.L., Mordes, J.P., Handler, E.S., Angelillo, M., Nakamura, N. and Rossini, A.A. (1987). Depletion of RT6$^+$ T lymphocytes induces diabetes in resistant BioBreeding (BB/W) rats. *J. Exp. Med.* **166**, 461.

Groen, H. (1996). T cell development in the diabetes-prone BB rat. A phenotypic analysis. Thesis, Rijksuniversiteit Groningen, Vakgroep Histologie en Celbiologie.

Grouard, G., Durand, I., Filgueira, L., Banchereau, J. and Liu, Y-J. (1996). Dendritic cells capable of stimulating T cells in germinal centres. *Nature* **384**, 364–367.

Gu, D., O'Reilly, L., Molony, L., Cooke, A. and Sarvetnick, N. (1995). The role of infiltrating macrophages in islet destruction and regrowth in a transgenic model. **8**, 483–492.

Hadzija, M., Semple, J.W. and Delovitch, T.L. (1991). Influence of antigen processing on thymic T cell selection. *Res. Immunol.* **142**, 421–424.

Hala, K., Malin, G., Dietrich, H., Loesch, U., Boeck, G., Wolf, H., Kaspers, B., Geryk, J., Falk, M. and Boyd, R.L. (1996). Analysis of the initiation period of spontaneous autoimmune thyroiditis (SAT) in obese strain (OS) of chickens. *J. Autoimmun.* **9**, 129–138.

Hanninen, A., Taylor, C., Streeter, P.R., Stark, L.S., Sarte, J.M., Shizuru, J.A., Simell, O. and Michie, S.A. (1993). Vascular addressins are induced on islet vessels during insulitis in nonobese diabetic mice and are involved in lymphoid cell binding to islet endothelium. *J. Clin. Invest.* **92**, 2509–2515.

Hara, Y., Caspi, R.R., Wiggert, B., Dorf, M. and Streilein, J.W. (1992). Analysis of an in vitro-generated signal that induces systemic immune deviation similar to that elicited by antigen injected into the anterior chamber of the eye. *J. Immunol.* **149**, 1531–1538.

Hassman, R., Solic, N., Jasani, B., Hall, R. and McGregor, A.M. (1988). Immunological events leading to destructive thyroiditis in the AUG rat. *Clin. Exp. Immunol.* **73**, 410–416.

Hayakawa, H., Sato, A., Imokawa, S., Toyoshima, M., Chida, K. and Iwata, M. (1996) Bronchiolar disease in rheumatoid arthritis. *Am. J. Respir. Crit. Care Med.* **154**, 1531–1536.

Heiligenhaus, A., Dutt, J.E. and Foster, C.S. (1996). Histology and immunopathology of systemic lupus erythematosus affecting the conjunctiva. *Eye* **10**, 425–432.

Heino, J., Viander, M., Peltonen, J. and Kouri, T. (1987). Adherent cells from rheumatoid synovia: identity of HLA-DR positive stellate cells. *Ann. Rheum. Dis.* **46**, 114–120.

Hoek, A., van Kasteren, Y., de Haan-Meulman, M., Schoemaker, J. and Drexhage, H.A. (1995). Dysfunction of monocytes and dendritic cells in patients with premature ovarian failure. *Am. J. Reprod. Immunol.* **33**, 495–502.

Hoek, A., Allaerts, W., Leenen, P.J.M., Schoemaker, J. and Drexhage, H.A. (1997). Dendritic cell and macrophages in the pituitary and the gonads. Evidence for their role in the fine regulation of the reproductive endocrine response. *Eur. J. Endocrinol.* **136**, 8–24.

Hoekman, K., von Blomberg-vd Flier, B.M.E., Wagstaff, J., Drexhage, H.A. and Pinedo, H.M. (1991). Reversible thyroid dysfunction during treatment with GM-CSF. *Lancet* **338**, 541–542.

Hoijer, M.A., Melief, M.J., van Helden-Meeuwsen, C.G., Eulderink, F. and Hazenberg, M.P. (1995). Detection of muramic acid in a carbohydrate fraction of human spleen. *Infect. Immun.* **63**, 1652–1657.

Holmdahl, R., Tarkowski, A. and Jonsson, R. (1991). Involvement of macrophages and dendritic cells in synovial inflammation of collagen induced arthritis in DBA/1 mice and spontaneous arthritis in MRL/lpr mice. *Autoimmunity* **8**, 271–280.

Homo-Delarche, F. and Boitard, C. (1996). Autoimmune diabetes: the role of the islets of Langerhans. *Immunol. Today* **17**, 456–460.

Hutchings, P., Rosen, H., O'Reilly, L., Simpson, E., Gordon, S. and Cooke, A.V. (1990). Transfer of diabetes in mice prevented by blockade of adhesion-promoting receptor on macrophages. *Nature* **348**, 639–642.

Ignatowicz, L., Kappler, J. and Marrack, P. (1996). The repertoire of T cells shaped by a single MHC/peptide ligand. *Cell* **84**, 521–529.

Ihm, S.H., Lee, K.U. and Yoon, J.W. (1991). Studies on autoimmunity for initiation of beta-cell destruction. VII. Evidence for antigenic changes on beta-cells leading to autoimmune destruction of beta-cells in BB rats. *Diabetes* **40**, 269–274.

Imai, Y. and Yamakawa, M. (1996). Morphology, function and pathology of follicular dendritic cells. *Pathol. Int.* **46**, 807–833.

Imai, Y., Sato, T., Yamakawa, M., Kasajima, T., Suda, A. and Watanabe, Y. (1989). A morphological and immunohistochemical study of lymphoid germinal centers in synovial and lymph node tissues from rheumatoid arthritis patients with special reference to complement components and their receptors. *Acta Pathol. Jpn* **39**, 127–134.

Issa-Chergui, B., Yale, J.F., Vigeant, C. and Seemayer, T.A. (1988). Major histocompatibility complex gene product expression on pancreatic beta cells in acutely diabetic BB rats. *Am. J. Pathol.* **130**, 156–162.

Ito, A., Woo, H.J., Imai, Y. and Osawa, T. (1988). Functional deficiencies of spleen dendritic cells in autoimmune MRL/lpr mice. *Immunol. Lett.* **17**, 223–228.

Iwai, H., Kuma, S., Inaba, M.M., Good, R.A., Yamashita, T., Kumazawa, T. and Ikehara, S. (1989). Acceptance of murine thyroid allografts by pretreatment of anti-la antibody or anti-dendritic cell antibody in vitro. *Tranplantation* **47**, 45–49.

Izumi, T., Suzuki, K., Saeki, M., Ookura, Y. and Hirono, S. (1995). An ultrastructural study on experimental autoimmune myocarditis with special reference to effector cells. *Eur. Heart J.* **16** (suppl. O), 75–77.

Jansen, A., Voorbij, H.A.M., Jeucken, P.H.M., Bruining, G.J., Hooijkaas, H. and Drexhage, H.A. (1993). An immunohistochemical study on organized lymphoid cell infiltrates in fetal and neonatal pancreases. *Autoimmunity* **15**, 31–38.

Jansen, A., Homo-Delarche, F., Hooijkaas, H., Leenen, P.J.M., Dardenne, M. and Drexhage, H.A. (1994). Immunohistochemical characterization of monocytes-macrophages and dendritic cells involved in the initiation of the insulitis and β cell destruction in NOD mice. *Diabetes* **43**, 667–675.

Jansen, A., van Hagen, M. and Drexhage, H.A. (1995). Defective maturation and function of antigen-presenting cells in type 1 diabetes. *Lancet* **345**, 491–492.

Jansen, A., Rosmalen, J.G.M., Homo-Delarche, F., Dardenne, M. and Drexhage, H.A. (1996). Effect of prophylactic insulin treatment on the number of ER-MP23$^+$ macrophages in the pancreas of NOD mice. Is the prevention of diabetes based on β-cell rest? *J. Autoimmunity* **9**, 341–348.

Jaramillo, A., Gill, B.M. and Delovitch, T.L. (1994). Insulin dependent diabetes mellitus in the non-obese diabetic mouse: a disease mediated by T cell anergy? *Life Sci.* **55**, 1163–1177.

Jiang, Z., Handler, E.S., Rossini, A.A. and Woda, B.A. (1990). Immunopathology of diabetes in the RT6-depleted diabetes-resistant BB/Wor rat. *Am. J. Pathol.* **137**, 767.

Kabel, P.J., Voorbij, H.A.M., van der Gaag, R.D., Wiersinga, W.M., De Haan, M. and Drexhage, H.A. (1987). Dendritic cells in autoimmune thyroid disease. *Acta Endocrinol.* (*Copenh.*) **281**, 42–48.

Kabel, P.J., Voorbij, H.A.M., De Haan, M., van der Gaag, R.D. and Drexhage, H.A. (1988). Intrathyroidal dendritic cells in Graves' disease and simple goitre. *J. Clin. Endocrinol. Metab.* **65**, 199–207.

Kabel, P.J., Voorbij, H.A.M., de Haan-Meulman, M., Pals, S.T. and Drexhage, H.A. (1989a). High endothelial venules present in lymphoid cell accumulations in thyroid affected by autoimmune disease. A study in men and BB rat of functional activity and development. *J. Clin. Endocrinol. Metab.* **68**, 744–751.

Kabel, P.J., Haan-Meulman, M. de, Voorbij, H.A.M., Kleingeld, M., Knol, E.F. and Drexhage, H.A. (1989b). Accessory cells with a morphology and marker pattern of dendritic cells can be obtained from elutriator purified blood monocyte fractions. An enhancing effect of metrizamide in this differentiation. *Immunobiology* **179**, 395–411.

Kabel, P.J., van Dinther, A., de Haan-Meulman, M., Berghout, A., Voorbij, H.A.M. and Drexhage, H.A. (1990). A diminished adherence of blood lymphocytes of patients with thyroid autoimmune disease to high endothelial venules in the thyroid and the thyroid-draining lymph nodes. *Autoimmunity* **5**, 247–256.

Kalinski, P., Hilkens, C.M., Snijders, A., Snijdewint, F.G. and Kapsenberg, M.L. (1997). IL-12-deficient dendritic cells, generated in the presence of prostaglandin E2, promote type 2 cytokine production in maturing human naive T helper cells. *J. Immunol.* **159**, 28–35.

Kamperdijk, E.W.A., Vught van, E., Richters, C.D. and Beelen, R.H.J. (1994). Morphology of dendritic cells. In: *Immunopharmacology of Macrophages and Other Antigen-presenting Cells* (eds C.A.F.M. Bruijnzeel-Koomen and E.C.M. Hoefsmit). Academic Press Harcourt Brace and Co., New York, pp. 45–61.

Kanauchi, H., Furukawa, F. and Imamura, S. (1991). Characterization of cutaneous infiltrates in MRL/lpr mice monitored from onset to the full development of lupus erythematosus-like skin lesions. *J. Invest. Dermatol.* **96**, 478–483.

Kasajima, T., Yamakawa, M. and Imai, Y. (1987). Immunohistochemical study of intrathyroidal lymph follicles. *Clin. Immunol. Immunopathol.* **43**, 117–128.

Katagiri, T. (1992) The dysfunction of human peripheral blood dendritic cells on concanavalin A-induced T cell responses in patients with systemic lupus erythematosus. *Arerugi* **41**, 693–698 [in Japanese].

Kavanaugh, A.F. and Lipsky, P.E. (1996). Rheumatoid arthritis. In: *Clinical Immunology. Principles and Practice*, vol. II. (eds. R.R. Rich, T.A. Fleisher, B.D. Schwartz, W.T. Shearer, and W. Strober). Mosby Year Book, St. Louis, pp. 1093–1116.

Kelsall, B.L., Stuber, E., Neurath, M. and Strober, W. (1996). Interleukin-12 production by dendritic cells. The role of CD40–CD40L interactions in Th1 T cell responses. *Ann. NY Acad. Sci.* **795**, 116–126.

Khoury, S.J., Gallon, L., Chen, W., Betres, K., Russell, M.E., Hancock, W.W., Carpenter, C.B., Sayegh, M.H. and Weiner, H.L. (1995). Mechanisms of acquired thymic tolerance in experimental autoimmune encephalomyelitis: thymic dendritic-enriched cells induce specific peripheral T cell unresponsiveness in vivo. *J. Exp. Med.* **182**, 357–366.

Kitahama, S., Litaka, M., Shimizu, T., Serizawa, N., Fukasawa, N., Miura, S., Kawasaki, S., Yamanaka, K., Kawakami, Y., Murakami, S., Ishii, J. and Katayama, S. (1996). Thyroid involvement by malignant histiocytosis of Langerhans' cell type. *Clin. Endocrinol.* **45**, 357–363.

Klasen, I.S., Kool, J., Melief, M.J., Loeve, I., van den Berg, W.B., Severijnen, A.J. and Hazenberg, M.P. (1992). Arthritis by autoreactive T cell lines obtained from rats after injection of intestinal bacterial cell wall fragments. *Cell. Immunol.* **139**, 455–467.

Klasen, I.S., Melief, M.J., van Halteren, A.G.S., Schouten, W.R., van Blankenstein, M., Hoke, G, de Visser, H., Hooijkaas, H. and Hazenberg, M.P. (1994). The presence of peptidoglycan–polysaccharide complexes in the bowel wall and the cellular responses to these complexes in Crohn's disease. *Clin. Immunol. Immunopathol.* **71**, 303–308.

Knight, S.C., Hunt, R., Dore, C. and Medawar, P.B. (1985). Influence of dendritic cells on tumor growth. *Proc. Natl. Acad. Sci. USA* **82**, 4495–4497.

Knight, S.C., Farrant, J., Chan, J., Bryant, A., Bedford, P.A. and Bateman, C. (1988). Induction of autoimmunity with dendritic cells: studies on thyroiditis in mice. *Clin. Immunol. Immunopathol.* **48**, 277–289.

Kool, J., de Visser, H., Gerrits-Boeye, M.Y., Klasen, I.S., Melief, M.J., van Helden-Meeuwsen, C.G., van Lieshout, L.M., Ruseler-van Embden, J.G., van den Berg, W.B., Bahr, G.M. and Hazenberg, M.P. (1994). Detection of intestinal flora-derived bacterial antigen complexes in splenic macrophages of rats. *Histochem. Cytochem.* **42**, 1435–1441.

Krenn, V., Schalhorn, N., Greiner, A., Molitoris, R., Konig, A., Gohlke, F. and Muller-Hermelink, H.K. (1996). Immunohistochemical analysis of proliferating and antigen-presenting cells in rheumatoid synovial tissue. *Rheumatol. Int.* **15**, 239–247.

Krieg, A.M. (1995). CpG DNA: a pathogenetic factor in systemic lupus erythematosus? *J. Clin. Immunol.* **15**, 284–292.

Kronin, V., Winkel, K., Suss, G., Kelso, A., Heath, W., Kirberg, F., Von Boehmer, H. and Shortman, K. (1996). A subclass of dendritic cells regulates the response of naive CD8 T cell by limiting their IL-2 production. *J. Immunol.* **157**, 3819–3827.

Lee, M.S., Wilkinson, B., Doyle, J.A. and Kossard, S. (1996). A comparative immunohistochemical study of lichen planus and discoid lupus erythematosus. *Aust. J. Dermatol.* **37**, 188–192.

Lety, M-A., Coulaud, J., Bens, M., Dardenne, M. and Homo-Delarche, F. (1992). Enhanced metabolism of arachidonic acid by macrophages from nonobese diabetic (NOD) mice. *Clin. Immunol. Immunopathol.* **64**, 188–196.

Li, M., Eastman, C.J. and Boyages, S.C. (1993). Iodine induced lymphocytic thyroiditis in the BB/W rat: early and late immune phenomena. *Autoimmunity* **14**, 181–187.

Linn, T., Noke, M., Woehrle, M., Kloer, H.U., Hammes, H.P., Litzlbauer, D., Bretzel, R.G. and Federlin, K. (1989). Fish oil-enriched diet and reduction of low-dose streptozocin-induced hyperglycemia. Inhibition of macrophage activation. *Diabetes* **38**, 1402–1411.

Linn, T., Strate, C., Federlin, K. and Papaccio, G. (1994). Intercellular adhesion molecule-1 (ICAM-1) expression in the islets of the non-obese diabetic and low-dose streptozotocin-treated mouse. *Histochemistry* **102**, 317–321.

Lioté, F., Boval-Boizard, B., Weill, D. and Wautier, J.-L. (1996). Blood monocytes activation in rheumatoid arthritis: increased monocyte adhesiveness, integrin expression, and cytokine release. *Clin. Exp. Immunol.* **106**, 13–19.

Lo, D., Reilly, C.R., Scott, B., Liblau, R., McDevitt, H.O. and Burkly, L.C. (1993). Antigen-presenting cells in adoptively transferred and spontaneous autoimmune diabetes. *Eur. J. Immunol.* **23**, 1693–1698.

Lo, D., Reilly, C., Marconi, L.A., Ogata, L., Wei, Q., Prud'homme, G., Kono, D. and Burkly, L. (1995). Regulation of CD4 T cell reactivity to self and non-self. *Int. Rev. Immunol.* **13**, 147–160.

Macatonia, S.E., Hosken, N.A., Litton, M., Vieira, P., Hsieh, C.S., Culpepper, J.A., Wysocka, M., Trinchieri, G., Murphy, K.M. and O'Garra, A. (1995). Dendritic cells produce IL-12 and direct the development of Th1 cells from naive $CD4^+$ T cells. *J. Immunol.* **154**, 5071–5079.

Mageed, R.A., Kirwan, J.R. and Holborow, E.J. (1991). Localization of circulating immune complexes from patients with rheumatoid arthritis in murine spleen germinal centres. *Scand. J. Immunol.* **34**, 323–331.

Maile, S. and Merker, H.J. (1995). The interstitial space of the thyroid gland of marmosets (*Callithrix jacchus*). *Anat. Anz.* **177**, 347–359.

Mandrup-Poulsen, T., Bendtzen, K., Nerup, J., Dinarello, C.A. Svenson, M. and Nielsen, J.H. (1987). Affinity-purified human interleukin-I is cytotoxic to isolated islets of Langerhans. *Diabetologia* **29**, 63–67.

Manjo, G., Joris, I., Handler, E.S., Desemone, J., Mordes, J.P. and Rossini, A.A. (1987). A pancreatic venular defect in the BB/Wor rat. *Am. J. Pathol.* **128**, 210–215.

Many, M.C., Maniratunga, S., Varis, I., Dardenne, M., Drexhage, H.A. and Denef, J-F. (1995). Two-step development of Hashimoto-like thyroiditis in genetically autoimmune prone non-obese diabetic mice: effects of iodine-induced cell necrosis. *J. Endocrinol.* **147**, 311–320.

Marazuela, M., Postigo, A.A., Acevedo, A., Diaz-Gonzalez, F., Sanchez-Madrid, F. and de Landazuri, M.O. (1994). Adhesion molecules from the LFA-1/ICAM-1,3 and VLA-4/VCAM-1 pathways on T lymphocytes and vascular endothelium in Graves' and Hashimoto's thyroid glands. *Eur. J. Immunol.* **24**, 2483–2490.

March, L.M. (1987). Dendritic cells in the pathogenesis of rheumatoid arthritis. *Rheumatol. Int.* **7**, 93–100.

Markholst, H. (1997). Characterization of the autosomal recessive T cell lymphopenic trait of DP-BB rats. *Exp. Clin. Endocrinol. Diabetes* **105**, 23.

Marth, T., Strober, W., Seder, R.A. and Kelsall, B.L. (1997). Regulation of transforming growth factor-beta production by interleukin-12. *Eur. J. Immunol.* **27**, 1213–1220.

Matyszak, M.K. and Perry, V.H. (1996). The potential role of dendritic cells in immune-mediated inflammatory diseases in the central nervous system. *Neuroscience* **74**, 599–608.

McCombe, P.A., de Jersey, J. and Pender, M.P. (1994). Inflammatory cells, microglia and MHC class II antigen-positive cells in the spinal cord of Lewis rats with acute and chronic relapsing experimental autoimmune encephalomyelitis. *J. Neuroimmunol.* **51**, 153–167.

McKeever, U., Mordes, J.P., Greiner, D.L., *et al.* (1990). Adoptive transfer of autoimmune diabetes and thyroiditis to athymic rats. *Proc. Natl Acad. Sci. USA* **87**, 7618–7622.

Melief, M.J., Hoijer, M.A., Paasen van, H.C. and Hazenberg, M.P. (1995). Presence of bacterial flora-derived antigen in synovial tissue macrophages and dendritic cells. *Br. J. Rheumatol.* **34**, 1112–1116.

Mooij, P. and Drexhage, H.A. (1993). Autoimmune thyroid disease. *Clin. Lab. Med.* **13**, 683–697.

Mooij, P., de Wit, H.J. and Drexhage, H.A. (1993). An excess of dietary iodine accelerates the development of a thyroid-associated lymphoid tissue in autoimmune prone BB rats. *Clin. Immunol. Immunopathol.* **69**, 189–198.

Mooij, P., de Wit, H.J., Bloot, A.M., Wilders-Truschnig, M.M. and Drexhage, H.A. (1993). Iodine deficiency induces thyroid autoimmune reactivity in Wistar rats. *Endocrinology* **133**, 1197–1204.

Mooij, P., Simons, P.J., de Haan-Meulman, M., de Wit, H.J. and Drexhage, H.A. (1994). Effect of thyroid hormones and other iodinated compounds on the transition of monocytes into veiled/dendritic cells: role of GM-CSF, TNF-α and IL-6. *J. Endocrinol.* **140**, 503–512.

Mori, M., Pimpineli, N., Romagnoli, P., Bernacchi, E., Fabbri, P. and Giannotti, B. (1994). Dendritic cells in cutaneous lupus erythematosus: a clue to the pathogenesis of lesions. *Histopathology* **24**, 311–321.

Neu, N., Pummerer, C., Rieker, T. and Berger, P. (1993). T cells in cardiac myosin-induced myocarditis. *Clin. Immunol. Immunopathol.* **68**, 107–110.

Nossal, G.J., Herold, K.C. and Goodnow, C.C. (1992). Autoimmune tolerance and type 1 (insulin-dependent) diabetes mellitus. *Diabetologia* **35**, S49–59.

O'Garra, A., Steinman, L. and Gijbels, K. (1997). $CD4^+$ T cell subsets in autoimmunity. *Curr. Opin. Immunol.*, in press.

Ohashi, P., Oehen, S., Buerki, K., Pircher, H., Ohashi, C., Odermatt, B., Malissen, B., Zinkernagel, R. and Hengartner, H. (1991). Ablation of tolerance and induction of diabetes by virus infection in viral antigen transgenic mice. *Cell* **65**, 305–317.

Oldstone, M.B.A., Nerenberg, M., Southern, P., Price, J. and Lewicki, H. (1991). Virus infection triggers insulin-dependent diabetes mellitus in a transgenic model: role of anti-self (virus) immune response. *Cell* **65**, 319–331.

Pallis, M., Robson, D.K., Haskard, D.O. and Powell, R.J. (1993). Distribution of cell adhesion molecules in skeletal muscle from patients with systemic lupus erythematosus. *Ann. Rheum. Dis.* **52**, 667–671.

Peters, J.H., Ruhl, S. and Friedrichs, D. (1987). Veiled accessory cells deduced from monocytes. *Immunobiology* **176**, 154.

Petri, M. (1996). Systemic lupus erythematosus. In: *Clinical Immunology. Principles and Practice*, vol. II (eds. R.R. Rich, T.A. Fleisher, B.D. Schwartz, W.T. Shearer and W. Strober). Mosby Year Book, St. Louis, pp. 1072–1092.

Petzelbauer, P., Fodinger, D., Rappersberger, K., Volc-Platzer, B. and Wolff, K. (1993). CD68 positive epidermal dendritic cells. *J. Invest. Dermatol.* **101**, 256–261.

Pilstrom, B. and Bohme, J. (1997). Alleviation of insulitis in NOD mice is associated with expression of transgenic MHC E molecules on primary antigen-presenting cells. *Immunology* **90**, 483–488.

Postigo, A.A., Marazuela, M., Sanchez-Madrid, F. and de Landazuri, M.O. (1994). B lymphocyte binding to E- and P-selectins is mediated through the de novo expression of carbohydrates on in vitro and in vivo activated human B cells. *J. Clin. Invest.* **94**, 1585–1596.

Radosevic, K., Drexhage, H.A., Ewijk van, W. and Leenen, P.J.M. (1997). Dendritic cells from diabetes-prone NOD mice induce a prolonged proliferative response of memory-like T cells. *Immunol. Lett.* **56**, 220 (abstract).

Ridderstad, A., Abedi-Valugerdi, M. and Moller, E. (1991). Cytokines in rheumatoid arthritis. *Ann. Med.* **23**, 219–223.

Robinson, C.P., Yamamoto, H., Peck, A.B. and Humphreys-Beher, M.G. (1996). Genetically programmed development of salivary gland abnormalities in the NOD (nonobese diabetic)-scid mouse in the absence of detectable lymphocytic infiltration: a potential trigger for sialoadenitis of NOD mice. *Clin. Immunol. Immunopathol.* **79**, 50–59.

Rose, L.M., Latchman, D.S. and Isenberg, D.A. (1997). Apoptosis in peripheral lymphocytes in systemic lupus erythematosus: a review. *Br. J. Rheumatol.* **36**, 158–163.

Sakaguchi, S., Takahashi, T. and Nishizuka, Y. (1982). Study on cellular events in postthymectomy autoimmune oophoritis in mice. 1. Requirement of Lyt-1 effector cells for oocytes damage after adoptive transfer. *J. Exp. Med.* **156**, 1565–1576.

Salisbury, A.K., Duke, O. and Poulter, L.W. (1987). Macrophage-like cells of the pannus area in rheumatoid arthritic joints. *Scand. J. Rheumatol.* **16**, 263–272.

Sallusto, F., Cella, M., Danieli, C. and Lanzavecchia, A. (1995). Dendritic cells use macropinocytosis and the mannose receptor to concentrate macromolecules in the major histocompatibility complex class II compartment: downregulation by cytokines and bacterial products. *J. Exp. Med.* **182**, 283–288.

Santiago-Schwarz, F., Sullivan, C., Rappa, D. and Carsons, S.E. (1996). Distinct alterations in lineage committed progenitor cells exist in the peripheral blood of patients with rheumatoid arthritis and primary Sjögren's syndrome. *J. Rheumatol.* **23**, 439–446.

Sasano, M., Goto, M. and Nishioka, K. (1990). Production of prostaglandin E2 induced by histamine by cloned rheumatoid synovial cells. *Ann. Rheum. Dis.* **49**, 504–506.

Sato, A., Hayakawa, H., Uchiyama, H. and Chida, K. (1996). Cellular distribution of bronchus-associated lymphoid tissue in rheumatoid arthritis. *Am. J. Respir. Crit. Care Med.* **154**, 1903–1907.

Savino, W., Carnaud, C., Luan, J.J., Bach, J.F. and Dardenne, M. (1993). Characterization of the extracellular matrix-containing giant perivascular spaces in the NOD mouse thymus. *Diabetes* **42**, 134–140.

Scherak, O., Kolarz, G., Popp, W., Wottawa, A. and Ritschka, L. (1993). Lung involvement in rheumatoid factor-negative arthritis. *Scand. J. Rheumatol.* **22**, 225–228.

Schwartz, R.S. (1996). Mechanisms of autoimmunity. In: *Clinical Immunology, Principles and Practice* (eds R.R. Rich, T.A. Fleisher, B.D. Schwartz, W.T. Shearer and W. Strober). Mosby Year Book, St. Louis, pp. 1053–1061.

Serreze, D.V., Gaedeke, J.W. and Leiter, E.H. (1993a). Hematopoietic stem-cell defects underlying abnormal macrophage development and maturation in NOD/Lt mice: defective regulation of cytokine receptors and protein kinase C. *Proc. Natl. Acad. Sci. USA* **90**, 9625–9629.

Serreze, D.V., Gaskins, H.R. and Leiter, E.H. (1993b). Defects in the differentiation and function of antigen presenting cells in NOD/Lt mice. *J. Immunol.* **150**, 2534–2543.

Shimuzu, S., Shiozawa, S., Shiozawa, K., Imura, S., Ishikawa, H., Hirohata, K. amd Fujita, T. (1988). The restoration of proliferation and differentiation of peripheral blood mononuclear non-adherent cells into immunoglobulin-secreting cells by autologous synovial adherent cells from patients with rheumatoid arthritis. *Virchows Arch. B Cell. Pathol. Incl. Mol. Pathol.* **54**, 350–356.

Shimizu, J., Carrasco-Marin, E., Kanagawa, O. and Unanue, E.R. (1995). Relationship between beta cell injury and antigen presentation in NOD mice. *J. Immunol.* **155**, 4095–4099.

Shimojo, N., Kohno, Y., Yamaguchi, K-I., Kikuoka, S-I., Hoshioka, A., Nimi, H., Hirai, A., Tamura, Y., Saito, Y., Kohn, L.D. and Tahara, K. (1996). Induction of Graves-like disease in mice by immunization with fibroblasts transfected with the thyrotropin receptor and a class II molecule. *Proc. Natl. Acad. Sci. USA* **93**, 11074–11079.

Simons, P.J., Delemarre, F.G.A. and Drexhage, H.A. (1997). Dendritic cells as regulators of growth and function of thyrocytes: a role of IL-1β and IL-6. *Immunol. Lett.* **56**, 217 (abstract).

Simons, P.J., Delemarre, F.G.A., Jeucken, P.H.M. and Drexhage, H.A. (1998). Pre-autoimmune thyroid abnormalities in the biobreeding diabetes-prone (BB-DP) rat. A possible relation with the intrathyroidal accumulation of dendritic cells and the initiation of the thyroid autoimmune response. *J. Endocrinol.*, in press.

Singh, A.K. (1995). Lupus in the Fas lane? *J. R. Coll. Physicians Lond.* **29**, 475–478.

Smith, H., Sakamoto, Y., Kasai, K. and Tung, K.S.K. (1991.) Effector and regulatory cells in autoimmune oophoritis elicited by neonatal thymectomy. *J. Immunol.* **147**, 2928–2933.

Stagg, A.J., Harding, B., Hughes, R.A., Keat, A. and Knight, S.C. (1991). The distribution and functional properties of dendritic cells in patients with seronegative arthritis. *Clin. Exp. Immunol.* **84**, 66–71.

Stephanson, E. and Ross, A.M. (1993). Expression of intercellular adhesion molecule-1 (ICAM-1) and OKM5 in UVA- and UVB-induced lesions in patients with lupus erythematosus and polymorphous light eruption. *Arch. Dermatol. Res.* **285**, 328–333.

Strunk, D., Egger, C., Leitner, G., Hanau, D. and Stingl, G. (1997). A skin homing molecule defines the Langerhans cell progenitor in human peripheral blood. *J. Exp. Med.* **185**, 1131–1136.

Sundick, R.S. (1989). Target organ defects in thyroid autoimmune disease. *Immunol. Res.* **8**, 39–60.

Summers, K.L., Daniel, P.B., O'Donnell, J.L. and Hart, D.N. (1995). Dendritic cells in synovial fluid of chronic inflammatory arthritis lack CD80 surface expression. *Clin. Exp. Immunol.* **100**, 81–89.

Summers, K.L., O'Donnell, J.L., Williams, L.A. and Hart, D.N. (1996). Expression and function of CD80 and CD86 costimulator molecules on synovial dendritic cells in chronic arthritis. *Arthritis. Rheum.* **39**, 1287–1291.

Suss, G. and Shortman, K. (1996). A subclass of dendritic cells kills CD4 T cells via Fas/Fas-ligand-induced apoptosis. *J. Exp. Med.* **183**, 1789–1796.

Suzuki, K. (1995). A histological study on experimental autoimmune myocarditis with special reference to initiation of the disease and cardiac dendritic cells. *Virchows Arch.* **426**, 493–500.

Tafuri, A., Bowers, W.E., Handler, E.S., Appel, M., Lew, R., Greiner, D., Mordes, J.P. and Rossini, A.A. (1993). High stimulatory activity of dendritic cells from diabetes-prone BioBreeding/Worcester rats exposed to macrophage-derived factors. *J. Clin. Invest.* **91**, 2040–2048.

Taguchi, O. and Nishizuka, Y. (1980). Autoimmune oophoritis in the thymectomized mice: T cell requirement in the adoptive cell transfer. *Clin. Exp. Immunol.* **42**, 324–331.

Takahashi, M., Honeyman, M.C. and Harison, L.C. (1997). Defective monocyte-derived dendritic cells from high-risk IDDM relatives. *Diabetologia* **40**, A23 (abstract).

Tandon, N., Metcalfe, R.A., Barnett, D. and Weetman, A.P. (1994). Expression of the costimulatory molecule B7/BB1 in autoimmune thyroid disease. *Q. J. Med.* **87**, 231–236.

Tas, M.P.R., de Haan-Meulman, M., Kabel, P.J. and Drexhage, H.A. (1991). Defects in monocyte polarization and dendritic cell clustering in patients with Graves disease. A putative role of a nonspecific immunoregulatory factor related to retroviral p15E. *Clin. Endocrinol.* **34**, 441–448.

Terashma, K., Ukai, K., Tajima, K., Yuda, F. and Imai, Y. (1988). Morphological diversity of DRC-1 positive cells: human follicular dendritic cells and their relatives. *Adv. Exp. Med. Biol.* **237**, 157–163.

Thomas, R. and Lipsky, P.E. (1996). Could endogenous self-peptides presented by dendritic cells initiate rheumatoid arthritis? *Immunol. Today* **17**, 559–564.

Thomas, R. and Quinn, C. (1996). Functional differentiation of dendritic cells in rheumatoid arthritis: role of CD86 in the synovium. *J. Immunol.* **156**, 3074–3086.

Thomas-Vaslin, V., Damotte, D., Coltey, M., Le Douarin, N.M., Coutinho, A. and Salaün, J. (1997). Abnormal T cell selection on NOD thymic epithelium is sufficient to induce autoimmune manifestations in C57BL/6 athymic nude mice. *Proc. Natl Acad. Sci. USA* **94**, 4598–4603.

Todd, J.A. and Farrall, M. (1996). Panning for gold: genome wide scanning for linkage in type 1 diabetes. *Hum. Mol. Genet.* **5**,1443–1448.

Toussaint-Demylle, D., Many, M.C., Theisen, H., Kraal, G. and Denef, J.F. (1990). Effects of iodide on class II-MHC antigen expression in iodine deficient hyperplastic thyroid glands. *Autoimmunity* **7**, 51–62.

Travaglio-Encinoza, A., Chaoiuni, I., Dersimonian, H. Jorgensen, C., Simony-Lafontaine, J., Romagne, F., Sany, J., Dupuy d'Angeac, A.D., Brenner, M.B. and Reme, T. (1995). T cell receptor distribution in rheumatoid synovial follicles. *J. Rheumatol.* **22**, 394–399.

Trinchieri, G. (1997). Function and clinical use of interleukin-12. *Curr. Opin. Hematol.* **4**, 59–66.

Tsai, V. and Zvaifler, N.J. (1988). Dendritic cell–lymphocyte clusters that form spontaneously in rheumatoid arthritis synovial effusions differ from clusters formed in human mixed leukocyte reactions. *J. Clin. Invest.* **82**, 1731–1745.

Tung, K.S.K., Smith, S., Teuscher, C., Cook, C. and Anderson, R.E. (1987). Murine autoimmune oophoritis, epididymoorchitis, and gastritis induced by day 3 thymectomy. *Am. J. Pathol.* **126**, 293–302.

Vafiadis, P., Bennet, S.T., Todd, J.A., Nadeau, J., Grabs, R., Goodyer, C.G., Wickramasinghe, S., Colle, E. and Polychronakos, C. (1997). Insulin expression in human thymus is modulated by INS VNTR alleles at the IDDM 2 locus. *Nature Genetics* **15**, 289–292.

Vakkila, J., Sihvola, M. and Hurme, M. (1990). Human peripheral blood-derived dendritic cells do not produce interleukin 1-alpha, interleukin 1-beta or interleukin 6. *Scand. J. Immunol.* **31**, 345–352.

van Eden, W., Anderton, S.M., van der Zee, A., Prakken, B.J., Broeren, C.B. and Wauben, M.H. (1996). (Altered) self peptide and the regulation of self reactivity in the peripheral T cell pool. *Immunol. Rev.* **149**, 55–73.

van Furth, R. (1980). *Mononuclear Phagocytes. Functional Aspects*, part I. Martinus Nijhoff, Dordrecht.

van Haarst, J.M.W., Hoogsteden, H.C., de Wit, H.J., Verhoeven, G.T., Havenith, C.E.G. and Drexhage, H.A. (1994). Dendritic cells and their precursors isolated from the human bronchoalveolar lavage: immunocytological and functional properties. *Am. J. Respir. Cell. Mol. Biol.* **11**, 344–350.

van de Plassche-Boers, E.M., Drexhage, H.A. and Kokjé-Kleingeld, M. (1985). The use of somatic antigen of *H. influenzae* for the monitoring of T-cell mediated skintest reactivity in man. *J. Immunol. Methods* **83**, 353–361.

Vieten, G., Grams, B., Muller, M., Hartung, K. and Emmendorffer, A. (1996). Examination of the mononuclear phagocyte system in lupus-prone male BXSB mice. *J. Leukocyte Biol.* **59**, 325–332.

Vivino, F.B. and Schumacker H.R. (1989). Synovial fluid characteristics and the lupus erythematosus cell phenomenon in drug-induced lupus. Findings in three patients and review of pertinent literature. *Arthritis Rheum.* **32**, 560–568.

von Herrath, M.G. and Holz, A. (1997). Pathological changes in the islet milieu precede infiltration of islets and destruction of β-cells by autoreactive lymphocytes in a transgenic model of virus-induced IDDM. *J. Autoimmun.* **10**, 231–238.

von Herrath, M.G., Homann, D., Dyrberg, T. and Oldstone, M.B.A. (1997). Treatment of virus-induced autoimmune diabetes by oral administration of insulin: study on the mechanism by which oral antigens can abrogate autoimmunity. *Exp. Clin. Endocrinol. Diabetes* **105**, 24–25.

Voorbij, H.A.M., Jeucken, P.H.M., Kabel, P.J., de Haan, M. and Drexhage, H.A. (1989). Dendritic cells and scavenger macrophages in the pancreatic islets of prediabetic BB rats. *Diabetes* **38**, 1623–1629.

Voorbij, H.A.M., Jeucken, P.H.M. and Drexhage, H.A. (1990a). A DTH skintest system using the insulinoma cell line RinM5F to monitor beta cell specific cellular autoimmune reactivity in the spontaneously diabetic BB/O rat. *Clin. Exp. Immunol.* **82**, 542–547.

Voorbij, H.A.M., Kabel, P.J. and de Haan, M., Jeucken, P., van der Gaag, R.D., de Baets, M.H. and Drexhage, H.A. (1990b). Dendritic cells and class II MHC expression on thyrocytes during the autoimmune thyroid disease of the BB rat. *Clin. Immunol. Immunopathol.* **55**, 9–22.

Waalen, K., Forre, O., Pahle, J., Natvig, J.B. and Burmester, G.R. (1987a). Characteristics of human rheumatoid synovial and normal blood dendritic cells. Retention of class II major histocompatibility complex antigens and accessory function after short-term culture. *Scand. J. Immunol.* **26**, 525–533.

Waalen, K., Forre, O., Teigland, J. and Natvit, J.B. (1987b). Human rheumatoid synovial and normal blood dendritic cells as antigen presenting cell-comparison with autologous monocytes. *Clin. Exp. Immunol.* **70**, 1–9.

Wang, B., Gonzalez, A., Benoist, C. and Mathis, D. (1996). The role of $CD8^+$ T cells in the initiation of insulin-dependent diabetes mellitus. *Eur. J. Immunol.* **26**, 1762–1769.

Warfvinge, G., Warfvinge, K. and Larsson, A. (1994). Histochemical visualization of mercury in the oral mucosa, salivary and lacrimal glands of BN rats with $HgCl_2$-induced autoimmunity. *Exp. Toxicol. Pathol.* **46**, 329–334.

Weringer, E.J. and Like, A.A. (1988). Identification of T cell subsets and class I and class II antigen expression in islet grafts and pancreatic islets of diabetic BioBreeding/Worcester rats. *Am. J. Pathol.* **132**, 292–303.

Wick, G., Hu, Y., Schwarz, S. and Kroemer, G. (1993). Immunoendocrine communication via the hypothalamo-pituitary-adrenal axis in autoimmune diseases. *Endocr. Rev.* **14**, 539–563.

Wilder, R.L. (1996). Hormones and autoimmunity: animal models of arthritis. *Ballières Clin. Rheumatol.* **10**, 259–271.

Wilders, M.M., Drexhage, H.A., Weltevreden, E.F., *et al.* (1983). Large mononuclear Ia-positive veiled cells in Peyer's patches. I. Isolation and characterization in rat, guinea pig and pig. *Immunology* **48**, 453.

Wilders, M.M., Drexhage, H.A., Kokjé, M., *et al.* (1984). Veiled cells in chronic idiopathic inflammatory bowel disease. *Clin. Exp. Immunol.* **55**, 377.

Wilders-Truschnig, M.M., Kabel, P.J., Drexhage, H.A., Beham, A., Leb, G., Eber, O., Heberstreit, J., Loidolt, D., Dohr, G., Lanzer, G. and Kreys, G.J. (1989). Intrathyroidal dendritic cells, epitheloid cells and giant cells in iodine deficient goiter. *Am. J. Pathol.* **135**, 219–225.

Wilders-Truschnig, M.M., Drexhage, H.A., Leb, G., Eber, O., Brezinschek, H.P., Dohr, G., Lanzer, G. and Kreys, G.J. (1990). Chromatographically purified IgG of endemic and sporadic goiter patients stimulates FRTL-5 cell growth in a mitotic arrest assay. *J. Clin. Endocrinol. Metab.* **70**, 444–452.

Wilkinson, L.S., Worrall, J.G., Sinclair, H.D. and Edwards, J.C. (1990). Immunohistochemical reassessment of accessory cell populations in normal and diseased human synovium. *Br. J. Rheumatol.* **29**, 259–263.

Witmer, M.D. and Steinman, R.M. (1984). The anatomy of peripheral lymphoid organs with emphasis on accessory cells: light microscopic immunocytochemical studies of mouse spleen, lymph node, and Peyer's patch. *Am. J. Anat.* **170**, 465–481.

Wu, L., Li, C.L. and Shortman, K. (1996). Thymic dendritic cell precursors: relationship to the T lymphocyte lineage and phenotype of the dendritic cell progeny. *J. Exp. Med.* **184**, 903–911.

Ziegler, A.G., Erhard, J., Lampeter, E.F., Nagelkerken, L.M. and Standl, E. (1992). Involvement of dendritic cells in early insulitis of BB rats. *J. Autoimmun.* **5**, 571–579.

CHAPTER 22
Interaction of Dendritic Cells with Bacteria

M. Rescigno[1], M. Rittig[2], S. Citterio[1], M.K. Matyszak[1], M. Foti[1], F. Granucci[1], M. Martino[1], U. Fascio[2], P. Rovere[4] and P. Ricciardi-Castagnoli[1]

[1]CNR Center of Cellular and Molecular Pharmacology, Milan, Italy; [2]Department of Anatomy, University of Erlangen, Germany; [3]Department of Biology, University of Milan, Italy; [4]HSR, Department of Internal Medicine, Milan, Italy

DENDRITIC CELLS AS SENTINELS TO ALERT THE ADAPTIVE IMMUNE RESPONSE

Initiation of an adaptive immune response to infectious agents is mediated by a class of sentinel phagocytic leukocytes termed dendritic cells (DC), the primary function of which is to capture, process and present antigens to unprimed T cells (Steinman, 1991; Ibrahim *et al.*, 1995). There are members of this family in most tissues, especially in those tissues that provide an environmental interface such as the skin, the gut and the lungs (Nelson *et al.*, 1994; Nestle *et al.*, 1993; Sertl *et al.*, 1986). Owing to this wide tissue distribution, DC can act as sentinels during bacterial infections. Uptake of pathogens induces a state of activation which eventually leads to the migration of the antigen-loaded DC to the lymphoid organs where the cells of the adaptive immune response can be alerted (Moll *et al.*, 1993). Thus, understanding the interaction of bacteria with DC, and the early molecular events resulting from this interaction may shed some light on the mechanisms of initiation of the immune response to infectious agents and on aspects of invasiveness, pathogenicity, and the persistence of certain bacteria.

ACTIVATED DC MATURE FROM A 'PROCESSING' TO A 'PRESENTING' PHENOTYPE

When activated by cytokines, DC undergo a process of maturation which has been described extensively (Schuler and Steinman, 1985; Inaba *et al.*, 1994; Roake *et al.*, 1995; Witmer-Pack *et al.*, 1987; Heufler *et al.*, 1988; Winzler *et al.*, 1997). We have previously shown that immature DC, grown *in vitro* as growth factor-dependent cell lines, preserve an immature phenotype (Winzler *et al.*, 1997) that is functionally defined as a 'processing phenotype'. *In vitro* proliferation and survival of such immature DC cells is strictly dependent upon the presence of exogenous GM-CSF and conditioned medium (Winzler *et al.*, 1997). However, they can be driven *in vitro* to differentiate and

Dendritic Cells: Biology and Clinical Applications
ISBN 0-12-455860-7

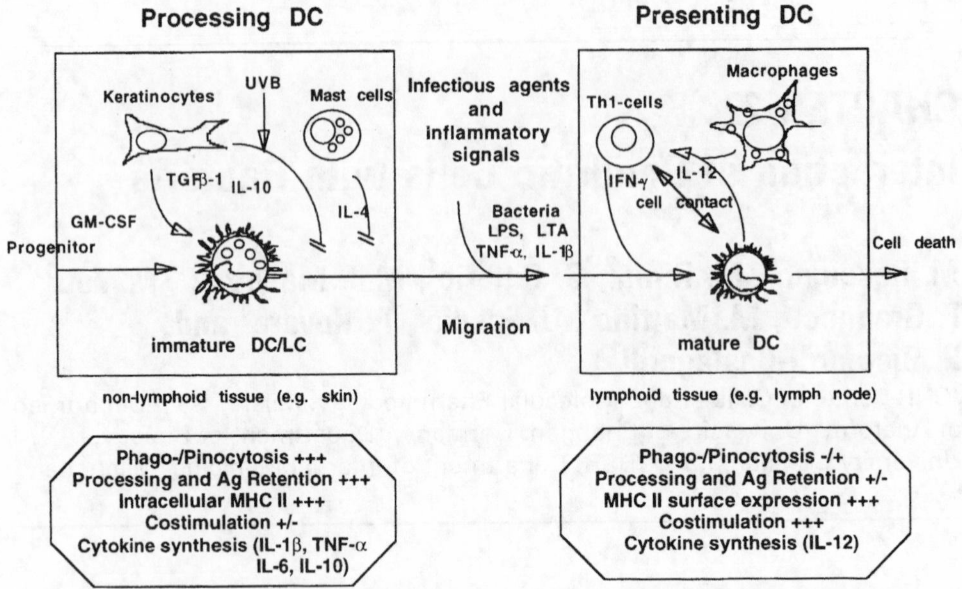

Fig. 1. Maturation stages of mouse DC.

to acquire the 'presenting phenotype' (Fig. 1). This maturation can be induced by infectious agents (bacteria, viruses, etc.), their products (LTA, LPS etc.) or by pro-inflammatory cytokines such as TNF-α.

During DC maturation induced by TNF-α, most intracellular class II molecules are translocated to the cell surface (Winzler *et al.*, 1997). MHC class I molecules and the costimulatory molecule B7.2 are also strongly upregulated (Fig. 2A). As a result, mature DC become the most efficient antigen-presenting cells (APC) able to polarize antigen-specific T cells by producing biologically active IL-12 (Winzler *et al.*, 1997), a key cytokine skewing the T cell response toward a T_H1-phenotype. Interestingly, maturation of DC is not accompanied by a significant modulation of molecules of the β_2-integrin family (CD11a, b and c; Fig. 2B).

Using this *in vitro* DC differentiation system, it is possible to analyze early and late molecular events of functional DC maturation induced by bacterial infection.

THE COMPLEXITY OF MICROORGANISMS AND THEIR STRATEGIES TO AVOID RECOGNITION

The interactions of DC with microorganisms are extremely complex. The reasons for this complexity are to be discovered in two characteristics of bacteria: their antigenic complexity, and the strategy developed by bacteria to evade the immune response of the host. This chapter aims to bring together some of the unifying principles governing the interaction of bacteria and DC. It will do so by reference to a limited number of microorganisms which have been chosen as representatives of three major bacterial groups according to their cell envelope, viz. Gram-positive, Gram-negative, and

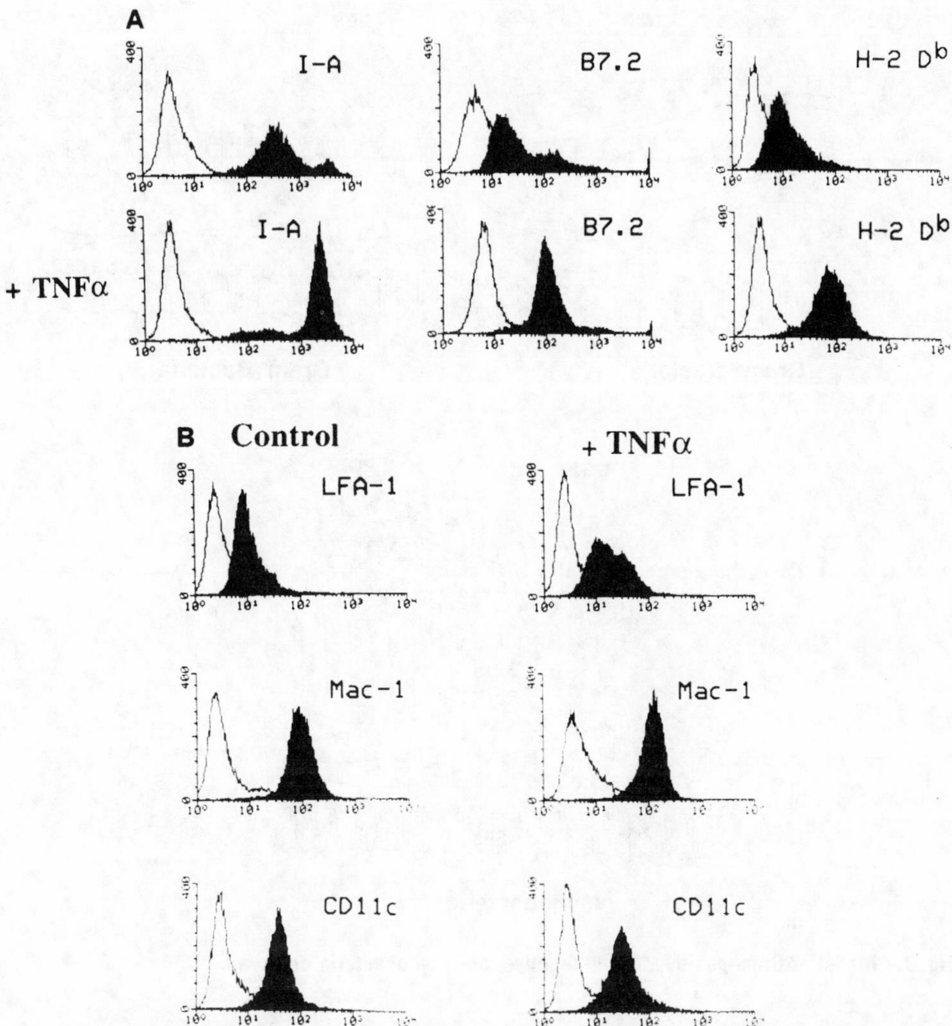

Fig. 2. Upregulation of MHC class I (D^b) and class II (I-A^b and B7.2) molecules on D1 cells after TNF-α treatment as shown by FACS analysis (A). In contrast, no significant upregulation of β_2-integrins is observed (B). Filled histograms show binding of specific antibodies, whereas isotype-matched control antibodies or secondary reagents are represented by open histograms. FcR blocking was performed before all labeling experiments.

mycobacteria. A common feature of the three groups is the inner protoplasmic membrane (PM) and a peptidoglycan (PG) cell wall. In addition, Gram-negative bacteria, exemplified here by *Salmonella typhimurium*, have an outer membrane containing proteins and lipopolysaccharides (LPS) which are antigenic. The outer membrane often contains pili, or fimbriae formed of type-specific protein antigens which can mediate attachment to the host cell surface or be anti-phagocytic (Fig. 3). Mycobacteria have an outer membrane of mycolic acid (MA) residues and phenolic glycolipids (PGL) linked through arabinogalactan (AG) to the inner peptidoglycan layer; the bacterial antigens

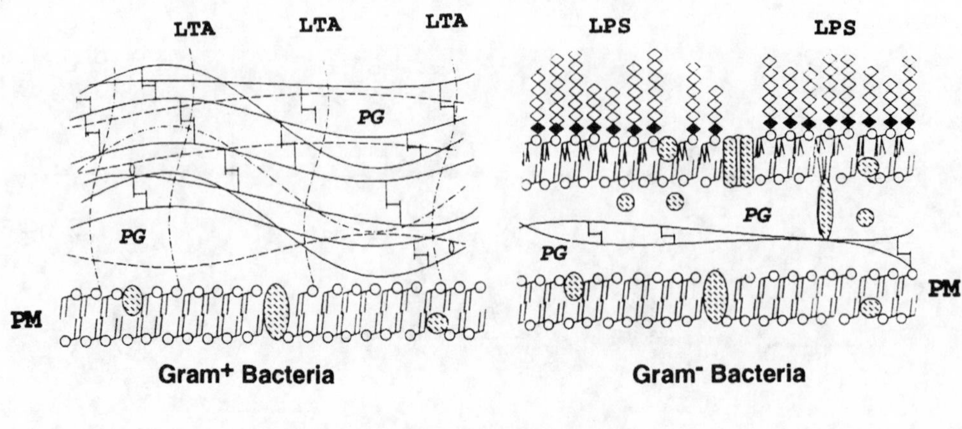

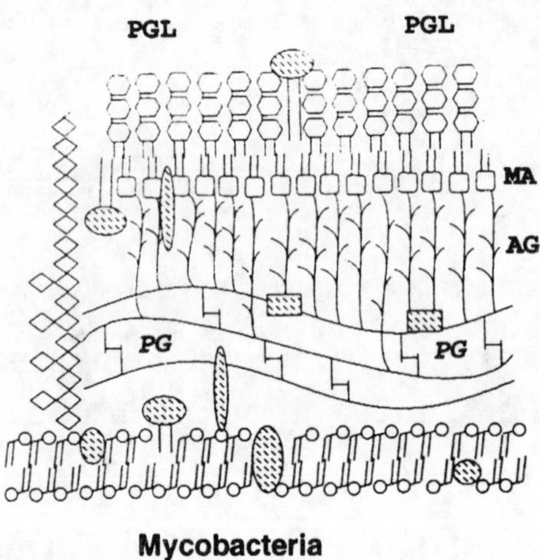

Fig. 3. Model of Gram-positive, Gram-negative, and mycobacteria cell wall.

are carbohydrate-based lipoarabinomannans which extend from the protoplasmic membrane to the bacterial surface. Finally, Gram-positive bacteria, exemplified here by *Streptococcus gordonii*, have a cell wall composed predominantly of peptidoglycan (PG), and lipoteichoic acids (LTA) attached directly to phospholipids of the protoplasmic membrane. LTA protrude to the cell surface where they form surface antigens for cell adhesion (Fig. 3).

Antigenic Complexity

The antigenic complexity of bacteria is the result of a number of several distinct epitopes, often repeated (as in the case of carbohydrates); however, bacterial protective structures, such as the capsule, may limit epitope recognition. In addition, antigen accessibility can vary because internal antigens may become accessible only after the bacterium has been killed.

Bacterial Strategies

Bacteria have developed strategies either to avoid immune effector mechanisms or even to adapt to them, and these may be as diverse as the pathogens themselves. They include anti-phagocytic capsules, resistance to microbicidal systems, anti-chemotactic products, the ability to release enzymes or cytokine analogs, and the subversion or exploitation of host cell functions.

IMMATURE DC ARE READILY PHAGOCYTIC

Since DC are essential for priming the immune system to antigens, it is important that they are present in tissues where they may encounter bacteria soon after invasion. This is indeed the case. DC have a privileged distribution in tissues which interface with the external environment and therefore they can serve as efficient sentinels for the uptake of invading microorganisms. Since both the bacterial cell and DC have a net negative charge, specific molecular interactions including bridging molecules are involved in the uptake process.

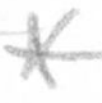

Despite several early reports on the uptake of particulate material and cells by DC (reviewed in Austyn, 1996), the phagocytic capacity of DC has long been denied. One reason for this was the technical difficulty, until recently, of growing DC in their immature phenotype. Earlier DC purification, and *in vitro* cell growth procedures were such that the enriched DC were in most cases terminally differentiated and had a mature phenotype and function. Maturation stages of DC were recognized only recently and it then became possible for immature 'processing DC' to be grown and maintained *in vitro* (Winzler *et al.*, 1997). At this functional stage, DC have phagocytic activity (Fig. 4) which decreases with DC differentiation *in vitro*. Indeed, several studies have shown that DC can internalize not only latex and zymosan beads (Inaba *et al.*, 1993; Reis e Sousa *et al.*, 1993; Austyn *et al.*, 1994; Matsuno *et al.*, 1996) but also apoptotic bodies (Parr *et al.*, 1991) as well as microbes such as *Bacillus Calmette-Guerin* (BCG) (Inaba *et al.*, 1993; Henderson *et al.*, 1997), *Saccharomyces cerevisiae*, *Corynebacterium parvum*, *Staphylococcus aureus* (Reis e Sousa *et al.*, 1993), *Leishmania* spp. (Blank *et al.*, 1993), and *Borrelia burgdorferi* (Filgueira *et al.*, 1996).

Both Gram-positive and Gram-negative bacteria, as well as their respective bacterial cell wall components (LPS, LTA), function as DC activators (Riva *et al.*, 1996; Thurnher *et al.*, 1997). The ability of DC to phagocytose particulates or bacteria is greatest in immature, processing DC, whereas this capacity is reduced, but not abolished, in mature presenting DC (Henderson *et al.*, 1997).

Upon attachment, DC engulf a bacterium by actively surrounding it with pseudopodia. This process is started intrinsically when phagocytosis-promoting receptors of the Fc-type are involved, but in the case of complement-type receptors it is dependent on complementary signals. The movement of the pseudopodia in activated DC involves actin-binding proteins, and it can be blocked by the drug cytochalasin D which stops the polymerization of actin and inhibits phagocytosis. The rearrangement of the cytoskeleton is associated with DC motility (Winzler *et al.*, 1997). The movement of activated DC can be observed by time-lapse video microscopy as shown in Fig. 5. Here it can be seen that in less than one minute (frames are 6 s apart) a cell completed the movement of one of its 'veils', thus indicating very intense motility.

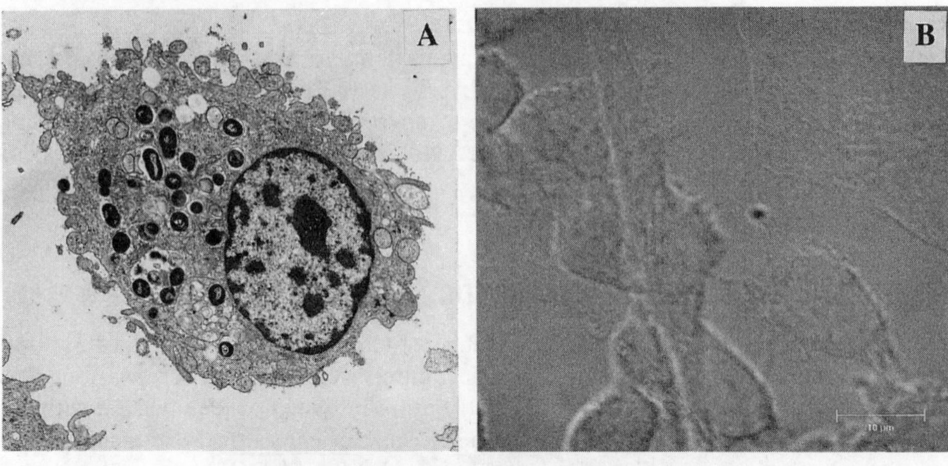

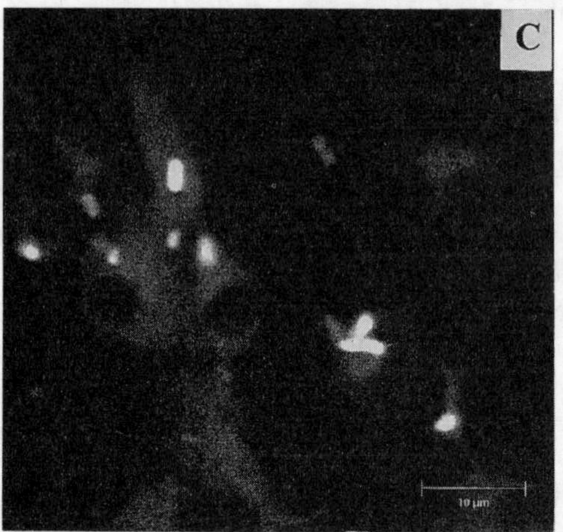

Fig. 4. Phagocytosis of bacteria. Phagocytosis of *S. gordonii* by D1 cells (A) as detected by EM: GFP (green fluorescent protein)-expressing *S. typhimurium* (C) as detected by confocal microscopy (nuclear section). DC cell shape is shown by phase contrast (B).

Once a bacterium has been fully internalized in the phagosome, fusion of the phagosome with other intracellular vacuoles or granules takes place. Processing of bacterial molecules for antigen presentation occurs in lysosomes following their fusion with phagosomes (see Fig. 6.). This process may take several hours, as antigen presentation of bacterial antigens is not observed earlier than 6 h following infection (Rescigno *et al.*, 1998). In addition to the conventional zipper-type phagocytosis, there are a number of other mechanisms by which phagocytes may engulf bacteria. From the various unconventional uptake mechanisms known (Swanson and Baer, 1995; Fig. 7), DC have been found to use macropinocytosis and coiling phagocytosis (as shown in Fig. 8), simultaneously with conventional phagocytosis for the uptake of bacteria (Rittig *et al.*, 1995; Rittig *et al.*, 1996). These alternative routes of internalization will almost certainly result in different routes of antigen processing and presentation. This is because

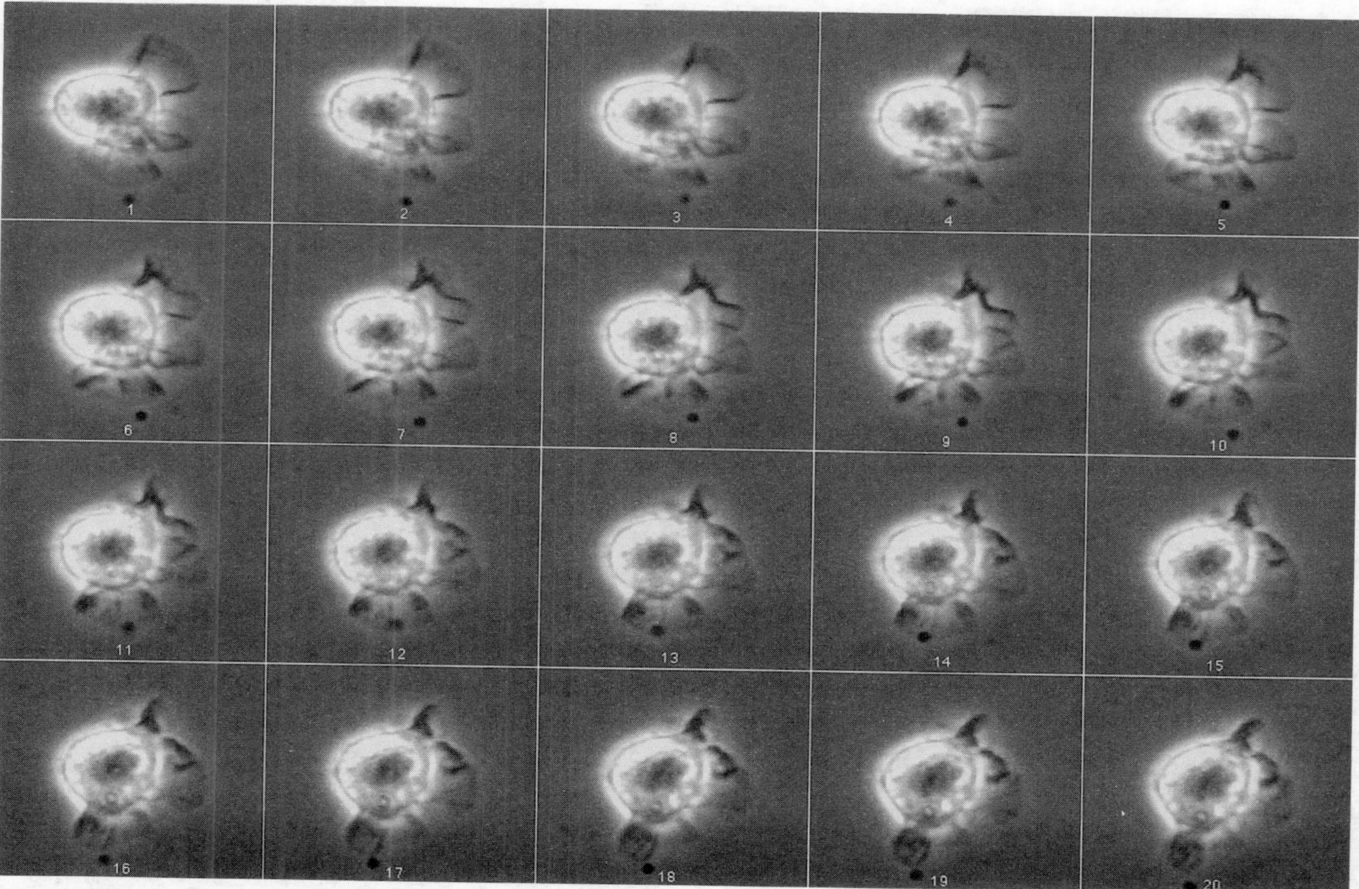

Fig. 5. High motility of TNF-α-activated D1 cells. Time-lapse video microscopy with frames 6 s apart for a total of 2 min of video recording.

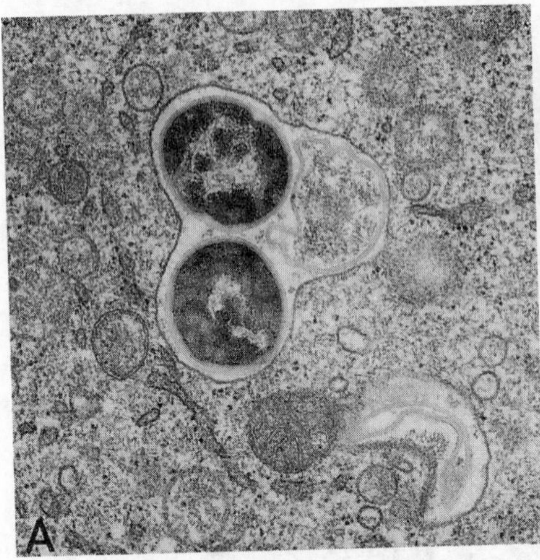

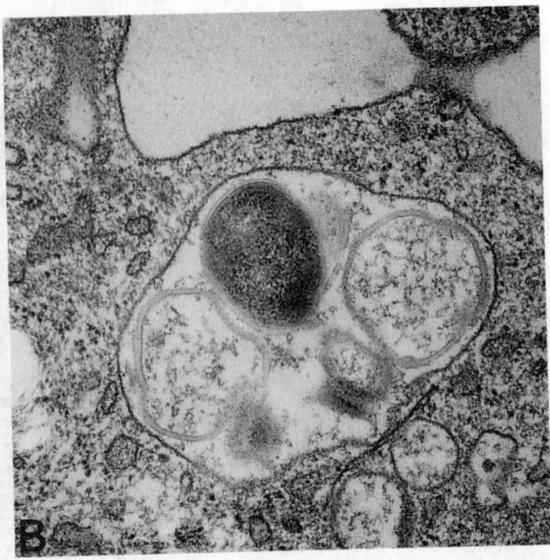

Fig. 6. Electron micrographs showing conventional phagocytosis of bacteria. Partial (A) and complete (B) degradation of bacteria in phagolysosomes.

macropinosomes are built differently from phagosomes (Swanson and Watts, 1995) and coiling phagocytosis of *Borrelia burgdoferi* delivers these spirochetes into the cytosol (Rittig *et al.*, 1992) from where spirochetal antigens can join the endogenous route of MHC class I presentation (Rittig *et al.*, 1994). Indeed, Lyme borreliosis is one of the bacterial infections which also elicit a cytotoxic CD8 response against the pathogen (Busch *et al.*, 1996).

DC SURFACE MOLECULES WHICH CAN MEDIATE THE UPTAKE OF BACTERIA

To be internalized, bacteria have first to be attached to phagocytosis-promoting receptors (Fig. 9). This may take place either via a direct interaction between microbial adhesins and phagocytic receptors (nonopsonic uptake); or indirectly via opsonins, for example antibody or complement. These act as bridging molecules between the microbial surface and opsonin receptors of the phagocytes (opsonic uptake). The fusion (zipper model) of the phagosome to form a discrete vacuole is probably under the control of specific fusogenic proteins which have still not been identified.

DC express a moderate level of Fc receptors (FcR) which is not modulated during maturation. Figure 10 shows the expression of FcR in immature and TNF-α-activated DC. The FcR was detected with the 2.4G2 mAb antibody, which recognizes both the mouse type II and type III FcgRs. As can be seen, the level of FcR expression in both immature and mature cells is similar. DC also express the Mac-1 molecule (CD11b/CD18; $\alpha_M\beta_2$-integrin) which is the CR3 complement receptor used for the phagocytosis of complement-coated bacteria. As with FcR, the surface expression of Mac-1 molecules is not changed during activation of DC (Fig. 10). This is in contrast to monocytes and neutrophils, which strongly upregulate Mac-1 expression during differentiation and in the presence of inflammatory stimuli. As well as having a role in receptor-mediated internalization, the Mac-1 molecule also mediates adhesion and chemotaxis (Anderson

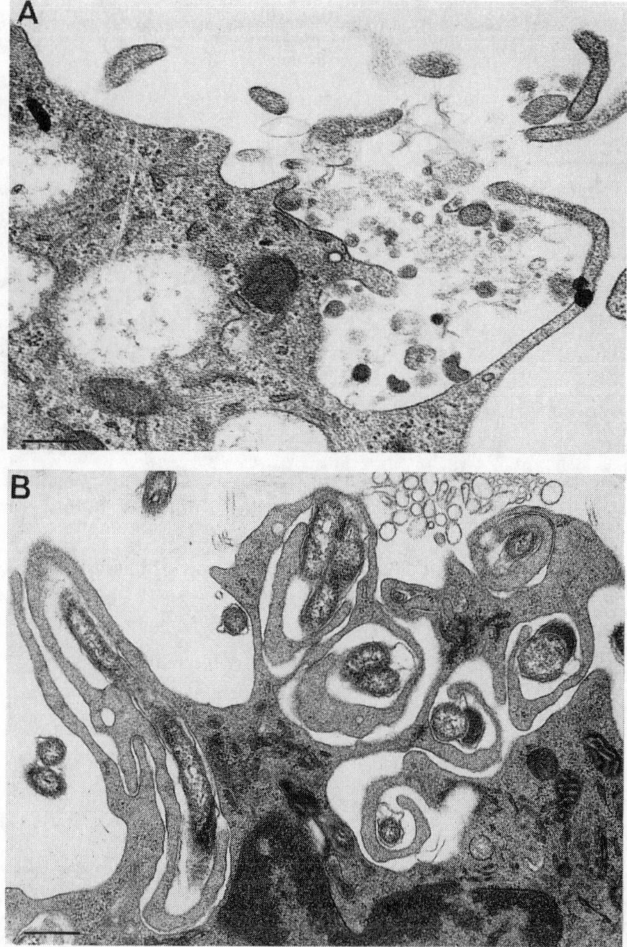

Fig. 7. DC ingestion of bacteria. Electron micrographs showing the morphological appearance of DC macropinocytosis (A) and coiling phagocytosis (B) of bacteria. Bars represent 0.3 μm (A) and 0.6 μm (B).

et al., 1986). Recent studies have shown that Mac-1 is stored in intracellular vesicles which are rapidly mobilized to the cell surface in response to chemoattractants (Miller *et al.*, 1987).

DC may also internalize bacteria through the mannose receptor. This is a 175 kDa C-type lectin which is expressed predominantly on macrophages and dendritic cells, including immature DC. It has a high affinity for carbohydrates, being involved in the internalization and presentation of mannosylated proteins (Agnes *et al.*, 1997). The high mannan content in the bacterial oligosaccharide cell envelope in both Gram-positive and Gram-negative bacteria assures efficient molecular recognition. Therefore it is likely that bacteria use the mannose receptor pathway for internalization; although this question remains to be definitely answered. Bacterial cell products, such as LPS, are certainly inducing activation of DC both *in vivo* (Roake *et al.*, 1995) and *in vitro*

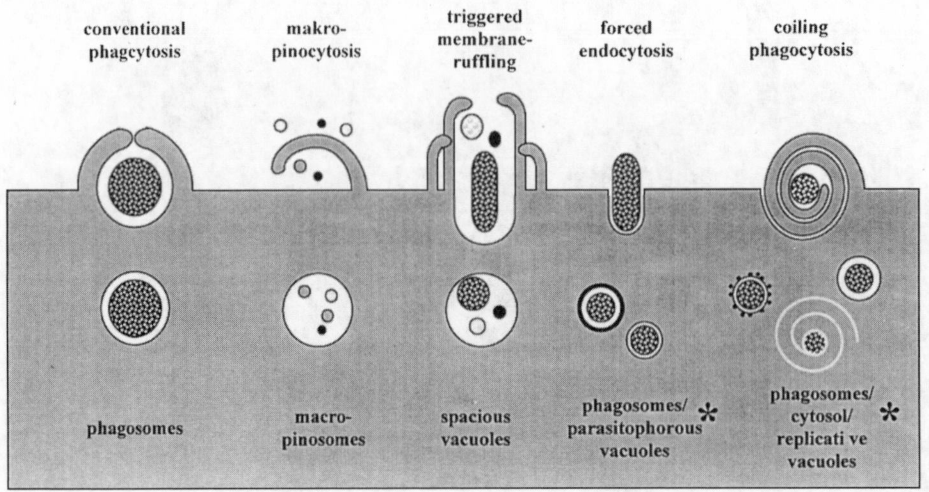

Fig. 8. Model of conventional and unconventional mechanisms of bacterial uptake.

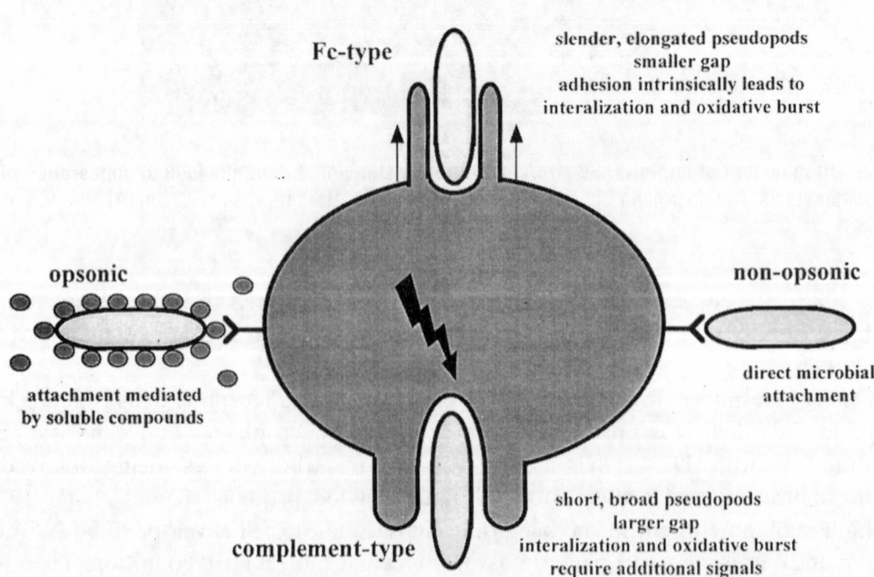

Fig. 9. Model of different types of conventional phagocytosis (Fc-type, opsonic, complement-type, and nonopsonic).

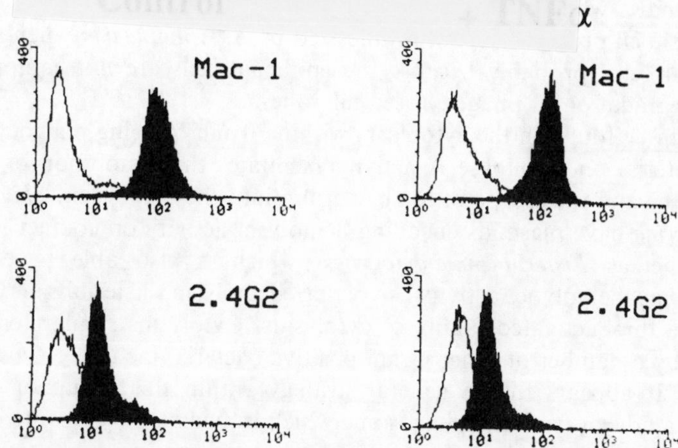

Fig. 10. Expression of FcR and integrins (CD11a, CD11b, and CD11c) on D1 cells following TNF-α-induced DC maturation, as detected by FACS analysis. Filled histograms show binding of specific antibodies, whereas isotype matched control antibodies or secondary reagents are represented by open histograms. FcR blocking was performed before all labeling experiments.

(Verhasselt *et al.*, 1997), but the molecular identity of the LPS receptor in the mouse is still controversial (Verhasselt *et al.*, 1997; Wright, 1995).

Finally, a recent study has shown the existence of a 'danger' receptor (Toll protein) (Medzhitov *et al.*, 1997). Although original studies have described Toll protein in *Drosophila*, the human homolog has now been cloned. Toll signals through the NF-κB pathway and induces the expression of NF-κB-controlled genes for inflammatory cytokines such as IL1, IL6, and IL8. It induces the expression of the costimulatory molecule B7.1. As yet the cellular distribution of this receptor in mammalian cells has not been characterized, and it would be of interest to find out whether it is expressed on DC.

INTRACELLULAR GROWTH AND SURVIVAL OF BACTERIA

In the normal course of events, the phagocytic vacuole containing the bacteria fuses with a second type of vacuole, the lysosome, giving rise to a hybrid vacuole termed the phagolysosome (Fig. 6). A number of bacteria have learned to escape lysosomal killing. Three different strategies for enhancing intracellular bacterial survival are known: (1) resistance to the killing action of the lysosomal enzymes; (2) rapid escape from the phagocytic vacuole into the cytoplasm; and (3) prevention of phagolysosomal fusion. The precise molecular basis by which the bacterium interferes with the host cell metabolism is largely unknown.

Salmonella typhimurium survives within the intracellular vacuole even after fusion with potentially lethal lysosomes, and a number of genes involved in this resistance have been identified. Following internalization by macrophages, *S. typhimurium* increases the synthesis of over 30 different bacterial proteins, including the heat shock proteins

GroEL and DnaK, which are also the immunodominant antigens. Interestingly, the bacterial heat shock proteins are not synthesized by *S. typhimurium* when the bacteria infect epithelial cells, probably because the epithelial cells are not equipped for the intracellular degradation of phagocytosed microbes.

Rickettsia can be found in the cytoplasm within 30 min of being phagocytosed. This is because bacterial phopholipase A activity facilitates the dissolution of the phagosomal membrane and the escape of the bacterium into the cytoplasm. *Shigella flexneri* and *S. dysenteriae* have plasmids encoding hemolysin activity on contact with the cell membrane, whereas *Listeria monocytogenes*—which is also able to escape from the vacuole—has hemolytic activity involving hemolysin, listeriolysin O (LLO) a member of the thiol-activated family of cytolysins. Cytolysins similar to listeriolysin are produced by a number of other Gram-positive bacteria, including *Clostridium* and *Streptococcus*. It appears that a general strategy within this group of cytoplasmic parasites is a rapid exit from the phagosome which is mediated by a controlled contact lysis of the membrane.

The bacteria which prevent fusion of the endocytic vacuole with the lysosome include *M. tuberculosis*, which preferentially infects macrophages. However, if the phagocytosed *M. tuberculosis* are coated with antibody, phagolysosomal fusion does take place, and the bacteria continue to multiply. This resistance is related to the structure of the mycobacterial envelope, which contains peptidoglycolipids not found in Gram-positive bacteria. The mycobacteria produce polyanionic glycolipids and sulfatides, which seem to interact specifically with the lysosomal membrane. This causes a reduction in vacuole mobility within the cytoplasm, and this may reduce the chances of lysosome and phagosome fusion.

Although precisely how bacteria and DC interact is not known, and needs to be elucidated, most of the mechanisms already described for the bacteria/macrophage interaction probably also apply to DC. Bacterial proteins can be processed and presented by DC on both MHC class I and class II through the exogenous pathway (Svensson, 1997; Rescigno *et al.*, 1998), but the mechanisms of MHC class I loading of phagocytosed material remain unclear in both systems (Carbone and Bevan, 1990; Rittig *et al.*, 1994; Reis e Sousa and Germain, 1995; Bachmann *et al.*, 1996; Norbury *et al.*, 1997; Wick and Pfeifer, 1996).

BACTERIAL INFECTION OF DC RESULTS IN CYTOKINE PRODUCTION AND FUNCTIONAL MATURATION

A few hours after bacterial infection, DC synthesize a number of cytokines and chemokines (Rescigno *et al.*, 1997). As shown in Fig. 11, the production of both TNF-α and IL-6 was readily detected in DC infected with either Gram-positive or Gram-negative bacteria. TNF-α production is rapidly induced following infection. It is likely that the phenotypical and the functional maturation which occurs in DC within 24 h of uptake of bacteria is the result of cytokine amplification during this response. Indeed, DC activation by TNF-α alone mimics the phenotypical maturation observed after bacterial infection, although the addition of anti-TNF-α antibodies only partly inhibits DC phenotypical and functional maturation.

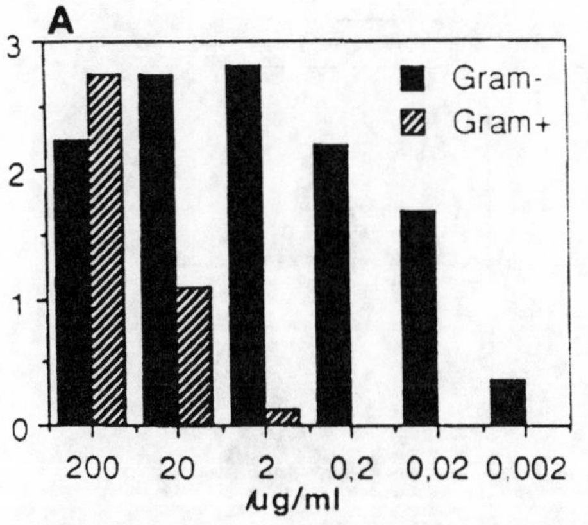

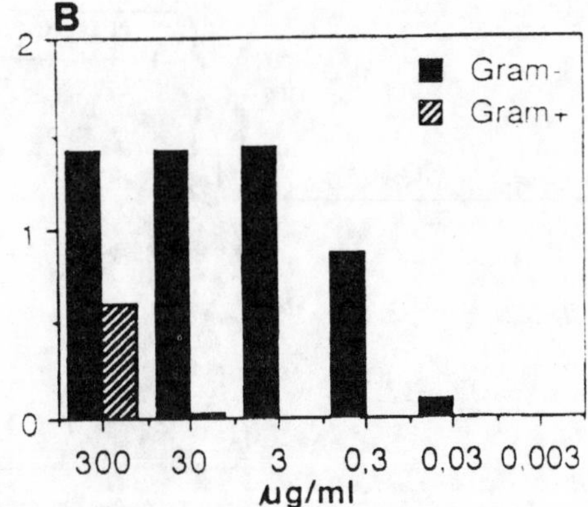

Fig. 11. TNF-α (A) and IL-6 (B) production by DC following bacterial stimulation as detected by standard ELISA assays. Cytokine values are expressed in ng/ml.

Furthermore, incubation of DC with several strains of bacteria resulted in a clear modification of cell surface activation markers. Consistent with acquisition of costimulatory activity during maturation is the upregulation of B7.2 (CD86) and CD40 molecules. This phenomenon is dose-dependent, and it is already maximal at a bacteria:DC ratio of 10:1 (Table 1). The upregulation of B7.2 and CD40 molecules has also been observed with BCG (Thurnher *et al.*, 1997) and *Mycobacterium tuberculosis* (Henderson *et al.*, 1997), but it was not observed following the use of inert latex beads of various sizes (Fig. 12). This is relevant when considering the rational design of new vaccines intended to target and activate DC. In fact, the upregulation of the costimulatory molecule B7.2 and the coordinated translocation of MHC molecules at the cell surface are essential molecular events for the subsequent antigen presentation and activation of both $CD4^+$ and $CD8^+$ T cells.

Table 1. Bacterial-induced upregulation of costimulatory molecules on DC

	CD40	B7.2
Uninfected D1 cells	+/−	+/−
D1 cells infected with		
Salmonella typhi	+++	+++
E. coli	++	++++
Lactobacillus	++	+++
Staphyloccus	++	+++
Staphylococcus aureus	++	+++
Streptococcus pyogenes	++	+++
Pneumococcus R6 (not capsulated)	++	++
Streptococcus	++	++
Lactococcus	++	+++
Streptococcus gordonii	++	++
Mycobacterium smegmatis	++	+++
Listeria monocytogenes	++	+++

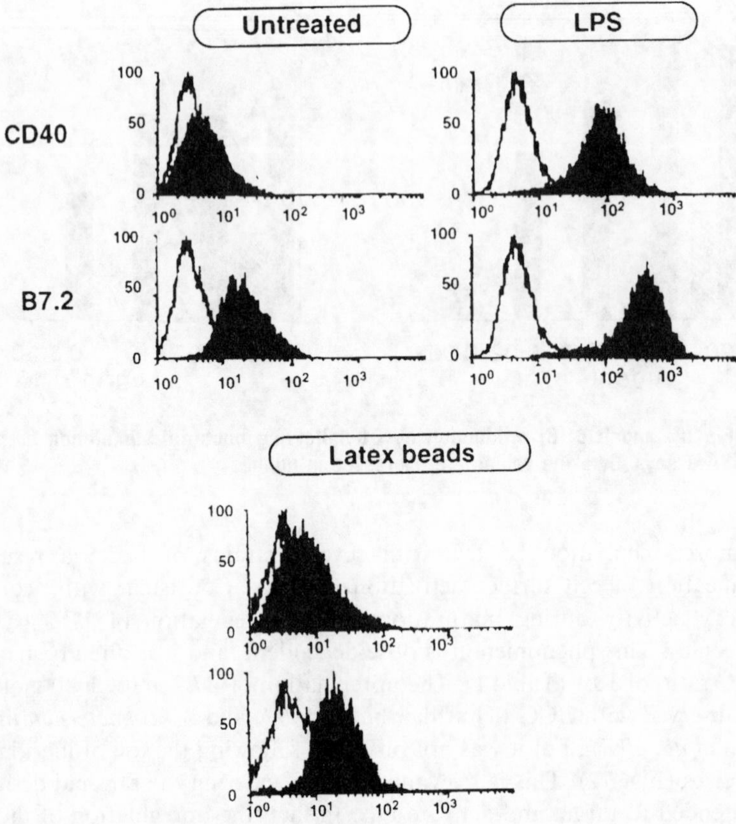

Fig. 12. Bacterial products induce DC maturation. Upregulation of the costimulatory molecules (CD40 and B7.2) on D1 cells is detected following LPS activation but not after latex beads phagocytosis (1 or 2 μm diameter).

DENDRITIC CELLS AS IMMUNIZATION TARGETS FOR THE RATIONAL DESIGN OF MUCOSAL VACCINES

In recent years it has become clear that antigen delivery is a crucial field of research for vaccine development. Appropriate targeting of an antigen to the immune system can affect the type of response (local/systemic, humoral/cellular, class I/class II-restricted, T_H1/T_H2) and can also be effective with low antigen doses. The delivery of vaccine antigens to mucosal surfaces is of particular interest, because it can generate local immunity at the major portals of pathogen entry. Vaccination strategies based on mucosal immunization can also be safer, minimize adverse effects, and make administration easier. Delivery systems based on live microorganisms, such as recombinant bacterial vectors, are especially relevant for mucosal immunization. Indeed, the most effective mucosal vaccines are based on killed or attenuated live pathogens such as *Vibrio cholera*, *Salmonella typhi*, and poliovirus.

Although much still has to be done to fully understand the interaction between DC and different bacteria, some common features have already been identified. All tested bacterial strains (pathogenic and nonpathogenic) lead to functional and phenotypical activation of DC. Thus, bacteria induce a host immune response mainly when they reach DC, or in other words, when they pass the epithelial barrier. Furthermore, according to how they enter the DC, i.e., conventional versus unconventional phagocytosis, there are different efficiencies of MHC class I and II presentation. Likewise, the capacity of microorganisms to escape the phagolysosome can result in reduced MHC II but increased MHC I presentation. All this has to be considered when developing live bacterial delivery systems for vaccines. Indeed, many laboratories are currently working on generating efficient carriers using attenuated pathogens so that they do not lose the capacity to enter host cells but their pathogenicity is weakened.

ACKNOWLEDGMENTS

We thank Donata Medaglini and Gianni Pozzi for providing the bacteria used in this study and Jürgen Wehland and Antonio Sechi for time lapse video microscopy. GFP-expressing *Salmonella typhimurium* was a kind gift of J.P. Kraehenbuhl. This work was supported by the EC grant no. ERB FMRX CT 960053 as part of the TMR program.

REFERENCES

Anderson, D.C., Miller, L.J., Schmalstieg, F.C., Rothlein, R. and Springer, T.A. (1986). Contributions of the Mac-1 glycoprotein family to adherence-dependent granulocyte functions: structure–function assessments employing subunit-specific monoclonal antibodies. *J. Immunol.* **137**, 15–27.

Austyn, J.M. (1996). New insights into the mobilization and phagocytic activity of dendritic cells. *J. Exp. Med.* **183**, 1287–1292.

Austyn, J.M., Hankins, D.F., Larsen, C.P., Morris, P.J., Rao, A.S. and Roake, J.A. (1994). Isolation and characterization of dendritic cells from mouse heart and kidney. *J. Immunol.* **152**, 2401–2410.

Bachmann, M., Lutz, M.B., Layton, G.T., Harris, S.J., Fehr, T., Rescigno, M. and Ricciardi-Castagnoli P. (1996). Dendritic cells process exogenous viral proteins and virus-like particles for MHC class I presentation to $CD8^+$ cytotoxic T lymphocytes. *Eur. J. Immunol.* **26**, 2595–2600.

Blank, C., Fuchs, H., Rappersberger, K., Rollinghoff, M. and Moll, H. (1993). Parasitism of epidermal Langerhans cells in experimental cutaneous leishmaniasis with *Leishmania major. J. Infect. Dis.* **167**, 418–425.

Busch, D.H., Jassoy, C., Brinckmann, U., Girschick, H. and Huppertz, H.I. (1996). Detection of *Borrelia burgdorferi*-specific $CD8^+$ cytotoxic T cells in patients with Lyme arthritis. *J. Immunol.* **157**, 3534–3541.

Carbone, F.R. and Bevan, M.J. (1990). Class I-restricted processing and presentation of exogenous cell-associated antigen in vivo. *J. Exp. Med.* **171**, 377–387.

Filgueira, L., Nestle, F.O., Rittig, M., Joller, H.I. and Groscurth, P. (1996). Human dendritic cells phagocytose and process *Borrelia burgdorferi. J. Immunol.* **157**, 2998–3005.

Henderson, R.A., Watkins, S.C. and Flynn, J.L. (1997). Activation of human dendritic cells following infection with *Mycobacterium tuberculosis. J. Immunol.* 159, 635–643.

Heufler, C., Koch, F. and Schuler, G. (1988). Granulocyte/macrophage colony-stimulating factor and interleukin 1 mediate the maturation of epidermal Langerhans cells into potent immunostimulatory dendritic cells. *J. Exp. Med.* **167**, 700–712.

Ibrahim, M.A.A., Chain, B.M. and Katz, D.R. (1995). The injured cell: the role of the dendritic cell system as a sentinel receptor pathway. *Immunol Today* **6**, 181–186.

Inaba, K., Inaba, M., Naito, M. and Steinman, R.M. (1993). Dendritic cell progenitors phagocytose particulates, including bacillus Calmette-Guerin organisms, and sensitize mice to mycobacterial antigens in vivo. *J. Exp. Med.* **178**, 479–488.

Inaba, K., Witmer-Pack, M., Inaba, M., Hathcock, K.S., Sakuta, H., Azuma, M., Yagita, H., Okumura, K., Linsley, P.S., Ikehara, S., Maramatsu, S., Hodes, R.J. and Steinman, R.M. (1994). The tissue distribution of the B7-2 costimulator in mice: abundant expression on dendritic cells in situ and during maturation in vitro. *J. Exp. Med.* **180**, 1849–1860.

Matsuno, K., Ezaki, T., Kudo, S. and Uehara, Y. (1996). A life stage of particle-laden rat dendritic cells in vivo: their terminal division, active phagocytosis, and translocation from the liver to the draining lymph [see comments]. *J. Exp. Med.* **183**, 1865–1878.

Medzhitov, R., Preston, H.P. and Janeway, C.J. (1997). A human homologue of the *Drosophila* Toll protein signals activation of adaptive immunity. *Nature* **388**, 394–397.

Miller, L.J., Bainton, D.F., Borregaard, N. and Springer, T.A. (1987). Stimulated mobilization of monocyte Mac-1 and p150,95 adhesion proteins from an intracellular vesicular compartment to the cell surface. *J. Clin. Invest.* **80**, 535–544.

Moll, H., Fuchs, H., Blank, C. and Röllinghoff, M. (1993). Langerhans cells transport *Leishmania major* from infected skin to the draining lymph node for presentation to antigen-specific T cells. *Eur. J. Immunol.* **23**, 1595–1601.

Nelson, D.J., McMenamin, C., McWilliam, A., Brenan, M. and Holt, P.G. (1994). Development of the airway intraepithelial dendritic cell network in the rat from class II major histocompatibility (Ia)-negative precursors: differential regulation of Ia expression at different levels of the respiratory tract. *J. Exp. Med.* **179**, 203–210.

Nestle, F.O., Zheng, X.G., Thompson, C.B., Turka, L.A. and Nickoloff, B.J. (1993). Characterization of dermal dendritic cells obtained from normal human skin reveals phenotypic and functionally distinctive subsets. *J. Immunol.* **151**, 6535–6540.

Norbury, C.C., Chambers, B.J., Prescott, A.R., Ljunggren, H.G. and Watts, C. (1997). Constitutive macropinocytosis allows TAP-dependent major histocompatibility complex class I presentation of exogenous soluble antigen by bone marrow-derived dendritic cells. *Eur. J. Immunol.* **27**, 280–288.

Parr, M.B., Kepple, L. and Parr, E.L. (1991). Langerhans cells phagocytose vaginal epithelial cells undergoing apoptosis during the murine estrous cycle. *Biol. Reprod.* **45**, 252–260.

Reis e Sousa, C. and Germain, R.N. (1995). Major histocompatibility complex class I presentation of peptides derived from soluble exogenous antigen by a subset of cell engaged in phagocytosis. *J. Exp. Med.* **182**, 841–851.

Reis e Sousa, C., Stahl, P.D. and Austyn, J.M. (1993). Phagocytosis of antigens by Langerhans cells in vitro. *J. Exp. Med.* **178**, 509–519.

Rescigno, M., Citterio, S. and Ricciardi-Castagnoli, P. (1997). Dendritic cells as targets for mucosal immunization. In: *Gram-positive Bacteria as Vaccine Vehicles for Mucosal Immunization* (eds G. Pozzi and J. Wells). Landes Bioscience, Berlin.

Rescigno, M., Citterio, S., Théry, C., Rittig, M., Medaglini, D., Pozzi, G., Amigorena, S. and Ricciardi-Castagnoli, P. (1998). Bacteria-induced neo-biosynthesis, stabilization and surface expression of functional class I molecules in mouse dendritic cells. *Proc. Natl Acad. Sci. USA* **95**, 5229–5234.

Rittig, M., Krause, A., Haupl, T., Schaible, U., Modolell, M., Kramer, M., Lutjen-Drecoll, E., Simon, M. and Burmester, G. (1992). Coiling phagocytosis is the preferential phagocytic mechanism for *Borrelia burgdorferi*. *Infect. Immun.* **60**, 4205–4212.

Rittig, M., Haupl, T. and Burmester, G.R. (1994). Coiling phagocytosis—a way for MHC class I presentation of bacterial antigens? *Int. Arch. Allergy Immunol.* **103**, 4–10.

Rittig, M.G., Filgueira, L., Dechant, C.A., Ricciardi-Castagnoli P., Groscurth, P. and Burmester, G.R. (1995). Dendritic cells use two different phagocytic mechanisms: possible consequences for antigen processing. *J. Cell. Biochem.* (*Suppl.*) **21**A, 30.

Rittig, M.G., Kuhn, K., Dechant, C., Gauckler, A., Modolell, M., Ricciardi-Castagnoli, P., Krause, A. and Burmester, G.R. (1996). Phagocytes from both vertebrate and invertebrate species use coiling phagocytosis. *Dev. Comp. Immunol.* **20**, 393–406.

Riva, S., Nolli, M.L., Lutz, M.B., Citterio, S., Girolomoni, G., Winzler, C. and Ricciardi-Castagnoli P. (1996). Bacteria and bacterial cell wall constituents induce the production of regulatory cytokines in dendritic cell clones. *J. Inflamm.* **46**, 98–105.

Roake, J.A., Rao, A.S., Morris, P.J., Larsen, C.P., Hankins, D.F. and Austyn, J.M. (1995). Dendritic cell loss from nonlymphoid tissues after systemic administration of lipopolysaccharide, tumor necrosis factor, and interleukin 1. *J. Exp. Med.* **181**, 2237–2247.

Schuler, G. and Steinman, R.M. (1985). Murine epidermal Langerhans cells mature into potent immunostimulatory dendritic cells *in vitro*. *J. Exp. Med.* **161**, 526–546.

Sertl, K., Takemura, T., Tschachler, E., Ferrans, V.J., Kaliner, M.A. and Shevach, E.M. (1986). Dendritic cells with antigen-presenting capability reside in airway epithelium, lung parenchyma, and visceral pleura. *J. Exp. Med.* **163**, 436–443.

Steinman, R.M. (1991). The dendritic cell system and its role in immunogenicity. *Annu. Rev. Immunol.* **9**, 271–296.

Svensson, M., Stockinger, B. and Wick, M.J. (1997). Bone marrow-derived dendritic cells can process bacteria for MHC-I and MHC-II presentation to T cells. *J. Immunol.* **158**, 4229–4236.

Swanson, J.A. and Baer, S.C. (1995). Phagocytosis by zippers and triggers. *Trends Cell Biol.* **5**, 89–93.

Swanson, J. and Watts, C. (1995). Macropynocytosis. *Trends Cell Biol.* **5**, 424–428.

Tan, M.C., Mommaas, A.M., Drijhout, J.W. *et al.* (1997). Mannose receptor-mediated uptake of antigens strongly enhances HLA class II-restricted antigen presentation by cultured dendritic cells. *Eur. J. Immunol.* **27**, 2426–2435.

Thurnher, M., Ramoner, R., Gastl, G., Radmayr, C., Böck, G., Herold, M., Klocker, H. and Bartsch, G. (1997). Bacillus Calmette-Guérin mycobacteria stimulate human blood dendritic cells. *Int. J. Cancer* **70**, 128–134.

Verhasselt, V., Buelens, C., Willems, F., De Groote, D., Haeffner-Cavaillon, N. and Goldman, M. (1997). Bacterial lipopolysaccharide stimulates the production of cytokines and the expression of costimulatory molecules by human peripheral blood dendritic cells. *J. Immunol.* **158**, 2919–2925.

Wick, M.J. and Pfeifer, J.D. (1996). Major histocompatibility complex class I presentation of ovalbumin peptide 257-264 from exogenous sources: protein context influences the degree of TAP-independent presentation. *Eur. J. Immunol.* **26**, 2790–2799.

Winzler, C., Rovere, P., Rescigno, M., Granucci, F., Penna, G., Adorini, L., Zimmermann, V.S., Davoust, J. and Ricciardi-Castagnoli, P. (1997). Maturation stages of mouse dendritic cells in growth factor-dependent long-term cultures. *J. Exp. Med.* **185**, 317–328.

Witmer-Pack, M.D., Olivier, W., Valinsky, J., Schuler, G. and Steinman, R.M. (1987). Granulocyte/macrophage colony-stimulating factor is essential for the viability and function of cultured murine epidermal Langerhans cells. *J. Exp. Med.* **166**, 1484–1498.

Wright, S.D. (1995). CD14 and innate recognition of bacteria. *J. Immunol.* **155**, 6–8.

CHAPTER 23
Dendritic Cells during Infection with HIV-1 and SIV

Ralph M. Steinman[1], Angela Granelli-Piperno[1], Klara Tenner-Racz[2], Paul Racz[2], Sarah Frankel[3], Elena Delgado[1], Ralf Ignatius[1] and Melissa Pope[1]

[1]Laboratory of Cellular Physiology and Immunology, Rockefeller University, New York, New York, USA; [2]Department of Pathology and Körber Laboratory for AIDS Research, Bernhard-Nocht-Institute for Tropical Medicine, Hamburg, Germany; [3]Division of Retrovirology, and the Division of AIDS and Emerging Infectious Disease Pathology, Walter Reed Army Institute of Research, Rockville, Maryland, USA

INTRODUCTION

The theme of this review is that dendritic cells (DC) drive the replication of HIV-1 and SIV, particularly in concert with $CD4^+$ T cells. DC probably have another major function, i.e., to elicit resistance to HIV-1 and SIV via stimulation of $CD8^+$ T cells. The latter can secrete anti-viral chemokines that block infection, and can give rise to specific cytolytic T lmphocytes (CTLs) that kill infected cells and prevent virus spread from cell to cell. However, the role of DC in $CD8^+$ T cell responses to HIV-1/SIV has yet to be analyzed in detail, so that we will concentrate on the DC–$CD4^+$ T cell interaction. Recent work will be discussed, since several reviews of this field already have appeared (Weissman and Fauci, 1997; Knight and Patterson, 1997; Cameron *et al.*, 1996; Grouard and Clark, 1997).

The immunodeficiency viruses, HIV-1 and SIV, target cells that express CD4 and chemokine receptors. These receptors are found on different types of leukocytes, especially T cells, macrophages, and DC. Here we emphasize the capacity of DCs to capture HIV-1 and SIV and to transmit infection to T cells. To do so, we try to bring together two sets of findings: experiments on the interaction of HIV-1 and SIV with different populations of human and macaque DC *in vitro*, and observations on the localization of viral RNA and protein *in situ* in the two species.

The function of the DC system during infection with HIV-1 and SIV will be analyzed in three different sites: body surfaces, especially stratified squamous epithelia; peripheral lymph nodes; and mucosal associated lymphoid organs (MALT) and overlying epithelium. In each site, there is evidence that DC can accelerate the replication of immunodeficiency viruses.

Dendritic Cells: Biology and Clinical Applications
ISBN 0-12-455860-7

DENDRITIC CELLS FROM SKIN: A MODEL FOR BODY SURFACES THAT ARE INVOLVED IN THE SEXUAL TRANSMISSION OF HIV-1 AND SIV

Maturation and Migration of DC at Body Surfaces

The prototype for the study of DC function at body surfaces is skin, where the DC are called Langerhans cells (LC). However, DC that are similar to epidermal LC are found in the epithelial tissues that cover the vagina, ectocervix, and anus; i.e., surfaces involved in the sexual transmission of HIV-1 and SIV. The dermis and subepithelial regions contain additional DC (Lenz *et al.*, 1993). These lack the Birbeck granules and CD1a antigens of LC but nonetheless give rise to typical immunostimulatory DC in culture. Thus both epidermal and dermal-derived DC are nonadherent and nonphagocytic cells that extend motile processes in several directions from the cell body. DC express very high levels of MHC class II, the costimulator CD86, and markers of unknown function, CD83 and p55 (Pope *et al.*, 1994; Pope *et al.*, 1995a; Pope *et al.*, 1997a).

Studies of skin DC have lead to the concept that there are two stages in their function (Romani *et al.*, 1991; Schuler and Steinman, 1985; Witmer-Pack *et al.*, 1987; Witmer-Pack *et al.*, 1988; Romani *et al.*, 1989a,b; Streilein and Grammer, 1989; Inaba *et al.*, 1989; Pure *et al.*, 1990; Pierre *et al.*, 1997). Skin and other tissues (e.g., blood, lung, marrow) contain immature or antigen-capturing DC that with appropriate stimuli (e.g., lipopolysaccharide (LPS) or TNF) become mature or T cell-stimulatory DC. In both human (Pope *et al.*, 1994; Pope *et al.*, 1995) and macaque (Pope *et al.*, 1997a) skin, the mature DC express much higher levels of antigen-presenting MHC class I and II products and high levels of membrane costimulators like B7-2/CD86. Mature DC can produce large amounts of IL-12, and they develop two markers whose function is still unknown: the immunoglobulin superfamily member CD83 (Zhou and Tedder, 1995), and a presumptive actin-bundling protein p55 (Mosialos *et al.*, 1996). Immature DC, in contrast, have the capacity to endocytose antigens by a variety of routes and process them within intracellular MHC II compartments (MIIC) (Sallusto and Lanzavecchia, 1994; Sallusto and Lanzavecchia, 1995; Sallusto *et al.*, 1996; Pierre *et al.*, 1997; Cella *et al.*, 1997; Kleijmeer *et al.*, 1994; Kleijmeer *et al.*, 1995; Nijman *et al.*, 1995; De Smedt *et al.*, 1996).

Two recent reports describe the regulation of intracellular MIICs during DC maturation (Pierre *et al.*, 1997; Talmor *et al.*, 1998). Over the course of 1–12 h, MHC II molecules within lysosomal MIICs sort away from the lysosomes to produce MHC II-rich, peripheral, nonlysosomal vesicles and MHC II-poor, perinuclear, lysosomes. By 24 h, most of the MHC II is on the cell surface (Plate 23.1). Using monoclonal antibodies to MHC–peptide complexes, we are finding that the complexes form within the cell as expected and then move to the surface. Therefore the very high levels of MHC II molecules on DC reflect their correspondingly large numbers of MIIC, in which internalized antigens can be successfully processed to form stable MHC II–peptide complexes. The reason for mentioning these new findings here is twofold: first to show that immature DC at body surfaces are specialized to capture antigens, including viruses, and second, to illustrate the major changes that are occurring in the physiology of maturing DC, given new evidence that these cells are permissive to HIV-1 infection (see below).

DC undergo another important change during maturation, which is that the cells begin to migrate (Larsen *et al.*, 1990; Lukas *et al.*, 1996; Pope *et al.*, 1994; Steinman *et al.*, 1995) (Plate 23.1). The DC leave the epidermis and dermis and enter the afferent lymphatics.

In vivo, DC in afferent lymphatics will access the lymph nodes, while in organ cultures of skin the DC migrate into the medium and are accessible for experimentation.

Immature DC Capture and Replicate M-tropic Strains of HIV-1

To determine the capacity of skin DC to capture HIV-1, Paul Cameron's group in Melbourne, Australia have taken sheets of skin (epidermis and dermis), abraded the epidermal surface, applied M-tropic and T-tropic HIV-1, and cultured the skin explants for 2 days (Reece *et al.*, 1998). The emigrating DC were collected and tested for the capacity to transmit an infection to activated T blasts. When M-tropic virus, e.g., Ba-L, was added to the abraded epidermis, the emigrating DC could transmit an infection to T cells. In contrast, T-tropic virus was not captured by the migrating DC if the virus was applied to the epidermis.

Zaitseva and coworkers have made somewhat analogous findings with LC in epidermis (Zaitseva *et al.*, 1997). They used polyclonal antisera specific for CCR5 and CXCR4, and found only the former to be expressed on the surface of immature LC. When M-tropic and T-tropic HIV-1 were added to isolated LC, M-tropic virus fused with the LC, whereas T-tropic virus only fused after the LC had been cultured for a short period, when CXCR4 also began to be expressed at the cell surface.

Another more accessible system that has been used to compare immature and mature DC involves cytokine-treated monocytes. Maturation was begun by culturing the cells for 6 days in GM-CSF and IL-4 (Sallusto and Lanzavecchia, 1994; Romani *et al.*, 1994), and then the cells were further differentiated by culture in a monocyte conditioned medium (Bender *et al.*, 1996; Romani *et al.*, 1996; Reddy *et al.*, 1997). Both the blood monocytes and mature DC were difficult to infect with HIV-1, but immature, GM-CSF/IL-4 DC were productively infected (Granelli-Piperno *et al.*, 1998). At the level of viral DNA, blood monocytes only formed early transcripts that could be amplified with primers for the RU5 region. In contrast, immature DC completed reverse transcription, showing strong signals when primers for the LTR and gag regions were used.

Only M-tropic virus replicated in immature, cytokine-driven DC. Placing the V-3 loop from the Ba-L M-tropic isolate into a T-tropic virus also allowed for replication. The immature DC reacted with monoclonal antibodies to CCR5 and CXCR4, the receptors for entry of M-tropic and T-tropic HIV-1, respectively, and both receptors could be signaled with their respective ligands, RANTES and SDF-1 (Delgado *et al.*, 1998). It is not clear whether the inability to replicate T-tropic isolates reflects a lack of entry via CXCR4 or some postreceptor event.

These findings on immature DC are relevant to transmission of HIV-1 *in vivo*, since M-tropic strains of HIV-1 are predominantly transmitted during clinical infection (van't Wout *et al.*, 1994; Zhu *et al.*, 1993). Immature DC at body surfaces and in blood may be the principal cells that are responsible for this phenomenon. Monocytes, in contrast, do not replicate HIV-1, while macrophages are not known to home to the T cell areas to transmit the virus to T cells.

Replication of HIV-1 and SIV in Mixtures of Mature DC and T Cells from Body Surfaces

The cells that emigrate from skin explants in standard 2–4-day culture protocols are actually mixtures of mature DC and T cells (Plate 23.1). The T cells are almost entirely of a memory phenotype (CD45R0$^+$, CD45RA$^-$, CD62L$^-$), and the emigrated DC are mature with very high levels of HLA-DR, CD86, p55, and CD83. Mature DC do not replicate virus, but the DC–T cell mixtures are permissive to both M-tropic and T-tropic HIV-1 (Pope *et al.*, 1994; Pope *et al.*, 1995b; Pope *et al.*, 1997b) and SIV (Pope *et al.*, 1997a).

The T cells that interact with DC to support viral replication can be syngeneic and need not proliferate (Pope *et al.*, 1994; Pope *et al.*, 1995b; Granelli-Piperno *et al.*, 1995). No mitogen, IL-2, or fetal calf serum is added to the culture, and cell staining with the Ki-67 cell cycle antigen is infrequent. However, skin T cells do express the activation antigen, CD69.

In the monkey, it has been possible to obtain DC and T cells from different sites and then determine the extent to which the findings with skin extend to other tissues. SIV-permissive mixtures of leukocytes have been isolated from other body surfaces of the macaque, such as the vagina and tonsillar epithelium (Pope *et al.*, 1997a). DC also can be obtained by cytokine stimulation of precursors in monkey blood (O'Doherty *et al.*, 1997) in a similar way to what is done with human blood (Bender *et al.*, 1996; Romani *et al.*, 1996; Reddy *et al.*, 1997). It has been found that mature DC can collaborate with T cells to drive SIV replication (O'Doherty *et al.*, 1997; Ignatius *et al.*, 1998). The DC can be obtained from either skin, blood, spleen, or lymph node. Interestingly the CD45RA$^-$ memory cells are much more permissive when cultured with DC than are CD45RA$^+$ naive populations.

Two standard SIV isolates have been evaluated for replication in DC–T cell mixtures. SIVmac239, which fails to replicate in macrophages, and the dual tropic SIVmac251 isolates, both replicate actively in DC–T cell mixtures (Pope *et al.*, 1997a; Ignatius *et al.*, 1998). Since SIVmac239 does infect macaques via the vaginal route, the findings suggest that SIVmac239 must be captured by DC rather than macrophages during transmission *in situ*.

Summary

Two sets of findings have been made with DC that have been isolated from body surfaces or derived from blood monocytes by stimulation with cytokines. Immature DC directly replicate HIV-1, but only M-tropic isolates. Mature DC do not replicate HIV-1 or SIV, but mixtures of mature DC and CD4$^+$ T cells are permissive without the addition of mitogens or IL-2. The findings suggest that when transmission is analyzed *in vivo*, migrating immature DC will be infected early on. Then, as the cells mature, DC will be able to transmit virus to T cells in draining lymphoid tissues.

DENDRITIC CELLS IN PERIPHERAL LYMPH NODES

Distinct Dendritic Cells in the T and B Cell Areas of Lymph Nodes

Lymph nodes are known to be a major depot for both HIV-1 and SIV RNA (Tenner Racz *et al.*, 1988; Schuurman *et al.*, 1988; Fox *et al.*, 1991) and gag protein (Biberfeld *et al.*, 1985; Tenner-Racz *et al.*, 1986; Tenner Racz *et al.*, 1988). To understand this finding, one must consider that there are at least two broad classes of DC in lymphoid

Table 1. Two types of dendritic cells in lymph nodes

Follicular dendritic cells (FDC)
B cell areas (especially in germinal centers)
Not a leukocyte (? fibroblast), CD45 negative
Retain antigens as immune complexes on FcR, C3R
Present native antigens to B cells
Hematopoietic-derived dendritic cells (DC)
T cell areas
Bone marrow-derived leukocyte, CD45 positive
Retain antigens as MHC–peptide complexes
Present processed antigens to T cells

organs (Table 1). Follicular dendritic cells (FDC) are mesenchymal-type cells that retain antigens in a native form, as extracellular immune complexes bound to Fc and C3 receptors. In contrast, marrow-derived DC retain processed antigens as MHC–peptide complexes on their cell surfaces. Retention of antigens as immune complexes on FDC was first visualized many years ago (Nossal *et al.*, 1968; Chen *et al.*, 1978b; Szakal *et al.*, 1989). Recently, it has been possible to visualize large amounts of processed antigen in MHC II–peptide complexes on T cell area DC as well (Inaba *et al.*, 1997). There is now direct evidence that DC present alloantigens (Kudo *et al.*, 1997), antigens (Ingulli *et al.*, 1997), and superantigens (Luther *et al.*, 1997) to T cells in the T cell areas.

The sharp distinction between the types of dendritic cells in B and T cell areas (Table 1) has changed very recently with the report of leukocyte-type DC in the germinal centers (GCs) of stimulated or secondary B cell follicles (Grouard *et al.*, 1996). These GCDC were visualized by Grouard *et al.* as $CD11c^+$, $CD3^-$, $CD4^+$, large, irregularly shaped cells. Upon isolation, the cells were not fully mature but developed high levels of costimulatory molecules within a day of culture. The GCDC also carried surface κ and λ light chains, indicating a capacity to carry immune complexes. Most importantly, GCDC were powerful stimulators of T cells in the mixed leukocyte reaction, while GC B cells had no detectable activity.

The origin of FDC, whose numbers increase in association with GC development (Chen *et al.*, 1978a), remains unclear. GCDC may arise from $CD11c^+$ cells in blood, but there is still no direct evidence for this, mainly because GCDC have to date been described in human tissue rather than the more accessible rodent systems. For DC in the T cell area, it is clear that at least some of these can originate from cells that have picked up antigens in the periphery and migrated to the lymph node (Steinman, 1991; Steinman *et al.*, 1995; Inaba *et al.*, 1990; Liu and MacPherson, 1993; Austyn *et al.*, 1988; Bujdoso *et al.*, 1989).

Transfer of Virus to T Cells when DC are Presenting Antigens and Superantigens

A model for what might happen when DC capture virus at a body surface, and then migrate as mature cells to lymph node T cell areas to present antigen, was provided by the work of Cameron some years ago (Cameron *et al.*, 1992; Cameron *et al.*, 1994). When mature DC were pulsed with HIV-1 and then used to present either superantigen or alloantigen, the virus only replicated when T cells were added. This was also the case during immune responses to tetanus toxoid (Weissman *et al.*, 1996). In these stimulated cultures, the DC:T cell ratio was small (1:30 to 1:100) relative to that in syngeneic, antigen-independent mixtures from skin that were described above (1:3 to 1:10).

When virus-pulsed DC stimulated a T cell response, the productive infection that took place occurred primarily in the responding T cells; i.e., most of the viral gag protein was found in MHC class II weak T cells rather than MHC II strong DC (Cameron *et al.*, 1992; Cameron *et al.*, 1994). Therefore, the prediction would be that in acute HIV-1 and SIV infection, DC would transmit virus to T cells, especially HIV-1/SIV-specific T cells, in the T cell areas.

Lymph Nodes during Acute SIV Infection: Active Infection in T Cell Areas

During acute infection in the SIV macaque model (Reimann *et al.*, 1994), virus replicates primarily in the T cell areas (Plate 23.2). The cells that show strong in-situ hybridization signals for viral RNA are primarily T cells, since most do not double label for macrophage and DC markers. One possibility is that virus is brought via DC to the T cells, as described in the previous section, particularly $CD4^+$ T cells trying to respond to the virus as antigen. An alternative would be that free virus simply infects any activated T cells in the node. The latter seems less plausible to us, since free virus is more likely to encounter resting, nonpermissive T cells than activated ones. In otherwords, the carriage of virus by DC ensures that virus is brought to T cells that are permissive for a productive infection.

Lymph Nodes during Chronic Infection with HIV-1 and SIV: Active Infection in B Cell Areas

In chronic HIV and SIV infection, a very different picture is seen in the lymph nodes. Now the cells with the most abundant viral mRNA by in-situ hybridization are found in the B cell areas, especially in GC. Viral RNA is found in two sites using radiolabeled antisense probes and autoradiography (Tenner Racz *et al.*, 1988; Schuurman *et al.*, 1988; Fox *et al.*, 1991; Tenner-Racz *et al.*, 1997) (Plate 23.3). One site consists of diffuse labeling over the FDC network. This labeling likely represents extracellular, antibody–virion complexes and is enhanced by protease treatment of the tissue section prior to in-situ hybridization (Tenner-Racz *et al.*, 1997). The other depot of viral RNA consists of small, $CD4^+$ cells that label intensely with antisense probes. This labeling represents actively infected T cells primarily, and is enhanced by heating the tissue sections prior to hybridization. The productively infected cells for the most part fail to double label for the CD68 antigen that is expressed in high amounts in macrophages and in lower amounts in DC.

What are the driving forces for viral replication within T cells of the germinal center? One possibility is that GC T cells are infected by virus that is deposited on the surface of FDC, since there is evidence that FDC-associated virus can be infectious (Heath *et al.*, 1995). Another possibility relates to the newly recognized, marrow-derived GCDC (Grouard *et al.*, 1996) (see above). These have human immunoglobulin on their surfaces and would be expected to capture HIV–anti-HIV complexes, although this has not been studied directly. Upon presenting antigens to $CD4^+$ helper cells in the GC, the HIV-1 that is picked up as immune complexes may be transmitted, thereby driving the replication of virus that is observed in GC T cells. The GCDC pathway may be a more effective way of transmitting virus to GC T cells since these cells interact with activated T cells, whereas FDCs are not known to.

Mechanism of Virus Transfer from Mature DC to T Cells

We have summarized above the capacity of mature DC to transfer HIV-1 and SIV to T cells, and described that this may occur in both the acute and chronic phases of virus replication in lymph nodes. This transmission is enhanced during antigen presentation but also can occur in the ostensible absence of antigen presentation, as with syngeneic memory T cells and with T cell lines (manuscript in preparation). Is the DC simply trapping virus, or must virus enter the DC prior to transmission and replication in T cells?

The latter seems to be the case, as indicated by recent experiments in which the DC and T cells were obtained from normal or CCR5 mutant donors. The CCR5 mutant cells do not allow entry of M-tropic strains like Ba-L into DC (Granelli-Piperno *et al.*, 1996). We found that CCR5 mutant DC could not be pulsed successfully with Ba-L, and likewise, normal, virus-pulsed DC could not transmit virus to CCR5 mutant T cells (Granelli-Piperno *et al.*, 1998). Therefore, both DC and T cells have to express functioning CCR5 receptors to support virus replication in cocultures. A nice internal control for these experiments is that IIIB T-tropic virus is infectious when either CCR5 mutant DC or T cells are studied.

The HIV-1 life cycle is known to be blocked in mature DC. For both M-tropic and T-tropic isolates, virus seems to enter the DC via CD4 and chemokine receptors; reverse transcription then begins but is not completed (Granelli-Piperno *et al.*, 1996). We suspect that, following entry via chemokine receptors, the virus can remain in an uncoated state close to the mature DC surface. Upon T cell contact, the virus-infected DC could direct virus to the T cell, as diagrammed in Plate 23.4.

Summary

HIV-1 and SIV replicate continuously in lymph nodes. In acute infection, replication is primarily in the T cell areas, while in chronic infection, actively infected cells predominate in the B cell areas. In both, it is possible that virus is being transmitted to the T cell via DC, and that the interaction of DC and T cells drives viral replication in the latter. A challenging feature is to understand how mature DC can capture but not replicate virus, but then transmit an active infection to T cells.

MUCOSAL-ASSOCIATED LYMPHOID TISSUE (MALT)

DC at the Surfaces of MALT

MALT is abundant in the gut, including the rectal mucosa. MALT exhibits many of the principles of a lymph node with B and T cell areas and two types of dendritic cells: FDC in the large germinal centers and DC in the T cell areas. However, one of the major distinctions in MALT is the presence of a specialized pathway for antigen delivery that utilizes M cells within the apical or dome epithelium. These M cells function to allow transit of antigens into the underlying lymphoid tissue (Neutra *et al.*, 1996; Frey *et al.*, 1996). Light and electron microscopy also routinely show lymphocytes forming a so-called 'lymphoepithelium'.

The special anatomy of the antigen-transporting lymphoepithelium of MALT is magnified in the tonsils at the upper end of the GI tract. These include the adenoid or nasopharyngeal tonsil at the back of the nose, the palatine tonsils at the back at the throat, and the sublingual tonsils in the rear of the tongue. In each case the tonsil surface invaginates to form clefts or crypts. Along these invaginations, the epithelium is very different from that seen at the remainder of the tonsil or pharyngeal surface. Most of the pharynx is lined by a multilayered skin-like epithelium in which there are few lymphocytes. In the crypts, however, the epithelium becomes much thinner and more ramified, there are antigen-transporting M cells, and there are many more lymphocytes, with most having the surface markers of memory cells (Plate 23.5).

It has only become apparent in this past year that there can be many DC lying beneath the M cells (Plate 23.5). In the mouse these cells are MHC II and CD11c positive, but lack macrophage markers like the F4/80 antigen and sialoadhesin (Kelsall and Strober, 1996). In human, S100 labels the presumptive DC in the crypt epithelium (Frankel *et al.*, 1996; Frankel *et al.*, 1997). Because DC in lymphoepithelium are chronically exposed to activation or maturation stimuli like LPS, and because lymphocytes seem to traffic chronically through this region, a cellular environment is set up that resembles the leukocytes that emigrate from skin explants and are so permissive to HIV-1 and SIV (see above).

Productive Infection of S100$^+$ Syncytia at the Surfaces of MALT

At the Armed Forces Institute of Pathology, an examination was made of a series of adenoids and tonsils that were removed because of hypertrophy, but in the absence of tonsilitis. Lymphoma was ruled out, and then a search was made for various infectious agents that might be causing the tonsil hypertrophy. In other words, most of these enlarged tonsils were examined as a diagnostic problem and not as a manifestation of HIV-1 infection. Infections like measles, EBV, and CMV were not found. However, HIV-1 gag protein was evident in large stellate cells at the surface of the MALT (Table 2). These HIV-1-infected cells were only found in the lymphoepithelium (Frankel *et al.*, 1997).

What was striking in these tonsils was that HIV-1 was identified using a stain for viral gag protein; in-situ hybridization was not required (Frankel *et al.*, 1996; Frankel *et al.*,

Table 2. Tonsils from HIV-1-infected individuals

- 28 specimens removed because of hypertrophy or diagnosis (no acute tonsilitis, and only 2 with HIV-1 OI)
- CD4 counts were 200–900/μl
- Several specimens were from donors who were known to be infected for 2–10 years prior to tonsilectomy

1997). This suggests that the cells were producing very high levels of virus. Further studies showed that the HIV-1-infected cells were multinucleated and could be labeled for the antigen S100. Anti-S100 strongly labels DC but not most populations of other leukocytes, such as multinucleated macrophage giant cells in leprosy and tuberculosis. Furthermore, S100$^+$ infected giant cells are quickly produced and abundant whenever HIV-1 is added to DC–T cell cocultures (Pope *et al.*, 1994; Pope *et al.*, 1995b; Frankel *et al.*, 1997; Pope *et al.*, 1997a), whereas giant cells are infrequent in infected macrophage cultures.

The findings of Frankel and colleagues were made on enlarged tonsils. It remains to be determined whether similar heavily infected cells occur routinely in tonsils and other mucosal lymphoid organs in chronically infected individuals. We think this will be the case. At mucosal surfaces, the DC are probably being activated chronically by stimuli entering from the environment via M cells, and these DC have ready access to memory lymphocytes. Therefore, the cellular milieu should resemble that seen with the permissive DC-T cell mixtures that are isolated from body surfaces (see above). However, it will be important to obtain large samples of MALT, since the infected cells may only be present in scattered foci in the lymphoepithelium.

Summary

In the study of HIV-1 and SIV pathogenesis, more attention has been given to peripheral lymph nodes than MALT. However, MALT may be very important in quantitative terms, not only because of the content of typical B cell and T cell areas, but because of the chronic activation stimuli in the lymphoepithelium that contains both DC and lymphocytes. High-level virus production in multinucleated cells derived from DC can occur in the lymphoepithelium of nasopharyngeal and palatine tonsils.

THE OTHER SIDE OF THE COIN: DENDRITIC CELLS MEDIATE RESISTANCE TO HIV-1, ESPECIALLY AT THE LEVEL OF CD8$^+$ T CELLS

We have considered here the role of DC in the replication of immunodeficiency viruses. DC also may have important roles in resistance, particularly in the stimulation of virus-specific CD8$^+$ T cells. HIV-1 and SIV infections behave as battlegrounds, that is, the virus replicates actively at all times, yet the levels of plasma viremia and CD4$^+$ T cells can remain steady for months and years. This 'stalemate' may depend on the fact that DC are driving virus replication via CD4$^+$ T cells and anti-viral resistance via CD8$^+$ T cells.

There may be many ways in which DC could capture viral antigens and induce the strong CD8$^+$ T cell responses that can be observed in HIV-1 infection. The first is by direct infection as described above, particularly at mucosal surfaces. However, there could be other pathways that do not require active infection of the DC. In influenza, DC are able to present nonreplicating virus (Bender *et al.*, 1995; Bender *et al.*, 1996), and there is an abundance of noninfectious virus in the plasma of HIV-1-infected individuals (Piatak *et al.*, 1993). DC can also present antigens from apoptotic cells, so called cross-priming (Albert *et al.*, 1998). In HIV-1 infection, many infected T cells die and possibly these are presented by DC. These latter presentation pathways, i.e., nonreplicating virus and dying infected cells, would allow DC to present HIV-1, but one would not necessarily detect active infection of the DC.

Table 3. Potential roles of DC in HIV-1/SIV infection

Body surfaces
- Immature migrating DC capture and replicate M-tropic virus.

Lymph nodes
- In acute infection, DC are infected in blood and at body surfaces and transmit virus to $CD4^+$ T cells, especially HIV-specific T cells.
- In chronic infection, germinal center DC capture antibody–virus complexes and transmit infection to $CD4^+$ T cells.

Mucosal surfaces
- Activated DC within the lymphoepithelium can support virus replication and transmit virus to adjacent T cells.

The identification of vaccine strategies for HIV-1 is one of the highest priorities. One approach is genetic immunization or DNA vaccines. It has recently been shown that DC are presenting the antigens encoded by DNA vaccines and are even carrying small amounts of vaccine DNA (Casares *et al.*, 1997). This finding suggests that if DNA targeting to DC could be amplified during vaccination, stronger anti-viral responses might be generated.

SUMMARIZING THE POSSIBLE ROLES OF DENDRITIC CELLS IN PROMOTING THE REPLICATION OF IMMUNODEFICIENCY VIRUSES

This chapter has considered some of the more recent literature on the potential roles of DC in promoting the replication of immunodeficiency viruses, HIV-1 and SIV. Additional reviews summarizing earlier work are available (Weissman and Fauci, 1997; Knight and Patterson, 1997; Cameron *et al.*, 1996; Grouard and Clark, 1997). We have divided the recent literature into anatomical compartments, and tried to relate observations with DC in culture to morphological studies of the virus *in situ*. The mechanisms whereby DC promote HIV-1/SIV replication may vary in different sites (Table 3). At body surfaces, immature DC may directly replicate virus. During acute infection, virus may be transmitted via DC to T cells that are responding to viral antigens in the T cell areas. In chronic infection, virus may be produced primarily via DC interacting with T cells in germinal centers of lymphoid organs and in the lymphoepithelium of MALT. Therefore, DC could be a major driving force or catalyst for viral replication in several pertinent anatomical compartments. In addition, the T cells die during their infection via DC, thereby leading to the critical loss of helper T cells during infections with immunodeficiency viruses.

ACKNOWLEDGMENT

Supported by grants from the NIH (AI40045 and AI40877), the Fogarty Foundation (TW00792), the German Ministry of Education and Research (#BMBF 01-K19469), the Körber Foundation (Hamburg), and Hoffman-LaRoche (Germany). The authors thank Judy Adams for help with the drawings. The work does not represent the opinion of the US Government.

REFERENCES

Albert, M.L., Sauter, B. and Bhardwaj, N. (1998). Dendritic cells acquire antigens from apoptotic cells and induce class-I restricted CTL responses. *Nature* **392**, 86–89.

Austyn, J.M., Kupiec-Weglinski, J.W., Hankins, D.F. and Morris, P.J. (1988). Migration patterns of dendritic cells in the mouse. Homing to T cell-dependent areas of spleen, and binding within marginal zone. *J. Exp. Med.* **167**, 646–651.

Bender, A., Bui, L.K., Feldman, M.A.V., Larsson, M. and Bhardwaj, N. (1995). Inactivated influenza virus, when presented on dendritic cells, elicits human CD8$^+$ cytolytic T cell responses. *J. Exp. Med.* **182**, 1663–1671.

Bender, A., Sapp, M., Schuler, G., Steinman, R.M. and Bhardwaj, N. (1996). Improved methods for the generation of dendritic cells from nonproliferating progenitors in human blood. *J. Immunol. Methods* **196**, 121–135.

Biberfeld, P., Porwit-Ksiazek, A., Bottiger, B., Morfeldt-Mansson, L. and Biberfeld, G. (1985). Immunohistopathology of lymph nodes in HTLV-III infected homosexuals with persistant adenopathy or AIDS. *Cancer Res.* **45**, 4665–4670.

Bujdoso, R., Hopkins, J., Dutia, B.M., Young, P. and McConnell, I. (1989). Characterization of sheep afferent lymph dendritic cells and their role in antigen carriage. *J. Exp. Med.* **170**, 1285–1302.

Cameron, P.U., Freudenthal, P.S., Barker, J.M., Gezelter, S., Inaba, K. and Steinman, R.M. (1992). Dendritic cells exposed to human immunodeficiency virus type-1 transmit a vigorous cytopathic infection to CD4$^+$ T cells. *Science* **257**, 383–387.

Cameron, P.U., Pope, M., Gezelter, S. and Steinman, R.M. (1994). Infection and apoptotic cell death of CD4$^+$ T cells during an immune response to HIV-1 pulsed dendritic cells. *Aids Res. Hum. Retroviruses* **10**, 61–71.

Cameron, P., Pope, M., Granelli-Piperno, A. and Steinman, R.M. (1996). Dendritic cells and the replication of HIV-1. *J. Leukocyte Biol.* **59**, 158–171.

Casares, S., Inaba, K., Brumeanu, T., Steinman, R.M. and Bona, C.A. (1997). Antigen presentation by dendritic cells following immunization with DNA encoding a class II-restricted viral epitope. *J. Exp. Med.* **186**, 1481–1486.

Cella, M., Engering, A., Pinet, V., Pieters, J. and Lanzavecchia, A. (1997). Inflammatory stimuli induce accumulation of MHC class II complexes on dendritic cells. *Nature* **388**, 782–787.

Chen, L.L., Adams, J.C. and Steinman, R.M. (1978a). Anatomy of germinal centers in mouse spleen with special reference to 'follicular dendritic cells'. *J. Cell Biol.* **77**, 148–164.

Chen, L.L., Frank, A.M., Adams, J.C. and Steinman, R.M. (1978b). Distribution of horseradish peroxidase (HRP)–anti HRP immune complexes in mouse spleen, with special reference to follicular dendritic cells. *J. Cell Biol.* **79**, 184–199.

Delgado, E., Finkel, V., Baggiolini, M., Clark-Lewis, I., Mackay, C.R., Steinman, R.M. and Granelli-Piperno, A. (1998). Mature dendritic cells respond to SDF-1, but not to several β chemokines. *Immunobiology* **198**, 490–500.

De Smedt, T., Pajak, B., Muraille, E., Lespagnard, L., Heinen, E., De Baetselier, P., Urbain, J., Leo, O. and Moser, M. (1996). Regulation of dendritic cell numbers and maturation by lipopolysaccharide in vivo. *J. Exp. Med.* **184**, 1413–1424.

Fox, C.H., Tenner-Racz, K., Racz, P., Firpo, A., Pizzo, P.A. and Fauci, A.S. (1991). Lymphoid germinal centers are reservoirs of human immunodeficiency virus type 1 RNA. *J. Infect. Dis.* **164**, 1051–1057.

Frankel, S.S., Wenig, B.M., Burke, A.P., Mannan, P., Thompson, L.D.R., Abbondanzo, S.L., Nelson, A.M., Pope, M. and Steinman, R.M. (1996). Replication of HIV-1 in dendritic cell-derived syncytia at the mucosal surface of the adenoid. *Science* **272**, 115–117.

Frankel, S.S., Tenner-Racz, K., Racz, P., Wenig, B.M., Hansen, C.H., Listinsky, C., Heffner, D., Nelson, A.M., Pope, M. and Steinman, R.M. (1997). Active replication of HIV-1 at the lymphoepithelial surface of the tonsil. *Am. J. Pathol.* **151**, 89–96.

Frey, A., Giannasca, K.T., Weltzin, R., Giannasca, P.J., Reggio, H.R., Lencer, W.I. and Neutra, M.R. (1996). Role of the glycocalyx in regulating access of microparticles to apical plasma membranes of intestinal epithelial cells: implications for microbial attachment and oral vaccine targeting. *J. Exp. Med.* **184**, 1045–1059.

Granelli-Piperno, A., Pope, M., Inaba, K. and Steinman, R.M. (1995). Coexpression of REL and SP1 transcription factors in HIV-1 induced, dendritic cell-T cell syncytia. *Proc. Natl Acad. Sci. USA* **92**, 10944–10948.

Granelli-Piperno, A., Moser, B., Pope, M., Chen, D., Wei, Y., Isdell, F., O'Doherty, F., Paxton, W., Koup, R., Mojsov, S., Bhardwaj, N., Clark-Lewis, I., Baggiolini, M. and Steinman, R.M. (1996). Efficient interaction of HIV-1 with purified dendritic cells via multiple chemokine coreceptors. *J. Exp. Med* **184**, 2433–2438.

Granelli-Piperno, A., Delgado, E., Finkel, V., Paxton, W. and Steinman, R.M. (1998). Immature dendritic cells selectively replicate M-tropic HIV-1, while mature cells efficiently transmit both M- and T-tropic virus to T cells. *J. Virol.* **72**, 2733–2737.

Grouard, G. and Clark, E.A. (1997). Role of dendritic and follicular dendritic cells in HIV infection and pathogenesis. *Curr. Opin. Immunol.* **9**, 563–567.

Grouard, G., Durand, I., Filgueira, L., Banchereau, J. and Liu, Y.-J. (1996). Dendritic cells capable of stimulating T cells in germinal centres. *Nature* **384**, 364–367.

Heath, S.L., Tew, J.G., Szakal, A.K. and Burton, G.F. (1995). Follicular dendritic cells and human immunodeficiency virus infectivity. *Nature* **377**, 740–744.

Ignatius, R., Isdell, F., O'Doherty, U. and Pope, M. (1998). Dendritic cells from skin and blood of macaques both promote SIV replication with T cells from different anatomical sites. *J. Med. Primatol.*, in press.

Inaba, K., Romani, N. and Steinman, R.M. (1989). An antigen-independent contact mechanism as an early step in T-cell-proliferative responses to dendritic cells. *J. Exp. Med.* **170**, 527–542.

Inaba, K., Metlay, J.P., Crowley, M.T. and Steinman, R.M. (1990). Dendritic cells pulsed with protein antigens in vitro can prime antigen-specific, MHC-restricted T cells in situ. *J. Exp. Med.* **172**, 631–640.

Inaba, K., Pack, M., Inaba, M., Sakuta, H., Isdell, F. and Steinman, R.M. (1997). High levels of a major histocompatibility complex II–self peptide complex on dendritic cells from lymph node. *J. Exp. Med.* **186**, 665–672.

Ingulli, E., Mondino, A., Khoruts, A. and Jenkins, M.K. (1997). In vivo detection of dendritic cell antigen presentation to $CD4^+$ T cells. *J. Exp. Med.* **185**, 2133–2141.

Kelsall, B.L. and Strober, W. (1996). Distinct populations of dendritic cells are present in the subepithelial dome and T cell regions of the murine Peyer's patch. *J. Exp. Med.* **183**, 237–247.

Kleijmeer, M.J., Oorschot, V.M.J. and Geuze, H.J. (1994). Human resident Langerhans cells display a lysosomal compartment enriched in MHC class II. *J. Invest. Dermatol.* **103**, 516–523.

Kleijmeer, M.J., Ossevoort, M.A., Van Veen, C.J.H., Van Hellemond, J.J., Neefjes, J.J., Kast, W.M., Melief, C.J.M. and Geuze, H.J. (1995). MHC class II compartments and the kinetics of antigen presentation in activated mouse spleen dendritic cells. *J. Immunol.* **154**, 5715–5724.

Knight, S.C. and Patterson, S. (1997). Bone marrow-derived dendritic cells, infection with human immunodeficiency virus, and immunopathology. *Annu. Rev. Immunol.* **15**, 593–615.

Kudo, S., Matsuno, K., Ezaki, T. and Ogawa, M. (1997). A novel migration pathway for rat dendritic cells from the blood: hepatic sinusoids–lymph translocation. *J. Exp. Med.* **185**, 777–784.

Larsen, C.P., Steinman, R.M., Witmer-Pack, M., Hankins, D.F., Morris, P.J. and Austyn, J.M. (1990). Migration and maturation of Langerhans cells in skin transplants and explants. *J. Exp. Med.* **172**, 1483–1493.

Lenz, A., Heine, M., Schuler, G. and Romani, N. (1993). Human and murine dermis contain dendritic cells: isolation by means of a novel method and phenotypical and functional characterization. *J. Clin. Invest.* **92**, 2587–2596.

Liu, L.M. and MacPherson, G.G. (1993). Antigen acquisition by dendritic cells: intestinal dendritic cells acquire antigen administered orally and can prime naive T cells in vivo. *J. Exp. Med.* **177**, 1299–1307.

Lukas, M., Stoessel, H., Hefel, L., Imamura, S., Fritsch, P., Sepp, N.T., Schuler, G. and Romani, N. (1996). Human cutaneous dendritic cells migrate through dermal lymphatic vessels in a skin organ culture model. *J. Invest. Dermatol.* **106**, 1293–1299.

Luther, S.A., Gulbranson-Judge, A., Acha-Orbea, H. and Maclennan, I.C.M. (1997). Viral superantigen drives extrafollicular and follicular B differentiation leading to virus-specific antibody production. *J. Exp. Med.* **185**, 551–562.

Mosialos, G., Birkenbach, M., Ayehunie, S., Matsumura, F., Pinkus, G.S., Kieff, E. and Langhoff, E. (1996). Circulating human dendritic cells differentially express high levels of a 55-kd actin-bundling protein. *Am. J. Pathol.* **148**, 593–600.

Neutra, M.R., Pringault, E. and Kraehenbuhl, J.-P. (1996). Antigen sampling across epithelial barriers and induction of mucosal immune responses. *Annu. Rev. Immunol.* **14**, 275–300.

Nijman, H.W., Kleijmeer, M.J., Ossevoort, M.A., Oorschot, V.M.J., Vierboom, M.P.M., van de Keur, M., Kenemans, P., Kast, W.M., Geuze, H.J. and Melief, C.J.M. (1995). Antigen capture and MHC class II compartments of freshly isolated and cultured human blood dendritic cells. *J. Exp. Med.* **182**, 163–174.

Nossal, G.J.V., Abbot, A., Mitchell, J. and Lummus, Z. (1968). Antigen in immunity. XV. Ultrastructural features of antigen capture in primary and secondary lymphoid follicles. *J. Exp. Med.* **127**, 277–296.

O'Doherty, U., Ignatius, R., Bhardwaj, N. and Pope, M. (1997). Generation of monocyte-derived dendritic cells from precursors in rhesus macaque blood. *J. Immunol. Methods* **207**, 185–194.

Piatak, M., Saag, M.S., Yang, L.C., Clark, S.J., Kappes, J.C., Luk, K.-C., Hahn, B.H., Shaw, G.M. and Lifson, J.D. (1993). High levels of HIV-1 in plasma during all stages of infection determined by competitive PCR. *Science* **259**, 1749–1754.

Pierre, P., Turley, S.J., Gatti, E., Hull, M., Meltzer, J., Mirza, A., Inaba, K., Steinman, R.M. and Mellman, I. (1997). Developmental regulation of MHC class II transport in mouse dendritic cells. *Nature* **388**, 787–792.

Pope, M., Betjes, M.G.H., Romani, N., Hirmand, H., Cameron, P.U., Hoffman, L., Gezelter, S., Schuler, G. and Steinman, R.M. (1994). Conjugates of dendritic cells and memory T lymphocytes from skin facilitate productive infection with HIV-1. *Cell* **78**, 389–398.

Pope, M., Betjes, M.G.H., Hirmand, H., Hoffman, L. and Steinman, R.M. (1995a). Both dendritic cells and memory T lymphocytes emigrate from organ cultures of human skin and form distinctive dendritic–T cell conjugates. *J. Invest. Dermatol.* **104**, 11–18.

Pope, M., Gezelter, S., Gallo, N., Hoffman, L. and Steinman, R.M. (1995b). Low levels of HIV-1 in cutaneous dendritic cells initiate a productive infection upon binding to memory $CD4^+$ T cells. *J. Exp. Med.* **182**, 2045–2056.

Pope, M., Elmore, D., Ho, D. and Marx, P. (1997a). Dendritic cell–T cell mixtures, isolated from the skin and mucosae of macaques, support the replication of SIV. *AIDS Res. Hum. Retroviruses* **13**, 819–827.

Pope, M., Frankel, S.S., Mascola, J.R., Trkola, A., Isdell, F., Birx, D.L., Burke, D.S., Ho, D.D. and Moore, J.P. (1997b). HIV-1 strains from subtypes B and E replicate in cutaneous dendritic cell–T cell mixtures without displaying subtype-specific tropism. *J. Virol.* **71**, 8001–8007.

Pure, E., Inaba, K., Crowley, M.T., Tardelli, L., Witmer-Pack, M.D., Ruberti, G., Fathman, G. and Steinman, R.M. (1990). Antigen processing by epidermal Langerhans cells correlates with the level of biosynthesis of major histocompatibility complex class II molecules and expression of invariant chain. *J. Exp. Med.* **172**, 1459–1469.

Reddy, A., Sapp, M., Feldman, M., Subklewe, M. and Bhardwaj, N. (1997). A monocyte conditioned medium is more effective than defined cytokines in mediating the terminal maturation of human dendritic cells. *Blood* **90**, 3640–3646.

Reece, J.C., Handley, A., Anstee, J., Morrison, W., Crowe, S.M. and Cameron, P.U. (1998). HIV-1 selection by epidermal dendritic cells during transmission across human skin. *J. Exp. Med.* **187**, 1623–1631.

Reimann, K.A., Tenner-Racz, K., Racz, P., Montefiori, D.C., Yasutomi, Y., Lin, W., Ransil, B.J. and Letvin, N.L. (1994). Immunopathogenic events in acute infection of rhesus monkeys with simian immunodeficiency virus of macaques. *J. Virol.* **68**, 2362–2370.

Romani, N., Inaba, K., Pure, E., Crowley, M., Witmer-Pack, M. and Steinman, R.M. (1989a). A small number of anti-CD3 molecules on dendritic cells stimulate DNA synthesis in mouse T lymphocytes. *J. Exp. Med.* **169**, 1153–1168.

Romani, N., Koide, S., Crowley, M., Witmer-Pack, M., Livingstone, A.M., Fathman, C.G., Inaba, K. and Steinman, R.M. (1989b). Presentation of exogenous protein antigens by dendritic cells to T cell clones: intact protein is presented best by immature, epidermal Langerhans cells. *J. Exp. Med.* **169**, 1169–1178.

Romani, N., Witmer-Pack, M., Crowley, M., Koide, S., Schuler, G., Inaba, K. and Steinman, R.M. (1991). Langerhans cells as immature dendritic cells. In: *Epidermal Langerhans Cells* (ed. G. Schuler) CRC Press, Boca Raton, pp. 191–216.

Romani, N., Gruner, S., Brang, D., Kampgen, E., Lenz, A., Trockenbacher, B., Konwalinka, G., Fritsch, P.O., Steinman, R.M. and Schuler, G. (1994). Proliferating dendritic cell progenitors in human blood. *J. Exp. Med.* **180**, 83–93.

Romani, N., Reider, D., Heuer, M., Ebner, S., Eibl, B., Niederwieser, D. and Schuler, G. (1996). Generation of mature dendritic cells from human blood: an improved method with special regard to clinical applicability. *J. Immunol. Methods* **196**, 137–151.

Sallusto, F. and Lanzavecchia, A. (1994). Efficient presentation of soluble antigen by cultured human dendritic cells is maintained by granulocyte/macrophage colony-stimulating factor plus interleukin 4 and downregulated by tumor necrosis factor α. *J. Exp. Med.* **179**, 1109–1118.

Sallusto, F. and Lanzavecchia, A. (1995). Dendritic cells use macropinocytosis and the mannose receptor to concentrate antigen in the MHC class II compartment. Downregulation by cytokines and bacterial products. *J. Exp. Med.* **182**, 389–400.

Sallusto, F., Nicolo, C., De Maria, R., Corinti, S. and Testi, R. (1996). Ceramide inhibits antigen uptake and presentation by dendritic cells. *J. Exp. Med.* **184**, 2411–2416.

Schuler, G. and Steinman, R.M. (1985). Murine epidermal Langerhans cells mature into potent immunostimulatory dendritic cells in vitro. *J. Exp. Med.* **161**, 526–546.

Schuurman, H.J., Krone, W.J., Broekhuizen, R. and Goudsmit, J. (1988). Expression of RNA and antigens of human immunodeficiency virus type-1 (HIV-1) in lymph nodes from HIV-1 infected individuals. *Am. J. Pathol.* **133**, 516–524.

Steinman, R.M. (1991). The dendritic cell system and its role in immunogenicity. *Annu. Rev. Immunol.* **9**, 271–296.

Steinman, R.M., Hoffman, L. and Pope, M. (1995). Maturation and migration of cutaneous dendritic cells. *J. Invest. Dermatol.* **105**, 2S–8S.

Streilein, J.W. and Grammer, S.F. (1989). In vitro evidence that Langerhans cells can adopt two functionally distinct forms capable of antigen presentation to T lymphocytes. *J. Immunol.* **143**, 3925–3933.

Szakal, A.K., Kosco, M.H. and Tew, J.G. (1989). Microanatomy of lymphoid tissue during humoral immune responses: structure function relationships. *Annu. Rev. Immunol.* **7**, 91–109.

Talmor, M., Mirza, A., Turley, S., Mellman, I., Hoffman, L.A. and Steinman, R.M. (1998). Cytokine requirements for the generation of large numbers of immature and mature dendritic cells from rat bone marrow cultures. *Eur. J. Immunol.* **28**, 811–817.

Tenner-Racz, K., Bofill, M., Schulz-Meyer, A., Dietrich, M., Weber, J., Pinching, A.J., Veronese-Dimarzo, F., Popovic, M., Klatzmann, D., Gluckman, J.C. and Janossy, G. (1986). HTLV-III/LAV viral antigens in lymph nodes of homosexual men with persistent generalized lymphadenopathy and AIDS. *Am. J. Pathol.* **123**, 9–15.

Tenner Racz, K., Racz, P., Schmidt, H., Dietrich, M., Kern, P., Louie, A., Gartner, S. and Popovic, M. (1988). Immunohistochemical, electron microscopic and in situ hybridization evidence for the involvement of lymphatics in the spread of HIV-1. *AIDS* **2**, 299–309.

Tenner-Racz, K., Stellbrink, H., van Lunzen, J., Schneider, C., Jacobs, J., Raschodorff, B., Groβschupff, G., Steinman, R.M. and Racz, P. (1998). The unenlarged lymph nodes of HIV-1 infected, asymptomatic patients with high CD4 T cell counts are sites for virus replication and CD4 T cell proliferation. The impact of active antiretroviral therapy. *J. Exp. Med.* **187**, 949–959.

van't Wout, A.B., Kootstra, N.A., Mulder-Kampinga, G.A., Albrect-van Lent, N., Scherpbier, H.J., Veenstra, J., Boer, K., Coutinho, R.A., Miedema, F. and Schuitemaker, H. (1994). Macrophage-tropic variants initiate human immunodeficency virus type 1 infection after sexual, parenteral, and vertical transmission. *J. Clin. Invest.* **94**, 2060–2067.

Weissman, D. and Fauci, A.S. (1997). Role of dendritic cells in immunopathogenesis of human immunodeficiency virus infection. *Clin. Microbiol. Rev.* **10**, 358–367.

Weissman, D., Barker, T.D. and Fauci, A.S. (1996). The efficiency of acute infection of $CD4^+$ T cells is markedly enhanced in the setting of antigen-specific immune activation. *J. Exp. Med.* **183**, 687–692.

Witmer-Pack, M.D., Olivier, W., Valinsky, J., Schuler, G. and Steinman, R.M. (1987). Granulocyte/macrophage colony-stimulating factor is essential for the viability and function of cultured murine epidermal Langerhans cells. *J. Exp. Med.* **166**, 1484–1498.

Witmer-Pack, M.D., Valinsky, J., Olivier, W. and Steinman, R.M. (1988). Quantitation of surface antigens on cultured murine epidermal Langerhans cells: rapid and selective increase in the level of surface MHC products. *J. Invest. Dermatol.* **90**, 387–394.

Zaitseva, M., Blauvelt, A., Lee, S., Lapham, C.K., Klaus-Kovtun, V., Mostowski, H., Manischewitz, J. and Golding, H. (1997). Expression and function of CCR5 and CXCR4 on human Langerhans cells and macrophages: implications for HIV primary infection. *Nature Medicine* **3**, 1369–1375.

Zhou, L.-J. and Tedder, T.F. (1995). Human blood dendritic cells selectively express CD83, a member of the immunoglobulin superfamily. *J. Immunol.* **154**, 3821–3835.

Zhu, T., Mo, H., Wang, N., Nam, D.S., Cao, Y., Koup, R.A. and Ho, D.D. (1993). Genotypic and phenotypic characterization of HIV-1 in patients with primary infection. *Science* **261**, 1179–1181.

CHAPTER 24
Dendritic Cells in Allergy

A.E. Semper, J.A. Hartley, I.G. Reischl and S.T. Holgate
University Medicine, Southampton General Hospital, Southampton, UK

INTRODUCTION

In modern society, the term allergy is frequently used loosely to describe human intolerance to a wide variety of environmental agents and toxins, even to such ubiquitous factors as water and sunlight. However, a more restricted definition is that of Gell and Coombes (1962), namely, 'immune responses which give rise to irritant or harmful reactions'. Although these workers recognized four types of such 'hypersensitivity' reactions, most of the classical allergic responses fall into the category of 'immediate' or 'type 1' hypersensitivity. It is these type 1 allergic reactions that are the subject of this chapter.

The allergic response is typically triggered at interfaces between the external environment and the internal milieu, giving rise to allergic asthma in the lungs, to perennial and seasonal rhinitis (hayfever) in the upper airways, to allergic conjunctivitis in the eye, and to allergic eczema (allergic dermatitis) in the skin. At its most acute, the allergic response manifests itself as the life-threatening condition of anaphylaxis. Despite this variety of target sites, allergic diseases share a common triggering mechanism, namely immunoglobulin E (IgE). Although IgE is present in the serum of all individuals, its levels are typically raised in those who express allergic diseases. Furthermore, this IgE is directed against specific, normally innocuous, environmental antigens (allergens). Indeed, it is the genetic tendency to develop allergen-specific IgE antibodies, termed atopy, that typifies all allergic or 'atopic' diseases.

In an individual previously sensitized to an allergen, allergen-specific IgE antibodies are present bound to high-affinity IgE receptors (FcεRI) on the surface of mast cells in target tissues such as the skin or lung. Upon re-exposure to allergen, receptor-bound IgE molecules on the sensitized mast cells are cross-linked, causing mast cell degranulation and release of mediators such as histamine, tryptase, prostaglandins and leukotrienes. These mediators cause increased vascular permeability, local oedema and itching resulting, for example, in the weal and flare reaction that occurs within 10–20 min of introducing allergen into the skin. This acute immediate allergic response is frequently followed by late-phase reactions (LPR) which typically peak at 6–12 h following allergen exposure then gradually decline over the next 12–24 h. During the late-phase response, the site of allergen exposure shows marked infiltration, notably by eosinophils and $CD4^+$ T helper (T_H) cells (Azzawi *et al.*, 1992). These cells are thought

Dendritic Cells: Biology and Clinical Applications
ISBN 0-12-455860-7

to contribute not only to continued hypersensitivity during the LPR, but also to disease chronicity (Zweiman, 1993).

The realization that there is an underlying persistent chronic inflammation in the target organs of allergic diseases has only been made in the past decade. This chronic allergic inflammation is characterized by the same cell types as the LPR, namely eosinophils (Bruijnzeel-Koomen *et al.*, 1988a; Djukanovic *et al.*, 1990) and $CD4^+$ T cells (Frew and O'Hehir, 1992; Poston *et al.*, 1992; Metz *et al.*, 1996). Both cell types show signs of activation (Azzawi *et al.*, 1990; Bradley *et al.*, 1991; Wilson *et al.*, 1992; Robinson *et al.*, 1993). Whereas the activated eosinophils probably contribute to disease chronicity by damaging epithelial and epidermal barriers, thus rendering these interfaces with the external milieu more vulnerable to environmental antigens, much attention has focused on the presence of activated T cells as the possible orchestrators of the chronic allergic immune response.

THE HELPER T CELL AS THE ORCHESTRATOR OF THE ALLERGIC INFLAMMATORY RESPONSE

In addition to identifying increased numbers of activated ($CD25^+$) $CD4^+$ T_H cells in the target organs of atopic diseases, evidence has accumulated to suggest that the $CD4^+$ cells present at sites of allergic inflammation (Del Prete, 1992; Robinson *et al.*, 1992; Thepen *et al.*, 1996) and allergen-specific $CD4^+$ T cells cloned from these sites (Wierenga *et al.*, 1990; Van Reijsen *et al.*, 1992), are skewed towards the T_H2 phenotype. In man, T_H2 cells are characterized by production of interleukins (IL) -3, -4, -5, -10 and 13 and low to negligible amounts of IFN-γ. These are indeed the cytokines expressed at the sites of allergic disease (Kapsenberg *et al.*, 1991; Kay *et al.*, 1991; Bentley *et al.*, 1993) and their production has been attributed to allergen-activated T cells (Krishnaswamy *et al.*, 1993; Ying *et al.*, 1993; Huang *et al.*, 1995). The cytokine products of T_H2-like cells are thought to be responsible for much of the pathophysiology of allergic diseases, with particular attention being focused on IL-4 and IL-5 (Drazen *et al.*, 1996). IL-4 (and IL-13) switch B cell immunoglobulin isotype production to IgE and thus contribute to the atopic element of allergic diseases. Furthermore, IL-4 promotes the differentiation of T_H cells along the T_H2 pathway, hence sustaining its own overproduction and that of other T_H2-like cytokines. IL-5, together with IL-3 and GM-CSF, enhances eosinophil differentiation and migration, leading to eosinophilia, and also contributes to the priming of eosinophils for the release of cytotoxic mediators. The key role played by IL-5 in the pathophysiology of pulmonary allergic responses has been highlighted by recent studies using IL-5 knockout mice (Foster *et al.*, 1996) and mice expressing the IL-5 transgene in the lung epithelium (Lee *et al.*, 1997).

ANTIGEN PRESENTATION AND T CELL ACTIVATION IN ALLERGIC DISEASE

Sensitization

To induce a primary immune response of a naive T cell to an environmental antigen, the antigen must be presented to the T cell in the context of MHC class II on the surface of an antigen-presenting cell (APC), together with potent costimulatory signals

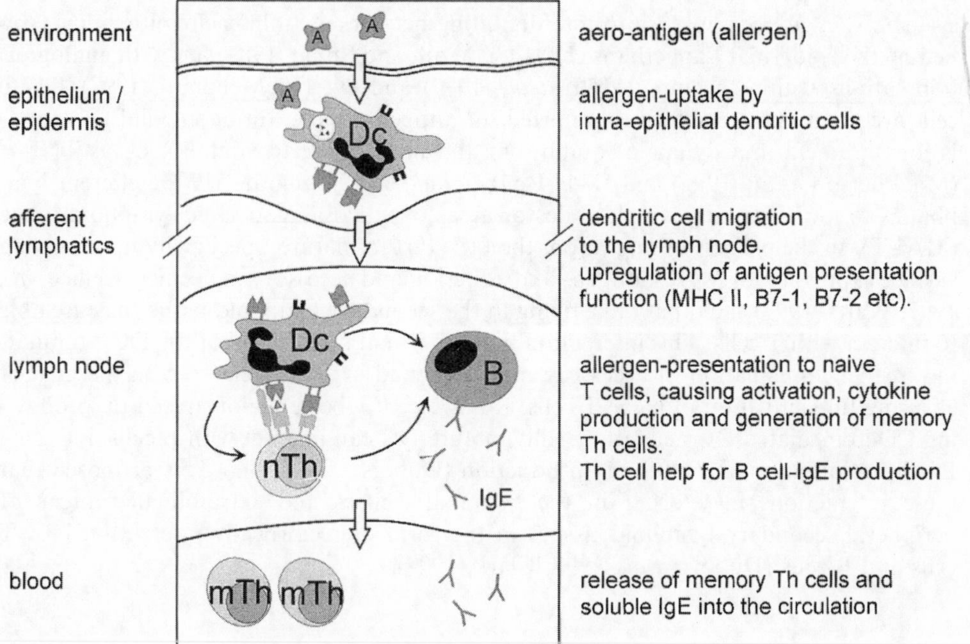

Fig. 1. Events leading to allergic sensitization to an environmental antigen (allergen). Intraepithelial dendritic cells take up antigen arriving from the environment, process it and transport it to the secondary lymphoid tissue for presentation to naive T helper cells (nTh). Naive T cells are activated to generate allergen-specific memory T cells (mTh) and to produce cytokines for B cell help. Providing sufficient IL-4 (or IL-13) is released on this first round of activation, B cells will switch to IgE production. Otherwise, immunoglobulin isotype switching to IgE may occur during a subsequent round of allergen-dependent activation.

Key	IgE	Allergen	FcεRI	Peptide
MHC II	B7-1/B7-2	CD28	CD4	TCR

provided by the APC (Lenschow *et al.*, 1996). Current dogma dictates that this function can only be fulfilled by dendritic cells (DC). Sensitization of new cohorts of naive T cells to environmental allergens is probably an on-going process contributing to the chronicity of allergic inflammation. The pathway for this sensitization (Fig. 1) is best characterized in the skin, although analogous processes probably occur in other target organs of allergic disease such as the lungs and eyes. The epithelial and epidermal interfaces between the body and the environment are the point of entry for allergens. These epithelia are patrolled by DC which are thought to act as sentinels of the immune system. They are organized into interdigitating networks within each epithelium, typified by the epidermal Langerhans cell (LC) (Wolff and Stingl, 1983) but with analogous populations within the lung (Holt *et al.*, 1989) and eye (McMenamin, 1997). These cells are in an immature form, optimized for antigen uptake. Intraepithelial DC populations are held in a dynamic equilibrium and in response to stimuli such as TNF-α (MacPherson *et al.*, 1995) and IL-1 (Roake *et al.*, 1995), migrate via the efferent lymphatics to local draining lymph nodes or areas of mucosal-associated lymphoid tissue (MALT). In the process of migration, the DC start to mature, specifically upregulating surface expression of MHC antigens and adhesion and accessory molecules (Cella *et al.*, 1997; Watts, 1997) such that on arriving in the secondary lymphoid tissue they are able to interact with T cells. This interaction induces a final maturation of the DC, stimulating further upregulation of accessory molecules and cytokine release with the goal of ensuring full activation of naive T cells. It has recently been demonstrated that following CD40-mediated DC activation, fully mature DC can interact with B cells, inducing B cell proliferation and antibody production (Dubois *et al.*, 1997). It is proposed that these interactions may occur in the germinal centres and extrafollicular areas of peripheral secondary lymphoid tissues in the form of reciprocally interacting DC, T cells and B cells (Dubois *et al.*, 1997; Clark, 1997).

Secondary Allergic Immune Responses

Memory T cells resulting from the expansion of activated naive T cells enter the blood, whence they can extravasate into target organs. It is questionable how dependent these memory T_H cells are on receiving CD28-mediated accessory signals for allergen-dependent activation (Gause *et al.*, 1997). Thus, it may be that they can be activated by interaction with a range of APC within the target tissue. The outcome of local antigen presentation is the activation and proliferation of resident memory $CD4^+$ T_H cells to yield T_H2 effector cells with concomitant release of T_H2-like cytokines which lead to B cell IgE production and recruitment of eosinophils and more memory T cells from the blood, thus perpetuating the allergic inflammation (Fig. 2). Using an *in vitro* allergen challenge model it has recently been shown that the T cells resident within asthmatic endobronchial biopsies release IL-5 during the first 24 h of allergen stimulation (Jaffar *et al.*, 1998). It is probable that newly arrived memory T_H cells are not fully differentiated down the T_H2 pathway and that this phenotype is reinforced locally upon subsequent, perhaps repeated, exposure to allergen.

Candidate APC for the stimulation of memory T_H cells in allergic inflammatory reactions are monocytes/macrophages, B cells and DC. Although monocytes/macrophages are present within allergic inflammatory infiltrates, it seems they are unable to induce full and sustained T cell activation (see later). Like DC, B cells are capable of allergen focusing, mediated in the case of the B cell through FcεRII (CD23), theoretically resulting in enhanced allergen presentation. However, B cells are present at only very low frequency in human airway mucosa (Graeme-Cook *et al.*, 1993). It is therefore tempting to speculate that, following allergic sensitization, the DC play a continued role in the local stimulation of memory T cells at the sites of allergic

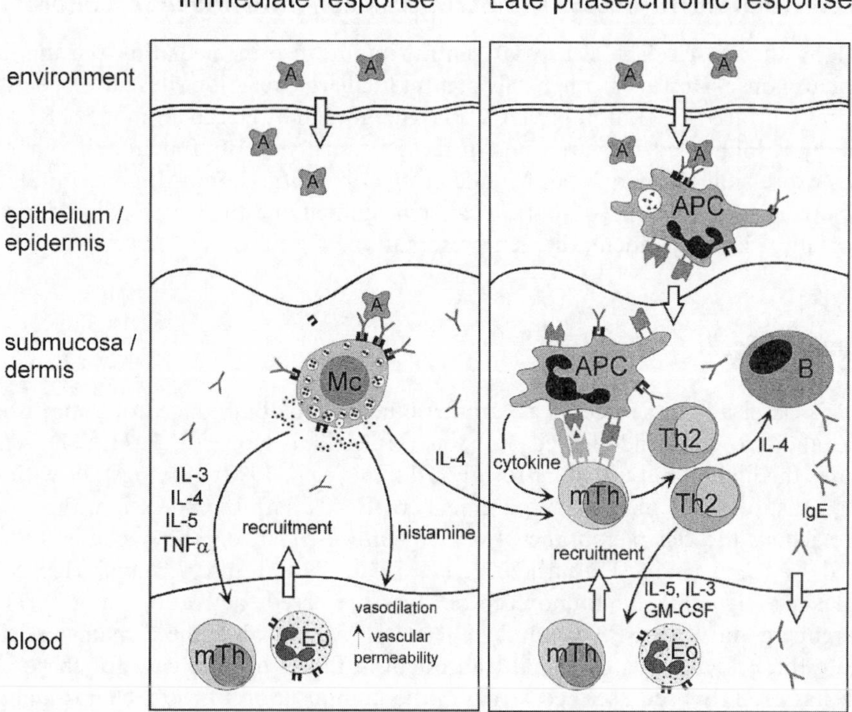

Fig. 2. The cellular mechanisms underlying the immediate allergic response (mast cell mediated) and the late-phase response (T cell mediated). The latter contributes to the generation of chronic allergic inflammation. See text for explanation. Note the central role played by the high-affinity IgE (FcεRI) receptors. In the immediate response, allergen cross-links IgE bound to FcεRI on the mast cell, causing degranulation. In the late-phase response, allergen and specific IgE are bound to receptors on the surface of antigen-presenting cells, most probably to FcεRI on dendritic cells. This leads to allergen focusing and increased activation of allergen-specific T helper cells.

Key

IgE Allergen FcεRI Peptide

MHC II B7-1/B7-2 CD28 CD4 TCR

inflammation. Support for this hypothesis comes from two observations. First, in atopic asthmatics, it has been shown that, *in vitro*, pulmonary DC can activate allergen-specific memory T_H2 cells (Bellini *et al.*, 1993); second, numbers of intra-epithelial DC are increased in the lungs of asthmatics (Bellini *et al.*, 1993; Tunon-de-Lara *et al.*, 1996) and hayfever sufferers (Fokkens *et al.*, 1989) compared to normal healthy controls.

FCεRI ON DENDRITIC CELLS: A MOLECULE MEDIATING DISEASE CHRONICITY

FcεRI on the mast cell is clearly of central importance in mediating the immediate allergic response. However, other cells present at allergic reaction sites have been shown to express surface FcεRI, notably DC. It is emerging that the function of FcεRI on DC in allergy is influenced by variations in receptor structure, its functional competency and its expression (Bieber, 1996; Mudde *et al.*, 1996; Stingl and Maurer, 1997), all of which are, in turn, influenced by the local environment and the very mediators released as a result of DC-dependent allergen presentation.

Structure of FcεRI

FcεRI is classically described as a tetrameric immunoglobulin-receptor comprising an α, a β and two disulphide-linked γ chains (Hulett and Hogarth, 1994). The α chain mediates the high-affinity binding to IgE (Hakimi *et al.*, 1990) and together with the γ chains constitutes the minimal requirement for FcεRI surface expression, the receptor only reaching the cell membrane after a retention signal on the γ chains has been masked by the α chain (Letourneur *et al.*, 1995). The β and γ chains each carry a cytoplasmic signalling immunoreceptor tyrosine-based activation motif (ITAM) (Scharenberg and Kinet, 1994; Cambier *et al.*, 1995), but while the γ chains are clearly obligate for FcεRI-mediated signal transduction, this is not the case for the β chain, which has recently been ascribed a role in the amplification of the γ chain signal (Lin *et al.*, 1996). Interestingly, genetic linkage of the β chain locus on chromosome 11q13 to atopy has been hypothesized for a subgroup of atopics (Shirakawa *et al.*, 1994). Mutations in this gene might augment the signalling by the β chain, thus further amplifying FcεRI signalling on mast cells and maybe also on DC.

FcεRI Expression by Dendritic Cells

Early studies demonstrated that LC from subjects with atopic dermatitis carried surface-bound IgE (Bruijnzeel-Koomen *et al.*, 1986), which was subsequently shown to be bound to FcεRI (Bruijnzeel-Koomen *et al.*, 1988b; Bieber *et al.*, 1992; Klubal *et al.*, 1997). FcεRI-bearing DC have now been described in various tissue sites including normal skin (Bieber and Ring, 1992; Wang *et al.*, 1992), the lung (Semper *et al.*, 1995b; Tunon-de-Lara *et al.*, 1996) and the nasal mucosa (Rajakulasingam *et al.*, 1997), and also on circulating DC (Fig. 3) (Maurer *et al.*, 1996; Hartley *et al.*, manuscript in preparation). In allergic disease, the numbers of FcεRI-positive DC are increased, as shown in the asthmatic lung (Semper *et al.*, 1995b; Tunon-de-Lara *et al.*, 1996), as are the numbers of cell surface FcεRI molecules, clearly demonstrated on LC isolated from atopic dermatitis lesions (Wollenberg *et al.*, 1996). In atopic dermatitis, levels of FcεRI on LC are significantly higher at lesional sites compared to uninvolved areas, although LC at nonlesional sites still bear higher receptor numbers than in nondiseased skin (Wollenberg *et al.*, 1996). Indeed, it has been suggested that, among skin diseases, high expression of FcεRI on epidermal LC may be a diagnostic marker of atopic dermatitis (Wollenberg *et al.*, 1995).

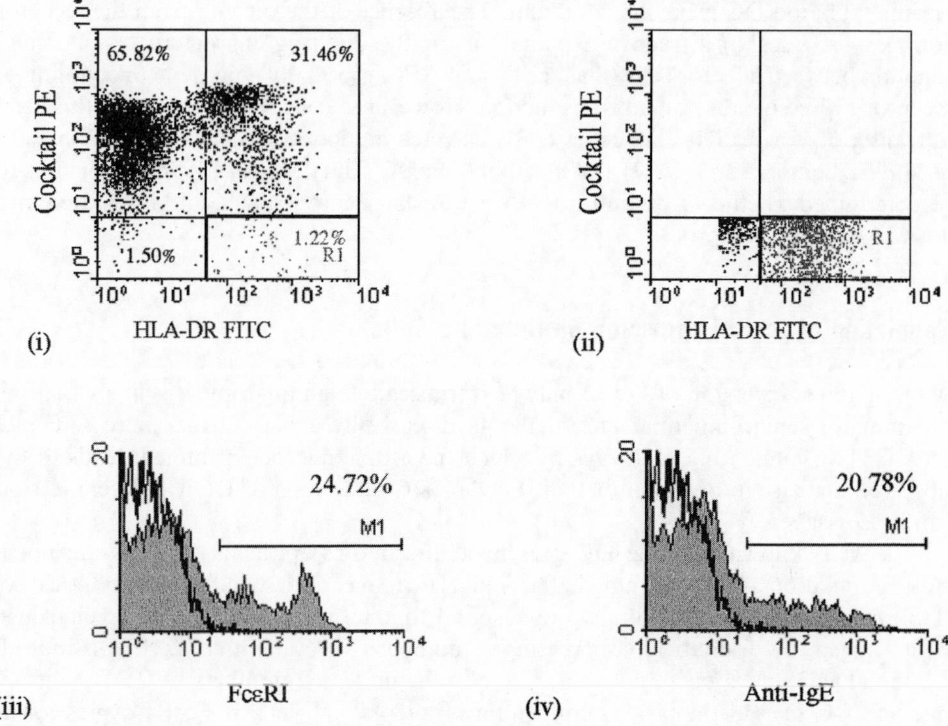

Fig. 3. Flow cytometric detection of surface FcεRI and IgE on peripheral blood DC. Peripheral blood mononuclear cells were stained with a cocktail of R-phycoerythrin (PE)-conjugated antibodies against CD3, CD19, CD14 and CD56 and with fluorescein (FITC)-labelled anti-HLA-DR. (i) Dendritic cells were identified as cells staining brightly for HLA-DR but negative for the antibody cocktail (region 1; R1); (ii) 5000 events were collected in region 1 and analysed (iii) for expression of FcεRI-α using an antibody that will only bind to unoccupied receptor or (iv) for the presence of surface bound IgE using anti-IgE. Note the presence of both free FcεRI and surface-bound IgE.

Structure of FcεRI on Dendritic Cells

FcεRI on mast cells and basophils comprises an $\alpha\beta\gamma\gamma$ tetramer. However, studies of rat-basophilic leukaemia (RBL) cells transfected with human FcεRI-α (Blank *et al.*, 1989) showed that, unlike its rodent counterpart, human FcεRI-α does not need to be associated with the β subunit to be expressed at the cell surface. Thus, transfectants expressing both $\alpha\beta\gamma\gamma$ and $\alpha\gamma\gamma$ FcεRI molecules were identified. It has since emerged that, *in vivo*, cells may also express FcεRI in the form of $\alpha\gamma\gamma$, most notably APC.

Messenger RNAs for FcεRI α and γ subunits were detected by RT-PCR analysis of LC (Jürgens *et al.*, 1995), circulating DC (Maurer *et al.*, 1996) and monocytes (Maurer *et al.*, 1994). However, as reported for monocytes (Maurer *et al.*, 1995), transcripts for the β chain could not be detected in circulating DC (Maurer *et al.*, 1996) and were only detected in LC in a minority of donors (Jürgens *et al.*, 1995). This suggests that DC might express FcεRI as an $\alpha\gamma\gamma$ complex. Indeed, Maurer and co-workers (1996) have shown that FcεRI immunoprecipitated from the surface of human peripheral blood DC lacks the β subunit. The absence of the β chain from the receptor complex provides an attractive explanation for the differing characteristics of FcεRI function between effector cells (mast cells) and APC, especially a possible uncoupling of receptor expression and signal transduction. However, recent results challenge this idea, as transcripts for FcεRI-β are consistently detected in monocyte-derived DC (Semper *et al.*, 1995a; Semper *et al.*, 1997) and in circulating DC (Hartley *et al.*, 1996). It remains to be determined whether β subunit mRNA is translated into protein, and integrated into an $\alpha\beta\gamma\gamma$ surface receptor.

Regulation of FcεRI Expression on Dendritic Cells

Although the expression of FcεRI may be intrinsically high in atopy, it is likely that the inflammatory environment at sites of allergic disease also acts to further increase FcεRI on DC. Two interacting pathways by which the atopic microenvironment leads to the observed increase in both numbers of FcεRI$^+$ DC and levels of DC FcεRI expression can be envisaged.

First, it is known that the DC present at the body's epithelial surfaces are not a static population and, in the lung in particular, turn over with a half-life of about 2 days (Holt *et al.*, 1994). These populations respond to external stimuli, including challenge with antigen, by dramatically increasing in number (McWilliam *et al.*, 1996). Indeed, continual antigen exposure may contribute to the increased numbers of CD1a$^+$ intraepithelial DC seen in the airway epithelium of allergic subjects. If FcεRI expression is intrinsically high in the circulation in atopy, the enhanced recruitment of DC in response to chemokines generated at sites of allergic inflammation would bring FcεRI-positive DC into the tissue.

Second, the allergic cytokine milieu may upregulate surface FcεRI on DC within the tissue. Data in support of this possibility are now emerging, although the investigation of *ex vivo* receptor expression on LC and other DC is complicated by the fact that these cells are prone to rapidly change their phenotype upon isolation (Reischl *et al.*, 1996), with FcεRI expression being particularly affected by some cell isolation protocols (Bieber, 1996; Reischl *et al.*, 1996). In spite of these difficulties, two factors have recently been identified as having a modulatory role on FcεRI expression, namely the receptor's own ligand IgE and IL-4, both of which are key molecules characteristic of allergic inflammation.

Although it is well established that the amount of total IgE in the serum correlates with receptor expression and IgE loading on monocytes (Maurer *et al.*, 1994) and LC (Bruijnzeel-Koomen *et al.*, 1986; Wollenberg *et al.*, 1996), the same trend has not yet conclusively been shown for DC in sites other than the epidermis. It is recognized that on mast cells (Yamaguchi *et al.*, 1997), basophils (Malveaux *et al.*, 1978) and monocytes (Reischl *et al.*, 1996), interaction of FcεRI with its ligand can upregulate expression of this receptor. Whether the same regulatory mechanism exists for FcεRI expression by DC remains to be elucidated.

A major advance in understanding the regulation of FcεRI expression was the discovery of the receptor-inducing effect of IL-4. IL-4 directly induces FcεRI α chain mRNA production by eosinophils (Terada *et al.*, 1995) and increases surface expression of the receptor on the pro-monocytic cell line THP1 (Reischl *et al.*, 1997a). Both the

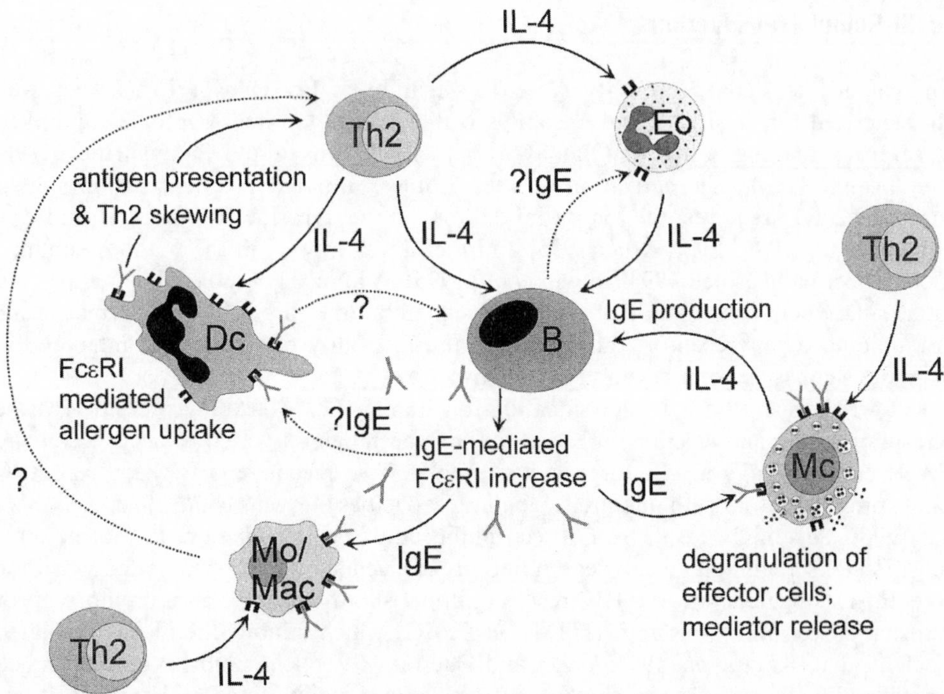

Fig. 4. The interconnecting pathways regulating FcεRI expression in allergic inflammation. IL-4-mediated upregulation of FcεRI has been reported for dendritic cells, monocytes, mast cells and eosinophils. FcεRI upregulation by IgE remains to be demonstrated for dendritic cells and eosinophils. The known function of FcεRI on dendritic cells is to enhance allergen uptake and activation of allergen-specific T helper (T_H) cells. It may also contribute to the skewing of the T_H response, thus exacerbating the production of IL-4 resulting in further FcεRI upregulation. Whether FcεRI-mediated allergen focusing on dendritic cells has consequences for B cell function remains to be demonstrated.

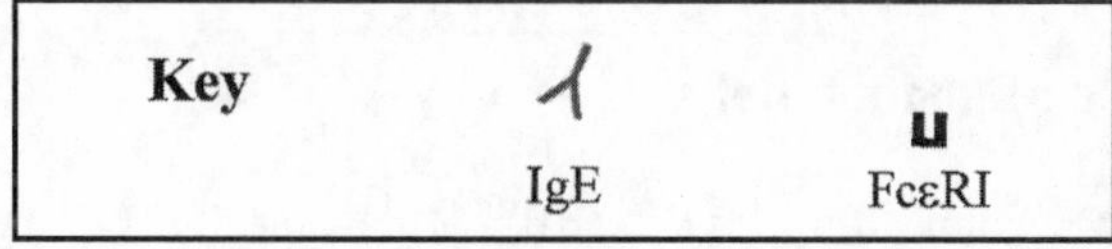

transcription of FcεRI-α and surface expression of the receptor complex are markedly increased by IL-4 in human mast cells (Toru *et al.*, 1996; Xia *et al.*, 1997) and LC (Bieber, 1996). During the differentiation of DC from monocytes, an increase of FcεRI α and β mRNA and protein occurs, possibly induced by the IL-4 required to suppress macrophage differentiation in these cultures (Semper *et al.*, 1997). Further studies are needed to examine the effect of IL-4 and IgE on DC, focusing in particular on the modulation of FcεRI subunits, the composition of the surface receptor and the possibility of counter-regulatory mechanisms.

These results link IgE, IL-4 and FcεRI in a vicious circle (Fig. 4), adding to the enormous complexity of allergic disease. It seems that once the dynamic balance of the immune system is perturbed by the allergic response, the progression of the disease becomes self-perpetuating.

FcεRI Signal Transduction

The cascade of signalling events caused by ligation of FcεRI by IgE has been well characterized for mast cells and basophils with evidence for the receptor being linked to several signalling pathways (Hamawy *et al.*, 1995; Beaven and Baumgartner, 1996; Choi *et al.*, 1996). The activation of these routes, initiated by the cross-linking of surface FcεRI, requires the phosphorylation of the tyrosine kinases *lyn* and *syk* (Jouvin *et al.*, 1994, Field *et al.*, 1995) and the ITAM motifs on the β and γ subunits (Scharenberg and Kinet, 1994; Jouvin *et al.*, 1995). A number of molecules are involved in the subsequent propagation of the FcεRI signal, but they are neither cell type-specific nor unique to this receptor, thus reducing the feasibility of therapeutic intervention once the signal has gone beyond *lyn* and *syk*.

Little is known about FcεRI signalling on human DC. Certainly protein tyrosine phosphorylation and calcium mobilization have been demonstrated to occur following FcεRI cross-linking on LC (Jürgens *et al.*, 1995). Two recent reports claim that APC can express receptors with impaired signalling capacities (Jürgens *et al.*, 1995; Reischl *et al.*, 1996). This might result from direct inhibition of FcεRI function. In murine mast cells, FcεRI signalling and cell degranulation has been shown to be inhibited when the receptor is coligated with FcγRII, resulting in phosphorylation of an immunoreceptor tyrosine-based inhibition motif (ITIM) on FcγRII which inhibits the ITAM-mediated FcεRI signal (Katz *et al.*, 1996; Vivier and Daeron, 1997). It remains to be determined whether ITIM-bearing receptors can control FcεRI signalling on DC. However, it has been demonstrated that co-cross-linking of FcεRI with the tyrosine phosphatase CD45 interferes with signal transduction on LC and monocytes (Bieber *et al.*, 1995; Reischl *et al.*, 1997b; Neel and Tonks, 1997). This and other as yet unidentified mechanisms probably interact to determine the outcome of FcεRI engagement on APC. Elucidating the molecular mechanisms underlying inhibition of FcεRI signalling by DC may identify means of therapeutically inhibiting FcεRI on DC.

Function of FcεRI on Dendritic Cells

FcεRI binds IgE with high affinity ($K_a = 10^{10}\,M^{-1}$). Specific IgE bound to FcεRI on DC can in turn bind allergen which is then subsequently internalized by receptor-mediated endocytosis (Jürgens *et al.*, 1995). Uptake of allergen via this route is of superior efficiency and specificity to the alternative antigen capture modes of non-specific adsorption, fluid-phase pinocytosis and macropinocytosis, thus 'focusing' antigen uptake. In the allergic process, antigen can be focused through IgE bound not only to FcεRI (Maurer and Stingl, 1995) but also to the low-affinity IgE receptor CD23 (Heyman *et al.*, 1993, van der Heijden *et al.*, 1993; Mudde *et al.*, 1996). When compared to FcγRII (CD32), FcεRII on B cells has been shown to be the dominant structure for allergen uptake (Bheekha Escura *et al.*, 1995). Therefore, it seems reasonable to suppose that, in an atopic environment with elevated levels of IgE where FcεRI is clearly the dominant IgE receptor on DC (Wollenberg *et al.*, 1996), allergen focusing via FcεRI will be more efficient than uptake mediated by Fcγ receptors. It should be noted that FcεRI-mediated allergen uptake seems to occur despite the $\alpha\gamma\gamma$ structure of this receptor on DC and monocytes (Maurer *et al.*, 1995; Maurer *et al.*, 1996).

In allergic disease, the consequence of antigen focusing through FcεRI is preferential uptake of allergens to which an individual is presensitized. After proteolytic processing, peptides derived from these allergens will occupy a greater proportion of surface MHC class II molecules on the DC surface. This is thought to enhance the activation of allergen-specific T cells as has been shown *in vitro* when IgE-dependent antigen presentation is mediated by FcεRI on either monocytes or peripheral blood DC (Maurer *et al.*, 1995; Maurer *et al.*, 1996). On a per-cell basis, Maurer and coworkers (1996) have suggested that DC are approximately 10 times more potent than monocytes at FcεRI-mediated IgE-dependent allergen presentation. Compared to allergen taken up by bulk-phase pathways alone, FcεRI-mediated uptake enhanced the activation of allergen-specific T cells 100- to 1000-fold (Maurer *et al.*, 1995).

Cross-linking FcεRI on the DC surface induces tyrosine phosphorylation of several proteins in a manner directly proportional to the density of surface receptor expression (Jürgens *et al.*, 1995). However, for LC, tyrosine phosphorylation did not necessarily lead to an increase in free intracellular calcium that would be indicative of cell activation, although cells activated by FcεRI cross-linking tended to display higher FcεRI expression and cells from atopic dermatitis lesional skin were consistently activated by FcεRI cross-linking (Jürgens *et al.*, 1995). Cell activation probably induces the synthesis and release of as yet undefined mediators from DC at allergic reaction sites. These mediators might further contribute to the vicious circle of events that lead to chronic allergic inflammation.

DC AND IMMUNE DEVIATION TOWARDS A T_H2 PHENOTYPE IN ALLERGY

It is tempting to speculate that the presence of FcεRI on DC could directly influence the differentiation of helper T cells along the T_H2 pathway. For example, allergen–IgE complexes internalized by FcεRI-mediated endocytosis may enter different proteolytic processing pathways in the DC to allergen taken up in the bulk phase. This might give rise to different peptide repertoires, possibly with differing TCR affinities. Alternatively, mediators released by DC activated by FcεRI cross-linking may favour the development of T_H2 cells. However, the existence of such mechanisms has not yet been demonstrated.

Consideration of FcεRI apart, considerable interest has focused on the possibility that T cell phenotype may be determined during the interaction between a T cell and an APC, as a result of antigen dose, the costimulatory signals received by the T cell, or the paracrine effects of cytokines released by the APC (Romagnani, 1996; Umetsu and DeKruyff, 1997).

Although in some systems high doses of antigenic peptide cause naive T cells to differentiate into T_H1-like cells, while low doses of the same peptide induce T_H2 differentiation (Constant *et al.*, 1995), in other systems the relationship between antigen dose and helper T cell differentiation is more complex (Hosken *et al.*, 1995). The same antigen dose need not necessarily lead to the same level of antigen presentation in different antigen-presenting cell types. For example, DC equipped with highly efficient mechanisms of macropinocytosis and receptor-mediated endocytosis for antigen, together with high levels of MHC class II surface expression and the capacity for serial triggering of T cell receptors by individual MHC–peptide complexes (Valitutti *et al.*, 1995), may activate more T cell receptors than the equivalent dose of antigen given to a macrophage. It should also be remembered that in addition to antigen availability, peptide affinity for MHC class II or the T cell receptor can affect T cell differentiation (Pearson *et al.*, 1997).

Much work has focused on the role of the B7 family of costimulatory molecules in the determination of T cell phenotype. Interestingly, B7-1 (CD80) and B7-2 (CD86) are differentially expressed and regulated on DC (Kawamura and Furue, 1995). However, although early studies suggested that engagement of CD28 can direct naive T cells to differentiate along a T_H2 pathway (Webb and Feldmann, 1995) and even that the preferential differentiation of T_H1 or T_H2 cells from uncommitted T_H precursors is induced by ligation of CD28 with B7-1 or B7-2, respectively (Kuchroo *et al.*, 1995), it now appears that the importance of the CD28 costimulatory pathway in determining T cell phenotype may be secondary to the role of the local cytokine environment (Seder *et al.*, 1994) and most probably varies depending on the system under investigation. Interactions between other receptor–ligand pairs, notably CD30 (T cell) and CD30 ligand (APC) may also be involved in determining the preferential development of T_H2 cells (Del Prete *et al.*, 1995; but also Hamann *et al.*, 1996) as may other, as yet unknown receptor/counter-receptor interactions.

DC have traditionally been regarded as poor cytokine producers (Steinman, 1991). However, under appropriate stimulation conditions, for example the cross-linking of CD40 by CD40 ligand that occurs during the interaction between DC and T cells, DC may be induced to produce cytokines, notably IL-12 (Cella *et al.*, 1996; Koch *et al.*, 1996). The IL-12 produced by DC directs both murine (Macatonia *et al.*, 1995) and human (Heufler *et al.*, 1996) naive T cells to differentiate towards a T_H1 phenotype. T_H2 cells are unresponsive to IL-12 (Hilkens *et al.*, 1996), probably owing to a lack of surface expression of the IL-12 receptor β_2 subunit by T_H2 cells (Rogge *et al.*, 1997). Together, this evidence suggests that DC are potent stimulators of T_H1 differentiation but maybe not of the T_H2 differentiated state seen in allergy. However, data are emerging suggesting at least two exogenous factors present at sites of allergic inflammation, IL-10 and prostaglandin E2 (PGE_2), can change DC phenotype away from potent IL-12 production (DeSmedt *et al.*, 1997; Kalinski *et al.*, 1997; Liu *et al.*, 1997), resulting *in vitro* in the development of T_H2 cells from naive helper T cells (Kalinski *et al.*, 1997). Furthermore, DC exposed to PGE_2 also produce increased levels of IL-10 (Kalinski *et al.*, 1997), suggesting a possible autocrine feedback loop to further inhibit IL-12. Similar processes may be acting *in vivo* since IL-12 production by monocytes is reduced in patients with allergic asthma (van der Pouw Kraan *et al.*, 1997).

The other known potent polarizing signal for T_H2 cell differentiation is IL-4 (Ohshima and Delespesse, 1997). However, DC are not known to produce this cytokine, so it must act in a paracrine fashion. The most important cellular source of IL-4 is a subject of debate in the field of allergy research, with possible candidates being the mast cell, the eosinophil and the T_H2 cell. In established allergic inflammation all three cell types may contribute to the available pool of IL-4. However, during the development of the first primary allergic response, before B cells have been class-switched to IgE production, what is the source of IL-4?

In the mouse, attention has been drawn to an $NK1.1^+$ TCR-α/β^+ $CD4^+$ T cell population found in the spleen and lymph nodes that is a potent and rapid producer of IL-4 upon TCR ligation *in vitro* (Yoshimoto and Paul, 1994) and facilitates increased IL-4 and IgE production *in vivo* (Yoshimoto *et al.*, 1995; Bendelac *et al.*, 1996). A $CD4^-$

$CD8^-$ TCR-α/β^+ population is thought to be the human homologue of these cells (do Carmo Leite-de-Moraes *et al.*, 1995). In both the mouse and man these cells recognize CD1 in conjunction with novel peptides; indeed, they can be activated by cells expressing CD1 (Bendelac *et al.*, 1995). Hence, in the presence of appropriate antigen, $CD1^+$ DC may be able to induce the IL-4 needed for T_H2 differentiation. Unfortunately, this hypothesis now seems less attractive since recent evidence suggests that activated $NK1.1^+$ $CD4^+$ T cells can efficiently produce IL-4 and the T_H1-promoting cytokine IFN-γ (Chen and Paul, 1997).

It may not be necessary to invoke novel T cell subsets as the source of IL-4 needed for the primary induction of T_H2 responses. IL-6, probably derived from APC, induces IL-4 production by naive T cells, polarizing their development towards T_H2 effector cells (Rincón *et al.*, 1997). Thus, by providing either IL-12 needed for T_H1 development or IL-6 required for polarization towards the T_H2 phenotype, DC may be able independently to supply the key polarizing signals for T_H cell differentiation. It remains to be determined whether DC are a potent source of IL-6 during antigen presentation and whether IL-6 production by DC at sites of allergic inflammation is elevated compared to normal subjects.

Finally, it must be said that atopy may be associated with a genetic tendency to preferentially express T_H2-like cytokines. The cytokines IL-3, -4, -5, -6, -9, -13 all map to the IL-4 gene cluster on chromosome 5q31.1. Genetic linkage has been shown between markers around this gene cluster and several parameters of allergy (Marsh *et al.*, 1994).

FAILURE OF MECHANISMS FOR MUCOSAL T CELL UNRESPONSIVENESS IN ALLERGY

In normal healthy individuals, soluble antigens entering the body through the mucosal surfaces characteristically elicit transient local secretory immunity that is replaced by long-term peripheral unresponsiveness. The mechanisms responsible for T cell unresponsiveness vary, partly as a result of antigen dose. In both the gut and the respiratory tract, high doses of antigen tend to induce anergy (or even clonal deletion in the case of oral tolerance), whereas low-dose, soluble antigen may cause immune deviation or active suppression by immunoregulatory T cells (Hoyne and Lamb, 1997). In the respiratory tract, the induction of T cell anergy is preceded by normal T cell activation and cytokine secretion (Hoyne *et al.*, 1996). This implies that the mucosal APC is not inherently tolerogenic, owing, for example, to a failure of costimulation. Instead it has been suggested that, in addition to inducing TCR ligation and T cell costimulation, mucosal APC may supply a third signal during the activation of a naive T cell causing it to differentiate into an immunoregulatory T cell (Hoyne and Lamb, 1997). Although appearing anergic *in vivo*, these cells probably persist *in vitro* and exert a suppressive effector function when activated upon subsequent exposure to the tolerizing antigen.

Possible candidates for the immunoregulatory $CD4^+$ T cell proposed in the model of Hoyne and Lamb are the 'regulatory/suppressor' T_H2 ('T_H3') subset of $CD4^+$ T cells. These have much in common with T_H2 cells, sharing similar cytokine profiles, with the exception that they produce characteristically high levels of the immunosuppressive cytokine TGF-β. This similarity is further reinforced by the fact that just as T_H1

cytokines inhibit T_H2 differentiation, IL-12 and IFN-γ block the induction of TGF-β producing immunoregulatory cells (Strober *et al.*, 1997).

Unpaired $CD4^+$ T cells?

Allergic diseases may result from impaired development of immunoregulatory $CD4^+$ T cells (Umetsu and DeKruyff, 1997), with T cell differentiation in the presence of low antigen dose then defaulting to the conventional T_H2 effector cell pathway. Since immunoregulatory $CD4^+$ T cells are probably terminally differentiated, it is thought unlikely that they can revert to conventional T_H2 cells. The ligand and receptor for the proposed 'third signal' required for the differentiation of immunoregulatory T cells from naive $CD4^+$ cells remain to be identified. However, owing to the requirement for sensitization of naive T cells in the model proposed by Hoyne and Lamb, it is tempting to speculate that in normal mucosae the ligand may be present on DC or be upregulated during DC–T cell interactions. Allergy might thus result from loss of either ligand expression on the DC or receptor expression on the T cell.

In the respiratory mucosa, other methods for the suppression of T cell activation have been identified that probably act to restrict the local activation of memory T_H cells. Alveolar macrophages, and to a lesser extent interstitial macrophages, fail to stimulate antigen-dependent T cell proliferation, although they do support cytokine secretion (Strickland *et al.*, 1996). This may be due to as yet unidentified receptor–ligand interactions, similar to the proposed signal needed for the generation of immunoregulatory $CD4^+$ cells from naive T_H cells. Alternatively, in rodents, the induction of apparent T cell anergy by alveolar macrophages has been attributed to NO released by the macrophages which inhibits the phosphorylation of kinases associated with intracellular signalling pathways in T cells (Bingisser *et al.*, 1997). In normal lung, macrophages also downregulate DC-mediated T cell activation (Holt *et al.*, 1993). It has again been suggested that the release of NO by alveolar macrophages leads to suppression of local DC maturation, holding them in a relatively immature form optimized for antigen uptake rather than antigen presentation (Holt *et al.*, 1993). It is easy to speculate that in allergic disease a change in macrophage phenotype or a proportionate increase in recently recruited monocytes may release DC from the suppressive macrophage environment, allowing their maturation and enabling local T cell activation. Similarly, the inhibition of T cell activation by alveolar macrophages is removed by pre-exposing the macrophages to GM-CSF (Bilyk and Holt, 1993), TNF-α or TGF-β (Bilyk and Holt, 1995), all of which are cytokines elevated at the sites of allergic inflammation.

FUTURE DIRECTIONS

Much of the recent upsurge in understanding in the field of human DC biology has been facilitated by the discovery that DC can be generated *in vitro* from either $CD34^+$ progenitors in the bone marrow (Reid *et al.*, 1992) or cord blood (Santiago-Schwarz *et al.*, 1992) or from adherent peripheral blood monocytes (Romani *et al.*, 1994; Sallusto and Lanzavecchia, 1994). This has allowed DC to be generated in sufficient numbers for functional experiments to be performed and has led to the identification of critical elements in the interaction between DC and T cells during antigen presentation.

Despite the technical difficulties of isolating a minority cell population from both control and diseased tissue, the relevance of particular molecular mechanisms and regulatory pathways in DC to the pathophysiological processes underlying human allergic diseases will ultimately only be elucidated by studying DC derived from relevant human tissues. This done, it is to be hoped that relevant targets for therapeutic intervention can be identified. Certainly, DC in the skin and other interface epithelia are easily accessible to therapeutic intervention. Based on the current state of knowledge, in allergic disease one possible therapeutic target in DC is FcεRI, where manipulations aimed at inhibiting FcεRI internalization or signal transduction can be envisaged.

Such targets might help to halt or delay the progression of disease chronicity. However, with atopic diseases already affecting 20–30% of the general population and, particularly in Western societies, increasing in prevalence (Holgate, 1997) it may be more relevant to develop prophylactic treatments for allergic diseases with the aim of preventing the disease ever becoming fully established. The perinatal period, that is late fetal and early postnatal life, is probably a critical time for shaping the immune response (Holt, 1996). Aeroallergen-specific T cells that proliferate *in vitro* in an allergen-dependent manner are present in neonatal umbilical cord blood (Piccini *et al.*, 1993). This implies that the fetus is exposed to trace amounts of food and aeroallergen via the mother and is sensitized to them *in utero*, a response that is presumably driven by DC somewhere in the fetus. However, the proliferative response of cord blood T cells to innocuous environmental antigens can be demonstrated for most neonates, irrespective of whether they go on to develop atopy. This suggests that although T cells are primed perinatally to innocuous environmental antigens, immune deviation to an inappropriate T_H2 allergic response towards these antigens occurs early in postnatal life. Environmental allergen load and an inherited genetic tendency to atopy will be important factors shaping the antigen-driven T cell selection process at this time. However, it is argued that, at least in the case of allergic lung disease, qualitative and quantitative differences in the kinetics of postnatal maturation of the airway intraepithelial DC network (Nelson *et al.*, 1994, Nelson and Holt, 1995) may be of paramount importance in driving the immune deviation process that determines T_H2-skewed T cell memory leading to allergy. If postnatal DC recruitment and maturation is a feature of early development in other anatomical locations, such as the skin and eye, it may be that this offers a common mechanism whereby the fate of sites that will be affected by allergy in later life is determined during the first few months of life.

REFERENCES

Azzawi, M., Bradley, B., Jeffery, P.K., Frew, A.J., Wardlaw, A.J., Knowles, G., Assoufi, B., Collins, J.V., Durham, S. and Kay, A.B. (1990). Identification of activated T lymphocytes and eosinophils in bronchial biopsies in stable atopic asthma. *Am. Rev. Resp. Dis.* **142**, 1407–1413.

Azzawi, M., Johnston, P.W., Majumdar, S., Kay, A.B. and Jeffery, P.K. (1992). T lymphocytes and activated eosinophils in airway mucosa in fatal asthma and cystic fibrosis. *Am. Rev. Resp. Dis.* **145**, 1477–1482.

Beaven, M.A. and Baumgartner, R.A. (1996). Downstream signals initiated in mast cells by FcεRI and other receptors. *Curr. Opin. Immunol.* **8**, 766–772.

Bellini, A., Vittori, E., Marini, M., Ackerman, V. and Mattoli, S. (1993). Intraepithelial dendritic cells and selective activation of Th2-like lymphocytes in patients with atopic asthma. *Chest* **103**, 997–1005.

Bendelac, A., Lantz, O., Quimby, M.E., Yewdell, J.W., Bennink, J.R. and Brutkiewicz, R.R. (1995). CD1 recognition by mouse NK1$^+$ T lymphocytes. *Science* **268**, 863–865.

Bendelac, A., Hunziker, R.D. and Lantz, O. (1996). Increased interleukin 4 and immunoglobulin E production in transgenic mice overexpressing NK1 T cells. *J. Exp. Med.* **184**, 1285–1293.

Bentley, A.M., Meng, Q., Robinson, D.S., Hamid, Q., Kay, A.B. and Durham, S.R. (1993). Increases in activated T lymphocytes, eosinophils and cytokine mRNA expression for interleukin-5 and granulocyte/macrophage colony-stimulating factor in bronchial biopsies after allergen challenge in atopic asthmatics. *Am. J. Respir. Cell Mol. Biol.* **8**, 35–42.

Bheekha Escura, R., Wasserbauer, E., Hammerschmid, F., Pearce, A., Kidd, P. and Mudde, G. C. (1995). Regulation and targeting of T-cell immune responses by IgE and IgG antibodies. *Immunology* **86**, 343–350.

Bieber, T. (1996). FcεRI on antigen presenting cells. *Curr. Opin. Immunol.* **8**, 773–777.

Bieber, T. and Ring, J. (1992). In vivo modulation of the high-affinity receptor for IgE (FcεRI) on human epidermal Langerhans' cells. *Int. Arch. Allergy Immunol.* **99**, 204.

Bieber, T., de la Salle, H., Wollenberg, A., Hakimi, J., Chizzonite, R., Ring, J., Hanau, D. and de la Salle, C. (1992). Human epidermal Langerhans cells express the high affinity receptor for immunoglobulin E (FcεRI). *J. Exp. Med.* **175**, 1285–1290.

Bieber, T., Jürgens, A., Wollenberg, A., Sander, E., Hanau, D. and de la Salle, H. (1995). Characterization of the protein tyrosine phosphatase CD45 on human epidermal Langerhans' cells. *Eur. J. Immunol.* **25**, 317–321.

Bilyk, N. and Holt, P. G. (1993). Inhibition of the immunosuppressive activity of resident pulmonary alveolar macrophages by granulocyte/macrophage colony-stimulating factor. *J. Exp. Med.* **177**, 1773–1777.

Bilyk, N. and Holt, P.G. (1995). Cytokine modulation of the immunosuppressive phenotype of pulmonary alveolar macrophage populations. *Immunology* **86**, 231–237.

Bingisser, R., Tilbrook, P.A., Holt, P.G. and Kees, U.R. (1997). Alveolar macrophages suppress T-cell activation by inhibiting tyrosine phosphorylation of JAK5 and CDC2 via nitric oxide. *Am J. Respir. Crit. Care Med.* **155**, A875.

Blank, U., Ra, C., Miller, L., White, K., Metzger, H. and Kinet, J-P. (1989). Complete structure and expression in transfected cells of high affinity IgE receptor. *Nature* **337**, 187–189.

Bradley, B.L., Azzawi, M., Jacobson, M., Assoufi, B., Collins, J.V., Irani, A.M.A., Schwartz, L.B., Durham, S.R., Jeffery, P.K. and Kay, A.B. (1991). Eosinophils, T-lymphocytes, mast cells, neutrophils, and macrophages in bronchial biopsy specimens from atopic subjects with asthma—comparison with biopsy specimens from atopic subjects without asthma and normal control subjects and relationship to bronchial hyperresponsiveness. *J. Allergy Clin. Immunol.* **88**, 661–674.

Bruijnzeel-Koomen, C., van Wichen, D.F., Toonstra, J., Berrens, L. and Bruijnzeel, P.L.B. (1986). The presence of IgE molecules on epidermal Langerhans' cells from patients with atopic dermatitis. *Arch. Dermatol. Res.* **278**, 199–205.

Bruijnzeel-Koomen, C.A.F.M., van Wichen, D.F., Spry, C.J., Venge, P. and Bruijnzeel, P.L.B. (1988a). Active participation of eosinophils in patch test reactions to inhalant allergens in patients with atopic dermatitis. *Br. J. Dermatol.* **118**, 229–238.

Bruijnzeel-Koomen, C., van den Donk, E.M.M., Bruijnzeel, P.L.B., Capron, M., de Gast, G.C. and Mudde, G.C. (1988b). Association and expression of CD1 antigen and the Fc receptor for IgE on epidermal Langerhans' cells from patients with atopic dermatitis. *Clin. Exp. Immunol.* **74**, 137–142.

Cambier, J.C., Daeron, M., Fridman, W., Gergely, J., Kinet, J-P., Klausner, R., Lynch, R., Malissen, B., Pecht, I., Reinherz, E., Ravetch, J., Reth, M., Samelson, L., Sandor, M., Schreiber, A., Seed, B., Terhorst, C., van der Winkel, J.G.J. and Weiss, A. (1995). New nomenclature for the reth motif. *Immunol. Today* **16**, 110.

Cella, M., Scheidegger, D., Palmer-Lehmann, K., Lane, P., Lanzavecchia, A. and Alber, G. (1996). Ligation of CD40 on dendritic cells triggers production of high levels of interleukin-12 and enhances T cell stimulatory capacity: T–T help via APC activation. *J. Exp. Med.* **184**, 747–752.

Cella, M., Engering, A., Pinet, V., Pieters, J. and Lanzavecchia, A. (1997). Inflammatory stimuli induce accumulation of MHC class II complexes on dendritic cells. *Nature* **388**, 782–787.

Chen, H. and Paul, W. E. (1997). Cultured NK1.1$^+$ CD4$^+$ T cells produce large amounts of IL-4 and IFN-γ upon activation by anti-CD3 or CD1. *J. Immunol.* **159**, 2240–2249.

Choi, O.H., Kim, J.H. and Kinet, J-P. (1996). Calcium mobilisation via sphingosine kinase in signalling by the FcεRI antigen receptor. *Nature* **380**, 634–636.

Clark, E.A. (1997). Regulation of B lymphocytes by dendtritic cells. *J. Exp. Med.* **185**, 801–803.

Constant, S., Pfeiffer, C., Woodard, A., Pasqualini, T. and Bottomly, K. (1995). Extent of T cell receptor ligation can determine the functional differentiation of naive $CD4^+$ T cells. *J. Exp. Med.* **182**, 1591–1596.

Del Prete, G. (1992). Human Th1 and Th2 lymphocytes: their role in the pathophysiology of atopy. *Allergy* **47**, 450–455.

Del Prete, G., De Carli, M., D'Elios, M.M., Daniel, K.C., Almerigogna, F., Alderson, M., Smith, C.A., Thomas, E. and Romagnani, S. (1995). CD30-mediated signaling promotes the development of human T helper type 2-like T cells. *J. Exp. Med.* **182**, 1655–1661.

DeSmedt, T., VanMechelen, M., DeBecker, G., Urbain, J., Leo, O. and Moser, M. (1997). Effect of interleukin-10 on dendritic cell maturation and function. *Eur. J. Immunol.* **27**, 1229–1235.

Djukanovic, R., Wilson, J.W., Britten, K.M., Wilson, S.J., Walls, A.F., Roche, W.R., Howarth, P.H. and Holgate, S.T. (1990). Quantitation of mast cells and eosinophils in the bronchial mucosa of symptomatic atopic asthmatics and healthy control subjects using immunohistochemistry. *Am. Rev. Respir. Dis.* **142**, 863–871.

do Carmo Leite-de-Moraes, M., Herbelin, A., Machavoine, F., Vicari, A., Gombert, J-M., Papiernik, M. and Dy, M. (1995). MHC class I-selected $CD4^-CD8^-TCR$-$\alpha\beta^+$ T cells are a potential source of IL-4 during primary immune response. *J. Immunol.* **155**, 4544–4550.

Drazen, J.M., Arm, J.P. and Austen, K.F. (1996). Sorting out the cytokines of asthma. *J. Exp. Med.* **183**, 1–5.

Dubois, B., Vanbervliet, B., Fayette, J., Massacrier, C., Van Kooten, C., Brière, F., Banchereau, J. and Caux, C. (1997). Dendritic cells enhance growth and differentiation of CD40-activated B lymphocytes. *J. Exp. Med.* **185**, 941–951.

Field, K.A., Holowka, D. and Baird, B. (1995). FcεRI-mediated recruitment of p53/p56 lyn to detergent-resistant membrane domains accompanies cellular signaling. *Proc. Natl Acad. Sci. USA* **92**, 9201–9205.

Fokkens, W.J., Vroom, T.M., Rijntjes, E. and Mulder, P.G.H. (1989). Fluctuation of the number of CD-1 (T6)-positive dendritic cells, presumably Langerhans cells, in the nasal mucosa of patients with an isolated grass-pollen allergy, before, during and after the grass-pollen season. *J. Allergy Clin. Immunol.* **84**, 39–43.

Foster, P.S., Hogan, S.P., Ramsay, A.J., Matthaei, K.I. and Young, I.G. (1996). Interleukin-5 deficiency abolishes eosinophilia, airways hyperreactivity, and lung damage in a mouse asthma model. *J. Exp. Med.* **183**, 195–201.

Frew, A.J. and O'Hehir, R.E. (1992). What can we learn from studies of lymphocytes present in allergic-reaction sites? *J. Allergy Clin. Immunol.* **89**, 783–788.

Gause, W.C., Mitro, V., Via, C., Linsley, P., Urban, J.F. and Greenwald, R.J. (1997). Do effector and memory T helper cells also need B7 ligand costimulatory signals? *J. Immunol.* **159**, 1055–1058.

Gell, P.G.H. and Coombes, R.R.A. (1962). *Clinical Aspects of Immunology.* Blackwell Scientific, Oxford.

Graeme-Cook, F., Bhan, A.K. and Harris, N.L. (1993). Immunohistochemical characterization of intra-epithelial and subepithelial mononuclear cells of the upper airways. *Am. J. Pathol.* **143**, 1416–1422.

Hakimi, J., Seals, C., Kondas, J. A., Pettine, L., Danho, W. and Kochan, J. (1990). The α subunit of the human IgE receptor (FcεRI) is sufficient for high affinity IgE binding. *J. Biol. Chem.* **265**, 22079–22081.

Hamann, D., Hilkens, C.M.U., Grogan, J.L., Lens, S.M.A., Kapsenberg, M.L., Yazdanbakhsh, M. and Vanlier, R.A.W. (1996). CD30 expression does not discriminate between human Th1-type and Th2-type T-cells. *J. Immunol.* **156**, 1387–1391.

Hamawy, M.M., Mergenhagen, S.E. and Siraganian, R.P. (1995). Protein tyrosine phosphorylation as a mechanism of signalling in mast cells and basophils. *Cell. Signal.* **7**, 535–544.

Hartley, J.A., Semper, A.E. and Holgate, S.T. (1996). In vivo and in vitro expression of FcεRI in human peripheral blood. *Immunology* **89**, 41.

Heufler, C., Koch, F., Stanzl, U., Topar, G., Wysocka, M., Trinchieri, G., Enk, A., Steinman, R.M., Romani, N. and Schuler, G. (1996). Interleukin-12 is produced by dendritic cells and mediates T-helper 1 development as well as interferon-gamma production by T-helper-1 cells. *Eur. J. Immunol.* **26**, 659–668.

Heyman, B., Tianmin, L. and Gustavsson, S. (1993). In vivo enhancement of the specific antibody response via the low-affinity receptor for IgE. *Eur. J. Immunol.* **23**, 1739–1742.

Hilkens, C.M.U., Messer, G., Tesselaar, K., Vanrietschoten, A.G.I., Kapsenberg, M.L. and Wierenga, E.A. (1996). Lack of IL-12 signaling in human allergen-specific Th2 cells. *J. Immunol.* **157**, 4316–4321.

Holgate, S.T. (1997). *The Rising Trend in Asthma.* Ciba Foundation Bulletin No. 206. Wiley, Chichester.

Holt, P.G. (1996). Primary allergic sensitization to environmental antigens—perinatal T-cell priming as a determinant of responder phenotype in adulthood. *J. Exp. Med.* **183**, 1297–1301.

Holt, P.G., Schon-Hegrad, M.A., Phillips, M.J. and McMenamin, P.G. (1989). Ia-positive dendritic cells form a tightly meshed network within the human airway epithelium. *Clin. Exp. Allergy* **19**, 597–601.

Holt, P.G., Oliver, J., Bilyk, N., McMenamin, C., McMenamin, P.G., Kraal, G. and Thepen, T. (1993). Downregulation of the antigen presenting cell function(s) of pulmonary dendritic cells in vivo by resident alveolar macrophages. *J. Exp. Med.* **177**, 397–407.

Holt, P.G., Haining, S., Nelson, D.J. and Sedgwick, J.D. (1994). Origin and steady-state turnover of class II MHC-bearing dendritic cells in the epithelium of the conducting airways. *J. Immunol.* **153**, 256–261.

Hosken, N.A., Shibuya, K., Heath, A.W., Murphy, K.M. and O'Garra, A. (1995). The effect of antigen dose on $CD4^+$ T helper cell phenotype development in a T cell receptor-$\alpha\beta$-transgenic model. *J. Exp. Med.* **182**, 1579–1584.

Hoyne, G.F. and Lamb, J.R. (1997). Regulation of T cell function in mucosal tolerance. *Immunol. Cell Biol.* **75**, 197–201.

Hoyne, G.F., Askonas, B.A., Hetzel, C., Thomas, W.R. and Lamb, J.R. (1996). Regulation of house dust mite responses by inhaled peptide: transient activation precedes the development of tolerance in vivo. *Int. Immunol.* **8**, 335–342.

Huang, S-K., Xiao, H-Q., Kleine-Tebbe, J., Paciotti, G., Marsh, D.G., Lichtenstein, L.M. and Liu, M.C. (1995). IL-13 expression at the sites of allergen challenge in patients with asthma. *J. Immunol.* **55**, 2688–2694.

Hulett, M.D. and Hogarth, P.M. (1994). Molecular basis of Fc receptor function. *Adv. Immunol.* **57**, 1–127.

Jaffar, Z.H., Roberts, K., Pandit, A., Linsley, P., Djukanovic, R. and Holgate, S.T. (1998). B7 costimulation is required for IL-5 and IL-13 secretion by bronchial biopsy tissue of atopic asthmatics in response to allergen stimulation. *Am. J. Respir. Cell Mol. Biol.*, in press.

Jouvin, M.H., Adamczewski, M., Numerof, R., Letourneur, O., Valle, A. and Kinet, J.P. (1994). Differential control of the tyrosine kinases Lyn and Syk by the two signaling chains of the high affinity immunoglobulin E receptor. *J. Biol. Chem.* **269**, 5918–5925.

Jouvin, M-H., Numerof, R.P. and Kinet, J-P. (1995). Signal transduction through the conserved motifs of the high affinity IgE receptor FcεRI. *Semin. Immunol.* **7**, 29.

Jürgens, M., Wollenberg, A., Hanau, D., de la Salle, H. and Bieber, T. (1995). Activation of human epidermal Langerhans cells by engagement of the high affinity receptor for IgE, FcεRI. *J. Immunol.* **155**, 5184–5189.

Kalinski, P., Hilkens, C.M.U., Snijders, A., Snijdewint, F.G.M. and Kapsenberg, M.L. (1997). IL-12-deficient dendritic cells, generated in the presence of prostaglandin E-2, promote type 2 cytokine production in maturing human naive T helper cells. *J. Immunol.* **159**, 28–35.

Kapsenberg, M.L., Wierenga, E.A., Bos, J.D. and Jansen, H.M. (1991). Functional subsets of allergen-reactive human $CD4^+$ T cells. *Immunol. Today* **12**, 392–395.

Katz, H.R., Vivier, E., Castells, M.C., McCormick, M.J., Chambers, J.M. and Austen, K.F. (1996). Mouse mast cell gp49B1 contains two immunoreceptor tyrosine-based inhibition motifs and suppresses mast cell activation when coligated with the high-affinity Fc receptor for IgE. *Proc Natl Acad Sci USA* **93**, 10809–10814.

Kawamura, T. and Furue, M. (1995). Comparative analysis of B7-1 and B7-2 expression in Langerhans cells: differential regulation by T helper type 1 and T helper type 2 cytokines. *Eur. J. Immunol.* **25**, 1913–1917.

Kay, A.B., Ying, S., Varney, V., Gaga, M., Durham, S.R., Moqbel, R., Wardlaw, A.J. and Hamid, Q. (1991). Messenger RNA expression of the cytokine gene cluster interleukin 3 (IL-3), IL-4, IL-5 and granulocyte/macrophage colony stimulating factor, in allergen-induced late-phase cutaneous reactions in atopic subjects. *J. Exp. Med.* **173**, 775–778.

Klubal, R., Maurer, D. and Stingl, G. (1997). The abundant expression of FcεRI in lesional atopic dermatitis skin is due to upregulation of FcεRI on epidermal Langerhans cells and to accumulation of FcεRI-bearing dermal dendritic cells. *J. Invest. Dermatol.* **108**, 436.

Koch, F., Stanzl, U., Jennewein, P., Janke, K., Heufler, C., Kämpgen, E., Romani, N. and Schuler, G. (1996). High level IL-12 production by murine dendritic cells: upregulation via MHC class II and CD40 molecules and downregulation by IL-4 and IL-10. *J. Exp. Med.* **184**, 741–746.

Krishnaswamy, G., Liu, M.C., Su, S-N., Kumai, M., Xiao, H-Q., Marsh, D.G. and Huang, S.K. (1993). Analysis of cytokine transcripts in the bronchoalveolar lavage cells of patients with asthma. *Am. J. Respir. Cell Mol. Biol.* **9**, 279–286.

Kuchroo, V.K., Das, M.P., Brown, J.A., Ranger, A.M., Zamvil, S.S., Sobel, R.A., Weiner, H.L., Nabavi, N. and Glimcher, L.H. (1995). B7-1 and B7-2 costimulatory molecules activate differentially the Th1/Th2 developmental pathways: application to autoimmune disease therapy. *Cell* **80**, 707–718.

Lee, J.J., McGarry, M.P., Farmer, S.C., Denzler, K.L., Larson, K.A., Carrigan, P.E., Brenneise, I.E., Horton, M.A., Haczku, A., Gelfand, E.W., Leikauf, G.D. and Lee, N.A. (1997). Interleukin-5 expression in the lung epithelium of transgenic mice leads to pulmonary changes pathognomonic of asthma. *J. Exp. Med.* **185**, 2143–2156.

Letourneur, F., Hennecke, S., Démollière, C. and Cosson, P. (1995). Steric masking of a dilysine endoplasmic reticulum retention motif during assembly of the human high affinity receptor for immunoglobulin. *J. Cell Biol.* **129**, 971–978.

Lenschow, D.J., Walunas, T.L. and Bluestone J.A. (1996). CD28/B7 system of T cell costimulation. *Annu. Rev. Immunol.* **14**, 233–258.

Lin, S., Cicala, C., Scharenberg, A.M. and Kinet, J-P. (1996). The FcεRIβ subunit functions as an amplifier of FcεRIγ-mediated cell activation signals. *Cell* **85**, 985–995.

Liu, L.M., Rich, B.E., Inobe, J., Chen, W.J. and Weiner, H.L. (1997). A potential pathway of Th2 development during primary immune response—IL-10 pretreated dendritic cells can prime naive CD4(+) T cells to secrete IL-4. *Adv. Exp. Med. Biol.* **417**, 375–381.

Macatonia, S., Hosken, N.A., Litton, M., Vieira, P., Hsieh, C-S., Culpepper, J.A., Wysocka, M., Trinchieri, G., Murphy, K.M. and O'Garra, A. (1995). Dendritic cells produce IL-12 and direct development of Th1 cells from naive $CD4^+$ T cells. *J. Immunol.* **154**, 5071–5079.

MacPherson, G.G., Jenkins, C.D., Stein, M.J. and Edwards, C. (1995). Endotoxin-mediated dendritic cell release from the intestine: characterization of released dendritic cells and TNF dependence. *J. Immunol.* **154**, 1317–1322.

Malveaux, F.J., Conroy, M.C., Adkinson, N.F. and Lichtenstein, L.M. (1978). IgE receptors on human basophils. Relationship to serum IgE concentration. *J. Clin. Invest.* **62**, 176.

Marsh, D.G., Neely, J.D., Breazeale, D.R., Ghosh, B., Freidhoff, L.R., Ehrlich-Kautzky, E., Schou, C., Krishnaswamy, G. and Beaty, T.H. (1994). Linkage analysis of IL-4 and other chromosome 5q31.1 markers and total serum immunoglobulin E concentrations. *Science* **264**, 1152–1156.

Maurer, D. and Stingl, G. (1995). Immunoglobulin E-binding structures on antigen-presenting cells present in skin and blood. *J. Invest. Dermatol.* **104**, 707–710.

Maurer, D., Fiebiger, E., Reininger, B., Wolff-Winiski, B., Jouvin, M-H., Kilgus, O., Kinet, J.-P. and Stingl, G. (1994). Expression of functional high affinity immunoglobulin E receptors (FcεRI) on monocytes of atopic individuals. *J. Exp. Med.* **179**, 745–750.

Maurer, D., Ebner, C., Reininger, B., Fiebiger, E., Kraft, D., Kinet, J-P. and Stingl, G. (1995). The high affinity IgE receptor (FCcRI) mediates IgE-dependent allergen presentation. *J. Immunol.* **154**, 6285–6290.

Maurer, D., Fiebiger, E., Reininger, B., Fischer, G., Wichlas, S., Jouvin, M.H., Schmitt-Egenolf, M., Kraft, D., Kinet, J.P. and Stingl, G. (1996). Peripheral blood dendritic cells express FcεRI as a complex composed of FcεRIα- and FcεRIγ-chains and can use this receptor for IgE-mediated allergen presentation. *J. Immunol.* **157**, 607–616.

McMenamin, P.G. (1997). The distribution of immune cells in the uveal tract of the normal eye. *Eye* **11**, 183–193.

McWilliam, A.S., Napoli, S., Marsh, A.M., Pemper, F.L., Nelson, D.J., Pimm, C.L., Stumbles, P.A., Wells, T.N.C. and Holt, P.G. (1996). Dendritic cells are recruited into the airway epithelium during the inflammatory response to a broad spectrum of stimuli. *J. Exp. Med.* **184**, 2429–2432.

Metz, D.P., Bacon, A.S., Holgate, S. and Lightman, S.L. (1996). Phenotypic characterization of T-cells infiltrating the conjuctivas in chronic allergic eye disease. *J. Allergy Clin. Immunol.* **98**, 686–696.

Mudde, G.C., Reischl, I.G., Corvaia, N., Hren, A. and Poellabauer, E.M. (1996). Antigen presentation in allergic sensitization. *Immunol. Cell Biol.* **74**, 167–173.

Neel, B.G. and Tonks, N.K. (1997). Protein tyrosine phosphatases in signal transduction. *Curr. Opin. Cell Biol.* **9**, 193–204.

Nelson, D.J. and Holt, P.G. (1995). Defective regional immunity in the respiratory-tract of neonates is attributable to hyporesponsiveness of local dendritic cells to activation signals. *J. Immunol.* **155**, 3517–3524.

Nelson, D.J., McMenamin, C., McWilliam, A.S., Brenan, M. and Holt, P.G. (1994). Development of the airway intraepithelial dendritic cell network in the rat from class II major histocompatibility (Ia)-negative precursors: differential regulation of Ia expression at different levels of the respiratory tract. *J. Exp. Med.* **179**, 203–212.

Ohshima, Y. and Delespesse, G. (1997). T cell-derived IL-4 and dendritic cell-derived IL-12 regulate the lymphokine-producing phenotype of alloantigen-primed naive human CD4 T cells. *J. Immunol.* **158**, 629–636.

Pearson, C.I., van Ewijk, W. and McDevitt, H.O. (1997). Induction of apoptosis and T helper 2 (Th2) responses correlates with peptide affinity for the major histocompatability complex in self-reactive T cell receptor transgenic mice. *J. Exp. Med.* **185**, 583–599.

Piccini, M-P., Mecacci, F., Sampognaro, S., Manetti, R., Parronchi, P., Maggi, E. and Romagnani, S. (1993). Aeroallergen sensitisation can occur during fetal life. *Int. Arch. Allergy Immunol.* **102**, 301–303.

Poston, R.N., Chanez, P., Lacoste, J.Y., Litchfield, T., Lee, T.H. and Bousquet, J. (1992). Immunohistochemical characterisation of the cellular infiltration in asthmatic bronchi. *Am. Rev. Respir. Dis.* **145**, 918–921.

Rajakulasingam, K., Durham, S.R., O'Brien, F., Humbert, M., Barata, L. T., Reece, L., Kay, A.B. and Grant, A.J. (1997). Enhanced expression of high-affinity IgE receptor (FcεRI) α chain in human allergen-induced arthritis with co-localization to mast cells, macrophages, eosinophils, and dendritic cells. *J. Allergy Clin. Immunol.* **100**, 78–86.

Reid, C.D.L., Stackpoole, A., Meager, A. and Tikerpae, J. (1992). Interactions of tumor necrosis factor with granulocyte-macrophage colony-stimulating factor and other cytokines in the regulation of dendritic cell growth in vitro from early bipotent $CD34^+$ progenitors in human bone marrow. *J. Immunol.* **149**, 2681–2688.

Reischl, I.G., Corvaia, N., Effenberger, F., Wolffwiniski, B., Kromer, E. and Mudde, G.C. (1996). Function and regulation of FcεRI expression on monocytes from nonatopic donors. *Clin. Exp. Allergy* **26**, 630–641.

Reischl, I.G., Bjerke, T., Brown, K., Peiritsch, S., Woisetschlager, M., Corvaia, N. and Mudde, G.C. (1997a). Characteristics of FcεRI expression on human monocytes and monocytic cell lines: Establishment of an in vitro model. *Int. Arch. Allergy Immunol.* **113**, 266–268.

Reischl, I.G., Corvaia, N., Unger, J., Woisetschlager, M. and Mudde, G.C. (1997b). Characterization of FcεRI expressing human monocytic cell lines. 1. The role of CD45 on signal transduction in primary monocytes and cell lines. *Int. Arch. Allergy Immunol.* **113**, 444–453.

Rincón, M., Anguita, J., Nakamura, T., Fikrig, E. and Flavell, R.A. (1997). Interleukin (IL)-6 directs the differentiation of IL-4-producing $CD4^+$ T cells. *J. Exp. Med.* **185**, 461–469.

Roake, J.A., Rao, A.S., Morris, P.J., Larsen, C.P., Hankins, D.F. and Austyn, J.M. (1995). Dendritic cell loss from non-lymphoid tissues after systemic administration of lipopolysaccharide, tumor necrosis factor, and interleukin 1. *J. Exp. Med.* **181**, 2237–2247.

Robinson, D.S., Hamid, Q., Ying, S., Tsicopoulos, A., Barkans, J., Bentley, A.M., Corrigan, C., Durham, S.R. and Kay, A.B. (1992). Predominant T-H2 like bronchoalveolar T-lymphocyte population in atopic asthma. *N. Engl. J. Med.* **326**, 298–304.

Robinson, D.S., Bentley, A.M., Hartnell, A., Kay, A.B. and Durham, S.R. (1993). Activated memory T helper cells in bronchoalveolar lavage fluid from patients with atopic asthma: relation to asthma symptoms, lung function, and bronchial responsiveness. *Thorax* **48**, 26–32.

Rogge, L., Barberis-Maino, L., Biffi, M., Passini, N., Presky, D.H., Gubler, U. and Sinigaglia, F. (1997). Selective expression of an interleukin-12 receptor component by human T helper 1 cells. *J. Exp. Med.* **185**, 825–831.

Romagnani, S. (1996). Development of Th1- or Th2-dominated immune responses: what about the polarizing signals? *Int. J. Clin. Lab. Res.* **26**, 83–98.

Romani, N., Gruner, S., Brang, D., Kämpgen, E., Lenz, A., Trockenbacher, B., Konwalinka, G., Fritsch, P.O., Steinman, R.M. and Schuler, G. (1994). Proliferating dendritic cell progenitors in human blood. *J. Exp. Med.* **180**, 83–93.

Sallusto, F. and Lanzavecchia, A. (1994). Efficient presentation of soluble antigen by cultured human dendritic cells is maintained by granulocyte/macrophage colony-stimulating factor plus interleukin 4 and downregulated by tumor necrosis factor α. *J. Exp. Med.* **179**, 1109–1118.

Santiago-Schwarz, F., Belilos, E., Diamond, B. and Carsons, S.E. (1992). TNF in combination with GM-CSF enhances the differentiation of neonatal cord blood stem cells into dendritic cells and macrophages. *J. Leukocyte Biol.* **52**, 274–281.

Scharenberg, A.M. and Kinet, J-P. (1994). Initial events in FcεRI signal transduction. *J. Allergy Clin. Immunol.* **94**, 1142–1146.

Seder, R.A., Germain, R.N., Linsley, P.S. and Paul, W.E. (1994). CD28-mediated costimulation of interleukin 2 (IL-2) production plays a critical role in T cell priming for IL-4 and interferon γ production. *J. Exp. Med.* **179**, 299–304.

Semper, A.E., Hartley, J.A. and Holgate, S.T. (1995a). Regulation of dendritic cell FcεRI subunit expression *in vitro. Immunology* **86**, 14.

Semper, A.E., Hartley, J.A., Tunon-de-Lara, J.M., Bradding, P., Redington, A.E., Church, M.K. and Holgate, S.T. (1995b). Expression of the high affinity receptor for immunoglobulin E (IgE) by dendritic cells in normals and asthmatics. *Adv. Exp. Med. Biol.* **378**, 136–138.

Semper, A.E., Hartley, J.A. and Holgate, S.T. (1997). Expression of FcεRI subunits during the in vitro differentiation of human dendritic cells. *Immunol. Lett.* **56**, 419.

Shirakawa, T., Li, A., Dubowitz, M., Dekker, J.W., Shaw, A.E., Faux, J.A., Ra, C., Cookson, W.O.C.M. and Hopkin, J.M. (1994). Association between atopy and variants of the β subunit of the high affinity immunogobulin E receptor. *Nature Genetics* **7**, 125–129.

Steinman, R.M. (1991). The dendritic cell system and its role in immunogenicity. *Annu. Rev. Immunol.* **9**, 271–296.

Stingl, G. and Maurer, D. (1997). IgE-mediated allergen presentation via Fc epsilon RI on antigen-presenting cells. *Int. Arch. Allergy Immunol.* **113**, 24–29.

Strickland, D., Kees, U.R. and Holt, P.G. (1996). Regulation of T-cell activation in the lung—alveolar macrophages induce reversible T-cell anergy in vitro associated with inhibition of interleukin-2 receptor signal-transduction. *Immunology* **87**, 250–258.

Terada, N., Konno, A., Terada, Y., Fukuda, S., Yamashita, T., Abe, T., Shimada, H., Ishida, K., Yoshimura, K., Tanaka, Y., Ra, C., Ishikawa, K. and Togawa, K. (1995). IL-4 upregulates FcεRIα-chain messenger RNA in eosinophils. *J. Allergy Clin. Immunol.* **96**, 1161–1169.

Thepen, T., Langeveld-Wildschut, E.G., Bihari, I.C., Van Wichen, D.F., Van Reijsen, F.C., Mudde, G.C. and Bruijnzeel-Koomen, C.A.F.M. (1996). Bi-phasic response against aeroallergen in atopic dermatitis showing a switch from an initial Th2 response into a Th1 response in situ. An immunocytochemical study. *J. Allergy Clin. Immunol.* **97**, 828–837.

Toru, H., Ra, C., Nonoyama, S., Suzuki, K., Yata, J-I. and Nakahata, T. (1996). Induction of the high-affinity receptor (FcεRI) on human mast cells by IL-4. *Int. Immunol.* **8**, 1367–1373.

Tunon-de-Lara, J.M., Redington, A.E., Bradding, P., Church, M.K., Hartley, J.A., Semper, A.E. and Holgate, S.T. (1996). Dendritic cells in normal and asthmatic airways: expression of the α subunit of the high affinity immunoglobulin E receptor (FcεRI-α). *Clin. Exp. Allergy* **26**, 648–655.

Umetsu, D.T. and DeKruyff, R.H. (1997). Th1 and Th2 $CD4^+$ cells in human allergic disease. *J. Allergy Clin. Immunol.* **100**, 1–6.

Valitutti, S., Müller, S., Cella, M., Padovan, E. and Lanzavecchia, A. (1995). Serial triggering of many T-cell receptors by a few peptide–MHC complexes. *Nature* **375**, 148–151.

van der Heijden, F.L., van Neerven, R.J.J., van Katwijk, M., Bos, J.D. and Kapsenberg, M.L. (1993). Serum-IgE-facilitated allergen presentation in atopic disease. *J. Immunol.* **150**, 3643–3650.

van der Pouw Kraan, T.C.T.M., Boeije, L.C.M., de Groot, E.R., Stapel, S.O., Snijders, A., Kapsenberg, M.L., van der Zee, J.S. and Aarden, L.A. (1997). Reduced production of IL-12 and IL-12-dependent IFN-gamma release in patients with allergic asthma. *J. Immunol.* **158**, 5560–5565.

van Reijsen, F.C., Bruijnzeel-Koomen, C.A.F.M., Kalthoff, F.S., Maggi, E., Romagnani, S., Westland, J.K.T. and Mudde, G.C. (1992). Skin-derived aeroallergen-specific T-cell clones of Th2 phenotype in patients with allergic dermatitis. *J. Allergy Clin. Immunol.* **90**, 184–192.

Vivier, E. and Daeron, M. (1997). Immunoreceptor tyrosine-based inhibition motifs. *Immunol. Today* **18**, 286–291.

Wang, B., Rieger, A., Kilgus, O., Ochiai, K., Maurer, D., Födinger, D., Kinet, J-P. and Stingl, G. (1992). Epidermal Langerhans' cells from normal human skin bind monomeric IgE via FcεRI. *J. Exp. Med.* **175**, 1353–1365.

Watts, C. (1997). Inside the gearbox of the dendritic cell. *Nature* **388**, 724–725.

Webb, L.M.C. and Feldmann, M. (1995). Critical role of CD28/B7 costimulation in the development of human Th2 cytokine-producing cells. *Blood* **86**, 3479–3486.

Wierenga, E.A., Snoek, M., De Groot, C., Chretien, I., Bos, J.D., Jansen, H.M. and Kapsenberg, M.L. (1990). Evidence for compartmentalization of functional subsets of $CD4^+$ T lymphocytes in atopic patients. *J. Immunol.* **144**, 4651–4656.

Wilson, J.W., Djukanovic, R., Howarth, P.H. and Holgate, S.T. (1992). Lymphocyte activation in bronchoalveolar lavage and peripheral blood in atopic asthmatics. *Am. Rev. Respir. Dis.* **145**, 958–960.

Wolff, K. and Stingl, G. (1983). The Langerhans cell. *J. Invest. Dermatol.* **80**, 17S–26S.

Wollenberg, A., Wen, S.P. and Bieber, T. (1995). Langerhans' cell phenotyping: a new tool for differential diagnosis of inflammatory skin diseases. *Lancet* **346**, 1626–1627.

Wollenberg, A., Kraft, S., Hanau, D. and Bieber, T. (1996). Immunomorphological and ultrastructural characterisation of Langerhans' cells and a novel, inflammatory dendritic epidermal cell (IDEC) population in lesional skin of atopic eczema. *J. Invest. Dermatol.* **106**, 446–453.

Xia, H-Z., Du, Z., Craig, S., Klisch, G., Noben-Trauth, N., Kochan, J.P., Huff, T.H., Irani, A-M.A. and Schwartz, L.B. (1997). Effect of recombinant human IL-4 on tryptase, chymase, and Fcε receptor type I expression in recombinant human stem cell factor-dependent fetal liver-derived human mast cells. *J. Immunol.* **159**, 2911–2921.

Yamaguchi, M., Lantz, C.S., Oettgen, H.C., Katona, I.M., Fleming, T., Miyajima, I., Kinet, J-P. and Galli, S.J. (1997). IgE enhances mouse mast cell FcεRI expression in vitro and in vivo: evidence for a novel amplification mechanism in IgE-dependent reactions. *J. Exp. Med.* **185**, 663–672.

Ying, S., Durham, S.R., Barkans, J., Masuyama, K., Jacobson, M., Rak, S., Löwhagen, O., Moqbel, R., Kay, A.B. and Hamid, Q.A. (1993). T cells are the principal source of interleukin-5 mRNA in allergen-induced rhinitis. *Am. J. Respir. Cell Mol. Biol.* **9**, 356–360.

Yoshimoto, T. and Paul, W.E. (1994). CD4pos, NK1.1pos T cells promptly produce interleukin 4 in response to in vivo challenge with anti-CD3. *J. Exp. Med.* **179**, 1285–1295.

Yoshimoto, T., Bendelac, A., Watson, C., Hu-Li, J. and Paul, W.E. (1995). Role of $NK1.1^+$ T cells in a Th2 response and in immunoglobulin E production. *Science* **270**, 1845–1847.

Zweiman, B. (1993). The late-phase reaction: role of IgE, its receptor and cytokines. *Curr. Opin. Immunol.* **5**, 950–955.

V DC-BASED THERAPIES

CHAPTER 25
Dendritic Cell Therapy of Cancer and HIV Infection

Michael T. Lotze, Hassan Farhood, Cara C. Wilson and Walter J. Storkus
University of Pittsburgh Medical Center, Pittsburgh, Pennsylvania, USA

> In addition to granulocytes, lymphocytes and mononuclear phagocytes, there is a fourth variety of adherent nucleated cell whose morphological features are quite distinct... The cytoplasm of this large cell is arranged in pseudopods of varying length with form and number resulting in a variety of cell shapes ranging from bipolar elongate cells to elaborate stellate or dendritic ones. Most pseudopods are long, uniform in width, and have blunt terminations, but smaller spinous processes are also evident. The cytoplasm contains many large circular phase-dense granules as well as infrequent refractile granules, probably lipid. There is no morphological evidence of active endocytosis even if the cells are cultivated for several hours in high concentrations (40% volume/volume) of serum, conditions known to stimulate endocytosis in macrophages *in vitro*.
>
> Ralph M. Steinman and Zanvil A. Cohn (1973)

INTRODUCTION

Evaluation of the use of dendritic cells (DC) as a component of cancer and HIV vaccine therapeutic approaches is a relatively recent development (Lotze, 1997). There is a century-long history of studies demonstrating how the immune system develops specific antibody responses to immunogens foreign to the host, such as viral antigens (Bibel, 1988). However, it is only recently becoming clear how we can assist the immune system in developing an immune response to antigens that are not foreign to the body, such as those produced by preexisting tumor cells or by T cells infected with the HIV virus. The means by which to immunize to T cell targets and, in particular, to ones which were already present in the host, has only recently been addressed. Our own entry into this field was prompted by the rapid identification of many human and murine tumor antigens (Itoh *et al.*, 1994; Frassanito *et al.*, 1995) recognized by T-lymphocytes over the course of the past seven years (Van der Bruggen *et al.*, 1991, 1994; Traversari *et al.*, 1992; Zakut *et al.*, 1993; Brichard *et al.*, 1993; Gaugler *et al.*, 1994; Bakker *et al.*, 1994; Robbins *et al.*, 1994; Kawakami *et al.*, 1994a, 1994b; Cox *et al.*, 1994; Coulie *et al.*,

Dendritic Cells: Biology and Clinical Applications
ISBN 0-12-455860-7

1994; Wolfel *et al.*, 1994; Castelli *et al.*, 1995; Van den Eynde *et al.*, 1995; Wang *et al.*, 1995; Jochmus *et al.*, 1997). It became clear that our mechanistic insights into how to integrate these targets of cellular immunity into vaccines were poorly evolved and required novel immunization strategies. Dendritic cells, recognized as cells uniquely capable of priming immune responses when used to present tumor-derived peptides, were clearly surveyed as the most successful adjuvant strategy. DC-peptide based vaccines were effective in promoting the expansion of antigen-specific T cells *in vitro*, and more importantly *in vivo*, resulting in T cell responses capable of either treating or preventing the outgrowth of a tumor challenge (Mayordomo *et al.*, 1995, 1996a, 1996b; Zitvogel *et al.*, 1996; Celluzzi *et al.*, 1996).

It is now abundantly clear that tumors of diverse histologic origins and etiologies (viral, oncogene, etc.) are susceptible to DC-based therapies. This chapter will focus on issues related to optimizing the use of DC in therapy as recently reviewed in part by others (Steinman, 1991; Grabbe *et al.*, 1995; Caux *et al.*, 1995; Zitvogel *et al.*, 1996; Thurnher *et al.*, 1997; Schuler and Steinman, 1997; van Schooten *et al.*, 1997; Gilboa *et al.*, 1998).

There are five primary goals of the biologic therapist seeking to treat cancer:

(1) *The induction of an effective anti-tumor immune response, largely mediated by effector T cells.* DC are notably efficient at recruiting, selecting, and expanding naive T cells with antigen specificity within lymphoid organs. These T cells may subsequently be exported into tumor sites as immune effectors capable of directly killing targets and releasing cytokines that facilitate additional immunocyte infiltration.

(2) *The promotion of effector T cells to migrate efficiently across vascular endothelial barriers into tumor lesions*. This issue has received limited study by tumor immunologists to date but represents a critical obstacle to the recruitment of sufficient immune effector cells to mediate clinical responsiveness. Tumor-associated or vaccine-delivered DC may play a role in this process by producing cytokines or chemokines that secondarily recruit T cells and additional blood/tissue-associated DC to the tumor site (Romani *et al.*, 1990; Mohamadzadeh *et al.*, 1996a; Hieshima *et al.*, 1997).

(3) *Maintaining a state of effectiveness of T cells at the tumor site*. It has recently become clear that both T cells and DC are susceptible to tumor-induced dysfunction and death (Griffith *et al.*, 1995; Hahne *et al.*, 1996; Shurin *et al.*, 1997b, c; Walker *et al.*, 1997; Zeytun *et al.*, 1997). Reciprocal interactions between these cells may provide survival factors (Anderson *et al.*, 1997; Wong *et al.*, 1997) necessary for the maintenance of the chronic inflammatory response.

(4) *Developing a state of long-lived memory*. Just as chronic responses to microbial pathogens are maintained, in part, by retention of antigens in follicular and perhaps other DC, it seems that a robust and durable T cell response may require DC provision of survival factors and possibly antigen.

(5) *Modifying the provision of angiogenic substances to the tumor*. It seems likely that DC, due to their ability to deliver antiangiogenic (IL-12, interferon-α) and possibly proangiogenic factors (Numasaki *et al.*, 1997), impact tumor progression.

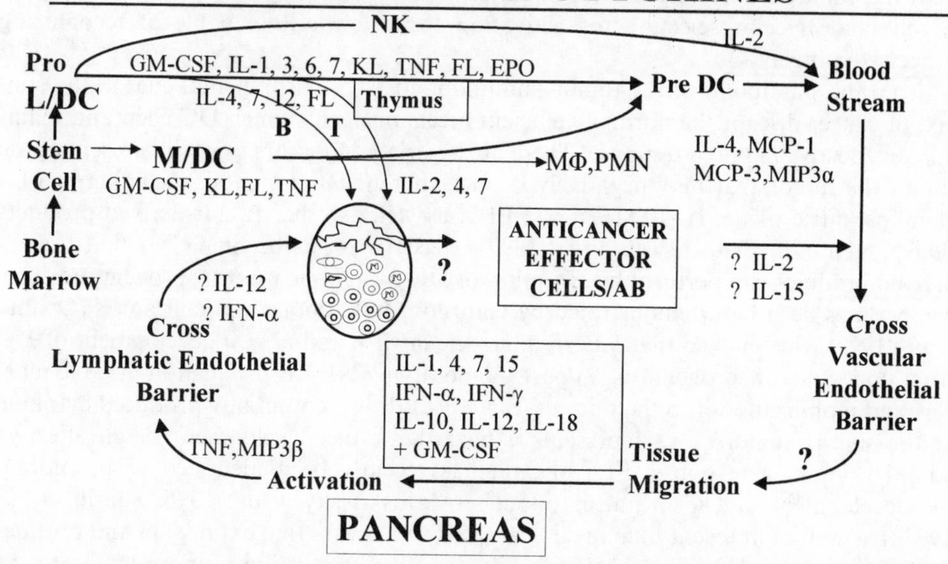

Fig. 1. Potential applications of DC in the setting cancer and HIV. DC are generated in the bone marrow and migrate into tissues after crossing a vascular endothelial barrier. This includes tumor sites shown above. Following inflammation, these DC are capable of acquiring tumor antigen, maturing and migrating across a second endothelial barrier, specifically the lymphatics, and trafficking to nodal sites. In lymph nodes, DC stimulate antigen-specific T cells and B cells in an evolving adaptive immune response.

The application of DC in therapy requires a detailed understanding of their complex biologic functions, which vary significantly depending on their state of maturation and anatomical location (Fig. 1). Indeed, DC are the track stars of immunology, arising in the bone marrow and maturing in the periphery following their diapedesis into tissues. Several individuals identify this phagocytic, low costimulatory molecule-expressing cell within tissues as the immature phenotype. It is quite likely, particularly in the setting of both normal and abnormal Langerhans cells, that there is an even earlier progenitor of DC in the tissues, one that is nonphagocytic and perhaps without any conventional DC markers (Katz *et al.*, 1979; Galy *et al.*, 1995; Favara *et al.*, 1997). Certainly the tissue macrophage's major role is to degrade damaged cells and eliminate apoptotic cells and debris. In the absence of inflammation, these cells remain solely phagocytic. In the setting of inflammation or tissue injury associated with production of inflammatory cytokines including IL-1, TNF-α, and IL-18, some of the cells undergo dramatic changes to assume the phenotype and function of a DC, particularly when GM-CSF and IL-4 are present. Its function, however, in the setting of tumor may be aberrant, unable to make this phenotypic conversion, making this antigen-presenting cell more tolerogenic than immunogenic (Watson *et al.*, 1995). Under normal conditions it undergoes a series of remarkable changes whereby it becomes actively macropinocytotic and capable of responding to TNF signals (Cumberbatch *et al.*, 1995; Grewal *et al.*, 1996; Caux *et al.*, 1996) prompting DC migration across the lymphatic endothelium and allowing for transport to draining nodal sites where the DC may present antigen to T cells and B cells, selecting for activation those few cells capable of recognizing processed antigen.

From the standpoint of the tumor immunobiologist, environmental cues in the context of cancer disrupt the normally efficient mechanisms by which DC elicit and maintain an effective immune response. There are a variety of factors typically present at the site of the tumor that may negatively impact afferent DC function, including prostaglandins, nitric oxide, IL-10, TGF-β, EBI-3, as well as other tumor-derived products (Davergne *et al.*, 1996; Esway *et al.*, 1997). Recently it has become clear that tumor-derived products can perturb the evolution of DC from bone marrow progenitors. This has perhaps been best demonstrated by Gabrilovich, Carbone and colleagues (Oyama *et al.*, 1998) who showed that VEGF alters the *in vitro* and *in vivo* development of DC from bone marrow progenitors, in part by modifying NF-κB production in bone marrow and mobilization into the nucleus. Since VEGF is a commonly produced cytokine at the site of tumors, this represents a hazard for the development of an effective adaptive immune response. FLT3-ligand has recently been identified as promoting the development of DC in murine models (Maraskovsky *et al.*, 1996; Shurin *et al.*, 1997a) as well as in recent human clinical trials. It appears that expression and production of this molecule in normal tissues may elicit the production of more DC from the bone marrow.

We have performed a number of studies that suggest that intravenous administration of high-dose interleukin-2 is associated with profound alterations in DC production and traffic (Elder *et al.*, 1997a). Furthermore, IL-2 may function to modify DC development directly or indirectly through activated T-cells (Mohamadzadeh *et al.*, 1996b; Bykovskaja *et al.*, 1998). It is likely that the initial notion of cytokines acting at a distance to regulate hematopoietic development will become a generalizable one, particularly in the setting of DC generation. Furthermore, we have recently been able to demonstrate that there is a marked increased in circulating DC during surgical trauma, perhaps reflecting the ability of stress hormones and cytokines to enhance either production or mobilization of these cells into the circulation (Lotze, unpublished).

TWO FUNDAMENTAL APPROACHES TO UTILIZING DC FOR THERAPY

Delivery of Tumor Antigen into DC

What is the best way to deliver tumor antigen into DC to elicit an effective immune response (Fig. 2)? We (Mayordomo *et al.*, 1995, 1996a, 1996b; Zitvogel *et al.*, 1996; Celluzzi *et al.*, 1996), and others (Porgador *et al.*, 1995), have pulsed synthetic peptides derived from tumor antigen protein precursors including the melanoma-associated antigens MART 1/Melan A, tyrosinase, or gp100, in order to load MHC complexes expressed by DC as well as the genes encoding these antigens (Alters *et al.*, 1997) to genetically modify DC to present their peptide epitopes to the immune system in a particularly immunogenic format. Some peptides when used alone can induce tolerance,

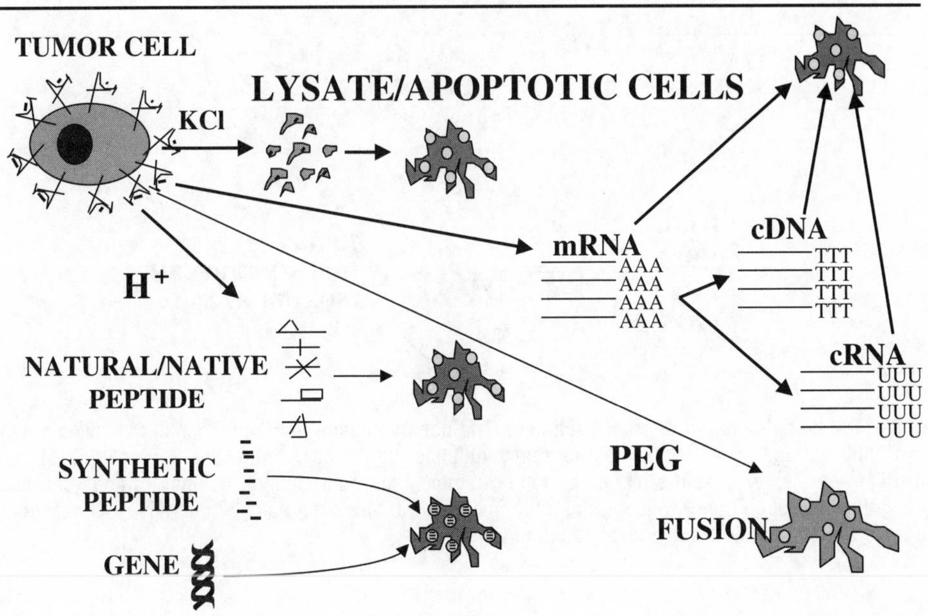

Fig. 2. Approaches to delivering antigen into DC. There are many strategies designed to deliver either peptides, proteins, lysates, mRNA or cDNA into DC. It is also conceivable that simple combinations of DC and tumor in coincubating approaches may be sufficient to yield immunologic complexes capable of promoting immune response.

unless presented by mature DC (Toes *et al.*, 1996). When the antigens are not known, a variety of alternative approaches have been described that provide a rational form of 'tumor antigen' for delivery to DC. These range from using tumor lysates (Ashley *et al.*, 1997), messenger RNA (mRNA) derived from the tumor itself (Boczkowski *et al.*, 1996), or stripped peptides (Storkus *et al.*, 1993a, 1993b; Zeh *et al.*, 1994; Zitvogel *et al.*, 1996c, d; Tjandrawan *et al.*, 1998) (acid-eluted from class I MHC or class II molecules on the tumor cell surface), or, alternatively, even fusing the tumor with DC to generate immunogenic heteroconjugates (Hart and Colaco, 1997; Celluzzi and Falo, 1998). Given the small size of some human tumors when they are resected, this seems technically a difficult approach. An alternative strategy is to deliver DC into tumors. The tumor environment is immunoinhibitory (Fig. 3) and protocols designed to stimulate DC using costimulation (Cella *et al.*, 1996; Flores-Romo *et al.*, 1997; Wilson *et al.*, 1997), cytokines (Sallusto and Lanzavecchia, 1994; Lu *et al.*, 1994, 1995; Caux *et al.*, 1996; Strobl *et al.*, 1996; Chapuis *et al.*, 1997; Esche *et al.*, 1997; Winzler *et al.*, 1997), small mitogenic molecules (Czernicki, 1997), or bacterial antigen (Sallusto *et al.*, 1995; Thurnher *et al.*, 1997) may be necessary to overcome the local inhibitory environment *in situ*.

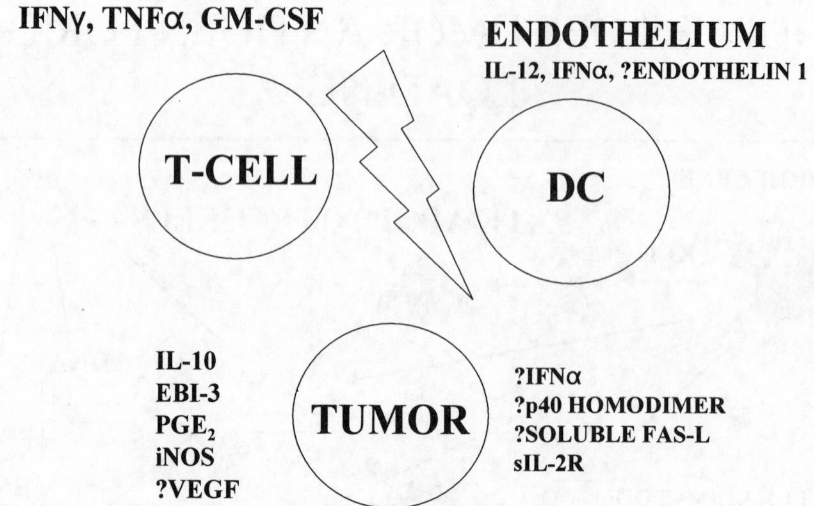

Fig. 3. The complex tumor microenvironment. The complex tumor microenvironment involves a number of different cell types. This almost certainly includes the tumor endothelium, across which T cells and DC transit, as well as the means by which tumor gains nourishment. DC may critically regulate angiogenesis through their production of antiangiogenic factors such as IL-12 and IFN-α. Other proangiogenic factors are also likely to be identified in DC.

Nongenetic strategies

There have been many strategies for delivering antigen into DC that have been established in murine models and are now undergoing evaluation in clinical trials. These include the use of synthetic peptide where the tumor antigen is known (Mayordomo *et al.*, 1995; Porgador and Gilboa *et al.*, 1995; Celluzzi *et al.*, 1996), stripped peptide coming from class I molecules from murine tumors (Zitvogel 1996c, d), use of recombinant protein, or tumor lysates. Alternative strategies that have also been utilized include direct fusion of DC with tumor, allowing provision of tumor antigen in the context of DC costimulatory molecules including production of cytokines. Most recently Falo and colleagues (Celluzzi and Falo, 1998) have demonstrated that simple coincubation of DC with tumor for several hours *ex vivo* yields an effective immunogen in prophylactic murine tumor models. The role of this 'vaccine' in therapy in murine or human tumors has not yet been clearly defined. This approach appears to be particularly germane physiologically since the preferred source of antigen for DC appears to be apoptotic bodies and apoptotic cells (Albert *et al.*, 1998; Bender *et al.*, 1998). Strategies designed to exploit the delivery of tumor antigen in this format would be predicted to be highly effective. This could include the use of radiation therapy, adenoviral delivery of p53 (DeLeo, 1998), or chemotherapeutic approaches, all designed to enhance tumor cell apoptosis and subsequent processing ('malting') of cellular debris/apoptotic bodies by DC *in situ*.

Genetic Modification of DC

Both viral and nonviral vectors have been employed to transfect human and murine DC (Lotze, 1996b; Davis and Lotze, 1997; Tüting, 1997a, 1997b, 1977c). We initially performed studies implementing bioballistic gene transfer using the gene gun and validated (Condon *et al.*, 1996; Tüting, 1998) the effective delivery of cytokine genes into DC that resulted in modified APC capable of promoting enhanced *in vitro* and *in vivo* anti-tumor responses. As the efficiency of these approaches is quite low (i.e., 1–5% transfection efficiency), we and others have assessed DC transduction using viral vectors (Brossart *et al.*, 1997). These have included retroviral vectors (Reeves *et al.*, 1996; Bello-Fernanadez *et al.*, 1997; Specht *et al.*, 1997; Nishioka *et al.*, 1997; McArthur and Mulligan, 1998), adenoviral vectors (Ribas *et al.*, 1997; Wan *et al.*, 1997), and pox viral vectors (Kim *et al.*, 1997; Bronte *et al.*, 1997). These vectors efficiently deliver cDNA encoding tumor antigens and/or immunostimulatory molecules (or in the setting of transplantation, inhibitory molecules) directly into DC. We have recently observed that genetically modified DC expressing the genes for IL-12 markedly enhance anti-tumor immune responses in murine models (Zitvogel *et al.*, 1995, 1996a, b; Nishioka *et al.*, 1997). Given the extraordinary ability of DC to initiate and elicit an effective immune response, it is quite likely that viral coat proteins may not only stimulate DC activation but also serve as a source of immunogenic peptide. Whether adenoviral vectors or vaccinia vectors that have been shown to be quite effective *in vitro* will be effective with repeated *in vivo* application remains to be seen.

Delivery of DC into Tumor

An alternative approach has been to deliver DCs directly into tumor. This can be done most generally by applying DC-mobilizing cytokines, such as FLT3-ligand, which have been shown in murine models (Lynch *et al.*, 1997, 1998; Esche *et al.*, 1997; Chen *et al.*, 1997; Peron *et al.*, 1997)) to enhance systemic and tumor-associated frequencies of DC, resulting in improved anti-tumor effects. DC increase in percentage in the spleen from <0.1% to as many as 25% of cells with FL treatment. In humans, increases from <0.3% in the peripheral blood to over 12% have been noted in early clinical trials. An alternative mobilizing strategy is to deliver the two cytokines, GM-CSF and IL-4, systematically, which has been employed to mature DC from macrophage progenitors or from CD34 progenitors. Our limited studies with this approach in animal models have demonstrated anti-tumor effects in a highly immunogenic tumor, the HPV-16-induced C3 sarcoma (Shurin, unpublished data). Recent clinical applications suggest an increase in DC number in the peripheral blood. Early, potentially promising results in prostate cancer and other tumors (Murphy *et al.*, 1996; Hall *et al.*, 1997; Tjoa *et al.*, 1997; Nestle *et al.*, 1998; Salgaller *et al.*, 1998a, b) with adoptive transfer of antigen-laden DC would suggest that this alternative strategy should also be evaluated in these tumor types.

We have also evaluated the impact of direct injection of DC into the tumor in three separate tumor models and have demonstrated anti-tumor effects. DC transfected with the cytokine genes encoding IL-12 have proven effective as a therapy, while we have seen only modest effects when limited numbers of unmodified DC are directly injected into the tumor itself (Nishioka *et al.*, 1997). We are also evaluating inducible promoters driving expression of cytokine genes only when the DC encounter antigen-specific T cells in nodal sites (Baar and Lotze, 1997).

One additional parameter that needs to be considered in adoptive approaches is how to deliver DC. It has been argued that the optimal means is to deliver DC subcutaneously vs. intravenous approaches, but such evaluations have frequently had a nontherapeutic endpoint (Barratt-Boyes *et al.*, 1997a, 1997b; 1998). In our own studies, comparable, and perhaps superior, effects were noted with intravenous administration vs. subcutaneous or intraperitoneal delivery approaches (Tüting *et al.*, 1997a, 1997b, 1997c, 1997d). A further interesting notion, initially delivering immunogenic DC directly into lymph nodes identified under ultrasound guidance, has been evaluated by Nestle and colleagues (Nestle *et al.*, 1998) in a series of 16 patients with metastatic melanoma with five partial or complete responses observed. DC generated from macrophage precursors and pulsed with specific melanoma-associated peptides or tumor lysates were used in this study. Similar types of procedures are ongoing at our institution (Hall *et al.*, 1997) and others.

WHICH DC SHOULD BE UTILIZED?

We now recognize (Fig. 1) that there are multiple means of generating DC from cytokine-treated individuals from CD34$^+$ progenitors or macrophage precursors. The major question currently being addressed by DC biologists is how to use these cells most effectively in therapy. The first question pertains to the source of the DC. The two predominant sources that clinicians have contemplated are CD34$^+$ precursors obtained from the bone marrow or G-CSF-mobilized stem cells obtained from the peripheral blood. An alternative approach is to perform a leukapheresis in order to obtain a sufficient number of macrophages that may be matured *in vivo* by 5–7-day culture in the cytokines, GM-CSF and IL-4, alone or with the addition of soluble CD40L or TNF-α (Fig. 4).

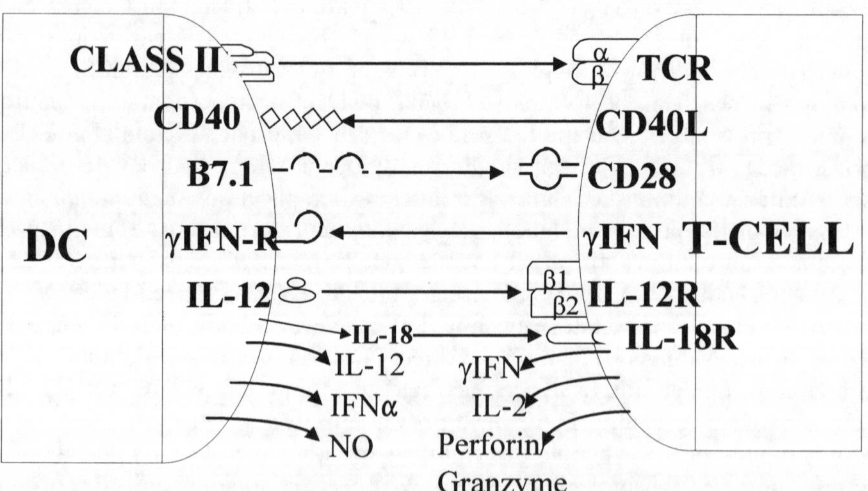

Fig. 4. Socratic interaction among T cells and DC. Sequential interactions between T cells and DC require an ongoing dialogue which allows development of the mature T cell response. Following these sequential activation steps, a naive T cell can exit the lymph node, having been expanded to encounter antigen in the periphery. It is envisioned that DC in the periphery also provide costimulation and cytokines during the effector phase of the immune response to tumor.

An important principle is that these different types of DC have not yet been adequately compared and contrasted in either murine or human clinical trials. In our early studies (Mayordomo *et al.*, 1995) we demonstrated that GM-CSF plus IL-4 cultured DC were superior in anti-tumor effects to those derived from CD34 precursors cultured in GM alone or GM-CSF plus TNF. In fact, anti-tumor responses were only observed in the cells that had been cultured with GM-CSF and IL-4, which exhibit an immature phenotype and may have different trafficking properties vs. GM-CSF- and TNF-treated cells. In addition, the notion of terminally maturing DC, so that reversion to cells of a macrophage phenotype is prevented (Romani *et al.*, 1996; Reddy *et al.*, 1997), has yet to be shown to be important in either murine or human studies. These critical questions can only be addressed in prospective trials to be carried out over the next few years. Currently there are more than thirty different ongoing clinical trials around the world in cancer therapy.

CLINICAL STUDIES IN CANCER

The first reported clinical trial of DC-based cancer therapy was initiated in 1994 (Chu *et al.*, 1996). In this protocol, patients underwent a 48-hour DC purification procedure with precursors obtained from peripheral blood mononuclear cells after a series of gradient density centrifugations. Isolated DC were pulsed with idiotype protein and administered intravenously in six patients with B cell lymphoma. Four therapeutic vaccines were applied. All vaccinated patients gave evidence of immune responsiveness in the form of lymphocytic proliferation and/or cytolytic activity against lymphocytic targets. Interestingly, one patient had a complete tumor regression, a second showed a partial response, and a third patient is tumor-free at a molecular detection level.

Other reported clinical trials include those performed in the setting of prostate cancer in which patients have been immunized using a similar approach with macrophage precursors (Murphy *et al.*, 1996). In these studies patients were vaccinated with prostate-specific antigen (PSA) or PMSA. The third study is a remarkable one which reported a 42% response rate in patients with melanoma who received $1\text{–}3 \times 10^6$ DC injected directly into inguinal lymph nodes using ultrasound guidance. In this trial, 16 patients were treated with DC pulsed with autologous tumor lysate or synthetic HLA-A1 or HLA-A2-presented melanoma by Nestle and associates (Nestle *et al.*, 1998). Visceral responses were noted in the lung and pancreas; showing that systematic immunity results from such inventions bodes well for the future of this therapy. Our own current results support one complete response and two partial responses as well as two patients with stable disease in over 20 patients treated (Hall *et al.*, 1997) using systemic administration of $1\text{–}3 \times 10^6$ 'dendriphages' (DC derived from macrophage precursors) weekly for 4 weeks.

CLINICAL STUDIES IN HIV

HIV-1 infection is characterized by progressive immune dysfunction, marked by depletion of $CD4^+$ lymphocytes and destruction of lymphoid organs (Pantaleo *et al.*, 1995). As a result of this immune dysfunction, the majority of HIV-infected persons develop opportunistic infections and malignancies associated with the acquired immunodeficiency syndrome (AIDS). Traditional approaches for treating HIV-1 infection have focused on the use of antiretroviral agents, alone and in combination. Antiretroviral monotherapy with nucleoside analogs such as AZT has had some clinical benefit in delaying the onset of HIV-related disease, although the clinical benefit, as well as the ability to raise $CD4^+$ T cell count and lower viral load, has been temporary. Therapy with combinations of antiretroviral nucleoside analog has had a more pronounced effect on suppressing viral load and raising peripheral $CD4^+$ T cell counts in infected persons. However, despite their well-documented antiviral effect, nucleoside analogs and other agents used in combination have not been shown to reverse the immune deterioration associated with HIV infection has not been shown. Therefore, combining therapeutic modalities designed to restore immune function with those aimed at suppressing viral replication may prove to be the most effective method of treating HIV infection.

Limitations of Antiretroviral Therapy and Rationale for Adjuvant DC Vaccines

New antiretroviral therapies, which include potent protease inhibitors in combination with nucleoside analog reverse-transcriptase (RT) inhibitors, have been shown to effectively lower viral load and increase peripheral $CD4^+$ T cell counts in a majority of HIV-infected patients. Despite the initial success of these drugs (termed HAART, for highly active antiretroviral therapy) in controlling HIV replication in many patients, there is increasing evidence that such therapeutic combinations have limitations. Many patients who respond to HAART with an absent or transient decrease in viral load show evidence of resistance to one or more of the drugs (Shafer *et al.*, 1998). Failure has also been attributed to lack of compliance due to drug toxicities as well as inadequate drug exposure as a result of pharmacologic factors. Even in cases of significant viral suppression and increases in CD4 counts, it is unclear whether complete immunologic recovery can occur in patients with more advanced disease. Autran *et al.* investigated the extent to which HAART could reverse the immunologic abnormalities associated with advanced HIV infection (Autran *et al.*, 1997). They reported a significant rise in peripheral $CD4^+$ T cells (memory, then later naive) and a decrease in lymphocyte activation markers on both $CD4^+$ and $CD8^+$ T cells. The numbers of peripheral $CD4^+$ T cells and the $CD4^+:CD8^+$ T cell ratio, however, did not normalize. Furthermore, although significant increases in proliferative responses to recall antigens were seen in these patients following therapy, no enhancement of HIV-specific proliferation was noted. We have also begun to characterize HIV-specific T cell responses before and after HAART, and find that although there may be increases in preexisting responses after initiating therapy, the breadth of CTL reactivities is not enhanced by therapy (Ferbas *et al.*, 1995; Klein *et al.*, 1995; Rinaldo *et al.*, 1995; and unpublished observations). In the setting of lowered viral replication resulting from HAART, a more effective HIV-specific cellular immune response can be generated using cultured DC as antigen-presenting cells. Generating broader, more potent HIV-specific immunity may be critical in maintaining a low viral load in the event of drug resistance or noncompliance.

Dendritic cells are likely the principal cells involved in priming HIV-specific T cell responses *in vivo*. An understanding of the factors involved in DC presentation of HIV-1 antigens to naive and memory T cells is crucial to the development of vaccines and immune-based therapies for HIV-1 infection. DC dysfunction *in vivo*, among other factors such as cytokine dysregulation, may contribute to the T cell defects characteristic of HIV disease. DC dysfunction might be corrected, and a more effective cellular immune response to HIV-1 generated, through the therapeutic use of appropriately-primed, cultured autologous DC in the setting of viral suppression with HAART.

There is increasing evidence that a potent cell-mediated immune response against HIV-1 may be beneficial in suppressing viral replication and delaying disease progression. There are data to suggest that individuals who are infected with HIV-1 but who have successfully controlled viral replication have a vigorous CTL response to HIV-1 antigens (Cao *et al.*, 1995) as well as strong HIV-specific T helper responses (Rosenberg, 1997). Early after HIV-1 infection, patients receiving antiretroviral interventions that suppress viral load may subsequently develop strong HIV-specific T helper responses similar to those associated with nonprogressors (Rosenberg *et al.*, 1997) or HIV-exposed but uninfected individuals. Unfortunately, it does not appear that these responses are spontaneously generated in chronically infected patients following suppression of viral load with potent antiretroviral agents (HAART) (Autran *et al.*, 1997; Vial *et al.*, 1997; Young *et al.*, 1997). One might argue that reconstituting a strong HIV-specific immune response in both the T helper and cytotoxic T cell effector arms in such individuals would lead to a more effective and longer lasting suppression of HIV-1. We have found that cultured DC are potent stimulators of both MHC class I- and II-restricted antigen-specific T cell responses. Furthermore, we have shown that when this potent APC is grown from the peripheral blood of HIV-infected individuals, it maintains its immunostimulatory characteristics, and stimulates HIV-specific T cells *in vitro* (Mellors *et al.*, 1997).

Although investigations of DC therapies in the setting of cancer suggest that the therapies appear to be safe and induce anti-tumor effects *in vivo*, to date only a single pilot study involving the administration of antigen-loaded DC to HIV-infected persons has been performed (Kundu *et al.*, 1998). This phase I clinical trial, carried out by Drs S. K. Kundu and T. C. Merigan at the Center for AIDS Research at Stanford University Medical Center, assessed the safety and antigen-presenting properties of allogeneic or autologous DC pulsed with recombinant gp160 or synthetic peptides administered to six HIV-infected donors. DC were isolated from leukapheresed PBMC from the recipient (one case) or HLA-matched siblings (five cases) using stepwise centrifugation and a short culture period with antigen, without exogenous cytokines. DC were incubated with HIV-1 gp160 or synthetic peptides corresponding to HLA-A2-restricted CTL epitopes (in env, gag, pol of HIV-1) and infused intravenously to HLA-A2^{+} HIV-infected donors 6–9 times at monthly intervals. Study subjects had CD4 counts ranging from 300 to 700/mm^3 at the initiation of the study and viral loads ranging from 3 to 5 log plasma RNA copies/ml. Following infusions, patients were monitored for changes in viral load and HIV-specific immune responses. No clinically significant adverse effects were seen in any patient, and plasma HIV-1 RNA and CD4^{+} T cell numbers were stable during the study period. The DC therapy appeared to enhance the HIV-specific CTL and/or lymphoproliferative response of patients who had initial CD4 counts of over 410/mm^3. The size of this pilot study precluded any conclusions as to clinical benefit of this approach, but the infusions were well tolerated and enhanced HIV-specific immune responses were observed in 50% of patients.

USE OF DC TO GENERATE T CELLS RECOGNIZING OCCULT TUMOR ANTIGENS

Tumor antigens capable of yielding target epitopes for T cell reactivity have been identified in the setting of various human malignancies: melanoma, colorectal cancer, pancreatic cancer, and leukemia. A number of groups, including our own, are utilizing DC to generate T cells recognizing occult tumor antigens *ex vivo* (Bakker *et al.*, 1995; Cardoso *et al.*, 1997; Peiper *et al.*, 1997; Tsai *et al.*, 1997; Brossart *et al.*, 1998; Choudhury *et al.*, 1998; Tjandrawan *et al.*, 1998) or to expand T cells for therapy without direct identification of antigens. Whether this will be a successful approach will remain speculative until clinical trials are reported.

USE OF DC TO ENHANCE T CELL SURVIVAL

Failure of immunotherapy may be due to the recently documented 'counterattack' by the tumor against pivotal immune effector cells including lymphocytes (O'Connell *et al.*, 1997; Walker *et al.*, 1997; Zeytun *et al.*, 1997) and DC (Shurin, 1997), a process we have termed tumor-induced cell death (TICD). Furthermore, the identification of Fas-signaling as the predominant mechanism of activation-induced cell death (AICD) (Alderson *et al.*, 1995) suggests that this is in part a natural biological phenomenon that controls the number of activated lymphocytes during an immune response. To enhance the effectiveness of DC-based therapies, alternative approaches designed to delay AICD or TICD are in order. An expected outcome of this approach is an enhanced quality and duration of effective immune responses. We have developed strategies to evaluate the role of tumor cells in the destruction of melanoma-specific $CD4^+$ and $CD8^+$ T cells and the role of antigen-laden DC in providing protection. This is an important area for research, we believe, that is largely unexplored and is expected to have a major impact on the future design of effective biological therapy approaches to cancer. In addition, DC that are not appropriately activated may induce a state of immune tolerance (Steptoe and Thomson, 1996). Although the phenomenon of improved cancer prognosis in patients with increased numbers of DC within the tumor site has been recognized for several years (Bigotti *et al.*, 1991; Lotze, 1997), the interpretation of this finding and its importance are largely unknown. In addition to this surmised afferent immunologic functions, DC may also exhibit an effector function in providing protection to antigen-specific T cells against premature programmed cell death induced by tumors *in vitro* (Daniel *et al.*, 1997; Lu, 1997) and *in vivo* (Finn *et al.*, 1996; Evans *et al.*, 1997).

Available literature suggests improved prognosis for cancer patients in relationship to tumor infiltration by DC. This finding applies to a variety of tumor origins and suggests a positive therapeutic outcome if DC are delivered to tumor sites (Grabbe *et al.*, 1995; Nishioka *et al.*, 1997). Preclinical murine models (Celluzzi, 1996; Young and Inaba, 1996) and initial clinical trials, including our own, using cultured DC are promising with objective responses, but the major issue is how DC mediate to these effects. The dynamic relationship between tumor cells, DC, and TIL within the tumor microenvironment is complex. Strategies directed at enhancing DC number and preventing their premature apoptotic death at tumor sites could be therapeutic. AICD, for example, is an apoptic program induced following cognate antigen recognition in activated immune cells (Alderson *et al.*, 1995). This natural termination of an immune response is a powerful negative feedback mechanism that insures removal of preactivated lymphocytes to avoid unwanted tissue injury. Tumor cells, as well as normal cells, express molecules capable of modifying immunity. What was not previously expected was that tumors could not only induce AICD that eliminated effete and presumably unnecessary specific effector lymphocytes but also could eliminate or tolerize other non-specific T cells. A diverse range of human and mouse tumor cells have been shown to induce rapid lymphocyte cell death by apoptosis following tumor cell/lymphocyte interaction. TICD, which does not require cognate recognition, is a plausible means by which immune suppression is unduced by tumor cells. To date, the most frequently implicated death mechanism mediating TICD is the Fas/Fas ligand apoptotic pathway (O'Connell *et al.*, 1997; Walker *et al.*, 1997; Zeytun *et al.*, 1997). Prevention of premature AICD of T cells has not been well studied but is believed to occur as a result of activation of CD28 on T cells. CD28-mediated anti-apoptosis presumably occurs due to upregulation of bcl-x_L, a member of the bcl-2 family of anti-apoptotic proteins (Boise *et al.*, 1993, 1995; Hawkins and Vaux, 1997). Balancing the anti-apoptotic activity of bcl-2 and bcl-x_L are a number of pro-apoptotic members of the bcl-2 family of apoptosis-related proteins such as bax, bad, bak, and bik, among others. Interestingly, IL-12 is protective of apoptotic death in activated T cells (Lotze, 1996), making the presence of DC, the major source of IL-12, at the tumor site potentially critical for expansion and protection of anti-tumor effector T cells.

FUTURE DIRECTIONS

It seems likely that combinations of FLT3-ligand, IL-2, interferon-α, or IL-12 may optimize DC-based clinical applications via their direct or indirect effects on DC. Given the high rate of spontaneous apoptotic death observed in T cells in the periphery of patients with a variety of neoplasms, such combination therapies would be envisioned to enhance T cell survival. It has taken over two decades to refine our approaches to utilizing T cells in the therapy of cancer; although they have yet to be demonstrated to predictably impact disease prognosis in patients with most tumor types, it is clear that in many patients clinical responsiveness is linked to enhanced T cellular immunity. It has now also become clear that DC may play an important supportive role in promoting and maintaining antigen-specific T cells *in vivo*. It is fully anticipated that DC will become a mainstay for inclusion in biological therapies for patients with cancer or HIV in the future.

REFERENCES

Agger, R., Crowley, M.T. and Witmer-Pack, M.D. (1990). The surface of DCs in the mouse as studied with monoclonal antibodies. *Int. Rev. Immunol.* **6**, 89–101.

Akbar, A.N., and Salmon, M. (1997). Cellular environments and apoptosis: tissue microenvironments control activated T-cell death. *Immunol. Today* **18**, 72–76.

Albert, M.L., Sauter, B. and Bhardwaj, N. (1998). Dendritic cells acquire antigen from apoptotic cells and induce class I-restricted CTLs. *Nature* **392**(6671), 86–89.

Alderson, M.R., Tough, T.W., Davis-Smith, T., Braddy, S., Falk, B., Schooley, K.A., Goodwin, R.G., Smith, C.A., Ramsdell, F. and Lynch, D.H. (1995). Fas ligand mediates activation-induced cell death in human T lymphocytes. *J. Exp. Med.* **181**, 71–77.

Alters, S.E., Gadea, J.R. and Philip, R. (1997). Immunotherapy of cancer. Generation of CEA specific CTL using CEA peptide pulsed dendritic cells. *Adv. Exp. Med. Biol.* **417**, 519–524.

Anderson, D.M., Maraskovsky, E., Billingsley, W.L., Dougall, W.C., Tometsko, M.E., Roux, E.R, Teepe, M.C., DuBose, R.F., Cosman, D. and Galibert, L. (1997). A homologue of the TNF receptor and its ligand enhance T-cell growth and dendritic-cell function. *Nature* **390**, 175–179.

Arai, H., Chan, S.Y., Bishop, D.K. and Nabel, G.J. (1997) Inhibition of the alloantibody response by CD95 ligand. *Nature Medicine* **3**, 843–848.

Ashley, D.M., Faiola, B., Nair, S., Hale, L.P., Bigner, D.D., and Gilboa. E. (1997). Bone marrow-generated dendritic cells pulsed with tumor extracts or tumor RNA induce antitumor immunity against central nervous system tumors. *J. Exp. Med.* **186**, 1177–1182.

Austyn, J.M. (1993). The dendritic cell system and anti-tumour immunity. *In Vivo* **7**, 193–202.

Autran, B., Carcelain, G., Li, T.S., Blanc, C., Mathez, D., Tubiana, R., Katlama, C., Debre, P. and Leibowitch, P. (1997). Positive effects of combined antiretroviral therapy on $CD4^+$ T cell homeostasis and function in advanced HIV disease. *Science* **277**, 112–116.

Baar, J. and Lotze, M.T. (1997). Interferon gamma inducible cytokine gene expression in plasmid-transfected dendritic cells. *J. Immunother.* **20**, 403.

Bakker, A.B.H., Schreurs, M.W.J., de Boer A.J., Kawakami, Y., Rosenberg, S.A., Adema, G.J. and Figdor, C.G. (1994). Melanocyte lineage-specific antigen gp100 is recognized by melanoma derived tumor infiltrating lymphocytes. *J. Exp. Med.* **179**, 1005–1009.

Bakker, A.B., Marland, G., de Boer, A.J., Huijbens, R.J., Danen, E.H., Adema, G.J. and Figdor, C.G. (1995). Generation of antimelanoma cytotoxic T lymphocytes from healthy donors after presentation of melanoma-associated antigen-derived epitopes by dendritic cells in vitro. *Cancer Res.* **55**(22), 5330–5334.

Barratt-Boyes, S.M., Kao, H. and Finn, O.J.(1998). Chimpanzee dendritic cells derived in vitro from blood monocytes and pulsed with antigen elicit specific immune responses in vivo. *J. Immunother.* **1**(2), 142–148.

Barratt-Boyes, S.M., Watkins, S.C. and Finn, O.J. (1997a). In vivo migration of dendritic cells differentiated in vitro: a chimpanzee model. *J. Immunol.* **158**(10), 4543–4547.

Barratt-Boyes, S.M., Watkins, S.C. and Finn, O.J. (1997b). Migration of cultured chimpanzee dendritic cells following intravenous and subcutaneous injection. *Adv. Exp. Med. Biol.* **417**, 71–75.

Bellgrau, D., Gold, D., Selawry, H., Moore, J., Franzusoff, A. and Duke, R.C. (1995). A role for CD95 ligand in preventing graft rejection. *Nature* **377**, 630–632.

Bello-Fernandez, C., Matyash, M., Strobl, H., Pickl, W.F., Majdic, O., Lyman, S.D. and Knapp, W. (1997). Efficient retrovirus-mediated gene transfer of dendritic cells generated from $CD34^+$ cord blood cells under serum-free conditions. *Hum. Gene Ther.* **8**, 1651–1658.

Bender, A., Albert, M., Reddy, A., Feldman, M., Sauter, B., Kaplan, G., Hellman, W., and Bhardwaj, N. (1997). The distinctive features of influenza virus infection of dendritic cells. *Immunobiology* **198**(5), 552–567.

Bernhard, H., Disis, M.L., Heimfeld, S., Hand, S., Gralow, J.R. and Cheever, M.A. (1995) Generation of immunostimulatory dendritic cells from human $CD34^+$ hematopoietic progenitor cells of the bone marrow and peripheral blood. *Cancer Res.* **55**, 1099–1104.

Bernhard, H., Maeurer, M.J., Jäger, E., Wölfel, T., Schneider, J., Karbach, J., Seliger, B., Huber, C., Storkus, W.J., Lotze, M.T., Meyer zum Büschenfelde, K.-H. and Knuth, A.. (1996) Recognition of human renal cell carcinoma and melanoma by HLA-A2-restricted cytotoxic T lymphocytes is mediated by shared peptide epitopes and up-regulated by interferon-γ. *Scand. J. Immunol.* **44**, 285–292.

Bibel, D.J. (1988) *Milestones in Immunology. A Historical Exploration.* Science Tech Publishers. Madison, WI.

Bigotti, G., Coli, A. and Castagnola, D. (1991). Distribution of Langerhans cells and HLA class II molecules in prostatic carcinomas of different histopathological grade. *Prostate* **19**(1), 73–87.

Bissonnette, R.P., Brunner, T., Lazarchik, S.B., Yoo, N.J., Boehm, M.F., Green, D.R. and Heyman, R.A. (1995). 9-*cis* Retinoic acid inhibition of activation-induced apoptosis is mediated via regulation of fas ligand and requires retinoic acid receptor and retinoid X receptor activation. *Mol. Cell. Biol.* **15**, 5576–5585.

Bjorkdahl, O., Wingren, A.G., Hedhund, G., Ohlsson, L. and Dohlsten, M. (1997). Gene transfer of a hybrid interleukin-1 beta gene to B16 mouse melanoma recruits leucocyte subsets and reduces tumour growth in vivo. *Cancer Immunol. Immunother.* **44**(5), 273–281.

Boczkowski, D., Nair, S.K., Snyder, D. and Gilboa, E. (1996). Dendritic cells pulsed with RNA are potent antigen-presenting cells in vitro and in vivo. *J. Exp. Med.* **184**(2), 465–472.

Boel, P., Wildmann, C.; Sensi, M.L., Brasseur, R., Renauld, J.C., Coulie, P., Boon, T. and van der Bruggen, P. (1995). BAGE: a new gene encoding an antigen recognized on human melanomas by cytolytic T lymphocytes. *Immunity* **2**, 167–75.

Boise, L.H., Gonzalez-Garcia, M., Postema, C.E., Ding, L., Lindsten, T., Turka, L.A., Mao, X., Nunez, G. and Thompson, C.B. (1993). Bcl-x, a bcl-2-related gene that functions as a dominant regulator of apoptotic cell death. *Cell* **74**, 597–608.

Boise, L.H., Minn, A.J., Noel, P.J., June, C.H., Accavitti, M.A., Linsten, T. and Thompson, C.B. (1995). CD28 costimulation can promote T cell survival by enhancing the expression of Bcl-xl. *Immunity* **3**, 87–98.

Boldin, M.P., Varfolomeev, E.E., Pancer, Z., Mett, I.L., Camonis, J.H. and Wallach, D. (1995). A novel protein that interacts with the death domain of Fas/APO1 contains a sequence motif related to the death domain. *J. Biol. Chem.* **270**, 7795–7798.

Boldin, M.P., Gpncharov, T.M., Goltsev, Y.V. and Wallach, D. (1996). Involvement of MACH, a novel MORT1/FADD-interacting protease in Fas/APO-1-and TNF receptor-induced cell death. *Cell* **85**, 803–815.

Brichard, V., Van Pel, A., Wolfel, T., Wolfel, C., De Plaen, E. Lethe, B., Coulie, P. and Boon, T. (1993). The tyrosinase gene codes for an antigen recognized by autologous cytolytic T lymphocytes on HLA- A2 melanomas. *J. Exp. Med.* **178**, 489–495.

Bronte, V., Carroll, M.W., Goletz, T.J., Wang, M., Overwijk, W.W., Marincola, F., Rosenberg, S.A., Moss, B. and Restifo, N.P. (1997). Antigen expression by dendritic cells correlates with the therapeutic effectiveness of a model recombinant poxvirus tumor vaccine. *Proc. Natl. Acad. Sci. USA* **94**(7), 3183–3188.

Brossart, P., Goldrath, A.W., Butz, E.A., Martin, S. and Bevan, M.J. (1997). Virus-mediated delivery of antigenic epitopes into dendritic cells as a means to induce CTL. *J. Immunol.* **158**, 3270–3276.

Brossart, P., Stuhler, G., Flad, T., Stevanovic, S., Rammensee, H.G., Kanz, L. and Brugger, W. (1998). Her-2/neu-derived peptides are tumor-associated antigens expressed by human renal cell and colon carcinoma lines and are recognized by in vitro induced specific cytotoxic T lymphocytes. *Cancer Res.* **58**(4), 732–736.

Brunner, T., Mogil, R.J., LaFace, D., Yoo, N.J., Mahboubi, A., Echeverri, F., Martin, S.J., Force, W.R., Lynch, D.H., Ware, C.F. and Green, D.R. (1995). Cell-autonomous Fas (CD95)/Fas-ligand interaction mediates activation-induced apoptosis in T-cell hybridomas. *Nature* **373**, 441–444.

Burkly, L., Hesslon, C., Ogata, L., Reilly, C., Marconi, L.A., Olson, D., Tizard, R., Cate, R. and Lo, D. (1995). Expression of *rel*B is required for the development of thymic medulla and dendritic cells. *Nature* **373**, 531–536.

Bykovskaja, S.N, Buffo, M.J, Bunker, M., Zhang, H., Majors, A., Herbert, M., Lokshin, A., Levitt, M.L, Jaja, A., Scalise, D., Kosiban, D., Evans, C., Marks, S. and Shogan, J. (1998). Interleukin-2 induces development of dendritic cells from cord blood CD34$^+$ cells. *J. Leukocyte Biol.* **63**, 620–630.

Campbell, R.L., Repasky, E.A. and Lotze, M.T. (1997). T-cell spectrin (fodrin) aggregation and uropod formation following dendritic cell encounter. *J. Immunother.* **20**, 405.

Cao, Y., Qin, L., Zhang, L., Safrit, J. and Ho, D.D., (1995). Virologic and immunologic characterization of long-term survivors of human immunodeficiency virus type 1 infection. *N. Engl. J. Med.* **332**, 201–208.

Cardoso, A.A., Seamon, M.J., Afonso, H.M., Ghia, P., Boussiotis, V.A., Freeman, G.J., Gribben, J.G., Sallan, S.E. and Nadler, L.M. (1997). Ex vivo generation of human anti-pre-B leukemia-specific autologous cytolytic T cells. *Blood* **90**(2), 549–561.

Casciola-Rosen, L., Nicholson, D.W., Chong, T., Rowan, K.R., Thornberry, N.A., Miller, D.K. and Rosen, A. (1996). Apopain/CPP32 cleaves proteins that are essential for cellular repair: a fundamental principle of apoptotic death. *J. Exp. Med.* **183**, 1947–1951.

Casiano, C.A., Martin, S.J., Green, D.R. and Tan, E.M. (1996). Selective cleavage of nuclear autoantigens during CD95 (Fas/APO-1)-mediated T cell apoptosis. *J. Exp. Med.* **184**, 765–770.

Castelli, C., Storkus, W.J., Maeurer, M.J., Martin, D.M., Huang, E.C., Pramanik, B.N., Nagabhushan, T.L., Parmiani, G. and Lotze, M.T. (1995). Mass spectrometric identification of a naturally-processed melanoma peptide recognized by CD8$^+$ cytotoxic T lymphocytes. *J. Exp. Med.* **181**, 363–368.

Caux, C., Vandervliet, B., Massacrier, C. *et al.* (1996). CD34$^+$ hematopoietic progenitors from human cord blood differentiate along two independent dendritic cell pathways in response to GM-CSF+TNFα, *J. Exp. Med.* **184**, 695–706.

Caux, C., Liu, Y.-J. and Banchereau, J. (1995). Recent advances in the study of dendritic cells and follicular dendritic cells. *Immunol. Today* **16**, 2–5.

Cella, M., Scheidegger, D., Palmer-Lehman, K., Lane, P., Lanzavecchia, A. and Alber, G. (1996). Ligation of CD40 on dendritic cells triggers production of high levels of interleukin-12 and enhances T cell stimulatory capacity: T-T help via APC activation. *J. Exp. Med.* **184**, 747–752.

Celluzzi, C.M., Mayordomo, J.I., Storkus, W.J., Lotze, M.T. and Falo, L.D. (1996). Peptide-pulsed dendritic cells induce antigen specific CTL-mediated protective tumor immunity. *J. Exp. Med.* **183**, 283–287.

Celluzzi, C.M. and Falo, L.D Jr (1998). Physical interaction between dendritic cells and tumor cells results in an immunogen that induces protective and therapeutic tumor rejection. *J. Immunol.* **160**(7), 3081–3085.

Chapuis, F., Rosenzwajg, M., Yagello, M., Ekman, M., Biberfeld, P. and Gluckman, J.C. (1997). Differentiation of human dendritic cells from monocytes *in vitro. Eur. J. Immunol.* **27**, 431–441.

Chaux, P., Favre, N., Martin, M. and Martin, F. (1997). Tumor-infiltrating dendritic cells are defective in their antigen-presenting function and inducible B7 expression in rats. *Int. J. Cancer.* **72**, 619–624.

Chen, K., Braun, S., Lyman, S., Fan, Y., Traycoff, C.M., Wiebke, E.A., Gaddy, J., Sledge, G., Broxmeyer, H.E. and Cornetta, K. (1997). Antitumor activity and immunotherapeutic properties of Flt3-ligand in a murine breast cancer model. *Cancer Res.* **57**, 3511–3516.

Chervonsky, A.V., Wang, Y., Wong, S.F., Visintin, I., Flavell, R.A., Janeway, C.A. Jr. and Matis, L.A. (1997). The role of Fas in autoimmune diabetes. *Cell* **89**, 7–24.

Choudhury, A., Toubert, A., Sutaria, S., Charron, D., Champlin, R.E. and Claxton, D.F. (1998). Human leukemia-derived dendritic cells: ex-vivo development of specific antileukemic cytotoxicity. *Crit. Rev. Immunol.* **18**(1–2), 121–131.

Condon, C., Watkins, S.C., Celluzzi, C.M., Thompson, K. and Falo, L.D. (1996) DNA-based immunization by *in vivo* transfection of dendritic cells. *Nature Medicine* **2**, 1122–1128.

Coulie, P.G., Brichard, V., VanPel, A., Wolfel, T., Schneider, J., Traversari, C., Mattei, S., De Plaen, E., Lurquin, C., Szikora, J.-P, Renauld, J.-C. and Boon, T. (1994). A new gene coding for a differentiation antigen recognized by autologous cytolytic T lymphocytes on HLA-A2 melanomas. *J. Exp. Med.* **180**, 35–42.

Cox, A.L, Skipper, J., Chen, Y., Henderson, R.A., Darrow, T.L., Shabanowitz, J., Engelhard, V.H., Hunt, D.F. and Slingluff, C.L. (1994). Identification of a peptide recognized by five melanoma-specific human cytotoxic T cell lines. *Science* **264**, 716–719.

Cumberbatch, M. and Kimber, I. (1995). Tumour necrosis factor-α is required for accumulation of dendritic cells in draining lymph nodes and for optimal contact sensitization. *Immunology* **84**, 31–35.

Czernicki, B.J., Carter, C., Rivoltini, L., Asoki, G.K., Kim, H.I., Weng, D.E., Roros, J.G., Hijazi, Y.M., Xu, S., Rosenberg, S.A. and Cohen, P.A. (1997). Calcium ionophore treated peripheral blood monocytes and dendritic cells rapidly display characteristics of activated dendritic cells. *J. Immunol.*, **159**, 3823–3837.

Daniel, P.T., Kroidl, A., Cayeux, S., Bargou, R., Blankenstein, and Dörken, B. (1997) Costimulatory signals through B7.1/CD28 prevent T cell apoptosis during target cell lysis. *J. Immunol.* **159**, 3808–3815.

Davis, I.D. and Lotze, M.T. (1997). Cytokine gene therapy. In *The Cytokine Handbook,* 3rd edn (ed. A Thomson). Academic Press, London.

De Maria, R., Lenti, L., Malisan, F., d'Agostino, F., Tomassini, B., Zeuner, A., Rippo, M.R. and Testi, R. (1997). Requirement for GD3 ganglioside in CD95- and ceramide-induced apoptosis. *Science* **277**, 1652–1655.

DeLeo, A.B. (1998). p53-based immunotherapy of cancer. *Crit. Rev. Immunol.* **18**(1–2), 29–35.

Devergne, O., Hummel, M., Koeppen, H., Le Beau, M.M., Nathanson, E.C., Kieff, E. and Birkenbach, M. (1996). A novel interleukin-12 p40-related protein induced by latent Epstein–Barr virus infection in B lymphocytes. *J. Virol.* **70**, 1143–1153.

Dhein, J., Walczak, H., Baumler, C., Debatin, K.M. and Krammer, P.H. (1995). Autocrine T-cell suicide mediated by APO1. *Nature* **373**, 438–441.

DiRosa, F. and Matzinger, P. (1996). Long-lasting CD8 T cell memory in the absence of CD4 T cells or B cells. *J. Exp. Med.* 2153–2163.

Donnenberg, A.D., Margolick, J.B., Beltz, L.A., Donnenberg, V.S. and Rinaldo, C.R. Jr. (1995). Apoptosis parallels lymphopoiesis in bone marrow of transplantation and HIV disease. *Rev. Immunol.* **146**, 11–21.

Drappa, J., Vaishnaw, A.K., Sullivan, K.E., Chu, J.-L. and Elkon, K.B. (1996). Fas gene mutations in the Canale–Smith syndrome, an inherited lymphoproliferative disorder associated with autoimmunity. *N. Engl. J. Med.* **335**, 1643–1649.

Elder, E.M., Stolinski, L.A., Whiteside, T.L. and Lotze, M.T. (1997a). Changes in DC precursor numbers during in vivo IL-2 adminstration. *J. Immunother.* **20**, 407.

Elder, E.M., Lotze, M.T. and Whiteside, T.L. (1997b). Culture of human dendritic cells (DC) for the therapy of patients with cancer. *J. Immunother.* **20**, 407.

Ellem, K.A., O'Rourke, M.G., Johnson, G.R,, Parry. G,, Misko, I.S., Schmidt, C.W., Parsons, P.G., Burrows, S.R., Cross, S., Fell, A., Li, C.L., Bell, J.R., Dubois, P.J., Moss, D.J., Good, M.F., Kelso, A., Cohen, L.K., Dranoff, G. and Mulligan, R.C. (1997). A case report: immune responses and clinical course of the first human use of granulocyte/macrophage-colony-stimulating-factor-transduced autologous melanoma cells for immunotherapy. *Cancer Immunol. Immunother.* **44**(1), 10–20.

Esche, C., Shurin, M.R., Haluszczak, C., Peron, J.M. and Lotze, M.T. (1997). Generation of human dendritic cells from $CD34^+$ precursors for human clinical trials. *J. Immunother.* **20**, 403.

Esway, J., Shurin, G.V., Lotze, M.T. and Barksdale, E.M. (1997). Creating immune privilege: neuroblastoma soluble factors cause apoptosis of Fas-sensitive targets. *J. Immunother.* **20**, 402.

Evans, E.M., Man, S., Evans, A.S. and Borysiewicz, L.K. (1997). Infiltration of cervical cancer tissue with human papillomavirus-specific cytotoxic T-lymphocytes. *Cancer Res.* **57**(14), 2943–2950.

Falo, L.D. and Lotze, M.T., (1997). Cancer vaccines. In *Manual of Clinical Laboratory Immunology*, 5th edn, chapter 133. (volume ed. Everly Conway de Macario; section ed. T. Whiteside). American Society for Microbiology Press.

Favara, B.E., Feller, A.C., Pauli, M., Jaffe, E.S., Weiss, L.M., Arico, M., Bucsky, P., Egeler, R.M., Elinder, G., Gadner, H., Gresik, M., Henter, J.I., Imashuku, S., Janka, Schaub, G., Jaffe, R., Ladisch, S., Nezelof, C. and Pritchard, J. (1997). Contemporary classification of histiocytic disorders. The WHO Committee on Histiocytic/Reticulum Cell Proliferations. Reclassification Working Group of the Histiocyte Society. *Med. Pediatr. Oncol.* **29**, 157–166.

Ferbas, J., Kaplan, A.H., Hausner, M.A., Hultin, L.E., Matud, J.L., Liu, Z., Paniculi, D.L., Nerng-Ho, H., Detels, R. and Giorgi, J.V. (1995). Virus burden in long-term survivors of human immunodefiency virus (HIV) infection is a determinant of anti-HIV $CD8^+$ lymphocytic activity. *J. Infect. Dis.* **172**, 329–339.

Finn, O.J., McKolanis, J.R., Nalesnik, M.A., Clarke, M.R., Lotze, M.T. and Ochoa, A.C. (1996). T cell defects in advanced breast, pancreatic, and colon cancer and improvements after vaccination with a mucin peptide. *Proc. Am. Ass. Cancer Res.* **37**, 475 (3344).

Flores-Romo, L. Björck, P., Duvert, V., van Kooten, C., Sailand, S. and Banchereau, J. (1997). CD40 ligation on human cord blood $CD34^+$ hematopoietic progenitors induces their proliferation and differentiation into functional dendritic cells. *J. Exp. Med.* **185**, 341–349.

Fonseca, R., Tefferi, A. and Strockler, J.G. (1997). Follicular dendritic cell sarcoma mimicking diffuse large cell lymphoma: a case report. *Am. J. Hematol.* **55**(3), 148–155.

Frassanito, M.A., Mayordomo, J.I., DeLeo, R.M., Storkus, W.J., Lotze, M.T. and DeLeo, A.B. (1995). Identification of Meth A sarcoma-derived class I major histocompatibility complex-associated peptides recognized by a specific $CD8^+$ cytolytic T lymphocyte. *Cancer Res.* **55**, 124–128.

French, L.E., Hahne, M., Viard, I., Radlgruber, G., Zanone, R., Becker, K., Muller, C. and Tschopp, J. (1996). Fas and Fas ligand in embryos and adult mice: ligand expression in several immune-privileged tissues and coexpression in adult tissues characterized by apoptotic cell turnover. *J. Cell. Biol.* **133**, 335–343.

Galy, A., Travis, M., Cen, D. and Chen, B. (1995). Human T, B, natural killer, and dendritic cells arise from a common bone marrow progenitor cell subset. *Immunity* **3**, 459–473.

Gaugler, B., Van den Eynde, B., van der Bruggen, P., Romerao, P., Gaforio, J.J., De Plaen, E., Lethe, B., Brasseur, F. and Boon, T. (1994). Human gene MAGE-3 codes for an antigen recognized on a melanoma by autologous cytolytic T lymphocytes. *J. Exp. Med.* **179**, 921–930.

Gilboa, E., Nair, S.K. and Lyerly, H.K. (1998). Immunotherapy of cancer with dendritic-cell-based vaccines. *Cancer Immunol. Immunother.* **46**(2), 82–87.

Goldman, S.A., Baker, E., Weyent, R.J., Lotze, M.T., Clarke, M.R. and Myers, J. (1998). Peritumoral CD1a-positive dendritic cells are associated with survival, recurrence and tumor stage in oral tongue squamous cell carcinoma. *Arch. Otolaryngol. Head Neck Surg.* **124**, 641–646.

Grabbe, S., Beissert, S., Schwarz, T. and Granstein, R.D. (1995). Dendritic cells as initiators of tumor immune responses: a possible strategy for tumor immunotherapy? *Immunol. Today* **16**, 117–121.

Grewal, I.S., Grewal, K.D., Wong, F.S., Picarella, D.E., Janeway, C.A. and Flavell, R.A. (1996). Local expression of transgene encoded TNFα in islets prevents autoimmune diabetes in nonobese diabetic (NOD) mice by preventing the development of auto-reactive islet specific T cells. *J. Exp. Med.* **184**, 1963–1974.

Griffith, T.S., Brunner, T., Fletcher, S.M., Green, D.R. and Ferguson, T.A. (1995). Fas ligand-induced apoptosis as a mechanism of immune privilege. *Science* **270**, 1189–1192.

Hahne, M., Rimoldi, D., Schroter, M., Romero, P., Schreier, M., French, L.E., Schneider, P., Bornand, T., Fontana, A.. Lienard, D., Cerottini, J.-C. and Tschopp, J. (1996). Melanoma cell expression of Fas (Apo-1/CD95) ligand: implications for tumor immune escape. *Science* **274**, 1363–1366.

Hall, T.D., Kinzler, D.M., Elder, E.M., Whiteside, T.L., Storkus, W.J. and Lotze, M.T. (1997). Evaluation and response of patients immunized to HLA-A2 polyepitope peptide mixture in patients with metastatic melanoma using autologous dendritic cells cultured with IL-4 and GM-CSF. *J. Immunother.* **20**, 405.

Haluszczak, C., Lotze, M.T. and Shurin, M.R. (1997). IL-12 and FLT3 ligand differentially stimulate lymphoid and myeloid dendropoiesis in vivo. *J. Immunother.* **20**, 406.

Hart, I. and Colaco, C. (1997). Immunotherapy. Fusion induces tumour rejection. *Nature* **388**, 626–627.

Hawkins, C.J. and Vaux, D.L. (1997). The role of the Bcl-2 family of apoptosis regulatory proteins in the immune system. *Semin. Immunol.* **9**, 25–33.

Hermans, I.F., Daish, A., Moroni, Rawson, P. and Ronchese, F. (1997). Tumor-peptide-pulsed dendritic cells isolated from spleen or cultured in vitro from bone marrow precursors can provide protection against tumor challenge. *Cancer Immunol. Immunother.* **44**, 341–347.

Herrmann, M., Lorenz, H.M., Voll, R., Grunke, M., Woith, W. and Kalden, J.R. (1994). A rapid and simple method for the isolation of apoptotic DNA fragments. *Nucleic Acids Res.* **22**, 5506–5507.

Hieshima, K., Imai, T., Baba, M., Shoudai, K., Ishizuka, K., Nakagawa, T., Tsuruta, J., Takeya, M., Sakaki, Y., Takatsuki, K., Miura, R., Opdenakker, G., Van Damme, J., Yoshie, O. and Moniyama, H. (1997). A novel human CC chemokine PARC that is most homologous to macrophage-inflammatory protein-1 alpha/LD78 alpha and chemotactic for T lymphocytes, but not for monocytes. *J. Immunol.* **159**(3), 1140–1149.

Hooper, N.M., Karran, E.H. and Turner, A.J. (1997). Membrane protein secretases. *Biochem. J.* **321**, 265–279.

Hsu, F.J., Benike, C., Fagnoni, F., Liles, T.M., Czerwinski, D., Taidi, B., Engleman, E.G. and Levy R. (1996). Vaccination of patients with B-cell lymphoma using autologous antigen-pulsed dendritic cells. *Nature Medicine* **2**, 52–58.

Huang, A.Y.C., Golumbek, P., Ahmadzadeh, M., Jaffee, E., Pardoll, D. and Levitsky, H. (1994). Role of bone marrow-derived cells in presenting MHC class I-restricted tumor antigens. *Science* **264**, 961–965.

Hunter, O., Haluszczak, C., Subbotin, V.M., Lotze, M.T. and Shurin, M.R. (1997). Administration of IL-12 and FLT3 ligand enhances murine dendritic cell generation. *J. Immunother.* **20**, 401.

Imamichi, H., Zhang, Y.-M., Lane, H.C., Falloon, J. and Salzman, N.P. (1997). Continued evolution of HIV-1 during combination therapy despite levels of HIV-1 RNA <500 copies/ml. *International Workshop on HIV Drug Resistance, Treatment Strategies and Eradication, St. Petersburg, FL. 1997.* Abstract 63.

Inaba, K., Inaba, M., Deguchi, M., Hagi, K., Yasumizu, R., Ikehara, S., Muramatsu, S. and Steinman, R.M. (1993). Granulocytes, macrophages, and dendritic cells arise from a common major histocompatibility complex class II-negative progenitor in mouse bone marrow. *Proc. Natl Acad. Sci. USA* **90**, 3038–3042.

Itoh, T, Storkus, W.J., Gorelik, E. and Lotze, M.T. (1994). Partial purification of murine tumor-associated peptide epitopes common to histologically distinct tumors, melanoma and sarcoma, which are presented by H-$2K^b$ molecules and recognized by $CD8^+$ tumor infiltrating lymphocytes. *J. Immunol.* **153**, 1202–1215.

Jochmus, I., Osen, W., Altmann, A., Buck, G., Hofmann, B., Schneider, A., Gissman, L. and Rammensee, H.G. (1997). Specificity of human cytotoxic T lymphocytes induced by a human papillomavirus type 16 E7-derived peptide. *J. Gen. Virol.* **78**(Pt 7), 1689–1695.

Ju, S.T., Panka, D.J., Cui, H., Ettinger, R., El-Khatlb, M., Sherr, D.H., Stanger, B.Z. and Marshak-Rothstein, A.. (1995). Fas(CD95)/FasL interactions required for programmed cell death after T-cell activation. *Nature* **373**, 444–448.

Katz, S.I., Tamaki, K. and Sachs, D.H. (1979). Epidermal Langerhans cells are derived from cells originating in bone marrow. *Nature* **282**, 324–326.

Kawakami, Y., Eliyahu, S., Delgado, CH., Robbins, P.F., Sakkaguchi, K., Appella, E., Yanelli, J.R., Adema, G.J., Kimi, T. and Rosenberg, S.A. (1994a). Identification of melanoma antigens recognized by tumor infiltrating lymphocytes associated with in vivo tumor rejection. *Proc. Natl Acad. Sci. USA* **91**, 6458–6462.

Kawakami, Y., Eliyahu, S., Delgado, C.H., Robbins P.F., Rivoltini, L., Topalian, S.L., Miki, T. and Rosenberg, S.A. (1994b). Cloning of the gene coding for a shared human melanoma antigen recognized by autologous T cells infiltrating into tumor. *Proc. Natl Acad. Sci. USA* **91**, 3515–3519.

Kayagaki, N., Kawasaki, A., Ebata, T., Ohmoto, H., Ikeda, S., Inoue, S., Yoshino, K., Okumura, K. and Yagita, H. (1995). Metalloproteinase-mediated release of human Fas ligand. *J. Exp. Med.* **182**, 1777–1783.

Keane, M.M., Ettenberg, S.A., Lowrey, G.A., Russell, E.K. and Lipkowitz, S. (1998). Fas expression and function in normal and malignant breast cell lines. *Cancer Res.* **56**, 4791–4798.

Kiener, P.A., Davis, P.M., Rankin, B.M., Klebanoff, S.J., Ledbetter, J.A., Starling, G.C. and Liles, W.C. (1997). Human monocytic cells contain high levels of intracellular Fas ligand: rapid release following cellular activation. *J. Immunol.* **159**, 1594–1598.

Kim, C.J., Prevette, T., Cormier, J., Overwijk, W., Roden, M., Restifo, N.P., Rosenberg, S.A. and Marincola, F.M. (19970) Dendritic cells infected with poxviruses encoding MART1/Melan A sensitize T lymphocytes in vitro. *J. Immunother.* **20**(4), 276–286.

Kinzler, D., Tahara, H., Elder, E., Johnson, C., Nguyen, N., Hanan, S., Thomas, R., Vu, H., Duran, P., Kirkwood, J. and Lotze, M. (1997). Patient recruitment onto a Phase I clinical trial of Interleukin 12 (IL-12) gene therapy for cancer. *J. Immunother.* **20**, 400.

Kischkel, F.C., Hellbardt, S., Behrmann, I., Germer, M., Pawlita, M., Krammer, P.H. and Peter, M.E. (1995). Cytotoxicity-development APO-1 (Fas/CD95)-associated proteins form a death-inducing signaling complex (DISC) with the receptor. *EMBO J.* **14**, 5579–5588.

Klein, M.R., van Baalen, C.A., Holwerda, A.M., Kerkhof Garde, S.R., Bende, R.J., Keet, I.P., Eeftinck-Schattenkerk, J.K., Osterhaus, A.D., Schuitemaker, H. and Miedema, F. (1995). Kinetics of gag-specific cytotoxic T lymphocyte responses during the clinical course of HIV-1 infection: a longitudinal analysis of rapid progressors and long-term asymptomatics. *J. Exp. Med.* **181**, 1365–1372.

Koch, F., Stanzl, U., Jennewein, P., Janke, K., Heufler, C., Kämpgen, Romani N. and Schuler G. (1996). High level IL-12 production by murine dendritic cells: Upregulation via MHC class II and CD40 molecules and downregulation by IL-4 and IL-10. *J. Exp. Med.* **184**, 741–746.

Kundu, S.K., Engleman, E., Benike, C., Shapero, M.H., Dupuis, M., van Schooten, W., Eibl, M. and Merigan, T.C. (1998). A pilot clinical trial of HIV antigen pulsed allogeneic and autologous dendritic cell therapy in HIV-infected patients. *AIDS Res. Hum. Retrov.* **14**(7).

Latinis, K.M., Carr, L.L., Peterson, E.J., Norian, L.A., Eliason, S.L. and Koretzky, G.A. (1997). Regulation of CD95 (Fas) ligand expression by TCR-mediated signaling events. *J. Immunol.* **158**, 4602–4611.

Lau, H.T., Yu, M., Adriano, F., Stoeckert, J. and Christian, J. (1996). Prevention of islet allograft rejection with engineered myoblasts expressing FasL in mice. *Science* **273**, 109–112.

Leithauser, F., Dhein, J., Mechtersheimer, G., Koretz, K., Bruderlein, S., Henne, C., Schmidt, A., Debatin, K.M., Krammer, P.H. and Moller, P. (1993). Constitutive and induced expression of APO-1, a new member of the nerve growth factor/tumor necrosis factor receptor superfamily, in normal and neoplastic cells. *Lab. Invest.* **69**, 415–429.

Lotze, M.T. (1966a). Introduction. *Interleukin 12: Cellular and Molecular Immunology of an Important Regulatory Cytokine.* (eds. M.T. Lotze, G. Trinchieri, M.K. Gately, and S.F. Wolf). New York Academy of Sciences, New York. [*Proc. N.Y. Acad. Sci.* **795**, xiii–xix].

Lotze, M.T. (1996b). A new perspective: *Cytokine Gene Therapy of Cancer. Cancer J from Scientific American* **2**:63–72.

Lotze, M.T. (1997). Getting to the source: dendritic cells as therapeutic reagents for the treatment of patients with cancer. *Ann. Surg.* **226**(1): 1–5.

Lotze, M.T. and Finn, O.J. (1990). Current paradigms in cellular immunity: implications for immunity to cancer. *Immunol. Today* **11**, 190–193.

Lotze, M.T. and Finn, O.J. (1993). Cellular immunity and the immunotherapy of cancer. *J. Immunother.* **14**, 79–87.

Lotze, M.T, Shurin, M., Davis, I., Amoscato, A. and Storkus, W.J. (1997). Dendritic cell based therapy of cancer. *Adv. Exp. Med. Biol.* **417**, 551–569.

Lu, L., Woo, J., Rao, A.S., Li, Y. Watkins, S.C., Qian S., Starzl, T.E., Demetris, A.J. and Thomson, A.W. (1994). Propagation of dendritic cell progenitors from normal mouse liver using GM-CSF and their natural maturational development in the presence of type 1 collagen. *J. Exp. Med.* **179**, 1823–1834.

Lu, L., Hsieh, M., Oriss, T.B., Morel, P.A., Starzl, T.E., Rao, A.S. and Thomson, A.W. (1995). Generation of dendritic cells from mouse spleen cell cultures in response to GM-CSF: immunophenotypic and functional analyses. *Immunology.* **84**, 127–134.

Lu, L., Qian, S., Rudert, W.A., Hershberger, P.A., Lynch, D.H. and Thomson, A.W. (1997). Fas ligand (CD95L) and B7 expression on dendritic cells provide counter-regulatory signals for T cell survival and proliferation. *J. Immunol.* **158**, 5676–5684.

Lynch D.H. (1998). Induction of dendritic cells (DC) by Flt3 Ligand (FL) promotes the generation of tumor-specific immune responses in vivo. *Crit. Rev. Immunol.* **18**(1–2), 99–107.

Lynch, D.H., Ramsdell, F. and Alderson, M.R. (1995). Fas and FasL in the homeostatic regulation of immune responses. *Immunol. Today* **16**, 569.

Lynch, D.H., Andreasen, A., Maraskovsky, E., Whitmore, J., Miller, R.E. and Schuh, J.C. (1997). Flt3 ligand induces tumor regression and antitumor immune responses in vivo. *Nature Medicine* **3**(6), 625–631.

Maeurer, M.J., Martin, D.M., Storkus, W.J., Hurd, S. and Lotze, M.T. (1995a). Cytolytic T cell clones define HLA-A2 restricted human cutaneous melanoma peptide epitopes: Correlation with T cell receptor usage. *Cancer J.* **1**, 162-170.

Maeurer, M.J., Martin, D.M., Storkus, W.J. and Lotze, M.T. (1995b). TCR usage in CTLs recognizing melanoma/melanocyte antigens. *Immunol. Today* **16**, 603–604.

Maeurer, M.J., Martin, D., Elder, E., Storkus, W.J. and Lotze, M.T. (1966). Detection of naturally processed and HLA-A1 presented melanoma T-cell epitopes defined by GM-CSF release, but not by cytolysis. *Clin. Cancer Res.* **2**, 87–95.

Maraskovsky, E., Brasel, K., Teepe, K., Teepe, M., Roux, E.R,, Lyman. S.D., Shortman, K. and McKenna, H.J. (1996). Dramatic increases in the numbers of functionally mature dendritic cells in Flt3 ligand-treated mice: multiple dendritic cell subpopulations identified. *J. Exp. Med.* **184**, 1953–1962.

Mariani, S.M., Matiba, B., Baumler, C. and Krammer, P.H., (1995). Regulation of cell surface APO-1/Fas (CD95) ligand expression by metalloproteases. *Eur. J. Immunol.* **25**, 2303–2307.

Matiba, B., Mariani, S.M. and Krammer, P.H. (1997). The CD95 system and the death of a lymphocyte. *Semin. Immunol.* **9**, 59–68

Matzinger, P. (1991). The JAM test. A simple assay for DNA fragmentation and cell death. *J. Immunol. Methods* **145**, 185–192.

Mayordomo, J.I., Zorina, T., Storkus, W.J., Zitvogel, L., Celluzzi, C., Falo, L.D., Melief, C.J., Ildstad, S.T., Kast W.M., DeLeo A. and Lotze, M.T. (1995). Bone marrow-derived dendritic cells pulsed with synthetic tumour peptides elicit protective and therapeutic anti-tumour immunity. *Nature Medicine* **1**, 1297–1302.

Mayordomo, J.I, Loftus, D.J, Sakamoto, H., Lotze, M.T., Storkus, W.J., Appella, E. and DeLeo, AB. (1996a). Therapy of murine tumors with dendritic cells pulsed with p53 wild type and mutant sequence peptides. *J. Exp. Med.* **183**, 1357–1365.

Mayordomo, J.I., Zitvogel, L., Tjandrawan, T., Lotze, M.T. and Storkus, W.J. (1996b). Dendritic cells presenting tumor peptide epitopes stimulate effective anti-tumor CTL in vitro and in vivo. In: *Melanoma Biology: Experimental Therapies.* IOC Press, Amsterdam.

McArthur, J.G. and Mulligan, R.C. (1998). Induction of protective anti-tumor immunity by gene-modified dendritic cells. *J Immunother.* **21**(1), 41–47.

Mellors, J.W., Munoz, A., Giorgi, J.V., Margolick, J.B., Tassoni, C.J., Gupta, P., Kingsley, L.A., Todd, J.A., Saah, A.J., Detels, R., Dhair, J.P. and Rinaldo, C.R. (1997). Plasma viral load and $CD4^+$ lymphocytes as prognostic markers of HIV-1 infection. *Ann. Intern. Med.* **126**, 983–985.

Mohamadzadeh, M., Poltorak, A.N., Bergstresser, P.R. and Beutler, B., Takashima, A. (1996a). Dendritic cells produce macrophage inflammatory protein-1γ, a new member of the CC chemokine family. *J. Immunol.* **156**, 3102–3106.

Mohamadzadeh, M., Ariizumi, K., Sugamura, K., Bergstresser, P.R. and Takashima, A. (1996b). Expression of the common cytokine receptor gamma chain on murine dendritic cells including epidermal Langerhans cells. *Eur. J. Immunol.* **26**, 156–160.

Moller, P., Koretz, K., Leithauser, F., Bruderlein, .S, Henne, C., Quentmeier, A. and Krammer, P.H. (1994). Expression of APO-1 (CD95), a member of the NGF/TNF receptor superfamily, in normal and neoplastic colon epithelium. *Int. J. Cancer* **57**, 371–77.

Moretta, A. (1997). Molecular mechanisms in cell-mediated cytotoxicity. *Cell* **90**, 13–18.

Morse, M.A., Zhou, L.J., Tedder, T.F., Lyerly, H.K. and Smith, C. (1997). Generation of dendritic cells in vitro from peripheral blood mononuclear cells with granulocyte-macrophage-colony-stimulating factor, interleukin-4, and tumor necrosis factor-alpha for use in cancer immunotherapy. *Ann. Surg.* **226**(1), 6–16.

Mortarini, R., Anichini, A., Di Nicola, M., Siena, S., Bregni, M., Belli, F., Molla, A., Gianni, A.M. and Parmiani, G. (1997). Autologous dendritic cells derived from CD34$^+$ progenitors and from monocytes are not functionally equivalent antigen-presenting cells in the induction of melan-A/Mart-1(27-35)-specific CTLs from peripheral blood lymphocytes of melanoma patients with low frequency of CTL precursors. *Cancer Res.* **57**(24), 5534–5541.

Murphy, G., Tjoa, B., Ragde, H., Kenny, G.and Boynton, A. (1996). Phase I clinical trial: T-cell therapy for prostate cancer using autologous dendritic cells pulsed with HLA-A0201-specific peptides from prostate-specific membrane antigen. *Prostate* **29**(6), 371–380.

Muzio, M., Chinnaiyan, A.M., Kischkel, F.C., O Rouke, K., Shevchenko, A.N., Ni, J., Scaffidi, C., Bredtz, J.E., Zhang, M., Gentz, R., Mann, M., Krammer, P.H., Peter, M.E. and Dixit, V.M., (1996). FLICE, a novel FADD-homologous ICE/CED-3-like protease, is recruited to the CD95 (Fas/APO-1) death-inducing signaling complex. *Cell* **85**, 817–827.

Nagata, S. and Golstein, P. (1995). The Fas death factor. *Science* **267**, 1449–1456.

Nagata, S. and Suda, T. (1995). Fas, and Fas ligand: lpr and gld mutations. *Immunol. Today* **16**, 39–43.

Nair, S.K., Snyder, D., Rouse, B.T. and Gilboa, E. (1997). Regression of tumors in mice vaccinated with professional antigen-presenting cells pulsed with tumor extracts. *Int. J. Cancer* **70**(6), 706–715.

Nastala, C.N., Edington, H.D., McKinney, T.G., Tahara, H., Nalesnik, M., Brunda, M.J., Gately, K.K., Wolf, S.F., Schreiber, R., Storkus, W.J. and Lotze, M.T. (1994). Recombinant interleukin-12 (IL-12) administration induces tumor regression in association with interferon-γ production. *J. Immunol.* **153**, 1697–1706.

Navabi, H., Jasani, B., Adams, M., Evans, A.S., Mason, M., Crosby, T. and Borysiewicz, L. (1997). Generation of in vitro autologous human cytotoxic T-cell response to E7 and HER-2/neu oncogene products using ex-vivo peptide loaded dendritic cells. *Adv. Exp. Med. Biol.* **417**, 583–589.

Nestle, F.O., Alijagic, S., Gilliet, M., Sun, Y., Grabbe, S., Dummer, R., Burg, G. and Schadendorf, D. (1988). Vaccination of melanoma patients with peptide- or tumor lysate-pulsed dendritic cells. *Nature Medicine* **4**(3), 328–332.

Nicoletti, I., Migliorati, G., Pagliacci, M.C., Grignani, F. and Riccardi, C. (1991). A rapid and simple method for measuring thymocyte apoptosis by propidium iodide staining and flow cytometry. *J. Immunol. Methods* **139**, 271–279.

Niehans, G.A., Brunner, T., Frizelle, S.P., Liston, J.C., Salerno, C.T., Knapp, D.J., Green, D.R. and Kratzke, R.A. (1997). Human lung carcinomas express Fas ligand. *Cancer Res.* **57**, 1007–1012.

Nishioka, Y., Shurin, M., Robbins, P.D., Storkus, W.J., Lotze, M.T. and Tahara, H. (1997). Effective tumor immunotherapy using bone marrow-derived dendritic cells (DC)'s genetically engineered to express Interleukin 12. *J. Immunother.* **20**, 419.

Nishioka, Y., Robbins, P.D., Lotze, M.T. and Tahara, H. Induction of systemic and therapeutic antitumor immunity using intratumoral injection of bone marrow-derived dendritic cells genetically engineered to express interleukin-12 (IL-12). (Submitted for publication).

Numasaki, M., Lotze, M.T. and Tahara, H. (1997). Interleukin 17 gene transfection into murine fibrosarcoma cell line MCA 205 increases tumorigenicity correlated with enhanced tumor microvascularity. *J. Immunother.* **20**, 399.

O'Connell, J., O'Sullivan, G.C., Collins, J.K. and Shanahan, F. (1996). The Fas counterattack: Fas-mediated T cell killing by colon cancer cells expressing Fas ligand. *J. Exp. Med.* **184**, 1075–1082.

O'Connell, J., Bennett, M.W., O'Sullivan, G.C., Collins, J.K. and Shanahan, F. (1997). The Fas counterattack: a molecular mechanism of tumor immune privilege. *Mol. Med.* **3**, 294–300.

Ohshima, Y. and Delespesse, G. (1997). T cell-derived IL-4 and dendritic cell-derived IL-12 regulate the lymphokine-producing phenotype of alloantigen-primed naive human CD4 T cells. *J. Immunol.* **158**, 629–636.

Ossevoort, M.A., Kleijmeer, M.J., Nijman, H.W., Geuze, H.J., Kast, W.M. and Melief, C.J.M. (1995). Functional and ultrastructural aspects of antigen processing by dendritic cells. In: *Dendritic Cells in Fundamental and Clinical Immunology* (eds. J. Banchereau and D. Schmitt). Plenum Press, New York, pp. 227–231.

Oyama, T., Ran, S., Ishida, T., Nadaf, S., Kerr, L., Carbone, D.P. and Gabrilovich, D.I. (1998). Vascular endothelial growth factor affects dendritic cell maturation through the inhibition of nuclear factor-κB activation in hemopoietic progenitor cells. *J. Immunol.* **160**, 1224–1232.

Pantaleo, G., Menzo, S., Vaccarezza, M., Graziosi, C., Cohen, O.J., Demarest, J.F., Montefiori, D., Orenstein, J.M., Fox, C., Shrager, L.K., Margolick, J.B., Buchbinder, S., Giorgi, J.V. and Fauci, A.S.

(1995). Studies in subjects with long-term nonprogressive human immunodeficiency virus infection. *N. Engl. J. Med.* **332**, 209–216.

Peiper, M., Goedegebuure, P.S. and Eberlein, T.J. (1997). Generation of peptide-specific cytotoxic T lymphocytes using allogeneic dendritic cells capable of lysing human pancreatic cancer cells. *Surgery* **122**, 235–241.

Peron, J.M., Esche, C., Hunter, O., Subbotin, V.M., Lotze, M.T. and Shurin, M.R. (1997). Effective treatment of murine liver metastases using FLT3 ligand (FL) and IL-12. *J. Immunother.* **20**, 400.

Pinkus, G.S., Pinkus, J.L., Langhoff, E., Matsumura, F., Yamashiro, S., Mosialos, G. and Said, J.W. (1997). Fascin, a sensitive new marker for Reed-Sternberg cells of Hodgkin's disease. *Am. J. Pathol.* **150**, 543–562.

Porgador, A. and Gilboa, E. (1995). Bone marrow-generated dendritic cells pulsed with a class I-restricted peptide are potent inducers of cytotoxic T lymphocytes. *J. Exp. Med.* **182**, 255–260.

Puck, J.M. and Sneller, M.C. (1997). ALPS: an autoimmune human lymphoproliferative syndrome associated with abnormal lymphocyte apoptosis. *Semin. Immunol.* **9**, 77–84.

Qin, Z., Noffz, G., Mohaupt, M. and Blankenstein, T. (1997). Interleukin-10 prevents dendritic cell accumulation and vaccination with granulocyte-macrophage colony-stimulating factor gene-modified tumor cells. *J Immunol.* **159**(2), 770–776.

Reddy, A., Sapp, M., Feldman, M., Subklewe, M. and Bhardwaj, N. (1997). A monocyte conditioned medium is more effective than defined cytokines in mediating the terminal maturation of human dendritic cells. *Blood* **90**(9), 3640–3646.

Reeves, M.E., Royal, R.E., Lam, J.S., Rosenberg, S.A. and Hwu, P. (1996). Retroviral transduction of human dendritic cells with a tumor-associated antigen gene. *Cancer Res.* **56**(24), 5672–5677.

Reichert, T.E., Rabinowich, H., Johnson, J.T. and Whiteside, T.L. (in press) Human immune cells in the tumor microenvironment: mechanisms responsible for signaling and functional defects. *J. Immunother.*

Reis, S., Stahl, P.D. and Austin, J.M. (1993). Phagocytosis of antigens by Langerhans cells in vitro. *J. Exp. Med.* **178**, 509–519.

Ribas, A, Butterfield, L.H., McBride, W.H., Jiliani, S.M., Bui, L.A., Vollmer, C.M., Lau, R., Dissette, V.B., HU, B., Chen, A.Y., Glaspy, J.A. and Economou, J.S. (1997). Genetic immunization for the melanoma antigen MART1/MelanA using recombinant adenovirus-transduced murine dendritic cells. *Cancer Res.* **57**(14), 2865–2869.

Rinaldo, C.R., Huang, X.-L., Fan, Z., Ding, M., Beltz, A., Logar, A., Paniculi, D., Mazzara, G., Liebmann, J., Cottrill, M. and Gupta, P. (1995). High levels of anti-HIV-1 memory cytotoxic T lymphocytic activity and low viral load are associated with lack of disease in HIV-1-infected long-term nonprogressors. *J. Virol.* **69**, 5838–5842.

Robbins, P.F., El-Gamil, M., Kawakami, Y. and Rosenberg, S.A. (1994). Recognition of tyrosinase by tumor-infiltrating lymphocytes from a patient responding to immunotherapy. *Cancer Res.* **54**, 3124–3126.

Robinson, D., Shibuya, K., Mui, A., Zonin, F., Murphy, E., Sana, T., Hartley, S.B., Menon, S., Kastelein, R., Bazan, F. and O'Garra, A. (1997). IGIF does not drive Th1 development but synergizes with IL-12 for interferon-gamma production and activates IRAK and NFκB. *Immunity* **7**, 571–581.

Rodriguez, I., Katsuura, K., Ody, C., Nagata, S. and Vassalli, P. (1996). Systemic injection of a tripeptide inhibits the intracellular activation of CPP32-like proteases in vivo and fully protects mice against Fas-mediated fulminant liver destruction and death. *J. Exp. Med.* **184**, 2067–2072.

Romani, N., Koide, S., Crowley, M., Witmer-Pack, M., Livingstone, A., Fayhman, C.G., Inaba, K. and Steinman, R.M. (1989). Presentation of exogenous protein antigen by dendritic cells to T cell clones. Intact protein is presented best by immature, epidermal Langerhans cells. *J. Exp. Med.* **169**, 1169–1178.

Romani, N., Reider, D., Heuer, M., Ebner, S., Kampgen, E., Eibl, B., Niederwieser, D. and Schuler, G. (1996). Generation of mature dendritic cells from human blood. An improved method with special regard to clinical applicability. *J. Immunol. Methods* **196**(2), 137–151.

Romani, N., Gruner, S., Brang, D., Kampgen, E., Lenz, A., Trockenbacher, B., Konwalinka, G., Fritsch, P.O., Steinman, R.M. and Schuler, G. (1994). Proliferating dendritic cell progenitors in human blood. *J. Exp. Med.* **180**, 83–93.

Romani, N., Kampgen, E., Koch, F., Heufler, C. and Schuler, G. (1990). Dendritic cell production of cytokines and responses to cytokines. *Int. Rev. Immunol.* **6**, 151.

Rosenberg, E.S., Billingsley, J.M., Caliendo, A.M., Boswell, S.L., Sax, P.E., Kalams, S.A. and Walker, B.D. (1997). Vigorous HIV-1-specific CD4$^+$ T cell responses associated with control of viremia. *Science* **278**(5342), 1447–1450.

Rosenberg, S.A., Yang, J.C., Schwartzentruber, D.J., Hwu, P., Marincola, F.M., Topalian, S.L., Restifo, N.P., Dudley, M.E., Schwarz, S.L., Spiess, P.J., Wunderlich, J.R., Parkhurst, M.R., Kawakami, Y., Seipp, C.A., Einhorn, J.H. and White, D.E. (1998). Immunologic and therapeutic evaluation of a synthetic peptide vaccine for the treatment of patients with metastatic melanoma. *Nature Medicine* **4**(3), 321–327.

Saas, P., Walker, P.R., Hahne, M., Quiquerez, AL., Schnuriger, V., Perrin, G., French, L., Van Meir, E.G., de Tribolet, N., Tschopp, J. and Dietrich, P.Y. (1997). Fas ligand expression by astrocytoma in vivo: maintaining immune privilege in the brain? *J Clin. Invest.* **99**, 1173–1178.

Salgaller, M.L., Tjoa, B.A., Lodge, P.A., Ragde, H., Kenny, G., Boynton, A. and Murphy, G.P. (1998a). Dendritic cell-based immunotherapy of prostate cancer. *Crit. Rev. Immunol.* **18**(1–2), 109–119.

Salgaller, M.L., Lodge, P.A., McLean, J.G., Tjoa, B.A., Loftus, D.J., Ragde, H., Kenny, G.M., Rogers, M., Boynton, A.L. and Murphy, G.P. (1998b). Report of immune monitoring of prostate cancer patients undergoing T-cell therapy using dendritic cells pulsed with HLA-A2-specific peptides from prostate-specific membrane antigen (PSMA). *Prostate* **35**(2), 144–151.

Sallusto, F. and Lanzavecchia, A. (1994). Efficient presentation of soluble antigen by cultured human dendritic cells is maintained by granulocyte/macrophage colony-stimulating factor plus interleukin-4 and downregulated by tumor necrosis factor alpha. *J. Exp. Med.* **179**, 1109.

Sallusto, F., Cella, M., Danieli, C. and Lanzavecchia, A. (1995). Dendritic cells use macropinocytosis and the mannose receptor to concentrate macromolecules in the major histocompatibility complex class II compartment: Downregulation by cytokines and bacterial products. *J. Exp. Med.* **182**, 389–400.

Savary, C.A., Grazziutti, M.L., Melichar, B., Przepiorka, D., Freedman, R.S., Cowart, R.E., Cohen, D.M., Anaissie, E.J., Woodside, D.G., McIntyre, B.W., Pierson, D.L., Pellis, N.R. and Rex, J.H. (1988). Multi-dimensional flow-cytometric analysis of dendritic cells in peripheral blood of normal donors and cancer patients. *Cancer Immunol. Immunother.* **45**(5), 234–240.

Scheicher, C., Mehlig, M., Dienes, H.-P. and Reske, K. (1995). Uptake of microparticle-absorbed protein antigen by bone marrow-derived dendritic cells results in up-regulation of interleukin-1α and interleukin-12 p40/p35 and triggers prolonged, efficient antigen presentation. *Eur. J. Immunol.* **25**, 1566–1572.

Schuler, F. and Steinman, R.M. (1997). Dendritic cells as adjuvants for immune-mediated resistance to tumors. *J. Exp. Med.* **186**(8), 1183–1187.

Seino, K.-I., Kayagaki, N., Okumura, K. and Yagita, H. (1997). Antitumor effect of locally produced CD95 ligand. *Nature Medicine* **3**, 165–170.

Shafer, R.W., Winters, M.A., Palmer, S. and Merigan, T.C. (1998). Multiple concurrent reverse transcriptase and protease mutations and multidrug resistance of HIV-1 isolates from heavily treated patients. *Ann. Intern. Med.* **128**, 906–911.

Shima, Y., Nishimoto, N., Ogata, A., Fujii, Y., Yoshizaki, K. and Kishimoto, T. (1995). Myeloma cells express Fas antigen/APO-1 (CD95) but only some are sensitive to anti-Fas antibody resulting in apoptosis. *Blood* **85**, 757–764.

Shiraki, K., Tsuji, N., Shioda, T., Isselbacher, K.J. and Takahashi, H. (1997). Expression of Fas ligand in liver metastases of human colonic adenocarcinomas. *Proc. Natl Acad. Sci. USA* **94**, 6420–6425.

Shurin, M.R., Pandharipande, P.P., Zorina, T.D., Haluszczak, C., Subbotin, V.M., Hunter, O., Brumfield, A., Storkus, W.J., Maraskovsky, E. and Lotze, M.T. (1997a). FLT3 ligand induces the generation of functionally active dendritic cells in mice. *Cell Immunol.* **179**(2), 174–184.

Shurin, G.V., Esway, J., Subbotin, V.M., Lotze, M.T. and Barksdale, E.M. (1997b). Functional Fas ligand is expressed on neuroblastoma cells. *J. Immunother.* **20**, 403.

Shurin, M.R., Esche, C., Lokshin, A. and Lotze, M.T. (1997c). Tumors induce apoptosis of dendritic cells in vitro. *J. Immunother.* **20**, 403.

Smith, M.C., Pendelton, C.D., Maher, V.E., Kelley, M.J., Carbone, D.P. and Berzofsky, J.A.. (1997). Oncogenic mutations in ras create HLA-A2.1 binding peptides but affect their extracellular antigen processing. *Int. Immunol.* **9**(8), 1085–1093.

Song, W., Kong, H.L., Carpenter, H., Torii, H., Granstein, R., Rafii, S., Moore, M.A. and Crystal, R.G. (1997). Dendritic cells genetically modified with an adenovirus vector encoding the cDNA for a model antigen induce protective and therapeutic antitumor immunity. *J. Exp. Med.* **186**(8), 1247–1256.

Sorg, U.R., Morse, T.M., Patton, W.N., Hock, B.D., Angus, H.B., Robinson, B.A., Colls, B.M. and Hart, D.N. (1997). Hodgkin's cells express CD83, a dendritic cell lineage associated antigen. *Pathology* **29**(3), 294–299.

Specht, J.M., Wang, G., Do, M.T., Lam, J.S., Royal, R.E., Reeves, M.E., Rosenberg, S.A. and Hwu, P. (1997). Dendritic cells retrovirally transduced with a model antigen gene are therapeutically effective against established pulmonary metastases. *J. Exp. Med.* **186**, 1213–1221.

Steinman, R.M. (1991). The dendritic cell system and its role in immunogenicity. *Annun. Rev. Immunol.* **9**, 271-296.

Steinman, R. and Cohn, Z.A. (1973). Identification of a novel cell type in peripheral lymphoid organs of mice. I. Morphology, quantitation, tissue distribution. *J. Exp. Med.* **137**, 1142–1162.

Steptoe, R.J. and Thomson, A.W. (1996). Dendritic cells and tolerance induction. *Clin. Exp. Immunol.* **105**, 397–402.

Stingl, G. and Bergstresser, P.R. (1993). Dendritic cells: a major story unfolds. *Immunol. Today* **16**, 330–333.

Storkus, W.J., Zeh III, H.J., Salter, R.D. and Lotze, M.T. (1993a). Identification of T cell epitopes: rapid isolation of class I-presented peptides from viable cells by mild acid elution. *J Immunother.* **14**, 94–103.

Storkus, W.J., Zeh III, H.J., Salter, R.D. and Lotze, M.T. (1993b). Isolation of human melanoma peptides recognized by class I restricted tumor infiltrating T lymphocytes. *J. Immunol.* **151**, 3719–3727.

Strand, S., Hofmann, W.J., Hug, H., Müller, M., Otto, G., Strand, D., Mariani, S.M., Stremmel, W., Krammer, P.H. and Galle, P.R. (1996). Lymphocyte apoptosis induced by CD95 (APO-1/Fas) ligand-expressing tumor cells—a mechanism of immune evasion? *Nature Medicine* **2**, 1361–1366.

Strobl, H., Riedl, E., Scheinecker, C., Bello-Fernandez, C., Pickl, W.F., Rappersberger, K., Majdic, O. and Knapp, W. (1996). TGF-β1 promotes in vitro development of dendritic cells from CD34$^+$ hemopoietic progenitors. *J. Immunol.* **157**, 1499–1507.

Stuber, G., Leder, G., Storkus, W.J., Lotze, M.T., Modrow, S., Klein, E., Karre, K. and Klein, G. (1994). Identification of wild-type and mutant p53 peptides capable of binding to HLA-A2 class I molecules assessed by the T2 stabilization assay and a novel class I reconstitution assay. *Eur. J. Immunol.* **24**, 765–768.

Szabolcs, P., Moore, M.A.S. and Young, J.W. (1995). Expansion of immunostimulatory dendritic cells among the myeloid progeny of human CD34$^+$ bone marrow precursors cultured with c-*kit* ligand, granulocyte-macrophage colony-stimulating factors, and TNF-α *J. Immunol.* **154**, 5851–5861.

Tahara, H., Zeh, H.J., Storkus, W.J., Pappo, I., Watkins, S.C., Gubler, U., Wolf, S.F., Robbins, P.D. and Lotze, M.T. (1994). Fibroblasts genetically engineered to secrete interleukin 12 can suppress tumor growth and induce antitumor activity to a murine melanoma in vivo. *Cancer Res.* **54**, 182–189.

Tahara, H., Zitvogel, L., Storkus, W.J., Zeh, H.J., III, McKinney, T.G., Schreiber, R.D., Gubler, U., Robbins, P.D. and Lotze, M.T. (1995). Effective eradication of established murine tumors with interleukin 12 (IL-12) gene therapy using a polycistronic retroviral vector. *J. Immunol.* **154**, 6466–6474.

Tahara, H., Zitvogel, L., Storkus, W.J., Elder, E.M., Kinzler, D., Whiteside, T.L., Robbins, P.D. and Lotze, M.T. (1997). Antitumor effects in patients with melanoma, head and neck and breast cancer in a phase I/II clinical trial of interleukin-12 (IL-12) gene therapy. *Proc. ASCO* **16**, 438a (1568).

Tanaka, M., Suda, T., Takahashi, T. and Nagata, S. (1995). Expression of the functional soluble form of human fas ligand in activated lymphocytes. *EMBO J* **14**, 1129–1135.

Tanaka, M., Suda, T., Haze, K., Nakamura, N., Sato, K., Kimura, F., Motoyoshi, K., Mizuki, M., Tagawa, S., Ohga, S., Hatake, K., Drummond, A.H. and Nagata, S. (1996) Fas ligand in human serum. *Nature Medicine* **2**, 317–322.

Tanguay, S. and Killion, J.J. (1994). Direct comparison of ELISPOT and ELISA-based assays for detection of individual cytokine-secreting cells. *Lymphokine Cytokine Res.* **1994**, 259–263.

Tarte, K., Lu, Z.Y., Fiol, G., Legouffe, E., Rossi, J.F. and Klein, B. (1997). Generation of virtually pure and potentially proliferating dendritic cells from non-CD34 apheresis cells from patients with multiple myeloma. *Blood* **90**(9), 3482–3495.

Tazi, A., Bouchonnet, F., Grandsaigne, M., Boumsell, L., Hance, A.J. and Soler, P. (1993). Evidence that granulocyte macrophage-colony-stimulating factor regulates the distribution and differentiated state of dendritic cells/Langerhans cells in human lung and lung cancers. *J. Clin. Invest.* **91**, 566–576.

Thome, M., Schneider, P., Hofmann, K., Fickenscher, H., Meinl, E., Neipel, F., Mattmann, C., Burns, K., Bodmer, J.L., Schroter, M., Scaffidi, C., Krammer, P.H., Peter, M.E. and Tschopp. (1997). Viral FLICE-inhibitory proteins (FLIPs) prevent apoptosis induced by death receptors. *Nature* **386**, 517–521.

Thurnher, M., Klocker, H., Papesh, C., Ramoner, R., Radmayr, C., Hobisch, A., Gastl, G., Romani, N., Ebner, S., Bock, G. and Bartsch, G. (1997a). Dendritic cells for the immunotherapy of renal cell carcinoma. *Urol. Int.* **59** 1–5.

Thurnher, M., Ramoner, R., Gastl, G., Radmayr, C., Böck, G., Herold, M., Klocker, H. and Bartsch, G. (1997b). Bacillus Calmette-Guérin mycobacteria stimulate human blood dendritic cells. *Int. J. Cancer* **70**, 128–134.

Tjandrawan, T., Martin, D.M., Maeurer, M.J., Castelli, C., Lotze, M.T. and Storkus, W.J. (1998). Autologous human dendriphages pulsed with synthetic or natural tumor peptides elicit tumor-specific CTLs in vitro. *J Immunother.* **21**(2), 149–157.

Tjoa, B., Erickson, S., Barren, R. 3rd., Ragde, H., Kenny, G., Boynton, A. and Murphy, G. (1995). In vitro propagated dendritic cells from prostate cancer patients as a component of prostate cancer immunotherapy. *Prostate* **27**(2), 63–69.

Tjoa, B., Boynton, A., Kenny, G., Ragde, H., Misrock, S.L. and Murphy, G. (1996). Presentation of prostate tumor antigens by dendritic cells stimulates T-cell proliferation and cytotoxicity. *Prostate* **28**(1), 65–69.

Tjoa, B.A., Erickson, S.J., Bowes, V.A., Ragde, H., Kenny, G.M., Cobb, O.E. and Ireton, R.C., Troychak, M.J., Boynton, A.L. and Murphy, G.P. (1997). Followup evaluation of prostate cancer patients infused with autologous dendritic cells pulsed with PSMA peptides. *Prostate* **32**(4), 272–278.

Toes, R.E.M., Blom, R.J.J., Offringa, R., Kast, W.M. and Melief, C.J.M. (1996). Enhanced tumor outgrowth after peptide vaccination. Functional deletion of tumor-specific CTL induced by peptide vaccination can lead to the inability to reject tumors. *J. Immunol.* **156**, 3911–3918.

Trauth, B.C., Klas, C., Peters, A.M., Matzku, S., Moller, P., Falk, W., Debatin, K.M. and Krammer, P.H. (1989). Monoclonal antibody-mediated tumor regression by induction of apoptosis. *Science* **245**, 301–305.

Traversari, C., van der Bruggen, P., Luescher, I.F. et al. (1992). A nonapeptide encoded by human gene MAGE-1 is recognized on HLA-A1 by cytolytic T-lymphocytes directed against tumour antigen MZ2-E. *J. Exp. Med.* **176**, 1453–1458.

Tsai, V., Southwood, S., Sidney, J., Sakaguchi, K., Kawakami, Y., Appella, E., Sette, A. and Celis E. (1997). Identification of subdominant CTL epitopes of the gp100 melanoma-associated tumor antigen by primary in vitro immunization with peptide-pulsed dendritic cells. *J. Immunol.* **158**(4), 1796–1802.

Tüting, T., DeLeo, A.B., Lotze, M.T. and Storkus, W.J. (1997a). Genetically modified bone marrow-derived dendritic cells expressing tumor-associated viral or "self" antigens induce antitumor immunity in vivo. *Eur. J. Immunol.* **27**(10), 2702–2707.

Tüting, T., Storkus, W.J. and Lotze, M.T. (1997b). Gene-based strategies for the immunotherapy of cancer. *J. Mol. Med.* **75**(7), 478–491.

Tüting, T., Zorina, T., Ma, D.I., Wilson, C.C., De Cesare, C.M., De Leo, A.B., Lotze, M.T. and Storkus, W.J. (1997c). Development of dendritic cell-based genetic vaccines for cancer. *Adv. Exp. Med. Biol.* **417**, 511–518.

Tüting, T., Baar, J., Gambotto, A., David, I.D., Storkus, W.J., Zavodny, P., Narula, S., Tahara, H., Robbins, P.D. and Lotze, M.T. (1997d). Inteferon-α gene therapy for cancer: retroviral transduction of fibroblast and particle-mediated transfection of tumor cells are equally effective strategies for gene delivery in murine tumor models. *Gene Ther.* **4**, 1053–1060.

Tüting, T., Wilson, A., Marman, D.M., Kasamon, Y.L., Rowles, J., Ma, D.I., Slingluff, D.L. Jr., Wagner, S.N., Van der Bruggen, P., Baar, J., Lotze, M.T. and Storkus, W.J. (1998). Autologous human-derived dendritic cells genetically modified to express melanoma antigens elicit primary cytotoxic T cell responses in vitro: enhancement by cotransfecting of genes encoding the T_H1 biasing cytokines IL-12 and IFNα. *J. Immunol.* **160**, 1139–1147.

van Schooten, W.C., Strang, G. and Palathumpat, V. (1997). Biological properties of dendritic cells: implications to their use in the treatment of cancer. *Mol. Med. Today* **3**(6), 254–260.

Van den Eynde, B., Peeters, O., De Backer, O., Gaugler, B., Lucas, S. and Boon, T. (1995). A new family of genes coding for an antigen recognized by cytolytic T lymphocytes on a human melanoma. *J. Exp. Med.* **182**, 689–698.

Van der Bruggen, P., Traversari, C., Chomez, P., Lurquin, C., De Plaen, E., Van Den Eynde, B., Knuth, A. and Boon, T. (1991). A gene encoding an antigen recognized by cytolytic T lymphocytes on a human melanoma. *Science* **254**, 1643-1047.

Van der Bruggen, P., Szikora, J.-P., Boel, P., Wildmann, C., Somville, M., Sensi, M. and Boon, T. (1994a). Autologous cytolytic T lymphocytes recognize a MAGE-1 nonapeptide on melanomas expressing HLA-Cw*16018. *Eur. J. Immunol.* **24**, 2134–2140.

Van der Bruggen, P., Bastin, J., Gajewski, T., Coulie, P.G., Boel, P., De Smet, C., Traversari, C., Townsend, A. and Boon, T. (1994b). A peptide encoded by human gene MAGE-3 and presented by HLA-A2 induces cytolytic T lymphocytes that recognize tumor cells expressing MAGE-3. *Eur. J. Immunol.* **24**, 3038–3043.

Vial, P.A., Liegmann, K., Noriega, L.M., Vial, C., Acuna, G., Marcotti, A., Palacios, O. and Bean, P. (1997). HIV-1 pol genotyping by DNA sequencing in patients with triple combination antiretroviral treatment in whom viral load remains high after 6 months of therapy. *International Workshop on HIV Drug Resistance, Treatment Strategies and Eradication, St. Petersburg, FL. 1997.* Abstract 1997.

Walker, P.R., Saas, P. and Dietrich, P.Y. (1997). Role of Fas ligand (CD95L) in immune escape: the tumor cell strikes back. *J. Immunol.* **158**, 4521–4524.

Wan, Y., Bramson, J., Carter, R., Graham, F. and Gauldie, J. (1997). Dendritic cells transduced with an adenoviral vector encoding a model tumor-associated antigen for tumor vaccination. *Hum. Gene Ther.* **8**, 1355–1363.

Wang, R.-F., Robbins, P.F., Kawakami, Y., Kang, X.-Q. and Rosenberg, S.A. (1995). Identification of a gene encoding a melanoma tumor antigen recognized by HLA-A31-restricted tumor-infiltrating lymphocytes. *J. Exp. Med.* **181**, 799–804.

Watson, G.A. and Lopez, D.M. (1995). Aberrant antigen presentation by macrophages from tumor-bearing mice is involved in the down-regulation of their T cell responses. *J. Immunol.* **155**, 3124–3134.

Weih, F., Carrasco, D., Durham, S.K., Barton, D.S., Rizzo, C.A., Ryseck, R.-P., Lira, S.A. and Bravo, R. (1995). Mutiorgan inflammation and hematopoietic abnormalities in mice with a targeted disruption of RelB, a member of the NF-κB/Rel family. *Cell* **80**, 331–340.

Weiner, G.J., Liu, Wooldridge, J.E., Dahle, C.E. and Krieg, A.M. (1997). Immunostimulatory oligodeoxynucleotides containing the CpG motif are effective as immune adjuvants in tumor antigen immunization. *Proc. Natl Acad. Sci. USA* **94**, 10833–10837.

Wilson Cara, C., Tueting, T., Ma, D.I., Haluszczak, C., Lotze, M. and Storkus, W. (1997). Activation of dendritic cells by surrogate T cell interactions leads to enhanced costimulation, secretion of TH1-associated cytokines, and CTL inductive capacity. In: *Procedings of the IV International Symposium on Dendritic Cells in Fundamental and Clinical Immunology* (Vol 3). (ed. P. Ricciardi-Castagnoli). Plenum Press, New York.

Winzler, C., Rovere, P., Rescigno, M., Granucci, F., Penna, G., Adorini, L., Zimmermann, V.S., Davoust, J. and Ricciardi-Castagnoli, P. (1997). Maturation stages of mouse dendritic cells in growth factor-dependent long-term cultures. *J. Exp. Med.* **185**, 317–328.

Wolfel, T., Van Pel, A., Brichard, V., Schneider, J., Seliger, B., Meyer zum Buschenfelde K.-H. and Boon, T. (1994). Two tyrosinase nonapeptides recognized on HLA-A2 melanomas by autologous cytolytic T lymphocytes. *Eur. J. Immunol.* **24**, 759–764.

Wong, B.R., Josien, R., Lee, S.Y., Sauter, B., Li, H.L., Steinman, R.M. and Choi, Y. (1997). TRANCE (tumor necrosis factor [TNF]-related activation-induced cytokine), a new TNF family member predominantly expressed in T cells, is a dendritic cell-specific survival factor. *J. Exp. Med.* **186**, 2075–2080.

Yang, S., Darrow, T.L., Vervaert, C.E. and Seigler, H.F. (1997). Immunotherapeutic potential of tumor antigen-pulsed and unpulsed dendritic cells generated from murine bone marrow. *Cell. Immunol.* **179**(1), 84–95.

Yang, Y., Minucci, S., Ozato, K., Heyman, R.A. and Ashwell, J.D. (1995). Efficient inhibition of activation-induced Fas ligand up-regulation and T cell apoptosis by retinoids requires occupancy of both retinoid X receptors and retinoic acid receptors. *J. Biol. Chem.* **270**, 18672–18677.

Yano, H., Fukuda, K., Haramaki, M., Momosaki, S., Ogasawara, S., Higaki, K. and Kojiro, M. (1996). Expression of Fas and anti-Fas-mediated apoptosis in human hepatocellular carcinoma cell lines. *J. Hepatol.* **25**, 454–464.

Young, B., Johnson, S., Bakhtiari, M., Shugarts, D., Young, R., Allen, M. and Kuritzkes, D. (1997).Genotypic analysis of HIV-1 protease from patients failing highly active antiretroviral therapy: preliminary analysis. *International Workshop on HIV Drug Resistance, Treatment Strategies and Eradication, St. Petersburg, FL. 1997.* Abstract 65.

Young, J.W. and Inaba, K. (1996). Dendritic cells as adjuvants for Class I major histocompatibility complex-restricted antitumor immunity. *J. Exp. Med.* **183**, 7–11.

Zakut, R., Topalian, S.L., Kawakami, Y., Mancini, M., Eliyahu, S. and Rosenberg, S.A. (1993). Differential expression of MAGE-1, -2, -3 messenger RNA in transformed and normal cell lines. *Cancer Res.* **53**, 54–47.

Zeh, H.J., Hurd, S., Storkus, W.J. and Lotze, M.T. (1993). Interleukin 12 promotes the proliferation and cytolytic maturation of immune effectors: implications for the immunotherapy of cancer. *J. Immunother.* **14**, 155–161.

Zeh, H.J. III, Salter, R.D., Lotze, M.T. and Storkus, W.J. (1994). Flow cytometric determination of peptide-class I complex formation. *Hum. Immunol.* **39**, 79-86.

Zeh, H.J., Tahara, H. and Lotze, M.T. (1995). Interleukin-12. In: *Cytokine Handbook* (ed. A. Thomson). Academic Press, London.

Zeytun, A., Hassuneh, M., Nagarkatti, M. and Nagarkatti, P.S. (1997). Fas–Fas ligand-based interactions between tumor cells and tumor-specific cytotoxic T lymphocytes: a lethal two-way street. *Blood* **90**, 1952–1959.

Zhou, L.-J. and Tedder, T.F. (1995a). Human blood dendritic cells selectively express CD83, a member of the immunoglobulin superfamily. *J. Immunol.* **154**, 3821–3835.

Zhou, L.-J. and Tedder, T.F. (1995b). A distinct pattern of cytokine gene expression by human CD83$^+$ blood dendritic cells. *Blood* **86**, 3295–3301.

Zitvogel, L., Tahara, H.T., Robbins, P.D., Storkus, W.J., Clarke, M.R., Nalesnik, M.A. and Lotze, M.T. (1995). Cancer immunotherapy of established tumors with interleukin-12 (IL-12): effective delivery by genetically engineering fibroblasts. *J. Immunol.* **155**, 1393–1403.

Zitvogel, L., Couderc, B., Mayordomo, J.I., Robbins, P.D., Lotze, M.T. and Storkus, W.J. (1996a). IL-12-engineered dendritic cells serve as effective tumor vaccine adjuvants *in vivo*. In: *Interleukin 12: Cellular and Molecular Immunology of an Important Regulatory Cytokine.* (ed. M.T. Lotze, G. Trinchieri, M.K. Gately and S.F. Wolf). New York Academy of Sciences, New York. [*Proc. N.Y. Acad. Sci.* **795**, 284–293.]

Zitvogel, L., Robbins, P.F., Clarke, M.R., Abe, R., Davis, C.G., Storkus, W.J. and Lotze, M.T. (1996b). B7.1 costimulation markedly enhances IL-12 mediated antitumor immunity *in vivo*. *Eur. J. Immunol.* **26**, 1335–1341.

Zitvogel, L., Mayordomo, J.I., Tjandrawan, T., DeLeo, A.B., Clarke, M.R., Lotze, M.T. and Storkus, W.J. (1996c). Therapy of murine tumors with tumor peptide pulsed dendritic cells: dependence on T-cells, B7 costimulation, and Th1-associated cytokines. *J. Exp. Med.* **183**, 87–98.

Zitvogel, L., Le Cesne, A., Cordier, L., Lotze, M.T., Escudier, B., Haddada, H., Tursz, T. and Kourilsky, F. (1996d). Specific active immunotherapy for cancer. gene or dendritic cell-based tumor vaccines. In: *Sourcebook on Asbestos Diseases*, (ed. vol 13). G.A. and B.J. Peters), The Michie Company/ Butterworth, Borough Green.

CHAPTER 26
Dendritic Cell Tolerogenicity and Prospects for Dendritic Cell-based Therapy of Allograft Rejection and Autoimmunity

Lina Lu[1,2], Samia J. Khoury[4], Mohamed H. Sayegh[5] and Angus W. Thomson[1,2,3]

[1]Thomas E. Starzl Transplantation Institute, and Departments of [2]Surgery and [3]Molecular Genetics and Biochemistry, University of Pittsburgh, Pittsburgh, Pennsylvania, USA; [4]Center for Neurologic Diseases and [5]Laboratory of Immunogenetics and Transplantation, Brigham and Women's Hospital, Harvard Medical School, Boston, Massachusetts, USA

> Emerging evidence points towards a role for DCs in tolerance, and it will therefore be imperative to pursue DCs more vigourously in allergy, transplantation and autoimmunity.
>
> Jacques Banchereau and Ralph M. Steinman (1998). *Nature* **392**, 245–252

INTRODUCTION

Other chapters in this book have reviewed extensively the properties of immunostimulatory dendritic cells (DC). Extensive recent studies that have improved our understanding of DC lineage development, differentiation, activation, and function, have revealed that myeloid DC progenitors (Thomson *et al.*, 1995a), lymphoid DC (Süss and Shortman, 1996), and even 'classic' myeloid DC (Inaba *et al.*, 1997) have potential to exhibit tolerogenic activity (see also reviews by Steptoe and Thomson, 1996; and Ni and O'Neill, 1997). This is manifested by suppression of T cell responses in models of T cell ontogeny, transplant rejection, tumors and autoimmunity. Several agents, e.g. IL-10, transforming growth factor-β (TGF-β) or the chimeric fusion protein cytotoxic T lymphocyte antigen 4 (CTLA4)-Ig can render DC tolerogenic. In addition, genetically engineered DC expressing immunosuppressive molecules, such as viral (v)IL-10 or TGF-β may offer potential for the 'silencing' of alloantigen- or autoantigen-specific T cells, with implications for tolerance induction.

The concept of tolerogenic DC is not new. Indeed, a role for DC in central tolerance induction was recognized initially in the context of self-tolerance within the thymus

Dendritic Cells: Biology and Clinical Applications
ISBN 0-12-455860-7

(Jenkinson *et al.*, 1985; Matzinger and Guerder, 1989). DC were shown subsequently to be able to induce peripheral, antigen-specific unresponsiveness in certain experimental models, or implicated as having a role in self-tolerance. Thus, DC lacking sufficient cell surface expression of costimulatory molecules, in particular CD80 (B7-1) and CD86 (B7-2), can induce alloantigen-specific anergy *in vitro* (Lu *et al.*, 1995a), and prolong donor-specific survival of heart or pancreatic islet cell allografts in non-immunosuppressed hosts. The cytokines IL-10 and TGF-β can downregulate costimulatory molecule or major histocompatibility complex (MHC) class II antigen expression on DC, such that the proliferation of $CD4^+$ T helper cells and the cytotoxic activity of $CD8^+$ T cells induced by these DC is clearly inhibited (Moore *et al.*, 1993; Caux *et al.*, 1994a). In addition, it has been reported recently that either lymphoid (Süss and Shortman, 1996) or myeloid DC that express Fas ligand (CD95 L) (Lu *et al.*, 1997b) can induce programmed cell death (apoptosis) in alloactivated T cells.

DC AND TOLERANCE INDUCTION

Tolerance is a fundamental property of the immune system and underlies selective unresponsiveness to self-autoantigens. It is the ultimate goal of transplant immunologists seeking permanent, drug-free, donor alloantigen-specific immunological unresponsiveness in humans, and of those seeking to restore tolerance to the autoantigens implicated in the pathogenesis of autoimmune diseases. The principal mechanisms by which tolerance is thought to be induced and maintained are clonal deletion, anergy, and suppression by regulatory cells. One of the principal determining factors in these processes is the function of the antigen-presenting cells (APC) that is critical in the initiation of the primary immune response. DC can present antigen in either a tolerogenic or immunogenic fashion (Finkelman *et al.*, 1996) depending on the inoculation regimen used. Evidence has accumulated from a variety of studies that DC may play a key role in determining the balance between tolerance and immunity (Thomson *et al.*, 1996). Upsetting this balance, for example, as the result of striking augmentation of functional DC in transplanted organs by donor treatment with Flt-3 ligand, can switch tolerance to rejection (Steptoe *et al.*, 1997). Observations of the tolerogenic capacity of DC in many diverse experimental systems are summarized in Table 1 and include reports of a role for DC both in central and peripheral tolerance.

DC have consistently been identified as prominent donor cells in the multilineage hematopoietic cell microchimerism that is observed in long-surviving rodent and human organ allograft recipients (Demetris *et al.*, 1993; Qian *et al.*, 1994; Starzl *et al.*, 1992; Starzl *et al.*, 1993; Starzl *et al.*, 1996), whether or not immunosuppressive therapy is used to promote graft survival. This finding, together with the well-known properties of DC as highly effective APC (Steinman, 1991), prompted our investigation of the significance and possible mechanistic role of donor-derived DC in organ transplant tolerance.

Compared with the heart or kidney, the liver is comparatively rich in DC, yet is generally regarded as the least immunogenic of transplanted whole organs. In the mouse, liver transplant tolerance is achieved in virtually all MHC-incompatible mouse strain combinations without the need for immunosuppression (Qian *et al.*, 1994). Using techniques established to propagate DC progenitors from normal mouse liver (Lu *et al.*, 1994), it was found that DC progenitors of donor origin could be propagated from the bone marrow of mice that spontaneously accepted

Table 1. Observations of the tolerogenic capacity of dendritic cells (DC)

Dendritic cell type	Tolerogenic effect reported	Reference
Thymic DC	Encephalitogen pulsing and adoptive transfer prevents EAE.[a]	Khoury *et al.* (1995)
	Tolerance acquired to host MHC in chimeric thymuses.	Jenkinson *et al.* (1985)
Langerhans cells	Deletion enhances effector phase of CH.[b]	Grabbe *et al.* (1995)
Pancreatic lymph node DC	Transfer reduces incidence of diabetes in NOD[c] mice *in vivo.*	Clare-Salzler *et al.* (1992)
Splenic DC	Reconstitution of DC-depleted thymuses restores ability to delete thymocytes *in vivo.*	Matzinger and Guerder (1989)
	Large numbers of DC reduce local HVG[d] reaction *in vivo.*	Knight *et al.* (1983)
	Large numbers of DC/high antigen load inhibit antitumor immunity.	Knight *et al.* (1985)
	$CD8^+$/$Fas\text{-}L^+$ DC induce apoptosis in activated T cells *in vitro.*	Süss and Shortman (1996)
	$CD8^+$ deregulates the response of naive CD8 T cells by limiting their IL-2 production.	Kronin *et al.* (1996)
Costimulator-deficient DC progenitors	Induction of alloantigen-specific unresponsiveness *in vitro.*	Lu *et al.* (1996)
	Adoptive transfer prolongs allograft survival.	Fu *et al.* (1996) Rastelliniet *al.* (1995)
Renal interstitial DC	Discordant expression of MHC class II and invariant chain may be a regulatory mechanism for peripheral T cell tolerance.	Saleem *et al.* (1997)
Cervical lymph node DC	Adoptive transfer delays the onset of lymphocytic thyroiditis.	Delemarre *et al.* (1995)
Mouse DC	Injection of rat anti-DC mAbs induces rat Ig-specific tolerance.	Finkelman *et al.* (1996)
Mouse DC	Induction of T cell anergy by tumor-associated antigen.	Grohmann *et al.* (1997)

[a]Experimental allergic encephalomyelitis.
[b]Contact hypersensitivity.
[c]Nonobese diabetic.
[d]Host versus graft.

MHC-mismatched liver allografts. Donor-derived DC could not, however, be propagated from the marrow of mice that acutely rejected heart grafts from the same donor strain (Lu *et al.*, 1995b; Thomson *et al.*, 1995c) (Fig. 1). Donor-derived DC progenitors can also be propagated from the blood of human liver allograft recipients given adjunctive donor bone marrow (Thomson *et al.*, 1995a; Rugeles *et al.*, 1997). This suggests that allogeneic DC might play a role in the induction of allotolerance, rather than simply be a consequence of it. Evidence from recent immunohistochemical studies of Demetris *et al.* (1997) further suggests that persistence of donor-derived DC may be important in the long-term maintenance of transplantation tolerance and the prevention of (chronic) organ allograft rejection.

Central Tolerance Induced by DC

The thymus plays a major role in immune homeostasis by the deletion of self-reactive T cells, thus contributing to the maintenance of self-tolerance. A number of cell types

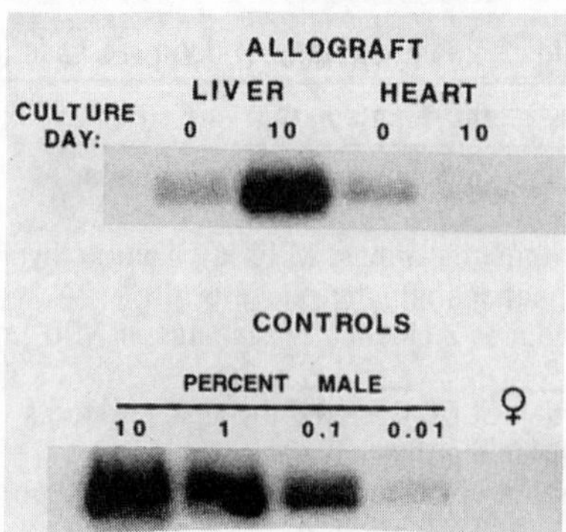

Fig. 1. Microchimerism in the bone marrow. Detection of the donor Y chromosome in freshly isolated (day 0) and 10-day cultured bone marrow cells from female (C3H) recipients of male (B10) livers or hearts. The animals were sacrificed 14 days or 8 days, respectively, after transplantation. In this strain combination, liver allografts are accepted spontaneously, whereas heart grafts are rejected with a median survival time of 8 days. Growth of donor-derived cells is evident in the DC cultures propagated from the bone marrow of liver allograft recipients, whereas there is little evidence of survival of male cells in the cultures from heart graft recipients. The results are representative of 3 separate experiments. For further details, see Lu *et al.*, 1995b.

present within the thymus, including DC, may potentially provide signals responsible for the negative selection of T cells. There is direct evidence, from studies of autoimmunity and allograft rejection, that tolerance exhibited following intrathymic inoculation of exogenous antigen is dependent on thymic DC (Oluwole *et al.*, 1995). Matzinger and Guerder (1989) outlined the critical role of DC in central tolerance by demonstrating that the tolerogenic properties of the APC-depleted mouse thymus could be restored by reconstitution with purified splenic DC. Intrathymic injection of Mls-incompatible spleen or thymic DC can induce tolerance via clonal anergy (Inaba *et al.*, 1991). Similar results have been reported in parent → F_1 bone marrow chimeras, and in transgenic mice (Gao *et al.*, 1990; Widera *et al.*, 1987). Strong T cell tolerance in parent → F_1 bone marrow chimeras prepared with supralethal irradiation was evident at the level of mature thymocytes, and presumably occurred in the thymus itself. It was demonstrated that T cell contact with thymic epithelial cells (including DC) induced clonal deletion of most of the host-reactive T cells, but also spared a proportion of these cells (possibly low-affinity cells). These findings indicate that the role of DC in deletion of autoreactive T cells in the thymus is not dependent upon unique characteristics of the thymic DC, but may also be mediated by signaling provided by DC from other tissue sites.

More recently, Ridge and Matzinger (1996) have reexamined neonatal tolerance induction in mice with a focus on DC as the allogeneic APC. Reexamination of the classic neonatal tolerance experiments of Billingham, Brent, and Medawar (1953) showed that tolerance was not an intrinsic property of the newborn immune system, but that the nature of the APC determined whether the outcome was neonatal tolerance or immunization. These studies demonstrated that the presentation of specific antigen by DC prior to the development of a mature immune system would allow developing T cells to recognize these antigens as if they were self.

Intrathymic injection of donor DC may provide a therapeutic approach for neonatal tolerance induction. Because the thymus is the primary site for central tolerance induction, a direct approach to tolerance by clonal deletion is injection of donor cells into the thymus. Since Posselt *et al.* (1990) used pancreatic islet cells as the donor tissue, intrathymic injection of donor spleen cells (Ohzato *et al.*, 1992) bone marrow, renal glomeruli (Remuzzi *et al.*, 1991), or DC (Ridge and Matzinger, 1996) to induce tolerance has been reported. While intrathymic injection has been a very effective strategy for inducing tolerance in rodents, no studies in large animals have been reported. In humans, the disadvantages of the technique are that (1), there is no effective method to eliminate mature donor-reactive T cells in large animals, and (2), the thymus of adult large animals including man is involuted, making it difficult to determine whether it still functions.

Peripheral Tolerance Induced by DC

It is now evident that DC can provide both stimulatory and downregulatory signals for immune reactions. Recent studies suggest that *in vitro* generated myeloid DC with an 'appropriate' surface phenotype ('immature' or 'costimulatory molecule deficient'), or $CD8^+$ lymphoid DC (in mice) can subvert allogeneic T cell responses. In addition, adoptive transfer of autoantigen-pulsed thymic DC (Khoury *et al.*, 1995) or splenic DC whose costimulatory (B7) molecule expression has been blocked by the chimeric fusion protein CTLA4-Ig (Khoury *et al.*, 1995), can inhibit development of autoimmune disease (experimental allergic encephalomyelitis, EAE) in rodents. The tolerogenicity of DC, and the possible mechanisms involved are summarized as follows.

Selective Activation of T_H2-like T Cell Subsets

Acquired thymic tolerance, induced by injecting antigen into the thymus, has been demonstrated for a number of autoimmune diseases (Gerling *et al.*, 1992; Goss *et al.*, 1994; Khoury *et al.*, 1993; Koevary and Blomberg, 1992). We have shown that injection of the immunodominant peptide of myelin basic protein in the thymus of Lewis rats, protects the animals from EAE (Khoury *et al.*, 1993). Thymic DC isolated from animals injected intrathymically with the peptide can transfer protection to naive Lewis rats, suggesting that DC mediate the effects of acquired thymic tolerance (Khoury *et al.*, 1993). Moreover, thymic but not splenic DC pulsed *ex vivo* with peptide protect recipients from EAE when injected systemically into naive Lewis rats. Interestingly, animals that underwent thymectomy before systemic injection of the *ex vivo* pulsed APC were not protected, raising the question of site-specific homing of DC.

Splenic APC, particularly DC, can mediate protection from EAE if they are pulsed with peptide *in vitro* in the presence of CTLA4-Ig (Fig. 2) (Khoury *et al.*, 1996). The mechanism of protection in this case is probably by causing a T_H2 switch, since immunohistology of the CNS demonstrated almost complete inhibition of T_H1 cytokines, IL-2 and IFN-γ, with upregulation of T_H2 cytokines IL-4 and IL-13 (Khoury *et al.*, 1996). Splenic DC pretreated with TGF-β and peptide were also tolerogenic (unpublished observations). Thus, nontolerogenic DC may become tolerogenic by blocking their ability to provide costimulatory signals or by modification with suppressive cytokines.

Other investigators have observed that antigen-specific suppression of delayed-type hypersensitivity responses can be achieved by intravenous administration of

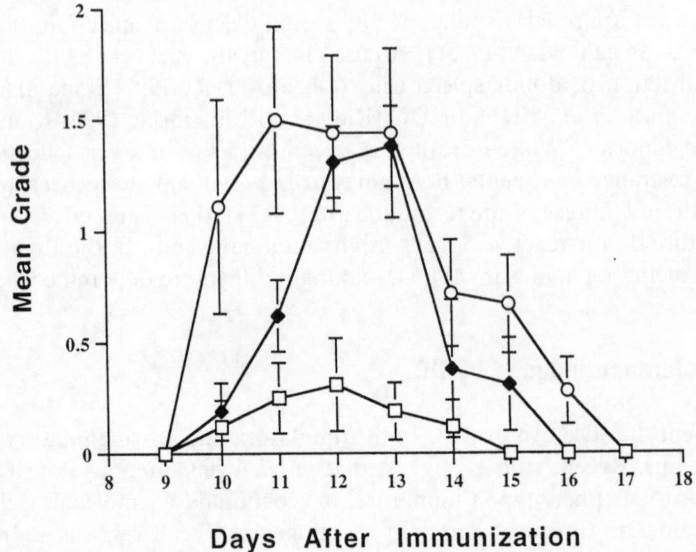

Fig. 2. Inhibition of EAE by DC treated *ex vivo* with peptide and CTLA-4Ig. Splenic DC were isolated by plastic adherence and incubated *in vitro* with peptide 71–90 (the encephalitogenic peptide of MBP) in the presence of CTLA4-Ig. After washing, 4.5×10^6 cells of the DC preparation were injected intravenously into Lewis rats, which were then immunized. Animals were graded for disease severity. Control animals (open circles) and animals treated with infusion of DC + peptide (filled symbols) showed the usual course of EAE with disease starting on day 10 after immunization and recovery by day 18. Animals treated with DC + peptide + CTLA-4Ig (open squares) had very mild disease.

antigen-pulsed Langerhans cells (LC) (Morikawa *et al.*, 1992) or splenic DC (Morikawa *et al.*, 1993), possibly via a mechanism involving selective activation of T_H2-like T cell subsets (Morikawa *et al.*, 1995).

Induction of Regulatory T Cells

Protection of prediabetic nonobese diabetic (NOD) mice from development of type-1 diabetes by transfer of DC isolated from pancreatic lymph nodes of diabetic NOD mice (Clare-Salzler *et al.*, 1992) may possibly be mediated by a mechanism involving the enhanced induction of regulatory T cells. Similarly, Delemarre *et al.* (1995) have reported that transferring cervical node DC from autoimmune lymphocytic thyroiditis (LT) resistant BB/Wor rats to LT-prone BB/Wor recipients delays the onset of LT.

Induction of T Cell Anergy

Costimulatory signals delivered by APC (e.g., via CD40, CD80, CD86) have been proposed to regulate the induction of immune responses. Antigen-specific tolerance can be achieved under conditions in which T cell receptor (TCR) triggering (signal 1) occurs without sufficient costimulation (signal 2), a process leading to anergy or apoptosis. Therefore, selective blockade of costimulatory signals is a promising strategy for therapeutic immunosuppression (Larsen *et al.*, 1996; Kirk *et al.*, 1997). We and

Table 2. Experimental manipulations rendering DC tolerogenic

Dendritic cell type	Tolerogenic effect reported	Reference
CTLA4-Ig-treated splenic DC	Protection from EAE[a]	Verberg *et al.* (1996)
IL-10 treated Langerhans cells	Antigen-specific anergy cells induction *in vitro*	Enk *et al.* (1993)
IL-10 treated splenic DC	Induce T_H2 response *in vivo*	De Smedt *et al.* (1997)
Immature DC exposed to IL-10	Induction of alloantigen- or peptide-specific anergy in T cells	Steinbrink *et al.* (1997)
DC grown in PGE_2	Promote T_H2 development	Kalinski *et al.* (1997)
Ultraviolet-B irradiated Langerhans cells	Antigen-specific unresponsiveness of T_H1 cells *in vitro*	Simon *et al.* (1991)

[a]EAE = experimental allergic encephalomyelitis.

others have demonstrated that DC whose allostimulatory function is impaired, by incomplete maturation, selective blockade of B7 family costimulatory molecules (using CTLA4-Ig), the influence of specific cytokines (i.e., IL-10), or ultraviolet B irradiation, can either induce alloantigen-specific hyporesponsiveness or apoptosis *in vitro* or suppress *in vivo* immune reactivity (Tables 1 and 2). Grohmann *et al.* (1997) reported that a tumor-associated and self-antigen peptide presented by DC could induce T cell anergy *in vivo*, but that IL-12 could prevent or revert the anergic state.

Intrathymic injection of antigen mediates peripheral tolerance through interaction of thymic DC with activated peripheral T cells that circulate to the thymus. This interaction leads to peripheral T cell anergy (Chen *et al.*, 1997a). There is also evidence that intrathymic injection of antigen leads to apoptosis of T cells, as we demonstrated in a TCR transgenic murine system (Chen *et al.*, 1998).

Induction of Activated T Cell Apoptosis

The expression by DC of some molecules associated with the inhibition of T cell growth or the induction of T cell apoptosis (i.e. nitric oxide [NO], or FasL) may render DC capable of subverting T cell responses. Mouse splenic $CD8^+$ lymphoid DC that strongly express FasL induce apoptosis in activated allogeneic $CD4^+$ T cells, resulting in diminished T cell proliferation in mixed leukocyte reactions (MLR) (Süss and Shortman, 1996). These DC can also impair IL-2 production by $CD8^+$ T cells. DC exposed to interferon-γ (IFN-γ), bacterial endotoxin (lipopolysaccharide, LPS), or allogeneic T cells can synthesize NO synthase (NOS). NO production suppresses allogeneic T cell proliferation in MLR, and also induces apoptosis both in activated T cells and in the DC themselves (Lu *et al.*, 1996; Bonham *et al.*, 1996a). Highly purified myeloid DC grown from mouse bone marrow in GM-CSF + IL-4 have been found to express FasL mRNA by reverse transcriptase polymerase chain reaction (RT-PCR), and to uniformly express FasL by both flow cytometric and immunocytochemical analysis. These cells, but not DC propagated from FasL-deficient (*gld*) mice, induced dose-dependent increases in DNA fragmentation in Fas^+ Jurkat T cells. The same DC also induced apoptosis of alloactivated T cells once the CD28/B7 pathway was blocked using CTLA4-Ig (Lu *et al.*, 1997b). It is interesting to speculate that $FasL^+$ donor liver DC progenitors might be responsible for host T cell deletion observed in murine spontaneous liver allograft acceptance (Qian *et al.*, 1997a). Cell interactions resulting in the apoptosis of liver graft-infiltrating T cells might be mediated by $FasL^+$ donor liver DC that are located in portal areas (Woo *et al.*, 1994). It has yet to be determined, however, whether there is selective deletion of donor-reactive T cells in the mouse orthotopic liver transplant model (Qian *et al.*, 1997b) associated with spontaneous acceptance in most combinations.

Downregulation of the Clonal Expansion of B Cells by Follicular DC

In germinal centers, B-lymphocytes are intimately associated with follicular dendritic cells (FDC). It has been hypothesized that FDC are involved in the regulation of B-cell growth and differentiation through cell–cell interaction. Highly enriched preparations of human follicular DC (FDC) were cultured with mitogen-stimulated B cells in the absence of T cells, and B cell [^{3}H]TdR uptake was inhibited by up to 80% (Freedman *et al.*, 1992). Furthermore, supernatants from cultured FDC were also able to inhibit B cell proliferation. These results demonstrated that FDC may downregulate the clonal expansion of B cells that occurs within lymphoid follicles as part of the normal physiologic immune response.

Route of Administration of DC

It is likely that the nature of ongoing immune responses is dependent on the signals provided by APC. Under experimental conditions, DC exhibit a dichotomous potential to regulate immune responsiveness, depending on the route of *in vivo* administration, the number of cells injected, the amount of antigen presented, and the source or population of DC. Thus, *in vivo* experimental studies have indicated that administration of DC loaded with low doses of tumor antigen can enhance tumor rejection in mice, while administration of DC loaded with high doses of tumor antigen, or administration of large numbers of tumor antigen-pulsed DC inhibited the antitumor effect of DC (Knight *et al.*, 1985). BM-derived DC propagated *in vitro* with GM-CSF + IL-4 accelerate donor-specific kidney allograft rejection if delivered intravenously, but can prolong graft survival when administrated via the portal vein (Gorczynski *et al.*, 1996). Liver-derived DC progenitors have been shown to prolong islet allograft survival, whereas splenic DC propagated from the same mice, using the same technique, induce rejection of pancreatic islet allografts in diabetic recipients (Rastellini *et al.*, 1995). There is also considerable evidence that specific components of the local tissue microenvironment, e.g., the cytokine TGF-β, may be responsible for imparting tolerogenic activity to DC that migrate from the anterior chamber of the eye to regional lymphoid tissue (Streilein *et al.*, 1992).

In summary, DC are capable of eliciting positive (sensitizing) and negative (tolerizing) responses in the immune system. This reflects the molecular regulation of the immunological activity of DC, including expression of first and second signal for T helper cell activation, stimulatory cytokines (IL-12, IL-6), and death-inducing ligands by DC (reviewed later). The ability to generate immunoregulatory DC in sufficient number, under well-defined conditions, has considerable implications for the development of effective DC-based therapy of cancer, infectious disease, autoimmunity, and allograft rejection.

MOLECULAR BASIS OF DC TOLEROGENICITY

The potent capacity of DC to activate immunologically naïve (resting) T cells is related to their high constitutive expression of MHC class II molecules, and T cell costimulatory molecules, such as CD40, CD80, and CD86. Deficiency or absence of expression of these molecules reduces the APC function of DC and may render them potentially tolerogenic. Thus, DC residing in peripheral tissues (e.g. skin) express relatively low levels of co-stimulatory molecules and are poor T cell stimulators when freshly isolated (Larsen *et al.*, 1994). Others have observed that LC precursors in the epidermis function poorly as T cell stimulators (Romani *et al.*, 1986), and there is even evidence that LC may provide downregulatory signals during elicitation of cutaneous (contact sensitivity) inflammatory reactions (Grabbe *et al.*, 1995). MHC class II^- DC precursors in the airway epithelium of rats (Nelson and Holt, 1995), freshly isolated heart or kidney DC (Austyn *et al.*, 1994), and DC progenitors propagated from the mouse liver (Lu *et al.*, 1994) are also poor allostimulators. Absence of expression of invariant chain by interstitial DC within nonlymphoid tissue (Saleem *et al.*, 1997) may also be a significant factor in the regulation of self-tolerance.

Presentation of antigen to T cells by APC in the absence of costimulatory molecules induces T cell anergy (Schwartz, 1990). The importance of costimulatory molecule deficiency on DC in peripheral tolerance induction has been emphasized by the fact that CTLA4-Ig, a potent blocker of the costimulatory B7-CD28 pathway, significantly prolongs the survival of allografts in various animal organ transplantation models (Lin *et al.*, 1993; Sayegh *et al.*, 1995). Studies in our laboratory have demonstrated that DC propagated *in vitro* from mouse BM in the presence of suboptimal concentrations of GM-CSF express only low levels of costimulatory molecules, i.e., MHC class II^+, $CD80^{low}$, $CD86^-$. These cells not only induce specific donor T cell unresponsiveness *in vitro* (Lu *et al.*, 1995a), but also prolong donor strain cardiac (Fu *et al.*, 1996) or pancreatic islet allograft survival (Rastellini *et al.*, 1995) when administered systemically one week before allograft transplantation. Likewise, in an autoimmune disease model, MBP-pulsed DC on which the expression of CD80 and CD86 has been blocked by CTLA4-Ig protect rats from the induction of experimental allergic encephalomyelitis (EAE) (Khoury *et al.*, 1996). It has also been suggested that rhesus monkey bone marrow-derived DC progenitors (MHC class $II^{-/dim}$) may exert tolerance-promoting activity both *in vivo* and *in vitro* (Thomas *et al.*, 1994). These observations have led to speculation that costimulatory molecule-deficient DC could play a role in peripheral T cell tolerance induction.

It has been proposed that expression of the CD8 molecule by a DC subpopulation in the mouse thymus and spleen (lymphoid DC) (Vremec *et al.*, 1992; Welsh and Kripke, 1990) may enable these cells to express a 'veto' function (Hambor *et al.*, 1990; Sambhara and Miller, 1991). Further work has demonstrated that $CD8^+$ DC isolated from the spleen express FasL and are capable of killing activated $CD4^+$ T cells via the Fas/FasL pathway (Süss and Shortman, 1996). However, recent evidence indicates that CD8 is not important in the 'veto' function of these murine lymphoid DC (Kronin *et al.*, 1997). We have also demonstrated in a recent study (Lu *et al.*, 1997b) that DC propagated from mouse bone marrow in GM-CSF + IL-4 (myeloid DC; MHC class II^{hi}, $CD80^{hi}$, $CD86^{hi}$) express functional FasL, but induce only a low level of apoptosis in alloantigen-activated T cells. Once the B7/CD28

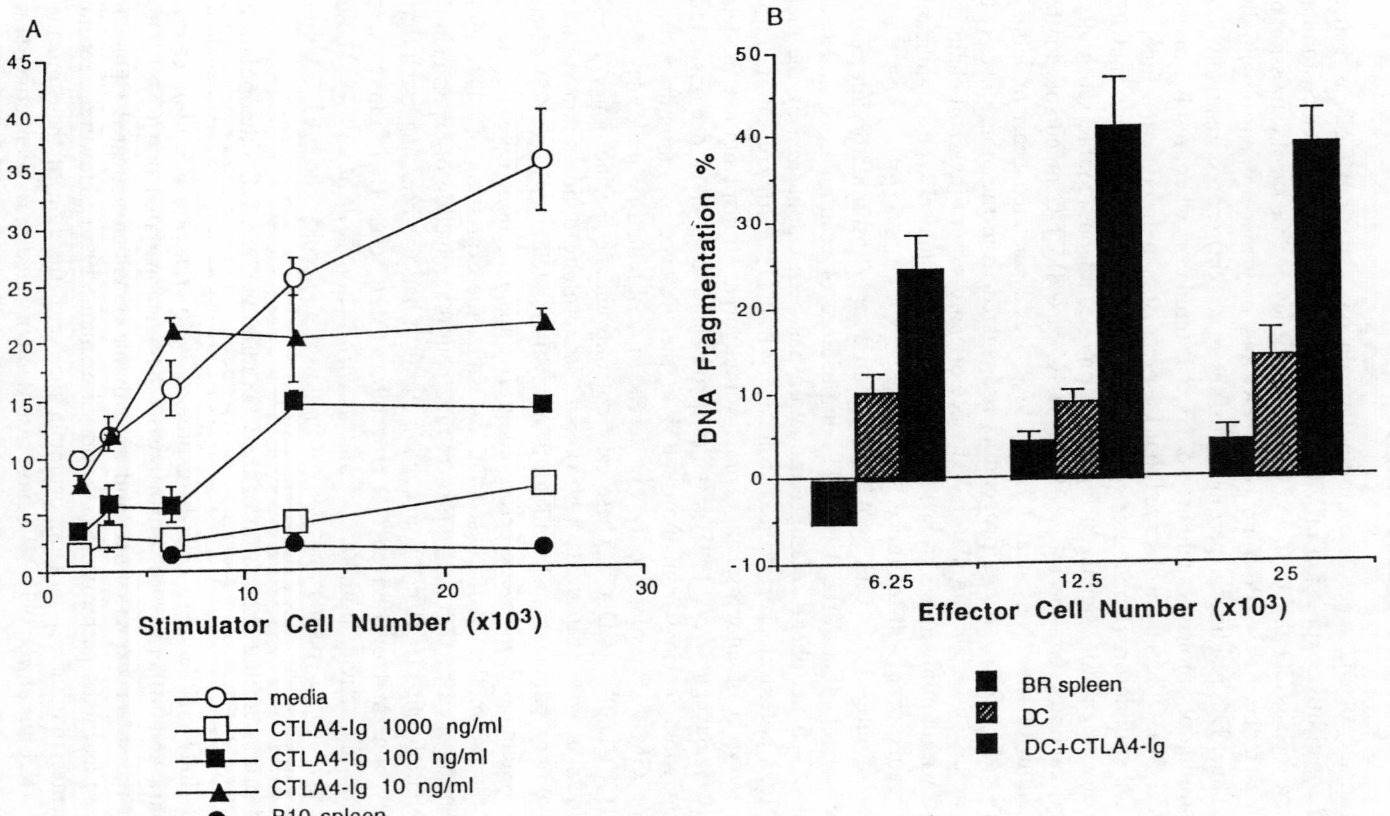

Fig. 3. Blockade of the B7–CD28 pathway augments apoptosis induced in allogeneic T cells by DC. MLR cultures were established with graded concentrations of bone marrow-derived DC (B10.BR) and allogeneic (C57BL/10) splenic T cells (2×10^5). (A) Blockade of B7–CD28 interactions with 1000 ng/ml CTLA4-Ig was effective in providing almost complete inhibition of T cell proliferation. (B) Blockade of B7–CD28 interactions by treatment of DC with 1000 ng/mL CTLA4-Ig also resulted in a marked increase in DNA fragmentation of activated allogeneic T cells in MLR cultures, compared with untreated DC.

pathway is blocked with CTLA4-Ig, however, significantly increased apoptosis of T cells can be detected, indicating that FasL and B7 molecules on DC may play counter-regulatory roles in proliferation and survival of T cells following DC–T cell interaction (Fig. 3). It appears that Fas/FasL interaction is probably not the only death-inducing pathway that exists in DC–T cell interaction, because a high level of T cell apoptosis can also be induced by DC propagated from the bone marrow of FasL-deficient (*gld*) mice in the presence of CTLA4-Ig (Lu *et al.*, 1997b). These studies suggest that other molecules expressed by DC could contribute to DC-induced apoptosis. Candidate molecular pathways include tumor necrosis factor (TNF)/TNF-R, TRAIL/TRAIL-R, or 4-1BB/4-1BBL (Lynch *et al.*, 1995; Wiley *et al.*, 1995). There is, however, no direct evidence to date whether these molecules are expressed on DC.

Studies of LPS-treated mice have suggested that NO production by presumptive intrathymic DC may be responsible for thymocyte apoptosis and possibly self-tolerance (Fehsel *et al.*, 1995). These findings are consistent with our observation of NO production by a subpopulation of DC following treatment *in vitro* with IFN-γ or LPS, or interaction with allogeneic T cells (Bonham *et al.*, 1996a; Lu *et al.*, 1996). Thus, the special properties of DC (surface expression of costimulatory/regulatory molecules, responsiveness to immunosuppressive cytokines, T cell interaction and *in vivo* homing to T-dependent areas of lymphoid tissues (Austyn and Larsen, 1990)) make their manipulation to maximize their tolerogenic potential an attractive approach for cell-based therapy of immune-mediated disorders (allograft rejection and autoimmune disease).

CULTURE OF TOLEROGENIC DC FOR THERAPEUTIC APPLICATION—THE INFLUENCE OF CYTOKINES, OTHER MICROENVIRONMENTAL FACTORS AND SIGNIFICANCE OF THE CELL SOURCE

Only trace numbers of DC can be obtained from normal tissue with extensive processing procedures. Since Inaba *et al.* (1992a,b) first described a method to propagate DC progenitors from normal mouse bone marrow or blood with GM-CSF, the availability of large numbers of myeloid DC has opened up possibilities for immunotherapy using DC as vaccines. Several groups have subsequently described methods for culture of large numbers of highly stimulatory human, nonhuman primate, mouse, or rat DC derived from different tissues using GM-CSF, most often in combination with IL-4. More limited studies have reported the propagation of DC with tolerogenic properties.

It has been well demonstrated that cytokines play a key role in the regulation of DC maturation and activation. TNF-α enhances the development of mature DC from human progenitors (Caux *et al.*, 1992; Szabolcs *et al.*, 1995), whereas IL-1β inhibits the function of LC (Grabbe *et al.*, 1994b). Monocytes represent an abundant source of precursors that can polarize towards either DC or macrophages 'dendrophages' depending on the external stimuli. This polarization can be driven *in vitro* by the addition of appropriate cytokines (GM-CSF + IL-4 or macrophage colony-stimulating factor-1; M-CSF). Monocyte-derived DC generated in culture with GM-CSF and IL-4 have a very high level of cell surface MHC class II and costimulatory molecules. In addition, they express the low-affinity receptor for Fcγ, FcγRII (CD32) (Sallusto *et al.*, 1995).

Rather conflicting results have been obtained concerning the effects of IFN-γ on the antigen-presenting function of DC and on the expression of costimulatory or MHC class II molecules by DC (Grabbe *et al.*, 1994a; Lutz *et al.*, 1996). IL-10 has been reported to reduce the expression of HLA-DR or CD86 molecules, but not CD80 or intercellular adhesion molecule-1 (ICAM-1; CD54) on human peripheral blood DC (Buelens *et al.*, 1995), and to downregulate both CD80 and CD86 expression on murine LC (Kaeamura and Furue, 1995). It inhibits the upregulation of CD83, CD86 and CD58 on *in vitro* generated human DC (Steinbrink *et al.*, 1997). IL-10 also suppresses production of IL-8 and TNF-α by DC activated by LPS (Buelens *et al.*, 1997). There is also evidence that IL-10 pretreatment strongly inhibits the DC-induced responses of naive and primed $CD4^+$ T cells in allogeneic MLR and anti-CD3 assays (Steinbrink *et al.*, 1997). In addition, IL-10-pretreated immature human DC induce alloantigen- or peptide-specific anergy in $CD4^+$ T cells (Steinbrink *et al.*, 1997). IL-10 can skew the T_H1/T_H2 balance to T_H2 cells by blocking IL-12 synthesis by DC (De Smedt *et al.*, 1997; Buelens *et al.*, 1997). It has also been reported that IL-10 accelerates murine Langerhans cell apoptosis in culture (Ludewig *et al.*, 1995). Interestingly, Kalinski and coworkers reported that DC grown in the presence of prostaglandin (PG) E_2 are unable to secrete IL-12, and when they present antigen to T_Hp cells they promote the development of T_H2 cells (Kalinski *et al.*, 1997).

DC propagated from different tissues may exhibit different phenotypes and functions. Experiments using adult mice have shown that the liver harbors stem cells and DC progenitors that can be propagated using GM-CSF but that only acquire functional maturation when exposed to extracellular matrix protein (collagen type-1) with which DC are spatially associated in normal liver (Lu *et al.*, 1994). Recipients treated 7 days before transplant with donor-derived liver DC progenitors exhibit prolonged survival of pancreatic islet allografts from the same donor strain (Rastellini *et al.*, 1995). Clearly, it is possible to propagate tolerogenic DC from different sources of precursors under well-defined laboratory conditions. *In vitro* manipulations that may render DC tolerogenic are summarized in Table 2.

Here we summarize several methods for obtaining sufficient numbers of 'tolerogenic' DC. The most critical feature of cell propagation for determination of DC function is the removal of contaminating cells, including granulocytes, macrophages, and B cells. Granulocytes, which are nonadherent cells, can be rinsed away during the culture. Macrophages remain firmly affixed to the culture plates. Most B cells, which represent a major component of starting bone marrow cell suspensions, can be removed initially by depletion with antibody and complement, or using immunomagnetic beads.

Propagation of Tolerogenic DC from Mouse Liver

Liver-derived DC progenitors can be propagated in liquid culture in the presence of GM-CSF, using a similar approach to that adopted by Inaba and colleagues for the generation of mouse blood or bone marrow-derived DC (Inaba *et al.*, 1992a,b). Approximately 2.5×10^6 loosely attached or floating cells with dendritic morphology can be harvested from a single mouse liver after 7–10 days of culture. These cells are poor stimulators of naive T cells, with a surface immunophenotype corresponding to DC progenitors (negative for lymphoid lineage markers, positive for the DC markers DEC-205 and CD11c, MHC class II^{low}, B7-2^{low} and positive for F4/80, and CD32). These liver-derived DC progenitors are poor allostimulators, elicit low levels of CTL alloresponses *in vitro*, and significantly prolong islet allograft survival if given intravenously (2×10^6) 7 days before donor islet cell transplantation in streptozotocin-diabetic mice. Large numbers of DC progenitors can be propagated from the livers of mice treated with the hematopoietic growth factor Flt-3 ligand (Drakes *et al.*, 1997).

Propagation of Tolerogenic DC Using Suboptimal Concentrations of GM-CSF

GM-CSF is a key cytokine for myeloid DC propagation from proliferating precursors or hematopoietic stem cells, and its effect on the maturation of DC appears to be dose-related. DC progenitors deficient in cell surface costimulatory molecules can be propagated from the bone marrow of normal or nonobese diabetic (NOD) mice using an appropriate low concentration of GM-CSF, with removal of contaminating granulocytes by antibody + complement depletion or gradient separation. The cells are characterized as DEC-205^+, MHC class II^+, $CD80^{dim}$, $CD86^{-/dim}$, $CD40^{dim}$ (Fig. 4), poor stimulators of naive allogenic T cells in MLR and with a high level of endocytotic

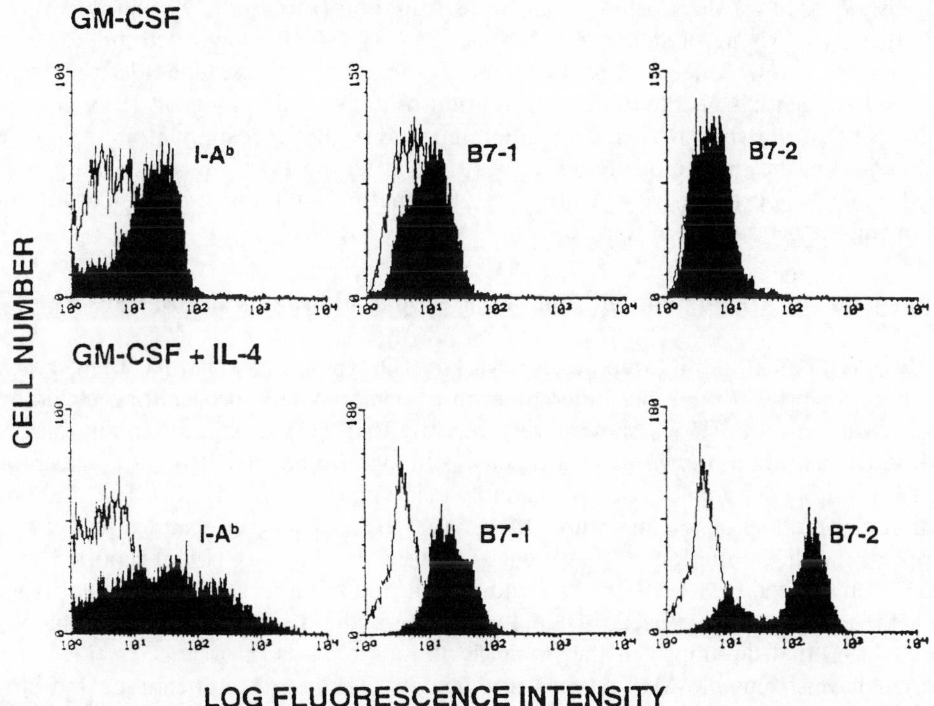

Fig. 4. Expression of MHC class II (I-A^b), B7-1 and B7-2 on (top) 8-day GSM-CSF and (bottom) 8-day GM-CSF + IL-4-stimulated B10 BM-derived bone marrow cells. The result is representative of three separate experiments. For further details see Lu *et al.* (1995a).

Table 3. Influence of donor-specific GM-CSF-stimulated DC progenitors (B7-2$^-$) on B10 cardiac allograft survival in C3H mice[a]

Group	Cells injected day −7	*n*	Graft survival time (days)	MST
A	None (media control)	8	8(×3), 12, 13(×2), 9, 10	9.5
B	Fresh B10 bone marrow cells (allogeneic)	4	12(×4)	12
Cultured cells				
C	B10 (B7-2$^+$) (allogeneic)	17	4(×5), 5(×3), 7(×2), 8(×2), 9, 10, 14(×2), 15	7[b]
D	B10 (B7-2$^-$) (allogeneic)	15	7, 19(×4), 20, 22(×2), 23 26, 27, 29, 30, 35, 67	22[c,d]
E	C3H (B7-2$^-$) (syngeneic)	4	12(×2), 13(×2)	12.5
F	BALB/c (B7-2$^-$) (third party)	9	7, 12, 16(×2), 17(×3), 19, 20	16.5

[a]Cells (2×10^6 i.v.) were injected 7 days before heterotopic (B10 → C3H) heart transplantation. MST = median survival time. MSTs were compared using the Kruskal–Wallis test. Pairwise comparison was done using the Wilcoxon sum rank test.
[b]$P < 0.01$ compared with groups D and F.
[c]$P < 0.003$ compared with groups C and E.
[d]$P < 0.01$ compared with group F.

activity. These 'immature' DC induce alloantigen-specific hyporesponsiveness in allogeneic T cells (Lu *et al.*, 1995a), and prolong heart allograft survival if given intravenously (2×10^6) 7 days before organ transplantation (Fu *et al.*, 1996) (Table 3). *In vivo* therapy of young prediabetic NOD mice with GM-CSF-propagated 'tolerogenic' DC grown in low concentration GM-CSF and pulsed with peptides derived from islet cell antigen has resulted in the prevention of diabetes development (P.A. Morel, University of Pittsburgh, personal communication). Both costimulatory molecule expression on the surface of these DC and their allostimulatory function are upregulated, and phagocytic activity (a property of immature DC) is lost upon maturation following further culture of these cells in GM-CSF + IL-4.

Propagation of 'Tolerogenic' DC from Mouse Bone Marrow with GM-CSF + TGF-β_1

TGF-β_1 is a potent immunosuppressive cytokine (Derynck, 1994) that has been shown to affect the proliferation and differentiation of hematopoietic progenitors, including DC. Yasunori *et al.* (1997) showed very recently that TGF-β_1 almost totally blocks mouse DC maturation *in vitro*. This effect was thought to be mediated via Fc-receptor (CD32)-bearing suppressor cells, presumably macrophages. However, TGF-β_1 did not inhibit the production of immature, MHC class II$^+$, CD86$^-$ DC, and also did not suppress the differentiation of these cells. Recently, Strobl *et al.* (1996) reported that TGF-β_1 promoted GM-CSF, TNF-α and c-kit ligand-induced DC development from CD34$^+$ hematopoietic progenitors in human cord blood. The human cord blood-derived DC that developed in the presence of additional TGF-β_1 were CD1a$^+$, and did not have strong allo-MLR stimulatory activity. Their surface phenotype and biological function were similar to that of fresh epidermal LC (immature DC). We have used TGF-β_1 in conjunction with GM-CSF to facilitate the generation of mouse bone marrow-derived DC deficient in costimulatory molecule expression and with potential tolerogenic activity. Compared with propagation of DC in low concentrations of

Table 4. Prolongation of cardiac allograft[a] survival by donor GM/TGF-β-DC

Group (n)	Treatment	Cell number ($\times 10^{-6}$)	Survival (days)	MST
A (7)	Media	0	6, 10($\times$3), 11, 12, 13	10
B (6)	Fresh BM	2	12($\times$4), 14, 15	12
C (6)	GM/IL-4-DC	2	5($\times$3), 6($\times$3)	5[c]
D (6)	GM/TGF-β-DC	1	12, 13($\times$3), 15, 46	13
E (10)	GM/TGF-β-DC	2	19, 20, 22, 23, 26, 27, 29, 30, 35, 67	26[d]

[a]B10 (H-2^b)$\rightarrow$ C3H (H-2^k) heart transplantation was performed at day 0.
[b]BM or DC from B10 mice were i.v. injected at day −7; GM = GM-CSF.
[c]$P < 0.01$ compared with group A.
[d]$P < 0.01$ compared with group A.

GM-CSF, relatively high yields and purity of potentially tolerogenic cells can be obtained from normal mouse bone marrow using GM-CSF plus TGF-β_1. The blocking effect of TGF-β on DC maturation can, however, be reversed either by adding TNF-α or IL-4, or by removing inhibitory cells (CD32$^+$ adherent cells).

DC propagated in the presence of GM-CSF + TGF-β_1 can significantly prolong survival of vascularized heart allografts from the same donor strain (Lu *et al.*, 1997a) if given 7 days before organ (cardiac) transplantation (Table 4). There is also evidence that TGF-β_1 impairs the antigen-presenting function of human BM-derived APC, including DC (Bonham *et al.*, 1996b). In the context of these and other reports, TGF-β has been strongly implicated as a key microenvironmental factor, acting on APC, in the generation of immune deviation and immunological privilege, such as occurs in the anterior chamber of the eye (Streilein *et al.*, 1992; Wilbanks and Streilein, 1992).

THERAPEUTIC APPLICATION OF TOLEROGENIC DC

Achievement of long-term, donor-specific acceptance of grafted tissue in the absence of immunosuppressive therapy (transplantation tolerance) remains an elusive goal in humans, although it has been achieved in rodent models using a variety of approaches. The mechanisms underlying graft acceptance vary according to the means used to create the state of acceptance. The key to transplantation tolerance is the control of graft-specific T cell responses. If donor antigen is presented in a nonimmunogenic manner by the graft (e.g., owing to modification of the graft tissue by culture), peripheral T cells of the recipient may ignore the graft. Nonstimulatory presentation of donor antigens on the graft can induce a state of unresponsiveness in recipient T cells, instead of activation. Several strategies have been demonstrated to achieve peripheral transplant tolerance in rodent models, and warrant further investigation both in nonhuman primates and humans. These include the blockade of receptor–ligand interactions essential to the functional activation of T cells via DC–T cell interaction (e.g., use of CTLA4-Ig in combination with anti-CD40L) (Larsen *et al.*, 1996; Kirk *et al.*, 1997).

Several approaches in which B7 costimulatory molecules have been targeted using CTLA4-Ig, or use of donor resting B cells, or macrophage infusions have demonstrated that antigen-specific tolerance can be achieved under conditions in which T cell receptor (TCR) triggering occurs without sufficient costimulation. We have reported that significant prolongation of heart allografts can be achieved by pretreatment of the recipient with 'tolerogenic' donor strain-derived DC propagated from mouse bone marrow using either GM-CSF (Fu *et al.*, 1996) or GM-CSF combined with TGF-β_1 (TGF-β-DC) (Lu *et al.*, 1997a). Donor (B10) DC (1–8 $\times$ 10^6) were injected intravenously into C3H ($H2^k$) recipients 7 days before B10 ($H2^b$) heart transplantation. The DC propagated using GM-CSF + IL-4 (mature DC; IL-4-DC) accelerated rejection of subsequent heart grafts from the B10 donor strain. Median graft survival time was strikingly reduced from 10 days to 5 days in the IL-4 DC pretreatment group. By contrast, TGF-β-DC (2 $\times$ 10^6 i.v., 7 days before organ transplantation) significantly prolonged heart allograft (median survival time from 10 to 26 days) (Table 4). This therapeutic effect was correlated with inhibited proliferation of recipient T cells stimulated with alloantigen *in vitro*, and with low CTL responses to donor targets. If C3H recipients were treated with TGF-β-DC from the bone marrow of either B10 (donor), C3H (recipient) or BALB/c (third party), the prolongation of graft survival was achieved only using donor strain DC. TGF-β-DC of the B10 strain were unable to prolong BALB/c heart graft (third party) survival. These studies indicated that the effect of the TGF-β-DC was antigen-specific. The inhibition of cardiac allograft rejection by TGF-β-DC was also dependent on the timing of donor DC administration. B10 TGF-β-DC (2 $\times$ 10^6) were given intravenously once only on either days −14, −7, −3, or +2 in relation to B10 heart transplantation performed on day 0. Only administration of the DC on day −7 significantly prolonged subsequent heart allograft survival. Furthermore, increases in the number of TGF-β-DC above 2 $\times$ 10^6 (to 8 $\times$ 10^6) did not significantly affect median graft survival time, indicating the importance of donor-specific antigen, timing, and amount of antigen delivered by the DC.

Other investigators have shown that resting B cells can induce tolerance, and that macrophages can also exert inhibitory activity on immune responses. There is as yet no clear explanation why DC should be more effective in the prolongation of graft survival than donor-specific B cells or monocytes/macrophages. No direct comparative studies have been reported. The expression of MHC class II on the DC surface, and the remarkable homing capacity of DC-lineage cells to T-dependent areas of host lymphoid tissue (Larsen *et al.*, 1990; Thomson *et al.*, 1995b), may contribute to their capacity to determine the balance between tolerance and immunity. Thus, donor-derived DC progenitors (MHC class II^+, B7-1^-, B7-2^{dim}) that interdigitate with T cells in secondary lymphoid tissues could provide sufficient first signal, but inadequate costimulation, predisposing to T cell tolerance.

BLOCKADE OF THE CD40/CD40 LIGAND PATHWAY POTENTIATES THE THERAPEUTIC EFFECT OF DC PROGENITORS

Although costimulatory molecule-deficient DC can prolong allograft survival, they cannot induce permanent allograft acceptance in nonimmunosuppressed recipients. The failure of these cells to induce allograft tolerance may be due to the 'late' upregulation of costimulatory molecules on the DC following their interaction with host T cells. This hypothesis is supported by the observation that coculture of B10 TGFβ-DC and C3H spleen T cells for 18 h induces CD40 and B7 expression on the DC. In order to induce long-term graft acceptance, it seems important to prevent the 'late' upregulation of costimulatory molecules, or to block the upregulated costimulatory signal with exogenous reagents, such as CTLA4-Ig.

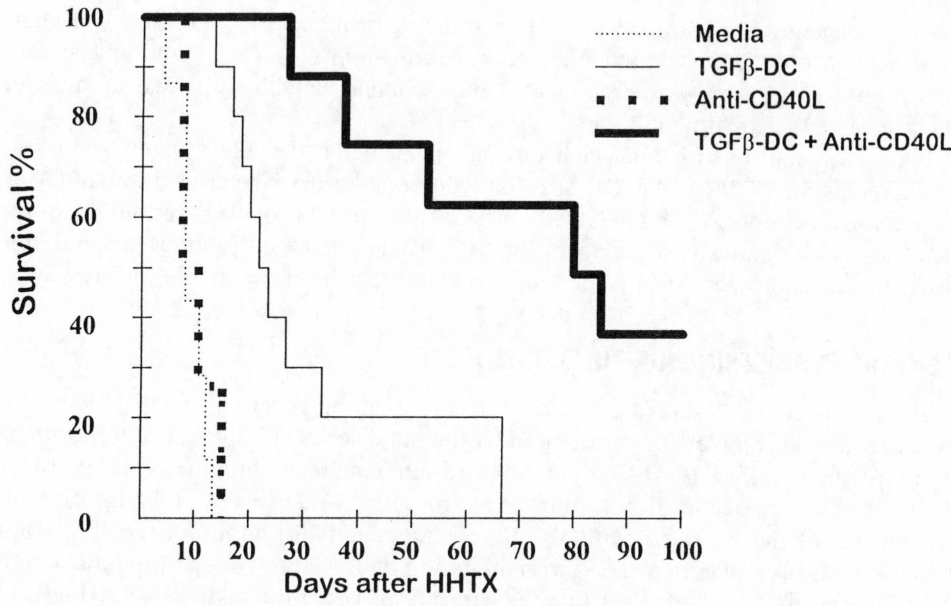

Fig. 5. DC enhance graft survival. Prolongation of B10 ($H2^b$) vascularized cardiac allografts in C3H ($H2^k$) recipients by TGF-β_1-DC and potentiation of the therapeutic effect by anti-CD40L mAb. GM-CSF + TGF-β_1-cultured DC (2×10^6) from B10 mice were administered intravenously either alone or together with anti-CD40L mAb 7 days before B10 heterotopic cardiac transplantation.

The CD40/CD40L (gp 39) pathway has been shown to play an important role in DC activation, and is crucial for the establishment of primary and secondary responses to T-dependent antigens (Armitage *et al.*, 1992; Yang and Wilson, 1996). Thus CD40 engagement upregulates the expression of CD80 and CD86 on DC, providing a link between the CD40/CD40L and CD80:CD86/CD28:CTLA-4 pathway (McLellan *et al.*, 1996; Caux *et al.*, 1994b). Ligation of CD40 on DC also induces production/secretion of IL-12, an important T_H1 cell activating cytokine. Combination of allogeneic donor DC progenitors with blockade of the CD40/CD40L pathway using anti-CD40L mAb 7 days before cardiac transplantation resulted in long-term graft survival (Fig. 5). However, a single injection of anti-CD40L mAb alone failed to prolong heart allograft survival. In a different model, Parker *et al.* (1995) have shown that anti-CD40L mAb combined with donor small lymphocytes blocks rejection of islet allografts. Hancock *et al.* (1996) have also found that treatment of recipients with donor spleen cells and anti-CD40L mAb leads to indefinite survival of mouse cardiac allografts, although repeated administration of the antibody was required.

The mechanisms by which administration of anti-CD40L mAb together with costimulator-deficient donor DC, or resting B cells, induces long-term graft survival are not clear. It was noted in the resting B cell studies that long-term graft survival was associated with striking inhibition of intragraft T_H1 cytokine and IL-12 expression, with reciprocal upregulation of T_H2 cytokines. We have demonstrated that anti-donor CTL activity of freshly isolated, heart graft-infiltrating cells is dramatically diminished in mice given combined TGF-β-DC/anti-CD40L mAb therapy (Lu *et al.*,

1997a). Generation of anti-donor CTL from recipient spleens was also markedly depressed. Moreover, increased apoptosis of graft-infiltrating cells and spleen cells was found in the combined treatment group, compared with untreated animals or those given either treatment alone.

In conclusion, the manner in which antigen is presented by DC plays an important role in the regulation of allogeneic DC–T cell interactions *in vivo*. The critical role of CD40 expression on donor DC, and of CD40L in T cell activation, provides a rational basis for blockade of this pathway to augment the tolerogenic potential of donor costimulator-deficient DC and other APC in the long-term suppression of organ allograft rejection.

GENETIC ENGINEERING OF TOLEROGENIC DC

Previous reports have shown that the antigen-presenting function of DC is impaired either by their incomplete maturation under the influence of suboptimal concentrations of a specific cytokine (GM-CSF) or by anti-inflammatory cytokines, i.e., IL-10 or TGF-β, or by blockade of costimulatory molecules (i.e., using CTLA4-Ig, or anti-CD40L mAb) that interfere with DC–T cell interaction. In addition, the expression by DC of key molecules associated with inhibition of T cell growth or with induction of T cell apoptosis (i.e., NO, FasL) or the capacity of certain cytokines (e.g., IL-10) to inhibit DC function, suggests that transfer of genes (cDNAs) encoding these molecules may render DC tolerogenic in models of transplantation or autoimmune disease.

There are recent reports that DC can be genetically modified using retroviral or adenoviral vectors (Song *et al.*, 1997; Specht *et al.*, 1997; see Chapter 32), or transfected with particulate/plasmid-based vectors that take advantage of the highly phagocytic nature of DC progenitors. Thus, Song *et al.* (1997), Specht *et al.* (1997), and Wan *et al.* (1997) have demonstrated that transfer of genes enocoding model antigens to mouse bone marrow-derived DC renders these cells capable of inducing protective and/or therapeutic antitumor immunity. Storkus and colleagues have observed that DC progenitors from mouse bone marrow transfected with vIL10-encoding plasmids via gene gun synthesize vIL-10 and exhibit substantially reduced capacity for the induction of allogeneic T cell proliferation (W. Storkus and T. Tüting, personal communication). vIL-10 production by DC was associated with significant reductions in cell surface expression of MHC class II and costimulatory molecules (CD80, CD86). We have also recently observed that retroviral transduction of mouse bone marrow-derived DC to produce vIL-10 substantially impairs their allostimulatory activity (T. Takayama, Y. Nishioka, L. Lu, M.T. Lotze, H. Tahara and A.W. Thomson, submitted for publication).

In principle, the potential tolerogenic activity of DC could be augmented or maximized by the transfer (alone or in combination) of genes encoding 'immunosuppressive' molecules that DC either do not make or may make only in insignificant amounts. The suggested candidate genes to achieve peripheral transplant tolerance include vIL-10, TGF-β, CTLA4-Ig, inducible NOS, EBI-3, IFN-γdR (defective IFN-γ receptor) and FasL (Table 5), the latter possibly in conjunction with bcl2 transfection to prevent premature death of the DC.

Viral vectors, especially adenoviral vectors (if transgene expression is required for short periods), are likely to provide higher frequencies of gene transduction into DC than particulate-cDNA insertion methods. The inherent immunogenicity of adenoviral

Table 5. Candidate genes as modulators of DC tolerogenicity

Gene	Possible effect
(v)IL-10	Inhibition of expression of CD80, CD86 and MHC II; suppression of IL-12; induction of T_H2 response
TGF-β	Inhibition of T cell proliferation
IFN-γdR	Neutralizes IFN-γ
EBI-3	Competitive intracellular binder of IL-12-p35
iNOS	Apoptosis-inducing activity for T cells
CTLA4-Ig	Blockade of B7 costimulatory signal
Fas Ligand	Apoptosis-inducing activity for T cells
TRAIL (TNF family)	Apoptosis-inducing activity for T cells

antigen displayed by transduced DC is, however, a significant potential problem. It could be overcome by use of modified viral vectors. Interestingly, Wan *et al.* (1997) have observed that although direct injection of retrovirus-encoding genes into mice elicits high levels of anti-viral antibodies, anti-retrovirus Ab cannot be detected in the serum once the retrovirus-encoding gene is introduced via transduced DC (Y. Wan, University of Toronto, personal communication). Clearly, an important concern for DC-based therapy will be the efficiency and stability of gene expression by DC *in vivo*.

ACKNOWLEDGMENTS

The authors' work is supported by National Institutes of Health grants DK 49745 and AI 41011. We thank our many colleagues, and in particular Drs Lotze, Robbins, Storkus and Tahara, who have made significant contributions to these studies.

REFERENCES

Armitage, R.J., Fanslow, W.C., Strockbine, L, Sato, T.A., Clifford, K.N., Macduff, B.M., Anderson, D.M., Gimpel, S.D., Davis-Smith, T., Maliszewski, C.R., Clark, E.A., Smith, C.A., Grabstein, K.H., Cosman, D. and Spriggs, M.K. (1992). Molecular and biological characterization of murine ligand for CD40. *Nature* **357**, 80–82.

Austyn, J.M. and Larsen, C.P. (1990) Migration patterns of dendritic leukocytes. Implications for transplantation. *Transplantation* **49**, 1–7.

Austyn, J.M., Hankins, D.F., Larsen, C.P., Morris, P.J., Rao, A.S. and Roake, J.A. (1994). Isolation and characterization of dendritic cells from mouse heart and kidney. *J. Immunol.* **52**, 2401–2410.

Billingham, R.E., Brent, L. and Medawar, P.B. (1953). 'Actively acquired tolerance' of foreign cells. *Nature* **172**, 603–606.

Bonham, C.A., Lu L., Li, Y., Hoffman, R.A., Simmons, R.L. and Thomson, A.W. (1996a). Nitric oxide production by mouse marrow-derived dendritic cells. *Transplantation* **62**, 1709–1714.

Bonham, C.A., Lu, L., Banas, A.R., Fontes, P., Rao, A.S., Zeevi, A. and Thomson, A.W. (1996b). TGF-β1 impairs the allostimulatory function of GM-CSF stimulated antigen presenting cells propagated from human bone marrow. *Transplant. Immunol.* **4**, 186–191.

Buelens, C., Willems, E., Delvaux, A., Pierard, G., Delville, J.P., Velu, T. and Goldman, M. (1995). Interleukin-10 differentially regulates B7-1 (CD80) and B7-2 (CD86) expression on human peripheral blood dendritic cells. *Eur. J. Immunol.* **25**, 2668–2672.

Buelens, C., Verhasselt, V., De Groote, D., Thielemans, K., Goldman, M. and Willems, F. (1997). Human dendritic cell responses to lipopolysaccharide and CD40 ligation are differentially regulated by interleukin-10. *Eur. J. Immunol.* **27**, 1848–1852.

Caux, C, Dezutter-Dambuyant, C., Schmitt D. and Banchereau, J. (1992). GM-CSF and TNFα cooperate in the generation of dendritic Langerhans cells. *Nature* **360**, 258–226.

Caux, C., Massacrier, B., Dervliet, V., Barthelemym C., Liu, Y. J. and Banchereau, J. (1994a). Interleukin-10 inhibits T cell alloreaction induced by human dendritic cells. *Int. Immunol.* **6**, 1177–1185.

Caux, C., Massacrier, C., Vanbervliet, B., Dubois, B., Van Koaten, C., Durand, I. and Banchereau, J. (1994b). Activation of human dendritic cells through CD40 cross-linking. *J. Exp. Med.* **180**, 1263–1272.

Chen, W., Issazadeh, S., Sayegh, M.H. and Khoury, S.J. (1997). In vivo mechanisms of acquired thymic tolerance. *Cell Immunol* **179**, 165–173.

Chen, W., Sayegh, M.H. and Khoury, S.J. (1998). Mechanisms of acquired thymic tolerance in vivo: intrathymic injection of antigen induces apoptosis of thymocytes and peripheral T cell anergy. *J. Immunol.* in press.

Clare-Salzler, M.J., Brooks, J., Chai, A.K. and Anderson, C. (1992). Prevention of diabetes in nonobese diabetic mice by dendritic cell transfer. *J. Clin. Invest.* **90**, 741–748.

Delemarre, F.G.A., Simons, P.J. and Drexhage, H.A. (1995). Class II expression and function of dendritic cells from thyroid gland lymph nodes of the BB rat. *Thyroid., Suppl.* **55**, S24.

Demetris, A.J., Murase, N., Fujisaki, S., Fung, J.J., Rao, A.S. and Starzl, T.E. (1993). Hematolymphoid cell trafficking, microchimerism, and GVHD reactions after liver, bone marrow, and heart transplantation. *Transplant. Proc.* **25**, 3337–3344.

Demetris, A.J., Murase, N., Ye, Q., Galvao, H.H.F., Richert, C., Saad, R., Pham, S., Duquesnoy, R.J., Zeevi, A., Fung, J.J. and Starzl, T.E. (1997). Analysis of chronic rejection and obliterative arteriopathy. *Am. J. Pathol.* **150**, 563–578.

De Smedt, T., Van Mechelen, M., De Becker, G., Urbain, J., Leo, O. and Moser, M. (1997). Effect of interleukin-10 on dendritic cell maturation and function. *Eur. J. Immunol.* **27**, 1229–1235.

Derynck, R. (1994). Transforming growth factor-beta. In *The Cytokine Handbook* (ed. A.W. Thomson) 2nd edn. Academic Press, San Diego, pp. 319–342.

Drakes, M.L., Lu, L., Subbotin, V.M. and Thomson, A.W. (1997). In vivo administration of flt3 ligand markedly stimulates generation of dendritic cell progenitors from mouse liver. *J. Immunol.* **159**, 4268–4278.

Enk, A.H., Angeloni, V.L., Udey, M.C. and Katz. S.I. (1993). Inhibition of Langerhans cell antigen-presenting function by IL-10. A role for IL-10 in induction of tolerance. *J. Immunol.* **151**, 2390–2398.

Fehsel, K., Kroncke, K.D., Meyer, K.L., Huber, H., Wahnm V. and Kolb-Bachofen, V. (1995) Nitric oxide induces apoptosis in mouse thymocytes. *J. Immunol.* **155**, 2858–2865.

Finkelman, F.D., Lees, A., Bimbaum, R., Gause, W.C. and Morris, S.C. (1996). Dendritic cells can present antigen in vivo in a tolerogenic or immunogenic fashion. *J. Immunol.* **157**, 1406–1414.

Freedman, A.S., Munro, J.M., Rhynhart, K., Schow, P., Daley, J., Lee, N., Svahn, J., Elisoeo, L. and Nadler, L.M. (1992). Follicular dendritic cells inhibit human B-lymphocyte proliferation. *Blood* **80**, 1284–1288.

Fu, F., Li, Y., Qian, S., Lu, L., Chambers, F., Starzl, T.E., Fung, J.J. and Thomson, A.W. (1996). Costimulatory molecule-deficient dendritic cell progenitors (MHC class II^{+}, $B7\text{-}1^{dim}$, $B7\text{-}2^{-}$) prolong cardiac allograft survival in non-immunosuppressed recipients. *Transplantation* **62**, 659–665.

Gao, E.K., Lo, D. and Sprent, J. (1990). Strong T cell tolerance in parent$\rightarrow$F1 bone marrow chimeras prepared with supralethal irradiation. Evidence for clonal deletion and anergy. *J. Exp. Med.* **171**, 1101–1112.

Gerling, I.C., Serreze, D.V., Christianson, S.W. and Leiter, E.H. (1992) Intrathymic islet cell transplantation reduces β-cell autoimmunity and prevents diabetes in NOD/Lt mice. *Diabetes* **41**, 1672–1676.

Gorczynski, R.M., Cohen, Z., Fu, X., Hua, Z., Sun, Y. and Chen, Z. (1996) Interleukin-13 in combination with anti-interleukin-12, increases graft prolongation after portal venous immunization with cultured allogeneic bone marrow-derived dendritic cells. *Transplantation* **62**, 1592–1600.

Goss, J.A., Nakafusa, Y., Roland, C.R., Hickey, W.F. and Flye, M.W. (1994). Immunological tolerance to a defined myelin basic protein antigen administered intrathymically. *J. Immunol.* **153**, 3890–3897.

Grabbe, S., Bruver, S., Beissert, S. and Granstein, R.D. (1994a). Interferon-γ inhibits tumor antigen presentation by epidermal antigen presenting cells. *J. Leukocyte Biol.* **55**, 695–701.

Grabbe, S., Bruvers, S. and Granstein, R.D. (1994b). Interleukin 1β but not transforming growth factor inhibits tumor antigen presentation by epidermal antigen-presenting cells. *J. Invest. Dermatol.* **102**, 67–73.

Grabbe, S., Steinbrink, K., Steinert, M., Luger, T.A. and Schwarz, T. (1995). Removal of the majority of epidermal Langerhans cells by topical or systemic steroid application enhances the effector phase of murine contact hypersensitivity. *J. Immunol.* **155**, 4207–4217.

Grohmann, U., Bianchi, R., Ayroldi, E., Belladonna, M.L., Surace, D., Fioretti, M.C. and Puccetti, P. (1997). A tumor-associated and self antigen peptide presented by dendritic cells may induce T cell anergy in vivo, but IL-12 can prevent or revert the anergic state. *J. Immunol.* **158**, 3593–3602.

Hambor, J.E., Kaplan, D.R. and Tykocinski, M.L. (1990). CD8 functions as an inhibitory ligand in mediating the immunoregulatory activity of $CD8^+$ cells. *J. Immunol.* **145**, 1644–1652.

Hancock, W.W., Sayegh, M.H., Zheng, X.G., Peach, R., Linsley, P.S. and Turka, L.A. (1996). Costimulatory function and expression of CD40 ligand, CD80, and CD86 in vascularized murine cardiac allograft rejection. *Proc. Natl Acad. Sci. USA* **93**, 139–167.

Inaba, M., Inaba, K., Hosono, M., Kumamoto, T., Ishida, T., Muramatsu, S., Masuda, T. and Ikehara, S. (1991). Distinct mechanisms of neonatal tolerance induced by dendritic cells and thymic B cells. *J. Exp. Med.* **173**, 549–559.

Inaba, K., Inaba, M., Romani, N., Aya, H., Deguchi, M., Ikehara, S., Muramatsu, S. and Steinman, R.M. (1992a). Generation of large numbers of dendritic cells from mouse bone marrow cultures supplemented with granulocyte/macrophage colony-stimulating factor. *J. Exp. Med.* **176**, 1693–1702.

Inaba, K., Steinman, R.M., Pack, M.W., Aya, H., Inaba, M., Sudo, T., Wolpe, S. and Schuler, G. (1992b). Identification of proliferating dendritic cell precursors in mouse blood. *J. Exp. Med.* **175**, 1157–1167.

Inaba, K., Pack, M., Inaba, M., Sakuta, H., Isdell, F. and Steinman, R.M. (1997). High levels of a major histocompatibility complex II-self peptide complex on dendritic cells from the T cell areas of lymph nodes. *J. Exp. Med.* **186**, 665–672.

Jenkinson, E.J., Jhittay, P., Kingston, R. and Owen, J.J.T. (1985). Studies of the role of the thymic environment in the induction of tolerance to MHC antigens. *Transplantation* **39**, 331–333.

Kaeamura, T. and Furue, M. (1995). Comparative analysis of B7-1 and B7-2 expression in Langerhans cells: differential regulation by T helper type 1 and T helper type 2 cytokines. *Eur. J. Immunol.* **25**, 1913–1917.

Kalinski, P., Hilkens, C.M., Snijders, A., Snijdewint, F. G. and Kapsenberg, M.L. (1997). IL-12-deficient dendritic cells, generated in the presence of prostaglandin E2, promote type 2 cytokine production in maturing human naive T helper cells. *J. Immunol.* **159**, 28–35.

Khoury, S.J., Sayegh, M.H., Hancock, W.W., Gallon, L., Carpenter, C.B. and Weiner, H.L. (1993). Acquired tolerance to experimental autoimmune encephalomyelitis by intrathymic injection of myelin basic protein or its major encephalitogenic peptide. *J. Exp. Med.* **178**, 559–566.

Khoury, S.J., Gallon, L., Chen, W., Betres, K., Russell, M.E., Hancock, W.W., Carpenter, C.B., Sayegh, M.H. and Weiner, H.L. (1995). Mechanisms of acquired thymic tolerance in experimental autoimmune encephalomyelitis: thymic dendritic-enriched cells induce specific peripheral T cell unresponsiveness in vivo. *J. Exp. Med.* **182**, 357–366.

Khoury, S.J., Gallon, L., Verburg, R.R., Chandraker, A., Peach, R. et al. (1996). Ex-vivo treatment of antigen presenting cells with CTLA4-Ig and encephalitogenic peptide prevents experimental autoimmune encephalomyelitis in the Lewis rat. *J. Immunol.* **157**, 3700–3705.

Kirk, A.D., Harlan, D.M., Armstrong, N.N., Davis, T.A., Dong, V., Gray, G.S., Hong, X., Thomas, D., Fechner, J.H. Jr. and Knechtle, S.J. (1997). CTLA4-Ig and anti-CD40 ligand prevent renal allograft rejection in primates. *Proc. Natl Acad. Sci. USA* **94**, 8789–8794.

Knight, S.C., Hunt, R., Dore, C. and Medawar, P.B. (1985). Influence of dendritic cells on tumor growth. *Proc. Natl Acad. Aci. Sci. USA* **82**, 4495–4497.

Knight, S.C., Mertin, J. and Clark, J. (1983). Induction of immune responses *in vivo* with small numbers of veiled (dendritic cells). *Proc. Natl Acad. Sci. USA* **80**, 6032–6035.

Koevary, S. and Blomberg, M. (1992). Prevention of diabetes in BB/Wor rats by intrathymic islet injection. *J. Clin. Invest.* **89**, 512–516.

Kronin, V., Winkel, K., Suss, G., Kelso, A., Heath, W., Kirberg, J., Boehmer, H.V. and Shortman, K. (1996). A subclass of dendritic cells regulates the response of naive CD8 T cells by limiting their IL-2 production. *J. Immunol.* **157**, 3819–3827.

Kronin, V., Vremec, D., Winkel, K., Classon, F.J., Miller, R.G., Mak, T.W., Shortman, K. and Suss, G. (1997). Are $CD8^+$ dendritic cells veto cells? The role of CD8 on dendritic cells in the regulation of CD4 and CD8 T cell responses. *Int. Immunol.*, In press.

Larsen, C.P., Morris, P.J. and Austyn, J.M. (1990). Migration of dendritic leukocytes from cardiac allografts into host spleens: a novel route for initiation of rejection. *J. Exp. Med.* **171**, 307–314.

Larsen, C.P., Ritchie, S.C., Hendrix, R., Linsley, P.S., Hathcock, K.S., Hodes, R.J., Lowry, R.P. and Pearson, T.C. (1994). Regulation of immunostimulatory function and costimulatory molecule (B7-1 and B7-2) expression on murine dendritic cells. *Immunol.* **152**, 5208–5219.

Larsen, C.P., Elwood, E.T., Alexander, D.Z., Ritchie, S.C., Hendrix, R., Tucker-Burden, C., Cho, H.R., Aruffo, A., Hollenbaugh, D., Linsley, P.S., Winn, K.J. and Pearson, T.C. (1996) Long-term acceptance of skin and cardiac allografts after blocking CD40 and CD28 pathways. *Nature* **381**, 434–438.

Lin, H., Bolling, S.F., Linsley, P.S., Wei, R.Q., Gordon, D., Thompson, C.B. and Turka, L.A. (1993). Long term acceptance of major histocompatibility complex mismatched cardiac allografts induced by CTLA4-Ig plus donor-specific transfusion. *J. Exp. Med.* **178**, 1801–1806.

Lu, L., Woo, J., Rao, A.S., Li, Y., Qian, S., Watkins, S.C., Starzl, T.E., Demetris, A.J. and Thomson, A.W. (1994). Propagation of dendritic cell progenitors from normal mouse liver using granulocyte/macrophage colony-stimulating factor and their maturational development in the presence of type-1 collagen. *J. Exp. Med.* **179**, 1823–1834.

Lu, L., McCaslin, D., Starzl, T.E. and Thomson, A.W. (1995a). Mouse bone marrow-derived dendritic cell progenitors (NLDC145$^+$, MHC class II$^+$, B7-1^{dim}, B7-2$^-$) induce alloantigen-specific hyporesponsiveness in murine T lymphocytes. *Transplantation* **60**, 1539–1545.

Lu, L., Rudert, W.A., Qian, S., McCaslin, D., Fu, F., Rao, A.S., Trucco, M., Fung, J.J., Starzl, T.E. and Thomson, A.W. (1995b). Growth of donor-derived dendritic cells from the bone marrow of murine liver allograft recipients in response to granulocyte/macrophage colony-stimulating factor. *J. Exp. Med.* **182**, 379–387.

Lu, L., Bonham, C.A., Chambers, F.D., Watkins, S.C., Hoffman, R.A., Simmons, R.L. and Thomson, A.W. (1996). Induction of nitric oxide synthase in mouse dendritic cells by interferon-γ, endotoxin and interaction with allogeneic T cells: nitric oxide production is associated with dendritic cell apoptosis. *J. Immunol.* **157**, 3577–3785.

Lu, L., Li, W., Fu, F., Chambers, F.G., Qian, S., Fung, J.J. and Thomson, A.W. (1997a). Blockade of the CD40–CD40L pathway potentiates the capacity of donor-derived dendritic cell progenitors to induce long-term cardiac allograft survival. *Transplantation* **64**, 1808–1815.

Lu, L., Qian, S., Hershberger, P.A., Rudert, W.A., Li, Y., Chambers, F.G., Lynch, D.H. and Thomson, A.W. (1997b). Fas ligand (CD95L) and B7 expression on dendritic cells provide counter-regulatory signals for T cell survival and proliferation. *J. Immunol.* **158**, 5676–5684.

Ludewig, B., Graf, D., Gelderblom, H.R., Becker, Y., Kroczek, R.A. and Pauli, G. (1995). Spontaneous apoptosis of dendritic cells in efficiently inhibited by TRAP (CD40-ligand) and TNF-α, but strongly enhanced by interleukin-10. *Eur. J. Immunol.* **25**, 1943–1950.

Lutz, M.B., Assmann, C.U., Girolomoni, G. and Ricciardi-Castagnoli, P. (1996). Different cytokines regulate antigen uptake and presentation of a precursor dendritic cell line. *Eur. J. Immunol.* **26**, 586–594.

Lynch, D.H., Ramsdell, F. and Alderson, M.R. (1995). Fas FasL in the homeostatic regulation of immune responses. *Immunol. Today* **16**, 569–574.

Matzinger, P. and Guerder, S. (1989). Does T cell tolerance require a dedicated antigen-presenting cell? *Nature* **338**, 74–76.

McLellan, A.D., Sorg, R.V., Williams, L.A. and Hart, D.N.J. (1996). Human dendritic cells activate T lymphocytes via a CD40:CD40 ligand-dependent pathway. *Eur. J. Immunol.* **26**, 1204–1210.

Moore, K.W., O'Garra, A., Malefyt, D.E.W., Vieram P. and Mosman, T.R. (1993). Interleukin-10. *Annu. Rev. Immunol.* **11**, 165–190.

Morel, A.S., Quaratino, S., Douek, D.C. and Londei, M. (1997). Split activity of interleukin-10 on antigen capture and antigen presentation by human dendritic cells: definition of a maturative step. *Eur. J. Immunol.* **27**, 26–34.

Morikawa, Y., Furotani, M., Kuribayashi, K., Marsuura, N. and Kakudo, K. (1992). The role of antigen-presenting cells in the regulation of delayed-type hypersensitivity. 1. Spleen dendritic cells. *Immunology* **77**, 81–87.

Morikawa, Y., Furotani, M., Mastsuura, N. and Kakudo, K. (1993). The role of antigen-presenting cells in the regulation of delayed-type hypersensitivity II. Epidermal Langerhans cells and peritoneal exudate macrophages. *Cell Immunol.* **152**, 200–210.

Morikawa, Y., Tohya, K., Matsuura, N. and Kakudo, K. (1995). Different migration patterns of antigen-presenting cells correlate with T_H1/T_H2-type responses in mice. *Immunology* **85**, 575–581.

Nelson, D.J. and Holt, P.G. (1995). Defective regional immunity in the respiratory tract of neonates is attributable to hyporesponsiveness of local dendritic cells to activation signals. *J. Immunol.* **155**, 3517–3524.

Ni, K. and O'Neill, H.C. (1997). The role of dendritic cells in T cell activation. *Immunol. Cell Biol.* **75**, 223–230.

Ohzato, H. and Monaco, A.P. (1992). Induction of specific unresponsiveness (tolerance) to skin allografts by intrathymic donor-specific splenocyte injection in antilymphocyte serum-treated mice. *Transplantation* **54**, 1090–1095.

Oluwole, S.J., Jin, M.X., Chowdhury, N.C., Engelstad, K., Ohajekwe, O.A. and James, T. (1995). Induction of peripheral tolerance by intrathymic inoculation of soluble alloantigens: evidence for the role of host antigen-presenting cells and suppressor cell mechanism. *Cell Immunol.* **162**, 33–41.

Parker, D.C., Greiner, D.L., Phillips, N.E., Appel, M.C., Steele, A.W., Durie, F.H., Noelle, R.J., Mordes, J.P. and Rossini, A.A. (1995). Survival of mouse pancreatic islet allograft recipients treated with allogeneic small lymphocytes and antibody to CD40 ligand. *Proc. Natl Acad. Sci. USA* **92**, 9560–9564.

Posselt, A.M., Barker, C.F., Tomaszewski, J.E., Markmann, J.F., Choti, M.A. and Man, A. (1990). Induction of donor-specific unresponsiveness by intrathymic islet transplantation. *Science* **249**, 1293–1295.

Qian, S., Demetris, A.J., Murase, N., Rao, A.S., Fung, J.J. and Starzl, T.E. (1994). Murine liver allograft transplantation: tolerance and donor cell chimerism. *Hepatology* **19**, 916–924.

Qian, S., Lu, L., Li, Y., Fu, F. Li, W. Starzl, T.E., Fung, J.J. and Thomson, A.W. (1997a). Apoptosis within spontaneously accepted mouse liver allografts: evidence for deletion of cytotoxic T cells and implications for tolerance induction. *J. Immunol.* **158**, 4654–4661.

Qian, S., Thai, N.L., Lu, L., Fung, J.J. and Thomson, A.W. (1997b). Liver transplant tolerance: mechanistic insights from animal models, with particular reference to the mouse. *Transplant. Rev.* **11**, 151–164.

Rastellini, C., Lu, L., Ricordi, C., Starzl, T.E., Rao, A.S. and Thomson, A.W. (1995). GM-CSF stimulated hepatic dendritic cell progenitors prolong pancreatic islet allograft survival. *Transplantation* **60**, 1366–1370.

Remuzzi, G., Rossini, M., Imberti, O. and Perico, N. (1991). Kidney graft survival in rats without immunosuppressants after intrathymic glomerular transplantation. *Lancet* **337**, 750–752.

Ridge, J.P. and Matzinger, P. (1996). Neonatal tolerance revisited: turning on newborn T cells with dendritic cells. *Science* **271**, 1723–1726.

Romani, N., Schuler, G. and Frisch, P. (1986). Ontogeny of Ia-positive and Thy-1-positive leukocytes of murine epidermis. *J. Invest. Dermatol.* **86**, 129–133.

Rugeles, M.T., Aitouche, A., Zeevi, A., Fung, J.J., Watkins, S.C., Starzl, T.E. and Rao, A.S. (1997). Evidence for the presence of multilineage chimerism and progenitors of donor dendritic cells in the peripheral blood of bone marrow-augmented organ transplant recipients. *Transplantation* **64**, 735–741.

Saleem, M., Sawyer, G.J., Schofield, R.A., Seymour, N.O., Gustafsson, K. and Fabre, J.W. (1997). Discordant expression on major histocompatibility complex class II antigen and invariant chain in interstitial dendritic cells. *Transplantation* **64**, 1134–1138.

Sallusto, F., Cella, M., Danieli, C. and Lanzavecchia, A. (1995). Dendritic cells use macropinocytosis and the mannose receptor to concentrate macromolecules in the major histocompatibility complex class II compartment: downregulation by cytokines and bacterial products. *J. Exp. Med.* **182**, 398–400.

Sambhara, S.R. and Miller, R.G. (1991). Programmed cell death of T cells signaled by the T cell receptor and $\alpha 3$ domain of MHC class I. *Science* **252**, 1424–1427.

Sayegh, M.H., Akalin, E., Hancock, W.W., Russell, M.E., Carpenter, C.B., Linsley, P.S. and Turka, L.A. (1995). CD28-B7 Blockade after alloantigenic challenge in vivo inhibits T_H1 cytokines but spares T_H2 *J. Exp. Med.* **181**, 1869–1874.

Schwartz, R.H. (1990). A cell culture model for T lymphocyte clonal anergy. *Science* **248**, 1349–1356.

Shapiro, R., Rao, A.S., Fontes, P., Jordan, M., Scantlebury, V.P., Vivas, C., Demetris, A.J., Zeevi, A., Rybka, W. and Carroll, P. (1995). Combined kidney/bone marrow transplantation—evidence of augmentation of chimerism. *Transplantation* **59**, 306–309.

Simon, J.C., Tigelaar, R.E., Bergstresser, P.R., Edelbaum, D. and Cruz, P.D. (1991). Ultraviolet B radiation converts Langerhans cells from immunogenic to tolerogenic antigen-presenting cells. Induction of specific clonal anergy in CD4 T helper cells. *J. Immunol.* **146**, 485–491.

Song, W., Kong, H.-L., Carpenter, H., Torii, H., Granstein, R., Rafii, S., Moore, M.A.S. and Crystal, R.G. (1997). Dendritic cells genetically modified with an adenovirus vector encoding the cDNA for a model antigen induce protective and therapeutic antitumor immunity. *J. Exp. Med.* **186**, 1247–1256.

Specht, J.M., Wang, G., Do, M.T., Lam, J.S., Royal, R.E., Reeves, M.E., Rosenberg, S.A. and Hwu, P. (1997) Dendritic cells retrovirally transduced with a model antigen gene are therapeutically effective against established pulmonary metastases. *J. Exp. Med.* **186**, 1213–1221.

Starzl, T.E., Demetris, A.J., Murase, N., Ildstad, S., Ricordi, C. and Trucco, M. (1992). Cell migration, chimerism, and graft acceptance. *Lancet* **339**, 1579–1582.

Starzl, T.E., Demetris, A.J., Trucco, M., Murase, N., Ricordi, C., Ildstad, S., Ramos, H., Todo, S., Tzakis, A., Fung, J.J., Nalesnik, M., Zeevi, A., Rudert, W.A. and Kocova, M. (1993). Cell migration and chimerism after whole organ transplantation: the basis of graft acceptance. *Hepatology* **17**, 1127–1152.

Starzl, T.E., Demetris, A.J., Murase, N., Trucco, M., Thomson, A.W. and Rao, A.S. (1996). The lost chord: microchimerism and allograft survival. *Immunol. Today* **17**, 577–584.

Steinbrink, K., Wölfl, M., Jonuleit, H., Knop, J. and Enk, A.H. (1997). Induction of tolerance by IL-10-treated dendritic cells. *J. Immunol.* **159**, 4772–4780.

Steinman, R.M. (1991). The dendritic cell system and its role in immunogenicity. *Annu. Rev. Immunol.* **9**, 271–296.

Steptoe, R.J. and Thomson, A.W. (1996). Dendritic cells and tolerance induction. *Clin. Exp. Immunol.* **105**, 397–402.

Steptoe, R.J., Fu, F., Li, W., Drakes, M., Lu, L., Demetris, A.J., Qian, S., McKenna, H.J. and Thomson, A.W. (1997). Augmentation of dendritic cells in murine organ donors by treatment with flt-3 ligand alters the balance between transplant tolerance and immunity. *J. Immunol.* **159**, 5483–5491.

Streilein, J.W., Wilbanks, G.A. and Cousins, S.W. (1992). Immunoregulatory mechanisms of the eye. *J. Neuroimmunol.* **39**, 185–200.

Strobl, H., Riedl, E., Scheinecker, C., Bello-Fernandez, C., Pickl, W., Rappersberger, K., Majdic, O. and Knapp, W. (1996). TGF-β1 promotes in vitro development of dendritic cells from $CD34^+$ hematopoietic progenitors. *J. Immunol.* **157**, 1499–1507.

Süss, G. and Shortman, K. (1996). A subclass of dendritic cells kills CD4 T cells via Fas/Fas-ligand induced apoptosis. *J. Exp. Med.* **183**, 1789–1796.

Szabolcs, P., Moore, M.A. and Young, J.W. (1995). Expansion of immunostimulatory dendritic cells among the myeloid progeny of human $CD34^+$ bone marrow precursors cultured with c-kit ligand, granulocyte-macrophage colony-stimulating factor and TNFα. *J. Immunol.* **154**, 5851–5861.

Thomas, J.M., Carver, F.M., Kasten-Jolly, J., Haisch, C.E., Rebellato, L.M., Gross, U., Vore, S.J. and Thomas, F.T. (1994). Further studies of veto activity in rhesus monkey bone marrow in relation to allograft tolerance and chimerism. *Transplantation* **57**, 101–115.

Thomson, A.W., Lu, L., Murase, N., Demetris, A.J., Rao, A.S. and Starzl, T.E. (1995a). Microchimerism, dendritic cell progenitors and transplantation tolerance. *Stem Cells* **13**, 622–639.

Thomson, A.W., Lu, L, Subbotin, V.M., Li, Y., Qian, S., Rao, A.S., Fung, J.J. and Starzl, T.E. (1995b). In vitro propagation and homing of liver-derived dendritic cell progenitors to lymphoid tissues of allogeneic recipients. *Transplantation* **59**, 544–551.

Thomson, A.W., Lu, L., Wan, Y., Qian, S., Larsen, C.P. and Starzl, T.E. (1995c). Identification of donor-derived dendritic cell progenitors in bone marrow of spontaneously tolerant liver allograft recipients. *Transplantation* **60**, 1555–1559.

Thomson, A.W., Lu, L., Steptoe, R.J. and Starzl, T.E. (1996). Dendritic cells and the balance between transplant tolerance and immunity. In: *Immune Tolerance* (eds J. Banchereau, B. Dodet, R. Schwartz, E. Trannoy). Elsevier, Paris, pp. 173–185.

Verberg, R., Chandraker, A., Gallon, L., Hancock, W.W., Sayegh, M.H. and Khoury, S.J. (1996). Ex-vivo treatment of antigen-presenting cells with CTLA4Ig and peptide prevents EAE in the Lewis rat. *J. Immunol.* **157**, 3700–3705.

Vremec, D., Zorbas, M., Scollay, R., Saunders, J., Ardavin, C.F., Wu, L. and Shortman, K. (1992). The surface phenotype of dendritic cells purified from mouse thymus and spleen: investigation of the CD8 expression by a subpopulation of dendritic cells *J. Exp. Med.* **176**, 47–58.

Wan, Y., Branson, J., Carter, R., Graham, F. and Gauldie, J. (1997). Dendritic cells transduced with an adenoviral vector encoding a model tumor-associated antigen for tumor vaccination. *Hum. Gene Ther.* **8**, 1355–1363.

Welsh, E.A. and Kripke, M.L. (1990). Murine Thy-1$^+$ dendritic epidermal cells induce immunological tolerance in vivo. *J. Immunol.* **144**, 883–891.

Widera, G., Burkly, L.C., Pinkert, C.A., Botlger, E.C., Cowing, C., Palmiter, R.D. and Brinster, R.L. (1987). Transgenic mice selectively lacking MHC class II (I-E) antigen expression on B cells: an in vivo approach to investigate Ia gene function. *Cell* **51**, 175–187.

Wilbanks, G.A. and Streilein, J.W. (1992). Fluids from immune privileged sites endow macrophages with the capacity to induce antigen-specific immune deviation via a mechanism involving transforming growth factor-β. *Eur. J. Immunol.* **22**, 1031–1036.

Wiley, S.R., Schooley, K., Smolak, P.J., Din, W.S., Huang, C.P., Nicholl, J.K., Sutherland, G.R., Smith, T.D., Rauch, C. and Smith, C.A. (1995). Identification and characterization of a new member of the TNF family that induces apoptosis. *Immunity* **3**, 673–682.

Woo, J., Lu, L., Rao, A.W., Li, Y., Subbotin, V., Starzl, T.E. and Thomson, A.W. (1994). Isolation, phenotype, and allostimulatory activity of mouse liver dendritic cells. *Transplantation* **58**, 484–491.

Yang, Y. and Wilson, J.M. (1996). CD40 ligand-dependent T cell activation: requirement of B7-CD28 signaling through CD40. *Science* **273**, 1862–1864.

Yasunori, Y., Tsumura, H., Miwa, M. and Inaba, K. (1997). Contrasting effects of TGF-β1 and TNFα on the development of dendritic cells from progenitors in mouse bone marrow. *Stem Cells* **15**, 144–153.

VI TECHNIQUES AND OTHER TOPICS IN DC BIOLOGY

CHAPTER 27
A Guide to the Isolation and Propagation of Dendritic Cells

Gerold Schuler[1], Manfred Lutz[1], Armin Bender[1], Beatrice Thurner[1], Claudia Röder[1], James W. Young[2] and Nikolaus Romani[3]

[1]Department of Dermatology, University of Erlangen-Nuerenberg, Germany; [2]Memorial Sloan-Kettering Cancer Center, New York, New York, USA; [3]Department of Dermatology, University of Innsbruck, Innsbruck, Austria

SUBSETS OF DC AND CRITERIA FOR THEIR IDENTIFICATION

Dendritic cells (DC) are distinctive leukocytes specialized to activate naive T lymphocytes (Steinman, 1991; Hart, 1997). DC are a trace cell type (typically <1% in most lymphoid and nonlymphoid organs), and the isolation of substantial numbers of highly purified DC from tissues has, therefore, been difficult. It was this laborious isolation of DC that allowed researchers to unravel the basic biology of DC and later to develop methods for the generation of large numbers of DC from hematopoietic precursors. The latter techniques have given DC research an enormous boost, as the large numbers of DC that can now be produced *in vitro* for the first time allow researchers to study DC function at the molecular level and to explore DC for inducing immunity *in vivo*.

We outline in this chapter the generation of DC from precursors, and also the isolation of DC directly from tissues, which is, of course, still essential for study of the *in situ* situation. Owing to space limitations we cannot give here a step-by-step description of the various techniques. Rather we will focus on outlining the principles, and will refer the reader to key references. We trust that such a guideline will be useful to the many novices who in our experience are either overwhelmed by or do not appreciate the problems and complexities inherent to the rapidly evolving field of DC.

It is becoming increasingly clear that the DC system is constituted by multiple DC subsets with distinct developmental pathways, functional properties, and maturational stages. For a better understanding it is helpful to recapitulate how the concept of the DC evolved (Steinman, 1991; Hart, 1997). DC were first isolated from murine spleen cell suspensions following 1–2 days of culture. These DC display the features of what we nowadays call 'mature' DC (see also below). Such mature DC are specialized to sensitize T cells ('T cell stimulatory mode'), and in all species studied are characterized by the following features: (1) potent stimulation of naive, unprimed helper as well as killer T cells both *in vitro* and *in vivo* (this is the unique and key feature of mature DC

Dendritic Cells: Biology and Clinical Applications
ISBN 0-12-455860-7

that is evident with antigens, alloantigens and superantigens); (2) nonadherent large cells with many motile, sheet-like cytoplasmic processes ('veils'), (3) phenotype of a 'lineage-negative leukocyte', i.e., lack of certain markers of other lineages, such as CD19,20 for B cells, CD3 for T cells, CD16,56 for NK cells, and absence or low expression of macrophage markers; (4) high levels of MHC class I and II products; (5) high levels of adhesion and costimulator molecules important for T cell stimulation (e.g., CD86) and DC–T cross-talk (e.g., CD40); (6) presence of markers that are characteristic though not absolutely specific for mature DC/DC subsets (e.g., DEC-205/NLDC 145, and the cytoplasmic markers 2A1, M342, and MIDC-8 found on mature murine DC; in the mouse CD11c is another useful marker as it is expressed on most immature as well as mature DC (for review see Steinman *et al.*, 1997); CD83 (Zhou and Tedder, 1995) and the cytoplasmic marker p55/fascin (Mosialos *et al.*, 1997) are novel markers for mature human DC); and as a recently discovered trait, (7) production of high levels of bioactive IL-12. Studies of epidermal Langerhans cells suggested that in peripheral tissues DC are 'immature', i.e., in the so-called 'antigen-processing mode'. Such 'immature DC' in response to inflammatory stimuli take up antigen, for example, by macropinocytosis (elegantly demonstrable by FITC-dextran uptake) (Sallusto *et al.*, 1995) and to some extent by phagocytosis in case of particulates (Austyn, 1996), process antigens in abundant intracellular lysosomal MHC II-rich organelles (Pierre *et al.*, 1997), and generate large amounts of MHC II–peptide complexes or TCR ligands (as evident from potent stimulation of peptide-specific T cell hybridomas/clones/lines (Sallusto and Lanzavecchia, 1994; Romani *et al.*, 1989; Koch *et al.*, 1995) but lack costimulatory molecules and, therefore, lack the capacity to prime T cells. Upon exposure to inflammatory cytokines these immature DC develop *in vitro* into mature stellate DC with abundant surface MHC II and costimulatory molecules, sparse MHC II-negative lysosomes, and strong T cell sensitizing capacity. *In vivo* studies indicated that LC successively matured *in vivo* as well while emigrating from the epidermis into the afferent lymphatics, and, finally into the T areas of draining lymph nodes (for review see Austyn, 1996). Further studies showed that DC at other sites such as lung and the interstitium of solid organs also matured. *In vitro* immunostimulatory DC could be generated from myeloid precursors in both man and mouse in the presence of GM-CSF. These observations led to the view of a single (myeloid-derived) DC system in which immature DC picked up antigen in the periphery, and then matured during migration (from epithelia via afferent lymphatics and from interstitial spaces via blood) to the T areas (draining nodes and spleen, respectively) to finally become interdigitating dendritic cells (IDC) in the center of the T areas. Recent studies have shown, however, that under steady-state conditions in mouse spleen most DC are actually located at the periphery of the T cell area as scattered profiles in the marginal zone (representing DC immigrating from the periphery and/or immature DC residing in the spleen) (reviewed in Steinman *et al.*, 1997). These DC are functionally (antigen-processing strong, T cell-sensitization weak) and phenotypically (CD11c^{+}, but weak NLDC-145/DEC-205 and granular antigens recognized by M342, MIDC-8, and 2A1) immature, but 6 h after systemic LPS administration mature functionally (upregulation of T cell stimulating capacity, downregulation of antigen processing) as well as phenotypically (CD11c^{+}, and also NLDC-145/DEC-205^{++} and granular antigens $^{++}$) and move to the periarteriolar sheaths to become IDCs (De Smedt *et al.*, 1996). Seminal studies by Shortman's group have revealed that under steady-state conditions a substantial proportion of the IDC isolated in the steady state are not immunostimulatory myeloid-related DC but rather lymphoid-related immunoregulatory DC (Süss and Shortman, 1996; Kronin *et al.*, 1997). These DC develop in a GM-CSF-independent fashion from nonmyeloid precursors that give rise also to lymphocytes and, besides being CD11c$^+$ NLDC-145$^+$, express CD8 and Fas-L. Although they are also mature in that they stimulate unprimed T cells, the outcome after initial antigen-specific activation is Fas-L-mediated death of CD4$^+$ T cells, and limited proliferation of CD8$^+$ T cells due to downregulation of IL-2 production via an unidentified mechanism. It is unknown whether lymphoid-derived DC undergo a process of maturation as observed with myeloid-derived DC. The lymphoid-derived DC might represent the bulk of IDC in the steady state, and may function in the thymic medulla for central tolerance, and in the T cell areas of peripheral organs to maintain tolerance to self-antigens that are found at high levels on these cells *in vivo* (Inaba *et al.*, 1998a). Lymphoid-derived DC have been generated *in vitro* in man as well (see 'Generation of lymphoid DC from CD34$^+$ cells' later), but their function and *in situ* localization has yet to be reported. When discussing the isolation and propagation techniques, we will relate the isolated DC subsets and progeny—as far as possible—to the framework that we have outlined above.

We emphasize the use of certain standard criteria to characterize DC that are isolated from tissues or propagated *in vitro*. This is critical as the respective methods are often not fully standardizable or not yet standardized, but data nevertheless must be comparable between different research groups. As mentioned above, the identification of mature DC in general relies on a combination of morphological (nonadherent highly motile veiled cells), phenotypic (lineage negative, MHC II^{++}, CD86^{++}, and, as far as now available, the presence of specific DC markers), and functional (potent T cell sensitization) criteria, and is well established for myeloid-related DC while the characteristics of the novel lymphoid-related DC are still evolving. One should keep in mind that immunostimulatory (myeloid) mature DC are primarily defined functionally as cells that exhibit potent activation of naive T cells at low DC:T ratios (in the allo-MLR, typically strong stimulation at DC:T ratios of $<$1:200). It is important to recall that only mature, but not immature myeloid DC (as they share several markers with macrophages) can be reliably identified as DC, except that the development of immature DC into mature DC can be directly demonstrated *in vitro*.

MURINE DENDRITIC CELLS

Isolation of Murine DC from Nonlymphoid and Lymphoid Organs

DC isolated from skin and spleen have been most intensively studied, and standard procedures that are also applicable to thymus and spleen are now available. DC have also been sucessfully isolated from other sites such as afferent lymph, Peyer's patches, lung, heart, kidney, and gut. DC have not been isolated directly from murine blood as it is available only in small amounts, although mouse blood was first used to identify proliferating precursors to DC and to generate DC *in vitro* (Inaba *et al.*, 1992a). When isolating DC from murine tissues, in particular lymphoid ones, it is advantageous to use specific pathogen-free mice, to let the mice rest for at least 5 days after shipment, and to avoid stress prior to sacrifice in order to maximize yield and purity of DC.

Skin

DC can be isolated from the epidermis (i.e., so-called epidermal Langerhans cells or LC) or the dermis (so-called dermal dendritic cells or DDC). LC are the best studied nonlymphoid DC, and have been key to the understanding of how DC function, notably the 'concept of DC maturation' (reviewed in Schuler, 1991; Moll, 1995). Although LC can be prepared from body skin, the ears are clearly the best source for obtaining highly enriched LC. Following incubation in low concentrations of trypsin (or, alternatively, dispase), the epidermal sheets can be separated from the dermal ones. Rocking of the epidemal sheets releases epidermal cells, which then can be treated with anti-Thy-1 and complement to remove most keratinocytes and lymphocytes (notably the Thy-1^+ dendritic epidermal TCRγ/δ^+ T cells). This leaves one with an epidermal cell suspension containing about 10% LC, which then can be purified by positive selection either by a 'mismatched panning technique' (Koch *et al.*, 1992) (which is cheap and works well) or by sorting (by fluorescence-activated (FACS) or magnetic cell sorting (MACS); Miltenyi *et al.*, 1990), for example, for MHC class II-positive cells, i.e., LC (yield after panning about 1.0–2.5 × 10^4 LC/ear). Further enrichment of fresh LC is also possible by harvesting the low-density fraction following gradient centrifugation. This, however, selects for a subset of fresh LC since immature LC (as immature DC in general) have a variable bouyant density, and only about one-third have low density. LC are immature *in situ* and, following isolation, have already started to mature (Pierre *et al.*, 1997). Untreated or anti-Thy-1/C′ treated (i.e., LC preenriched) epidermal cell suspensions can be cultured for 2–4 days, after which the LC have matured and can be enriched to 60–90% by simple density gradient centrifugation of the nonadherent fraction and harvesting of the low-density fraction (since mature LC like mature DC in general exhibit a low bouyant density). By further enrichment via positive selection, for example, via 'mismatched panning', one can obtain pure LC (yield about 3.0–4.5 × 10^4 LC/mouse ear). Another simple approach to isolating (matured) skin DC is to culture ear halves floating on medium. Owing to production of inflammatory cytokines, the epidermal (i.e., LC) and dermal DC spontanously emigrate from the skin and drop into the culture medium, and can be harvested (about 1 × 10^4 DC/dorsal ear half) (Lenz *et al.*, 1993; Pope *et al.*, 1995). We have recently further improved this elegant approach that circumvents any exposure to enzymes or antibodies (Ortner *et al.*, 1996). For further information and technical details, the reader is referred to the references cited and reviews in which we have described the methods and their pitfalls in detail (Schuler and Koch, 1991; Romani *et al.*, 1996a).

Spleen

DC were discovered in murine spleen, and for years have been isolated from this organ by rather standardized procedures. It is now clear that by using these standard procedures most of the DC that are released from spleen emanate from the periphery of the white pulp (i.e., the marginal zone), but not the the central, IDC-rich periarterial sheaths. These marginal zone DC *in situ* strongly express CD11c, but little CD86, and lack markers found *in situ* on IDC, notably DEC-205 (NLDC-145) and granular antigens recognized by monoclonal antibodies (mAbs) M342, MIDC-8, and 2A1 (Steinman *et al.*, 1997). An optimized basic protocol starts with preparing a low-density fraction (e.g., by flotation of spleen cell suspensions over dense BSA columns) of a collagenase-digested (increases yield 2- to 3-fold over simple mechanical disruption) splenocyte suspension which is plated in 100 mm culture dishes. After 90 min culture at 37°C the DC and macrophages are adherent, and lymphocytes can be removed by washing. DC become nonadherent after overnight culture and can be harvested at 60–80% purity. By EA rosetting in which antibody-coated erythrocytes are used to remove contaminating Fc receptor$^+$ macrophages and B cells, the DC if needed can be enriched further to >95%; for a detailed description of this method, see Romani *et al.* (1996) and Inaba *et al.* (1992c). The final yield is from 2×10^5 to 7×10^5 DC per spleen. These DC are functionally mature (potent T cell stimulation, for example, in the allo-MLR 30–100 times more potent than bulk spleen cells; downregulated antigen-processing capacity), are CD11c$^+$, MHC class II^{++}, CD86^{++}, express granular antigens recognized by mAbs M342, MIDC-8, and 2A1, and in addition express the DC-specific marker 33D1. When DC were isolated from freshly isolated low-density fractions (rather than after overnight culture) by positive selection utilizing the N418 anti-CD11c mAb and FACS or MACS, it became clear that the DC were functionally immature (high antigen processing capacity, poor T cell stimulation), and had the phenotype of the marginal zone DC (Metlay *et al.*, 1990; Crowley *et al.*, 1990). Following overnight culture in the presence of GM-CSF, however, they developed into mature DC identical to those that are obtained by the standard procedure after culture of low-density fractions. This maturation *in vitro* fits well the *in vivo* observation that marginal zone DC following systemic LPS administration mature and move to the periarteriolar sheaths (De Smedt *et al.*, 1996).

An important recent discovery was the finding that collagenase digestion of spleen *and* use of Ca^{2+}-free media was required to release the central periarterial, or interdigitating, CD8$^+$ dendritic cells besides the peripheral marginal zone DC (Vremec *et al.*, 1992). Collagenase releases interdigitating DC that are associated with the stroma, and Ca^{2+}-free conditions/EDTA are required to disintegrate interdigitating DC–T clusters to allow accumulation in the low-density fraction. DC can then be isolated either by negative selection with antibodies (Vremec *et al.*, 1992) or by positive selection via CD11c (found *in situ* on marginal zone as well as interdigitating DC) from low-density fractions (Inaba *et al.*, 1992c). A substantial fraction of CD11c$^+$ DC isolated under these conditions carry the phenotype of IDC *in situ* (MHC class II^{++}, CD86^{++}, 2A1$^+$), and also express DEC-205 (recognized by mAb NLDC-145) and CD8$^+$. The latter DC represent the novel Fas-L$^+$ lymphoid-derived and immunoregulatory DC subset (Süss and Shortman, 1996) although in our hands (unpublished results) there is no complete overlap.

Lymph Node

Despite a high frequency of IDC in sections, it has been difficult to isolate DC from nodes. Only recently, by emphasizing collagenase treatment and Ca^{2+}-free media, could CD11c$^+$ DC carrying the same markers as IDC (MHC class II^{++}, CD86^{++}, DEC-205$^+$, 2A1$^+$) be effectively isolated from lymph nodes (Inaba *et al.*, 1998a). In contrast to spleen, CD8 expression was only very weak. The new method for isolating DC from lymph nodes is an important advance since it allows the study of DC in the major organs where immune responses are generated.

Thymus

Methods similar to those employed for the isolation of spleen DC are used for the isolation of thymic DC (Crowley *et al.*, 1989; Vremec *et al.*, 1992; Romani *et al.*,1996a).

In vivo Expansion of DC Prior to Isolation

Repeated injections of Flt3-L into mice resulted in a dramatically increased number of DC, including known and possibly novel DC subsets in various organs (Pulendran *et al.*, 1997). This proves to be a novel approach to studying DC that can be isolated in high numbers directly from tissues.

PROPAGATION OF MURINE DC FROM HEMATOPOIETIC PRECURSORS

Blood

The generation of (myeloid-related) mature DC from proliferating precursors under the aegis of GM-CSF was actually first described using mouse blood as a source (Inaba *et al.*, 1992a), and was then described for other sources (such as bone marrow, which is more easily accessible in mice than blood) and other species including man.

Bone Marrow

Myeloid DC with GM-CSF. The methodology for inducing DC growth from mouse blood (Inaba *et al.*, 1992a) was modified for MHC class II-negative precursors in bone marrow (Inaba *et al.*, 1992b) that in the presence of GM-CSF give rise to DC, macrophages and granulocytes. The protocol is described in detail by Inaba *et al.* (1998b). In brief, bone marrow cell suspensions, depleted of red cells (by ammonium chloride lysis) and lymphocytes, MHC class II^+ cells, and eventually granulocytes (by Ab/C'-mediated lysis), are cultured in 24-well plates in the presence of recombinant muGM-CSF (10–20 ng/ml) (or 3% v/v conditioned medium from a cell line transduced with the muGM-CSF gene) to obtain proliferating immature cells. It is critical to remove non-adherent, newly formed granulocytes by gentle washes during the first 2–4 days of culture. This leaves behind proliferating clusters that are loosely attached. At days 4–6 these clusters can then be dislodged, whereby inhibitory adherent macrophages are left behind (Yamaguchi, 1997), and maturation of DC is promoted. The yield is about 5×10^6 DC per animal (i.e., 2 femurs and tibias) of which about 40% are mature DC (for criteria see below). TNF-α when added during the last 2 days of culture significantly increases the percentage and yield of mature (MHC class II^{++}, $CD86^{++}$) DC (Yamaguchi *et al.* 1997). Instead of mAb/C'-treatment of bone marrow cells, it is also possible to deplete FcR^+ cells by panning on dishes coated with gamma globulin. Some authors have used GM-CSF + IL-4 rather than GM-CSF alone to generate mature DC from murine bone marrow (Lu *et al.*, 1995; Mayordomo *et al.*, 1997; Dillon, 1997). We have not found that the addition of IL-4 is needed in mouse, although in rat it is required to generate large numbers of DC from bone marrow (Talmor *et al.*, 1997). Scheicher *et al.* (1992) described an alternative protocol that relies on culturing bone marrow cell suspensions (without any depletion step except standard red cell lysis) in the presence of 10–20 ng/ml GM-CSF in 100 mm Petri dishes (rather than 24-well plates), and positive magnetic bead selection of MHC class II cells at the very end of culture. We have recently developed a strikingly simple method that has the additional advantage of an at least 20-fold higher yield of highly pure DC per mouse (Lutz *et al.*, 1998). The method can also be performed under serum-free conditions. It relies on culturing bone marrow cells at low density over a prolonged period. Briefly, unseparated bone marrow cells are cultured at low density (2×10^6/100 mm Petri dish/10 ml) in the presence of 20 ng/ml GM-CSF. Fresh medium and GM-CSF are exchanged several times. Under the conditions of low starting cell density and prolonged culture, contaminating lymphocytes and granulocytes die. Apoptosis of granulocytes is enhanced by reducing the GM-CSF concentration by half from day 8 onward. Virtually pure DC that consist of immature and mature subsets are found in suspension on days 10–12. Adding TNF-α (500 U/ml) or 1 μg/ml LPS for 24 h allows one to obtain homogenous and fully mature DC. Immature DC typically express low or intermediate levels of MHC class II on their surface (but contain ample MHC II in intracellular compartments or MIICs—most elegantly visualized by confocal microscopy; Pierre *et al.*, 1997), do not express CD86 or DEC-205, and are weak in sensitizing T cells but active in antigen uptake, processing, and presentation (as can be shown by the use of T cell hybridomas). Mature DC progeny, in contrast, have very high levels of MHC class II molecules (1–2 logs higher than typical B cells) and CD86, and express the multilectin receptor DEC-205 that is detected with mAb NLDC-145. The latter can be used to positively select mature DC by FACS, MACS, or panning.

Lymphoid DC with SCF, TNF-α, IL-1β, IL-3, IL-7, Flt3-L, and CD40L. Lymphoid lineage-related DC can be derived from thymic as well as bone marrow precursors *in vitro*. These lymphoid-derived DC develop in the absence of GM-CSF but with a cocktail of cytokines (SCF, TNF-α, IL-1β, IL-3, IL-7, Flt3-L, CD40L). Unlike the case for myeloid, immunostimulatory DC, there are no procedures yet available that allow the simple generation of large numbers of lymphoid-related DC (Saunders *et al.*, 1996).

HUMAN DENDRITIC CELLS

Isolation of Human DC from Nonlymphoid and Lymphoid Organs

In contrast to mouse studies, in man skin, blood, and tonsil are readily accessible, and methods for isolating DC from these sites have been elaborated.

Skin

DC from human epidermis (i.e., LC) and/or dermis can be isolated using the techniques established in mice. For a detailed description of the techniques that we use routinely, see Schuler and Koch (1991b) and Romani *et al.* (1996a). In short, as starting material one uses split-thickness skin that is obtained from patients undergoing reconstructive plastic surgery of breast or abdomen, or less preferably from cadaver skin (within 24 h of death). To enrich for LC, epidermal sheets are removed following incubation in low concentrations of trypsin, and epidermal cell suspensions are prepared. These primary epidermal cells have a viability of 85% and contain 1–3% LC. In contrast to mouse, there is no simple way to preenrich human LC by depletion of a majority of keratinocytes. Fresh, immature LC can be further enriched to 5–15% by gradient centifugation (e.g., over Lymphoprep), but as in the mouse this selects for a subset of fresh LC owing to the variable bouyant density of immature DC. It appears preferable, therefore, to isolate LC from fresh epidermal cell suspension by positive selection, for example, by using anti-CD1a mAb and either FACS, panning, or immunadsorption to magnetic beads. For the latter approach one can use, for example, anti-CD45 mAb and Dynabeads (Dynal, Oslo, Norway) (Morris *et al.*, 1992) or anti-CD1a and the MACS technique (Miltenyi Biotec GmbH, Bergisch Gladbach, Germany). As with all positive selection techniques, one has to keep in mind that binding of a mAb to a surface molecule will induce functional changes. In contrast to fresh LC, the preparation of cultured and mature LC is rather simple, reproducible, and straightforward. One simply has to culture the epidermal cells for 3 days, and then harvest the nonadherent cell suspension that contains mostly dead, fully differentiated keratinocytes and viable, 'hairy' or 'veiled' LC. Part of the LC are attached to T cells (see below). The mature LC have a low bouyant density and, therefore, enrich in the low-density fraction following density separation. Alternatively, cultured LC can be purified to virtually 100% by positive selection approaches as mentioned above. From 1 cm^2 epidermis one usually obtains 3×10^6 viable epidermal cells containing 1–3% LC. One-third to two-thirds of the initially plated fresh LC can be recovered as mature LC from the epidermal cell cultures. As in the mouse, mature human DC can also be obtained by emigration from 2–4-day human skin organ cultures. The emigrants consist almost exclusively of DC and memory T cells with some of the DC bound to T cells. If necessary (e.g., for studying HIV pathogenesis), free DC and T can be separated from the DC–T conjugates by anti-CD3 staining and FACS sorting (Lenz *et al.*, 1993; Pope *et al.*, 1995; Steinman *et al.*, 1995).

Blood

The beginner is often confused by the various isolation procedures published, and the DC subsets that are described therein. To avoid such confusion it may be best to start with stating that (1) there are two DC subsets circulating in blood, one being $CD11c^+$ and the other $CD11c^-$ (O'Doherty *et al.*, 1994), and (2) DC can be isolated either from fresh or from cultured blood. We have described the respective standard procedures that we use in detail in Romani *et al.* (1996a).

Isolation of DC from Cultured Human Blood. This is the classical method for isolating DC from human blood. First, peripheral blood mononuclear cells (PBMC) are prepared, and T cells are depleted by E rosetting. The ER^- (i.e., T depleted) fraction is then cultured for 36–48 h, and the nonadherent fraction is collected. Next, monocytes are removed by panning on human immunoglobulin-coated dishes (Romani *et al.*, 1996a), and the nonadherent cells are loaded onto a metrizamide gradient. The low-density fraction is harvested. It contains DC at 50–70% purity (yield $1–3 \times 10^6$ DC from one buffy coat, i.e., 500×10^6 PBMC). The main contaminants are B and NK cells (most of which have moved to the high-density fraction). This procedure is rather simple, and the partially purified DC populations are perfectly suited for functional studies such as CTL induction. The DC that are isolated by this procedure are primarily

CD11c$^+$ (80–90%), and correspond to the CD11c$^+$ DC subset found in fresh blood (see below) (only about 10–20% of the DC in these preparations constitute the CD11c$^-$ subset as this subset (50% of the DC in fresh blood) dies during culture (see below)). The CD11c$^+$ DC subset has matured during culture and exhibits the classical features of mature DC (nonadherence, veiled appearance, high levels of adhesion and costimulatory molecules, and potent T cell stimulatory capacity) including *de novo* expression of the novel marker CD83 by most DC (in contrast, only 0.1% mature CD83$^+$ DC are present in fresh blood, and in part cluster with T cells and are thus lost during the E rosetting step). Further enrichment can be achieved either by positive selection for CD11c$^+$ or CD83$^+$ cells (using panning, FACS or, preferably, immunomagnetic beads) or by depletion of B, NK, and T cells and monocytes by the same techniques.

Slightly modified versions of this basic approach are described in detail by Tedder and Jansen (1997). In short, an ER$^-$ PBMC fraction is prepared and plated. After overnight culture the nonadherent fraction is harvested, resuspended, and replated once or twice to remove remaining monocytes. The nonadherent, DC-enriched fraction is centrifuged over metrizamide. The low-density fraction contains 20–80% DC. Alternatively, PBMC are depleted by immunomagnetic beads using mAB to CD3, CD19, CD14, CD56, and then cultured overnight. The CD83$^+$ DC can then be enriched from the nonadherent fraction.

Isolation of DC from Fresh Human Blood. To isolate DC from fresh blood (containing about 1% DC), in a first step again an ER$^-$ (i.e., T depleted) fraction is prepared (Romani *et al.*, 1996a). The ER$^-$ fraction is then incubated with a cocktail of mouse mAbs against CD3, CD16, CD19, and CD11b, and then put onto Petri dishes coated with goat anti-mouse IgG in order to remove T, NK, and B cells and monocytes (instead of panning one can, of course, also use immunomagnetic depletion, e.g., by the Dynabead or MACS technology, although this approach is more expensive). The DC can then be isolated from the nonadherent (i.e. T, B, NK cell and monocyte depleted) cell fraction by two- or three-color sorting (for example, using a FACStar Plus Cell Sorter, Becton Dickinson) (O'Doherty *et al.*, 1994). For two-color sorting the nonadherent fraction is first incubated with FITC goat anti-mouse IgG + IgM antibody (to stain residual anti-CD3, anti-CD16, anti-CD19, or anti-CD11b labeled cells that escaped the panning step), then with mouse immunoglobulin (to quench free FITC goat anti-mouse IgG + IgM binding sites), and finally with PerCP-conjugated anti-HLA-DR (Becton Dickinson, Moutain View, CA). During all these steps it is essential to use a chelating washing medium (such as Hanks Balanced Salt Solution without Ca^{2+} and Mg^{2+} containing 1% bovine serum albumin and 1 mM EDTA to ensure optimal yields during cell sorting). DC are sorted as FITC cocktail-negative and PerCP-HLA-DR-positive cells (yield 1×10^6 virtually pure DC after sorting per 500×10^6 starting population). If in addition to PerCP-conjugated anti-HLA-DR one also includes PE-conjugated anti-CD11c in the final staining step, it becomes apparent by three color-staining/sorting that about half of the DC population (FITC cocktail-negative, PerCP-HLA-DR$^+$) prepared by this method represents the CD11c$^+$ and the CD11c$^-$ subset, respectively.

The CD11c$^+$ and CD11c$^-$ DC subsets (both HLA-DR$^+$, CD4$^+$, CD3/16/19/11b$^-$) were discovered by O'Doherty and colleagues (1994). Neither subset upon isolation from fresh blood exhibits the typical dendritic morphology of mature DC. The CD11c$^+$

subset (also CD45RA$^-$/RO$^+$, CD5$^+$, CD13^{++}, CD33^{++}) nevertheless has potent T cell stimulatory function immediately after isolation and, upon culture, spontaneously (i.e., without need for any additives) develops into typical mature DC. This subset expresses CD32, and escaped detection as long as immunoglobulin panning was used for fresh cells; upon culture CD32 disappears, so that in the conventional method (see above) this DC subset is not depleted. In contrast to CD11c$^+$ DC, the freshly isolated CD11c$^-$ subset (also CD45RA$^+$/RO$^-$, CD5$^-$, CD13$^-$, CD33^{dim}) is functionally immature, but develops into mature DC with typical dendritic morphology and potent T cell stimulatory function provided that monocyte-conditioned medium (prepared by culturing monocytes on immunoglobulin-coated dishes) or IL-3 (see below) is present. Without these additives the CD11c$^-$ subset dies (this is why in the traditional DC isolation method from cultured ER$^-$ fractions this subset is largely lost). The CD11c$^-$ DC do not convert, however, into CD11c$^+$ DC upon culture, and also remain CD45RA$^+$/RO$^-$, CD5$^-$, CD33^{dim}.

An alternative and rather simple method for isolating DC from fresh blood is based on the fact that both the CD11c$^+$ and CD11c$^-$ subsets express significant levels of CD4 (which are downregulated upon culture, so that cultured DC are no longer susceptible to HIV infection). A blood DC isolation kit is available from Miltenyi Biotec GmbH (Bergisch Gladbach, Germany). DC are enriched by depletion of T, B, and NK cells and then enriched using CD4 MicroBeads.

How do the CD11c$^+$ and CD11c$^-$ subsets identified by O'Doherty *et al.* (1994) relate to DC subsets identified by other authors? Thomas and coworkers have sorted fresh PBMC for CD13$^+$/CD33$^+$/CD14^{dim} cells (Thomas *et al.*, 1993) which contain the CD11c$^+$ (and likely other cells like basophils) but not the CD11c$^-$ subset which seem identical to the CD33^{dim} CD14$^-$ CD16$^-$ DC (Thomas and Lipsky, 1994). Strobl *et al.* (submitted) have recently shown that the CD11c$^-$ subset is CD68^{bright}, MPO (myeloperoxidase)$^-$, LZ (lysozyme)$^-$ (while the CD11c$^+$ DC subset is CD68^{dim}, MPO$^-$, LZ$^+$), and requires IL-3 for survival. Interestingly, Olweus *et al.* (1997) have recently identified CD11c$^-$/HLA-DR$^-$/lineage$^-$ (i.e. negative for CD3 (T cells); CD14 (monocytes); CD16 and CD56 (NK cells); CD19, CD20, and goat anti-human IgM (B cell)), and IL-3R (Receptor)^{high} DC precursors that upon culture in GM-CSF + IL-3 developed into potent T cell stimulators. These cells appear identical to the CD11c$^-$ DC subset described by O'Doherty, the CD11c$^-$CD68^{bright} DC subset described by Strobel *et al.* and the CD33^{dim} CD14$^-$ CD16$^-$ DC described by Thomas *et al.* The CD11c$^-$, HLA-DR$^+$, lineage$^-$, IL-3R^{high} DC subset in blood expresses the lymph node homing molecule L-selectin (CD62L) but otherwise appears identical to analogous DC precursors found in T areas of lymph nodes and tonsils (see below). These CD11c$^-$ DC are thus obviously identical to the CD4$^+$, CD11c$^-$, HLA-DR$^+$, lineage$^-$, CD45-RA$^+$ enigmatic 'plasmacytoid' T cells (or 'plasmacytoid' monocytes) that have recently been shown to require IL-3 (+CD40 ligand) for survival and differentiation into mature and potent T cell stimulatory DC (Grouard *et al.*, 1997). It has been suggested that these cells might represent the precursors of lymphoid-related DC in humans. Recent studies, however, show that these cells can be propagated *in vitro* from CD34^{++}M-CSFR$^+$ progenitors, indicating that they are of myeloid origin (Strobl *et al.*, 1998). The CD11c$^-$ DC subset found in blood may be constantly produced in bone marrow, and migrate in the steady state independently of inflammation and foreign antigen through blood to the T areas of tonsil and lymph nodes (by crossing the HEV) and possibly the

T areas of spleen as well (by crossing the marginal zone sinuses), and reside there as 'plasmacytoid T cells/plasmacytoid monocytes' without initiating immune responses. In case of an ongoing antigen-driven T cell activation (induced by DC of the LC type or the dermal DC type that have been mobilized from the periphery in response to antigen deposition and inflammation) CD11c$^-$ DC might be rescued and induced to mature by T cell signals (IL-3 + CD40 ligand). Alternatively, at inflammatory sites in peripheral tissues, these DC precurors may be attracted by chemokines and encounter CD40L$^+$ T cells or CD40L$^+$ mast cells. The role of these CD11c$^-$ DC (simple immunostimulation or immunoregulation?) is, however, not know to date.

Tonsil

Besides CD1a$^+$ DC of the LC type in the stratified epithelium, the following subsets of DC and DC precursors are discernible *in situ* by immunohistochemistry, and can be isolated from tonsils: (1) CD40$^+$, CD86$^+$, CD83$^+$ IDC (interdigitating cells) scattered in the T areas (Björck *et al.*, 1997); (2) CD4$^+$CD3$^-$CD11c$^+$ DC in the germinal centers (GCDC) (Grouard *et al.*, 1996), and (3) CD4$^+$CD3$^-$CD11c$^-$ plasmacytoid DC precursors in the T cell areas (within and around the HEV) (Grouard *et al.*, 1997). IDC are best isolated as lineage$^-$ CD40^{++} cells. Tonsils are cut into pieces and digested in collagenase and DNase I, and free cells are layered on a 50% Percoll gradient. Low-density fractions are obtained and are depleted of B cells and monocytes (eventually also of T and NK cells) by immunomagnetic beads. The depleted fraction is then labeled with appropriate mAb, and IDC are sorted as CD40$^+$CD3$^-$CD19$^-$CD20$^-$ cells. The IDC are HLA-DR^{+++}, CD1a$^-$ CD2$^-$ CD4$^\pm$, CD33$^-$, CD11c^{++}, CD86^{++}, and (about 50% only) also CD83^{++}, and represent mature DC. The isolation of the other two tonsillar DC subsets also starts with preparing T, B, NK cell and monocyte depleted tonsillar cells, which are then sorted into CD4$^+$CD11c$^+$ lineage$^-$ germinal center DC, and CD4$^+$CD11c$^-$ lineage$^-$ plasmacytoid DC precursors. The isolated germinal center DC exhibit a dendritic morphology, are potent stimulators of CD4$^+$ T cells, and are similar in phenotype to the CD11c$^+$ CD4$^+$ DC subset in peripheral blood from which they may derive. Germinal center DC are thought to contribute to the generation of memory B cells by activating germinal center T cells. CD11c$^-$CD4$^+$ plasmacytoid DC precursors may derive from the CD11c$^-$CD4$^+$ DC immature DC subset in blood described above.

Propagation of Human DC from Hematopoietic Precursors

In man, DC can either be generated from rare, proliferating CD34$^+$ precursors ($1.2 \pm 0.6\%$ in bone marrow, $0.06 \pm 0.02\%$ in peripheral blood of healthy adults, $0.29 \pm 0.17\%$ in cord blood) or from more frequent, nonproliferating CD14$^+$ monocytes (usually 5–10% of PMBC in healthy adults). The CD34$^+$ method uses GM-CSF$^+$ TNF-α as key cytokines, while the CD14$^+$ approach requires GM-CSF + IL-4. For experimental purposes, cord blood CD34$^+$ cells and CD14$^+$ monocytes are convenient and effective sources for propagating DC *in vitro*. For clinical use, adult blood is most accessible, but requires G-CSF ($\pm$ other cytokines) pretreatment of the patient to increase the otherwise minimal percentage of CD34$^+$ cells, while no such preteatment is needed if CD14$^+$ cells are used as the starting population. Most laboratories and published methods use culture medium that contains fetal calf serum (FCS) to generate DC. While this is sufficient for most experimental purposes, any method for generating DC for clinical use has to avoid FCS as well as any other nonhuman proteins. It also appears critical that the characteristics of the DC, notably their maturational stage, are well characterized in order to allow comparison of results obtained in clinical trials.

Generation of Myeloid DC from Monocytes

In 1994 it became apparent that the combined action of GM-CSF + IL-4 can direct $CD14^+$ monocytes to differentiate into DC (Sallusto and Lanzavecchia, 1994; Romani *et al.*, 1994). To produce stable, mature DC from $CD14^+$ precursors, it is, however, necessary to prime in GM-CSF and IL-4, and then to induce final differentiation and maturation. In standard cultures containing FCS, several types of inflammatory stimuli (including IL-1, TNF-α, LPS) or CD40L can induce DC maturation (Sallusto *et al.*, 1994; Zhou and Tedder, 1996). In the absence of FCS, these stimuli are, however, insufficient, and upon removal of cytokines the cells re-adhere and become monocytes/macrophages. We found that monocyte-conditioned medium (produced by monocytes attached to human immunoglobulin-coated dishes) induces optimal maturation of DC even in the absence of FCS while cytokines did not (Romani *et al.*, 1996b). It appears that this is because monocyte-conditioned medium, besides several inflammatory cytokines, contains in addition prostaglandins (Rieser *et al.*, 1997; Jonuleit *et al.*, 1997) which, quite surprisingly, also promote DC differentiation.

As a starting population for DC generation one can use partially enriched monocytes prepared from PBMC by simple plastic adherence (Sallusto *et al.*, 1994; Romani *et al.*, 1994); by adherence followed by metrizamide gradient centrifugation (Tedder and Jansen, 1997); by T cell depletion (via E rosetting) (Bender *et al.*, 1996) or B + T ± NK depletion (by immunomagnetic beads) of PBMC (this latter method is our preferred approach for experimental purposes (Romani *et al.*, 1996b); by multistep Percoll gradient centrifugation followed by immunomagnetic depletion of T + B ± NK cells ± residual erythrocytes (via anti-CD3, anti-CD19 ± anti-CD56 or anti-CD56 ± anti-glycophorin) from the low density fraction (Sallusto *et al.*, 1994); or by elutriation. Alternatively, for special purposes, monocytes can be purified by $CD14^+$ flow cytometry (FACS) (Bender *et al.*, 1996) or magnetic cells sorting (MACS) (Pickl *et al.*, 1996) (a kit is available from Miltenyi Biotec GmbH, Bergisch Gladbach, Germany). Monocytes/monocyte-enriched fractions are cultured at a density of about $3–5 \times 10^5$/ml in GM-CSF (800 U/ml) + IL-4 (1000 U/ml) for several (6–9) days; and following this 'priming phase' in a second step or 'differentiation phase' (2–3 days). They are then exposed, in the continued presence of GM-CSF ± IL-4, to either monocyte-conditioned medium or, alternatively, a cocktail (TNF-α ± IL-1 ± IL-6 + PGE_2) that mimics monocyte-conditioned medium (Rieser *et al.*, 1997; Jonuleit *et al.*, 1997). In the initial period, higher cell densities might be possible (Thurnher *et al.*, 1997), but maturation in the second phase requires densities below 5×10^5/ml. IL-4 can be used at lower concentrations. In our own experience, concentrations < 200 U/ml are variable, concentrations >200 U/ml work except with an occasional donor, and a concentration of 1000 U/ml never fails. Yield is between 50% and 95% of input $CD14^+$ cells, and usually in the higher range in FCS cultures as opposed to FCS-free cultures. For clinical use we have recently optimized our previously published FCS-free culture method for use with leukapheresis products (yield: 5×10^8 DC per leukapheresis product) (B. Thurner *et al.*, manuscript in preparation).

It is not clear at present whether the monocyte-derived DC that are generated *in vitro* have their equivalents *in vivo*. However, the DC generated by this method appear attractive for experimental purposes as well as for clinical use since virtually pure and homogeneous populations in two distinct stages can be generated. Following culture in GM-CSF and IL-4, the DC are immature, that is, relatively weak in priming T cells (weak stimulatory capacity for allogeneic naive (notably cord blood-derived) T cells in the MLR), but active in antigen uptake, processing, and presentation (as shown by high uptake of FITC-dextran by macropinocytosis, ample intracellular MHC II^+ organelles, and processing of tetanus toxoid and presentation to T cell clones) (Sallusto *et al.*, 1994; Sallusto *et al.*, 1995). Following induction of maturation, MHC class II molecules are translocated to the surface, long-lived specific peptide–MHC class II complexes are generated, costimulatory molecules (like CD86) are upregulated, and DC consequently acquire a strong capacity to prime naive T cells.

With respect to the maturational stage of DC that will prove optimal for immunization, the more potent mature DC should be prioritized because experiments that demonstrated striking efficacy of DC in mice have primarily used mature DC (Schuler and Steinman, 1997). This is also underscored by recent findings that the $CD14^+$ derived, fully mature DC (i) induce potent CTL responses and T_H1 responses even in the presence of IL-4 and anti-IL12 (H. Jonuleit *et al.*, manuscript in preparation), and (ii) unlike immature DC do not convert into tolerogenic DC in the presence of IL-10 (Steinbrink *et al.*, 1997). We feel that the following set of criteria is useful to document fully mature human DC (Romani *et al.*, 1996b). First, allogeneic MLR stimulatory activity should be strong at DC:T cell ratios of 1:1000 (rather than 1:10 as often used) with stimulation indices ≥ 20. Second, typical morphology with highly motile, large sheet-like processes or veils. Third, stable phenotype (i.e., DC stay nonadherent and viable for at least 2 days if recultured in the absence of any cytokines). Fourth, characteristic phenotype ($CD83^+$, $CD86^{++}$, $HLA\text{-}DR^{+++}$, $M\text{-}CSF\text{-}R^-$, intracellularly $p55^+$ or $fascin^+$). Fifth, resistance to the tolerizing effects of IL-10 (Steinbrink *et al.*, 1997).

Generation of Myeloid DC from Neutrophil Committed Granulocytes

Oehler and colleagues have recently demonstrated that highly purified lactoferrin-positive immediate precursors of endstage neutrophilic polymorphonuclear granulocytes can develop into DC in response to GM-CSF + IL-4 + TNF-α (Oehler *et al.*, 1998). Additional stimulation with CD40L induces CD83 expression. The DC are highly efficient both in the allogeneic MLR and in presenting soluble antigen to autologous T cells. These striking findings underline the potential complexity of the DC system, although as for the $CD14^+$ derived DC (see above) it is unclear whether this novel pathway of DC differentiation does occur *in vivo* as well.

Generation of Myeloid DC from Cord Blood $CD34^+$ Cells

Caux and colleagues first demonstrated that cord blood $CD34^+$ cells develop into DC in response to GM-CSF + TNF-α (Caux *et al.*, 1992). $CD34^+$ cells that are isolated, e.g., by the MACS technique and grown in liquid cultures in GM-CSF + TNF-α proliferate, and after 12–14 days give rise to $CD1a^+$, $CD14^-$, DC that in part (20%) express the so-called Birbeck granules that are characteristic of Langerhans cells (yield about $10–30 \times 10^6$ $CD1a^+$ cells at 50–80% purity per 1×10^6 $CD34^+$ input). A classical mature DC phenotype ($CD83^+$ etc.) was not demonstrated. Interestingly, it turned out that at day 5–7 two mutually exclusive subsets of DC precursors emerge independently, and give rise to distinct DC progeny, both of which are $CD1a^+$ $CD14^-$ but otherwise are different (Caux *et al.*, 1996a). Specifically, the $CD1a^+CD14^-$ precursor gives rise to $CD1a^+CD14^-$ DC of the Langerhans cell type (Birbeck granules$^+$, Lag antigen$^+$, E-cadherin$^+$). The $CD1a^-CD14^+$ precursor, in contrast, develops into $CD1^+CD14^-$ DC that are Birbeck granule$^-$, Lag antigen$^-$, E-cadherin$^-$ but express CD2, CD9, CD68, and factor XIIIa, thus resembling dermal or interstitial dendritic cells. The $CD1a^-CD14^+$, but not the $CD1a^+CD14^-$ one is bipotential, and in response to M-CSF develops into macrophages. Both DC progeny are potent stimulators of T cells, but the dermal/interstitial type DC is much more potent in taking up antigens via the mannose-R and macropinocytosis, expresses some nonspecific esterase, and has the striking capacity to induce naive, CD40-triggered B cells to differentiate into IgM-secreting cells if IL-2 is present. This implies a special role of this DC subset in initiating humoral immunity (Caux *et al.*, 1997). Instead of GM-CSF + TNF-α, one can also use IL-3 + TNF-α or even CD40L alone to propagate DC from $CD34^+$ cord cells (Caux *et al.*, 1996b; Flores-Romo *et al.*, 1997). CD40 ligation on human cord $CD34^+$ cells gives rise to $HLA\text{-}DR^+$ $CD1a^-$ $CD4^{\pm}$ $CD40^-$ $CD86^{++}$ DC that appear relatively weak in stimulating T cells. Immunohistochemically, DC exhibiting such a phenotype can be identified in T areas of tonsil, and may subserve particular (immunoregulatory?) functions.

Knapp's group has recently shown that TGF-β_1 is required for the generation of cord blood $CD34^+$ cell-derived DC under serum-free conditions (X-vivo 15 medium). TGF-β_1 enhanced DC generation by preventing apoptosis of precurors cells, and at the same time promoted the acquisition of the LC phenotype (i.e., Birbeck granules and associated Lag-antigen) (Riedl *et al.*, 1997). From 1×10^4 input $CD34^+$ cells, after 7 days of culture in TGF-β_1 + GM-CSF + TNF-α + SCF, about 8×10^4 $CD1a^+$ DC (but only 35% pure) developed. FLT3-ligand amplified DC/LC about 4.5-fold yet only if TGF-β_1 was present (Strobl *et al.*, 1997). The optimal protocol under serum-free conditions (X-vivo 15 medium), therefore, is to culture purified $CD34^+$ cord cells in TGF-β_1 + FLT3-L + GM-CSF + TNF-α + SCF. At day 10 of culture about 70% of cells generated were $CD1a^+$, and showed a phenotype (e.g. $HLA\text{-}DR^+$, $CD40^+$, $CD80^{\pm}$, $CD86^{\pm}$, $CD32^+$, $CD14^{\pm}$, $CD86^+$, MPO^-, LZ^-, Lag antigen^{++} (at least 15% of cells)) reminiscent of LC rather than fully mature DC. This protocol allows one to obtain large quantities of (immature) DC (38×10^4 $CD1a^+$ cells at 65% purity per 1×10^4 $CD34^+$ cells plated). It also showed that a surprisingly high 20% of singly seeded $CD34^+$ cells can give rise to pure DC colonies (CFU-DC) (with 63–91% of the cells expressing Lag antigen) besides bipotential monocyte/DC precursors.

Generation of Myeloid DC from Bone Marrow $CD34^+$ Cells

The generation of DC from bone marrow $CD34^+$ cells has been most extensively studied by Young and colleagues (Young *et al.*, 1995; Szabolcs *et al.*, 1995; Szabolcs, 1996). Upon suspension culture in GM-CSF + TNF-α + SCF for 12–14 days, an effective yield of about 1.7×10^6 mature DC per single ml of adult human bone marrow is obtained. In this culture system, monocytes/macrophages, granulocytic precursors, and DC developed concomitantly. Clonogenic assays revealed that—similarly to the situation in cord blood—DC arose either from pure DC colonies or from bipotential post-CFU intermediates that gave rise to either DC or macrophages. The generation of DC from bone marrow $CD34^+$ cells has yet to be optimized with respect to increasing the low percentage of DC in the bulk cultures and avoidance of FCS.

Generation of Myeloid DC from Peripheral Blood $CD34^+$ Cells

Stingl's group has shown that $CD1a^+$ DC (23% of all cells) arise from $CD34^+$ precursors in the peripheral blood of normal, healthy adults under the aegis of GM-CSF + TNF-$\alpha \pm$ IL-4 (Strunk *et al.*, 1996). A striking finding was that part of the DC progeny exhibited LC characteristics (Birbeck granules and Lag antigen), and that these cells all derived from the CLA^+CD34^+ cell subset while the CLA^-CD34^+ cells gave rise to $CD1a^+$ DC that were devoid of Birbeck granules (Strunk *et al.*, 1997). Several groups have described the generation of DC from $CD34^+$ cells mobilized into peripheral blood by G-CSF and/or other cytokines like IL-3. Mackensen and co-workers, for example, generated large numbers of DC of the LC type (Lag antigen$^+$) (up to 1.7×10^7 $CD1a^+$ cells at 45% purity per 1.0×10^6 $CD34^+$ input cells) by avoiding TNF-α (which in their system promoted macrophage development), and culturing $CD34^+$ cells in a combination of early-acting hematopoietic growth factors (SCF, EPO, IL-1β, IL-3, IL-6) and GM-CSF + IL-4 in FCS-containing cell culture medium (Herbst *et al.*, 1996). Siena *et al.* (1995), in contrast, substituted clinically inadequate FCS by autologous high-dose chemotherapy recovery serum, and generated DC by culturing $CD34^+$ cells in the presence of GM-CSF + TNF-α + SCF + FLT3 ligand. The stimulation of $CD34^+$ cells in a blood cell autograft (15×10^6 $CD34^+$ cells/kg) theoretically should provide up to 40×10^9 DC in an adult patient. The DC progeny generated from peripheral blood $CD34^+$ cells might be heterogeneous and are not yet as well characterized as DC derived from cord blood $CD34^+$ cells or $CD14^+$ monocytes in peripheral blood, but will undoubtedly prove useful in clinical studies. Given recent developments that might soon allow the massive *ex vivo* expansion of $CD34^+$ cells, notably the multipotential ones, the $CD34^+$ approach might become even more attractive (Petzer *et al.*, 1996; Fischer *et al.*, 1997).

Generation of Lymphoid DC from $CD34^+$ Cells

In mice, progenitors have been identified that give rise to T cells and lymphoid DC (Saunders *et al.*, 1996). Similar precursors (presumably $CD10^+$ $CD34^+$ cells) seem to exist also in humans (Galy *et al.*, 1995; Res *et al.*, 1996). While in mice an immunoregulatory function of lymphoid DC has been demonstrated at least *in vitro*, the function of human lymphoid-related DC remains to be determined.

ACKNOWLEDGEMENTS

We apologize to all colleagues whose work could not be cited here owing to space constraints. Our current research in the field of DC isolation and propagation is supported by grants from the German Ministry of Science (BMBF 01GE9601 to G.S.) and the German Science Foundation (DFG, SFB 263 to G.S.).

REFERENCES

Austyn, J.M. (1996). New insights into the mobilization and phagocytic activity of dendritic cells. *J. Exp. Med.* **183**, 1287–1292.

Bender, A., Sapp, M., Schuler, G., Steinman, R.M. and Bhardwaj, N. (1996). Improved methods for the generation of dendritic cells from nonproliferating progenitors in human blood. *J. Immunol. Methods* **196**, 121–135.

Björck, P., Flores-Romo, L. and Liu, Y.J. (1997). Human interdigitating dendritic cells directly stimulate CD40-activated naive B cells. *Eur. J. Immunol.* **27**, 1266–1274.

Caux, C., Dezutter-Dambuyant, C., Schmitt, D. and Banchereau, J. (1992). GM-CSF and TNF-α cooperate in the generation of dendritic Langerhans cells. *Nature* **360**, 258–261.

Caux, C., Vanbervliet, B., Massacrier, C., Dezutter-Dambuyant, C., De Saint-Vis, B., Jacquet, C., Yoneda, K., Imamura, S., Schmitt, D. and Banchereau, J. (1996a). CD34$^+$ hematopoietic progenitors from human cord blood differentiate along two independent dendritic cell pathways in response to GM-CSF + TNF-α. *J. Exp. Med.* **184**, 695–706.

Caux, C., Vanbervliet, B., Massacrier, C., Durand, I. and Banchereau, J. (1996b). Interleukin-3 cooperates with tumor necrosis factor α for the development of human dendritic Langerhans cells from cord blood CD34$^+$ hematopoietic progenitor cells. *Blood* **87**, 2376–2385.

Caux, C., Massacrier, C., Vanbervliet, B., Dbois, B., Durand, I., Cella, M., Lanzavecchia, A. and Banchereau, J. (1997). CD34$^+$ hematopoietic progenitors from human cord blood differentiate along two pathways in response to GM-CSF + TNF alpha: II. Functional analysis. *Blood* **90**, 1458–1470.

Crowley, M.T., Inaba, K., Witmer-Pack, M. and Steinman, R.M. (1989). The cell surface of mouse dendritic cells: FACS analyses of dendritic cells from different tissues including thymus. *Cell. Immunol.* **118**, 108–125.

Crowley, M.T., Inaba, K., Witmer-Pack, M.D., Gezelter, S. and Steinman, R.M. (1990). Use of the fluorescence activated cell sorter to enrich dendritic cells from mouse spleen. *J. Immunol. Methods* **133**, 55–66.

De Smedt, T., Pajak, B., Muraille, E., Heinen, E., De Baetselier, P., Urbain, J., Leo, O. and Moser, M. (1996). Positive and negative regulation of dendritic cell function by lipopolysaccharide in vivo. *J. Exp. Med.* **184**, 1413–1424.

Dillon, S.M., Hart, D.N.J., Abernethy, N., Watson, J.D., and Baird, M.A. (1997). Priming to mycobacterial antigen in vivo using antigen-pulsed antigen presenting cells generated in vitro is influenced by the dose and presence of IL-4 in APC cultures. *Scand. J. Immunol.* **46**, 1–9.

Fischer, M., Goldschmitt, J., Peschel, C., Brakenhoff, J.P.G., Kallen, K.-J., Wollmer, A., Grötzinger, J. and Rose-John, S. (1997). A bioactive designer cytokine for human hematopoietic progenitor cell expansion. *Nature Biotechnology* **15**, 142–145.

Flores-Romo, L., Björck, P., Duvert, V., Van Kooten, C., Saeland, S. and Banchereau, J. (1997). CD40 ligation on human cord blood CD34$^+$ hematopoietic progenitors induces their proliferation and differentiation into functional dendritic cells. *J. Exp. Med.* **185**, 341–349.

Galy, A., Travis, M., Cen, D. and Chen, B. (1995). Human T, B, natural killer, and dendritic cells arise from a common bone marrow progenitor cell subset. *Immunity* **3**, 459–473.

Grourard, G., Durand, I., Filgueira, L., Banchereau, J. and Liu, Y.J. (1996). Dendritic cells capable of stimulating T cells in germinal centers. *Nature* **384**, 364–367.

Grouard, G., Rissoan, M.-C., Filgueira, L., Durand, I., Banchereau, J. and Liu, Y.-J. (1997). The enigmatic plasmacytoid T cells develop into dendritic cells with interleukin (IL)-3 and CD40-Ligand. *J. Exp. Med.* **185**, 1101–1111.

Hart, D.N.J. (1997). Dendritic cells: unique leukocyte populations which control the primary immune response. *Blood* **90**, 3245–3287.

Herbst, B., Köhler, G., Mackensen, A., Veelken, H., Kulmburg, P., Rosenthal, F.M., Schaefer, H.E., Mertelsmann, R., Fisch, P. and Lindemann, A. (1996). In vitro differentiation of CD34$^+$ hematopoietic progenitor cells toward distinct dendritic cell subsets of the birbeck granule and MIIC-positive Langerhans cell and the interdigitating dendritic cell type. *Blood* **88**, 2541–2548.

Inaba, K., Inaba, M., Romani, N., Aya, H., Deguchi, M., Ikehara, S., Muramatsu, S. and Steinman, R.M. (1992a). Generation of large numbers of dendritic cells from mouse bone marrow cultures supplemented with granulocyte/macrophage colony-stimulating factor. *J. Exp. Med.* **176**, 1693–1702.

Inaba, K., Steinman, R.M., Pack, M.W., Aya, H., Inaba, M., Sudo, T., Wolpe, S. and Schuler, G. (1992b). Identification of proliferating dendritic cell precursors in mouse blood. *J. Exp. Med.* **175**, 1157–1167.

Inaba, K., Swiggard, W.J., Nonacs, R.M., Witmer-Pack, M.D. and Steinman, R.M. (1992c). Enrichment of dendritic cells by plastic adherence and EA rosetting, Unit 3.7, 3.7.1 - 3.7.11. In: *Current Protocols of Immunology* (series ed. R. Coico), Wiley, New York.

Inaba, K., Swiggard, W.J., Romani, N., Schuler, G. and Steinman, R.M. (1998a) Generation of dendritic cells from proliferating mouse bone marrow progenitors. Unit 3.7 In: *Current Protocols of Immunology* (eds R. Coico, A. Ranz, A. Kruisbeck). Wiley, New York, in press.

Inaba, K., Pack, M., Inaba, M., Sakuta, H., Isdell, F. and Steinman, R.M. (1998b). High levels of an MHC II–self peptide complex on dendritic cells from the T cell areas of lymph nodes. *J. Exp. Med.* **186**, 665–672.

Jonuleit, H., Kühn, U., Müller, G., Steinbrink, K., Paragnik, L., Schmitt, E., Knop, J. and Enk, A.H. (1997). Pro-inflammatory cytokines and prostaglandins induce maturation of potent immunostimulatory dendritic cells under fetal calf serum-free conditions. *Eur. J. Immunol.* **27**, 3135–3142.

Koch, F., Kämpgen, E., Schuler, G. and Romani, N. (1992). Effective enrichment of murine epidermal Langerhans cells by a modified—'mismatched'—panning technique. *J. Invest. Dermatol.* **99**, 803–807.

Koch, F., Trockenbacher, B., Kämpgen, E., Grauer, O., Stössel, H., Livingstone, A.M., Schuler, G. and Romani, N. (1995). Antigen processing in populations of mature murine dendritic cells is caused by subsets of incompletely matured cells. *J. Immunol.* **155**, 93–100.

Kronin, V., Vremec, D., Winkel, K., Classon, B.J., Miller, R.G., Mak, T.W., Shortman, K. and Süss, G. (1997). Are $CD8^+$ dendritic cells (DC) veto cells? The role of CD8 on DC in DC development and in the regulation of CD4 and CD8 T cell responses. *Int. Immunol.* **9**, 1061–1064.

Lenz, A., Heine, M., Schuler, G. and Romani, N. (1993). Human and murine dermis contain dendritic cells. *J. Clin. Invest.* **92**, 2587–2596.

Lu, L., McCaslin, D., Starzl, T.E. and Thomson, A.W. (1995). Bone marrow-derived dendritic cell progenitors (NLDC 145^+, MHC class II^+, B7-1^{dim}, B7-2^-) induce alloantigen-specific hyporesponsiveness in murine T lymphocytes. *Transplantation* **60**, 1539–1545.

Lutz, M.B., Kukutsch, N., Ogilvie, A.L.J., Rossner, S., Koch, F., Romani, N. and Schuler, G. (1998). An advanced culture method for generating large quantities of highly pure dendritic cells from mouse bone marrow. *J. Immunol. Methods*, in press.

Mayordomo, J.I., Zorina, T., Storkus, W.J., Zitvogel, L., Garcia-Prats, M.D., Deleo, A.B., and Lotze, M.T. (1997). Bone marrow-derived dendritic cells serve as potent adjuvants for peptide-based antitumor vaccines. *Stem Cells* **15**, 94–103.

Metlay, J.P., Witmer-Pack, M.D., Agger, R., Crowley, M.T., Lawless, D. and Steinman, R.M. (1990). The distinct leukocyte integrins of mouse spleen dendritic cells as identified with new hamster monoclonal antibodies. *J. Exp. Med.* **171**, 1753–1771.

Miltenyi, S., Müller, W., Weichel, W. and Radbruch, A. (1990). High gradient magnetic cell separation with MACS. *Cytometry* **11**, 231–238.

Moll, H. (1995). *The Immune Functions of Epidermal Langerhans Cells.* R.G. Landes/Springer-Verlag, Austin, New York, Berlin.

Morris, J., Alaibac, M., Jia, M.-H. and Chu, T. (1992). Purification of functional active epidermal Langerhans cells: a simple and efficient new technique. *J. Invest. Dermatol.* **99**, 237–240.

Mosialos, G., Birkenbach, M., Ayehurie, S., Matsumura, F., Pinkus, G.S., Kieff, E. and Langhoff, E. (1996). Circulating human dendritic cells differentially express high levels of a 55-kd actin-bundling protein. *Am. J. Pathol.* **148**, 593–600.

O'Doherty, U., Peng, M., Gezelter, S., Swiggard, W.J., Betjes, M., Bhardwaj, N. and Steinman, R.M. (1994). Human blood contains two subsets of dendritic cells, one immunologically mature and the other immature. *Immunology* **82**, 487–493.

Oehler, L., Majdic, O., Pickl, W.F., Stöckl, J., Riedl, E., Drach, J., Rappersberger, K., Geissler, K. and Knapp, W. (1998). Neutrophil granulocyte committed cells can be driven to acquire dendritic cell characteristics. *J. Exp. Med.* **187**, 1019–1028.

Olweus, J., BitMansour, A., Warnke, R., Thompson, P.A., Carballido, J., Picker, L.J. and Lund-Johansen, F. (1997). Dendritic cell ontogeny: a human dendritic cell lineage of myeloid origin. *Proc. Natl Acad. Sci. USA* **94**, 12551–12556.

Ortner, U., Inaba, K., Koch, F., Heine, M., Miwa, M., Schuler, G. and Romani, N. (1996). An improved isolation method for murine migratory cutaneous dendritic cells. *J. Immunol. Methods* **193**, 71–79.

Petzer, A.L., Zandstra, P.W., Piret, J.M. and Eaves, C.J. (1996). Differential cytokine effects on primitive ($CD34^+CD38^-$) human hematopoietic cells: novel responses to Flt3-ligand and thrombopoietin. *J. Exp. Med.* **183**, 2551–2558.

Pickl, W.F., Majdic, O., Kohl, P., Stöckl, J., Riedl, E., Scheinecker, C., Bello-Fernandez, C. and Knapp, W. (1996). Molecular and functional characteristics of dendritic cells generated from highly purified $CD14^+$ peripheral blood monocytes. *J. Immunol.* **157**, 3850–3859.

Pierre, P., Turley, S.J., Gatti, E., Hull, M., Meltzer, J., Mirza, A., Inaba, K., Steinman, R.M. and Mellman, I. (1997). Developmental regulation of MHC class II transport in mouse dendritic cells. *Nature* **388**, 787–792.

Pope, M., Betjes, M.G.H., Hirmand, H., Hoffman, L. and Steinman, R.M. (1995). Both dendritic cells and memory T lymphocytes emigrate from organ cultures of human skin and form distinctive dendritic–T-cell conjugates. *J. Invest. Dermatol.* **104**, 11–17.

Pulendran, B., Lingappa, J., Kennedy, M.K., Smith, J., Teepe, M., Rudensky, A., Maliszewski, C.R. and Maraskovsky, E. (1997). Developmental pathways of dendritic cells in vivo: distinct function, phenotype, and localization of dendritic cell subsets in FLT3 ligand-treated mice. *J. Immunol.* **159**, 2222–2231.

Res, P., Martínez-Cáceres, E., Jaleco, A.C., Staal, F., Noteboom, E., Weijer, K. and Spits, H. (1996). $CD34^+CD38^{dim}$ cells in the human thymus can differentiate into T, natural killer, and dendritic cells but are distinct from pluripotent stem cells. *Blood* **87**, 5196–5206.

Riedl, E., Strobl, H., Majdic, O. and Knapp, W. (1997). TGF-β1 promotes in vitro generation of dendritic cells by protecting progenitor cells from apoptosis. *J. Immunol.* **158**, 1591–1597.

Rieser, C., Böck, G., Klocker, H., Bartsch, G. and Thurnher, M. (1997). Prostaglandin E2 and tumor necrosis factor α cooperate to activate human dendritic cells: synergistic activation of interleukin 12 production. *J. Exp. Med.* **186**, 1603–1608.

Romani, N., Koide, S., Crowley, M., Witmer-Pack, M., Livingstone, A.M., Fathman, C.G., Inaba, K. and Steinman, R.M. (1989). Presentation of exogenous protein antigens by dendritic cells to T cell clones: intact protein is presented best by immature epidermal Langerhans cells. *J. Exp. Med.* **169**, 1169–1178.

Romani, N., Gruner, S., Brang, D., Kämpgen, E., Lenz, A., Trockenbacher, B., Konwalinka, G., Fritsch, P.O., Steinman, R.M. and Schuler, G. (1994). Proliferating dendritic cell progenitors in human blood. *J. Exp. Med.* **180**, 83–93.

Romani, N., Bhardwaj, N., Pope, M., Koch, F., Swiggard, W.J., O'Doherty, U., Witmer-Pack, M.D., Hoffman, L., Schuler, G., Inaba, K. and Steinman, R.M. (1996a). Dendritic cells. In: *Weir's Handbook of Experimental Immunology* (ed. L.A. Herzenberg), Blackwell Science, Oxford, pp. 156.1–156.14.

Romani, N., Reider, D., Heuer, M., Ebner, S., Kämpgen, E., Eibl, B., Niederwieser, D. and Schuler, G. (1996b). Generation of mature dendritic cells from human blood—an improved method with special regard to clinical applicability. *J. Immunol. Methods* **196**, 137–151.

Sallusto, F. and Lanzavecchia, A. (1994). Efficient presentation of soluble antigen by cultured human dendritic cells is maintained by granulocyte/macrophage colony-stimulating factor plus interleukin 4 and downregulated by tumor necrosis factor α. *J. Exp. Med.* **179**, 1109–1118.

Sallusto, F., Cella, M., Danieli, C. and Lanzavecchia, A. (1995). Dendritic cells use macropinocytosis and the mannose receptor to concentrate macromolecules in the major histocompatibility complex class II compartment: downregulation by cytokines and bacterial products. *J. Exp. Med.* **182**, 389–400.

Saunders, D., Lucas, K., Ismaili, J., Wu, L., Maraskovsky, E., Dunn, A. and Shortman, K. (1996). Dendritic cell development in culture from thymic precursor cells in the absence of granulocyte/macrophage colony-stimulating factor. *J. Exp. Med.* **184**, 2185–2196.

Scheicher, C., Mehlig, M., Zecher, R. and Reske, K. (1992). Dendritic cells from mouse bone marrow: in vitro differentiation using low doses of recombinant granulocyte-macrophage colony-stimulating factor. *J. Immunol. Methods* **154**, 253–264.

Schuler, G. (ed.) (1991). *Epidermal Langerhans Cells.* CRC Press, Boca Raton, FL.

Schuler, G. and Koch, F. (1991). Enrichment of epidermal Langerhans cells. In: *Epidermal Langerhans Cells* (ed. Schuler, G.). CRC Press, Boca Raton, FL, pp. 139–157.

Schuler, G. and Steinman R.M. (1997) Dendritic cells as adjuvants for immune-mediated resistance to tumors. *J. Exp. Med.* **186**, 1183–1187.

Siena, S., Di Nicola, M., Bregni, M., Mortarini, R., Anichini, A., Lombardi, L., Ravagnani, F., Parmiani, G. and Gianni, A.M. (1995). Massive ex vivo generation of functional dendritic cells from mobilized CD34$^+$ blood progenitors for anticancer therapy. *Exp. Hematol.* **23**, 1463–1471.

Steinbrink, K., Wolfl, M., Jonuleit, H., Knop, J. and Enk, A.H. (1997). Induction of tolerance by IL-10-treated dendritic cells. *J. Immunol.* **159**, 4772–4780.

Steinman, R.M. (1991). The dendritic cell system and its role in immunogenicity. *Annu. Rev. Immunol.* **9**, 271–296.

Steinman, R., Hoffman, L. and Pope, M. (1995). Maturation and migration of cutaneous dendritic cells. *J. Invest. Dermatol.* **105** (Suppl.), 2S–7S.

Steinman, R.M., Pack, M. and Inaba, K. (1997). Dendritic cells in the T-cell areas of lymphoid organs. *Immunol. Rev.* **156**, 25–37.

Strobl, H., Bello-Fernandez, C., Riedl, E., Pickl, W.F., Majdic, O., Lyman, S.D. and Knapp, W. (1997). Flt3 ligand in cooperation with transforming growth factor-beta1 potentiates in vitro development of Langerhans-type dendritic cells and allows single-cell dendritic cell cluster formation under serum-free conditions. *Blood* **90**, 1425–1434.

Strunk, D., Rappersberger, K., Egger, C., Strobl, H., Krömer, E., Elbe, A., Maurer, D. and Stingl, G. (1996). Generation of human dendritic cells/Langerhans cells from circulating CD34$^+$ hematopoietic progenitor cells. *Blood* **87**, 1292–1302.

Strunk, D., Egger, C., Leitner, G., Hanau, D. and Stingl, G. (1997). A skin homing molecule defines the Langerhans cell progenitor in human peripheral blood. *J. Exp. Med.* **185**, 1131–1136.

Süss, G. and Shortman, K. (1996). A subclass of dendritic cells kills CD4 T cells via Fas/Fas-ligand-induced apoptosis. *J. Exp. Med.* **183**, 1789–1796.

Szabolcs, P., Moore, M.A.S. and Young, J.W. (1995). Expansion of immunostimulatory dendritic cells among the myeloid progeny of human CD34$^+$ bone marrow precursors cultured with c-*kit* ligand, granulocyte-macrophage colony-stimulating factor, and TNF-α. *J. Immunol.* **154**, 5851–5861.

Szabolcs, P., Avigan, D., Gezelter, S., Ciocon, D.H., Moore, M.A.S., Steinman, R.M. and Young, J.W. (1996). Dendritic cells and macrophages can mature independently from a human bone marrow-derived, post-colony-forming unit intermediate. *Blood* **87**, 4520–4530.

Talmor, M., Mirza, A., Turley, S., Mellman, I., Hoffman, L.A. and Steinman, R.M. (1998). Cytokine requirements for the generation of large numbers of immature and mature dendritic cells from rat bone marrow cultures. *J. Exp. Med.*, in press.

Tedder, T.F. and Jansen, P.J. (1998). Isolation and generation of human dendritic cells, Unit 7.23, Supplement 23, 7.32.1-7.32.15. In: *Current Protocols of Immunology* (series ed. R. Coico). Wiley, New York.

Thomas, R., Davis, L.S. and Lipsky, P.E. (1993). Isolation and characterization of human peripheral blood dendritic cells. *J. Immunol.* **150**, 821–834.

Thomas, R. and Lipsky, J.J. (1994). Human peripheral blood dendritic cell subsets. Isolation and characterization of precursors and mature antigen-presenting cells. *J. Immunol.* **153**, 4016–4028.

Thurnher, M., Papesh, C., Ramoner, R., Gastl, G., Böck, G., Radmayr, C., Klocker, H. and Bartsch, G. (1997). In vitro generation of CD83$^+$ human blood dendritic cells for active tumor immunotherapy. *Exp. Hematol.* **25**, 232–237.

Vremec, D., Zorbas, M., Scollay, R., Saunders, D.J., Ardavin, C.F., Wu, L. and Shortman, K. (1992). The surface phenotype of dendritic cells purified from mouse thymus and spleen: Investigation of the CD8 expression by a subpopulation of dendritic cells. *J. Exp. Med.* **176**, 47–58.

Yamaguchi, Y., Tsumura, H., Miwa, M. and Inaba, K. (1997). Contrasting effects of TGF beta1 and TNF alpha on the development of dendritic cells from progenitors in mouse bone marrow. *Stem Cells* **15**, 144–153.

Young, J.W., Szaboles, P. and Moore, M.A.S. (1995). Identification of dendritic cell colony-forming units among normal human CD34$^+$ bone marrow progenitors that are expanded by c-kit ligand and yield pure dendritic cell colonies in the presence of granulocyte/macrophage colony-stimulating factor and tumor necrosis factor alpha. *J. Exp. Med.* **182**, 1111–1120.

Zhou, L.-J. and Tedder, T.F. (1995). Human blood dendritic cells selectively express CD83, a member of the immunoglobulin superfamily. *J. Immunol.* **154**, 3821–3835.

Zhou, L.J. and Tedder, T.F. (1996). CD14$^+$ blood monocytes can differentiate into functionally mature CD83$^+$ dendritic cells. *Proc. Natl Acad. Sci. USA* **93**, 2588–2592.

CHAPTER 28
Propagation and Culture of Dendritic Cells

Shannon J. Turley[1], Ralph M. Steinman[2], Ira Mellman[1] and Kayo Inaba[3]
[1]Department of Cell Biology, Yale University School of Medicine, New Haven, Connecticut, USA; [2]Laboratory of Cellular Physiology and Immunology, Rockefeller University, New York, USA; [3]Department of Zoology, Faculty of Science, Kyoto University, Kyoto, Japan

INTRODUCTION

Dendritic cells (DC) are attracting considerable attention as adjuvants for human immunization. This interest derives from several findings that are by now well known in the field. DC are more potent than other antigen-presenting cells (APC) at stimulating helper and cytotoxic T cells (Steinman and Witmer, 1978; Nussenzweig and Steinman, 1980; Nussenzweig *et al.*, 1980; Steinman *et al.*, 1983; Sunshine *et al.*, 1983; Inaba *et al.*, 1987). DC can cluster and activate naive T cells (Inaba and Steinman, 1984; Inaba and Steinman 1985; Adema *et al.*, 1997) and prime immune responses *in vivo* independently of other adjuvants (Inaba *et al.*, 1990). DC also process antigens to form MHC–peptide complexes more efficiently than other cell types, a feature that at least in part reflects their extraordinary ability to developmentally regulate the intracellular localization and transport of MHC molecules (Cella *et al.*, 1997; Pierre *et al.*, 1997).

The effectiveness of these cells in anti-tumor and anti-viral therapies, however, depends on the availability of large numbers of autologous DC of the appropriate lineage, developmental stage, and phenotypic stability. Precise biochemical and cell biological analyses also require an abundant cell source which cannot easily be obtained by isolating tissue DC. To overcome the obstacle of low DC numbers *in situ*, procedures have been designed to generate useful quantities of DC *in vitro*. The central aim of this chapter is to describe these culture methods, their starting populations, growth requirements, and DC progeny. Before doing this, we will first provide a historical review of the work that initially characterized DC development *in vivo*. We feel that a consideration of the early conceptual framework is important in understanding the recent evolution of DC propagation techniques as well as their end products and applications. We will then describe the current methods for growing DC, from both proliferating and nonproliferating progenitors, and conclude with a discussion of new insights into DC function obtained with these culture systems.

Dendritic Cells: Biology and Clinical Applications
ISBN 0-12-455860-7

EARLY DISCOVERIES IN DC BIOLOGY

Identification of a New Type of Mononuclear Leukocyte

In 1973, Steinman and Cohn described a novel population of cells present in peripheral lymphoid organs including spleen, lymph nodes, and Peyer's patches (Steinman and Cohn, 1973; Steinman and Cohn, 1974). The cells were distinct from phagocytes (mononuclear and polymorphonuclear), lymphocytes, and connective-tissue cells by morphological criteria and were most numerous in the spleen. Phase-contrast microscopy revealed a distinctive shape and motility in this cell population. Cytochemical stains showed sparse acid phosphatase-positive granules (lysosomes) and a lack of membrane ATPase. Electron-microscopic analysis demonstrated the absence of the well-developed endocytic system typical of primary phagocytes (Steinman and Cohn, 1973). Shortly thereafter, these 'dendritic cells', named for their irregular shape and formation of spiny processes, were distinguished by functional criteria (Steinman and Cohn, 1974). Notably, the DC were weakly endocytic *in vitro* (Steinman and Cohn, 1974) and *in vivo* (Steinman *et al.*, 1974) for a variety of ligands, including antigen–antibody complexes. The DC were also unresponsive to lymphocyte mitogens. Morphologically similar, Fc receptor-negative, nonphagocytic cells were soon identified in many other sites: several tissues of the rat (Klinkert *et al.*, 1982), and the afferent lymph from many species (Drexhage *et al.*, 1979; Knight, 1984; Spry *et al.*, 1980; Pugh *et al.*, 1983).

An Origin in the Bone Marrow

Like other blood-borne cells, DC were exquisitely radiosensitive and could be ablated from spleen by ionizing irradiation (Steinman *et al.*, 1974). This allowed Steinman and colleagues to restore DC in bone marrow chimeras and demonstrate that DC arise from a bone marrow progenitor. Several other laboratories made similar observations using bone marrow chimeras to replenish DC in the epidermis (Langerhans cells) (Frelinger *et al.*, 1979; Katz *et al.*, 1979), thymic medulla (interdigitating cells) (Barclay and Mayrhofer, 1981), interstitial spaces of many organs (interstitial DC) (Hart and Faber, 1981), and afferent lymph (veiled cells) (Pugh *et al.*, 1983). Collectively these studies provided ample evidence that DC are of hematopoietic origin.

A Proliferating Progenitor

To determine the replicative capacity of DC and/or their progenitors, [^{3}H]thymidine labeling experiments were carried out. [^{3}H]thymidine was not incorporated by spleen DC immediately after labeling *in vivo* or *in vitro*. However, significant labeling was detected after 2 or more days of an *in vivo* pulse, with peak incorporation occurring after 5 days (Steinman and Cohn, 1974; Steinman *et al.*, 1974). The delay in detecting labeled spleen DC indicated that this population originated from a proliferating progenitor, but that time was required for the cells to differentiate and/or migrate to the spleen. Similar findings were made by Pugh and colleagues with rat pseudoafferent lymph DC, i.e., the cells were not dividing while in the lymph but they derived from a progenitor that incorporated [^{3}H]thymidine at least 2 days earlier (Pugh *et al.*, 1983).

DCs Arise from Hematopoietic Progenitors

Together, these pioneering studies characterized a new family of cells that would turn out to be pivotal players in immune responses and potential therapeutic agents for treatment of disease. Using organ dissociation, these cells were identified in several different tissues. The criteria used to identify DC were considered carefully in order to distinguish this cell type from others, especially macrophages. Although not dividing themselves in their resident tissues, DC appeared to be the progeny of bone marrow-derived proliferating precursors located elsewhere. Today it is clear that DC form *in vitro* from mouse and rat bone marrow progenitors and in humans from the $CD34^+$ subset that represents $\sim 1\%$ of marrow cells (Caux *et al.*, 1992; Reid *et al.*, 1992; Santiago-Schwarz *et al.*, 1992; Szabolcs *et al.*, 1995).

DC DEVELOPMENT *IN VIVO*

Initial Conceptualization of a DC System

The DC identified in the first studies of lymphoid organs and afferent lymph were all rich in MHC class II molecules and potent stimulators of the mixed lymphocyte reaction (MLR), a reaction that was known to require expression of MHC class II on the stimulator cells. Thus, the first concept of the DC system was one in which all components were constitutively equipped to activate T cells (Steinman and Nussenzweig 1980; Tew *et al.*, 1982).

DC located in distant sites were suspected to be interconnected by a process of migration. Shelley reported that contact allergens, when applied to the epidermis for 1 h, were selectively engulfed by LC. Since phagocytes are generally not present in this site, the authors proposed that LC form a ‘reticuloendothelial trap’ in the skin, responsible for trapping antigen and initiating the classical T cell-mediated response of contact allergy (Shelley and Lennart, 1976). The mechanism by which the LC encountered the antigen-specific T cell, however, was still unknown. Silberberg-Sinakin *et al.* addressed this with EM analysis of ferritin-treated skin (Silberberg-Sinakin *et al.*, 1976). Using the presence of Birbeck granules as the diagnostic criterion, they noted an increase in ferritin-bearing LC in the dermal lymphatics and regional lymph nodes following intradermal injection of the allergen. These results suggested that LC pick up the allergen in the skin and migrate to nearby lymph nodes via afferent lymphatics in order to arouse contact allergy. Later it was discovered that LC, once thought to be neural, neuroectodermal, or mesenchymal in origin, expressed leukocyte markers such as Fc receptors (Stingl *et al.*, 1977, Tamaki *et al.*, 1979; Haines *et al.*, 1983; Schuler and Steinman 1985) and MHC class II products (Frelinger *et al.*, 1979; Tamaki *et al.*, 1979). Stingl found that LC could present protein antigens to primed cells and stimulate a secondary MLR (Stingl *et al.*, 1978). Drexhage and Hoefsmit, noting the findings with contact allergens and the cytological similarities of the DC in different tissues, proposed a linear relationship whereby epidermal LC became lymph veiled cells and then interdigitating cells in the T cell areas of lymph nodes (Drexhage *et al.*, 1979; Hoefsmit *et al.*, 1982).

Changes in Mouse Epidermal Langherhans Cells (LC)

A more intricate, developmentally-oriented picture of the DC system became evident with the work of Schuler and Steinman (1985) and Romani and colleagues (Romani *et al.*, 1989a; Romani *et al.*, 1989b). The approach was to monitor the features of epidermal LC in a 3-day culture, as either whole epidermal suspensions or purified LC. The LC were found to change significantly as a function of time *in vitro*. Importantly, the freshly isolated LC were weak accessory cells in the MLR and oxidative mitogenesis of T cells. An instructive example was the response to the anti-CD3 monoclonals, in which the mitogen was presented by FcR on the LC. The fresh LC had at least 10-fold higher levels of FcR than the cultured LC, but the latter were at least 10-fold more potent as accessory cells (Romani *et al.*, 1989c). In other words, the level of TCR ligand or signal 1 (see p. 545) was not the determining factor in DC function. Somehow the LC were maturing in ways other than presentation of TCR ligand, to become potent T cell stimulators. Shortly thereafter, Romani and colleagues showed that cultured LC bound and clustered T cells better than fresh LC (Romani *et al.*, 1989a). Fresh LC, on the other hand, were far more effective at capturing protein antigens for stimulation of T cell clones and hybridomas (Romani *et al.*, 1989b).

The cell surface of the cultured LC was also remodeled during culture. While Fc receptors, membrane ATPase, nonspecific esterase activity, and the macrophage antigen F4/80 were all downregulated, expression of MHC products (class I and II), and the CD80/86, CD40, and CD54 costimulators increased (Romani *et al.*, 1989a). Freshly isolated LC were also shown to actively synthesize MHC class II and invariant chain (Ii), whereas cultured LC did not (Pure *et al.*, 1990).

Together, these studies began to establish a developmental program whereby DC first sample antigens present in peripheral tissues and then deliver these to densely packed lymph nodes or spleen, where they have the greatest chance of interacting with the appropriate T-lymphocyte. According to this model, protective immune response begins with the capture of a threatening foreign antigen or pathogen by resident tissue DC. By unknown mechanisms, these antigen-bearing DC move out of the peripheral tissue and travel via lymphatics to draining lymph nodes. During this migration the internalized antigen is degraded into fragmented products including immunogenic peptides. Resulting peptides are presumably captured by newly synthesized MHC products, since treatment with cycloheximide reduces antigen presentation (Pure *et al.*, 1990). These antigen-capturing DC were termed 'immature' because they are destined to terminally differentiate into more powerful T cell stimulatory DC. T cell stimulatory DC are referred to as 'mature' DC since they carry out the second phase of DC function, induction of the T cell response. Mature DC no longer capture antigens but express *de novo* high levels of important adhesion and costimulatory molecules such as CD40, CD54, CD58, CD80, and CD86. An additional, intermediate stage of maturation has recently been identified and will be described later in this chapter.

Since DC have not been found exiting lymph nodes, their second functional phase also represents the final stage in their life history. In fact, DC have been shown to die by apoptosis after activating the appropriate T cells. A diagram of the DC life history highlighting the two main functional stages and the novel intermediate DC is provided in Plate 28.1. Although not discussed extensively here, there are many other changes that take place involving cytokine and chemokine production/responsiveness, expression of an array of DC specific markers (recognized by monoclonal antibodies to mouse, rat, and human antigens), cell size and shape, and the cytoskeleton.

Immature Cells are the Prototype DC in Many Tissues

Functional studies on DC freshly isolated from numerous nonlymphoid, peripheral tissues indicated that the cells underwent a large increase in T cell stimulatory capacity after 1–2 days of culture. The development of T cell stimulatory ability was associated with an upregulation of costimulatory molecules like CD86 (Larsen *et al.*, 1992; Inaba *et al.*, 1994). Therefore, in addition to epidermal LC, DC located in rat lung (Holt *et al.*, 1993), mouse spleen (Crowley *et al.*, 1990), human blood (O'Doherty *et al.*, 1993), and mouse kidney and heart (Austyn *et al.*, 1994) all qualified as immature DC.

Maturation *in vivo*

Transplanted and explanted skin experiments illustrated that a similar maturation process occurs *in vivo*. When Larsen and coworkers followed LC in transplants, both to syngeneic and to allogeneic recipients, the LC moved in large numbers out of the epidermis and into dermal lymphatics. When skin was placed in simple organ cultures, the LC migrated in a similar fashion, but this time out of the skin and into the culture medium (Larsen *et al.*, 1990). In all cases, the migrated cells exhibited features of maturing DC. For example, the cells were enlarging in size, expressing higher levels of MHC class II products and B7 molecules (Larsen *et al.*, 1994), and developing powerful T cell stimulatory capacity (Larsen *et al.*, 1990).

More detailed information has come from the work of De Smedt and colleagues on DC in spleen (De Smedt *et al.*, 1996). Most of the DC released into splenic suspensions are immature. These DC are marked by a high level of CD11c integrin but low levels of several antigens that are found on T cell area DC or interdigitating cells (IDC), such as DEC-205 antigen receptor, and the granule antigens identified by the monoclonal antibodies 2A1 and M342. Upon culture, the spleen DC upregulate the IDC markers. Cells with the markers of immature DC are abundant in the red pulp and also at the periphery of the white pulp, at regions where T cells first enter the white pulp nodule to form the periarterial sheaths. DeSmedt and coworkers found that the immature DC at the edge of the white pulp are capable of capturing protein antigens but weak at stimulating responses to superantigens. However, 6 h after administration of lipopolysaccharide (LPS), the DC in this site become functionally mature. Their protein capture capacity is dramatically reduced and presentation of superantigens is significantly enhanced. Also, the cells acquired higher levels of DEC-205 and M342. *In vivo*, the DC seemed to move *en masse* from the marginal zone into the deeper T cell areas (De Smedt *et al.*, 1996).

Mediators of Maturation

When maturation was studied with purified immature LC, it was found that GM-CSF and, to a lesser extent, IL-1 were critical (Witmer-Pack *et al.*, 1987; Heufler *et al.*, 1988). However, it was not clear whether the cytokine was functioning as a survival factor, a maturation factor, or both. M-CSF, a standard stimulus for macrophage survival and maturation, was inactive, as was G-CSF. It remains unclear why LC, or for that matter DC, in many different tissues (above), begin to mature when simply placed into culture or transplanted. However, it is important to stress that cell growth is not required; LC mature in epidermal culture even after exposure to 27 000 rads of ionizing irradiation (R.M. Steinman, personal observation). Molecules such as TNF-α (Caux *et al.*, 1992; Szabolcs *et al.*, 1995, Caux *et al.*, 1996), CD40L (Flores-Romo *et al.*, 1997), ceramide (Sallusto *et al.*, 1996), IL-1β and LPS (Sallusto and Lanzavecchia, 1995) are commonly known to drive maturation of immature DC. Other molecules, including CGRP (Hosoi *et al.*, 1993), IL-10 (Caux *et al.*, 1994; Buelens *et al.*, 1997), prostaglandins and nitric oxide (Steinman, 1998) may act to suppress maturation of nonlymphoid DC.

Mature DC *in vivo*

From a collection of morphological, phenotypic, and functional studies we know that DC in most tissues are immature. Although these DC begin to mature upon isolation, they only become potent T cell stimulators after overnight culture or longer. What DC are mature *in vivo*? The data are not extensive, but there are two likely possibilities: DC found in afferent lymph, especially when stimulated by transplantation or application of a contact allergen, and DC that are deep within the T cell area, the IDC. In these cases, the DC can be termed mature because they are large and rich in cell surface MHC–peptide complexes and CD86. Many other traits (Plate 28.1) still need to be identified.

The Life History of the DC Involves Multiple Stages

A key component in the development of DC is maturation of nonproliferating cells. During maturation, the DC shifts from a cell that is capturing and processing antigens to a terminally differentiated cell with reduced endocytic capacity, high levels of costimulators, and strong stimulatory potential for naive T cells. Experimentally, maturation takes place when DC are manually removed from their resident tissues and placed in culture, but it also occurs *in vivo*, for example, during inflammation or hypersensitivity or when skin is transplanted. However, maturation stimuli are poorly defined, with the exception of LPS which is a powerful *in vivo* inducer of the classical DC population in mouse spleen.

IN VITRO DEVELOPMENT OF DC FROM PROLIFERATING PROGENITORS

Proliferating Progenitors in Mouse Blood

It was not until 1992 that investigators were able to generate large numbers of DC from proliferating progenitors and essentially replicate the DC developmental program occuring *in vivo*. Inaba and colleagues applied GM-CSF to erythrocyte (RBC)-depleted mouse blood cells in culture, and after 1 week loosely adherent aggregates of proliferating cells became evident (Inaba *et al.*, 1992a). The aggregates were attached to a monolayer of tightly adherent stromal cells and were covered with spiny cells. When dislodged and replated in a new culture vessel, these aggregates gave rise to single, nonadherent DC with functional and morphological qualities of mature DC. The maturation process took 1–2 days and could not be redirected or stopped with phagocyte stimulants such as M-CSF and G-CSF.

Proliferating Progenitors in Mouse Bone Marrow

Initially, when mouse marrow was stimulated with GM-CSF, it was difficult to detect DC development amid the much larger numbers of resident marrow lymphocytes and proliferating phagocytes. However, the formation of distinctive DC aggregates became readily apparent when resident marrow RBC, MHC class II^+ cells, and lymphocytes (mainly B cells but also T cells) were depleted (before culture) and nonadherent granulocytes were washed away (during the first 4 days of culture). DC aggregates differed from those of developing phagocytes in that the macrophages developed in flattened, adherent colonies, while granulocytes developed in nonadherent aggregates of round cells.

Because the DC aggregates were loosely adherent, they could be dislodged and separated from the firmly adherent stroma by gentle pipetting. Just like the mouse blood cultures, reculturing of the dislodged cells for 1–2 days greatly enhanced formation of single, mature DC. Cells within the aggregates had a high [^{3}H]thymidine labeling index, whereas single, mature DC were nonproliferating. Additionally, cells within the aggregate expressed Fc receptors and could phagocytose particulates, including mycobacteria, whereas mature DC had very low levels of Fc receptors and were nonphagocytic (Inaba *et al.*, 1993). Importantly, the mature DC were powerful T cell stimulators in the MLR. Subsequent studies of cell surface phenotype indicated that the cells in the aggregates had low levels of CD86 while the mature cells released from the aggregate had high levels of this antigen at the cell surface (Inaba *et al.*, 1994). In addition mature DC progeny could not be redirected to the macrophage lineage with M-CSF owing to a lack of M-CSF receptor expression (Witmer-Pack *et al.*, 1987; Inaba *et al.*, 1992b).

In the 6 years that we have been stimulating mouse marrow with GM-CSF, it has not been necessary to add cytokines such as IL-4 and/or TNF-α. Other groups report the need to add IL-4 (Lu *et al.*, 1996). It is possible that TNF-α and IL-4, or their functional equivalents, are being produced in our cultures. In fact, when immature DC are isolated from the aggregates and depleted of macrophages, TNF-α is required for optimal maturation (Yamaguchi *et al.*, 1997). Nevertheless, the standard stimulus for DC maturation in marrow cultures is to dislodge the aggregates of growing cells and transfer these to a fresh culture vessel.

Proliferating Lines of Immature Mouse Spleen DC

Winzler and colleagues described a system for sustaining proliferating cultures of immature mouse spleen DC for more than one year (Winzler *et al.*, 1997). The cells grew in aggregates fed by a conditioned medium from a cell line stimulated with GM-CSF. These cultures are, therefore, supplemented with both the cytokines produced by the cell line and the supplemented GM-CSF. Maturation is induced in this system by culturing the cells with stimuli like LPS or a variety of bacteria, including Gram-positive or LPS-negative bacteria. Most of the features of immature and mature DCs derived from GM-CSF-driven bone marrow cultures can also be observed in this cell line.

$CD34^+$ Progenitors in Human Neonatal Cord Blood

In 1992, Caux and Banchereau succeeded in generating large numbers of DC from human $CD34^+$ precursors in cord blood (Caux *et al.*, 1992). This system required the addition of both GM-CSF and TNF-α. The DC developed in large aggregates, but there was no need to transfer the aggregates to observe DC development. Since TNF-α is applied exogenously in this system, it is possible that the TNF-α was inducing maturation of DC in addition to other effects (e.g., suppressing granulocyte formation). Many of the DC progeny had all the features of LC, including Birbeck granules. Subsequent studies by Caux and colleagues have shown that there are actually two pathways of DC development in these cultures. One pathway produces typical LC with Birbeck granules (LAG-1), E-cadherin, and CD1a (Caux *et al.*, 1996; Caux *et al.*, 1997). More evidence for the existence of this pathway comes from the phenotype of TGF-β knockout (KO) mice. All subsets of DC appear to be intact in these animals with the exception of LC, which are totally absent (Borkowski *et al.*, 1996). The other pathway involves a $CD14^+$ intermediate and yields progeny that express CD2 and CD9 but no LC markers. This second pathway provides cells that are similar to dermal or interstitial DC. The $CD14^+$ cell can be driven to form CD14-rich macrophages with M-CSF or $CD14^-$ DCs with GM-CSF and TNF-α (Caux *et al.*, 1996; Szabolcs *et al.*, 1996).

Proliferating Progenitors in Human Bone Marrow

Szabolcs and coworkers extended the work of Caux and Banchereau from cord blood to bone marrow, again starting with $CD34^+$ progenitors. It was essential to add both GM-CSF and TNF-α to generate DC. Stem cell factor (SCF), or c-kit ligand, increased the number of DC by acting on the proliferating progenitor (Szabolcs *et al.*, 1995). The progeny in these bone marrow cultures were diverse. Typical mature DC accounted for a small fraction of the population, about 10%. The other progeny included polymorphonuclear and mononuclear cells. The latter can be driven to form DC when Fc receptor-positive macrophages are removed from the cultures. The mononuclear cells can also form macrophages if M-CSF is added as a stimulus (Szabolcs *et al.*, 1996).

Proliferating Progenitors in Rat Bone Marrow

Although mouse bone marrow cultures require only GM-CSF and human bone marrow cultures require GM-CSF and TNF-α, neither regimen produces significant numbers of DC from rat bone marrow. Instead, IL-4 must be added concominantly with GM-CSF (Talmor *et al.*, 1998). The presence of TNF-α during the first 6 days of these cultures has no effect on DC yields. Nevertheless, the development of DC seems to occur in the same fashion as in mouse and human bone marrow cultures. Large proliferating aggregates appear in the culture, usually by days 5–8. When these are dislodged and transferred to a new culture vessel, single, mature DC develop within 1–2 days. The cells within the aggregates are MHC class II and CD86 low, and do not stimulate a MLR. The mature cells that develop from the aggregate are MHC class II and CD86 rich, are unresponsive to M-CSF, and are powerful MLR stimulators.

There are two unusual features of rat relative to mouse and human marrow. First, there is little contamination of the preparations with developing granulocytes. Second,

DC development seems to arrest rather tightly at the immature stage, since few single, mature DC are produced until one dislodges the aggregates and transfers them to a fresh culture vessel. The cause of these differences is not understood but may involve the presence of IL-4 in combination with the initial marrow inoculum. Unlike the human and mouse systems where the starting population is selected for by cell sorting or RBC lysis and complement-mediated depletion of T cells, B cells, and Ia^+ cells, the rat cultures begin with bulk marrow cells depleted only of RBC. In any case, the rat system has proven to be superior for studying immature DC and their transition into mature DC.

Propagating DC from Proliferating Progenitors—Cultural Differences?

Great efforts have been made to design methods for fostering extensive DC growth *in vitro*. Protocols are now available to propagate DC from numerous species and starting progenitor populations. Proliferating cultures of mouse, rat, and human DC exhibit some differences in terms of cytokine growth requirements (Plate 28.2) and the extent to which growing macrophages and granulocytes contaminate the preparation. It is also important to note that multiple pathways of DC development have been identified in human cultures, but not in rodent marrow. Studies are underway to sort out these variances and to establish a better understanding of DC ontogeny and growth requirements.

There are several important common features which make these methods both practical and powerful tools for studying DC development and function (Plate 28.2). In each of these methods, immature DC develop from and accumulate in distinct aggregates of proliferating cells. This allows for the convenient enrichment of the immature DC, a subset that is difficult to analyze *in situ* or *ex vivo*. DC grown from these cultures also seem to follow similar maturational programs. For example, when aggregates derived from all three species are dislodged and transferred to a fresh culture dish, maturation ensues. Maturation takes place over a day or two in a manner similar to that seen when nonproliferating immature DC are cultured from many sources, such as mouse epidermis and spleen, rat lung, and human blood. The hallmarks of maturation, expression of strong T cell stimulating activity and high levels of surface MHC and costimulatory molecules, are evident in the resulting populations after treatment with maturation stimuli and/or cluster dissociation and reculture.

IN VITRO DEVELOPMENT OF DC FROM NONPROLIFERATING PRECURSORS

Blood Monocytes Can Give Rise to DC

Given the capacity of GM-CSF to drive DC development in mouse blood and marrow, similar experiments were performed with adult human blood. Very few DC developed, however, unless the cells were cultured for 6–7 days in a combination of GM-CSF and IL-4 or IL-13 (Romani *et al.*, 1994; Sallusto and Lanzavecchia, 1994). Today, sorted $CD14^+$ cells or T-depleted, monocyte-enriched blood cells are used as starting populations in these cultures. This approach produces DC that are not fully mature and therefore do not resemble the classical, stellate DC associated with T cell stimulation.

For example, these DC still express the monocyte markers CD14 and CD32 Fc gamma receptor, although at considerably lower levels than their precursors. Much of the MHC class II lies within intracellular compartments (MIIC) that double label for the lysosomal marker, Lamp-1. The cells are active in endocytosis, utilizing both macropinocytosis and adsorptive uptake via the macrophage mannose receptor (MR) and Fc receptors. Maturation can be induced if these DC are cultured in additional stimuli such as TNF-α, IL-1β, LPS, CD40L, and/or a monocyte-conditioned medium for several days (Sallusto and Lanzavecchia 1994; Sallusto and Lanzavecchia, 1995; Romani *et al.*, 1996; Bender *et al.*, 1996). On the matured cells, MHC products and costimulatory molecules (e.g., CD40, CD54, CD86) are expressed at the surface although their levels may not be as high as in mature DC generated in other systems or isolated from lymphoid tissues. MHC class II in these cells is very long lived (Cella *et al.*, 1997). The DC restricted antigens p55, CD25 and CD83 also come up after addition of maturation stimuli (Reddy *et al.*, 1997). The mature products retain their DC features when cytokines are removed.

The DC precursor in these cultures is the blood monocyte. Cells undergoing differentiation do not enter the cell cycle according to Ki-67 (cell cycle antigen) labeling and propidium iodide staining for >2N levels of DNA (Granelli-Piperno *et al.*, 1998). In addition, the transformation from monocyte to DC is unaffected by irradiation.

The mechanism underlying the IL-4 effect is not clear. One possibility is that the IL-4 antagonizes the macrophage-stimulating actions of M-CSF (Jansen *et al.*, 1989), allowing monocyte differentiation into a DC instead of a macrophage. Upon removal of GM-CSF and IL-4, these cells lose the hallmarks of DC and revert back to adherent phagocytic cells.

The Monocyte Route—A Promising System

A new and accessible model for propagating immature and mature human DC has been developed. The culture system begins with blood monocytes, either purified CD14$^+$ cells or less pure populations that are monocyte-enriched by plastic adherence or T cell depletion. Development of immature DC from blood monocytes does not involve cell proliferation and is exquisitely dependent on the presence of IL-4 and GM-CSF. Immature DC generated in this culture system may be especially efficient in endocytosis owing to residual expression of antigens derived from their phagocyte precursors. Since progression from immature to mature DC is entirely dependent on exogenously added growth factors, the monocyte system may be advantageous for harnessing synchronized populations of immature DC for study or therapies.

Lymphoid Precursors Generate DC

DC can also be generated from progenitor cells identified in human thymus and bone marrow and in mouse thymus. These progenitors express low levels of CD4 and have restricted developmental potential, giving rise only to T cells, B cells, NK cells, and DC (Ardavin *et al.*, 1993; Wu *et al.*, 1996). Unlike the culture systems described above, the generation of lymphoid DC *in vitro* does not require GM-CSF and occurs within 4 days of culture (Saunders *et al.*, 1996). In fact, several combinations of growth agents can drive production of DC from CD4$^+$ thymic precursors. For example, IL-1β,

TNF-α, IL-7, SCF, Flt3L and anti-CD40 can drive significant DC differentiation, but 2-fold more DC result when this combination is accompanied by IL-3. In this system, DC may share a more immediate $CD25^+/CD44^+/c\text{-}kit^+$ precursor with T cells. These DC are termed lymphoid DC since they express lymphocyte markers such as CD8a and Thy-1 and their $CD4^+$ precursor cannot give rise to macrophages or granulocytes (Vremec *et al.*, 1992). Lymphoid DC are equipped with FasL for inducing apoptosis on Fas-expressing T cells (Süss and Shortman, 1996). Thymus-derived lymphoid DC may, therefore, be involved in negatively regulating T cell function. Another $CD4^+$ human DC precursor was recently described (Grouard *et al.*, 1997). This intermediate precursor cell, identified in blood and tonsils, requires IL-3 and CD40L to generate DC.

CELL BIOLOGY OF DC MATURATION

A Two-limb System

Although this multitalented cell has been implicated in a wide array of immunological mechanisms such as isotype switching (Dubois *et al.*, 1997), lymphoid organ construction (Winzler *et al.*, 1997), negative selection, and peripheral tolerance (Banchereau and Steinman, 1998), the chief role for this preeminent APC is the initiation of primary immune responses against dangerous agents. Activation of naive T cells into armed effector cells requires several molecular interactions that are often divided into two categories: *signal 1* and *signal 2*. In this oversimplified scheme of virgin T cell stimulation, the antigen-specific T cell receptor recognizes peptide–MHC complexes on the surface of the DC, constituting signal 1. Signal 2 interactions involve conjugates formed by costimulatory and adhesion molecules such as B7/CD28, ICAM-1/LFA-1, CD40/CD40L. IDC are perfectly equipped for activating T cells since they express high levels of the molecules needed to trigger signal 1 and signal 2. In order to generate the TCR ligand of signal 1, the DC must first internalize and process the antigen from which the peptide is derived, a task that mature DC are not designed to carry out (Steinman, 1991).

The *ex vivo* studies that linked peripheral, LC-like DC to lymphoid organ DC (IDC) in a precursor/product relationship lead to one of the most important concepts in the biology of these cells: DC exist in two distinct functional states (Schuler and Steinman, 1985; Romani *et al.*, 1989b). Through a process of maturation (and migration *in vivo*), immature DC, which are equipped for antigen interiorization and processing, give rise to mature DC specifically equipped to present antigen to and activate T cells. As described above, immature DC cannot effectively activate antigen-specific T cells owing to their lack of surface peptide–MHC complexes and costimulators but are quite proficient at ingesting antigens. On the other hand, mature DC cannot efficiently engulf macromolecules or pathogens but are potent stimulators of antigen-specific T cells. Immature DC irreversibly differentiate into mature DC when stimulated with inflammatory stimuli or when subjected to physical trauma (explantation/transplantation in the case of skin and cluster dissociation in proliferating DC cultures). This maturation is a complicated and tightly regulated process that may hold the key to the striking effectiveness of DC triggering immune responses. In principle, a two-limb developmental system allows DC carry out their immunological responsibilities while preventing overstimulation of the immune system and unwanted immunity against self-antigens.

Regulation of Antigen Internalization

The paradox that DC rigorously present antigen to T cells but cannot efficiently endocytose antigen has been resolved. The specific mechanisms by which DC ingest these antigens, however, are not fully understood. At a time when DC were considered poor endocytosers, two important studies revealed that freshly isolated but not cultured DC were proficient at phagocytosing mycobacteria, latex microspheres, yeast, and bacteria (Inaba *et al.*, 1993; Reis e Sousa *et al.*, 1993). LC were also shown to internalize the yeast cell wall derivative zymosan, via a mannan/β-glucan inhibitable receptor(s) (Reis e Sousa *et al.*, 1993). A few years ago, Sallusto and co-workers carefully investigated some of these mechanisms in an elegant study using human monocyte-derived immature DC. They found that this subset of immature DC depends largely on the mannose receptor (MR) and macropinocytosis for accumulation of antigen inside MHC class II cytoplasmic compartments and subsequent presentation to T cells. Most importantly, they indicated that macropinocytosis, the predominant endocytic pathway in their system, ceased after treatment with anti-inflammatory stimuli such as LPS, TNF-α, IL-1β, and also CD40L (Sallusto and Lanzavecchia, 1995). Winzler, using a mouse spleen cell line, showed that TNF-α treatment of immature DC induces dramatic rearrangement of actin cytoskeletal elements (Winzler *et al.*, 1997). It is, therefore, likely that macropinocytosis, an actin-dependent engulfment process, is downregulated as a result of treatment with molecules that transduce the same signaling cascade(s) as TNF-α. It will be important to confirm the occurence of these phenomena *in vivo*. The expression patterns of other molecules involved in antigen uptake, such as Fc receptor, DEC-205 antigen receptor, and transferrin receptor, have also been shown to change during DC maturation in several experimental systems. Today we can appreciate that DC are capable of endocytosing antigens by developmentally regulated mechanisms. The efficiency of these mechanisms relative to presentation capacity and internalization by other APC is currently being investigated.

Stages of Maturation

As indicated throughout this chapter, several groups have characterized specific events that occur during DC differentiation from bone marrow precursors to terminally differentiated cells. Given the complexity of the DC life history and the dearth of these cells in peripheral tissues, these investigators have opted to use *in vitro* culture systems that generate large numbers of developing DC from physiologically relevant progenitors. From studies using mouse (Pierre *et al.*, 1997) and rat bone marrow-derived DC Talmor, 1998), human stem cell-derived DC (Gatti and Velleca, manuscript in preparation), and monocyte-derived human DC (Cella *et al.*, 1997), we now know that the transport and turnover of MHC class II is developmentally regulated, changing dramatically during the development of these cells. Using patterns of MHC class II and lysosomal compartmentalization, determined by confocal laser scanning microscopy, FACS analysis, subcellular fractionation, and functional criteria assessed by antigen uptake and presentation assays, we established a three-stage developmental scheme.

This scheme is analagous to the maturational pattern of DC freshly isolated from mouse spleen and epidermis. Other groups have documented similar developmental changes occuring in DC derived from human monocytes (Cella *et al.*, 1997) as well as a spleen cell line (Winzler*et al.*, 1997), although slight variations are also noted.

In GM-CSF-driven bone marrow cultures, the majority of DC emerge from large, loosely adherent clusters of proliferating cells. These clusters are composed of dividing DC precursors along with abundant immature or 'early' DC. The DC precursors can be distinguished from their progeny since early DC do not incorporate BRDU but do express low levels of MHC class II, whereas the DC precursors do incorporate BRDU but do not express MHC class II. Early DC display distinctive intracellular MHC class II-rich compartments that are generally dispersed throughout the cytoplasm. At this stage, the MHC class II compartments, referred to as MIIC, contain Ii, the lysosomal glycoproteins LGP110 and LGP120, and the peptide-editing molecule H2-M. These compartments probably correspond to the late endosomes and lysosomes that are found in all cells but that accumulate MHC class II products in MHC class II-expressing cell types such as DC (Kleijmeer *et al.*, 1997). Nevertheless, MIIC/lysosomes are likely to host the formation of MHC class II–peptide complexes, although the ultimate fate of these complexes is unknown. In early DC MHC class II molecules reach the plasma membrane very inefficiently and instead are degraded with relatively short half-lives in both mouse and human cells ($< 10\,h$) (Pierre *et al.*, 1997; Cella *et al.*, 1997).

Early DC exhibit very low surface levels of the costimulators CD80, CD86, and CD40, and proficiency at internalizing soluble antigens as well as particulate matter, dying cells, and mycobacteria. Early DC remain associated with the cluster until a maturation signal is introduced. Inflammatory compounds such as LPS and TNF-α can provide this signal. The most powerful inducer of maturation *in vitro*, however, is the physical disruption and replating of the DC cluster. We suspect that a trauma or manipulation of this kind causes changes in putative stress kinases, resulting in the activation or inhibition of signaling pathways that regulate DC maturation.

When coerced to mature, early DC differentiate into 'intermediate' stage DC. The intermediate DC was only recently described as a cell of medium-large size with a rounded shape that develops within several hours of maturation from an early or immature DC. In these cells, intracellular MHC class II no longer localizes to lysosomes but can be found in peripherally situated vesicles called CIIV (MHC class II vesicles). CIIV are thought to serve as specialized processing or storage compartments for peptide–MHC class II complexes that deliver their cargo to the cell surface. Lysosomes begin clustering at the microtubule organizing center (MTOC) and expression of proteins such as DEC-205, 2A1, M342, CD54, CD40, and B7 becomes detectable at the intermediate stage. Intermediate DC can internalize antigens although their endocytic potential is reduced relative to early DC (Garrett and Mellman, manuscript in preparation).

Intermediate DC differentiate into 'late' stage DC which exhibit a phenotype typical of the classical mature DC. During the transition from intermediate to late stages, DC transport most of their newly synthesized MHC class II directly to the plasma membrane, resulting in a reduced rate of lysosomal MHC class II degradation. Lysosomes in late DC are tightly clustered in a perinuclear position. Whereas intermediate stage DC are round and relatively large (something like a sand dollar), late-stage DC exhibit long, spiny processes protruding from a greatly reduced cell body (something like a sea urchin). Owing to an interesting but poorly understood reconfiguration of their endocytic machinery, late DC can no longer internalize antigens efficiently using macropinocytosis (Cella *et al.*, 1997) or phagocytosis (Reis e Sousa *et al.*, 1993). Many of these physical changes are likely related to the rearrangements in actin filaments and microtubules observed during DC maturation (Winzler *et al.*, 1997). Late-stage DC exhibit very high levels of surface MHC products and costimulatory molecules and secretion of IL-12 (Cella *et al.*, 1996; Koch *et al.*, 1996). At maturity, mouse DC express high levels of the lineage markers 2A1 (Inaba *et al.*, 1992b), DEC-205 (Kraal *et al.*, 1986; Witmer-Pack *et al.*, 1995), MIDC-8 (Breel *et al.*, 1987), and M342 (Agger *et al.*, 1992) and human DC express p55 (Mosialos *et al.*, 1996) and CD83 (Zhou and Tedder, 1995). Increased expression of certain adhesion molecules is also detected in late DC and proposed to mediate migration as well as T cell clustering. Late-stage DC have been shown to undergo Fas-induced apoptosis, but precise mechanisms controlling DC death *in vitro* and *in vivo* remain unclear (Winzler *et al.*, 1997; Bjorck *et al.*, 1997).

CONCLUSION

DC comprise a complicated family of cells located in almost every tissue of the body. This family is strategically organized into a network of antigen-capturing and antigen-presenting subsets that are interconnected by maturation and migration. In order to truly understand their functional attributes, and thus their therapeutic applications, developing DC from all lineages must be accessible to the investigator. Unfortunately, adequate populations of immature tissue DC are troublesome to harvest because they are present in low frequencies and mature rapidly upon manipulation. The *in vitro*, culture systems described in this chapter have made the study of DC functional development and ontogeny feasible. While the field has already reaped many benefits from these tools, our understanding of this remarkable APC will be greatly enhanced by molecular and cell biological analyses of DC grown in normal and genetically manipulated propagation systems.

REFERENCES

Adema, G.J., Hartgers, F., Verstraten, R., De Vries, E., Marland, G., Menon, S., Forster, J., Xu, Y., Nooyen, P., McClanahan, T., Bacon, K.B. and Figdor, C.G. (1997). A dendritic-cell-derived C-C chemokine that preferentially attracts naive T cells. *Nature* **387**, 713–717.

Agger, R., Witmer-Pack, M.D., Romani, N., Stossel, H., Swiggard, W.J., Metlay, J.P., Storozynsky, E., Freimuth, P. and Steinman, R.M. (1992). Two populations of splenic dendritic cells detected with M342, a new monoclonal to an intracellular antigen of interdigitating cells and some B lymphocytes. *J. Leukocyte Biol.* **52**, 34–42.

Ardavin, C., Wu, L., Chung-Leung, L. and Shortman, K. (1993). Thymic dendritic cells and T cells develop simultaneously in the thymus from a common precursor population. *Nature* **362**, 761–763.

Austyn, J.M., Hankins, D.F., Larsen, C.P., Morris, P.J., Rao, A.S. and Roake, J.A. (1994). Isolation and characterization of dendritic cells from mouse heart and kidney. *J. Immunol.* **152**, 2401–2410.

Banchereau, J. and Steinman, R.M. (1998). Dendritic cells and the control of immunity. *Nature* **392**, 245–252.

Barclay, A.N. and Mayrhofer, G. (1981). Bone marrow origin of Ia-positive cells in the medulla of rat thymus. *J. Exp. Med.* **153**, 1666–1671.

Bender, A., Sapp, M., Schuler, G., Steinman, R.M., and Bhardwaj, N. (1996). Improved method for the generation of dendritic cells from nonproliferating progenitors in human blood. *J. Immunol. Methods* **196**, 121–135.

Bjorck, P., Banchereau, J. and Flores-Romo, L. (1997). CD40 ligation counteracts Fas-induced apoptosis in human dendritic cells. *Int. Immunol.* **9**, 365–372.

Borkowski, T.A., Letterio, J.J., Farr, A.G. and Udey, M.C. (1996). A role for endogenous transforming growth factor $\beta1$ in Langerhans cell biology: the skin of transforming growth factor $\beta1$ null mice is devoid of epidermal Langerhans cells. *J. Exp. Med.* **184**, 2417–2422.

Breel, M., Mebius, R.E. and Kraal, G. (1987). Dendritic cells of the mouse recognized by two monoclonal antibodies. *Eur. J. Immunol.* **17**, 1555–1559.

Buelens, C., Verhasselt, V., De Groote, D., Thielemans, K., Goldman, M. and Willems, F. (1997). Human dendritic cell responses to lipopolysaccharide and CD40 ligation are differentially regulated by interleukin-10. *Eur. Immunol.* **27**, 1848–1852.

Caux, C., Dezutter-Dambuyant, C., Schmitt, D. and Bachereau, J. (1992). M-CSF and TNF-α cooperate in the generation of dendritic Langerhans cells. *Nature* **360**, 258–261.

Caux, C., Massacrier, C., Vanbervliet, B., Barthelemy, C., Liu, Y.J. and Banchereau, J. (1994). IL-10 inhibits T cell alloreaction induced by human dendritic cells. *Int. Immunol.* **6**, 1177–1185.

Caux, C., Vanbervliet, B., Massacrier, C, Dezutter-Dambuyant, C., de Saint-Vis, B., Jacquet, C., Yoneda, K., Imamura, S., Schmitt, D. and Banchereau, J. (1996). CD34[+] hematopoietic progenitors from human cord blood differentiate alongside two independent dendritic cell pathways in response to GM-CSF+TNF-α. *J. Exp. Med.* **184**, 695–706.

Caux, C., Massacrier, C., Vanbervliet, B., Dubois, B., Durand, I., Cella, M., Lanzavecchia, A. and Banchereau, J. (1997). CD34[+] hematopoietic progenitors from human cord blood differentiate along two independent dendritic cell pathways in response to GM-CSF+TNF-α II. Functional analysis. *Blood* **90**, 1458–1470.

Cella, M., Scheideffer, D., Palmer-Lehmann, K., Lane, P., Lanzavecchia, A. and Alber, G. (1996). Ligation of CD40 on dendritic cells triggers production of high levels of interleukin-12 and enhances T cell stimulatory capacity. *J. Exp. Med.* **184**, 747–752.

Cella, M., Engering, A., Pinet, V., Pieters, J. and Lanzavecchia, A. (1997). Long-lived peptide–MHC class II complexes induced in dendritic cells by inflammatory stimuli. *Nature* **388**, 782–787.

Crowley, M.T., Inaba, K., Witmer-Pack, M.D., Gezelter, S. and Steinman, R.M. (1990). Use of the fluorescence activated cell sorter to enrich dendritic cells from mouse spleen. *J. Immunol. Methods* **133**, 55–66.

De Smedt, T., Pajak, B., Muraille, E., Lespagnard, L., Heinen, E., De Baetselier, P., Urbain, J., Leo, O. and Moser, M. (1996). Regulation of dendritic cell numbers and maturation by lipopolysaccharide *in vivo*. *J. Exp. Med.* **184**, 1413–1424.

Drexhage, H.A., Mullink, H., deGroot, J., Clarke, J. and Balfour, B.M. (1979). A study of cells present in peripheral lymph of pigs with special reference to a type of cell resembling the Langherhans cells. *Cell. Tiss. Res.* **202**, 407–430.

Dubois, B., Vandenabeele, S., Bridon, J.M., Vanbervliet, B., Durand, I., Banchereau, J., Caux, C. and Briere, F. (1997). Human dendritic cells skew isotype switching of CD40-activated naive B cells towards IgA1 and IgA2. *J. Exp. Med.* **185**, 1909–1918.

Flores-Romo, L., Bjorck, P., Duvert, V., Van Kooten, C., Saeland, S. and Banchereau, J. (1997). CD40 ligation on human CD34[+] hematopoietic progenitors induces their proliferation and differentiation into functional dendritic cells. *J. Exp. Med.* **185**, 341–349.

Frelinger, J.G., Hood, L., Hill, S., and Frelinger, J. A. (1979). Mouse epidermal Ia molecules have a bone marrow origin. *Nature* **282**, 321–323.

Galy, A., Travis, M., Cen, D. and Chen, B. (1995). Human T, B, natural killer, and dendritic cells arise from a common bone marrow progenitor cell subset. *Immunity* **3**, 459–473.

Granelli-Piperno, A., Delgado, E., Finkel, V., Paxton, W. and Steinman, R.M. (1998). Immature dendritic cells selectively replicate M-tropic HIV-1, while mature cells efficiently transmit both M- and T-tropic virus to T cells. *J. Virol.* **72**, 2733–2737.

Grouard, G., Rissoan, M-C., Filgueira, L., Durand, I., Banchereau, J. and Liu, Y-J. (1997). The enigmatic plasmacytoid T cells develop into dendritic cells with IL-3 and CD40-ligand. *J. Exp. Med.* **85**, 1101–1111.

Haines, K.A., Flotte, T.J., Springer, T.A., Gigli, I. and Thorbecke, G.J. (1983). Staining of Langerhans cells with monoclonal antibodies to macrophages and lymphoid cells. *Proc. Natl Acad. Sci. USA* **80**, 3448–3451.

Hart, D.N.J. and Fabre, J.W. (1981) Demonstration and characterization of Ia-positive dendritic cells in the interstitial connective tissues of rat heart and other tissues, but not brain. *J. Exp. Med.* **153**, 347–361.

Heufler, C., Koch, F. and Schuler, G. (1988) Granulocyte/macrophage colony-stimulating factor and interleukin 1 mediate the maturation of murine epidermal Langerhans cells into potent immunostimulatory dendritic cells. *J. Exp. Med.* **167**, 700–705.

Hoefsmit, E.C.M., Duijvestijn, A.M. and Kamperdijk, E.W.A. (1982). Relation between Langerhans cells, veiled cells, and interdigitating cells. *Immunobiology* **161**, 255–265.

Holt, P.G., Oliver, J., Bilyk, N., McMenamin, C., McMenamin, P.G., Kraal, G. and Thepen, T. (1993). Downregulation of the antigen presenting cell function(s) of pulmonary dendritic cells *in vivo* by resident alveolar macrophages. *J. Exp. Med.* **177**, 397–407.

Hosoi, J., Murphy, G.F., Egan, C.L., Lerner, E.A., Grabbe, S., Asahina, A. and Granstein, R.D. (1993). Regulation of Langerhans cell function by nerves containing calcitonin gene-related peptide. *Nature* **363**, 159–163.

Inaba, K. and Steinman, R.M. (1984). Resting and sensitized T lymphocytes exhibit distinct stimulatory [antigen-presenting cell] requirements for growth and lymphokine release. *J. Exp. Med.* **160**, 1717–1735.

Inaba, K. and Steinman, R.M. (1985). Protein-specific helper T lymphocyte formation initiated by dendritic cells. *Science* **229**, 475–479.

Inaba, K., Young, J.W. and Steinman, E.M. (1987). Direct activation of $CD8^+$ cytotoxic T lymphocytes by dendritic cells. *J. Exp. Med.* **166**, 182–194.

Inaba, K., Metlay, J.P., Crowley, M.T. and Steinman, R.M. (1990). Dendritic cells pulsed with protein antigens *in vitro* can prime antigen-specific, MHC-restricted T cells *in situ*. *J. Exp. Med.* **172**, 631–640.

Inaba, K., Steinman, R.M., Pack, M.W., Aya, H., Inaba, M., Sudo, T., Wolpe, S. and Schuler, G. (1992a). Identification of proliferating dendritic cell precursors in mouse blood. *J. Exp. Med.* **175**, 1157–1167.

Inaba, K., Inaba, M., Romani, N., Aya, H., Deguchi, M., Ikehara, S., Muramatsu, S. and Steinman, R.M. (1992b). Generation of large numbers of dendritic cells from mouse bone marrow cultures supplemented with granulocyte-macrophage colony-stimulating factor. *J. Exp. Med.* **176**, 1693–1702.

Inaba, K., Inaba, M., Naito, M. and Steinman, R.M. (1993). Dendritic cell progenitors phagocytose particulates, including bacillus Calmette-Guerin organisms, and sensitize mice to mycobacterial antigens *in vivo*. *J. Exp. Med.* **180**, 479–488.

Inaba, K., Witmer-Pack, M., Inaba, M., Hathcock, K.S., Sakuta, H., Azuma, M., Yagita, H., Okumura, K., Linsley, P.S., Ikehara, S., Muramatsu, S., Hodes, R.J. and Steinman, R.M. (1994). The tissue distribution of the B7-2 costimulator in mice: abundant expression on dendritic cells *in situ* and during maturation *in vitro*. *J. Exp. Med.* **180**, 1849–1860.

Jansen, J.H., Wientjens, G.J.H.M., Fibbe, W.E., Willemze, R. and Kluin-Nelemans, H.C. (1989). Inhibition of human macrophage colony stimulating formation by interleukin 4. *J. Exp. Med.* **170**, 577–582.

Katz, S.I., Tamaki, K. and Sachs, D.H. (1979). Epidermal Langerhans cells are derived from cells originating in bone marrow. *Nature* **82**, 324–326.

Kleijmeer, M.J., Morkowski, S., Griffith, J.M., Rudensky, A.Y. and Geuze, H.J. (1997). Major histocompatibility complex class II compartments in human and mouse B lymphoblasts represent conventional endocytic compartments. *J. Cell. Biol.* **139**, 639–649.

Klinkert, W.E., LaBadie, J.H. and Bowers, W.E. (1982). Accessory and stimulating properties of dendritic cells and macrophages isolated from various rat tissues. *J. Exp. Med.* **156**, 1–19.

Knight, S.C. (1984). Veiled cells—"dendritic cells" of the peripheral lymph. *Immunobiology* **168**, 349–361.

Koch, F., Stanzl, U., Jennewien, P., Janke, K., Heufler, C., Kampgen, E., Romani, N. and Schuler, G. (1996). High level IL-12 production by murine dendritic cells: upregulation via MHC class II and CD40 molecules and downregulation by IL-4 and IL-10. *J. Exp. Med.* **184**, 741–747.

Kraal, G., Breel, M., Janse, M. and Bruun, G. (1986). Langerhans cells, veiled cells, and interdigitating cells in the mouse recognized by a monoclonal antibody. *J. Exp. Med.* **163**, 981–997.

Larsen, C.P., Steinman, R.M., Witmer-Pack, M.D., Hankins, D.F., Morris, P.J. and Austyn, J.M. (1990). Migration and maturation of Langerhans cells in skin transplants and explants. *J. Exp. Med.* **172**, 1483–1494.

Larsen, C.P., Ritchie, S.C., Pearson, T.C., Linsley, P.S. and Lowry, R.P. (1992). Functional expression of the costimulatory molecules, B7/BB1, on murine dendritic cell populations. *J. Exp. Med.* **176**, 1215–1220.

Larsen, C.P., Ritchie, S.C., Hendrix, R., Linsley, P.S., Hathcock, R.J., Lowry, R.P. and Pearson, T.C. (1994). Regulation of immunostimulatory function and costimulatory molecule (B7-1 and B7-2) expression on murine dendritic cells. *J. Immunol. Methods* **52**, 5208–5219.

Lu, L., Bonham, C.A., Chambers, F.G., Watkins, S.C., Hoffman, R.A., Simmons, R.L. and Thomson, A.W. (1996). Induction of nitric oxide synthase in mouse dendritic cells by IFN-gamma, endotoxin, and interaction with allogeneic T cells: nitric oxide production is associated with dendritic cell apoptosis. *J. Immunol.* **157**, 3577–3586.

Mosialos, G., Birkenbach, M., Ayehunie, S., Matsumura, F., Pinkus, G.S., Kieff, E. and Langhoff, E. (1996). Circulating human dendritic cells differentially express high levels of a 55-kd actin-bundling protein. *Am. J. Pathol.* **148**, 593–600.

Nussenzweig, M.C. and Steinman, R.M. (1980). Contributions of dendritic cells to stimulation of the murine syngeneic mixed lymphocyte reaction. *J. Exp. Med.* **151**, 1196–1212.

Nussenzweig, M.C., Steinman, R.M., Gutchinov, B. and Cohn, Z.A. (1980). Dendritic cells are accessory cells for the development of anti-trinitrophenyl cytotoxic T lymphocytes. *J. Exp. Med.* **152**, 1070–1084.

O'Doherty, U., Steinman, R.M., Peng, M., Cameron, P.U., Gezelter, S., Kopeloff, I., Swiggard, W.J., Pope, M. and Bhardwaj, N. (1993). Dendritic cells freshly isolated from human blood express CD4 and mature into typical immunostimulatory dendritic cells after culture in monocyte-conditioned medium. *J. Exp. Med.* **178**, 1067–1078.

Pierre, P., Turley, S.J., Gatti, E., Hull, M., Meltzer, J., Mirza, A., Inaba, K., Steinman, R.M. and Mellman, I. (1997). Developmental regulation of MHC class II transport in mouse dendritic cells. *Nature* **388**, 787–792.

Pugh, C.W., Macpherson, G.G. and Steer, H.W. (1983). Characterization of nonlymphoid cells derived from rat peripheral lymph. *J. Exp. Med.* **157**, 1758–1779.

Pure, E., Inaba, K., Crowley, M.T., Tardelli, L., Witmer-Pack, M.D., Ruberti, G., Fathman, G. and Steinman, R.M. (1990). Antigen processing by epidermal Langerhans cells correlates with the level of biosynthesis of major histocompatibility complex class II molecules and expression of invariant chain. *J. Exp. Med.* **172**, 1459–1469.

Reddy, A., Sapp, M., Feldman, M., Subklewe, M. and Bhardwaj, N. (1997). A monocyte conditioned medium is more effective than defined cytokines in mediating the terminal maturation of human dendritic cells. *Blood* **90**, 3640–3646.

Reid, C.D., Stackpoole, A., Meager, A. and Tikerpae, J. (1992). Interactions of tumor necrosis factor with granulocyte-macrophage colony-stimulating factor and other cytokines in the regulation of dendritic cell growth *in vitro* from early bipotent CD progenitors in human bone marrow. *J. Immunol.* **149**, 2681–2688.

Reis e Sousa, C., Stahl, P. and Austyn, J. (1993). Phagocytosis of antigens by Langerhans cells *in vitro*. *J. Exp. Med.* **178**, 509-519.

Romani, N., Lenz, A., Glassel, H., Stossel, H., Stanzl, U., Majdic, O., Fritsch, P. and Schuler, G. (1989a). Cultured human Langerhans cells resemble lymphoid dendritic cells in phenotype and function. *J. Invest. Dermatol.* **93**, 600–609.

Romani, N., Koide, S., Crowley, M., Witmer-Pack, M., Livingstone, A.M., Fathman, C.G., Inaba, K. and Steinman, R.M. (1989b). Presentation of exogenous antigens by dendritic cells to T cell clones: intact protein is presented best by immature epidermal Langerhans cells. *J. Exp. Med.* **169**, 1169–1178.

Romani, N., Inaba, K., Pure, E., Crowley, M., Witmer-Pack, M. and Steinman, R. M. (1989c). A small number of anti-CD3 molecules on dendritic cells stimulate DNA synthesis in mouse T lymphocytes. *J. Exp. Med.* **169**, 1153–1168.

Romani, N., Gruner, S., Brang, D., Kampgen, E., Lenz, A., Trockenbacher, B., Konwalinka, G., Fritsch, P., Steinman, R. M. and Schuler, G. (1994). Proliferating dendritic cell progenitors in human blood. *J. Exp. Med.* **180**, 83–93.

Romani, N., Reider, D., Heuer, M., Ebner, S., Eibl, B., Niederwieser, D. and Schuler, G. (1996). Generation of mature dendritic cells from human blood: an improved method with special regard to clinical applicability. *J. Immunol. Methods* **196**, 137–151.

Sallusto, F. and Lanzavecchia, A. (1994). Efficient presentation of soluble antigen by cultured human dendritic cells is maintained by granulocyte/macrophage colony stimulating factor plus interleukin 4 and downregulated by tumor necrosis factor-α. *J. Exp. Med.* **179**, 1109–1118.

Sallusto, F. and Lanzavecchia, A. (1995). Dendritic cells use macropinocytosis and the mannose receptor to concentrate antigen in the MHC class II compartment. Downregulation by cytokines and bacterial products. *J. Exp. Med.* **182**, 389–400.

Sallusto, F., Nicolo, C., DeMaria, R., Cortini, S. and Testi, R. (1996). Ceramide inhibits antigen uptake and presentation by dendritic cells. *J. Exp. Med.* **184**, 2411–2416.

Santiago-Schwarz, F., Belilos, E., Diamond, B. and Carsons, S.E. (1992). TNF in combination with GM-CSF enhances the differentiation of neonatal cord blood stem cells into dendritic cells and macrophages. *J. Leukocyte Biol.* **52**, 274–281.

Saunders, D., Lucas, K., Ismaili, J., Wu, L., Maraskovsky, E., Dunn, A. and Shortman, K. (1996). Dendritic cell development in culture from thymic precursor cells in the absence of granulocyte/macrophage colony stimulating factor. *J. Exp. Med.* **184**, 2185–2196.

Schuler, G. and Steinman, R.M. (1985). Murine epidermal Langerhans cells mature into potent immunostimulatory dendritic cells *in vitro. J. Exp. Med.* **161**, 526–546.

Shelley, W.B. and Lennart, J. (1976). Langerhans cells form a reticuloepithelial trap for external contact antigens. *Nature* **261**, 46–47.

Silberberg-Sinakin, I., Thorbecke, G.J., Baer, R.L., Rosenthal, S.A. and Berezowsky, V. (1976). Antigen-bearing Langerhans cells in skin, dermal lymphatics and in lymph nodes. *Cell Immunol.* **25**, 137–151.

Spry, C.J., Pflug, A.J., Janossy, G. and Humphrey, J.H. (1980). Large mononuclear (veiled) cells with 'Ia-like' membrane antigens in human afferent lymph. *Clin. Exp. Immunol.*, **39**, 750–755.

Steinman, R. M. (1991). The dendritic cell system and its role in immunogenicity. *Annu. Rev. Immunol.* **9**, 271–296.

Steinman, R. M. (1998). In: *Fundamental Immunology* (ed. W. E. Paul). Lippincott-Raven, Philadelphia, in press.

Steinman, R.M. and Cohn, Z. A. (1973). Identification of a novel cell type in peripheral lymphoid organs of mice. I. Morphology, quantitation, tissue distribution. *J. Exp. Med.* **137**, 1142–1162.

Steinman, R.M. and Cohn, Z.A. (1974). Identification of a novel cell type in peripheral lymphoid organs of mice. II. Functional properties *in vitro. J. Exp. Med.* **139**, 380–397.

Steinman, R.M. and Nussenzweig, M.C. (1980). Dendritic cells: features and functions. *Immunol. Rev.* **53**, 127–147.

Steinman, R.M. and Witmer, M.D. (1978). Lymphoid dendritic cells are potent stimulators of the primary mixed leukocyte reaction in mice. *Proc. Natl Acad. Sci. USA* **75**, 5132–5136.

Steinman, R.M., Lustig, D.S. and Cohn, Z.A. (1974). Identification of a novel cell type in peripheral lymphoid organs of mice. III. Functional properties *in vivo. J. Exp. Med.* **139**, 1431–1445.

Steinman, R.M., Gutchinov, B., Witmer, M.D. and Nussenzweig, M.C. (1983). Dendritic cells are the principal stimulators of the primary mixed leukocyte reaction in mice. *J. Exp. Med.* **157**, 613–627.

Stingl, G., Wolff-Schreiner, E.C., Pichler, W.J., Gshnait, F., Knapp, W. and Wolff, K. (1977). Epidermal Langerhans cells bear Fc and C3 receptors. *Nature* **268**, 245–246.

Stingl, G., Katz, S.I., Clement, L., Green, I. and Shevach, E.M. (1978). Immunologic functions of Ia-bearing epidermal Langerhans cells. *J. Immunol.* **121**, 2005–2013.

Sunshine, G.H., Goldman, D.P., Wortis, H.H., Marrack, P. and Kappler, J.W. (1983). Mouse spleen dendritic cells present soluble antigens to antigen-specific T cell hybridomas. *J. Exp. Med.* **158**, 1745–1750.

Süss, G. and Shortman, K. (1996). A subclass of dendritic cells kills CD4 T cells via Fas/Fas-ligand-induced apoptosis. *J. Exp. Med.* **183**, 1789–1796.

Szabolcs, P., Moore, M.A.S., and Young, J.W. (1995). Expansion of immunostimulatory dendritic cells among the myeloid progeny of human $CD34^+$ bone marrow precursors cultured with c-kit ligand, granulocyte-macrophage colony stimulating factor, and TNF *J. Immunol.* **154**, 5851–5861.

Szabolcs, P., Avigan, D., Gezelter, S., Ciocon, D.H., Moore, M.A.S., Steinman, R.M. and Young, J.W. (1996). Dendritic cells and macrophages can mature independently from a human bone marrow-derived post-CFU intermediate. *Blood* **87**, 4520–4530.

Talmor, M., Mirza, A., Turley, S.J., Mellman, I., Hoffman, L.A. and Steinznan, R.M. (1998). Cytokine requirements for the generation of large numbers of dendritic cells from rat bone marrow cultures. *Eur. J. Immunol.* **28**, 811–817.

Tamaki, K., Stingl, G., Gullino, M., Sachs, D.H. and Katz, S.I. (1979). Ia antigens in mouse skin are predominantly expressed on Langerhans cells. *J. Immunol.* **123**, 784–787.

Tew, J.G., Thorbecke, J.S. and Steinman, R.M. (1982). Dendritic cells in the immune response: characteristics and recommended nomenclature (A report from the Reticuloendothelial Society Committee on Nomenclature). *J. Reticulo. Soc.* **31**, 371–380.

Vremec, D., Zorbas, M., Scollay, R., Saunders, D.C., Ardavin, C.F., Wu, L. and Shortman, K. (1992). The surface phenotype of dendritic cells purified from mouse thymus and spleen: investigation of the CD8 expression by a subpopulation of dendritic cells. *J. Exp. Med.* **176**, 47–58.

Winzler, C., Rovere, P., Rescigno, M., Citterio, S., Granucci, F., Mutini, C., Adorini, L., Penna, G., Delia, D., Zimmerman, V.S., Davoust, J. and Ricciardi-Castagnoli, P. (1997). Maturation steps of mouse dendritic cells in growth-factor dependent long-term cultures. *J. Exp. Med.* **185**, 317–328.

Witmer-Pack, M.D., Olivier, W., Valinsky, J., Schuler, G. and Steinman, R.M. (1987). Granulocyte/macrophage colony-stimulating factor is essential for the viability and function of cultured murine epidermal Langerhans cells. *J. Exp. Med.* **166**, 1484–1498.

Witmer-Pack, M.D., Swiggard, W.J., Mirza, A. and Steinman, R.M. (1995). Tissue distribution of the DEC-205 protein that is detected by the monoclonal antibody NLDC-145. II. Expression in situ in lymphoid and nonlymphoid tissues. *Cell. Immunol.* **163**, 157–162.

Wu, L., Li, C.L. and Shortman, K. (1996). Thymic dendritic cell precursors: relationship to the T lymphocyte lineage and phenotype of the dendritic cell progeny. *J. Exp. Med.* **184**, 903–911

Yamaguchi, Y., Tsumura, H., Miwa, M. and Inaba, K. (1997). Contrasting effects of TGFβ1 and TNFα on the development of dendritic cells from progenitors in mouse bone marrow. *Stem Cells* **15**, 144–153.

Zhou, L.J. and Tedder, T.F. (1995). Human blood dendritic cells selectively express CD83, a member of the immunoglobulin superfamily. *J. Immunol.* **154**, 3821–3835.

CHAPTER 29
Phenotypic Characterization of Dendritic Cells

Georgina J. Clark and Derek N.J. Hart
Mater Medical Research Institute, Mater Misericordiae Hospitals, South Brisbane, Queensland, Australia

INTRODUCTION

Definition of DC

Dendritic cells (DC) are a population of leukocytes with specialist antigen-presenting cell (APC) function. They were defined originally on morphological grounds but are now better defined by functional criteria as described earlier in this volume. These criteria include the ability (1) to take up, process and present antigen (Ag), (2) to migrate selectively through tissues and (3) to interact with, stimulate and direct primary T-lymphocyte responses (Hart, 1997). The basic surface membrane phenotype identifies DC as $CD45^+$ leukocytes that express high levels of MHC class II molecules in the absence of markers associated with other leukocyte lineages including CD3, CD15, CD16, CD56, CD19, CD20 and CD14. DC were thought to develop primarily from committed myeloid precursors derived from the pluripotent stem cell (Hart, 1997). However, lymphoid precursor-derived DC have now been described (Chapter 6) and include thymic DC and perhaps a subpopulation within other lymphoid tissues (Fairchild and Austyn, 1990). Their phenotype is described in a later section below. The production of DC-like cells from *in vitro* culture protocols has improved experimental productivity but further complicated the cellular populations that need consideration as DC. We have approached the phenotypic characterization of DC in two ways. First by describing the surface markers used to define DC populations, particularly human, and then by describing how the phenotype relates to DC function.

Differentiation Pathway

Studies on the differentiation pathway of myeloid lineage-derived DC (hereafter DC) have provided evidence for the existence of a number of phenotypically distinguishable populations related both to the stage of DC differentiation and their tissue of origin.

The DC originates in the bone marrow (BM) and migrates into the blood as an immature population before forming an extensive network of interstitial DC in most

Dendritic Cells: Biology and Clinical Applications
ISBN 0-12-455860-7

nonlymphoid organs except brain, parts of the eye and testes (Hart, 1997). Migration of these interstitial DC into the afferent lymphatic system and then to the T-lymphocyte areas of the lymphoid organs designated as the interdigitating DC (IDC), is induced by a variety of stimuli including inflammatory mediators, microbial antigens and other 'danger' signals. The phenotype of the cell changes throughout the differentiation and migration corresponding both to the location and functional state of each particular DC population.

Species Issues

Langerhans cells (LC) were originally identified in human skin on the basis of their morphology and ATPase staining. The morphological, cytochemical and functional description of DC following isolation from mouse spleen was a major step forward (Steinman and Cohn, 1973). Subsequently similar cells were identified in other organs of rat, pigs, rabbits, sheep and man (Hart, 1997; Drexhage *et al.*, 1979). However, it was difficult to define DC further owing to the lack of specific markers. Additional complications arose from the differential expression of some markers between species, making the criteria used to identify DC in one species not always relevant in others. For example, the expression of MHC class II is restricted to APC in the mouse but is expressed by APC, kidney tubules and activated T-lymphocytes in man. Certain critical reagents, e.g. CD14 and CD1 mAb, are not yet available for studying these molecules in mice.

One other major species difference relates to the DC population derived from lymphoid precursors which, apart from some *in vitro* data, has yet to be identified in man.

CELL SURFACE ANTIGENS ASSOCIATED WITH DC

Problems in the Production of mAb

The production of mAb which recognize DC-specific markers has been difficult. The 33D1, (Nussenzweig *et al.*, 1982), NLDC-148 (Kraal *et al.*, 1986) and N418 (Metlay *et al.*, 1990) mAb have assisted characterization of mouse DC populations. At least two cytoplasmic markers for mouse DC have also been described, M342 and MIDC-8, but are not widely used (Agger *et al.*, 1992). Despite the interest, there has been less success generating human DC-specific reagents. The difficulty in purifying large numbers of cells for immunization and screening protocols and the inevitable predominance of mAb recognizing the more immunogenic molecules including CD45 and HLA antigens has created the need to develop alternative strategies. Neonatal immunization with monocytoid cell lines has been used to induce tolerance to dominant antigens prior to immunization with DC. This has been somewhat successful in the generation of two novel mAb, CMRF-44 and CMRF-56, that show relative specificity for activated DC (see below).

Markers Used to Define Mouse and Rat DC

Three mAb recognize relatively DC-specific epitopes on mouse DC. Marginal zone spleen DC can be isolated by the 33D1 rat mAb (Nussenzweig *et al.*, 1982); however, the details on the structure of this antigen are unavailable. A second rat mAb, NLDC-145 (Kraal *et al.*, 1986), recognizes the DEC-205 Ag, expressed by DC in the T-lymphocyte areas including the splenic white pulp (and not the marginal zone DC or LC) and by thymic cortical epithelium and activated macrophage (Mϕ). A cDNA clone has been isolated encoding the mouse DEC-205 Ag (Jiang *et al.*, 1995), suggesting the molecule is related to the macrophage mannose receptors. The third mAb, the rat N418 mAb that binds a CD11c (β_2-integrin family) epitope (Metlay *et al.*, 1990), is expressed in high density on mouse DC but is also found on other leukocytes including Mϕ. A mouse mAb, OX62, has been produced that recognizes an integrin expressed predominantly on rat DC (Brenan and Puklavec, 1992).

Markers Used to Define Human DC Populations

The human DC surface phenotype depends on the cell origin, means of purification (if any) and the state of activation. Certain well-characterized surface markers that show selectivity for some DC populations in combination with more widely expressed molecules such as HLA-DR have proved useful.

Members of the CD1 family of molecules, which have structural similarity with MHC class I molecules, are expressed by cortical thymocytes and differentially by DC populations. LC express CD1a and variable amounts of CD1c (Davis *et al.*, 1988). Dermal or migrating LC are reported to express CD1b (Richters *et al.*, 1996). All three members of the CD1 gene family, CD1a, CD1b and CD1c, are probably expressed by the IDC draining the skin (Cattoretti *et al.*, 1987). Blood and tonsil DC do not express CD1a. Both the absence and expression of CD1c have been noted on blood DC and this remains controversial (Egner *et al.*, 1993a; Xu *et al.*, 1992; Hart and McKenzie, 1988).

A subset of activated freshly isolated blood DC, but not tonsil DC, has been reported to express CD11c, (Thomas and Lipsky, 1994; O'Doherty *et al.*, 1993). As this integrin is also expressed on monocytes (Mo) and Mϕ, it has not proved particularly useful for investigating human DC.

Three recently described mAb, CD83, CMRF-44 and CMRF-56, recognize antigens primarily expressed on activated, or cultured, human DC (Fig. 1). The CD83 mAb, HB15a, was raised against transfectants expressing the HB15 cDNA. It stains cultured human blood DC, LC and some IDC in the lymph node as well as showing limited reactivity with activated B-lymphocytes (Zhou and Tedder, 1995). Analysis of the cDNA indicated that this antigen is a member of the immunoglobulin gene superfamily (Zhou *et al.*, 1992); however, its function is unknown. Reagents to the mouse homologue are not yet available but are eagerly anticipated. A soluble form of the antigen has been reported in the supernatant of some cultured human cell lines (unpublished data) which may influence use of this marker for phenotypic analysis. The CMRF-44 mAb binds an antigen expressed at high density on cultured blood DC, a small number of freshly isolated DC and isolated LC (Hock *et al.*, 1994; Fearnley *et al.*, 1997). This marker has enabled positive selection for purification of DC and has been useful in tissue sections. The antigen, which has not been characterized biochemically as yet, is expressed at low levels by B-lymphocytes, and by Mo and Mϕ following treatment with high dose IFN-γ (above physiological levels).

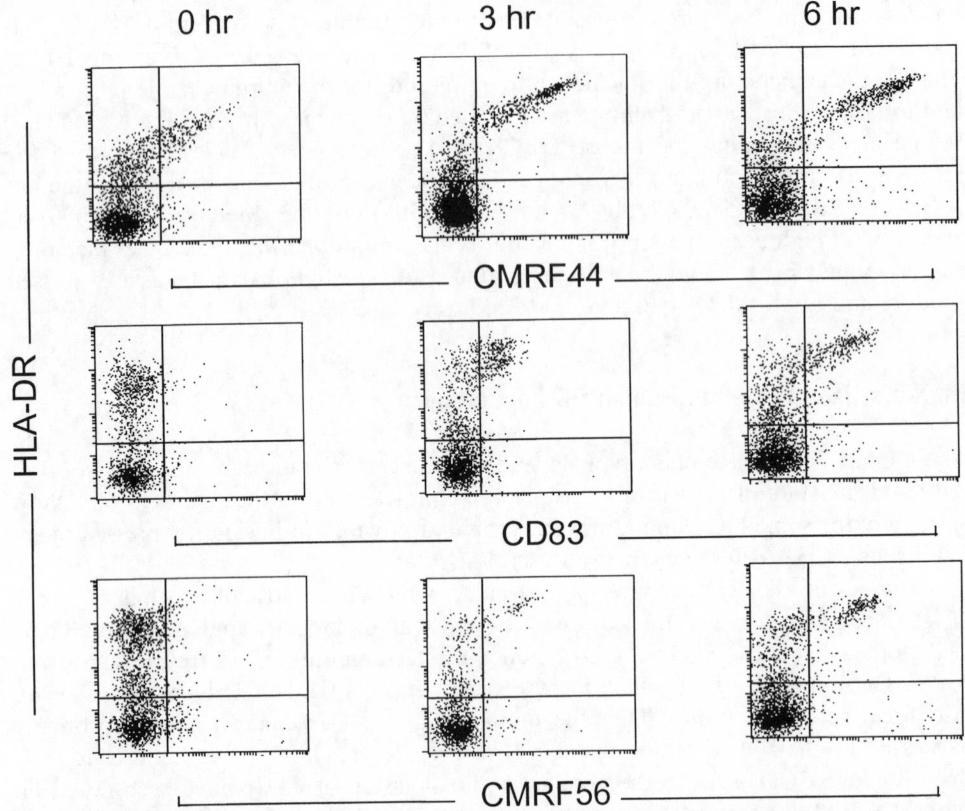

Fig. 1. DC antigens. Expression of the antigens recognized by CMRF-44, CD83 and CMRF-56 mAb on directly isolated DC. Directly isolated blood DC were cultured in medium for 0, 3, or 6 h then analysed by double labelling with CMRF-44, CD83 or CMRF-56 mAb and sheep anti-mouse FITC conjugate and HLA-DR conjugated to PE. The gates delineating positive staining shown have been set on isotype-matched negative control staining. This figure demonstrates the effect of short-term culture on the expression of some DC phenotypic markers.

The CMRF-56 mAb identifies another distinct differentiation/activation marker on cultured DC (Hock *et al.*, in preparation). Cocapping studies distinguish this antigen from those detected by the CMRF-44 and CD83 mAb but its further biochemical characterization is also awaited. Other potentially useful markers include a neoepitope of C9, described on human blood DC, which is recognized by the mAb X-11 (Wuerzner *et al.*, 1991) and the Lag mAb which identifies a molecule present within LC (Strunk *et al.*, 1997).

THE SURFACE PHENOTYPE OF DIFFERENT DC POPULATIONS

In common with other leukocytes, DC express CD45 isoforms (Prickett and Hart, 1990; Freudenthal and Steinman, 1990; Zhou and Tedder, 1995; Wood *et al.*, 1991; Hart and Fearnley, 1997). Other non-lineage-restricted antigens commonly found on the surface

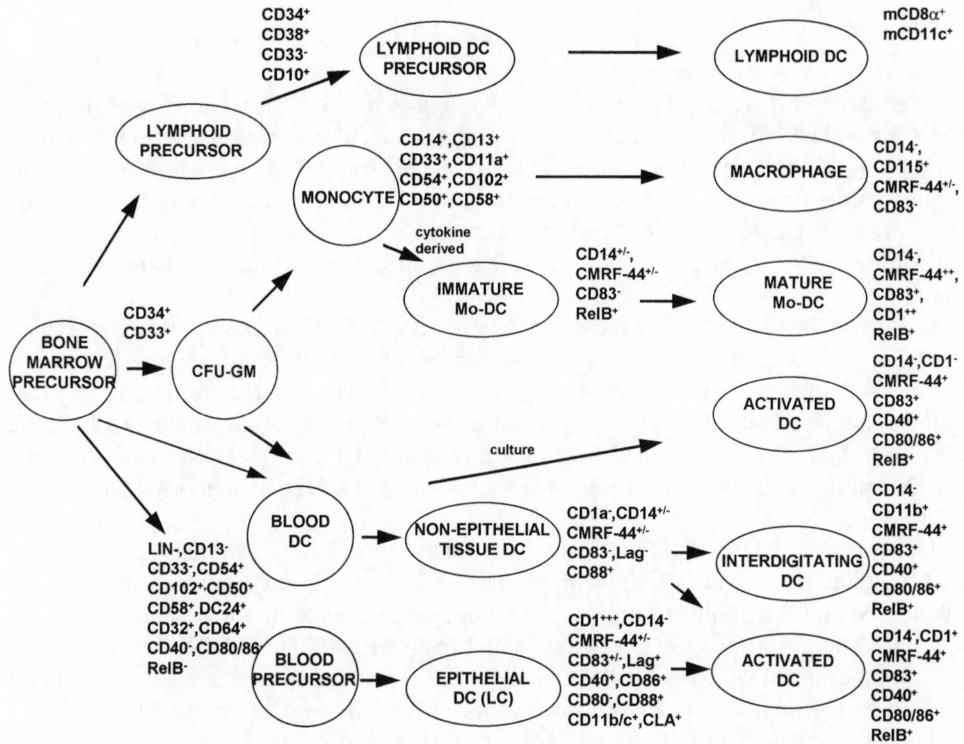

Fig. 2. A putative haemopoietic differentiation pathway for myeloid and lymphoid DC indicating phenotypic markers that are useful for defining the cell populations.

of DC (and other leukocytes) pertain to the migration and function of DC. Such markers are not useful in DC purification but help to phenotypically characterize a DC population (summarized in Fig. 2). The phenotype of DC populations is very dynamic. Exposure to small amounts of foreign substances and short periods of culture throughout the preparation dramatically influence the phenotype of the resulting population (Fig. 1). Thus one must clearly distinguish the method of purification and enrichment of a population under investigation.

Bone Marrow Precursors

A subpopulation of human CD34$^+$ BM cells are immunostimulatory and may represent a DC precursor (Egner *et al.*, 1993b). These cells appear still to have the capacity to differentiate into both the lymphoid and myeloid lineage, the predominant population of CD34$^+$, CD33$^+$ cells present in BM being the precursor population for the myeloid DC. The freshly isolated precursor appears to be CD14$^-$ but a CD14$^+$ precursor may evolve during *in vitro* culture. An alternative CD34$^+$ precursor is thought to differentiate along an independent pathway to provide Lag$^+$, CD1a$^+$ epithelial-associated LC (Strunk *et al.*, 1997).

Blood DC

Fresh Blood DC

As discussed earlier, the DC lineage is distinguished from other leukocyte populations by a lack of lineage-specific membrane molecules. Fresh blood DC express high levels of MHC molecules and CD45RA Ag (Hart, 1997). Immunoselection techniques using flow cytometry or magnetic bead technology can be used to isolate the lineage negative (lin^-) cells which, although heterogeneous, include most fresh (uncultured) DC. The phenotype of blood DC purified with minimal manipulation is immature.

Freshly isolated blood DC have low levels of CD11c (Thomas and Lipsky, 1994; O'Doherty *et al.*, 1993) but express a variety of adhesion molecules, few costimulatory molecules, (McLellan *et al.*, 1995; McLellan *et al.*, 1996; Freudenthal and Steinman, 1990; Hart *et al.*, 1993) and some Fc receptors (Fanger *et al.*, 1996; Davis *et al.*, 1988) as described later. Freshly isolated DC express the cross-reacting DC-24 epitope defined by IgM CD24 mAb but not the CD24 protein (Williams *et al.*, 1996).

The $CD13^+$, $CD33^+$, $CD14^{dim}$ DC precursor population isolated directly from PBMC differentiates, after culture, into cells with dendritic processes, a more mature phenotype and the ability to induce T-lymphocyte responses in an MLR or to soluble antigen (Thomas *et al.*, 1993; Thomas and Lipsky, 1994). The $CD2^+$, HLA-DR^{+++}, lin^- population of cells from PBMC is capable of processing and presenting nominal antigen to T-lymphocytes (Takamizawa *et al.*, 1997). The expression of CD2 on freshly isolated blood DC is rapidly downregulated during culture.

Cultured Blood DC

DC are commonly purified by virtue of their low density compared to other PBMC populations after a brief period of tissue culture. This characteristic allows the use of a variety of gradient media to enrich DC from other contaminating cells. BSA, metrizamide, Nycodenz and Percoll gradients have all been used successfully; however, their osmotic effects may induce phenotypic or functional changes in the purified cells. Morphologically these cultured cells have prominent cytoplasm and some dendritic processes, while phenotypically there is upregulation of surface antigen associated with DC activation. This allows purification by positive selection using the CMRF-44, CMRF-56 and CD83 reagents (Fearnley *et al.*, 1997) or double and triple labelling for phenotypic analysis. There is also upregulation of a number of critical functional cell surface antigens. The CD33, CD13 Ag (Thomas *et al.*, 1993; Fearnley *et al.*, 1997) and the novel DC-24 carbohydrate epitope (Williams *et al.*, 1996) are downregulated on this population.

Nonlymphoid Tissue-derived DC—the Interstitial DC

The first encounter of DC with either antigen or the 'danger' signals identifying a 'foreign' threat to the host occurs in the tissues. Thus these tissue-associated DC can be described as surveillance cells. The nonlymphoid tissue-derived DC can be separated into two phenotypically distinct populations.

Superficial Epithelial DC Populations

The DC populations in the superficial epithelial tissues include the LC and the cells in the gut, the urogenital tract and some in the respiratory tract. LC are identified as the MHC class II^{+++}, $CD1a^{+++}$, $CD14^{-}$ cell in the epidermis and the presence of Birbeck granules within them can be demonstrated by electron microscopy (Romani and Schuler, 1992). *In situ*, some cells express very low levels of the CMRF-44, CD83, CD40 and CD86 Ag but not the CD80 Ag. Isolated LC express higher levels of these antigens (except CD80), which may reflect upregulation during isolation (McLellan *et al.*, 1997). There is selective expression of certain β_1-integrins (VLA subfamily a1-a9, av). Rare $CD1a^{++}$ DC are identified in the epithelium of the gut but more extensive numbers are found in the lamina propria. $CD1a^{+}$ cells have recently been identified in the urothelium of bladder, ureter and kidney (Troy *et al.*, 1998b).

The respiratory mucosa hosts an extensive population of DC. Again few are located within the epithelial surface but an extensive network of DC is localized beneath the basement membrane (McWilliam *et al.*, 1995; McWilliam *et al.*, 1996). The phenotype of these cells reflects the influence of inflammatory and other mediators on DC activation.

Nonepithelial DC Populations

This population of cells includes the dermal DC (Davis *et al.*, 1988) and DC in the heart, kidney, lung and liver (Austyn *et al.*, 1994; Hart *et al.*, 1981) and perhaps deep epithelial glandular structures. Dermal DC do not have prominent Birbeck granules and are MHC class II^{+}, $CD1a^{+}$, $CD36^{+}$, Lag^{-} (Romani *et al.*, 1989). Staining for factor XIIIa also identifies a dermal cell with dendritic morphology (Cerio *et al.*, 1989). Further phenotypic analysis of these populations is required to distinguish these DC from $CD1a^{+++}$ LC. *In situ*, only a subpopulation of the dermal DC expresses the CMRF-44 and CD83 Ags (McLellan *et al.*, 1997) but these upregulate rapidly on isolated cells. Isolated mouse dermal DC are reported to be $N418^{-}$ and NLDC-145^{-} (Austyn *et al.*, 1994).

In situ phenotypic analysis of human liver DC distinguished these from Mϕ (Prickett *et al.*, 1988). Interstitial DC have been isolated from mouse heart and kidney (Austyn *et al.*, 1994), rat liver (Hart and Fabre, 1981), and the rat iris (Steptoe *et al.*, 1995). These cells express low-density MHC molecules (which upregulate in culture) and lack significant expression of the 33D1, N418 and DEC-205 Ags.

Lymphoid tissue-derived DC (IDC)

IDC from the lymphoid tissues are a heterogeneous population either representing activated and nonactivated populations or perhaps distinct populations derived from different lineages. This needs clarification and may be species dependent.

In man, lin^{-} DC associated with the T-lymphoid areas of tonsil are $CD13^{-}$, $CD33^{-}$, CMRF-44^{-} and $CD83^{-}$. A proportion of MHC class II^{+} DC in these areas is activated, expressing CMRF-44, CD83, CD11b and costimulatory molecules (manuscript in preparation). A population of CMRF-44^{-} tonsil IDC phenotypically resembles the $CD4^{+}$, $CD11c^{-}$ 'plasmacytoid T-lymphocytes' described by Grouard (Grouard *et al.*, 1996). It is likely that these cells represent the same population as the HLA-DR^{+}, lin^{-}, IL-$3R^{high}$ cells described by Olweus (Olweus *et al.*, 1997) and they may represent a DC lineage distinct from the LC pathway. No functional difference in the properties of the CMRF-44$^+$ and CMRF-44$^-$ IDC populations has been revealed as yet. A third population found predominantly in the germinal centres can be distinguished from the follicular DC by the absence of CD21 but expression of CD4, CD11c, CD11b, CD13, CD33 and CD45 (Grouard *et al.*, 1996).

Phenotypically distinct populations of IDC are also found in the mouse spleen. The mouse DC marker NLDC-145 reacts with cells in the inner periarteriolar lymphocyte sheath around the central arteriole and not in the follicular or marginal zone (Kraal *et al.*, 1986). A second population identified by the 33D1 mAb is found in the periphery of the T-lymphocyte area and marginal zone (Metlay *et al.*, 1990). More recently the analysis of flt-3L-stimulated mouse DC identified up to four populations from spleen based on staining by CD11c and NLDC-145 mAb (Maraskovsky *et al.*, 1996).

In vitro Cultured DC-like Cells

DC have been generated from a number of sources by culture of cells in the presence of a variety of cytokines and media supplements (Inaba *et al.*, 1992; Scheicher *et al.*, 1992; Inaba *et al.*, 1993a,b; Mayordomo *et al.*, 1995; Celluzzi *et al.*, 1996; Dillon *et al.*, 1997; Zitvogel *et al.*, 1996; Gabrilovich *et al.*, 1996; Mayordomo *et al.*, 1996). Again, there appear to be clear species differences.

Cultured Mouse Cells

Mouse MHC class II$^-$ BM cells cultured in the presence of GM-CSF develop into a complex cellular population. This includes a subpopulation of DC expressing high levels of MHC molecules, CD44 and CD11b, medium levels of CD24, CD45 and CD8 and low levels of NLDC-145, 33D1, CD11c as well as the Mϕ marker F4/80 and Fcγ receptors (Inaba *et al.*, 1992).

Cultured Human Cells

Various cultured human cell preparations have been exploited to provide large numbers of DC-like cells for basic studies and therapeutic administration. The starting populations of cells have included the CD34$^+$ BM, cord blood and GM-CSF mobilized peripheral blood cells. Although there are definite similarities with the 'gold standard' of directly purified blood DC populations, there are also notable differences. Generally these culture systems result in heterogeneous populations of cells, some of which undoubtedly have the true DC phenotype (accounting for the functional properties) but many may not. CD1a has commonly been used as a marker for DC progeny but the induction of CD1a on monocytic cells may confound the results.

Cells cultured from CD34$^+$ BM in the presence of GM-CSF with a variety of cytokines including IL-4, IL-13, TNF-α and SCF generate cells which include a CD14$^-$, HLA-DR$^-$ subpopulation of cells that coexpresses many of the accessory molecules and is able to stimulate allogeneic T-lymphocytes (Szabolcs *et al.*, 1995; Young *et al.*, 1995). These cultures include 10–15% CD1a$^+$ cells. The culture of CD34$^+$ cord blood cells with GM-CSF and TNF-α generates a subpopulation of cells with some characteristics of DC and LC including expression of CD1a, HLA-DR, costimulatory molecules and, in some cells, Birbeck granules (Caux *et al.*, 1992). Yields of 5–15% CD1a$^+$

cells are reported. Further characterization has suggested that DC are derived from the $CD13^{+++}$ cells (Rosenzwajg *et al.*, 1996).

Similarly, the generation of a $CD1a^+$, CLA^+ LC precursor from mobilized peripheral blood cells cultured with GM-CSF has been reported (Strunk *et al.*, 1997). Apparently higher yields of $CD1a^+$ cells (35–55%) are obtained from this source.

Mo-derived DC (Mo-DC) can be grown from either PBMC or $CD14^+$ monocytes in the presence of a combination of cytokines generally including GM-CSF and IL-4 (Sallusto and Lanzavecchia, 1994) or monocyte-conditioned medium. The presence of IL-4 may induce the downregulation of CD14 (Lauener *et al.*, 1990) and suppress monocyte development (Jansen *et al.*, 1989). The resulting populations are heterogeneous with respect to many markers including CD1a. The CMRF-44^+, $CD14^-$ cells isolated from such cultures indicated that the allostimulatory activity was present only in a subpopulation of the $CD1a^+$ cells (Vuckovic *et al.*, 1997). The CD83 Ag was upregulated on the $CD1a^+$ cell population of Mo-DC (Zhou and Tedder, 1996a) as is the Rel-B transcription factor (Akagawa *et al.*, 1996). The latter study also distinguished commitment to either Mϕ or DC differentiation by expression of the M-CSF receptor. Other studies have involved detailed analyses of Mo-DC derived from culture of $CD14^+$ monocytes with GM-CSF and IL-4 or TNF-α (Zhou and Tedder, 1996a; Pickl *et al.*, 1996). The resulting cells expressed CD1a/b/c, CD80 and CD5, and further upregulated CD40, MHC class II, CD4, CD11b/c, CD43, CD45, CD54, CD58 and CD59 whilst downregulating CD14, CD15s, CD64 and CDw65. The populations again were mixed and contained significant amounts of mRNA for myeloperoxidase and lysozyme suggesting that the resulting cells are different from DC purified without *in vitro* culture. Thus these cultures contain potent allostimulatory cells which are probably true DC, whilst at the same time containing a number of contaminating cell populations.

Lymphoid Lineage-derived DC

A lymphoid progenitor gives rise to the mouse thymic DC (Ardavin and Shortman, 1993; Fairchild and Austyn, 1990). The cells are characterized by the expression of CD8α, CD44, HSA, CD11a and MHC class II molecules in the absence of CD3 and rearranged TCR (Wu *et al.*, 1995; Vremec *et al.*, 1992). A similar cell identified in peripheral lymphoid tissues has a tolerogenic function rather than the allostimulatory function associated with the myeloid DC. The human $CD34^+$, $CD38^{dim}$ thymic precursor reportedly differentiates, in the presence of GM-CSF and TNF-α, into T lymphocytes, NK cells and DC (Res *et al.*, 1996). The DC resulting from this culture are $CD4^+$, $CD40^+$, MHC class II^+, $CD33^-$ with a subset expressing CD1a. They do not express other lineage markers including CD8. A second report observed *in vitro* a $CD10^+$ human lymphoid progenitor-derived DC (Galy *et al.*, 1995) that gives rise to T- and B-lymphocytes, NK cells and DC.

DC Derived from Diseased Tissue

Lin^- DC isolated from reactive sites of autoimmune diseases, e.g. chronic arthritic joints in rheumatoid arthritis, have a somewhat unexpected phenotype in that they lack high-density expression of the CD80/CD86 costimulator molecules (Summers *et al.*, 1995; Summers *et al.*, 1996). Otherwise the isolated cells are morphologically similar to activated DC with high-density expression of CD40 and adhesion molecules. A small number of the cells express the CMRF-44 activation marker but not the CD83 marker (Summers *et al.*, 1995). However, these markers and the costimulator molecules are induced after culture in the absence of synovial fluid.

Analysis of the DC found in tumour tissue has also revealed striking new information. First, relatively few DC are present in renal cell carcinoma and the majority of these have an unactivated phenotype (Troy *et al.*, 1998b). Only a small proportion (5–15%) of tumour-associated DC are CMRF-44$^+$ and few have upregulated the CD86 molecule. Similar results pertain to prostatic carcinoma (Troy *et al.*, 1998b). Likewise, phenotypically immature DC predominate in breast and bowel carcinoma and only a proportion are CD1a$^+$ (manuscript in preparation).

FUNCTIONAL PHENOTYPE OF DC

Many molecules useful for surface phenotyping and purification of DC populations have unknown functions. DC populations can also be phenotyped using molecules associated with specific functions.

Molecules Involved in Antigen Uptake, Processing and Presentation

Receptors involved in the uptake of antigens can be divided into a number of classes based on their mode of action. These include the pattern recognition receptors, the complement (C′) receptors and the Fc receptors.

Pattern Recognition Receptors

The pattern recognition receptors bind a range of molecules with structural patterns common to the surface of many microorganisms but absent from the surface of mammalian cells (Pearson, 1996). Such antigens tend to be complex carbohydrates that show some specificity in the terminal sugar residues. Mo-DC express surface molecules that are thought to bind these antigens including the macrophage mannose receptor (Sallusto *et al.*, 1995; Kraal *et al.*, 1986; Tan *et al.*, 1997; Engering *et al.*, 1997) and other lectin-like molecules, i.e. the NKRP1A molecule (Poggi *et al.*, 1997). Expression of these molecules on other DC populations remains to be established.

Functional studies on mouse DC suggest that LC (Reis e Sousa *et al.*, 1993) express mannose receptors. The DEC-205 Ag is related to the macrophage mannose receptor and probably acts as an antigen receptor (Jiang *et al.*, 1995). A cDNA clone encoding the human DEC-205 homologue has been isolated (Kato *et al.*, 1998) and initial tissue distribution studies by RT-PCR analysis suggest that the mRNA is predominantly expressed in activated DC populations. The expression of the protein and ligand specificity have yet to be studied. The significance of this late expression presents intriguing questions as to the functional role of this molecule in humans.

Complement (C′) Receptors

Some C′ receptors have been described on DC. Low levels of CD11b (Egner *et al.*, 1993a; Thomas and Lipsky, 1994; Weber-Matthiesen and Sterry, 1990) and CD11c

(Shibaki *et al.*, 1995) are found on blood DC and LC. Dermal DC and a subpopulation of LC express CD88 (C5a receptors) (Morelli *et al.*, 1996). DC do not express the CD21 (CR2) and CD35 (CR1) receptors (Hart and McKenzie, 1988). Protection of blood DC against C′-mediated lysis may be via the expression of CD55, CD59 and CD46 (Hart and Fearnley, 1997). CD46 Ag is also expressed by cytokine-derived DC (Grosjean *et al.*, 1997; Fugier-Vivier *et al.*, 1997).

Fc Receptors

FcR allow the specific uptake of opsonized antigens by various cells. Both CD32 and CD64 but not CD16 are expressed by fresh blood DC, early in their differentiation; however, careful cell preparation was required for this analysis. These two FcγR enable DC to phagocytose, although at a reduced rate, opsonized ox red blood cells (Fanger *et al.*, 1996; Fanger *et al.*, 1997). Human LC express CD32, CD64 and both the high and low receptors for IgE (Reiger *et al.*, 1992; Bieber *et al.*, 1992). However, the FcεRI complex on DC lacks the β chain required for activity (Maurer *et al.*, 1996). The CMRF-35 Ag is a molecule that has considerable similarity with the Fc receptor for polymeric IgA and IgM, although a ligand for CMRF-35 has not been identified (Jackson *et al.*, 1992). This antigen is expressed in different forms, on human blood DC, LC and tonsil DC (manuscript in preparation).

Migration and Adhesion of DC Populations

The phenotype of DC migrating through the tissues prior to interaction with T lymphocytes relates to adhesion molecule and chemokine receptor expression.

Adhesion Molecules

DC express a wide variety of adhesion molecules. The ligands for CD11a (LFA-1), i.e. CD54 (ICAM-1), CD50 (ICAM-2) and CD102 (ICAM-3), are all expressed on DC but show differential regulation. CD54 is expressed at low density on blood DC and LC but is quickly upregulated by activation (Starling *et al.*, 1995), whereas CD50 is expressed at high density, showing little change in expression level with activation (Hart and Prickett, 1993). CD102 is expressed in highest density on DC and may be the most important CD11a ligand involved in early DC–T lymphocyte adhesion (Starling *et al.*, 1995). LC also express high levels of CD102 (Vedel *et al.*, 1992; Zambruno *et al.*, 1995; Lee *et al.*, 1993).

E-cadherin has a role in migration and is expressed by mouse (Borkowski *et al.*, 1994) and human LC (Blauvelt *et al.*, 1995) and blood DC but downregulates from LC as the cells migrate. The presence of E-cadherin on LC may reflect their unique adhesive interaction with the squamous epithelium. Although selectins have yet to be described on DC, LC do express the E-selectin ligand or cutaneous lymphocyte-associated (CLA) antigen (Koszik *et al.*, 1994) which may be involved in cell interaction during trafficking. Interaction between DC and the connective tissue may be stabilized by isoforms of the CD44 molecule that is expressed in high density by DC (Prickett *et al.*, 1992). Detailed analysis of the expression of the isoforms has only been performed on Mo-DC which express the V3, V6 and V9 isoforms (Sallusto and Lanzavecchia,

1994). Other molecules that may play adhesive roles reportedly expressed on DC include syndecan (CD138), the endothelial molecule endoglin (CD105) and neurothelin (CD147) (Hart and Fearnley, 1997). In addition, subpopulations of DC express CD106 (V-CAM) (Norton *et al.*, 1992), and CD31 (PECAM-1) is expressed on blood and tonsil DC (Hancock and Atkins, 1984).

Receptors for Chemoattractants

As DC respond to chemokines they must express receptors for chemoattractant molecules that presumably influence their migration and antigen-presenting roles. Mo-DC differentiated in the presence of GM-CSF and IL-13 express the CCR1, CCR2, CCR5, CXCR1, CXCR2 and CXCR4 receptors but not the CCR3, CCR4 or CXCR3 receptors (Sozzani *et al.*, 1997). Lung DC express a receptor for the C-C chemokine MIP-3α (Power *et al.*, 1997). However, the expression of a particular receptor does not always indicate that DC demonstrate chemotaxis in response to all chemokines that bind that receptor. Sozzani *et al.* have shown that although these DC populations should bind IL-8 and MCP-1, they do not migrate in response (Sozzani *et al.*, 1997), while others showed that CD34$^+$-derived DC did migrate in response to MCP-1 (Xu *et al.*, 1996). Migration of Mo-DC is found in response to formylpeptides, C5a, SDF-1, MCP-3, MCP-4, MIP-1a, MIP-1b, MIP-5, RANTES and platelet-activating factor (Sozzani *et al.*, 1995). Low numbers of LC localized at the basement membrane of the epidermis express the C5aR (CD88), the expression of which is increased following culture of purified LC with GM-CSF. These cells were also shown to migrate in response to C5a (Morelli *et al.*, 1996).

Adhesion and Signalling

Direct adhesion between T lymphocytes and DC is probably mediated by CD2 (LFA-2) ICAM-3 on the T-lymphocyte and LFA-3/LFA-1/ICAM-3 on the DC (Prickett *et al.*, 1992) and results in phenotypic changes due to upregulation of costimulatory and other functional molecules.

Costimulatory Molecules

Following migration of DC to the T-lymphocyte areas of the lymphoid tissue, DC acquire a phenotype relating to their stimulatory properties. CD40, which is only present in low amounts on blood DC (McLellan *et al.*, 1996) and LC (Romani *et al.*, 1989) is upregulated following stimulation of the DC. It is present on the more mature tonsillar DC population (Hart and McKenzie, 1988). Likewise, CD80 and CD86 are not expressed by resting blood DC but are rapidly upregulated following activation (McLellan *et al.*, 1995; Hart *et al.*, 1993; Symington *et al.*, 1993). Reciprocal T-lymphocyte CD40L feedback after antigen recognition induces major CD40-mediated increases in DC CD80/CD86 expression (McLellan *et al.*, 1996). The immunoglobulin superfamily member SLAM (CDw150) has been identified on blood DC; it upregulates following activation and has a putative costimulatory role (Hart and Fearnley, 1997).

Cytokines may also modulate DC phenotype and function. Type I IL-1R are expressed by LC and IL-1α and IL-1β clearly induce CD40 expression on human blood DC (McLellan *et al.*, 1996). Both type I and type II TNFR are expressed on human blood DC (McKenzie *et al.*, 1995) and GM-CSFR has been demonstrated on human blood DC (Zhou and Tedder, 1996b) and tonsil DC (Hart and Calder, 1994).

Inhibition of DC Function

The expression on DC of cell surface molecules with inhibitory functions has been documented recently. The mouse CD8α^+ lymphoid DC population found in the thymus and spleen expresses high levels of FasL (Suss and Shortman, 1996). The possibility that myeloid-derived DC were regulated by Fas-mediated apoptosis after performing APC function is an intriguing one. Recent data suggests they do express Fas on their surface. They also express receptors for IL-10 and TGF-β, both cytokines known to downregulate DC function. Rat spleen DC express the NKR-P1 marker, a molecule associated with NK cell function (Josien *et al.*, 1997). Transcripts for a novel molecule (ILT3) were cloned from EBV-B cell lines using RT-PCR and primers designed to amplify immunoglobulin superfamily members (Samaridis and Colonna, 1997). An antibody to this molecule stained monocytes, CD83$^+$ DC and Mo-DC (Cella *et al.*, 1997). A putative immunotyrosine-based inhibitory motif is found in the cytoplasmic region of ILT3 and the ILT3-specific antibody prevented Ca^{2+} mobilization indicative of an inhibitory signal.

Other Molecules

The production of mAb recognizing DC-specific surface antigens has been frustrating and researchers have looked at alternative ways to characterize these cells. A number of mAb binding non-surface-expressed molecules have proved useful and a phenotypic profile of these secreted molecules may further characterize DC populations.

Secreted Molecules; Cytokines and Chemokines

Interaction with T-lymphocytes and signalling to other cells certainly involves cytokines (Chapter 37) and chemokines and DC may be further phenotyped by their limited production of either. Populations of DC may express small amounts of IL-1 (Hart and Calder, 1994; Zhou and Tedder, 1996b; Caux *et al.*, 1994), TNF-α (Zhou and Tedder, 1996b; McKenzie *et al.*, 1995), lymphotoxin and GM-CSF (Hart and Calder, 1994). Activated DC have been reported to produce IL-7 (Sorg *et al.*, 1997/8) and IL-12 (Yawalkar *et al.*, 1996), while Mo-DC produce IL-15 (Jonuleit *et al.*, 1997).

CD83$^+$ DC purified from blood as metrizamide low-density mononuclear cells were found to express mRNA for a variety of chemokines; Mip-1b, IL-8, low levels for MCP-1 and RANTES and on activation for Mip-1a (Zhou and Tedder, 1996b). Mo-DC differentiated in the presence of GM-CSF and IL-13 produce MCP-1, RANTES and MIP-1a and the recently described chemokine termed macrophage-derived chemokine (MDC). MDC acts as a chemoattractant for Mo, Mo-DC and NK cells (Godiska *et al.*, 1997). Expression of MDC by DC purified without exposure to cytokines has not been demonstrated. A second chemokine expressed by Mo-derived DC, DC-CK1 is a chemoattractant for CD45RA$^+$ T-lymphocytes, and *in situ* hybridization identified its expression in germinal centres and the T-lymphocyte areas of tonsil (Adema *et al.*,

1997). DC-CK1 expression appears to be induced by IL-4 but inhibited by GM-CSF, indicating that its expression will be markedly influenced by the cytokine combination used to differentiate the DC population.

Cytoskeletal Markers

A 55 kDa actin-bundling protein (p55, fascin) is expressed by the majority of human blood DC, IDC, cytokine-derived DC but not other leukocyte lineages (Mosialos *et al.*, 1996). Messenger RNA for a protein, restin, associated with the intermediate filament cytoskeletal network of Reed–Sternberg cells (RSC) in Hodgkin's disease has been detected in human DC populations (Bilbe *et al.*, 1992).

Cytoplasmic Markers

Enzyme reactivities are useful phenotypic markers distinguishing DC from other cells, particularly from classic Mo/Mϕ. The latter cell populations show myeloperoxidase activity (Steinman and Cohn, 1973; Witmer and Steinman, 1984; Egner *et al.*, 1993a,b; Buckley *et al.*, 1987), and low levels of 5′-nucleotidase, dipeptidyl peptidase and cathepsin B activity (Romani and Schuler, 1992; Knight *et al.*, 1986; Thomas *et al.*, 1993), whereas DC appear to lack these. DC also express low levels or show a different intracellular distribution of other enzymes such as nonspecific esterase (Arkema *et al.*, 1991), acid phosphatase or CD68, a lysosomal marker (Hart and McKenzie, 1988). The S100 mAb detects an intracellular isomer useful for histological studies on formalin-fixed sections (Takahashi *et al.*, 1982) but, because of its solubility, not in frozen sections. Recent data suggest that it is associated with activated DC (Troy *et al.*, 1997).

Transcription Factors

The expression of many surface molecules including CD80/CD86 and MHC class II is clearly regulated differently in DC compared with other cells, e.g. B-lymphocytes, in terms of basal activity, levels and kinetics. Transcription factors regulating the DC phenotype may provide a further level of phenotyping. However, it may be the pattern of expression of a variety of transcription factors and not the absolute presence or absence of any one factor that will provide the best distinction of DC from other cells.

The NF-κB transcription family member Rel-B shows some selective expression in mouse thymus, spleen and lymph node DC (Carrasco *et al.*, 1993) and mice with a deleted Rel-B gene show, among other phenotypes, a lack of mature functional DC (see Chapter 30) (Burkly *et al.*, 1995). Human DC grown from peripheral blood with GM-CSF express c-rel, rel-B, NF-κBp65 and NF-κBp50 (Granelli-Piperno *et al.*, 1995) but lack the widely expressed transcription factor SP-1. Rel-B has been identified in Mo-DC (Akagawa *et al.*, 1996) and human tonsil DC (Feuillard *et al.*, 1996). Peripheral blood DC purified following culture express Rel-B which is absent in freshly purified blood DC (manuscript submitted).

The specialized function of DC in processing and presentation of antigens suggests that other intracellular enzymes or regulatory proteins may be useful in identifying this cell lineage. The techniques of differential display are fast describing new DC molecules and a full repetoire of molecules expressed both at the DC surface and intracellularly is soon anticipated.

NEW STRATEGIES FOR DC MARKERS

There is clearly a need for other specific DC markers that recognize the DC populations found in different sites and at different stages of maturation and differentiation. Analysis of DC lysates by PAGE has demonstrated the presence of novel antigens not expressed in monocyte lysates (Hock and Hart, 1992), suggesting that the production of mAb is still a worthwhile, if time-consuming, strategy. The major limitation to this approach relates to obtaining sufficient material for immunization and screening. The presence of novel carbohydrate determinants on DC populations is another approach. The expression of members of the scavenger receptors and the pattern recognition receptors that bind different lectins led to the strategy presently being investigated in this laboratory that these lectins may identify novel DC associated molecules.

Molecular techniques are also proving rewarding in the isolation of novel markers, and the usefulness of intracellular markers should not be overlooked. Differential display technology has allowed isolation of a number of potentially useful molecules including a novel human AHCY-like molecule, DD4b5.3 (unpublished) and a disintegrin family member (Mueller *et al.*, 1997).The mRNA encoding the AHCY-like molecule appears to be expressed in LC and differentiated populations of DC but not in less mature cells. The disintegrin family member is expressed by Mo-DC but not in $CD14^+$ monocyte populations. Similar technology using mouse cell lines has isolated a cDNA for a DC-specific C-type lectin-1, Dectin, which appears to be involved in T-lymphocyte activation (Ariizumi *et al.*, 1996). It is expressed by LC and a subpopulation of $CD11c^+$ spleen cells.

APPLICATION OF PHENOTYPE

Detailed knowledge of the phenotype of DC is crucial to understanding the biology of the cells being studied. In addition, as many applications of DC for clinical treatments are being investigated, it is crucial that the most appropriate cell population to be used for each is identified.

Purification of homogeneous DC populations for particular uses is presently difficult for most populations except the activated $CD83^+$, CMRF-44^+, HLA class II^+, $CD14^-$ blood DC or $N418^{bright}$, DEC-205^{bright} mouse spleen DC. The ability to positively or negatively select a population for a particular purpose requires the availability of the necessary reagents. Drug targeting or antigen loading of cells for therapeutic purposes may be more readily achieved using immature DC that express antigen uptake receptors rather than cells with a more mature phenotype. The homogeneity of a population may influence the outcome particularly if DC populations that are able to tolerize (Matzinger and Guerder, 1989) are included in a tumour therapy protocol.

The availability of the CMRF-44 mAb which reacts with blood DC after a brief period of *in vitro* culture led us to exploit the DC phenotype to develop the first routine blood test for human DC. Using a method suitable for most diagnostic flow cytometers, reliable counts can be obtained from 5 ml EDTA blood samples. Initial clinical data suggest that it will be possible to obtain blood DC counts (mean absolute DC number 9×10^3/ml blood, range 3–15 $\times 10^3$/ml) as a routine from patients (manuscript submitted). Interpreting these data in relation to the patients' clinical state will, it is hoped, provide important new information which may affect their treatment.

Phenotypic characterization of DC can also be applied directly to certain potential DC malignancies. Class I histiocytosis is a rare childhood condition that is defined by CD1 staining suggesting a LC origin of this malignancy (Egeler *et al.*, 1993). This is further supported in one case by positive staining with the CMRF-44 and CD83 mAb (unpublished). A DC origin for the malignant cells in Hodgkin's disease has been suggested for a proportion of cases in which the malignant cell expresses a number of DC markers including CD83 (Sorg *et al.*, 1997) and p55 (Mosialos *et al.*, 1996).

The functions of molecules expressed specifically in DC populations is relevant to the ability to use DC in clinical strategies. Thus DEC-205 or the CMRF-35 Ags may be targets for antigen loading for tumour immunotherapy. The ability to specifically inhibit a particular enzyme or DNA-binding protein that is important to DC function may allow new immunosuppressive treatments that may lead to applications in clinical transplantation and autoimmune disease. An understanding of the function of the CD83, CMRF-44 and CMRF-56 antigens may likewise contribute to therapeutic interventions.

ACKNOWLEDGEMENTS

We acknowledge the Haematology/Immunology/Transfusion Medicine Research Group, Christchurch School of Medicine, The New Zealand Health Research Council, The Marsden Fund and The New Zealand Lotteries Grant Board.

REFERENCES

Adema, G.J., Hartgers, F., Verstraten, R., de Vries, E., Marland, G., Menon, S., Foster, J., Xu, Y., Nooyen, P., McClanahan, T., Bacon, K.B. and Figdor, C.G. (1997). A dendritic-cell-derived C-C chemokine that preferentially attracts naive T cells. *Nature* **387**, 713

Agger, R., Witmer-Pack, M., Romani, N., Stossel, H., Swiggard, W.J., Metlay, J.P., Storozynsky, E., Freimuth, P. and Steinman, R.M. (1992). Two populations of splenic dendritic cells detected with M342, a new monoclonal to an intracellular antigen of interdigitating dendritic cells and some B lymphocytes. *J. Leukocyte Biol.* **52**, 34–42.

Akagawa, K.S., Takasuka, N., Nozaki, Y., Komuro, I., Azuma, M., Ueda, M., Naito, M. and Takahasi, K. (1996). Generation of $CD1^+$ $RelB^+$ dendritic cells and tartrate-resistant acid phosphatase-positive osteoclast-like multinucleated giant cells from human monocytes. *Blood* **88**, 4029–4039.

Ardavin, C. and Shortman, K. (1993). Thymic dendritic cells and T cells develop simultaneously in the thymus from a common precursor population. *Nature* **362**, 761–763.

Ariizumi, K., Xu, S., Bergstresser, P.R. and Takashima, A. (1996). Identification of dendritic cell-specific C-type lectin-1 (Dectin-1) that is required for the activation of T cells. *4th International Symposium on Dendritic Cells in Fundamental and Clinical Immunology* (Abstract).

Arkema, J.M.S., Schadee-Eestermans, I.L., Beelen, R.H.J. and Hoefsmith, E.C.M. (1991). A combined method for both endogenous myeloperoxidase and acid phosphatase cytochemistry as well as immunoperoxidase surface labelling discriminating human peripheral blood-derived dendritic cells and monocytes. *Histochemistry* **95**, 573–578.

Austyn, J.A., Hankins, D.F., Larsen, C.P., Morris, P.J., Rao, A.S. and Roake, J.A. (1994). Isolation and characterization of dendritic cells from mouse heart and kidney. *J. Immunol.* **152**, 2401–2410.

Bieber, T., de la Salle, H., Wollenberg, A., Hakimi, J., Chizzonite, R., Ring, J., Hanau, D. and de la Salle, C. (1992). Human epidermal Langerhans cells express the high affinity receptor for immunoglobulin E (FcεRI). *J. Exp. Med.* **175**, 1285–1290.

Bilbe, G., Delabie, J., Bruggen, J., Richener, H., Asselbergs, F.A., Cerletti, N., Sorg, C., Odink, K., Tarcsay, L., Wiesendanger, W., de Wolf-Peeters, C. and Shipman, R. (1992). A novel intermediate filament-associated protein highly expressed in the Reed–Sternberg cells of Hodgkin's disease. *EMBO J.* **11**, 2103.

Blauvelt, A., Katz, S.I. and Udey, M.C. (1995). Human Langerhans cells express E-Cadherin. *J. Invest. Dermatol.* **104**, 293–296.

Borkowski, T.A., Van Dyke, B.J., Schwarzenberger, K., McFarland, V.W., Farr, A.G. and Udey, M.C. (1994). Expression of E-cadherin by murine dendritic cells: E-cadherin as a dendritic cell differentiation antigen characteristic of epidermal Langerhans cells and related cells. *Eur. J. Immunol.* **24**, 2767–2774.

Brenan, M. and Puklavec, M. (1992). The MRC OX-62 antigen: a useful marker in the purification of rat veiled cells with the biochemical properties of an integrin. *J. Exp. Med.* **175**, 1457–1465.

Buckley, P.J., Smith, M.R., Braverman, M.F. and Dickson, S.A. (1987). Human spleen contains phenotypic subsets of macrophages and dendritic cells that occupy discrete microanatomic locations. *Am. J Pathol.* **128**, 505–519.

Burkly, L., Hession, C., Ogata, L., Reilly, C., Marconi, L.A., Olson, D., Tizard, R., Cate, R. and Lo, D. (1995). Expression of relB is required for the development of thymic medulla and dendritic cells. *Nature* **373**, 531–536.

Carrasco, D., Ryseck, R. and Bravo, R. (1993). Expression of rel B transcripts during lymphoid organ development: specific expression in dendritic antigen-presenting cells. *Development* **118**, 1221–1231.

Cattoretti, G., Berti, E., Mancuso, A., D'Amato, L., Schiro, R., Soligo, D. and Delia, D. (1987). CD1, a MHC class I related family of antigens with widespread distribution on resting and activated cells. In: *Leucocyte Typing III* (ed. A.J.E. McMichael). Oxford University Press, Oxford, pp. 89–92.

Caux, C., Dezutter-Dambuyant, C., Schmitt, D. and Banchereau, J. (1992). GM-CSF and TNF cooperate in the generation of dendritic Langerhans cells. *Nature* **360**, 258–261.

Caux, C., Massacier, C., Vanbervliet, B., Dubois, B., Van Cooten, C., Durand, I. and Banchereau, J. (1994). Activation of human dendritic cells through CD40 cross-linking. *J. Exp. Med.* **180**, 1263–1272.

Cella, M., Dohring, C., Samaridis, J., Dessing, M., Brockhaus, M., Lanzavecchia, A. and Colonna, M. (1997). A novel inhibitory receptor (ILT3) expressed on monocytes, macrophages and dendritic cells involved in antigen processing. *J. Exp. Med. 185*, 1743–1751.

Celluzzi, C.M., Mayordomo, J.I., Storkus, W.J., Lotze, M.T. and Falo, L.D. (1996). Peptide-pulsed dendritic cells induce antigen-specific, CTL-mediated protective tumor immunity. *J. Exp. Med.* **183**, 283–287.

Cerio, R., Griffiths, C.E.M., Cooper, K.D., Nickoloff, B.J. and Headington, J.T. (1989). Characterization of factor XIIIa positive dermal dendritic cells in normal and inflamed skin. *Br. J Dermatol.* **121**, 421–431.

Davis, A.L., McKenzie, J.L. and Hart, D.N.J. (1988). HLA-DR positive leukocyte subpopulations in human skin include dendritic cells, macrophages and CD7-negative T cells. *Immunology* **65**, 573–581.

Dillon, S.M., Hart, D.N.J., Abernethy, N., Watson, J.D. and Baird, M.A. (1997). Priming to mycobacterial antigen in vivo using antigen pulsed antigen presenting cells generated in vitro is influenced by the dose and presence of IL-4 in APC cultures. *Scand. J. Immunol.* **46**, 1–9.

Drexhage, H.A., Mullink, H., de Groot, J., Clarke, J. and Balfour, B.M. (1979). A study of cells present in peripheral lymph of pigs with special reference to a type of cell resembling the Langerhans cell. *Cell Tissue Res.* **202**, 407–430.

Egeler, R.M., Neglia, J.P., Puccetti, D.M., Brennan, C.A. and Nesbit, M.E. (1993). Association of Langerhans cell histiocytosis with malignant neoplasms. *Cancer* **71**, 865–873.

Egner, W., Andreesen, R. and Hart, D.N.J. (1993a). Allostimulatory cells in fresh human blood: heterogeneity in antigen presenting cell populations. *Transplantation* **56**, 945–950.

Egner, W., McKenzie, J.L., Smith, S.M., Beard, M.E.J. and Hart, D.N.J. (1993b). Identification of potent mixed leucocyte reaction-stimulatory cells in human bone marrow. *J. Immunol.* **150**, 3043–3052.

Engering, A.J., Cella, M., Fluitsma, D., Brockhaus, M., Hoefsmit, E.C.M., Lanzavecchia, A. and Pieters, J. (1997). The mannose receptor functions as a high capacity and broad specificity antigen receptor in human dendritic cells. *Eur. J. Immunol.* **27**, 2417–2425.

Fairchild, P.J. and Austyn, J.M. (1990). Thymic dendritic cells: phenotype and function. *Int. Rev. Immunol.* **6**, 187–196.

Fanger, N.A., Wardwell, K., Shen, L., Tedder, T.F. and Guyre, P.M. (1996). Type I (CD64) and type II (CD32) Fc-gamma receptor-mediated phagocytosis by human blood dendritic cells. *J. Immunol.* **157**, 541–548.

Fanger, N.A., Voigtlaender, D., Liu, C., Swink, S., Wardwell, K., Fisher, J., Graziano, R.F., Pfefferkorn, L.C. and Guyre, P.M. (1997). Characterization of expression, cytokine regulation, and effector function of the high affinity IgG receptor FcγRI (CD64) expressed on human blood dendritic cells. *J. Immunol.* **158**, 3090–3098.

Fearnley, D.B., McLellan, A.D., Mannering, S.I., Hock, B.D. and Hart, D.N.J. (1997). Isolation of human blood dendritic cells using the CMRF-44 monoclonal antibody: implications for studies on antigen presenting cell function and immunotherapy. *Blood* **89**, 3708–3726.

Feuillard, J., Korner, M., Israel, A., Vassy, J. and Raphael, M. (1996). Differential nuclear localization of p50, p52 and RelB proteins in human accessory cells of the immune response *in situ. Eur. J Immunol.* **26**, 2547–2551.

Freudenthal, P.S. and Steinman, R.M. (1990). The distinct surface of human blood dendritic cells, as observed after an improved isolation method. *Proc. Natl Acad. Sci. USA* **87**, 7698–7702.

Fugier-Vivier, I., Servet-Delprat, C., Rivailler, P., Rissoan, M., Liu, Y. and Rabourdin-Combe, C. (1997). Measles virus suppresses cell-mediated immunity by interfering with the survival and functions of dendritic and T cells. *J. Exp. Med.* **186**, 813–823.

Gabrilovich, D.I., Nadaf, S., Corak, J., Berzofsky, J.A. and Carbone, D.P. (1996). Dendritic cells in antitumor immune responses. *Cell. Immunol.* **170**, 111–119.

Galy, A., Travis, M., Cen, D. and Chen, B. (1995). Human T, B, natural killer and dendritic cells arise from a common bone marrow progenitor cell subset. *Immunity* **3**, 459–473.

Godiska, R., Chantry, D., Raport, C.J., Sozzani, S., Allavena, P., Leviten, D., Mantovani, A. and Gray, P.W. (1997). Human macrophage-derived chemokine (MDC), a novel chemoattractant for monocytes, monocyte-derived dendritic cells and natural killer cells. *J. Exp. Med.* **185**, 1595–1604.

Granelli-Piperno, A., Pope, M., Inaba, K. and Steinman, R.M. (1995). Coexpression of NF-kB/Rel and Sp 1 transcription factors in human immunodeficiency virus 1-induced, dendritic cell–T-cell syncytia. *Proc. Natl Acad. Sci. USA* **92**, 10944–10948.

Grosjean, I., Caux, C., Bella, C., Berger, I., Wild, F., Banchereau, J. and Kaiserlian, D. (1997). Measles virus infects human dendritic cells and blocks their allostimulatory properties for $CD4^+$ T cells. *J. Exp. Med.* **186**, 801–812.

Grouard, G., Durand, I., Filgueira, L., Banchereau, J. and Liu, Y. (1996). Dendritic cells capable of stimulating T cells in germinal centres. *Nature* **384**, 364–367.

Hancock, W.W. and Atkins, R.C. (1984). Immunohistologic analysis of the cell surface antigens of human dendritic cells using monoclonal antibodies. *Transplant. Proc.* **16**, 963–967.

Hart, D.N.J. (1997). Dendritic cells: unique leucocyte populations which control the primary immune response. *Blood* **90**, 3245–3287.

Hart, D.N.J. and Calder, V.L. (1994). Human dendritic cells: function and cytokine production. Immunopharmacology of macrophages and other antigen-presenting cells. In: *Handbook of Immunopharmacology* (eds C.A.F.M. Bruijnzeel-Loomen and E.C.M. Hoefsmit), pp. 63–91.

Hart, D.N.J. and Fabre, J.W. (1981). Demonstration and characterization of Ia-positive dendritic cells in the interstitial connective tissues of rat heart and other tissues, not brain. *J. Exp. Med.* **153**, 347–361.

Hart, D.N.J. and Fearnley, D. (1997). Dendritic cell studies report. In: *Leucocyte Typing VI* (eds T. Kishimoto *et al.*) Garland Publishing, New York.

Hart, D.N.J. and McKenzie, J.L. (1988). Isolation and characterization of human tonsil dendritic cells. *J. Exp. Med.* **168**, 157–170.

Hart, D.N.J. and Prickett, T.C.R. (1993). Intercellular adhesion molecule-2 (ICAM-2) expression on human dendritic cells. *Cell. Immunol.* **148**, 447–454.

Hart, D.N.J., Fuggle, S.V. Williams, K.A., Fabre, J.W., Ting, A. and Morris, P.J. (1981). Localization of HLA-ABC and DR antigens in human kidney. *Transplantation* **31**, 428–433.

Hart, D.N.J., Starling, G.C., Calder, V.L. and Fernando, N.J. (1993). B7/BB-1 is a leucocyte differentiaion antigen on human dendritic cells induced by activation. *Immunology* **79**, 616–620.

Hock, B.D. and Hart, D.N.J. (1992). Cellular protein profiles of human dendritic cells; a comparative study. *Transplant. Proc.* **24**, 2323.

Hock, B.D., Starling, G.C., Daniel, P.B. and Hart, D.N.J. (1994). Characterisation of CMRF-44, a novel monoclonal antibody to an activation antigen expressed by the allostimulatory cells within peripheral blood, including dendritic cells. *Immunology* **83**, 573–581.

Inaba, K., Inaba, M., Romani, N., Hideki, A., Deguchi, M., Ikehara, S., Muramatsu, S. and Steinman, R.M. (1992). Generation of large numbers of dendritic cells from mouse bone marrow cultures supplemented with GM-CSF. *J. Exp. Med.* **176**, 1693–1702.

Inaba, K., Inaba, M., Deguchi, M., Hagi, K., Yasumizu, R., Ikehara, S., Muramatsu, S. and Steinman, R.M. (1993a). Granulocytes, macrophages and dendritic cells arise from a common MHC class II-negative progenitor in mouse bone marrow. *Proc. Natl Acad. Sci. USA* **90**, 3038–3042.

Inaba, K., Inaba, M., Naito, M. and Steinman, R.M. (1993b). Dendritic cell progenitors phagocytose particulates, including bacillus Calmette-Guerin organisms and sensitize mice to mycobacterial antigens in vivo. *J. Exp. Med.* **178**, 479–488.

Jackson, D.G., Hart, D.N.J., Starling, G.C. and Bell, J.I. (1992). Molecular cloning of a novel member of the immunoglobulin gene superfamily homologous to the polymeric immunoglobulin receptor. *Eur. J Immunol.* **22**, 1157–1163.

Jansen, J.H., Wientjens, G.H.M., Fibbe, W.E., Willemze, R. and Kluin-Nelemans, H.C. (1989). Inhibition of human macrophage colony formation by interleukin 4. *J. Exp. Med.* **170**, 577–582.

Jiang, W., Swiggard, W.J., Heufler, C., Peng, M., Mirza, A., Steinman, R.M. and Nussenzweig, M.C. (1995). The receptor DEC-205 expressed by dendritic cells and thymic epithelial cells is involved in antigen processing. *Nature* **375**, 151–154.

Jonuleit, H., Wiedemann, K., Muller, G., Degwert, J., Hoppe, U., Knop, J. and Enk, A.H. (1997). Induction of IL-15 messenger RNA and protein in human blood-derived dendritic cells. *J. Immunol.* **158**, 2610–2615.

Josien, R., Heslan, M., Soulillou, J. and Cuturi, M.C. (1997). Rat spleen dendritic cells express natural killer cell receptor protein 1 (NKR-P1) and have cytotoxic activity to select targets via a Ca^{2+} dependent mechanism. *J. Exp. Med.* **186**, 467–472.

Kato, M., Neil, T., Clark, G., Morris, C., Sorg, R. and Hart, D.N.J. (1997). The molecular cloning of human DEC-205, putative antigen-uptake receptor on DC. *Immunogenetics* **47**, 442–450.

Knight, S.C., Farrant, J., Bryant, A., Edwards, A.J., Burman, S., Lever, A., Clarke, J. and Webster, A.D.B. (1986). Non-adherent, low density cells from human peripheral blood contain dendritic cells and monocytes, both with veiled morphology. *Immunology* **57**, 595–603.

Koszik, F., Strunk, D., Simonitsch, I., Picker, L.J., Stingl, G. and Payer, E. (1994). Expressions of monoclonal antibody HECA-452-defined E-selectin ligands on Langerhans cells in normal and diseased skin. *J. Invest. Dermatol.* **102**, 773–780.

Kraal, G., Breel, M., Janse, M. and Bruin, G. (1986). Langerhans cells, veiled cells and interdigitating cells in the mouse recognised by a monoclonal antibody. *J. Exp. Med.* **163**, 981–997.

Lauener, R.P., Goyert, S.M., Geha, R.S. and Vercelli, D. (1990). Interleukin 4 down-regulates the expression of CD14 in normal human monocytes. *Eur. J Immunol.* **20**, 2375.

Lee, M.G., Borkowski, T.A. and Udey, M.C. (1993). Regulation of expression of B7 by murine Langerhans cells: a direct relationship between B7 mRNA levels and the level of surface expression of B7 by Langerhans cells. *J. Invest. Dermatol.* **101**, 883–886.

Maraskovsky, E., Brasel, K., Teepe, M., Roux, E.R., Lyman, S.D., Shortman, K. and McKenna, H.J. (1996). Dramatic increase in the numbers of functionally mature dendritic cells in Flt3 ligand-treated mice: multiple dendritic cell subpopulations identified. *J. Exp. Med.* **184**, 1953–1962.

Matzinger, P. and Guerder, S. (1989). Does T-cell tolerance require a dedicated antigen-presenting cell? *Nature* **338**, 74–76.

Maurer, D., Fiebiger, E., Ebner, C., Reininger, B., Fischer, G.F., Wichlas, S., Jouvin, M., Schmitt-Egenolf, M., Kraft, D., Kinet, J. and Stingl, G. (1996). Peripheral blood dendritic cells express FcεRI as a complex composed of FcεRIα- and FcεRI-gamma-chains and can use this receptor for IgE-mediated allergen presentation. *J. Immunol.* **157**, 607–616.

Mayordomo, J.I., Zorina, T., Storkus, W.J., Zitvogel, L., Celluzzi, C., Falo, L.D., Melief, C.J., Ildstad, S.T., Kast, W.M., DeLeo, A.B. and Lotze, M.T. (1995). Bone marrow-derived dendritic cells pulsed with synthetic tumour peptides elicit protective and therapeutic antitumour immunity. *Nature Medicine* **1**, 1297–1302.

Mayordomo, J.I., Loftus, D.J., Sakamoto, H., De Cesare, C.M., Appasamy, P.M., Lotze, M.T., Storkus, W.J., Appella, E. and De Leo, A.B. (1996). Therapy of murine tumors with p53 wild-type and mutant sequence peptide-based vaccines. *J. Exp. Med.* **183**, 1357–1365.

McKenzie, J.L., Calder, V.C., Starling, G.C. and Hart, D.N.J. (1995). Role of tumor necrosis factor α in dendritic cell mediated primary mixed leukocyte reactions. *Bone Marrow Transplant.* **15**, 163–171.

McLellan, A.D., Starling, G.C., Williams, L.A., Hock, B.D. and Hart, D.N.J. (1995). Activation of human peripheral blood dendritic cells induces the CD86 costimulatory molecule. *Eur. J Immunol.* **25**, 2064–2068.

McLellan, A.D., Sorg, R.V., Williams, L.A. and Hart, D.N.J. (1996). Human dendritic cells activate T lymphocytes via a CD40:CD40 ligand-dependent pathway. *Eur. J Immunol.* **26**, 1204–1210.

McLellan, A.D., Sorg, R.V., Heiser, A., Fearnley, D.B. and Hart, D.N.J. (1997). Dermal dendritic cells in the T cell areas of normal human skin display an activated $CD83^+$/$CMRF\text{-}44^+$ phenotype, in preparation.

McWilliam, A.S., Nelson, D.J. and Holt, P.G. (1995). The biology of airway dendritic cells. *Immunol. Cell Biol.* **73**, 405–413.

McWilliam, A.S., Napoli, S., Marsh, A.M., Pemper, F.L., Nelson, D.J., Pimm, C.L., Stumbles, P.A., Wells, T.M. and Holt, P.G. (1996). Dendritic cells are recruited into the airway epithelium during the inflammatory response to a broad spectrum of stimuli. *J. Exp. Med.* **184**, 2429–2431.

Metlay, J.P., Witmer-Pack, M.D., Agger, R., Crowley, M.T., Lawless, D. and Steinman, R.M. (1990). The distinct leucocyte integrins of mouse spleen DC as identified with new hamster mAb. *J. Exp. Med.* **171**, 1753–1771.

Morelli, A., Larregina, A., Chuluyan, E., Kolkowski, E. and Fainboim, L. (1996). Expression and modulation of C5a receptor (CD88) on skin dendritic cells. Chemotactic effect of C5a on skin migratory dendritic cells. *Immunology* **89**, 126–134.

Mosialos, G., Birkenbach, M., Ayehunie, S., Matsumura, F., Pinkus, G.S., Kieff, E. and Langhoff, E. (1996). Circulating human dendritic cells differentially express high levels of a 55-kd actin-bundling protein. *Am. J. Pathol.* **148**, 593–600.

Mueller, C.G.F., Rissoan, M., Salinas, B., Smina, A., Ravel, O., Bridon, J., Briere, F., Lebecque, S. and Liu, Y. (1997). Polymerase chain reaction selects a novel disintegrin proteinase from CD40-activated germinal center dendritic cells. *J. Exp. Med.* **186**, 655–663.

Norton, J., Sloane, J.P., Al-Saffar, N. and Haskard, D.O. (1992). Expression of adhesion molecules in human intestinal graft-versus-host disease. *Clin. Exp. Immunol.* **87**, 231–236.

Nussenzweig, M.C., Steinman, R.M., Witmer, M.D. and Gutchinov, B. (1982). A monoclonal antibody specific for mouse dendritic cells. *Proc. Natl Acad. Sci. USA* **79**, 161–165.

O'Doherty, U., Steinman, R.M., Peng, M., Cameron, P.U., Gezelter, S., Kopeloff, I., Swiggard, W.J., Pope, M. and Bardwaj, N. (1993). Dendritic cells freshly isolated from human blood express CD4 and mature into typical immunostimulatory dendritic cells after culture in monocyte-conditioned medium. *J. Exp. Med.* **178**, 1067.

Olweus, J., BitMansour, A., Warnke, R., Thompson, P.A., Carballido, J., Picker, L.J. and Lund-Johansen, F. (1997). Dendritic cell ontogeny: A human dendritic cell lineage of myeloid origin. *Proc. Natl Acad. Sci. USA* **94**, 12551–12556.

Pearson, A.M. (1996). Scavenger receptor in innate immunity. *Curr. Opin. Immunol.* **8**, 20–28.

Pickl, W.F., Majdic, O., Kohl, P., Stockl, J., Riedl, E., Scheinecker, C., Bello-Fernandez, C. and Knapp, W. (1996). Molecular and functional characteristics of dendritic cells generated from highly purified $CD14^+$ peripheral blood monocytes. *J. Immunol.* **157**, 3850–3859.

Poggi, A., Rubartelli, A., Moretta, L. and Zocchi, M.R. (1997). Expression and function of NKRP1A molecule on human monocytes and dendritic cells. *Eur. J. Immunol.* **27**, 2965–2970.

Power, C.A., Church, D.J., Meyer, A., Alouani, S., Proudfoot, A.E.I., Clark-Lewis, I., Sozzani, S., Mantovani, A. and Wells, T.N.C. (1997). Cloning and characterization of a specific receptor for the novel CC chemokine MIP-3a from lung dendritic cells. *J. Exp. Med.* **186**, 825–835.

Prickett, T.C.R. and Hart, D.N.J. (1990). Anti-leucocyte common (CD45) antibodies inhibit dendritic cell stimulation of CD4 and CD8 T lymphocyte proliferation. *Immunology* **69**, 250.

Prickett, T.C.R., McKenzie, J.L. and Hart, D.N.J. (1988). Characterization of human interstitial dendritic cells in liver. *Transplantation* **46**, 754.

Pricket, T.C.R., McKenzie, J.L. and Hart, D.N.J. (1992). Adhesion molecules on human tonsil dendritic cells. *Transplantation* **53**, 483.

Reiger, A., Wang, B., Kilgus, O., Ochiai, K., Maurer, D., Fodinger, D., Kinet, J. and Stingl, G. (1992). FcεRI mediates IgE binding to human epidermal Langerhans cells. *J. Invest. Dermatol.* **99**, 30s–32s.

Reis e Sousa, C., Stahl, P.D. and Austyn, J.M. (1993). Phagocytosis of antigens by Langerhans cells *in vitro*. *J. Exp. Med.* **178**, 509–519.

Res, P., Martinezcaceres, E., Jaleco, A.C., Staal, F., Noteboom, E., Weijer, K. and Spits, H. (1996). CD34(+) CD38 (dim) cells in the human thymus can differentiate into T, natural killer, and dendritic cells but are distinct from pluripotent stem cells. *Blood* **87**, 5196–5206.

Richters, C.D., Reits, E.A.J., Vanpelt, A.M., Hoekstra, M.J., Vanbaare, J., Dupont, J.S. and Kamperdijk, E.W.A. (1996). Effect of low dose UVB irradiation on the migratory properties and functional capacities of human skin dendritic cells. *Clin. Exp. Immunol.* **104**, 191–197.

Romani, N. and Schuler, G. (1992). The immunologic properties of epidermal Langerhans cells as a part of the dendritic cell system. *Springer Semin. Immunopathol.* **13**, 265–279.

Romani, N., Lenz, A., Glassel, H., Stossel, H., Stanzl, U., Majdic, O., Fritsch, P. and Schuler, G. (1989). Cultured human Langerhans cells resemble lymphoid dendritic cells in phenotype and function. *J. Invest. Dermatol.* **93**, 600–609.

Rosenzwajg, M., Canque, B. and Gluckman, J.C. (1996). Human dendritic cell differentiation pathway from CD34+ hematopoietic precursor cells. *Blood* **87**, 535–544.

Sallusto, F. and Lanzavecchia, A. (1994). Efficient presentation of soluble antigen by cultured human dendritic cells is maintained by granulocyte/macrophage colony-stimulating factor plus interleukin 4 and downregulated by tumour necrosis factor-α. *J. Exp. Med.* **179**, 1109.

Sallusto, F., Cella, M., Danieli, C. and Lanzavecchia, A. (1995). Dendritic cells use macropinocytosis and the mannose receptor to concentrate macromolecules in the major histocompatibility complex class II compartment: downregulation by cytokines and bacterial products. *J. Exp. Med.* **182**, 389–400.

Samaridis, J. and Colonna, M. (1997). Cloning of novel immunoglobulin superfamily receptors expressed on human myeloid and lymphoid cells: structural evidence for new stimulatory and inhibitory pathways. *Eur. J Immunol.* **27**, 660–665.

Scheicher, C., Mehlig, M., Zecher, R. and Reske, K. (1992). Dendritic cells from mouse bone marrow: in vitro differentiation using low doses of recombinant granulocyte-macrophage colony-stimulating factor. *J. Immunol. Methods* **154**, 253–264.

Shibaki, A., Meunier, L., Ra, C., Shimada, S., Ohkawara, A. and Cooper, K.D. (1995). Differential responsiveness of Langerhans cell subsets of varying phenotypic states in normal human epidermis. *J. Invest. Dermatol.* **104**, 42–46.

Sorg, U.R., Morse, T.M., Patton, W.N., Hock, B.D., Angus, H.B., Robinson, B.A., Colls, B.M. and Hart, D.N.J. (1997). Hodgkin's cells express CD83, a dendritic cell lineage associated marker. *Pathology* **29**, 294–299.

Sorg, R.V., McLellan, A.D., Hock, B.D., Fearnley, D.B. and Hart, D.N.J. (1997/8). Human dendritic cells express functional interleukin-7. *Immunobiology* **198**, 26–38.

Sozzani, S., Sallusto, F., Luini, W., Zhou, D., Piemonti, L., Allavena, P., Van Damme, J., Valitutti, S., Lanzavecchia, A. and Mantovani, A. (1995). Migration of dendritic cells in response to formyl peptides, C5a, and a distinct set of chemokines. *J. Immunol.* **155**, 3292–3295.

Sozzani, S., Luini, W., Borsatti, A., Polentarutti, N., Zhou, D., Piemonti, L., D'Amico, G., Power, C.A., Wells, T.N.C., Gobbi, M., Allavena, P. and Mantovani, A. (1997). Receptor expression and responsiveness of human dendritic cells to a defined set of CC and CXC chemokines. *J. Immunol.* **159**, 1993–2000.

Starling, G.C., Egner, W., McLellan, A.D., Fawcett, J., Simmons, D.L. and Hart, D.N.J. (1995). Intercellular adhesion molecule-3 is a costimulatory ligand for LFA-1 expressed on human blood dendritic cells. *Eur. J Immunol.* **25**, 2528–2532.

Steinman, R.M. and Cohn, Z.A. (1973). Identification of a novel cell type in peripheral lymphoid organs of mice. Morphology, quantitation; tissue distribution. *J. Exp. Med.* **137**, 1142.

Steptoe, R.J., Holt, P.G. and McMenamin, P.G. (1995). Functional studies of major histocompatibility class II-positive dendritic cells and resident tissue macrophages isolated from the rat iris. *Immunology* **85**, 630–637.

Strunk, D., Egger, C., Leitner, G., Hanau, D. and Stingl, G. (1997). A skin homing molecule defines the Langerhans cell progenitor in human peripheral blood. *J. Exp. Med.* **185**, 1131–1136.

Summers, K.L., Daniel, P.B., O'Donnell, J. and Hart, D.N.J. (1995). Dendritic cells in synovial fluid chronic inflammatory arthritis lack CD80 surface expression. *Clin. Exp. Immunol.* **100, 81–89.**

Summers, K., O'Donnell, J., Williams, L.A. and Hart, D.N.J. (1996). Expression and function of CD80 and CD86 costimulator molecules on synovial dendritic cells in chronic arthritic disease. *Arthritis Rheum.* **39**, 1287–1291.

Süss, G. and Shortman, K. (1996). A subclass of dendritic cells kills CD4 T cells via Fas/fas-ligand-induced apoptosis. *J. Exp. Med.* **183**, 1789–1796.

Symington, F.W., Brady, W. and Linsley, P.S. (1993). Expression and function of B7 on human epidermal Langerhans cells. *J. Immunol.* **150**, 1286–1295.

Szabolcs, P., Moore, M.A.S. and Young, J.W. (1995). Expansion of immunostimulatory dendritic cells among the myeloid progeny of human $CD34^+$ bone marrow precursors cultured with c-*kit* ligand, granulocyte-macrophage colony-stimulating factor, and TNF-α. *J. Immunol.* **154**, 5851–5861.

Takahashi, Y., Yamaguchi, H., Ishizeki, J., Nakajima, T. and Nakazota, Y. (1982). Immunohistochemical and immunoelectron microscopic localization of S-100 protein in the interdigitating reticulum cells of the human lymph node. *Virchows. Arch. B. Cell Pathol. Incl. Mol. Pathol.* **37**, 125–135.

Takamizawa, M., Rivas, A., Fagnoni, F., Benike, C., Kosek, J., Hyakawa, H. and Engelman, E.G. (1997). Dendritic cells that process and present nominal antigens to naive T lymphocytes are derived from $CD2^+$ precursors. *J. Immunol.* **158**, 2134–2142.

Tan, M.C.A.A., Mommaas, A.M., Drijfhout, J.W., Jordens, R., Onderwater, J.J.M., Verwoerd, D., Mulder, A.A., van der Heiden, A.N., Scheidegger, D., Oomen, L.C.J.M., Ottenhoff, T.H.M., Tulp, A., Neefjes, J.J. and Koning, F. (1997). Mannose receptor-mediated uptake of antigens strongly enhances HLA class II-restricted antigen presentation by cultured dendritic cells. *Eur. J. Immunol.* **27**, 2426–2435.

Thomas, R. and Lipsky, P.E. (1994). Human peripheral blood dendritic cell subsets: isolation and characterization of precursor and mature antigen presenting cells. *J. Immunol.* **153**, 4016.

Thomas, R., Davis, L.S. and Lipsky, P.E (1993). Isolation and characterization of human peripheral blood dendritic cells. *J. Immunol.* **150**, 821–834.

Troy, A., Davidson, P., Atkinson, C. and Hart, D. (1998a). Phenotypic characterization of the dendritic cell infiltrate in prostate cancer. *J. Urol.*, in press.

Troy, A.J., Summers, K.L., Davidson, P.J.T., Atkinson, C.A. and Hart, D.N.J. (1998b). Minimal recruitment and activation of dendritic cells within renal cell carcinoma. *Clin. Cancer Res.* **4**, 585–593.

Vedel, J., Vincendeau, P., Bezian, J.H. and Taieb, A. (1992). Flow cytometry analysis of adhesion molecules on human Langerhans cells. *Clin. Exp. Dermatol.* **17**, 240–245.

Vremec, D., Zorbas, M., Scollay, R., Saunders, D.J. and Ardavin, C.F. (1992). The surface phenotype of dendritic cells purified from mouse thymus and spleen: investigation of the CD8 expression by a subpopulation of dendritic cells. *J. Exp. Med.* **176**, 47–58.

Vuckovic, S., Fearnley, D.B., Whyte, L. and Hart, D.N.J. (1998). Generation of $CMRF\text{-}44^+$ monocyte derived dendritic cells. Insights into phenotype and function. *Exp. Haematol.*, in press.

Weber-Matthiesen, K. and Sterry, W. (1990). Organisation of the monocyte/macrophage system of normal human skin. *J. Invest. Dermatol.* **95**, 83–89.

Williams, L.A., McLellan, A.D., Summers, K.L., Sorg, R.V., Fearnley, D.B. and Hart, D.N.J. (1996). Identification of a novel dendritic cell surface antigen defined by carbohydrate specific CD24 antibody cross reactivity. *Immunology* **89**, 120–125.

Witmer, M.D. and Steinman, R.M. (1984). The anatomy of peripheral light-microscopic immunocytochemical studies of mouse spleen, lymph node and Peyers patch. *Am. J. Anat.* **170**, 465–481.

Wood, G.S., Freudenthal, P.S., Edinger, A., Steinman, R.M. and Warnke, R.A. (1991). CD45 epitope mapping of human $CD1^+$ dendritic cells and peripheral blood dendritic cells. *Am. J. Pathol.* **138**, 1451–1459.

Wu, L., Vremec, D., Ardavin, C., Winkel, K., Suss, G., Georgiou, H., Maraskovsky, E., Cook, W. and Shortman, K. (1995). Mouse thymus dendritic cells: kinetics of development and changes in surface markers during maturation. *Eur. J. Immunol.* **25**, 418–425.

Wuerzner, R., Xu, H., Franzke, A., Schulze, M., Peters, J.H. and Goetze, O. (1991). Blood dendritic cells carry terminal complement complexes on their cell surface as detected by newly developed neo-epitope-specific monoclonal antibodies. *Immunology* **74**, 132–138.

Xu, H., Friedrichs, U., Gieseler, R.K.H., Ruppert, J., Ocklind, G. and Peters, J.H. (1992). Human blood dendritic cells exhibit a distinct T-cell stimulating mechanism and differentiation pattern. *Scand. J. Immunol.* **36**, 689.

Xu, L.L., Warren, M.K., Rose, W.L., Gong, W. and Wang, J.M. (1996). Human recombinant monocyte chemotactic protein and other C-C chemokines bind and induce directional migration of dendritic cells in vitro. *J. Leukocyte Biol.* **60**, 365–371.

Yawalkar, N., Brand, C.U. and Braathen, L.R. (1996). IL-12 gene expression in human skin-derived CD1a(+) dendritic lymph cells. *Arch. Dermatol.* **288**, 79–84.

Young, J.W., Szabolcs, P. and Moore, M.A.S. (1995). Identification of dendritic cell colony-forming units among normal human $CD34^+$ bone marrow progenitors that are expanded by c-kit ligand and yield pure dendritic cell colonies in the presence of granulocyte/macrophage colony-stimulating factor and tumor necrosis factor-α. *J. Exp. Med.* **182**, 1120.

Zambruno, G., Cossarizza, A., Zacchi, V., Ottani, D., Luppi, A.M., Gianetti, A. and Girolomoni, G. (1995). Functional intercellular adhesion molecule-3 is expressed by frehsly isolated epidermal Langerhans cells and is not regulated during culture. *J. Invest. Dermatol.* **105**, 215–219.

Zhou, L.J. and Tedder, T.F. (1995). Human blood dendritic cells selectively express CD83, a member of the immunoglobulin superfamily. *J. Immunol.* **154**, 3821–3836.

Zhou, L. and Tedder, T.F. (1996a). $CD14^+$ blood monocytes can differentiate into functionally mature $CD83^+$ dendritic cells. *Proc. Natl Acad. Sci. USA* **93**, 2588–2592.

Zhou, L.J. and Tedder, T.F. (1996b). A distinct pattern of cytokine gene expression by human $CD83^+$ blood dendritic cells. *Blood* **86**, 3295–3301.

Zhou, L., Schwarting, R., Smith, H.M. and Tedder, T.F. (1992). A novel cell-surface molecule expressed by human interdigitating reticulum cells, Langerhans cells, and activated lymphocytes is a new member of the Ig superfamily. *J. Immunol.* **149**, 735–742.

Zitvogel, L., Mayordomo, J.I., Tjandrawan, T. and DeLeo, A.B. (1996). Therapy of murine tumors with tumor peptide-pulsed dendritic cells: dependence on T cells, B7 costimulation and T helper cell 1-associated cytokines. *J. Exp. Med.* **183**, 87–97.

CHAPTER 30
Targeted Gene Knockouts: Insights into Dendritic Cell Biology

Mary T. Crowley and David Lo
Department of Immunology, The Scripps Research Institute, La Jolla, California, USA

> "Hush, Dorothy," whispered the Tiger, "you'll ruin my reputation if you are not more discreet. It isn't what we are, but what folks think we are, that counts in this world."
>
> L. Frank Baum, *The Road to Oz*

INTRODUCTION

Dendritic cells (DC) are potent stimulators of naive T cells. This unique function of DC is a result of (1) their expression of important costimulatory molecules, (2) their residence in both lymphoid and nonlymphoid tissue, (3) their ability to migrate from sites of antigen entry to lymphoid organs, and (4) their efficient antigen processing and presentation of a wide variety of antigens. Recently, information gained from studies using knockout mice suggests that DC may have important activities distinct from but still related to their function as potent antigen-presenting cells. For example, DC may have a role in the development of secondary lymphoid organs and organization of splenic architecture (Koni *et al.*, 1997; Wang *et al.*, 1996). Still other studies have suggested that DC can organize lymphoid infiltrates within nonlymphoid tissue (Burkly *et al.*, 1995; Drijkoningen *et al.*, 1987; Krenn *et al.*, 1996; Mooij *et al.*, 1993).

Studies of DC have been hampered by the fact that DC are sparsely distributed in tissues and hence are difficult to isolate. Moreover, DC express distinct yet overlapping subsets of surface markers (Maraskovsky *et al.*, 1996; Steinman *et al.*, 1997; Vremec and Shortman, 1997; Wu *et al.*, 1996) and have different biological roles (Ardavin, 1997; Josien *et al.*, 1997), further complicating efforts to assign a discrete role to DC in immunobiology. Recently, however, it has been shown that large quantities of homogeneous populations of DC can be generated from precursors in both mice and humans (Inaba *et al.*, 1992). This has greatly facilitated studies characterizing DC phenotypes, gene expression, and physiology. Despite advances made in these *in vitro* studies, only limited knowledge exists about the factors and mechanisms which regulate ontogeny, cell cycle, homing, tissue distribution, functional activity and life

Dendritic Cells: Biology and Clinical Applications
ISBN 0-12-455860-7

span of DC. These aspects of DC biology are likely a result of DC-specific gene expression combined with the ability of DC and DC precursors to receive and respond to cues from the surrounding microenvironment.

KNOCKOUTS THAT AFFECT HEMATOPOIETIC LINEAGES INCLUDING DC

Targeted gene knockout mice have proven useful in examining the role of various transcription factors and growth factors in the control of hematopoiesis. TGF-β knockout mice possess a specific defect in epidermal Langerhans cell (LC); LC were not detected in epidermal cell suspensions or epidermal sheets prepared from TGF-β^{-} mice, although CD11c^{+} cells were detected in lymphoid organs (Borkowski *et al.*, 1996). These mice also exhibit widespread T cell autoreactivity and autoantibody production (Furukawa, 1997; Letterio *et al.*, 1997; Nakabayashi *et al.*, 1997). Mice lacking either lymphotoxin-α or lymphotoxin-β do not develop peripheral lymphoid tissue and have disorganized splenic architecture without defined B and T areas or follicular dendritic cells (Fu *et al.*, 1997; Koni *et al.*, 1997). RelB, a member of the NF-κB/Rel family, is highly expressed in DC and inducibly expressed in B cells and fibroblasts. RelB-knockout mice do not develop peripheral lymphoid tissue; they lack distinct thymic stromal components (Burkly *et al.*, 1995; Weih *et al.*, 1995) and exhibit poor cellular immunity, reduced splenic and thymic DC populations, multi-organ inflammation and splenomegaly as a result of inflammatory cell infiltrate (DeKoning *et al.*, 1997; Weih *et al.*, 1997). The transcription factor Ikaros is important for development of lymphoid compartments but not myeloid or erythroid development. Ikaros knockout mice lack B lymphocytes and fetal thymocytes; they exhibit reduced thymic DC populations and fail to develop peripheral lymphoid tissue (Wang *et al.*, 1996). The transcription factor PU.1 is a key element in the development of multipotent progenitors since cells deficient in this factor demonstrate a cell-autonomous block in lymphoid and myeloid but not erythroid development (Scott *et al.*, 1997).

To date, analyses of key knockout mice have provided important information on the impact of a variety of genes on multiple hematopoietic lineages. While DC are among the cells affected, detailed analysis is lacking in most cases. Perhaps the best-studied knockout mice with respect to DC development and function remain RelB-knockout mice. Therefore, the majority of results and discussion here will be concerned with these findings by ourselves and others. Interpretation of DC-deficiencies observed in other knockout mice and predictions about what other DC-related defects may be found in knockout and transgenic mice will draw largely from findings in RelB-deficient mice.

RelB-KNOCKOUT MICE

A Role for RelB In Dendritic Cells?

The early finding that RelB was highly expressed in DC (Carrasco *et al.*, 1993) prompted the suggestion that this factor had a role in some aspect of DC biology. Subsequent studies of RelB-knockout mice and cells have yielded a wealth of information about the importance of this factor in endotoxin responses of bone marrow stromal cells (Xia *et al.*, 1997), development and function of distinct thymic compartments

(Naspetti *et al.*, 1997), and the impact of a systemic inflammatory response on splenic DC. Additionally, characterization of DC populations found in mutant mice raises interesting issues regarding the influence of other cell types on DC fate.

DC Abnormalities in Tissues of RelB Knockouts

At least as early as 4 days of age, the lymphoid organs of RelB-deficient mice exhibit some differences from normal mice. Specifically, $CD11c^+$ DC in spleen are not evenly distributed as in normal spleens at this time (Fig. 1d–f) but instead are localized in T cell-rich foci (Fig. 1a–c). $CD11c^+$ thymic DC are greatly reduced in number. While the organization remains somewhat focal in nature, the DC appear to be more loosely 'packed' than the distribution found in normal thymuses at this age (Fig. 2a,b). There is an absence of UEA-1^+ medullary epithelial cells in RelB-knockout thymic medulla (Fig. 2c) (Burkly *et al.*, 1995). Another subset of medullary epithelial cells expressing the marker bound by the 95 antibody is present but fails to organize appropriately into discrete areas that would represent the thymic medulla; the cells remain scattered throughout the thymus (Naspetti *et al.*, 1997).

As the mice age, the phenotype of the RelB-mutant mice becomes more severe. At 2 weeks of age, RelB-knockout mice have disorganized splenic architecture characterized by a reduction in white pulp and an increase in red pulp due to the infiltration of granulocytic cells (Burkly *et al.*, 1995; Weih *et al.*, 1995). Despite the enlarged size, spleens from RelB-knockout animals contain only 15–20% the expected total number of dendritic cells. By FACS analysis these correspond to the subset of large, DEC-205^+, $CD11c^+$ DC normally found in the T areas of organized white pulp (Fig. 3, right). The DC deficiency is due to the complete absence of the major subset of DC: those bearing the antigen recognized by the 33D1 monoclonal antibody (Fig. 3, left).

In normal mice under nonpathological conditions, the majority of splenic DC are present in the red pulp and marginal zone and are phenotypically distinct from those that reside in the white pulp (Fig. 4b) (Steinman *et al.*, 1997). Immunohistochemical examination reveals that this distribution is absent from spleens of RelB-knockout mice; the DC are tightly packed into the small areas of organized white pulp (Fig. 4d). The RelB mutation in these mice results in the obliteration of the marginal zone normally delineated by $SER4^+$ metallophilic macrophages (Fig. 4a,c). Interestingly, the $SER4^+$ macrophages have an apparently normal distribution in the liver of RelB-knockout mice. However, it is unlikely that the mere absence of splenic $SER4^+$ cells is responsible for the disorganization of the spleen, since M-CSF-deficient mice, which do not develop this subset of macrophages, have normal DC populations in the spleen (Witmer-Pack *et al.*, 1993). Interactions between several cell types may instead be required for the organization of lymphoid tissues. For example, RelB-knockout mice have little or no thymic medulla and this is associated with an absence of UEA-1^+ medullary cells and greatly decreased numbers of thymic DC (Fig. 2c) (DeKoning *et al.*, 1997; Weih *et al.*, 1997).

Another dramatic defect in $RelB^-$ mice is the complete lack of peripheral lymph nodes and Peyer's patches. Rudimentary mesenteric nodes may occur in $RelB^-$ mice although they are largely depleted of lymphocytes and instead contain large numbers of macrophages and neutrophils (Weih *et al.*, 1997). In contrast to the situation in

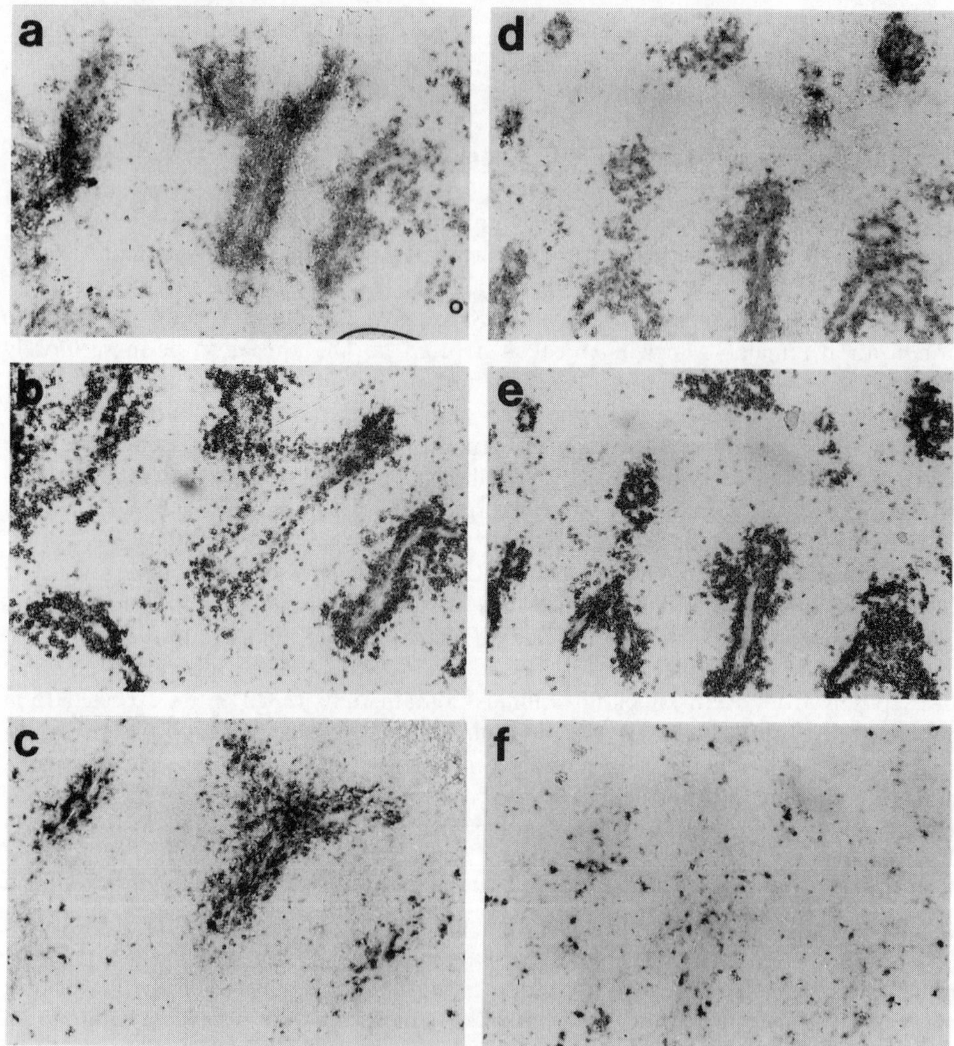

Fig. 1. Histology of 4-day-old RelB-mutant spleens showing abnormal distribution of CD11c$^+$ dendritic cells. RelB-mutant mice exhibit co-localization of T cells ((a) anti-TCR) and B cells ((b) anti-B220) in the neonatal spleen which is indistinguishable from T and B staining in normal mice ((d) and (e), respectively). In mutant spleens, the DC recognized by anti-CD11c monoclonal N418 (Metlay *et al.*, 1990) also remain co-localized with B and T cells (c). In normal spleens, CD11c$^+$ cells are found dispersed throughout the spleen (f). This unusual distribution may be due to retention of RelB$^-$ DC following entry into the spleen or an inability to migrate as normal cells.

lymphoid organs, the tissue distribution and phenotype of epidermal Langerhans cells does not appear to be compromised in RelB-knockout mice. LC appear to migrate normally from the epidermis of skin explant cultures (unpublished results). It is not known whether RelB-knockout LC will migrate normally from epidermal layers to the draining lymphatics in response to more physiological cues such as contact allergens, dermal TNF-α, tissue damage, or infection.

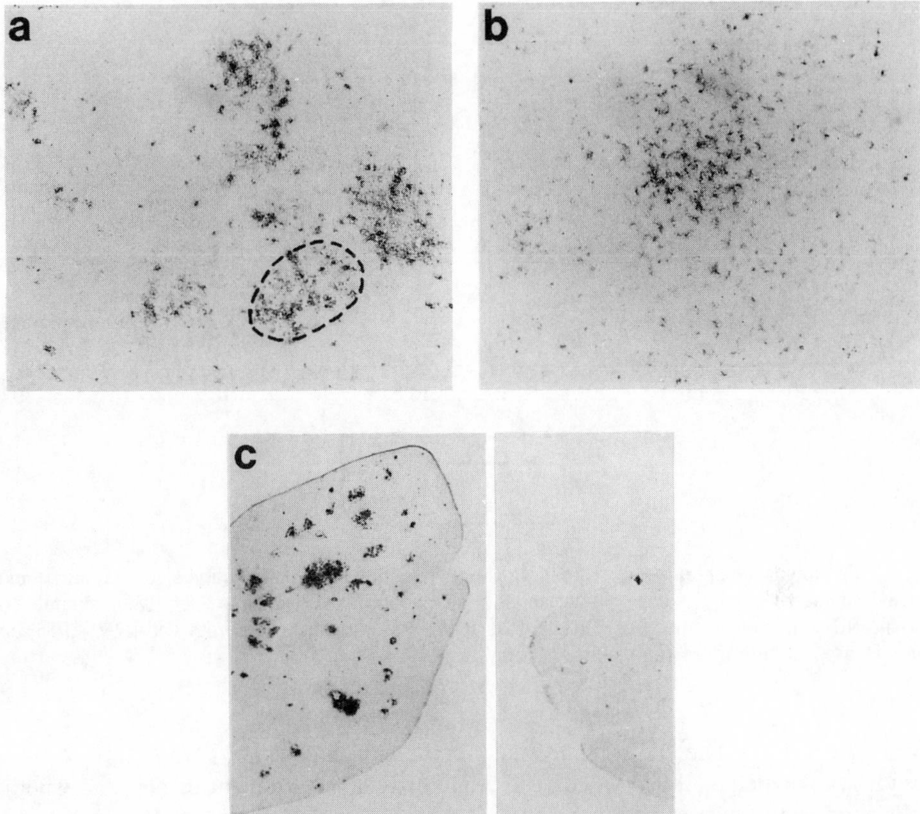

Fig. 2. Abnormal distribution of CD11c⁺ DC in 4-day-old RelB-mutant thymus. The CD11c⁺ staining pattern in the normal thymus (a) shows numerous concentrated pockets of DC with relatively few cells having migrated outside of these pockets (pocket 'border' indicated by broken line). It is not known whether these pockets represent CFU or aggregates of mature cells. In contrast, CD11c⁺ DC in the RelB-mutant thymus (b) do not remain concentrated in similar foci. RelB⁻ DC either were not effectively retained in discrete areas or perhaps were less capable of forming CFU. UEA-1⁺ medullary epithelial cells are present in 4-day-old normal thymus ((c), right side) but UEA-1 is not bound by cells in the RelB-deficient thymus ((c), left side).

Other Abnormalities Possibly Related to the RelB Knockout DC Deficiency

Positive selection and export of mature T cells appears normal despite the absence of a thymic medulla and paucity of thymic DC in RelB-knockout mice. However, the majority of peripheral T cells in mutant animals display the activation marker CD69 as well as high levels of CD44 (DeKoning *et al.*, 1997). This observation suggests that the systemic inflammation present in these animals may cause widespread T cell activation. T cell effector mechanisms, such as CTL activity and cytokine production, may in turn contribute to the sustained inflammatory response in the animals. In support of this view, Weih and colleagues demonstrated that RelB-deficient mice that also lack mature T cells (RAG⁻ × RelB⁻) fail to develop an inflammatory phenotype

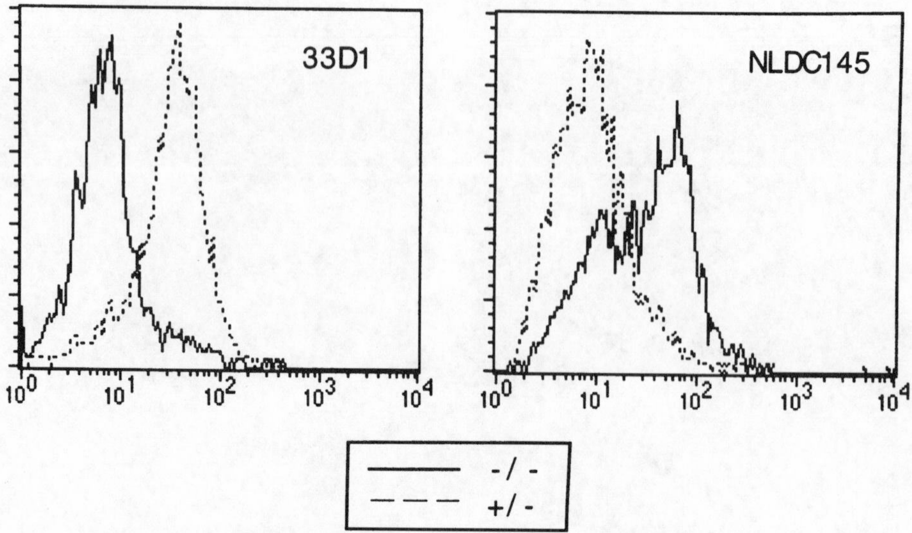

Fig. 3. Phenotype of splenic dendritic cells from RelB-deficient (solid curves) or normal (broken curves) animals. Dendritic cells were isolated as described (Crowley *et al.*, 1989), stained with the anti-DC monoclonal antibodies 33D1 and NLDC145 and counterstained with anti-B7-2 (CD86) antibody. Fluorescence profiles represent B7-2-bright cells.

(Weih *et al.*, 1996). The DC compartments in these mice have not been examined, so we do not know whether the absence of T cells impacts development of DC and whether RelB expression has any additional influence on DC development in the absence of T lymphocytes. Another explanation for the activated T cells is that they are autoreactive cells released inappropriately to the periphery as mature T cells. In this respect, the studies demonstrating that positive selection in the RelB mutants is normal also indicate that negative selection may be impaired (DeKoning *et al.*, 1997).

The defects described above might be due to the requirement for RelB in mature or progenitor DC or both. This would reflect a cell-autonomous role for RelB in DC biology. It is unlikely that RelB is required to permit early stages of DC development, since *in vitro* culture of bone marrow from RelB-knockout animals or normal animals gives rise to comparable numbers of DC that are phenotypically similar and functionally equivalent. RelB-knockout and normal bone marrow-derived DC exhibit similar allogeneic and antigen-specific T cell stimulation. An alternative explanation for deficiencies is that RelB-dependent events in other cell types may influence the developmental and differentiative events of DC. Finally, a combination of cell-autonomous and extrinsic RelB-dependent events may guide the development and fate of DC. One approach useful in distinguishing between these possibilities is the generation of chimeric animals.

In Vivo and *In Vitro* Studies on Bone Marrow Chimeras

Bone marrow from $RelB^-$ or $RelB^+$ animals can be transferred into lethally irradiated animals, giving rise to mice with a RelB deficiency limited to cells of hematopoietic

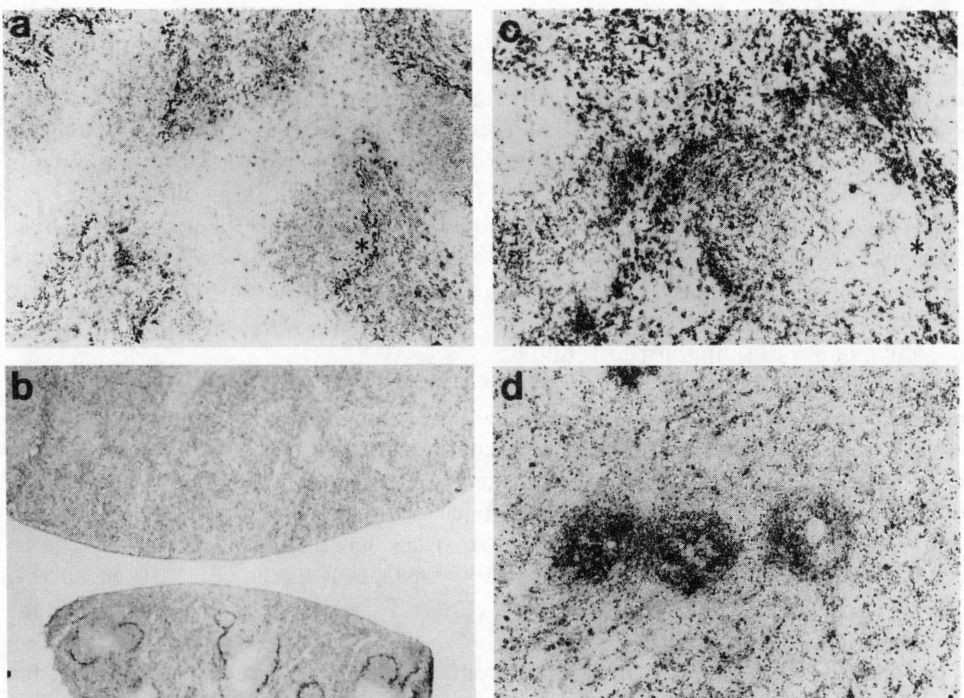

Fig. 4. CD11c$^+$ DCs and SER4$^+$ macrophages in RelB-deficient and normal spleens. In the normal spleen, SER4 stains macrophages that lie in the marginal zone around white pulp nodules (a). RelB-deficient animals lack this characteristic pattern ((b), RelB$^-$ at top, normal on bottom). In the resting state, splenic CD11c$^+$ cells occupy macrophage-free regions at the margins of white and red pulp and extend somewhat into the T area (c). Asterisks mark a single position on sequential sections. CD11c$^+$ cells are missing from the marginal areas in mutant spleens. Densely stained DC are found only around the central arteriole of the small areas of organized white pulp (d).

origin. RelB$^-$ $\rightarrow$ B6 chimeric animals do not develop the inflammatory phenotype found in the RelB knockouts. This is not unexpected in light of the recent discovery that deregulated chemokine expression by non-bone marrow-derived stromal cells mediates the systemic inflammatory response in mutant animals (Xia *et al.*, 1997). In contrast to mutant mice, all the subsets of DC can be isolated in equivalent numbers from spleen, thymus and peripheral lymph nodes of animals reconstituted with either RelB-knockout or control bone marrow. Upon histological examination of CD11c$^+$ cells, the distribution of dendritic cells, in the thymus and lymph nodes of these mice is indistinguishable from that in control chimeras. Thus, in the absence of a systemic inflammatory response, RelB$^-$ DC possess the capacity to populate tissues in a seemingly unimpaired fashion when a normal radioresistant infrastructure already exists within the tissue.

Curiously, even in the absence of an overt systemic inflammatory syndrome, studies reveal that T-lymphocytes from chimeric animals still contained a slightly higher percentage of cells bearing an activated phenotype CD69$^+$, CD44$^+$ (DeKoning *et al.*, 1997). Moreover, *in vitro* proliferative responses of T cells from RelB$^-$ $\rightarrow$ B6 bone marrow chimeras to syngeneic stimulators remained very high relative to T cells from control chimeras or relative to the response to allogeneic stimulators. The authors suggest that this high syngeneic response corresponded to 'self-recognition' by autoreactive T cells which escaped thymic negative selection. If negative selection is impaired in those chimeric mice, then the thymic DC compartment may be fingered as the likely culprit and it is possible that some aspect of APC function is impaired in RelB-knockout DC. It is important to test this possibility, although there are not very many *in vitro* assays that test the unique activities that DC may exhibit *in vivo*. Allogeneic and syngeneic stimulatory activities as well as presentation of specific peptides and whole protein by $RelB^-$ DC to transgenic TCR-bearing T cells do not appear to be different when measured *in vitro* via thymidine incorporation by responding T-lymphocytes (unpublished results).

Analysis of these chimeric mice does not establish whether the inflammatory infiltrate is due solely to the inducible chemokine production of the fibroblasts. Weih and colleagues bred RelB-knockout mice to recombinase-activating gene-1-deficient transgenic mice ($RAG\text{-}1^-$) in order to evaluate the roles of mature lymphocytes in the inflammatory syndrome. The $RelB^-$/RAG mice lack both B and T cells and are disease free. Thus, the inflammatory syndrome due to the deregulated fibroblast chemokine production seems to require T cells for the propagation of inflammatory signals. If thymic negative selection is impaired, autoreactive T cells may in fact be the trigger for fibroblast activation.

Unrelated studies directed at understanding thymic development suggest that the expansion of medullary epithelial cells correlates with the presence of thymocytes (Naspetti *et al.*, 1997). Therefore, the stromal components of thymus and other lymphoid organs may not progress normally in RAG × RelB or other lymphocyte-deficient mice. Consequently, if DC organization in thymus, spleen, and lymph nodes requires appropriate stromal architecture, DC distribution would be affected in these and other T-deficient mice. Analysis of the DC populations in these and other lymphocyte-deficient mice will provide useful information about the direct and indirect contributions of lymphocytes to DC development and presence in tissues.

It is clear that the lack of splenic and thymic DC is due in large part to the effects of a systemic inflammatory response in the animal. This is in agreement with observations made over 10 years ago on the effects of endotoxin on non-lymphoid splenic populations (Groeneveld *et al.*, 1986). Of note, a single 30 μg dose of LPS is sufficient to disrupt the marginal zone and cause the vast majority of DC to leave the spleen. Remaining $CD11c^+$ DC are found tightly clustered around the central arterioles in the T areas (Fig. 5). This is strikingly similar to the situation observed in RelB-knockout mice. We have noted, however, that a single LPS treatment does not result in the complete loss of $SER4^+$ macrophages from marginal zone as observed in RelB-knockout mice. Since persistent exposure to LPS reveals a splenic architecture more similar to that of the RelB knockout, it is possible that the dramatic phenotype found in RelB-knockout mice arises only during sustained inflammatory signals.

Implications

While the effects of the inflammatory syndrome clearly contribute to the deficiency in DC in lymphoid tissues of RelB mice, we cannot rule out other contributing factors. For example, since RelB is expressed in DC, it may be important for some aspect of DC

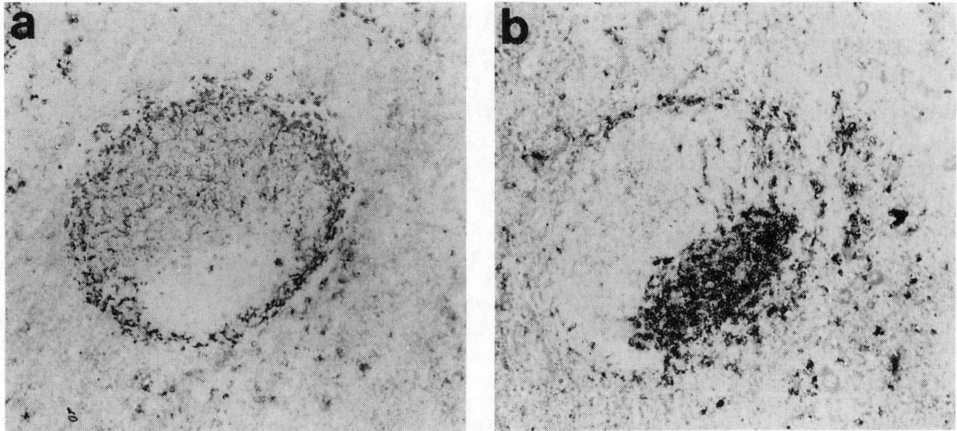

Fig. 5. LPS exposure results in redistribution and loss of splenic CD11c$^+$ DC. As early as 2 h after LPS exposure, CD11c$^+$ cells at the red pulp/white pulp border are reduced in number (not shown). By 24 h (pictured), N418 staining is found almost exclusively within the marginal zone in a compact core around the central arteriole. Compare to Fig. 4c. At that time, the yield of splenic DC from LPS-treated animals is 20–30% that of normal animals.

development and APC activity that has not yet been characterized. Additionally, non-bone marrow-derived cells may be important in orchestrating DC homing to tissues and organization within those tissues. As described above, stromal components are potentially very important in compartmentalizing the different areas of the spleen, thymus, and other lymphoid organs. The nature of this process has not been explained but it may be based upon migration via specific receptor–ligand interactions between two or more cell types. There is already evidence that stromal components important for thymic organization are RelB dependent (Naspetti *et al.*, 1997). The hypothesis that DC are dependent upon the appropriate organization of medullary epithelial cells is supported by the discovery of a normal distribution of CD11c$^+$ dendritic cells in the thymus of bone marrow chimeras. Some of the possible defects in cell–cell signaling and migration may involve poor chemokine production or recognition by stromal and dendritic cells. Recently a number of dendritic cell-derived chemokines have been described (Adema *et al.*, 1997; Greaves *et al.*, 1997; Mohamadzadeh *et al.*, 1996; Vicari *et al.*, 1997). It will be important to determine whether expression of key chemokines and their respective receptors are RelB dependent in DC or other cell types where expression occurs. In addition to further analysis of chimeric animals, examination of the architecture and cell populations present in developing organs in normal and RelB-mutant mice will increase our understanding of this issue.

OTHER KNOCKOUT MICE

A number of interesting questions about DC biology may be addressed by a more thorough examination of DC compartments in some of the other knockout mice that exhibit DC deficiencies. The findings from RelB-knockout mice may serve to focus questions and predictions about the cause of the various phenotypes observed in other knockout mice.

Ikaros-knockout mice do not exhibit a systemic inflammatory syndrome although they do have reduced numbers of thymic DC and several abnormalities in the T- and B-lymphocyte compartments. There is a dramatic defect in the development of cortical and medullary structures in the Ikaros$^-$ thymus. Structures do not appear until 1 week after birth, whereas normal newborns have elaborate epithelial networks and an actively differentiating thymus. There are no reports describing DC found in other tissues of these mice. Moreover, it has not been shown whether the decrease in thymic DC is due to the loss of a specific population (i.e., $CD8^+$ or $CD8^-$). Bearing in mind that several reports present evidence of a common precursor for T-lymphocytes and thymic DC (Ardavin, 1997; Galy *et al.*, 1995; Marquez *et al.*, 1995; Wu *et al.*, 1995), it is inviting to suggest that Ikaros has an intrinsic role in thymic DC biology. By extension, the thymic DC themselves may be important in the timely development of the cortical and medullary structures in the thymus. Thus, the Ikaros knockout may be a useful system for examining the development and role of these special DC. Some of the basic issues that need to be addressed include the following. Do Ikaros$^-$ bone marrow chimeras develop normal numbers of thymic DC as in RelB chimeras? Does the presence of mature thymic DC induce the normal development of medullary and stromal components in fetal thymic organ cultures from Ikaros$^-$ mice? Are there lymphoid-lineage DC in other tissues that may be affected as well? What are the roles of the lymphoid-lineage DC that distinguish it from other DC?

Another knockout mouse that may prove useful is the PU.1-deficient mouse (McKercher *et al.*, 1996; Tondravi *et al.*, 1997). PU.1 regulates genes important in early stages in both lymphoid and myeloid development. These animals have a severe phenotype consisting of abnormalities in multiple hematopoietic lineages and often suffer lethal infections shortly after birth. However, T-lymphocytes and neutrophils can develop if the animals are sustained with antibiotics. B-lymphocytes and macrophage lineages remained undetectable in these animals. Unfortunately, nothing is known about dendritic cell lineages in these animals. The selective impairment of some hematopoietic lineages in these mice could be useful for identifying dendritic cells and their progenitors which arise from different lineages.

The dendritic cell compartments have not been examined in mice lacking either lymphotoxin-α (LTα) or lymphotoxin-β (LTβ) (Fu *et al.*, 1997; Koni *et al.*, 1997). However, some defects observed in these mice are strikingly similar to those in RelB- and Ikaros-knockout mice, so the possibility exists that there are underlying defects in dendritic cells as well. These mice have a disorganized splenic architecture with leukocyte invasion into the red pulp areas and poorly defined B and T areas seemingly without follicular dendritic cells. As in RelB-knockout mice, LTβ-deficient mice lack splenic metallophilic macrophages and peripheral lymph nodes. One underlying cause for these similarities may involve the nonlymphoid architecture of the lymphoid organs. That is, without an effective epithelial architecture, the presence, interaction, and appropriate localization of DC, macrophages, and perhaps non-bone marrow-derived cells within the tissue may be disrupted. In such a case, lymphocytes may be unable to traffic and reside normally in these organs. For example, epidermal Langerhans cells bind LTα via TNF receptors (Borkowski *et al.*, 1996; Borkowski *et al.*, 1997; de Graaf *et al.*, 1996; Larregina *et al.*, 1996) and this interaction may be important for activities involved in migration to and localization within the draining nodes.

TGF-β-deficient mice are so far the most definitive example of a dendritic cell knockout in that there is a clear deficiency in one specific lineage of dendritic cells—the epidermal Langerhans cell. This deficiency is apparently due to a specific requirement of LC for TGF-β. TGF-β knockouts have massive system-wide inflammation due to SLE-like autoantibodies and Sjögren syndrome-like lymphoproliferation (Furukawa, 1997). However, the lack of LC is not a consequence of inflammation in the skin or other organs (Yaswen *et al.*, 1997); treatments that alleviate the inflammatory syndrome do not result in repopulation of the skin with LC. Studies with chimeric mice show that bone marrow-derived TGF-deficient LC can repopulate normal skin or even TGF-β-null skin engrafted onto nude recipients (Borkowski *et al.*, 1997). Thus TGF-β is not necessary for development of precursors, but it is necessary to permit migration of these cells in normal tissue. These results emphasize the importance of the tissue environment for the development of dendritic cells.

SUMMARY

The RelB-, Ikaros-, and lymphotoxin-knockout mice share certain phenotypic abnormalities such as a disorganized splenic architecture and a lack of peripheral lymph nodes. There are many factors important in the development and functioning of lymphoid organs. The disruption of one or more components by mutation or disease can be sufficient to derail the process. Whether DC deficiencies are a cause or effect of these and other abnormalities is not clear in each situation. Generation of chimeric mice is a useful technique to answer the question of whether the knockout directly affects the bone marrow-derived cells. Adoptive transfer of specific populations can further address the roles that individual cell types play in the phenotype of the knockout animal and in a normal biological response. For example, we now know that the gross DC deficiency observed in RelB-knockout mice is not just a direct consequence of gene loss in DC. Rather, it is a response to the inflammatory syndrome experienced by these animals. The abnormalities in early thymic and splenic DC resident in RelB-knockout organs are likely due to a failure of non-bone marrow-derived cells to create an appropriate environment where DC and other bone marrow-derived cells may function. Specifically, stromal, vascular, or epithelial elements may produce and release chemokines that attract DC. These elements may also express cell surface molecules which similarly guide receptor-bearing DC to the right location in tissues. These functions of stromal elements may be RelB dependent. Already evidence exists that one chemokine for mesangial cells and lymphocytes, TCA4, is poorly produced in RelB-knockout animals (Tanabe *et al.*, 1997). Unfortunately, the tissue microenvironment is often not considered in studies aimed at understanding DC biology.

Ideally, gene knockouts that adversely affect DC development and function should have some relevance to clinical disease states. One example has been discussed above. A chronic LPS-mediated inflammatory response will have devastating effects on the immune system (de Graaf *et al.*, 1996; De Smedt *et al.*, 1996; Herbst *et al.*, 1996; Roake *et al.*, 1995). Our own observations in RelB-knockout mice describe specific effects on the DC populations under such conditions. How the loss of splenic DC benefits the animal in this situation is not clear. It may be an attempt to downregulate the immune response during the systemic inflammatory response. Immunosuppression from chronic bacterial infection is a dangerous condition that occurs in tuberculosis and leprosy patients (Ellner, 1996; Maes *et al.*, 1996) as well as patients recovering from endotoxic shock (Junger *et al.*, 1996). The nature of the immunosuppression has not been characterized but it is plausible that the immunosuppression is a result of induced DC loss (Muraille *et al.*, 1997). One might envision immunotherapies that would replenish DC or block the factors that induce the loss in the first place. Of course there remain many questions regarding this particular phenomenon. Are the DC responding directly to LPS? Do DC respond to LPS-induced products of other cells? If the latter, what products? Assuming the DC do not die, where do they go after they leave the spleen? Have they acquired a new functional capacity?

Other transgenic and knockout mice which have symptoms similar to those observed in some human pathologies have been described. These include the BTK-deficient mouse model of XID and XLA (Tsukada *et al.*, 1993; Zhu *et al.*, 1994), the MRL-lpr/lpr mouse model of SLE and rheumatoid arthritis (Bond *et al.*, 1990; Koopman and Gay, 1988; Roark *et al.*, 1995), and other mouse models of atherosclerosis (Plump, 1997), mucosal inflammation (Strober *et al.*, 1997), and contact dermatitis (Burns and Gaspari, 1996; Sundberg and King, 1996). Characterization of the perturbed DC populations in such knockout mice may enable us to better understand the symptoms in human patients and redirect our thinking toward more effective treatments.

The purpose of this chapter is to convey the message that an enormous body of information on dendritic cell biology may be had by examining DC in various knockout animals. The concept of a DC-knockout mouse is attractive. That is, it would be desirable to have a mouse model where the consequences of the loss of DC can be studied without interference from effects induced in other cell types. In reality, however, it is unlikely that such 'DC-specific' candidates for gene deletion exist except for those products that are expressed in discrete subsets of mature DC. For example, RelB may have a different role in $33D1^+$ DC versus DEC-205^+ DC versus LC. Additionally, a knockout of DC-specific genes expressed in anything earlier than a committed DC would be difficult, since DC can apparently arise from progenitors of either lymphoid or myeloid potential. That is, knocking out a gene expressed in DC-progenitors may well affect other cell lineages. Most importantly, the commitment along a particular lineage from progenitor to DC may be guided by microenvironmental cues rather than genetic programming. Thus, for purposes of understanding DC biology, it is important to keep in mind that it is not necessarily relevant whether the particular gene is expressed in DC or not. Since dendritic cells are involved in antigen-specific and innate immunity, they must recognize and respond to a huge variety of signals from the environment and from other cells in the animal. It should be just as useful to study effects on DC populations due to changes in other cell types impacted by specific gene loss.

ACKNOWLEDGMENTS

We thank Dr Mary Pauza for helpful discussions and critical review of this manuscript. These studies were supported by grants from the NIH (AI29689, AI31583, AI38375), the Juvenile Diabetes Foundation International, and the International Human Frontier Science Program. This is manuscript No. 11197 from the Scripps Research Institute.

REFERENCES

Adema, G.J., Hartgers, F., Verstraten, R., de Vries, E., Marland, G., Menon, S., Foster, J., Xu, Y., Nooyen, P., McClanahan, T., Bacon, K.B. and Figdor, C.G. (1997). A dendritic-cell-derived C-C chemokine that preferentially attracts naive T cells. *Nature* **387**, 713–717.

Ardavin, C. (1997). Thymic dendritic cells. *Immunol. Today* **18**, 350–361.

Bond, A., Cooke, A. and Hay, F.C. (1990). Glycosylation of IgG, immune complexes and IgG subclasses in the MRL-lpr/lpr mouse model of rheumatoid arthritis. *Eur. J. Immunol.* **20**, 2229–2233.

Borkowski, T.A., Letterio, J.J., Farr, A.G. and Udey, M.C. (1996). A role for endogenous transforming growth factor beta 1 in Langerhans cell biology: the skin of transforming growth factor beta 1 null mice is devoid of epidermal Langerhans cells. *J. Exp. Med.* **184**, 2417–2422.

Borkowski, T.A., Letterio, J.J., Mackall, C.L., Saitoh, A., Wang, X., Roop, D.R., Gress, R.E. and Udey, M.C. (1997). A role for TGFbeta-1 in Langerhans cell biology. Further characterization of the epidermal Langerhans cell defect in TGFbetal null mice. *J. Clin. Invest.* **100**, 575–581.

Burkly, L., Hession, C., Ogata, L., Reilly, C., Marconi, L.A., Olson, D., Tizard, R., Cate, R. and Lo, D. (1995). Expression of RelB is required for the development of thymic medulla and dendritic cells. *Nature* **373**, 531–536.

Burns, R.P.J. and Gaspari, A.A. (1996). The use of transgenic mouse models to investigate the immune mechanisms of allergic contact dermatitis: an area of emerging opportunities. *Am. J. Contact Dermatitis* **7**, 120–130.

Carrasco, D., Ryseck, R.P and Bravo, R. (1993). Expression of RelB transcripts during lymphoid organ development: specific expression in dendritic antigen-presenting cells. *Development* **118**, 1221–1231.

Crowley, M., Inaba, K., Witmer-Pack, M. and Steinman, R.M. (1989). The cell surface of mouse dendritic cells: FACS analyses of dendritic cells from different tissues including thymus. *Cell. Immunol.* **118**, 108–125.

de Graaf, J.H., Tamminga, R.Y., Dam-Meiring, A., Kamps, W.A. and Timens, W. (1996). The presence of cytokines in Langerhans' cell histiocytosis. *J. Pathol.* **180**, 400–406.

De Smedt, T., Pajak, B., Muraille, E., Lespagnard, L., Heinen, E., De Baetselier, P., Urbain, J., Leo, O. and Moser, M. (1996). Regulation of dendritic cell numbers and maturation by lipopolysaccharide in vivo. *J. Exp. Med.* **184**, 1413–1424.

DeKoning, J., DiMolfetto, L., Reilly, C., Wei, Q., Havran, W.L. and Lo, D. (1997). Thymic cortical epithelium is sufficient for the development of mature T cells in RelB-deficient mice. *J. Immunol.* **158**, 2558–2566.

Drijkoningen, M., De Wolf-Peeters, C., Snauwaert, J., De Greef, H. and Desmet, V. (1987). Immunohistochemical study of epidermal Langerhans cells and dermal dendritic cells in benign and malignant skin lesions characterized by a dermal lymphoid infiltrate consisting either of B-cells or T-cells. *Virchows Archiv. A. Pathol. Anat. Histopathol.* **411**, 337–343.

Ellner, J.J. (1996). Immunosuppression in tuberculosis. *Infect. Agents Dis.* **5**, 62–72.

Fu, Y.X., Huang, G., Matsumoto, M., Molina, H. and Chaplin, D.D. (1997). Independent signals regulate development of primary and secondary follicle structure in spleen and mesenteric lymph node. *Proc. Natl Acad. Sci. USA* **94**, 5739–5743.

Furukawa, F. (1997). Animal models of cutaneous lupus erythematosus and lupus erythematosus photosensitivity. *Lupus* **6**, 193–202.

Galy, A., Travis, M., Cen, D. and Chen, B. (1995). Human T, B, natural killer, and dendritic cells arise from a common bone marrow progenitor cell subset. *Immunity* **3**, 459–473.

Greaves, D.R., Wang, W., Dairaghi, D.J., Dieu, M.C., Saint-Vis, B., Franz-Bacon, K., Rossi, D., Caux, C., McClanahan, T., Gordon, S., Zlotnik, A. and Schall, T.J. (1997). CCR6, a CC chemokine receptor that interacts with macrophage inflammatory protein 3alpha and is highly expressed in human dendritic cells. *J. Exp. Med.* **186**, 837–844.

Groeneveld, P.H., Erich, T. and Kraal, G. (1986). The differential effects of bacterial lipopolysaccharide (LPS) on splenic non-lymphoid cells demonstrated by monoclonal antibodies. *Immunology* **58**, 285–290.

Herbst, B., Kohler, G., Mackensen, A., Veelken, H., Kulmburg, P., Rosenthal, F.M., Schaefer, H.E., Mertelsmann, R., Fisch, P. and Lindemann, A.D. (1996). In vitro differentiation of $CD34^+$ hematopoietic progenitor cells toward distinct dendritic cell subsets of the Birbeck granule and MIIC-positive Langerhans cell and the interdigitating dendritic cell type. *Blood* **88**, 2541–2548.

Inaba, K., Inaba, M., Romani, N., Aya, H., Deguchi, M., Ikehara, S., Muramatsu, S. and Steinman, R.M. (1992). Generation of large numbers of dendritic cells from mouse bone marrow cultures supplemented with granulocyte/macrophage colony-stimulating factor. *J. Exp. Med.* **176**, 1693–1702.

Josien, R., Heslan, M., Soulillou, J.P. and Cuturi, M.C. (1997). Rat spleen dendritic cells express natural killer cell receptor protein 1(NKR-P1) and have cytotoxic activity to select targets via a Ca^{2+}-dependent mechanism. *J. Exp. Med.* **186**, 467–472.

Junger, W.G., Hoyt, D.B., Liu, F.C., Loomis, W.H. and Coimbra, R. (1996). Immunosuppression after endotoxin shock: the result of multiple anti-inflammatory factors. *J. Trauma* **40**, 702–709.

Koni, P.A., Sacca, R., Lawton, P., Browning, J.L., Ruddle, N.H. and Flavell, R.A. (1997). Distinct roles in lymphoid organogenesis for lymphotoxins alpha and beta revealed in lymphotoxin beta-deficient mice. *Immunity* **6**, 491–500.

Koopman, W.J. and Gay, S. (1988). The MRL-lpr/lpr mouse. A model for the study of rheumatoid arthritis. *J. Rheumatol.* Suppl. **75**, 284–289.

Krenn, V., Schalhorn, N., Greiner, A., Molitoris, R., Konig, A., Gohlke, F. and Muller-Hermelink, H.K. (1996). Immunohistochemical analysis of proliferating and antigen-presenting cells in rheumatoid synovial tissue. *Rheumatol. Int.* **15**, 239–247.

Larregina, A., Morelli, A., Kolkowski, E. and Fainboim, L. (1996). Flow cytometric analysis of cytokine receptors on human Langerhans' cells. Changes observed after short-term culture. *Immunology* **87**, 317–325.

Letterio, J.J., Geiser, A.G., Kulkarni, A.B., Dang, H., Kong, L., Nakabayashi, T., Mackall, C.L., Gress, R.E. and Roberts, A.B. (1997). Autoimmunity associated with TGF-beta-1-deficiency in mice is dependent on MHC class II antigen expression. *J. Clin. Invest.* **98**, 2109–2119.

Maes, H.H., Causse, J.E. and Maes, R.F. (1996). Mycobacterial infections: are the observed enigmas and paradoxes explained by immunosuppression and immunodeficiency? *Med. Hypotheses* **46**, 163–171.

Maraskovsky, E., Brasel, K., Teepe, M., Roux, E.R., Lyman, S.D., Shortman, K. and McKenna, H.J. (1996). Dramatic increase in the numbers of functionally mature dendritic cells in Flt3 ligand-treated mice: multiple dendritic cell subpopulations identified. *J. Exp. Med.* **184**, 1953–1962.

Marquez, C., Trigueros, C., Fernandez, E. and Toribio, M.L. (1995). The development of T and non-T cell lineages from $CD34^+$ human thymic precursors can be traced by the differential expression of CD44. *J. Exp. Med.* **181**, 475–483.

McKercher, S.R., Torbett, B.E., Anderson, K.L., Henkel, G.W., Vestal, D.J., Baribault, H., Klemsz, M., Feeney, A.J., Wu, G.E., Paige, C.J. and Maki, R.A. (1996). Targeted disruption of the PU.1 gene results in multiple hematopoietic abnormalities. *EMBO J.* **15**, 5647–5658.

Metlay, J., Witmer-Pack, M.D., Agger, R., Crowley, M.T., Lawless, D. and Steinman, R.M. (1990). The distinct leukocyte integrins of mouse spleen dendritic cells as identified with new hamster monoclonal antibodies. *J. Exp. Med.* **171**, 1753–1771.

Mohamadzadeh, M., Poltorak, A.N., Bergstressor, P.R., Beutler, B. and Takashima, A. (1996). Dendritic cells produce macrophage inflammatory protein-1 gamma, a new member of the CC chemokine family. *J. Immunol.* **156**, 3102–3106.

Mooij, P., de Wit, H.J. and Drexhage, H.A. (1993). An excess of dietary iodine accelerates the development of a thyroid-associated lymphoid tissue in autoimmune prone BB rats. *Clin. Immunol. Immunopathol.* **69**, 189–198.

Muraille, E., De Smedt, T., Andris, F., Pajak, B., Armant, M., Urbain, J., Moser, M. and Leo, O. (1997). Staphylococcal enterotoxin B induces an early and transient state of immunosuppression characterized by V beta-unrestricted T cell unresponsiveness and defective antigen-presenting cell functions. *J. Immunol.* **158**, 2638–2647.

Nakabayashi, T., Letterio, J.J., Geiser, A.G., Kong, L., Ogawa, N., Zhao, W., Koike, T., Fernandes, G., Dang, H. and Talal, N. (1997). Up-regulation of cytokine mRNA, adhesion molecule proteins, and MHC class II proteins in salivary glands of TGF-betal knockout mice: MHC class II is a factor in the pathogenesis of TGF-beta-1 knockout mice. *J. Immunol.* **158**, 5527–5535.

Naspetti, M., Aurrand-Lions, M., DeKoning, J., Malissen, M., Galland, F., Lo, D. and Naquet, P. (1997). Thymocytes and RelB-dependent medullary epithelial cells provide growth-promoting and organization signals, respectively, to thymic medullary stromal cells. *Eur. J. Immunol.* **27**, 1392–1397.

Plump, A. (1997). Atherosclerosis and the mouse: a decade of experience. *Ann. Med.* **29**, 193-198.

Roake, J.A., Rao, A.S., Morris, P.J., Larsen, C.P., Hankins, D.F. and Austyn, J.M. (1995). Dendritic cell loss from nonlymphoid tissues after systemic administration of lipopolysaccharide, tumor necrosis factor, and interleukin 1. *J. Exp. Med.* **181**, 2237–2247.

Roark, J.H., Kuntz, C.L., Nguyen, K.A., Caton, A.J. and Erikson, J. (1995). Breakdown of B cell tolerance in a mouse model of systemic lupus erythematosus. *J. Exp. Med.* **181**, 1157–1167.

Scott, E.W., Fisher, R.C., Olson, M.C., Kehrli, E.W., Simon, M.C. and Singh, H. (1997). PU.1 functions in a cell-autonomous manner to control the differentiation of multipotential lymphoid-myeloid progenitors. *Immunity* **6**, 437–447.

Steinman, R.M., Pack, M. and Inaba, K. (1997). Dendritic cells in the T-cell areas of lymphoid organs. *Immunol. Rev.* **156**, 25–37.

Strober, W., Kelsall, B., Fuss, I., Marth, T., Ludviksson, B., Ehrhardt, R. and Neurath, M. (1997). Reciprocal IFN-gamma and TGF-beta responses regulate the occurrence of mucosal inflammation. *Immunol. Today* **18**, 61–64.

Sundberg, J.P. and King, L.E.J. (1996). Mouse mutations as animal models and biomedical tools for dermatological research. *J. Invest. Dermatol.* **106**, 368–376.

Tanabe, S., Lu, Z., Luo, Y., Quackenbush, E.J., Berman, M.A., Collins-Racie, L.A., Mi, S., Reilly, C., Lo, D., Jacobs, K.A. and Dorf, M.E. (1997). Identification of a new mouse beta chemokine, TCA-4, with activity on T lymphocytes and mesangial cells. *J. Immunol.* **159**, 5671–5679.

Tondravi, M.M., McKercher, S.R., Anderson, K., Erdmann, J.M., Quiroz, M., Maki, R. and Teitelbaum, S.L. (1997). Osteopetrosis in mice lacking haematopoietic transcription factor PU.1. *Nature* **386**, 81–84.

Tsukada, S., Rawlings, D.J. and Witte, O.N. (1993). Role of Bruton's tyrosine kinase in immunodeficiency. *Curr. Opin. Immunol.* **6**, 623–630.

Vicari, A.P., Figueroa, D.J., Hedrick, J.A., Foster, J.S., Singh, K.P., Menon, S., Copeland, N.G., Gilbert, D.J., Jenkins, N.A., Bacon, K.B. and Zlotnik, A. (1997). TECK: a novel CC chemokine specifically expressed by thymic dendritic cells and potentially involved in T cell development. *Immunity* **7**, 291–301.

Vremec, D. and Shortman, K. (1997). Dendritic cell subtypes in mouse lymphoid organs: cross-correlation of surface markers, changes with incubation, and differences among thymus, spleen, and lymph nodes. *J. Immunol.* **159**, 565–573.

Wang, J.H., Nichogiannopoulou, A., Wu, L., Sun, L., Sharpe, A.H., Bigby, M. and Georgopoulos, K. (1996). Selective defects in the development of the fetal and adult lymphoid system in mice with an Ikaros null mutation. *Immunity* **5**, 537–549.

Weih, F., Carrasco, D., Durham, S.K., Barton, D.S., Rizzo, C.A., Ryseck, R.P., Lira, S.A. and Bravo, R. (1995). Multiorgan inflammation and hematopoietic abnormalities in mice with a targeted disruption of RelB, a member of the NF-kappa B/Rel family. *Cell* **80**, 331–340.

Weih, F., Durham, S.K., Barton, D.S., Sha, W.C., Baltimore, D. and Bravo, R. (1996). Both multiorgan inflammation and myeloid hyperplasia in RelB-deficient mice are T cell dependent. *J. Immunol.* **157**, 3974–3979.

Weih, F., Warr, G., Yang, H. and Bravo, R. (1997). Multifocal defects in immune responses in RelB-deficient mice. *J. Immunol.* **158**, 5211–5218.

Witmer-Pack, M.D., Hughes, D.A., Schuler, G., Lawson, L., McWilliam, A., Inaba, K., Steinman, R.M. and Gordon, S. (1993). Identification of macrophages and dendritic cells in the osteopetrotic (op/op) mouse. *Cell Sci.* **104**, 1021–1029.

Wu, L., Li, C.L. and Shortman, K. (1996). Thymic dendritic cell precursors: relationship to the T lymphocyte lineage and phenotype of the dendritic cell progeny. *J. Exp. Med.* **184**, 903–911.

Wu, L., Vremec, D., Ardavin, C., Winkel, K., Suss, G., Georgiou, H., Maraskovsky, E., Cook, W. and Shortman, K. (1995). Mouse thymus dendritic cells: kinetics of development and changes in surface markers during maturation. *Eur. J. Immunol.* **25**, 418–425.

Xia, Y., Pauza, M.E., Feng, L. and Lo, D. (1997). RelB regulation of chemokine expression modulates local inflammation. *Am. J. Pathol.* **151**, 375–387.

Yaswen, L., Kulkarni, A.B., Fredrickson, T., Mittleman, B., Schiffman, R., Payne, S., Longenecker, G., Mozes, E. and Karlsson, S. (1997). Autoimmune manifestations in the transforming growth factor-beta 1 knockout mouse. *Gastroenterology* **113**, 825–832.

Zhu, Q., Zhang, M., Rawlings, D.J., Vihinen, M., Hagemann, T., Saffran, D.C., Kwan, S.P., Nilsson, L., Smith, C.I. and Witte, O.N. (1994). Deletion within the Src homology domain 3 of Bruton's tyrosine kinase resulting in X-linked agammaglobulinemia (XLA). *J. Exp. Med.* **180**, 461-470.

CHAPTER 31
Mobilization, Migration, and Localization of Dendritic Cells

Simon M. Barratt-Boyes[1] and Louis D. Falo, Jr.[2]
[1]Department of Infectious Diseases and Microbiology, Graduate School of Public Health and [2]Department of Dermatology, University of Pittsburgh Medical Center, Pittsburgh, Pennsylvania, USA

Travel, in the younger sort, is a part of education ...

Francis Bacon (1561–1626)

INTRODUCTION

Dendritic cells (DC) play a pivotal role in the initiation and regulation of T cell-dependent immune responses. This function appears to require at least three important capabilities *in vivo*. First, dendritic cells are professional antigen-presenting cells. As such, they are capable of taking up and processing antigen, and presenting immunogenic epitopes in the context of MHC class I or class II molecules for recognition by T cells. Importantly, in addition to the formation of the antigenic ligand recognized by the T cell receptor, dendritic cells can present antigen in the context of a variety of costimulatory interactions necessary for optimal T cell activation. These antigen-presenting functions contribute to the defining function of dendritic cells—the extraordinarily potent capacity to stimulate T cells, including the ability to prime naive T cells *in vivo* (reviewed in Steinman, 1991).

In addition to their antigen-presentation function, dendritic cells serve a sentinel function. On the frontiers of the adaptive immune response, dendritic cells survey epithelial surfaces for agents or insults that may present a threat to the body's safety. In the presence of 'danger' or antigenic insult, they evolve into antigen chaperones, delivering antigens from the periphery to the central lymphoid organs, where they can be presented to T-lymphocytes in the appropriate context for the induction of effector T-lymphocyte responses (reviewed in Romani and Schuler, 1992). Through this chaperone function, dendritic cells both protect antigen from destruction, such as by degradation by extracellular proteases (Falo *et al.*, 1992; Kozlowski *et al.*, 1992), and direct antigen to the lymphatic tissues which are designed to maximize encounters between dendritic cells and lymphocytes. The importance of this chaperone function for the induction of immune responses is emphasized by studies demonstrating that transport of antigen into lymphoid organs is not only necessary, but can be sufficient for the

Dendritic Cells: Biology and Clinical Applications
ISBN 0-12-455860-7

induction of an antigen-specific immune response (Kundig *et al.*, 1995). Hence dendritic cell migration, especially movement from the periphery to lymphoid organs following antigen exposure, is a fundamental component of immune system function. Furthermore, it is becoming increasingly evident that an understanding of this process of dendritic cell migration and localization may be central to the success of dendritic cell-based approaches to immunotherapy.

NATURAL DENDRITIC CELL TRAFFICKING

Dendritic Cell Migration from the Skin

Natural trafficking refers to mobilization, migration, and localization of endogenous dendritic cells, which is physiological and potentially distinct from that of exogenously derived dendritic cells which have been extracted, manipulated *in vitro* and then readministered. Several years ago, it was demonstrated that epidermal Langerhans cells could mature during *in vitro* culture into cells with phenotypic and functional characteristics similar to those of dendritic cells found in lymph nodes, suggesting a link between dendritic cells in nonlymphoid tissue, and dendritic cells in the lymphoid organs (Schuler and Steinman, 1985). Much of the subsequent focus of natural dendritic cell trafficking has been on the movement of epidermal Langerhans cells from skin to draining lymph nodes in response to an exogenous stimulus, such as a contact sensitizer applied to the shaved skin of a mouse. Fluorescent compounds such as fluorescein isothiocyanate can serve both as antigen and cell marker and are ideal for these studies. Importantly, the identity of fluorescently labeled cells in draining lymph nodes can be confirmed by morphology and labeling with cell-specific antibodies.

Such studies have shown that dendritic cell influx into lymph nodes occurs as soon as 4 h after antigen exposure, peaking at 2 days after exposure and then gradually declining (Macatonia *et al.*, 1986; Macatonia *et al.*, 1987). Dendritic cells isolated from draining lymph nodes for up to 3 days after skin painting contained fluorescent particles and stimulated antigen-specific responses *in vitro*, suggesting that the migrating cells are responsible for initiating the delayed-type hypersensitivity seen in response to challenge by contact sensitizing agents. The numbers of MHC class II-positive Langerhans cells in the skin declined in accordance with dendritic cell influx into lymph nodes, but normalized within 2–5 days, indicating that there is active homeostasis of dendritic cell numbers in skin (van Wilsem *et al.*, 1994). Interestingly, not all antigen-bearing cells exit the epidermis following skin painting (van Wilsem *et al.*, 1994). The migration of cells out of sensitized skin can be significantly inhibited by administering antibodies to ICAM-1 and LFA-1, suggesting that these adhesion molecules play a critical role in dendritic cell movement *in vivo* (Ma *et al.*, 1994).

Migration of Langerhans cells has been studied in response to skin transplantation by examining epidermal and dermal sheets (Larsen *et al.*, 1990). As with contact sensitization, within 24 h of transplantation the numbers of Langerhans cells in allografts and isografts markedly decreased, and by 3 days after transplantation cords of Langerhans cells could be identified within dermal lymphatics. In association with this movement from the epidermis, isolated dendritic cells increased their ability to stimulate allospecific T cell responses, suggesting that the process of migration was accompanied by a functional maturation. This maturation may be incomplete, however, as further enhancement of immunostimulatory capacity can occur with short-term culture (Larsen *et al.*, 1990).

These studies suggested that dendritic cell migration and maturation is induced by a local inflammatory response associated with application of a contact sensitizer or transplantation, but the mechanisms involved with dendritic cell mobilization are not well understood. This interpretation is supported by the results of more direct experiments using pro-inflammatory factors administered *in vivo*. Intradermal injection of murine TNF-α into mice results in a dose-dependent accumulation of dendritic cells in draining lymph nodes which was detectable within 2–4 h (Cumberbatch and Kimber, 1992). Likewise, systemic administration of lipopolysaccharide can result in almost total depletion of dendritic cells from heart, kidney, and spleen in treated mice within 1–3 days (Roake *et al.*, 1995; De Smedt *et al.*, 1996). A functional maturation appears to precede this exodus, as splenic dendritic cells isolated 6 h after lipopolysaccharide administration have increased levels of B7 costimulator molecule expression, reduced capacity to process soluble antigen, and enhanced T cell stimulatory capacity *in vitro* as compared to cells from control animals. These functionally potent dendritic cells were transiently identified within T cell-rich areas of spleen; this area is devoid of dendritic cells 2 days after lipopolysaccharide injection (De Smedt *et al.*, 1996).

Langerhans cells have been demonstrated to express high levels of E-cadherin while in the epidermis, and E-cadherin has been shown to mediate high-affinity binding of Langerhans cells to keratinocytes *in vivo* (Tang *et al.*, 1993; Blauvelt *et al.*, 1995). It has recently been proposed that E-cadherin plays an important role in Langerhans cell keratinocyte adhesion and Langerhans cell localization in the epidermis *in vivo*, and that reduced E-cadherin expression as a consequence of Langerhans cell activation results in decreased Langerhans cell–keratinocyte adhesion (Jakob *et al.*, 1997). Evidence supporting this hypothesis has recently been reviewed (Udey, 1997).

Studies of natural dendritic cell trafficking have been limited by the indirect means of identifying cells, such as application of fluorescent marker to the skin with subsequent uptake or association of reagent by cells. However, Condon *et al.* (1996) have combined this classical labeling approach with the direct *in situ* transfection of Langerhans cells through cutaneous gene delivery of plasmid DNA encoding naturally fluorescent green fluorescent protein (GFP). After rhodamine painting and GFP gene delivery, dendritic cells expressing both markers were present in the draining lymph nodes of treated mice, identifying transfected cells as skin-derived dendritic cells. These studies directly demonstrate trafficking of *in vivo* transfected skin-derived dendritic cells to the draining lymph nodes, and have implications for the use of dendritic cells genetically engineered *in vivo* to induce or suppress antigen-specific immune responses in the host.

Natural dendritic cell trafficking studies have been done in sheep using a lymphatic cannulation technique. Migrating cells can be harvested prior to entry into the lymph node by first ablating the node and cannulating the pseudo-afferent lymphatic vessels that arise by anastomosis (Hall, 1967). Afferent lymph dendritic cells can be identified by expression of CD1, a marker expressed by epidermal Langerhans cells (Bujdoso *et al.*, 1989). The advantage of this system has been that the dynamics of dendritic cell migration in response to antigen challenge can be studied in individual animals. In sheep given repeated intradermal injections of antigen, the proportion of dendritic cells in afferent lymph remained constant (at 1–10%), although there was a transient

3- to 5-fold decrease in total cell output from 1 to 3 days after antigen exposure (Hopkins *et al.*, 1989). Dendritic cells taken from afferent lymph 5 days after antigen challenge expressed increased levels of MHC class II molecules and had enhanced ability to stimulate allogeneic T cells as compared to non-antigen-stimulated animals, reflecting a functional maturation of migrating cells (Hopkins *et al.*, 1989). Interestingly, however, the same cells stimulated antigen-specific autologous T cell lines more efficiently, suggesting that the capacity to process and present soluble antigen was not lost.

Taken together, these findings imply that epidermal dendritic cells are stimulated to migrate in response to nonspecific inflammatory signals, a logical stimulus given that infections invariably generate inflammation. The stimulated cells, laden with antigen sampled from the local inflamed tissue, enter lymphatics and begin the functional maturation into antigen-presenting cells which is completed in the lymphoid tissue. The observation that dendritic cells collected in dermal cords (Larsen *et al.*, 1990) or afferent lymph (Hopkins *et al.*, 1989) have properties intermediate between Langerhans cells and interdigitating lymph node dendritic cells is consistent with this model of maturation.

Interestingly, interruption of dendritic cell migration as a means of reducing immune responsiveness appears to be exploited by at least one pathogen, the murine retrovirus Rauscher leukemia virus. Systemic viral infection blocks dendritic cell migration from skin to lymph nodes in response to the contact sensitizer fluorescein isothiocyanate (Gabrilovich *et al.*, 1994). Viral DNA was identified in a proportion of skin and lymph node dendritic cells, suggesting that direct infection of dendritic cells may have been responsible. Though the precise mechanism for altered migration was not determined, a partial downregulation of ICAM-1 adhesion molecule expression on Langerhans cells may have played a role (Gabrilovich *et al.*, 1994).

Dendritic Cell Migration from Mucosal Surfaces and the Liver

Dendritic cell activity in intestine and lung has been studied in depth by MacPherson and Holt, who have authored separate chapters in this book, and trafficking from these tissues will be discussed only briefly here. Similarly to the peripheral lymphadenectomy technique in sheep, mesenteric lymph node ablation in the rat and subsequent cannulation of the thoracic duct allows collection of dendritic cells derived from small intestine (Pugh *et al.*, 1983). Oral or intraintestinal feeding of antigen then can be used to test the capacity of intestinal dendritic cells to acquire specific antigens. The onset of migration of dendritic cells from the gut is rapid following antigen exposure; lymphatic dendritic cells collected within 8 h of challenge were capable of stimulating antigen-primed splenocytes (Liu and MacPherson, 1991) and could initiate antigen-specific T cell responses when injected into naive mice (Liu and MacPherson, 1993). However, the kinetic response is relatively short compared to that reported for skin-derived dendritic cells, as lymphatic dendritic cells collected just 24 h after intraintestinal antigen exposure were ineffective at stimulating primed splenocytes (Liu and MacPherson, 1993). Systemic injection of endotoxin induced rapid dendritic cell exodus from intestine that peaked from 12 to 24 h (MacPherson *et al.*, 1995), in keeping with the notion that inflammatory mediators initiate dendritic cell migration. Interestingly, however, there was no detectable change from normal in the functional status of dendritic cells isolated after endotoxin administration, as the cells stimulated allogeneic T cell responses and presented soluble antigen to sensitized T cells normally (MacPherson *et al.*, 1995). This may reflect a difference in the maturation status of dendritic cells migrating from intestine as compared to skin and other tissues.

Recent studies on dendritic cells in the respiratory system have focused on the recruitment of cells into airway epithelium in response to inflammation. Work from Holt and colleagues demonstrated that dendritic cell recruitment into tracheal epithelium parallels that of neutrophils, peaking in number at 24 h after intranasal or aerosol challenge with bacteria, virus, or soluble protein (McWilliam *et al.*, 1994; McWilliam *et al.*, 1996). This indicates that antigen-presenting cells migrate into this epithelial surface in the early response to infection, in apparent contrast to the situation in skin, where a rapid exodus of resident dendritic cells is observed following antigen challenge or inflammation. This may reflect a difference in dendritic cell residency in different epithelial surfaces. For example, Langerhans cells may be present in skin in sufficient numbers to handle antigen exposure without the need for additional recruitment; in contrast, the dendritic cell population in airway epithelium may be limited and more transient (Holt *et al.*, 1988), hence the need to respond by cell influx following airway antigen challenge. Steroid administration inhibits the local recruitment of dendritic cells into airway epithelium (Holt and Thomas, 1997), a response which is consistent with the general immunosuppressive properties of corticosteroids.

There is a paucity of literature reporting on the natural migration of dendritic cells through internal organs, in part because of technical challenges related to studying migration outside of epithelial surfaces. A novel approach to address this problem has been taken by Matsuno *et al.* (1996). These workers used carbon particles injected intravenously into rats that had surgical ablation of the celiac lymph nodes which drain the liver (Matsuno *et al.*, 1995). Particle-laden dendritic cells were then collected via thoracic duct cannulation in a similar manner to that used for intestinal dendritic cell collection. These studies indicated that hepatic dendritic cells phagocytose intravascular particles, enter hepatic lymphatics and localize in T cell-dependent areas of draining lymph nodes (Matsuno *et al.*, 1996). The blood–lymph translocation of dendritic cells at the level of the hepatic sinusoids was confirmed by additional adoptive transfer experiments (Kudo *et al.*, 1997). This novel transfer mechanism of dendritic cells from blood to lymph is befitting of the role of the liver as a filter for gut-derived antigens and toxins, which arrive in the liver via the blood. We will come back to a discussion of dendritic cell migration from liver later in this chapter in the setting of whole-organ transplantation.

TRAFFICKING OF ADOPTIVELY TRANSFERRED DENDRITIC CELLS

There is considerable current interest in the development of immunotherapies utilizing adoptively transferred, antigen-loaded dendritic cells, as discussed elsewhere in this book. We and others have shown that antigen-loaded DC can induce antigen-specific CTL *in vivo*, and can initiate protective and therapeutic antitumor immunity in animal models (Celluzzi *et al.*, 1996; Mayordomo *et al.*, 1995; Ossevoort *et al.*, 1995; Porgador and Gilboa, 1995; Porgador *et al.*, 1996; Paglia, *et al.*, 1996). Importantly, results from a clinical trial suggest that antigen-pulsed DC can induce measurable antitumor immunity, including some degree of clinical response, in humans (Hsu *et al.*, 1996).

The Route of Administration Affects Dendritic Cell Homing

Adoptive transfer of purified cells to recipient animals provides an additional level of complexity to studies of dendritic cell migration. Early reports in this area focused on testing the assumption that interdigitating dendritic cells of peripheral lymphoid tissues arose from veiled cells found in afferent lymph. Afferent lymph dendritic cells were collected from the thoracic lymph of mesenteric lymphadenectomized rats, radiolabeled and administered via intradermal or intravenous injection to naive recipients (Fossum, 1988). Following intravenous injection, radiolabeled cells localized to spleen and liver but were excluded from peripheral lymph nodes and Peyer's patches. In contrast, cells injected into footpads were retained in popliteal lymph nodes, although a majority remained at the site of injection. Radiolabeled cells localized in T cell-dependent areas of spleen and lymph node following intravenous or intradermal injection, respectively. As predicted, in lymph nodes the injected cells were morphologically indistinct from endogenous interdigitating dendritic cells (Fossum, 1988). These findings were supported by similar studies in mice by Austyn and coworkers, who focused on adoptive transfer of purified splenic dendritic cells (Kupiec-Weglinski, 1988; Austyn *et al.*, 1988). The migration of cells from skin was dependent on cell viability, as fixed radiolabeled dendritic cells remained exclusively at the site of intradermal injection (Kupiec-Weglinski *et al.*, 1988), supporting the notion that migration is an active rather than passive event. The conclusions of these studies were that intravenous (systemic) injection of dendritic cells leads to homing to spleen, liver and lung, whereas intradermal (regional) administration results in localization in peripheral lymph nodes. Interestingly, the findings were similar whether the injected cells were derived from spleen or afferent lymph, suggesting that the route of administration, and not the tissue of origin, determined the eventual fate of injected dendritic cells.

There appear to be definite functional consequences of the differential dendritic cell homing following subcutaneous and intravenous injection. Morikawa *et al.* (1992) showed that murine splenic dendritic cells, when pulsed with keyhole limpet hemacyanin and administered subcutaneously, elicited delayed-type hypersensitivity responses in recipient mice when the antigen was subsequently injected into the ear. Conversely, intravenous transfer of antigen-pulsed cells did not result in delayed-type hypersensitivity responses, but induced serum antibodies specific for the antigen. This humoral response was dependent on an intact spleen (Morikawa *et al.*, 1992). Similar findings were reported when epidermal Langerhans cells were used as antigen-presenting cells (Morikawa *et al.*, 1993). Further studies showed that intravenous administration of keyhole limpet hemacyanin-pulsed dendritic cells resulted in increased levels of mRNA transcripts for IL-10 in spleen, whereas subcutaneous injection led to high levels of mRNA for IL-2 in draining lymph nodes (Morikawa *et al.*, 1995). *In vitro* studies tend to support these *in vivo* findings. Murine dendritic cells isolated from lymph nodes stimulated primary T cell responses to antigen, whereas dendritic cells isolated from blood failed to stimulate a response (Hill *et al.*, 1994). In additional studies, mitogen-treated murine dendritic cells isolated from spleen induced secretion of T_H1 cytokines from T cells, whereas Peyer's patch dendritic cells induced a T_H2 profile (Everson *et al.*, 1996).

In summary, these results suggest that the site of dendritic cell homing is crucial to the type of immune response elicited to antigen. Dendritic cells that home to lymph nodes following subcutaneous injection induce T_H1 responses, with IL-2 production and delayed-type hypersensitivity responses, whereas dendritic cells that home to spleen following intravenous injection elicit T_H2 responses, with IL-10 expression and production of antibodies. This regional influence of dendritic cell homing on the type of immune response elicited may be logical when one considers that different infections also tend to have a regional distribution. For example, helminth and nematode infections, which are most efficiently expelled with T_H2 immune responses, predominate in the gut. However, there does not appear to be direct evidence that dendritic cells that drain the gut home in significant numbers to spleen.

Presentation of Antigen Affects Dendritic Cell Persistence in Lymphatic Tissues

The above studies reinforce the principle that dendritic cells and T cells interact in an antigen-specific manner in lymphoid organs; however, they do not demonstrate this directly. Jenkins and coworkers have done just that by using T cells expressing a transgenic T cell antigen receptor. In this model, T cells have specificity for a defined antigen–MHC complex, in this case an ovalbumin peptide-I-A^d complex. Using this system, dendritic cells and ovalbumin-specific T cells were labeled with two different fluorochromes and injected into syngeneic recipients with or without pulsing the dendritic cells with the specific ovalbumin antigen. The homing behavior of the labeled cells was studied by confocal fluorescent microscopy of tissue sections (Ingulli *et al.*, 1997). As predicted, subcutaneous injection of dendritic cells that were not presenting ovalbumin resulted in accumulation of dendritic cells in the lymph node paracortex without association with labeled T cells. In contrast, when dendritic cells were first loaded with the specific ovalbumin peptide, the transgenic T cells formed large clusters around the individual fluorescent dendritic cells within the node. Consistent with other studies, this interaction led to a T_H1-type immune response with production of IL-2 *in vivo* and delayed-type hypersensitivity responses following subcutaneous ovalbumin injection (Ingulli *et al.*, 1997). However, an unexpected finding was that ovalbumin antigen-pulsed dendritic cells disappeared from the draining lymph nodes by 48 h after injection, whereas pulsed dendritic cells persisted (Ingulli *et al.*, 1997). These studies add another dimension to the understanding of dendritic cell trafficking as they suggest that the persistence of antigen-presenting dendritic cells within lymph nodes is influenced by the antigen-specific interaction with T cells. Activated T cells may transmit a signal which results in effective removal of the source of stimulating antigen and potentially opens the way for localization of other antigen-laden dendritic cells.

Trafficking of Dendritic Cells after Transplantation

It is believed that the migration of small numbers of donor leukocytes out of whole-organ allografts into recipient organs, a condition known as microchimerism, may be responsible for the high rate of acceptance of liver transplants observed in humans (Starzl *et al.*, 1992). Dendritic cells have been implicated in this process (Starzl *et al.*, 1993), as discussed at length elsewhere in this book. To study this phenomenon mouse liver dendritic cell precursors, expanded *in vitro* using low levels of GM-CSF to induce an immature dendritic cell phenotype (Lu *et al.*, 1994), were injected into allogeneic recipients. Tissue sections were taken at intervals after injection and donor cells were identified by reactivity with donor-specific antibodies (Thomson *et al.*, 1995a). As predicted by the studies we have described above, donor dendritic cells homed to T-dependent areas of secondary lymphoid organs where they upregulated expression of MHC class II molecules (Thomson *et al.*, 1995a). Interestingly, donor dendritic cells could be identified at least 2 months after injection into allogeneic recipients (Qian *et al.*, 1994; Thomson *et al.*, 1995a), reflecting the persistence of donor leukocytes seen in transplant patients (Starzl *et al.*, 1992). In additional studies, small numbers of donor-derived dendritic cells could be propagated from bone marrow of mice 14 days after successful allogeneic liver transplantation (Thomson *et al.*, 1995b), whereas no donor-derived dendritic cells could be isolated from the bone marrow of mice rejecting allogeneic cardiac transplants (Lu *et al.*, 1995). These studies provide strong correlative evidence that migration of dendritic cells from donor organs to recipient lymphoid tissue plays an important role in allograft acceptance.

Trafficking of *in Vitro* Derived Dendritic Cells

Before leaving the discussion of trafficking of adoptively transferred dendritic cells, we need to introduce a related but separate issue, that of migration of dendritic cells that have been derived *in vitro* for therapeutic use. As discussed elsewhere in this book, a burgeoning field has developed around the use of dendritic cells for immunotherapy of cancer and infectious diseases, based on the functional capacity of dendritic cells to associate with and stimulate T cells in T cell-rich lymphoid compartments. Dendritic cells intended for this use are being derived from precursor populations, such as $CD34^+$ bone marrow cells or peripheral blood monocytes, by culturing with various cytokine combinations *in vitro* (Caux *et al.*, 1992; Sallusto and Lanzavecchia, 1994). The fundamental question arises whether such *in vitro* derived dendritic cells have the capacity to migrate when administered back to the host. This issue has been addressed in a preclinical chimpanzee model using dendritic cells derived *in vitro* from blood monocytes using recombinant human cytokines (Barratt-Boyes *et al.*, 1996; Barratt-Boyes *et al.*, 1997). Dendritic cells were labeled with a lipophilic fluorescent marker and injected subcutaneously into donor chimpanzees. Injected skin and draining lymph nodes were collected at various times after injection and examined by fluorescence microscopy. Labeled dendritic cells migrated to lymph nodes where they remained for at least 5 days (Barratt-Boyes *et al.*, 1997). The injected cells associated with T cells in the paracortex, and, most importantly, retained high level expression of costimulatory and MHC molecules *in situ* (see Plate 31.1), indicating that the dendritic cell phenotype was maintained outside of the *in vitro* cytokine-rich environment. These results are encouraging as they suggest that cultured human dendritic cells can traffic normally when used therapeutically in patients. Whether the migratory behavior is retained in patients with profound disease is a perplexing question that has yet to be addressed.

MIGRATION OF HUMAN DENDRITIC CELLS

Several descriptive reports have been published on trafficking of dendritic cells in humans. As described above, the early reports of microchimerism in transplant recipients identified donor-derived leukocytes in lymphoid organs distant from the transplant organ; the donor cells were suspected of being dendritic cells based on immunohistochemistry and morphology (Starzl *et al.*, 1993). In separate studies, the influence of local secretion of GM-CSF on dendritic cell recruitment to human lung *in vivo* was studied using in-situ hybridization and immunohistochemistry (Tazi *et al.*, 1993). The authors found a close correlation between the production of GM-CSF in lung carcinomas and the presence of CD1a$^+$ dendritic cells infiltrating these tumors, indicating that this growth factor may be important in recruitment and perhaps differentiation of dendritic cells in the lung (Tazi *et al.*, 1993). Experimental manipulations of human dendritic cells *in vivo* have been done by grafting human skin onto nude mice and observing cell migration after application of a contact sensitizer (Hoefakker *et al.*, 1995). As predicted, the xenogeneic human epidermal dendritic cells in this model behaved in much the same way as allogeneic mouse dendritic cells, migrating to lymph nodes under the apparent influence of IL-1 and TNF-α produced by keratinocytes in the graft (Hoefakker *et al.*, 1995).

Finally, a developing area of research of great interest is the identification of novel chemokines that affect dendritic cell and T cell trafficking. Two recent studies warrant particular attention. Adema *et al.* (1997) have identified a C-C chemokine that is specifically expressed by human dendritic cells at high levels. Interestingly, the chemokine, designated as DC-CKl, is elaborated by dendritic cells present in the germinal centers and T cell areas of lymph nodes and preferentially attracts naive T cells of the CD45RA$^+$ phenotype. Hence DC-CK1 appears to be important in promoting the association of antigen-loaded dendritic cells with naive circulating T cells at the site of induction of immune responses. Conversely, Greaves *et al.* (1997) have identified a novel chemokine receptor which appears to be selectively expressed by human dendritic cells. This receptor was shown to interact only with the C-C chemokine macrophage inflammatory protein 3α and has been designated C-C chemokine receptor 6 (Greaves *et al.*, 1997). The function of macrophage inflammatory protein 3α is not presently known, but it has little structural homology with other known C-C chemokines. In addition, *in vitro* derived dendritic cells have been shown to be chemotactically responsive to the C-C chemokines RANTES, MIP-1α and monocyte chemotactic protein 3 (Sozzani *et al.*, 1995; Xu *et al.*, 1996). It is likely that chemokines play an important role in the migration of dendritic cells to secondary lymphoid organs and the interaction between dendritic cells and T cells within these organs. The identification and cloning of such chemokines may lead to the clinical application of chemokines in association with dendritic cell-based immunotherapy.

REFERENCES

Adema, G.J., Hartgers, F., Verstraten, R., de Vries, E., Marland, G., Menon, S., Foster, J., Xu, Y., Nooyen, P., McClanahan, T., Bacon, K.B. and Figdor, C.G. (1997). A dendritic cell-derived C-C chemokine that preferentially attracts naive T cells. *Nature* **387**, 713–717.

Austyn, J.M., Kupiec-Weglinski, J.W., Hankins, D.F. and Morris, P.J. (1988). Migration patterns of dendritic cells in the mouse: homing to T cell-dependent areas of spleen, and binding within marginal zone. *J. Exp. Med.* **167**, 646–651.

Barratt-Boyes, S.M., Henderson, R.A. and Finn, O.J. (1996). Chimpanzee dendritic cells with potent immunostimulatary function can be propagated from peripheral blood. *Immunology* **87**, 528–534.

Barratt-Boyes, S.M., Watkins, S.C. and Finn, O.J. (1997). *In vivo* migration of dendritic cells differentiated *in vitro*. A chimpanzee model. *J. Immunol.* **158**, 4543–4547.

Blauvelt, A., Katz, S.I. and Udey, M.C. (1995). Expression of E-cadherin by murine dendritic cells: E-cadherin as a dendritic cell marker characteristic of epidermal Langerhans cells and related cells. *Eur. J. Immunol.* **24**, 2767–2770.

Bujdoso, R., Hopkins, J., Dutia, B.M., Young, P. and McConnell, I. (1989). Characterization of sheep afferent lymph dendritic cells and their role in antigen carriage. *J. Exp. Med.* **170**, 1285–1302.

Caux, C., Dezutter-Dambuyant, C., Schmitt, D. and Banchereau, J. (1992). GM-CSF and TNF-α cooperate in the generation of dendritic Langerhans cells. *Nature* **360**, 258–261.

Celluzzi, C.M., Mayordomo, J.I., Storkus, W.J., Lotze, M.T. and Falo, L.D., Jr. (1996). Peptide-pulsed dendritic cells induce antigen-specific, CTL-mediated protective tumor immunity. *J. Exp. Med.* **183**, 283–287.

Condon, C., Watkins, S.C., Celluzzi, C.M., Thompson, K. and Falo, L.D. Jr. (1996). DNA-based immunization by *in vivo* transfection of dendritic cells. *Nature Medicine* **2**, 1122–1128.

Cumberbatch, M. and Kimber, I. (1992). Dermal tumor necrosis factor-α induces dendritic cell migration to draining lymph nodes, and possibly provides one stimulus for Langerhans' cell migration. *Immunology* **75**, 257–263.

De Smedt, T., Pajak, B., Muraille, E., Lespagnard, L., Heinen, E., De Baetselier, P., Urbain, J., Leo, O. and Moser, M. (1996). Regulation of dendritic cell numbers and maturation by lipopolysaccharide *in vivo*. *J. Exp. Med.* **184**, 1413–1424.

Everson, M.P., McDuffie, D.S., Lemak, D.G., Koopman, W.J., McGhee, J.R. and Beagley, K.W. (1996). Dendritic cells from different tissues induce production of different T cell cytokine profiles. *J. Leukocyte Biol.* **59**, 494–498.

Falo L.D. Jr., Colarusso, L.J., Benacerraf, B. and Rock, K.L. Serum proteases alter the antigenicity of peptides presented by class I major histocompatibility complex molecules. *Proc. Natl Acad. Sci. USA* **89**, 8347–8350.

Fossum, S. (1988). Lymph-borne dendritic leukocytes do not recirculate, but enter the lymph node paracortex to become interdigitating cells. *Scand. J. Immunol.* **27**, 97–105.

Gabrilovich, D.I, Woods, G.M., Patterson, S., Harvey, J.J. and Knight, S.C. (1994). Retrovirus-induced immunosuppression via blocking of dendritic cell migration and down-regulation of adhesion molecules. *Immunology* **82**, 82–87.

Greaves, D.R., Wang, W., Dairaghi, D.J., Dieu, M.C., de Saint-Vis, B., Franz-Bacon, K., Rossi, D., Caux, C., McClanahan, T., Gordon, S., Zlotnik, A. and Schall, T.J. (1997). CCR6, a CC chemokine receptor that interacts with macrophage inflammatory protein 3α and is highly expressed in human dendritic cells. *J. Exp. Med.* **186**, 837–844.

Hall, J.G. (1967). Studies of the cells in the afferent and efferent lymph of lymph nodes draining the site of skin homografts. *J. Exp. Med.* **125**, 737–754.

Hill, S., Coates, J.P., Kimber, I. and Knight, S.C. (1994). Differential function of dendritic cells isolated from blood and lymph nodes. *Immunology* **83**, 295–301.

Hoefakker, S., Balk, H.P., Boersma, W.J., van Joost, T., Notten, W.R. and Claassen, E. (1995). Migration of human antigen-presenting cells in a human skin graft onto nude mice model after contact sensitization. *Immunology* **86**, 296–303.

Holt, P.G. and Thomas, J.A. (1997). Steroids inhibit uptake and/or processing but not presentation of antigen by airway dendritic cells. *Immunology* **91**, 145–150.

Holt, P.G., Schon-Hegrad, M.A. and Oliver, J. (1988). MHC Class II antigen-bearing dendritic cells in pulmonary tissues of the rat: regulation of antigen presentation activity by endogenous macrophage populations. *J. Exp. Med.* **167**, 262–274.

Hopkins, J., Dutia, B.M., Bujdoso, R. and McConnell, I. (1989). *In vivo* modulation of CD1 and MHC class II expression by sheep afferent lymph dendritic cells: comparison of primary and secondary immune responses. *J. Exp Med.* **170**, 1303–1318.

Hsu, F.J., Benike, C., Fagnoni, F., Liles, T.M., Czerwiski, D., Taidi, B., Engleman, E.G. and Levy, R. (1996). Vaccination of patients with B-cell lymphoma using autologous antigen-pulsed dendritic cells. *Nature Medicine* **2**, 52–58.

Ingulli, E., Mondino, A., Khoruts, A. and Jenkins, M.K. (1997). *In vivo* detection of dendritic cell antigen presentation to $CD4^+$ T cells. *J. Exp. Med.* **185**, 2133–2141.

Jakob, T., Saitoh, A. and Udey, M.C. (1997). E-cadherin-mediated adhesion involving Langerhans cell-like dendritic cells expanded from murine fetal skin. *J. Immunol.* **159**, 2693–2701.

Kozlowski, S., Corr, M., Takeshita, T., Boyd, L.F., Pendleton, C.D., Germain, R.N., Berzofsky, J.A. and Margulies, D.H. (1992). Serum angiotensin-1 converting enzyme activity processes a human immunodeficiency virus 1 gp 160 peptide for presentation by major histocompatibility complex class I molecules. *J. Exp. Med.* **176**(6), 1417–1422.

Kudo, S., Matsuno, K., Ezaki, T. and Ogawa, M. (1997). A novel migration pathway for rat dendritic cells from the blood: hepatic sinusoids–lymph translocation. *J. Exp. Med.* **185**, 777–784.

Kundig, T.M., Bachmann, M.F., DiPado, C., Simard, J.J.L., Battegay, M., Lother, H., Gessner, A., Kühlcke, K., Ohashi, P.S., Hengartner, H. and Zinkernagel, R.M. (1995). Fibroblasts as efficient antigen-presenting cells in lymphoid organs. *Science* **268**, 1343–1347.

Kupiec-Weglinski, J.W., Austyn, J.M. and Morris, P.J. (1988). Migration patterns of dendritic cells in the mouse: traffic from the blood, and T cell-dependent and independent entry to lymphoid tissues. *J. Exp. Med.* **167**, 632–645.

Larsen, C.P., Steinman, R.M., Witmer-Pack, M., Hankins, D.F., Morris, P.J. and Austyn, J.M. (1990). Migration and maturation of Langerhans cells in skin transplants and explants. *J. Exp. Med.* **172**, 1483–1493.

Liu, L.M. and MacPherson, G.G. (1991). Lymph-borne (veiled) dendritic cells can acquire and present intestinally administered antigens. *Immunology* **73**, 281–286.

Liu, L.M. and MacPherson, G.G. (1993). Antigen acquisition by dendritic cells: Intestinal dendritic cells acquire antigen administered orally and can prime naive T cells in vivo. *J. Exp. Med.* **177**, 1299–1307.

Lu, L., Woo, J., Rao, A.S., Li, Y., Watkins, S.C., Qian, S., Starzl, T.E., Demitris, A.J. and Thomson, A.W. (1994). Propagation of dendritic cell progenitors from normal mouse liver using granulocyte/macrophage colony-stimulating factor and their maturational development in the presence of type-1 collagen. *J. Exp. Med.* **179**, 1823–1834.

Lu, L., Rudert, W.A., Qian, S., McCaslin, D., Fu, F., Rao, A.S., Trucco, M., Fung, J.J., Starzl, T.E. and Thomson, A.W. (1995). Growth of donor-derived dendritic cells from the bone marrow of murine liver allograft recipients in response to granulocyte/macrophage colony-stimulating factor. *J. Exp. Med.* **182**, 379–387.

Ma, J., Wang, J.-H., Guo, Y.-J., Sy, M.-S. and Bigby, M. (1994). *In vivo* treatment with anti-ICAM-1 and anti-LFA-1 antibodies inhibits contact sensitization-induced migration of epidermal Langerhans cells to regional lymph nodes. *Cell. Immunol.* **158**, 389–399.

Macatonia, S.E., Edwards, A.J. and Knight, S.C. (1986). Dendritic cells and the initiation of contact sensitivity to fluorescein isothiocyanate. *Immunology* **59**, 509–514.

Macatonia, S.E., Knight, S.C., Edwards, A.J., Griffiths, S. and Fryer, P. (1987). Localization of antigen on lymph node dendritic cells after exposure to the contact sensitizer fluorescein isothiocyanate: functional and morphological studies. *J. Exp. Med.* **166**, 1654–1667.

MacPherson, G.G., Jenkins, C.D., Stein, M.J. and Edwards, C. (1995). Endotoxin-mediated dendritic cell release from the intestine: characterization of released dendritic cells and TNF dependence. *J. Immunol.* **154**, 1317–1322.

Matsuno, K., Kudo, S., Ezaki, T. and Miyakawa, K. (1995). Isolation of dendritic cells in the rat lymph. *Transplantation* **60**, 765–768.

Matsuno, K., Ezaki, T., Kudo, S. and Uehara, Y. (1996). A life stage of particle-laden rat dendritic cells in vivo: their terminal division, active phagocytosis, and translocation from the liver to the draining lymph. *J. Exp. Med.* **183**, 1865–1878.

Mayordomo, J.I. *et al.* (1995). Bone marrow-derived dendritic cells pulsed with synthetic tumor peptides elicit protective and therapeutic antitumor immunity. *Nature Medicine* **1**, 1297.

McWilliam, A.S., Nelson, D., Thomas, J.A. and Holt, P.G. (1994). Rapid dendritic cell recruitment is a hallmark of the acute inflammatory response at mucosal surfaces. *J. Exp. Med.* **179**, 1331–1336.

McWilliam, A.S., Napoli, S., Marsh, A.M., Pemper, F.L., Nelson, D.J., Pimm, C.L., Stumbles, P.A., Wells, T.N.C. and Holt, P.G. (1996). Dendritic cells are recruited into the airway epithelium during the inflammatory response to a broad spectrum of stimuli. *J. Exp. Med.* **184**, 2429–2432.

Morikawa, Y., Furotani, M., Kuribayashi, K., Matsuura, N. and Kakudo, K. (1992). The role of antigen-presenting cells in the regulation of delayed-type hypersensitivity. I. Spleen dendritic cells. *Immunology* **77**, 81–87.

Morikawa, Y., Furotani, M., Matsuura, N. and Kakudo, K. (1993). The role of antigen-presenting cells in the regulation of delayed-type hypersensitivity. II. Epidermal Langerhans cells and peritoneal exudate macrophages. *Cell. Immunol.* **152**, 200–210.

Morikawa, Y., Tohya, K., Ishida, H., Matsuura, N. and Kakudo, K. (1995). Different migration patterns of antigen-presenting cells correlate with Th1/Th2-type responses in mice. *Immunology* **85**, 575–581.

Ossevoort, M.A., Feltkamp, M.C., van Veen, K.J., Melief, C.J. and Kast, W.M. (1995). Dendritic cells as carriers for a cytotoxic T-lymphocyte epitope-based peptide vaccine in protection against a human papillomavirus type 16 induced tumor. *J. Immunother.* **18**, 86–94.

Paglia, P., Chiodoni, C., Rodolfo, M. and Colombo, M.P. (1996). Murine dendritic cells loaded in vitro with soluble protein prime cytotoxic T lymphocytes against tumor antigen in vivo. *J. Exp. Med.* **183**, 317–322.

Porgador, A. and Gilboa, F. (1995). Bone marrow-generated dendritic cells pulsed with a class I-restricted peptide are potent inducers of cytotoxic T lymphocytes. *J. Exp. Med.* **182**, 255–260.

Porgador, A., Snyder, D. and Gilboa, E. (1996). Induction of antitumor immunity using bone marrow-generated dendritic cells. *J. Immunol.* **156**, 2918–2926.

Pugh, C.W., MacPhearson, G.G. and Steer, H.W. (1983). Characterization of nonlymphoid cells derived from rat peripheral lymph. *J. Exp. Med.* **157**, 1758–1779.

Qian, S., Demitris, A.J., Murase, N., Rao, A.S., Fung, J.J. and Starzl, T.E. (1994). Murine liver allograft transplantation: tolerance and donor cell chimerism. *Hepatology* **19**, 916–924.

Roake, J.A., Rao, A.S., Morris, P.J., Larsen, C.P., Hankins, D.F. and Austyn, J.M. (1995). Dendritic cell loss from nonlymphoid tissues after systemic administration of lipopolysaccharide, tumor necrosis factor, and interleukin 1. *J. Exp. Med.* **181**, 2237–2247.

Romani, N. and Schuler, G. (1992). The immunologic properties of epidermal Langerhans cells as a part of the dendritic cell system. *Springer Semin. Immunopathol.* **13**, 265–279.

Sallusto, F. and Lanzavecchia, A. (1994). Efficient presentation of soluble antigen by cultured human dendritic cells is maintained by granulocyte/macrophage colony-stimulating factor plus interleukin 4 and downregulated by tumor necrosis factor α. *J. Exp. Med.* **179**, 1109–1118.

Schuler, C. and Steinman, R.M. (1985). Murine epidermal Langerhans cells mature into potent immunostimulatory dendritic cells *in vitro. J. Exp. Med.* **161**, 526–531.

Sozzanni, S., Sallusto, F., Luni, W., Zhou, D., Piemnoti, L., Allavena, P., Van Damme, J., Valitutti, S., Lanzavecchia, A. and Mantovani, A. (1995). Migration of dendritic cells in response to formyl peptides, C5a and a distinct set of chemokines. *J. Immunol.* **155**, 3292–3295.

Starzl, T.E., Demitris, A.J., Murase, N., Ildstad, S., Ricordi, C. and Trucco, M. (1992). Cell migration, chimerism, and graft acceptance. *Lancet* **339**, 1579–1582.

Starzl, T.E., Demitris, A.J., Murase, N., Thomson, A.W., Trucco, M. and Ricordi, C. (1993). Donor cell chimerism permitted by immunosuppressive drugs: new view of organ transplantation. *Immunol. Today* **14**, 326–332.

Steinman, R.M. (1991). The dendritic cell system and its role in immunogenicity. *Annu. Rev. Immunol.* **9**, 271–296.

Tang, A., Amagai, L., Granger, G., Stanley, J.R. and Udey, M.C. (1993). Adhesion of epidermal Langerhans cells to keratinocytes is mediated by E-cadherin. *Nature* **361**, 82–84.

Tazi, A., Bouchonnet, F., Grandsaigne, M., Boumsell, L., Hance, A.J. and Soler, P. (1993). Evidence that granulocyte macrophage colony-stimulating factor regulates the distribution and differentiated state of dendritic cells/Langerhans cells in human lung and lung cancers. *J. Clin. Invest.* **91**, 566–576.

Thomson A.W., Lu, L., Wan, Y., Qian, S., Larsen, C.P. and Starzl, T.E. (1995a). Identification of donor-derived dendritic cell progenitors in bone marrow of spontaneously tolerant liver allograft recipients. *Transplantation* **60**, 1555–1559.

Thomson A.W., Lu, L., Subbotin, V.M., Li, Y., Qian, S., Rao, A.S., Fung, J.J. and Starzl, T.E. (1995b). In vitro propagation and homing of liver-derived dendritic cell progenitors to lymphoid tissues of allogeneic recipients: implications for the establishment and maintenance of donor cell chimerism following liver transplantation. *Transplantation* **59**, 544–551.

Udey M.C. (1997). Cadherins and Langerhans cell immunobiology. *Clin. Exp. Immunol.* **107** (Suppl. 1): 6–8.

van Wilsem, E.J.G., Breve, J., Kleijmeer, M. and Kraal, G. (1994). Antigen-bearing Langerhans cells in skin draining lymph nodes: phenotype and kinetics of migration. *J. Invest. Dermatol.* **103**, 217–220.

Xu, L.L., Warren, M.K., Rose, W.L., Gong, W.H. and Wang, J.M. (1996). Human recombinant monocyte chemotactic protein and other C-C chemokines bind and induce directional migration of dendritic cells in vitro. *J. Leukocyte Biol.* **60**, 365–371.

CHAPTER 32
Genetic Engineering of Dendritic Cells

Thomas Tüting[1,3], Laurence Zitvogel[2] and Yasuhiko Nishioka[3]
[1]J. Gutenberg-University, Mainz, Germany; [2]Institut Gustave-Roussy, Villejuif, France; [3]University of Pittsburgh School of Medicine, Pittsburgh, Pennsylvania, USA

DNA-BASED IMMUNIZATION IS AN EXCITING NEW FIELD FOR VACCINE DEVELOPMENT

Vaccination is one of the most efficacious medical interventions used to prevent infectious disease. Recent advances in immunology and molecular biology have allowed for the construction of subunit vaccines consisting of antigen-encoding cDNA incorporated into recombinant viruses. Recombinant viral vaccines efficiently induce both humoral and cell-mediated immune responses to the encoded transgene, often after a single inoculation [1]. Their major disadvantages are potential safety issues such as conversion to virulence or recombination with wild-type viruses and potential interference with preexisting immunity to the vaccine carrier. In 1992, Johnston and colleagues reported the surprising observation that particle-mediated gene transfer of an expression plasmid encoding human growth hormone into the skin of mice resulted not only in the systemic delivery of the molecule but also in the induction of antigen-specific antibody responses [2]. Subsequent studies revealed that immunization with purified plasmid DNA encoding influenza antigens elicited both humoral and cellular immune responses, including antigen-specific $CD8^+$ cytotoxic T cells and $CD4^+$ T helper cells, and protected mice against a lethal challenge with live influenza virus [3–7]. This has opened up an alternative field of DNA-based vaccine development that circumvents the major problems associated with the application of recombinant viral vaccines. Numerous studies have demonstrated that plasmid DNA, delivered either by particle bombardment or by needle injection into skin or muscle, can promote effective immune responses against different viruses, bacteria, and parasites in rodents [8]. With the molecular identification of tumor antigens [9], there has also been increasing interest in the development of DNA-based immunization strategies for tumor immunotherapy. Both recombinant viruses and plasmid DNA encoding model tumor antigens such as chicken ovalbumin [10], β-galactosidase [11–13], or CEA [14] induced protective immune responses in mice leading to rejection of a subsequent, normally lethal challenge with tumor cells expressing the respective antigen.

Dendritic Cells: Biology and Clinical Applications
ISBN 0-12-455860-7

PROFESSIONAL ANTIGEN-PRESENTING CELLS ARE CRITICAL FOR THE INITIATION OF CELLULAR IMMUNE RESPONSES

The ability of plasmid DNA immunization to elicit strong CTL responses was initially thought to be a consequence of the intracellular antigen synthesis in target cells *in vivo* following DNA immunization. Recently, studies have been performed to elucidate the mechanism of antigen presentation following plasmid DNA immunization in bone marrow-chimeric mice [15–18]. Parent ⇨F_1 bone marrow chimeras were generated in which H-$2^{b\times d}$ (C57BL/6 × BALB/c) recipient mice received bone marrow that expressed only H-2^b (CS7BL/6) or H-2^d (BALB/c) MHC molecules. Since H-2^b or H-2^d T cells are educated in an H-$2^{b\times d}$ thymus, cytotoxic T-lymphocytes (CTL) are capable of recognizing peptide antigens presented by both H-2^b and H-2^d [17]. Following intramuscular or intradermal immunization with plasmid DNA encoding influenza nucleoprotein (for which H-2^b and H-2^d-restricted CTL epitopes have been defined), CTL responses were restricted to the MHC haplotype of the bone marrow alone and not to the second haplotype expressed by the recipient's myocytes or keratinocytes. These results seem to rule out the possibility that keratinocytes or myocytes, the predominant transfected cell types after intradermal or intramuscular DNA immunization, can directly activate naive T cells. Instead, the initiation of cell-mediated immune responses appears to require presentation of immunogenic peptides derived from the encoded antigen by bone marrow-derived antigen-presenting cells (APC) such as dendritic cells (DC). Professional APC may acquire the antigen either through direct transfection or via antigen uptake from alternate transfected cell types. Cutaneous DNA immunization using the gene gun has been shown to result *in vivo* in direct transfection of skin-derived dendritic cells that localize in the T cell-rich areas of draining lymph nodes [10]. Consistent with these observations, DC migrating out of DNA-injected tissue appear to carry plasmid DNA and trigger immune responses to the transgene [19]. Furthermore, splenic DC have been implicated in the induction of immunity following intramuscular injection of retroviral vectors encoding an HIV protein or ovalbumin in mice [20]. DC isolated from the spleens of these mice were shown to contain provirus, to express retrovirally encoded proteins, to present ovalbumin to a specific T cell line, and to induce CTL specific for the HIV protein (i.e., as peptide–MHC complexes) after adoptive transfer to naive mice. However, it is unclear whether DC within the muscle were transduced prior to their migration into the spleen, or whether the retrovirus entered the blood after intramuscular injection and transduced DC within the spleen. Taken together, these and similar studies [21] point to a critical role for professional antigen-presenting cells in the initiation of primary cellular immunity following DNA-based immunization.

CULTURED DC AS A BIOLOGICAL ADJUVANT FOR DNA-BASED IMMUNIZATION

The establishment of culture conditions that allow for the *in vitro* generation of large numbers of immunostimulatory DC from precursor populations in bone marrow and blood has stimulated significant interest in the use of DC as a biological adjuvant for DNA-based vaccines [22–33]. Mouse DC have been isolated from spleen, or grown from bone marrow cells cultured with GM-CSF and IL-4. Human DC have been grown from cord blood or bone marrow $CD34^+$ progenitors or from peripheral

Table 1. Gene transfer strategies for *ex vivo* gene delivery into DC

Recombinant viral vectors	Nonviral gene transfer
• Retrovirus (including lentivirus)	• Liposomes
• Adenovirus	• Receptor-mediated endocytosis
• Herpes simplex virus	• Particle bombardment (gene gun)
• Vaccinia, fowlpox, canarypox virus	• Electroporation

blood mononuclear cells. Culture of $CD34^+$ progenitors with GM-CSF, TNF-α, and c-kit ligand (stem cell factor, SCF) supports the growth and differentiation of DC. DC can also be obtained by culture of plastic-adherent PBMC with GM-CSF and IL-4. Cultured murine bone marrow-derived DC, when adoptively transferred, can effectively present tumor peptide epitopes to the immune system, leading to the induction of prophylactic and therapeutic cell-mediated immunity against experimental murine tumors that express the same epitope [28–31]. Primary tumor antigen-specific T cell responses could also efficiently be induced in the human system *in vitro* using cultured, peptide-pulsed, autologous DC as stimulators and peripheral blood leukocytes from healthy donors or cancer patients as responders [32, 33]. Clinical trials using cultured, peptide-pulsed DC that are adoptively transferred for the treatment of metastatic melanoma have begun at multiple institutions this year.

Currently, a number of laboratories are exploring the insertion of cDNA encoding an entire tumor antigen into cultured DC as an alternative to the use of peptides for DC-based tumor immunotherapy. A major strength of such gene-based vaccines compared to peptide-based approaches is that their application does not require prior knowledge of the patient HLA-haplotype or of specific T cell epitopes. The fact that the induction of immune responses following plasmid DNA immunization has been shown to require antigen presentation by professional APC additionally provides the rationale for the adoptive transfer of cultured DC, *ex vivo* genetically modified to express tumor antigens. Endogenous antigen synthesis within DC ensures direct access to the MHC class I antigen processing pathway. After homing to T cell-rich areas of secondary lymphoid organs, appropriate MHC class I-binding epitopes should be presented to naive T cells in the context of high levels of costimulatory molecules. A number of approaches are currently being evaluated for the introduction of genes into cultured dendritic cells, particularly for the immunotherapy of cancer (Table 1).

THE ADOPTIVE TRANSFER OF ANTIGEN-TRANSDUCED DC PROMOTES CELL-MEDIATED IMMUNITY IN EXPERIMENTAL MURINE MODELS

Viral vectors have been used to genetically modify murine bone marrow-derived DC *ex vivo* to express model tumor antigens [34–39]. The adoptive transfer of these DC was able to promote tumor antigen-specific T cell responses and prophylactic as well as therapeutic cell-mediated immunity against tumors in experimental murine models. Recombinant retroviral vectors generally require that the target cells undergo cell division and must therefore be applied during the early stages of DC differentiation. Both coculture with irradiated retroviral producer cell lines [34] as well as repeated centrifugal transduction with retroviral supernatant on days 2, 3, and 4 of culture [35] have successfully been employed to transduce a large proportion of developing dendritic cells. Of importance is the use of ecotropic producer cells or ecotropic supernatant containing high-titers of recombinant retrovirus (>10^6 pfu/ml). The major advantage of retroviral DC transduction is the stable integration of the transgene into the chromosome leading to gene expression throughout the life of the cell and its progeny.

The use of recombinant adenovirus has been investigated as an alternative to retroviral transduction for gene transfer into DC. Adenoviral vectors allow transiently for strong transgene expression also in nondividing cells, but their utility may be limited by transient gene expression and immune responses against the virus itself. DC appear to be somewhat resistant to adenoviral infection and a high multiplicity of infection (MOI) is required to successfully express genes. The adoptive transfer of immortalized murine DC lines or cultured bone marrow-derived DC transduced with recombinant adenovirus expressing model tumor antigens such as β-galactosidase promotes antigen-specific CTL responses and prophylactic as well as therapeutic anti-tumor immunity [36–39]. Of importance, vaccination with cultured DC infected *ex vivo* with recombinant adenoviral vectors was shown to circumvent the problem of neutralizing antibodies that is known to severely limit the repeated application of adenoviruses alone for vaccination purposes in rodents [36]. Thus, cultured DC may be an ideal adjuvant for the implementation of adenoviral vectors in tumor vaccine strategies. However, none of the studies reported has employed tumor antigens similar to those found so far for human cancers, which all appear to derive from normal germline-encoded genes. It will be critical whether the inherent immunogenicity associated with the use of adenoviral vectors will help or suppress the induction of immune responses against 'self' antigens, which most likely will prove to be considerably less immunogenic.

Several studies have shown that nonviral gene transfer methods can also be used for the insertion of genes encoding tumor antigens into murine DC [40–42]. The adoptive transfer of bone marrow-derived DC *ex vivo* engineered to express tumor antigens using particle bombardment promotes antigen-specific CTL responses and protective tumor immunity *in vivo* despite the considerably lower transduction efficiency when compared to viral vectors. The adoptive transfer of freshly isolated murine splenic DC, lipofected with cDNA encoding an HSV antigen, protected mice against a subsequent challenge with live HSV-1 [41]. The resulting immune response appeared to be associated mainly with an increased T_H1 $CD4^+$ T cell response as demonstrated by the production of high titers of IgG2a but not IgG1 antibodies. Splenocytes from the vaccinated mice produced IFN-γ and IL-2, but not IL-4, when they were restimulated *in vitro*. The use of DC as an adjuvant for plasmid DNA immunization led to immune responses that were superior to those induced following direct intramuscular injection of DNA alone. Immunizations with splenic DC, lipofected with mRNA encoding the model tumor antigen chicken ovalbumin, also induced antigen-specific CTL responses and protective immunity against an ovalbumin-transfected tumor [42]. Nonviral gene delivery methods have several important advantages of potential clinical interest: (1) More than one gene can readily be transfected simultaneously, allowing for cotransfection of genes encoding distinct tumor antigens and/or immunostimulatory cytokines. (2) Only the gene of interest is transcribed, without immunological interference from viral proteins both *in vitro* and *in vivo*. (3) There is no risk of recombination associated with replication-deficient viral vectors. (4) Insertion of foreign DNA into the genome is less likely owing to the transient nature of gene transfer. (5) The approach uses highly purified DNA that can readily and economically be produced in large quantities and is very stable.

ANTIGEN-TRANSDUCED HUMAN DC PROMOTE CELL-MEDIATED IMMUNITY *IN VITRO*

Tumor antigens have also been expressed in human DC using various viral and nonviral gene transfer methods [43–50]. DC grown from proliferating $CD34^+$ progenitors have been transduced successfully using retroviral vectors. Such transductions have been performed with vectors encoding the tumor-associated antigen MUC-1 [43] or the melanoma-associated antigen MART-1/Melan-A [44]. MART-1-transduced DC were capable of stimulating IFN-γ release from MART-1-specific tumor-infiltrating lymphocytes. Importantly, these gene-modified DC were capable of inducing primary, tumor antigen-specific CTL responses *in vitro*. Another study carefully assessed the phenotype and function of retrovirally transduced DC developing in culture from bone marrow and cord blood $CD34^+$ progenitors using mouse CD2 as a reporter gene [45]. Transduction did not affect DC differentiation, since differentiated, marker gene-expressing DC exhibited a mature phenotype ($CD40^+$, $CD80^+$, $CD83^+$, $CD86^+$, $p55^+$, $S100^+$) and normal T cell-stimulatory capacity (allogeneic MLR and antigen-specific recall responses). Average transduction efficiencies of 11.5% for cells grown from bone marrow progenitors, and 21.2% for cord blood progenitors, were reported for the $CDla^+$ DC progeny. Retroviral transductions did not appear to differentially affect the proportion of DC in relation to other myeloid populations developing in the cultures. Human monocyte-derived DC have also been retrovirally transduced with the reporter genes LacZ and CAT [46]. Since retroviral transduction generally requires cell division for successful retroviral integration, it is somewhat surprising that transduction efficiencies of 42–60% were reported for $CD1a^+$ cells and that the gene products were still detectable after 20 days of culture.

Adenoviral vectors appear to be particularly attractive for gene transfer into PBMC-derived DC, since they readily express large amounts of gene products in nondividing cells. An E1-deleted, replication-incompetent AdV type 5 vector was used to transfer genes to human monocyte-derived DC [47]. To achieve gene expression in 95% or more of the cells, MOIs greater than 1000 were required, underscoring the low infectivity of DC for adenoviral vectors. However, while a melanoma cell line was more readily transduced, high viral loads resulted in cytopathic effects that were not seen for DC. Greater than 90% of the DC remained viable after exposure to virus at an MOI of 10 000, while 100% of the melanoma cells were killed. This report demonstrated that high level expression of reporter genes (LacZ and luciferase) and IL-2 and IL-7 could be achieved by adenovirus-mediated transduction at these high MOIs. In contrast, a variety of physical methods for gene transfer, including DNA/liposome complexes, electroporation and calcium phosphate precipitation, were relatively inefficient.

Plasmid DNA encoding reporter genes and melanoma-associated antigens can be introduced into human PBMC-derived DC using liposomes [48] or particle bombardment [49]. Similar to murine studies, these nonviral gene transfers are much less efficient. Low level expression of the reporter genes (CAT, and LacZ encoding

β-galactosidase) and tyrosinase were detected at the protein level. Furthermore, DC transfected with the tyrosinase gene were shown to cluster with a CTL line specific for a tyrosinase peptide and to induce secretion of TNF-α by these antigen-specific T cells, suggesting that the antigen-expressing DC were capable of antigen processing and presentation [48]. Transfection of PBMC-derived DC with plasmid DNA encoding melanoma antigens has also been performed using particle bombardment [49]. While only up to 5% of DC can be transduced with this gene transfer method, it consistently leads to low levels of antigen expression without interference from viral proteins. The induction of CTL using gene gun-transfected DC *in vitro* was shown using five different melanoma antigens: MART-1/Melan-A, pmel17/gp100, tyrosinase, MAGE-1, and MAGE-3. These studies suggest that a nonviral gene delivery system can also be used to present a given melanoma-associated antigen in an immungenic format by gene-modified DC and promote the induction of primary melanoma-reactive CTL.

GENETIC ENGINEERING OF DC WITH GENES ENCODING CYTOKINES AND COSTIMULATORY MOLECULES

Cytokines and costimulatory molecules are known to be involved in CTL generation. Thus, DC might become even more potent in generating CTL when they can be genetically engineered to overexpress appropriate cytokines or costimulatory molecules. Candidate genes include IFN-α, TNF-α, GM-CSF, CD40L, IL-1, IL-2, IL-4, IL-12 and IL-15. IL-12 and TNF-α have been reported to enhance the function of DC, including upregulation of MHC class I and class II molecules and costimulatory molecules [22, 50, 51]. GM-CSF, which is the essential cytokine for myeloid DC generation from bone marrow, is capable of enhancing the APC function of DC [22, 51, 53]. Addition of IL-4 in DC culture from PBMC with GM-CSF is reported to generate more potent DC [52]. Transduction with these cytokine genes would be expected to affect DC function as well as phenotype in an autocrine manner. On the other hand, paracrine effects on T cells by cytokines produced from gene-modified DC can be considered. IFN-α, IL-2, IL-12 and IL-15 [54] in particular are known to enhance CTL activity. Furthermore, IL-2 and IL-12 have the ability to increase the expression of cytotoxic molecules, perforin and granzyme B, in T and of NK cells [55, 56]. Transduction with these cytokine genes might therefore enhance the function of induced CTL. Further studies are needed to clarify the effects of cytokine transduction on DC function and induction of CTL.

FUTURE DEVELOPMENTS

Many viral and nonviral gene transfer strategies are currently being investigated for the expression of suitable antigens in DC. Recombinant poxviruses have been shown to efficiently transduce PBMC-DC [57]. At recent international meetings the use of recombinant Canary poxvirus, recombinant Semliki Forest virus, and HSV-derived viral vectors has been reported as a useful tool for genetic modification of DC. It is presently unclear which viral gene transfer system will be most useful for clinical applications. Retroviral vectors offer the advantage of stable gene expression combined with low or absent immunogenicity but are associated with safety concerns. Highly immunogenic viral vectors such as adenoviruses or poxviruses will be of little use for the induction of antigen-specific CTL in the human system *in vitro*, particularly if they are used more than once. However, it is unclear whether immune responses to components of immunogenic viral vectors will augment or suppress the induction of desired immune responses to the encoded antigen *in vivo* when virally transduced DC are adoptively transferred for immunization purposes. Nonviral strategies such as liposome-mediated transfer, particle-mediated transfer, electroporation or receptor-mediated endocytosis of plasmid DNA are being investigated intensively as an alternative to viral vectors and are modified to enhance transduction efficiency of DC. One such strategy, for example, exploits the capacity for cell entry by adenoviral particles [58, 59]. Plasmid DNA is complexed with adenoviral particles using polylysine and can be introduced into the cytoplasm of cells. UV-inactivation of the adenovirus circumvents the problem of endogenous adenoviral gene expression without compromising endocytosis, which is mediated by the adenoviral envelope proteins. Another strategy attempts to target the mannose receptor for DNA uptake into DC using mannosylated polylysine–DNA complexes. It would be desirable to find a simple, safe, and efficient way to express antigens in DC in the years to come.

The studies outlined above have made it clear that antigen-encoding genes can be delivered to DC by a variety of gene transfer methods, leading to expression in functional forms (e.g., enzymes and cytokines) or immunogenic forms (e.g., viral and tumor antigens). The relative efficiencies of these individual techniques for delivery and expression of defined genes have now to be assessed in systematic, comparative studies using standardized reagents and clearly defined protocols. The immune responses resulting from the adoptive transfer of cultured DC *ex vivo* gene-modified using different viral and nonviral vector systems must be characterized carefully in animal models and compared to those induced by direct inoculation of plasmid DNA *in vivo*. With further improvements in gene transfer technology, strategies may also be developed to target the delivery of genes directly to DC *in vivo*, thus obviating the requirement for *ex vivo* transduction of these cells prior to vaccination.

REFERENCES

1. Ertl, H.C.J. and Xiang, Z. (1996). Novel vaccine approaches. *J. Immunol.* **156**, 3579–3582.
2. Tang, D.C., DeVit, M.J. and Johnston, S.A. (1992). Genetic immunization: a simple method for eliciting an immune response. *Nature* **356**, 152–154.
3. Fynan, E.F., Webster, R.G., Fuller, D.H., Haynes, J.R., Santoro, J.C. and Robinson, H.L. (1993). DNA vaccines: protective immunizations by parenteral, mucosal, and gene-gun inoculations. *Proc. Natl Acad. Sci. USA* **90**, 11478–11482.
4. Ulmer, J.B., Donnelly, J.J., Parker, S.E., Rhodes, G.H., Felgner, P.L., Dwarki, V.J., Gromkowski, S.H., Deck, R.R., Dewitt, C.M., Friedman, A., Hawe, L.A., Leander, K.R., Martinez, D., Perry, H.C., Shiver, J.W., Montgomery, D.L., Liu, M.A. (1993). Heterologous protection against influenza by injection of DNA encoding a viral protein. *Science* **259**, 1745–1749.
5. Wang, B., Ugen, K.E., Srikantan, V., Agadjanyan, M.G., Dnag, K., Refaeli, Y., Sato, A.I., Boyer, J., Willams, W.V. and Weiner, D.B. (1993). Gene inoculation generates immune responses against human immunodeficiency virus type 1. *Proc. Natl Acad. Sci. USA* **90**, 4156–4160.
6. Robinson, H.L., Hunt, L.A. and Webster, R.G. (1993). Protection against a lethal influenza virus challenge by immunization with a hemagglutinin-expressing plasmid DNA. *Vaccine* **11**, 957–960.
7. Davis, H.L., Michel, M.L. and Whalen, R.G. (1993). DNA-based immunization induces continuous secretion of hepatitis B surface antigen and high levels of circulating antibody. *Hum. Mol. Genet.* **2**, 1847–1851.

8. Donnelly, J.J., Ulmer, J.B., Shiver, J.W. and Liu, M.A. (1997). DNA vaccines. *Annu. Rev. Immunol.* **15**, 617–648.
9. Boon, T. and Van der Bruggen, P. (1996). Human tumor antigens recognized by T lymphocytes. *J. Exp. Med.* **183**, 725–729.
10. Condon, C., Watkins, S.C., Celluzzi, C.M., Thompson, K. and Falo, L.D. (1996). DNA-based immunization by *in vivo* transfection of dendritic cells. *Nature Medicine* **2**, 1122–1128.
11. Wang, M., Bronte, V., Chen, P.W., Gritz, L., Panicali, D., Rosenberg, S.A. and Restifo, N.P. (1995). Active immunotherapy of cancer with a nonrepliating recombinant fowl poxvirus encoding a model tumor-associated antigen. *J. Immunol.* **154**, 4685.
12. Chen, P.W., Wang, M., Bronte, V., Zhai, Y., Rosenberg, S.A. and Restifo, N.P. (1996). Therapeutic antitumor response after immunization with a recombinant adenovirus encoding a model tumor-associated antigen. *J. Immunol.* **156**, 224–231.
13. Irvine, K.R., Rao, R.B., Rosenberg, S.A. and Restifo, N.P. (1996). Cytokine enhancement of DNA immunization leads to effective treatment of established pulmonary metastases. *J. Immunol.* **156**, 238–245.
14. Conry, R.M., Widera, G., LoBuglio, A.F., Fuller, J.T., Moore, S.T., Barlow, D.L., Turner, J., Yang, N-S. and Curiel, D.T. (1996). Selected strategies to augment polynucleotide immunization. *Gene Ther.* **3**, 67–74.
15. Corr, M., Lee, D.J., Carson, D.A. and Tighe, H. (1996). Gene vaccination with naked plasmid DNA: mechanism of CTL priming. *J. Exp. Med.* **184**, 1555–1560.
16. Doe, B., Selby, M., Barnett, S., Baenziger, J. and Walker, C.M. (1996). Induction of cytotoxic T lymphocytes by intramuscular immunization with plasmid DNA is facilitated by bone marrow-derived cells. *Proc. Natl Acad. Sci. USA* **93**, 8578–8583.
17. Fu T.-M., Ulmer, J.B., Caulfield, M.J., Deck, R.R., Friedman, A., Wang, S., Liu, X., Donnelly, J.J. and Liu, M.A. (1997). Priming of cytotoxic T lymphocytes by DNA vaccines: requirements for professional antigen presenting cells and evidence for antigen transfer from myocytes. *Mol. Med.* **3**, 362–371.
18. Iwasaki, A., Torres, C.A.T., Ohashi, P.S., Robbinson, H.L. and Barber, B.H. (1997). The dominant role of bone marrow-derived cells in CTL induction following plasmid DNA immunization at different sites. *J. Immunol.* **159**, 11–14.
19. Casares, S., Inaba, K., Brumeanu, T.-D., Steinman, R.M. and Bona, C.A. (1997). Antigen presentation by dendritic cells after immunization with DNA encoding a major histocomapatibility complex class II-restricted viral epitope. *J. Exp. Med.* **186**, 1481–1486.
20. Song, E.S., Lee, V., Surh, C.D., Lynn, A., Brumm, D., Jolly, D.J., Warner, J.F. and Chada, S. (1997). Antigen presentation in retroviral vector-mediated gene transfer *in vivo. Proc. Natl Acad. Sci. USA* **94**, 1943–1948.
21. Bronte, V., Carroll, M.W., Goletz, T.J., Wang, M., Overwijk, W.W., Marincola, F., Rosenberg, S.A., Moss, B. and Restifo, N.P. (1997). Antigen expression by dendritic cells correlates with the therapeutic effectiveness of a model recombinant poxvirus tumor vaccine. *Proc. Natl Acad. Sci. USA* **94**, 3183–3188.
22. Steinman, R.M. (1991). The dendritic cell system and its role in immunogenicity. *Annu. Rev. Immunol.* **9**, 271–296.
23. Cella, M., Sallusto, F. and Lanzavecchia, A. (1997). Origin, maturation and antigen presenting function of dendritic cells. *Curr. Opin. Immunol.* **9**, 10–16.
24. Schuler, G. and Steinman, R.M. (1997). Dendritic cells as adjuvants for immune-mediated resistance to tumors. *J. Exp. Med.* **186**, 1183–1187.
25. Inaba, K., Inaba, M., Romani, N., Aya, H., Deguchi, M., Ikehara, S., Muramatsu, S. and Steinman, R.M. (1992).Generation of large numbers of dendritic cells from mouse bone marrow cultures supplemented with granulocyte-macrophage colony-stimulating factor. *J. Exp. Med.* **176**, 1693–1702.
26. Romani, N., Gruner, S., Bran, D., Kämpgen, E., Lenz, A., Trockenbacher, B., Konwalinka, G., Gritsch, P.O., Steinman, R.M. and Schuler, G. (1994). Proliferating dendritic cell progenitors in human blood. *J. Exp. Med.* **180**, 83–93.
27. Young, J.W. and Inaba, K. (1996). Dendritic cells as adjuvants for class I major histocompatibility complex-restricted antitumor-immunity. *J. Exp. Med.* **183**, 7–11.
28. Mayordomo, J.I., Zorina, T., Storkus, W.J., Zitvogel, L., Celuzzi, C.M., Falo, L.D., Kast, W.M., Ildstad, S.T., DeLeo, A.B. and Lotze, M.T. (1995). Bone marrow-derived dendritic cells pulsed with tumor peptides elicit protective and therapeutic anti-tumor immunity. *Nature Medicine* **1**, 1297–1302.

29. Porgador, A., Snyder, D. and Gilboa, E. (1996). Induction of antitumor immunity using bone marrow-generated dendritic cells. *J. Immunol.* **56**, 2918–2926.
30. Zitvogel, L., Mayordomo, J.I., Tjandrawan, T., DeLeo, A.B., Clarke, M.R., Lotze, M.T. and Storkus, W.J. (1996). Therapy of murine tumors with tumor peptide pulsed dendritic cells: dependence on T cells, B7 costimulation, and Th1-associated cytokines. *J. Exp. Med.* **183**, 87–97.
31. Celluzi, C.M., Mayordomo, J.I., Storkus, W.J., Lotze, M.T. and Falo, L.D. (1996). Peptide-pulsed dendritic cells induce antigen-specific, CTL-mediated protective tumor immunity. *J. Exp. Med.* **183**, 283–287.
32. Bakker, A.B.H., Marland, G., de Boer, A.J., Huijbens, J.F., Danen, E.H.J., Adema, G.J. and Figdor, D.G.T. (1995). Generation of antimelanoma cytotoxic T lymphocytes from healthy donors after of melanoma-associated antigen-derived epitopes by dendritic cells *in vitro. Cancer Res.* **55**, 5330–5334.
33. Tjandrawan, T., Mäurer, M.J., Castelli, C., Lotze, M.T. and Storkus, W.J. (1998). Autologous dendritic cells with synthetic melanoma peptides elicit specific CTL effector cells *in vitro. J. Immunother.* **21**, 149–157.
34. Specht, J.M., Wang, G., Do, M.T., Lam, J.S., Royal, R.E., Reeves, M.E., Rosenberg, S.A. and Hwu, P. (1997). Dendritic cells retrovirally transduced with a model antigen gene are therapeutically effective against established pulmonary metastases. *J. Exp. Med.* **186**, 1213–1221.
35. Nishioka, Y., Shurin, M., Robbins, P.D., Storkus, W.J., Lotze, M.T. (1997). Effective tumor immunotherapy using bone marrow-derived dendritic cells genetically engineered to express interleukin 12. *J. Immunother.* **20**, 419.
36. Brossart, P, Goldrath, A.W., Butz, E.A., Martin, S. and Bevan, M.J. (1997). Virus-mediated delivery of antigenic epitopes into dendritic cells as a means to induce CTL. *J. Immunol.* **158**, 3270–3276.
37. Ribas, A., Butterfield, L.H., McBride, W.H., Jilani, S.M., Bui, L.A., Vollmer, C.M., Lau, R., Dissette, V.B., Hu, B., Chen, A.Y., Glaspy, J.A. and Economou, J.S. (1997). Genetic immunization for the melanoma antigen MART-1/Melan-A using recombinant adenovirus-transduced murine dendritic cells. *Cancer Res.* **57**, 2865–2869.
38. Wan, Y., Bramson, J., Carter, R., Graham, F. and Gauldie, J. (1997). Dendritic cells transduced with an adenoviral vector encoding a model tumor-associated antigen for tumor vaccination. *Hum. Gene Ther.* **8**, 1335–1363.
39. Song, W., Kong, H.-L., Carpenter, H., Torii, H., Granstein, R., Rafii, S., Moore, M.A.S. and Crystal, R.G. (1997). Dendritic cells genetically modified with an adenovirus vector encoding the cDNA for a model antigen induce protective and therapeutic antitumor immunity. *J. Exp. Med.* **186**, 1247–1256.
40. Tüting, T., DeLeo, A., Lotze, M.T. and Storkus, W.J. (1997). Bone marrow-derived dendritic cells genetically-modified to express tumor-associated antigens induce antitumor immunity *in vivo. Eur. J. Immunol.* **27**, 2702–2707.
41. Manickan, E., Kanangat, S., Rouse, R.J.D., Yu, Z. and Rouse, B.T. (1997). Enhancement of immune response to naked DNA vaccine by immunization with transfected dendritic cells. *J. Leukocyte Biol.* **61**, 125–132.
42. Boczkowski, D., Nair, S.K., Snyder, D. and Gilboa, E. (1996). Dendritic cells pulsed with RNA are potent antigen-presenting cells *in vitro* and *in vivo. J. Exp. Med.* **184**, 465–472.
43. Henderson, R.A., Nimgaonkar, M.T., Watkins, S.C., Robbins, P.D., Ball, E.D. and Finn, O.J. (1996). Human dendritic cells genetically engineered to express high levels of the human epithelial tumor antigen mucin (MUC-1). *Cancer Res.* **56**, 3763–3770.
44. Reeves, M.E., Royal, R.E., Lam, J.S., Rosenberg, S.A. and Hwu, P. (1996). Retroviral transduction of human dendritic cells with a tumor-associated antigen gene. *Cancer Res.* **56**, 5672–5677.
45. Szabols, P., Gallardo, H.F., Ciocon, D.H., Sadelein, M. and Young, J.W. (1997). Retrovirally transduced an dendritic cells express a normal phenotype and potent T cell stimulatory capacity. *Blood* **90**, 2160–2167.
46. Aicher, A., Westermann, J., Cayeux, S., Willimsky, G., Daemen, K., Blankenstein, T., Uckert, W., Dorken, B. and Pezzutto, A. (1997). Successful retroviral mediated transduction of a reporter gene in an dendritic cells: feasibility of therapy with gene-modified antigen presenting cells. *Exp. Hematol.* **25**, 39–44.
47. Arthur, J.F., Butterfield, L.H., Roth, M.D., Bui, L.A., Kiertscher, S.M., Lau, R., Dubinette, S., Glaspy, A., McBride, W.H. and Economou, J.S. (1997). A comparison of gene transfer methods in human dendritic cells. *Cancer Gene Ther.* **4**, 17–25.

48. Alijagic, S., Moller, P., Artuc, M., Jurgovsky, K., Czarnetzki, B.M. and Schadendorf, D. (1995). Dendritic cells generated from peripheral blood transfected with human tyrosinase induce specific T cell activation. *Eur. J. Immunol.* **25**, 3100–3107.
49. Tüting, T., Wilson, C.C., Martin, D., Kasamon, Y., Rowles, J., Ma, D.I., Slingluff, C.L., Wagner, S.N., van der Bruggen, P., Baar, J., Lotze, M.T. and Storkus, W.J. (1998). Autologous human monocyte-derived dendritic cells genetically modified to express melanoma antigens elicit primary cytotoxic T cell responses *in vitro*: enhancement by cotransfection of genes encoding the Th1-biasing cytokines IL-12 and IFN-α. *J. Immunol.* **160**, 1139–1147.
50. Koide, S.L., Inaba, K. and Steinman, R. (1987). Interleukin-1 enhances T dependent immune responses by amplifying the function of dendritic cells. *J. Exp. Med.* **165**, 515–530.
51. McLellan, A.D., Sorg, R.V., Williams, L.A. and Hart, D.N.J. (1996). Human dendritic cells activate T lymphocytes via a CD40 : D40 ligand-dependent pathway. *Eur. J. Immunol.* **26**, 1204–1210.
52. Sallusto, F. and Lanzavecchia, A. (1994). Efficient presentation of soluble antigen by cultured human dendritic cells is maintained by granulocyte/macrophage colony-stimulating factor plus interleukin 4 and downgregulated by tumor necrosis factor α *J. Exp. Med.* **179**, 1109–1118.
53. Larsen, C.P., Ritchie, S.C., Hendrix, R., Linsley, P.S., Hathcock, K.S., Hodes, R.J., Lowry, R.P. and Pearson, T.C. (1994). Regulation of immunostimulatory function and costimulatory molecules (B7-1 and B7-2) expression on murine dendritic cells. *J. Immunol.* **152**, 5208–5219.
54. Bhardwaj, N., Seder, R.A., Reddy, A. and Feldman, M.V. (1996). IL-12 in conjunction with dendritic cells enhances antiviral $CD8^+$ CTL responses *in vitro*. *J. Clin. Invest.* **98**, 715–722.
55. Chouaib, S. *et al.* (1994). Interleukin 12 induces the differentiation of major histocompatibility complex class I-primed cytotoxic T-lymphocyte precursors into allospecific cytotoxic effectors. *Proc. Natl Acad. Sci. USA* **91**, 12659–12663.
56. Mehrotra, P.T., Wu, D., Crim, J.A., Mostowski, H.S. and Siegel, J.P. (1993). Effect of IL-12 on the generation of cytotoxic activity in human $CD8^+$ T lymphocytes. *J. Immunol.* **151**, 2444–2452.
57. Kim, C.J., Prevette, T., Cormier, J., Overwijk, W., Roden, M., Restifo, N.P., Rosenberg, S.A. and Marincola, F.M. (1997). Dendritic cells infected with poxviruses encoding MART-1/Melan A 15 sensitize T lymphocytes *in vitro*. *J. Immunother.* **20**, 276–286.
58. Wagner, E., Zatloukal, K., Cotton, M., Kirlappos, H., Mechtler, K., Curiel, D.T. and Birnstiel, M.L. (1992). Coupling of adenovirus to transferrin-polylysine/DNA complexes greatly enhances receptor-mediated gene delivery and expression of transfected genes. *Proc. Natl Acad. Sci. USA* **89**, 6099–6103.
59. Mulders, P., Pang, S., Dannull, J., Kaboo, R., Hinkel, A., Michel, L., Tso, C.L., Roth, M. and Belldegrun, A. (1998). Highly efficient and consistent gene transfer into dendritic cells utilizing a combination of ultraviolet-irradiated adenovirus and poly (L-lysine) conjugates. *Cancer Res.* **58**, 956–961.

CHAPTER 33
Dendritic–Tumor Cell Fusions

Jianlin Gong[1], David Avigan[2] and Donald Kufe[1]
[1]Cancer Pharmacology, Dana-Farber Cancer Institute, [2]Department of Medicine, Beth Israel-Deaconess Medical Center, Harvard Medical School Boston, Massachusetts, USA

INTRODUCTION

Immunological recognition of tumor-specific antigens has been documented in patients with malignancy [1–9]. However, responses are thought to be ineffective because tumor cells present antigen in the absence of crucial secondary signals needed to generate primary immune responses [10, 11]. A recent focus of investigation has been the use of dendritic cells (DC) to reverse tumor-induced anergy. DC richly express class I, class II, and costimulating molecules essential for the initiation of T cell responses [12–14]. Manipulation of DC to express tumor antigens has led to immunological rejection of tumors in animal models. Such manipulation has been accomplished through the pulsing of DC with tumor-specific peptides, proteins, or cell extracts, as well as through transfection or transduction of DC with genes encoding tumor-specific or associated antigens [15–21]. For example, animal studies have shown that DC pulsed with tumor peptides are effective in protecting animals from tumor challenge and mediate tumor regressions in cancer-bearing hosts [22]. Also, a clinical study using idiotype-pulsed DC for the treatment of B cell lymphoma has demonstrated efficacy without significant morbidity [23].

Strategies using DC-based vaccines have several potential shortcomings. Loading of tumor-specific peptides is inefficient and requires the presence of a particular HLA haplotype. The nature of tumor-specific or associated proteins is unknown for many human malignancies and the immunogenicity of those that have been identified is uncertain. Furthermore, strategies based on responses to a single antigen are susceptible to resistance mechanisms in which the tumor cell evades immunological detection through down-regulating expression of that antigen.

We have employed an alternative strategy for creating an anti-tumor vaccine by fusing DC with tumor cells [24, 25]. Hybrid cells are thereby created that express tumor antigens while concomitantly expressing costimulatory and adhesion molecules normally found on DC. The advantage of this approach is that tumor antigens, identified or unidentified, are presented by DC to directly activate naive T-lymphocytes. We have developed this approach using MC38 murine adenocarcinoma cells transfected to express the MUC1 tumor-associated antigen.

Dendritic Cells: Biology and Clinical Applications
ISBN 0-12-455860-7

TECHNIQUE OF DC–TUMOR CELL FUSIONS

Selection of DC

DC [26–29] are generated from murine bone marrow by methods described by Inaba and coworkers [30]. Bone marrow is flushed from long bones and red cells are lysed with ammonium chloride. Lymphocytes, granulocytes, B cells and Ia^+ cells are depleted from the bone marrow cells by incubation with monoclonal antibodies (mAbs) (1) 2.43, anti-CD8 (TIB 210; ATCC, Rockville, MD, USA); (2) GK1.5, anti-CD4 (TIB 207); (3) RA3-3A1/6.1, anti-B220/CD45R (TIB 146); (4) B21-2, anti-Ia (TIB 229); and (5) RB6-8C5, anti-Gr-1 (Pharmingen, San Diego, CA, USA), and then rabbit complement. The cells are plated in six-well culture plates with RPMI 1640 medium supplemented with 5% heat-inactivated FCS, 50 mM 2-mercaptoethanol, 1 mM HEPES (pH 7.4), 2 mM glutamine, 10 U/ml penicillin, 100 μg/ml streptomycin and 500 U/ml recombinant murine GM-CSF (Boehringer Mannheim, IN, USA). After culture for 5 days, non-adherent and loosely adherent cells are collected and replated in 100 mm Petri dishes (10^6 cells/ml; 8 ml/dish). The nonadherent cells are washed away after incubation for 30 min and GM-CSF in RPMI medium is added to the adherent cells. After 18 h, DC harvested for subsequent fusion have a purity over 90% as determined by FACS analysis.

Selection of Tumor Cells

MC38 adenocarcinoma cells were used in a syngeneic C57BL/6 mouse model. The cells were stably transfected with a cDNA encoding the MUC1 tumor-associated antigen. The MUC1 cDNA was isolated from an MCF-7 cell cDNA library [31] and cloned into the pLNSX vector driven by the SV40 promoter. Cells transduced with the empty pLNSX vector have been designated MC38/Neo, and those expressing the DF3/MUC1 molecule as MC38/MUC1.

The DF3/MUCl antigen is a high-molecular-mass glycoprotein which is over-expressed in certain human carcinomas that include breast cancer [32, 33]. Aberrant glycosylation of the DF3 protein core in tumor cells results in the generation of distinct epitopes not found in normal tissue. Studies have demonstrated that these normally cryptic epitopes are recognized by cytotoxic T-lymphocytes in patients with breast cancer [34]. MUC1 was transfected into the MC38 cell line to determine whether an identifiable tumor antigen could be effectively presented by the fusion cell and induce an antigen-specific CTL response. In addition, the MUC1 antigen served as a marker to verify successful creation of a fusion cell expressing both DC and cell line specific antigens.

Cell Fusion [35, 36]

DC and MC38/MUC1 cells were fused with 50% polyethylene glycol (PEG) in Dulbecco's PBS without Ca^{2+} and Mg^{2+} at pH 7.4 and 37°C. The fusion protocol is outlined in Fig. 1. DC have a limited lifespan and the unfused DC die over several days in culture. To prevent growth of unfused MC38/MUCl tumor cells, cells were cultured in media containing 10% FCS, as well as hypoxanthine, aminopterin, and thymidine (HAT) after completion of the fusion. These tumor cells express low levels of hypoxanthine phosphoribosyltransferase (HPRT). Therefore, only tumor cells fused with DC were capable of long-term survival. The fusion cells became loosely adherent and were easily harvested. Of note, the success of selecting fusion cells is not dependent on using tumor cells that express low levels of HPRT. Whereas HAT exposure

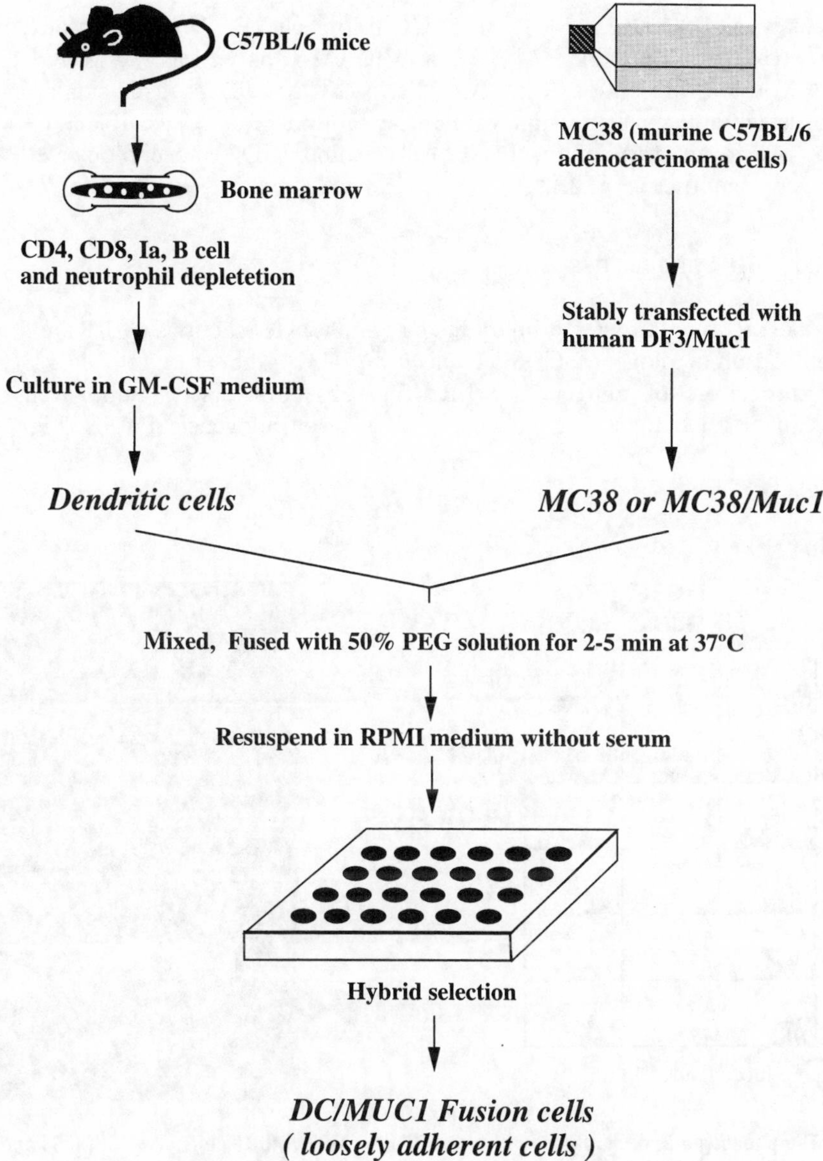

Fig. 1. Diagram of the fusion procedure.

represents one method of selection, tumor cells not sensitive to HAT can be removed by phenotypic characteristics such as their firm adherence to flasks or physical properties (i.e., size) that differ from those of fusion cells.

CHARACTERIZATION OF DC–TUMOR CELL FUSIONS

Phenotype and Morphology

FACS analysis of the DC and MC38/MUC1 fusion cells (FC/MUC1) revealed expression of MHC class I and II, B7-l, B7-2 and ICAM-1, as well as the MUC1 antigen (Fig. 2A). Fusion with untransfected MC38 cells (FC/MC38) results in similar patterns of cell surface antigen expression with the exception of no detectable DF3/MUC1 antigen. Moreover, most of the fusion cells exhibit a DC morphology with veiled processes or dendrites (Fig. 2B).

Activation of T-Lymphocytes

DC are potent stimulators of primary mixed lymphocyte reactions (MLR) and induce the proliferation of allogeneic $CD8^+$ T cells *in vitro* [37]. The fusion cells, like DC, were potent stimulators of allogeneic MLR (Fig. 3a). Conversely, tumor cells alone were incapable of inducing significant proliferation of allogeneic T cells (Fig. 3a). In

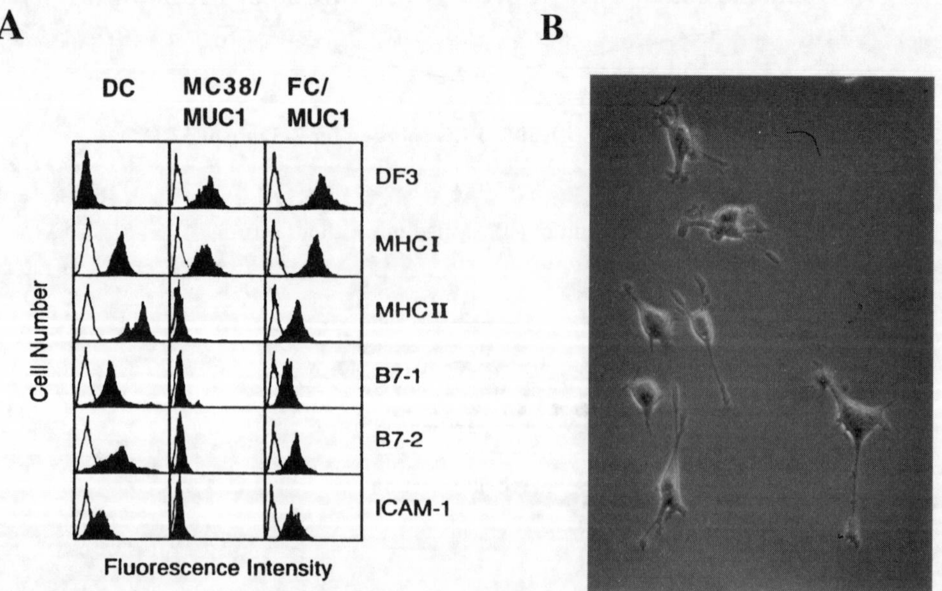

Fig. 2. The phenotype and morphology of fused DC and MC38/MUC1 cells. (A) DC, MC38 and fused cells (FC/MUC1) were analyzed by flow cytometry for the indicated antigens. (B) The morphology of fused cells was observed at 12 days.

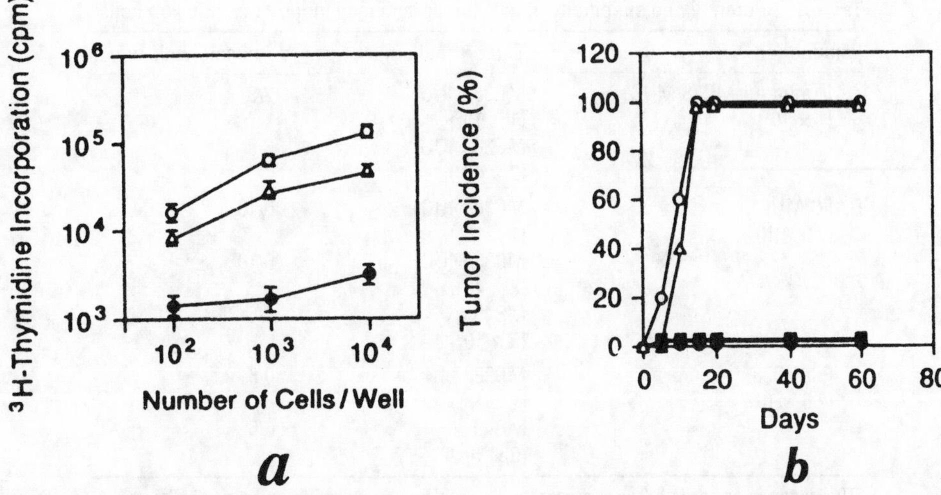

Fig. 3. Function of FC/MUC1 cells. (a) DC (○), MC38/MUC1 (●) and FC/MUC1 (△) were irradiated (30 Gy) and added at the indicated ratios to 1×10^5 allogeneic Balb/c T cells. Cells were cocultured for 5 days. [^{3}H]Thymidine uptake at 6 h of incubation is expressed as the mean ± SE of three determinations. Similar results were obtained in three separate experiments. (b) Female C57Bl/6 mice (10/group) were injected subcutaneously with: (i) 2×10^5 MC38/MUC1 cells (○); (ii) 2×10^6 DC mixed with 2×10^5 MC38/MUC1 cells (△); (iii) 2×10^5 FC/MUC1 cells (●); or (iv) 5×10^5 FC/MUC1 cells (■). Tumor incidence (≥3 mm in diameter) was monitored at the indicated days after injection. Similar results were obtained in three separate experiments.

tumorigenicity studies, inoculation of MC38/MUC1 cells into syngeneic mice results in the formation of subcutaneous tumors (Fig. 3b). Similar findings were obtained with DC mixed with MC38/MUC1 (Fig. 3b) or MC38 cells. However, no tumors developed in the mice injected with FC/MUC1 after 2–3 months of observation (Fig. 3b).

SPECIFIC ANTI-TUMOR IMMUNITY GENERATED WITH DC–TUMOR CELL FUSIONS

Assessment of Specific Anti-tumor Immunity

FC/MUC1 cells were examined for their ability to protect animals against challenge with tumor cells and for the generation of specific anti-tumor immunity *in vivo*. Syngeneic mice immunized twice with 10^6 irradiated MC38/MUC1 and then challenged with $1–2 \times 10^6$ MC38/MUC1 cells developed tumors (Table 1). Control animals immunized with DC alone or PBS and challenged subcutaneously with 2.5×10^5 MC38 or MC38/MUC1 cells exhibited tumor growth within 10–20 days (Fig. 4a). By contrast, mice immunized twice with 2.5×10^5 FC/MUC1 cells remained tumor-free after challenge with $1–2 \times 10^6$ MC38/MUC1 cells (Fig. 4a and Table 1). Similar findings were obtained after immunization with 2.5×10^5 FC/MC38 cells and then challenged

Table 1. Potency and specificity of anti-tumor immunity induced with fusion cells[a]

Immunogen	Tumor challenge	Animals with tumor
A. Irradiated MC38/MUC1 (1×10^6)	MC38/MUC1 (1×10^6)	2/3
	MC38/MUC1 (2×10^6)	3/3
B. FC/MUC1 (2.5×10^5)	MC38/MUC1 (1×10^6)	0/10
	MC38/MUC1 (2×10^6)	0/10
	MB49 (5×10^5)	6/6
C. FC/MC38 (2.5×10^5)	MC38 (1×10^6)	0/6
	MB49 (5×10^5)	6/6

[a]The numbers in parentheses represent cells used for immunization or tumor challenge.

with MC38 cells (Table 1). These findings indicate that the fusion cells are capable of inducing responses to tumor antigens other than MUC1. Moreover, immunization with FC/MUC1 or FC/MC38 cells had no detectable effect on growth of the unrelated syngeneic MB49 bladder carcinoma (Table 1).

Cytotoxic T-lymphocytes (CTLs) were isolated from mice immunized with FC/MUC1, DC alone, or PBS. CTLs from mice immunized with FC/MUC1 induced lysis of MC38/MUCl, but not MB49 cells (Fig. 4b and data not shown). By contrast, CTLs from mice immunized with DC or PBS exhibited no detectable lysis of the MC38/MUC1 targets (Fig. 4b). To further define the effectors responsible for anti-tumor activity, mice were injected intraperitoneally with antibodies against $CD4^+$ or $CD8^+$ cells before and after immunization with FC/MUC1. Depletion of the respective populations by 80–90% was confirmed with flow cytometric analysis of splenocytes (data not shown). The finding that injection of anti-CD4 and anti-CD8 antibodies increases tumor incidence indicated that both $CD4^+$ and $CD8^+$ T cells contribute to anti-tumor activity (Fig. 4c). Moreover, depletion of $CD4^+$ and $CD8^+$ T cells was associated with reduced lysis of MC38/MUC1 cells *in vivo* (Fig. 4d).

Prevention and Treatment of Pulmonary Metastases [38]

FC/MUC1 cells were examined for their ability to prevent tumor development and to eradicate established tumors. A murine model was used in which intravenous injection of MC38 cells produces widespread pulmonary metastases. Immunization with FC/MUC1 intravenously or subcutaneously completely protected against intravenous challenge with MC38/MUC1 cells (Fig. 5a). Control animals challenged with intravenous MC38/MUC1 cells developed over 250 pulmonary metastases (Fig. 5a). In the treatment model, MC38/MUC1 pulmonary metastases were established 4 days prior to immunization with FC/MUC1. While control mice treated with vehicle developed

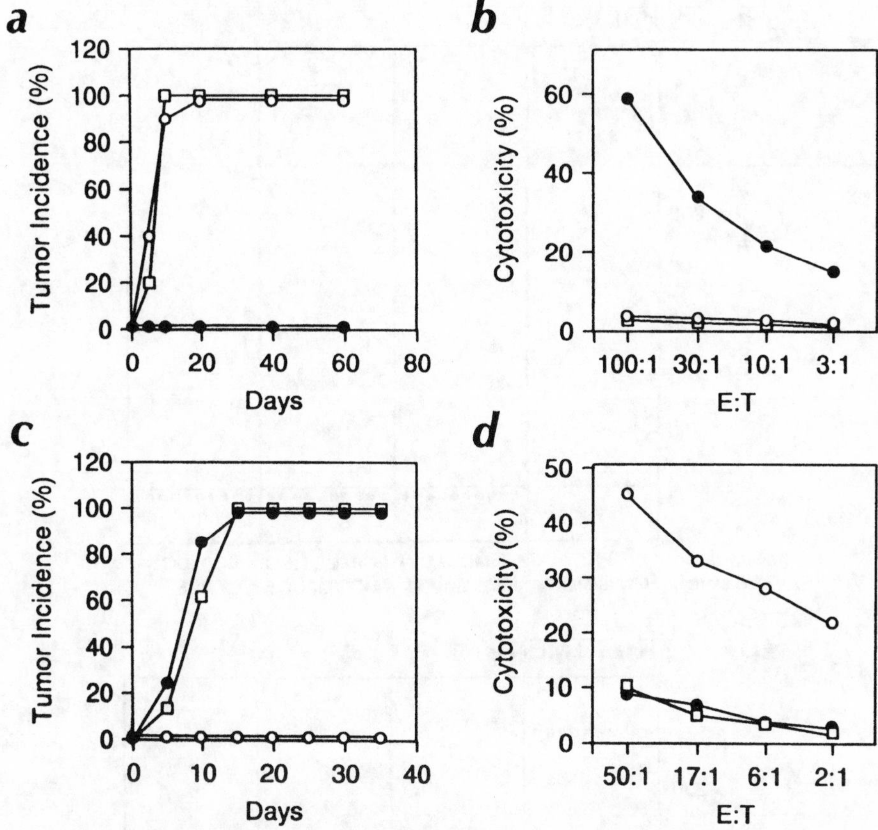

Fig. 4. Induction of anti-tumor activity by FC/MUC1. (a) Groups of 10 mice were immunized twice at 14-day intervals by subcutaneous injection of 3×10^5 DC (○) or FC/MUC1 cells (●). PBS was injected as a control (□). After 14 days, mice were challenged subcutaneously with 2.5×10^5 MC38/MUC1 cells. Tumors ≥3 mm in diameter were scored as positive. Similar results were obtained in three separate experiments. (b) Mice injected twice with DC (○), FC/MUC1 (●) or PBS (□) were challenged with 2.5×10^5 MC38/MUC1 tumor cells. Splenocytes were isolated at 20 days after challenge and incubated at the indicated E : T ratios with MC38/MUC1 target cells. CTL activity (mean ± SE) was determined by the 4 h LDH release assay. Similar results were obtained in three separate experiments. (c) Mice (8/group) were injected intravenously and intraperitoneally every other day with mAbs against $CD4^+$ (□) and $CD8^+$ (●) cells beginning 4 days before the first of two immunizations with FC/MUC1 and continuing until 4 days before challenge with 5×10^5 MC38/MUC1 cells. Rat IgG (○) was injected as a control. Tumors ≥3 mm were scored as positive. Similar results were obtained in two separate experiments. (d) Mice were treated as above with mAbs against $CD4^+$ (□) and $CD8^+$ (●) or rat IgG (○), immunized with FC/MUC1, and then challenged with MC38/MUC1 cells. Splenocytes were harvested at 20 days after tumor challenge and incubated with MC38/MUC1 cells. CTL activity (mean ± SE) was determined by the 4 h LDH release assay. Similar results were obtained in three separate experiments.

over 250 metastases, 9 of 10 mice treated with FC/MUC1 cells had no detectable metastases and one mouse had fewer than 10 nodules (Fig. 5b). Mice treated with FC/MC38 cells similarly had no detectable MC38 pulmonary metastases (Fig. 5b). These findings indicated that FC/MUC1 fused cells are effective in the treatment of established metastatic disease.

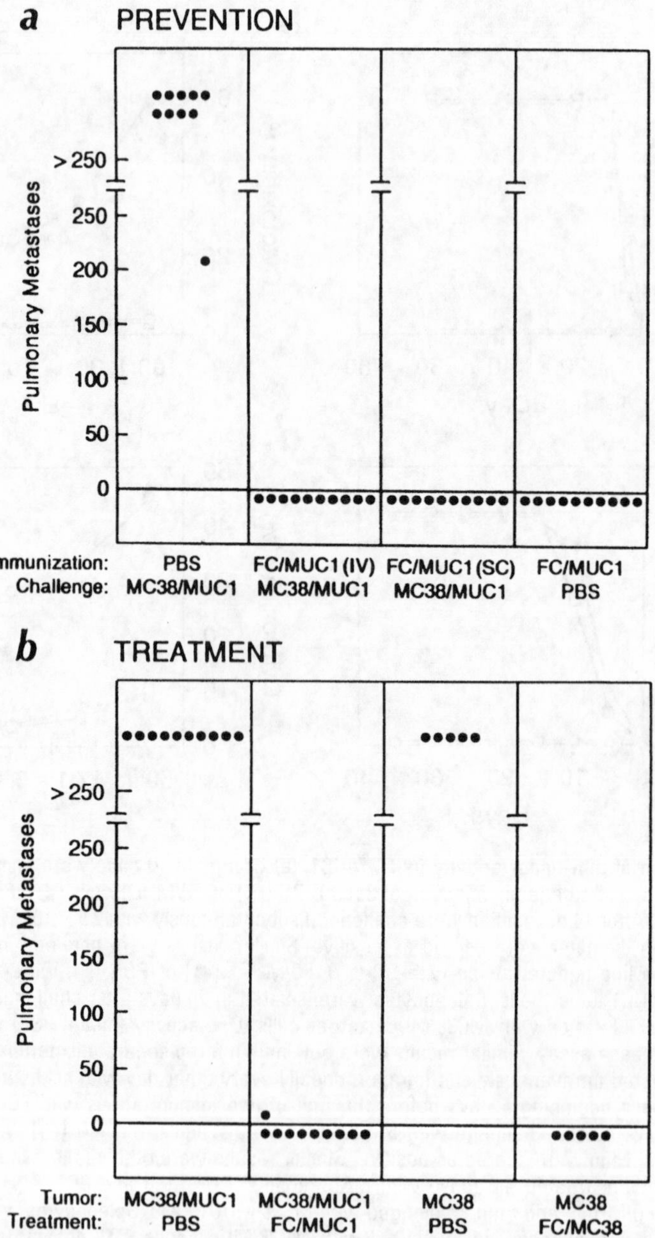

Fig. 5. Immunization with FC for prevention and treatment of pulmonary metastases. (a) Groups of 10 mice were injected twice with FC/MUC1 cells or PBS and then challenged after 14 days with intravenous administration of 1×10^6 MC38/MUC1 cells. The mice were sacrificed 28 days after challenge. Pulmonary metastases were enumerated after staining the lungs with india ink. (b) Groups of 10 mice were injected intravenously with 1×10^6 MC38/MUC1 or MC38 cells. The mice were immunized with 1×10^6 FC/MUC1 or FC/MC38 at 4 and 18 days after tumor challenge and then sacrificed after an additional 10 days. Pulmonary metastases were enumerated for each mouse. Similar results were obtained in two separate experiments (10/10 mice treated with FC/MUC1 had no pulmonary metastases in the second experiment).

DESIGN OF HUMAN DC–TUMOR CELL FUSIONS

Sources of Human Dendritic Cells

Recent efforts have focused on the development of successful fusions between human DC and tumor cells in an attempt to create effective anti-tumor vaccines for clinical use. However, the generation of large numbers of functionally active DC from patients with malignancy has remained a challenge. Mature DC are present in only trace amounts in the peripheral blood. DC have been successfully generated from $CD34^+$ cells in bone marrow and cord blood cultured in the presence of appropriate cytokines [39, 40]. DC have also been produced by isolation of intermediate precursor populations in the human blood [41]. Our group has recently found that peripheral blood progenitor cells (PBPC) collected from patients with advanced breast cancer undergoing autologous transplantation are rich in DC precursors [42]. Patients were treated with chemotherapy followed by GM/G-CSF or G-CSF alone, and PBPCs were collected upon WBC recovery following the nadir period. The cells were then cultured with GM-CSF and IL-4 for 1 week in the presence of human sera. One ml of PBPC generated $6–60 \times 10^6$ functionally active DC. On FACS analysis, the cells prominently expressed class II and costimulatory molecules, as well as CD83. The isolated cells were also potent stimulators of allogeneic MLR and were capable of processing and presenting tetanus antigen to autologous T cells. Thus, the isolation procedure provides a potential source of DC for human fusions.

Sources of Human Tumor Cells

Two sources of tumor cells for fusion have been explored.

Tumor cell lines. Tumor cell lines have been used for the initial human fusion studies because of their stability for *in vitro* growth. Specifically, we have used human MCF-7 breast cancer cells which express MUC1 and cytokeratin. The cells were maintained in DMEM supplemented with 10% heat-inactivated fetal calf serum (FCS), 2 mM glutamine, 100 U/ml penicillin, and 100 μg/ml streptomycin.

Primary tumor cells from patients. Patient-derived primary or metastatic breast tumor cells are separated from surgical specimens by digestion with collagenase, hyaluronidase and DNAse (C/H/D, 1 : 0.1 : 1 mg/ml) in Ca^{2+}/Mg^{2+}-free Hanks' balanced salt solution (pH 7.3–7.5). The cells are maintained short-term in suspension culture. Culturing of primary breast tumor cells can be difficult. However, we have found that fusion with DC can result in stable expression of the MUC1 tumor-associated antigen and therefore potentially others that are as yet unknown.

Human DC–Tumor Cell Fusions

Fusions of human DC (HuDC) with MCF-7 cells were accomplished following a similar protocol to that outlined above in murine model. Briefly, MCF-7 cells were mixed with HuDC and extensively washed in serum-free medium (RPMI 1640). 50% PEG was used for the fusion. After 5 min, the PEG was progressively diluted by slow addition of serum-free medium. The cells were washed free of PEG and resuspended in RPMI 1640 medium with 10% human serum and 100 U/ml of GM-CSF in 24-well

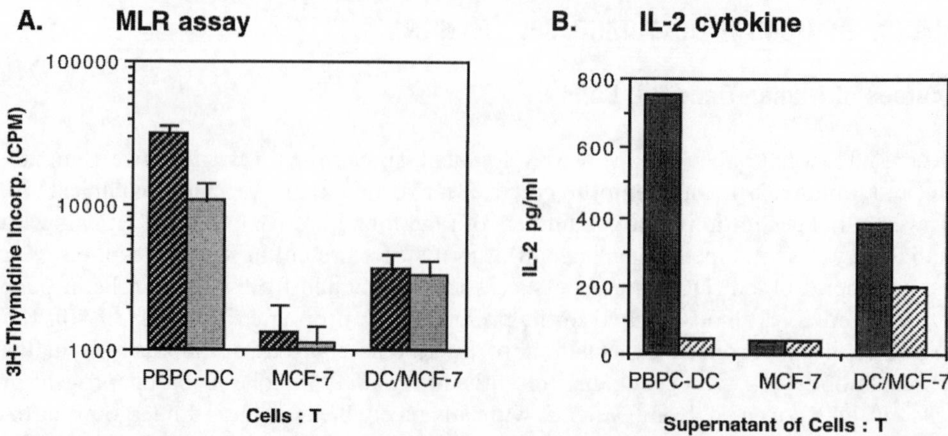

Fig. 7. Activation of T cells by HuDC/MCF7. (A) Patient DC generated from PBPC and fused with MCF-7 cells (HuDC/MCF-7) or irradiated MCF-7 cells were cocultured with 1 : 20, 1 : 40, 1 : 80, and 1 : 160 allogeneic (hatched bars) and syngeneic (grey bars) T cells. After 5 days, [^{3}H]thymidine uptake at 12 h of incubation is expressed at the mean ± SE of three determinations. (B) Supernatants collected from HuDC, MCF-7, and HuDC/MCF-7 fusion cells were cocultured with allogeneic (solid bars) and autologous (hatched bars) T cells at day 3 and analyzed for IL-2 by ELISA.

plates with 1×10^4 tumor cells number per well. After 1–2 weeks of culture, the loosely adherent fusion cells were assayed for the presence of DC and tumor markers and for functional characteristics.

The HuDC–MCF-7 fused cells (FC/MCF7) express MUC1 and cytokeratin, as well as costimulatory and MHC class I, II molecules (Plate 33.6A). Double immunoperoxidase staining revealed concurrent expression of MUC1 and DR (Plate 33.6C). Western blotting revealed the presence of the MUC1 protein in the fusion cells, but not in the DC alone (Plate 33.6B). The fusion cells were potent stimulators of allogeneic MLR at a level comparable to that obtained for DC alone. By contrast, MCF-7 cells were poor inducers of allogeneic T cell proliferation (Fig. 7A). Importantly, the fusion cells induced proliferative responses of autologous T cells associated with an increase in IL-2 production (Fig. 7B). No change in cytokine production was seen when DC isolated from normal volunteers were fused to MCF-7 cells and cocultured with autologous T cells. These results indicate that reactivity is not simply to allogeneic antigens and that breast cancer patients may have circulating T cells that have been primed against tumor-associated antigens.

Clinical Trial

The next phase of investigation will be the design of a clinical trial to determine whether DC–tumor fusion cells are capable of inducing anti-tumor responses *in vivo*. In adapting this strategy to the clinical setting, a reliable source of both tumor cells and DC will be required for serial vaccinations. Preclinical studies will focus on the use of both cell lines and primary tumor cells to generate HuDC–tumor fusions. While carcinoma cell lines offer a convenient and easily maintained source of tumor, their safety in clinical studies has not been well established. In addition, the use of tumor cell lines would potentially lead to the induction of allogeneic responses that may overwhelm tumor-specific reactions and may also result in unpredictable immunological sequelae. Therefore, primary autologous tumor cells will be used when possible in clinical trials.

In an initial experiment, we have shown that primary breast cancer cultures can be established from patient-derived tissue samples. Mastectomy specimens have been processed and placed into single-cell suspensions for 5 days. At the time of harvest, the tumor cells have demonstrated excellent viability with a minority of contaminating stromal cells. Immunocytochemical staining has revealed that the tumor cells express MUC1 and cytokeratin, but not DR. Fusions of the tumor cells and autologous DC have generated cells that express both MUC1 and DR.

Initial clinical studies will focus on defining the toxicity and optimal dosing of fusion vaccines and will involve patients with advanced breast cancer who have been unresponsive to conventional treatment. Subsequent trials will involve patients in a minimal disease setting, such as those with high-risk stage II disease or after autologous transplantation, where immunotherapy may prove to be crucial in eliminating minimal residual disease. Patients will undergo biopsy of lesions and tumor cells will be grown in primary culture. DC will be isolated from patient PBMC and fused with tumor cells as outlined above. Strategies for cryopreservation are currently being explored so that fusion cells can be stored. The fusion cells will be irradiated and serial vaccinations will be given. Toxicity profiles and immunological changes will be followed as primary end points. Initial studies will involve escalating doses of fusion cells to determine the relationship between dose, toxicity, and efficacy.

The use of DC–breast cancer fusion cells potentially allows for the presentation of multiple tumor antigens in the context of DC-mediated costimulation. If efficacious, this approach should result in the breaking of tumor-induced anergy and the activation and amplification of tumor-directed CTL clones. Immunological measurement of this effect will focus on the frequency of tumor-specific CTL in the patient's peripheral blood prior to and following vaccination.

SUMMARY

DC are potent antigen-presenting cells that prime naive CTL. In this chapter, we describe a DC-based strategy of fusing DC with carcinoma cells. The fusion cells are positive for MHC class I and II, costimulating molecules, and ICAM-1. The results show that the fusion cells stimulate naive T cells in the primary mixed leukocyte reaction (MLR) and induce tumor-specific CTL *in vivo*. Antibody-mediated depletion experiments demonstrate that induction of $CD4^+$ and/or $CD8^+$ CTL protects against challenge with tumor cells. Immunization with fusion cells induces rejection of established metastases. Results obtained in human DC–tumor fusion studies indicate that fusion cells could be evaluated in the clinical setting.

REFERENCES

1. Hellstrom, K.E. and Hellstrom, I. (1969). *Cellular Immunity Against Tumor Specific Antigens*. Academic Press, New York.
2. Hellstrom, I. and Hellstrom, K.E. (1968). Cell mediated reactivity to human tumor type associated antigens: does it exist? *J. Biol. Response Modif.* **2**, 1352–1355.

3. Boon, T. and Van der Bruggen. (1996). Human tumor antigens recognized by T lymphocytes. *J. Exp. Med.* **183**, 725–729.
4. Carrel, S. and Johnson, J.P. (1993). Immunologic recognition of malignant melanoma by autologous T lymphocytes. *Curr. Opin. Oncol.* **5**, 383–389.
5. Storkus, W.J., Zeh III, H.J., Maeurer, M.J., Salter, R.D. and Lotze, M.T. (1993). Identification of human melanoma peptides recognized by class I restricted tumor infiltrating T lymphocytes. *J. Immunol.* **151**, 3719–3727.
6. Cox, A.L., Skipper, J., Chen, Y., Henderson, R.A., Darrow, T.L., Shabanowitz, J., Engelhard, V.H., Hunt, D.F. and Slingluff Jr., C.L. (1994). Identification of a peptide recognized by five melanoma-specific human cytotoxic T cell lines. *Science* **264**, 716–719.
7. Patel, B.T., Lutz, M.B., Schlag, P. and Schirrmacher, V. (1992). An analysis of autologous T-cell antitumor responses in colon carcinoma patients following active specific immunization (ASI). *Int. J. Cancer.* **51**, 878–885.
8. Ioannides, C.G. and Freedman, R.S. (1991). T cell responses to ovarian tumor vaccines: identification and significance for future immunotherapy. *Int. Rev. Immunol.* **7**, 349–364.
9. Kawakami, Y., Eliyahu, S., Delgado, C.H., Robbins, P.F., Sakaguchi, K., Appella, E., Yannelli, J.R., Adema, G.J., Miki, T. and Rosenberg, S.A. (1994). Identification of a human melanoma antigen recognized by tumor-infiltrating lymphocytes associates with in vivo tumor rejection. *Proc. Natl Acad. Sci. USA* **91**, 6458–6462.
10. Townsend, S.E. and Allison, J.P. (1993). Tumor rejection after direct costimulation of $CD8^+$ T cells by B7 transfected melanoma cells. *Science* **259**, 368–370.
11. Speiser, D.E., Miranda, R., Zakarian, A., Bachmann, M.F., McKall-Faienza, K., Odermatt, B., Hanahan, D., Zinkernagel, R.M. and Ohashi, P.S. (1997). Self antigens expressed by solid tumors do not efficiently stimulate naive or activated T cells: implications for immunotherapy. *J. Exp. Med.* **186**, 645–653.
12. Steinman, R.M. (1991). The dendritic cell system and its role in immunogenicity. *Annu. Rev. Immunol.* **9**, 271–296.
13. Young, J.W., Koulova, L., Soergel, S.A., Clark, E.A., Steinman, R.M. and Dupont, B. (1992). The B7/BB1 antigen provides one of several costimulatory signals for the activation of $CD4^+$ T lymphocytes by human blood dendritic cells in vitro. *J. Clin. Invest.* **90**, 229–237.
14. Inaba, K., Witmer-Pack, M., Inaba, M., Hathcock, K. S., Sakuta, H., Azuma, M., Yagita, H., Okumura, K., Linsley, P.S., Ikehara, S., Muramatsu, S., Hodes, R.J. and Steinman, R.M. The tissue distribution of the B7-2 costimulator in mice: abundant expression on dendritic cells in situ and during maturation in vitro. *J. Exp. Med.* **180**, 1849–1860.
15. Young, J.W. and Inaba, K. (1996). Dendritic cells as adjuvants for class I major histocompatibility complex-restricted antitumor immunity. *J. Exp. Med.* **183**, 7–11.
16. Inaba, K., Metlay, J.P., Crowley, M.T. and Steinman, R.M. (1990). Dendritic cells pulsed with protein antigens in vitro can prime antigen-specific, MHC-restricted T cells in situ. *J. Exp. Med.* **172**, 631–640.
17. Flamand, V., Sornasse, T., Thielemans, K., Demanet, C., Bakkus, M., Bazin, H., Tielemens, F., Leo, O., Urbain, J. and Moser, M. (1994). Murine dendritic cells pulsed in vitro with tumor antigen induce tumor resistance in vivo. *Eur. J. Immunol.* **24**, 605–610.
18. Boczkowski, D., Nair, S.K., Snyder, D. and Gilboa, E. (1996). Dendritic cells pulsed with RNA are potent antigen-presenting cells in vitro and in vivo. *J. Exp. Med.* **184**, 465–472.
19. Celluzzi, C.M., Mayordomo, C.I., Storkus, W.J., Lotze, M.T. and Falo, L.D. (1996). Peptide-pulsed dendritic cells induce antigen-specific CTL-mediated protective tumor immunity. *J. Exp. Med.* **183**, 283–287.
20. Reeves, M.E, Royal, R.E, Lam, J.S, Rosenberg, S.A. and Hwu, P. (1996). Retroviral transduction of human dendritic cells with a tumor-associated antigen gene. *Cancer Res.* **56**, 5672–5677.
21. Gong, J.L., Chen, L., Chen, D., Kashiwaba, M., Manome, Y., Tanaka, T. and Kufe, D. (1997). Induction of antigen specific antitumor immunity with adenoviral transduced dendritic cells. *Gene Ther.* **4**, 1023–1028.
22. Mayordomo, J.I., Zorina, T., Storkus, W.J., Zitvogel, L., Celluzzi, C., Falo, L.D., Melief, C.J., Ildstad, S.T., Kast, W.M., Deleo, A.B. and Lotze, M.T. (1995). Bone marrow-derived dendritic cells pulsed with synthetic tumour peptides elicit protective and therapeutic antitumour immunity. *Nature Medicine* **1**, 1297–1302.

23. Hsu, F.J., Bennike, C., Fagnoni, F., Liles, T.M., Czerwinski, D., Taidi, B., Engleman, E.G. and Levy, R. (1996). Vaccination of patients with B-cell lymphoma using autologous antigen-pulsed dendritic cells. *Nature Medicine* **2**, 52–58.
24. Gong, J.L., Chen, D., Kashiwaba, M. and Kufe, D. (1997). Induction of antitumor activity by immunization with fusions of dendritic and carcinoma cells. *Nature Medicine* **3**, 558–561.
25. Hart, I. and Colaco, C. (1997). Fusion induces tumor rejection. *Nature* **388**, 626–627.
26. Freudenthal, P.S. and Steinman, R.M. (1990). The distinct surface of human blood dendritic cells, as observed after an improved isolation method. *Proc. Natl Acad. Sci. USA* **87**, 7698–7702.
27. Inaba, K., Inaba, M., Romani, N., Aya, H., Deguchi, M., Ikehara. S., Muramatsu, S. and Steinman. R.M. (1993). Granulocytes, macrophages and dendritic cells arise from a common major histocompatibility complex class II-negative progenitor in mouse bone marrow. *Proc. Natl Acad. Sci. USA* **90**, 3038–3042.
28. Gong, J.L., McCarthy, K.M., Rogers, R.A. and Schneeberger, E.E. (1994). Interstitial lung macrophages interact with dendritic cells to present antigenic peptides derived from particulate antigen to T cells. *Immunology* **81**, 343–351.
29. Romani, N., Koide, S., Crowley, M., Witmer-Pack, M., Livingstone, A.M., Fathman, C.G., Inaba, K. and Steinman, R.M. (1989). Presentation of exogenous protein is presented best by immature, epidermal Langerhans cells. *J. Exp. Med.* **169**, 1169–1178.
30. Inaba, K., Inaba, M., Romani, N., Aya, H., Deguch, M., Ikehara, S., Muramatsu, S. and Steinman, R.M. (1992). Generation of large numbers of dendritic cells from mouse bone marrow cultures supplemented with granulocyte/macrophage colony-stimulating factor. *J. Exp. Med.* **176**, 1693–1702.
31. Siddiqui, J., Abe, M., Hayes, D., Shani, E., Yunis, E. and Kufe, D. (1988). Isolation and sequencing of a cDNA coding for the human DF3 breast carcinoma-associated antigen. *Proc. Natl Acad. Sci. USA* **85**, 2320–2323.
32. Kufe, D.W., Ighirami, G., Abe, M., Hayes, D., Justi-Wheeler, H. and Schlom, J. (1984). Differential of a novel monoclonal antibody (DF3) with human malignant versus benign breast tumors. *Hybridoma* **3**, 223–232.
33. Hayes, D.F., Mesa-Teja, R., Papsidero, L.D., Croghan, G.A., Korzun, A.H., Norton, L., Wood, W., Holland, J., Grimes, M., Weiss, R.B., Ree, J.H., Thor, A.D., Koerner, F.C., Rice, M.A., Barcos, M. and Kufe, D.W. (1991). Prediction of prognosis in primary breast cancer by detection of a high molecular weight mucin-like antigen using monoclonal antibodies DF3, F36/22, and CU18: a cancer a leukemia Group B study. *J. Clin. Oncol.* **9**, 1113–1123.
34. Jerome, K.R., Brand, D.L., Bendt, K.M., Boyer, C.M., Taylor-Papadimitriou. J., McKenzie, I.F.C., Bast, R.C. Jr and Finn, O.J. (1991). Cytotoxic T-lymphocytes derived from patients with breast adenocarcinoma recognize an epitope present on the protein core of a mucin molecule preferentially expressed by malignant cells. *Cancer Res.* **51**, 2908–2916.
35. Galfre, G. and Milstein, C. (1981). Preparation of monoclonal antibodies: strategies and procedures. *Methods Enzymol.* **3**, 3–46.
36. Harlow, E.D. and Lane, D. (1988) *Antibodies. A Laboratory Manual.* Cold Spring Harbor Laboratory Press, Cold Spring Harbor, NY, chapter 6-7, pp. 139–281.
37. Inaba, K., Young, J.W. and Steinman, R.M. (1987). Direct activation of $CD8^+$ cytotoxic T lymphocytes by dendritic cells. *J. Exp. Med.* **166**, 182–194.
38. Wexler, H. (1966) Accurate identification of experimental pulmonary metastases. *J. Natl Cancer Inst.* **36**, 641–643.
39. Reid, C.D.L., Stackpoole, A., Meager, A. *et al.* (1992). Interactions of tumor necrosis factor with granulocyte-macrophage colony-stimulating factor and other cytokines in the regulation of dendritic cell growth in vitro from early bipotent $CD34^+$ progenitors in human bone marrow. *J. Immunol.* **149**, 2681–2688.
40. Young, J.W. and Steinman, R.M. (1996). The hematopoietic development of dendritic cells: A distinct pathway for myeloid differentiation. *Stem Cells* **14**, 376–387.
41. Romani, N., Gruner, S., Brang, D., Kampgen, E., Lenz, A., Trockenbacher, B., Konwalinka, G., Fritsch, P.O., Steinman, R.M. and Schuler, G. (1994). Proliferating dendritic cell progenitors in human blood. *J. Exp. Med.* **180**, 83–94.
42. Avigan, D., Gong, J., Chen, D., Anderson, K. and Kufe, D.W. Dendritic cells derived from unmanipulated peripheral blood stem cells harvested from patients undergoing autologous transplantation for advanced breast cancer, submitted.

CHAPTER 34
Regulation of Antigen Capture, MHC Biosynthesis and Degradation Optimizes Presentation of Infectious Antigens in Maturing Dendritic Cells

Marina Cella, Mariolina Salio, Doris Scheidegger, Anneke Engering, Jean Pieters, Federica Sallusto and Antonio Lanzavecchia
Basel Institute for Immunology, Basel, Switzerland

MONOCYTE-DERIVED DENDRITIC CELLS AS A MODEL FOR DENDRITIC CELL MATURATION

In the late 1980s, the ground-breaking work of Steinman and coworkers established that dendritic cells (DC) exist in two stages of differentiation (Kampgen *et al.*, 1991; Pure *et al.*, 1990; Romani *et al.*, 1989; Schuler and Steinman, 1985; Steinman, 1991). The immature DC are present in nonlymphoid tissues, where their function is to capture antigen and subsequently migrate to secondary lymphoid organs where they stimulate naive T cells. By the time they reach the lymph nodes they switch their properties, losing antigen-capturing capacity while acquiring the ability to stimulate T cells. From this early work it was clear that a better understanding of the mechanism of antigen capture, and of the signals that trigger DC maturation, is a key not only to understanding the biology of these cells, but also to exploiting them as therapeutic agents.

An *in vitro* model originally described by Sallusto and coworkers proved particularly useful for studying the life cycle of human DC (Sallusto *et al*, 1995; Sallusto and Lanzavecchia, 1994) (outlined in Fig. 1). By culturing human peripheral blood monocytes with GM-CSF and IL-4 it is possible to generate a virtually pure population of immature DC characterized by high endocytic activity but low T cell stimulatory capacity. These immature DC can be driven to mature rapidly by stimulation with TNF-α, IL-1, or LPS, which results in downregulation of the endocytic activity while increasing the expression of adhesion and costimulatory molecules. The resulting mature DC can be activated to an even greater stimulatory level by stimulation with CD40L, which results in further upregulation of costimulatory molecules as well as in the production of the T_H1-polarizing cytokine IL-12 (Cella *et al.*, 1996; Heufler *et al.*, 1996). These results formally established the importance of inflammatory stimuli and T cell help in activation of antigen-presenting cells (APC) and provided a novel model of T–T cell collaboration via the activation of DC. Below we summarize a series of experiments that

Dendritic Cells: Biology and Clinical Applications
ISBN 0-12-455860-7

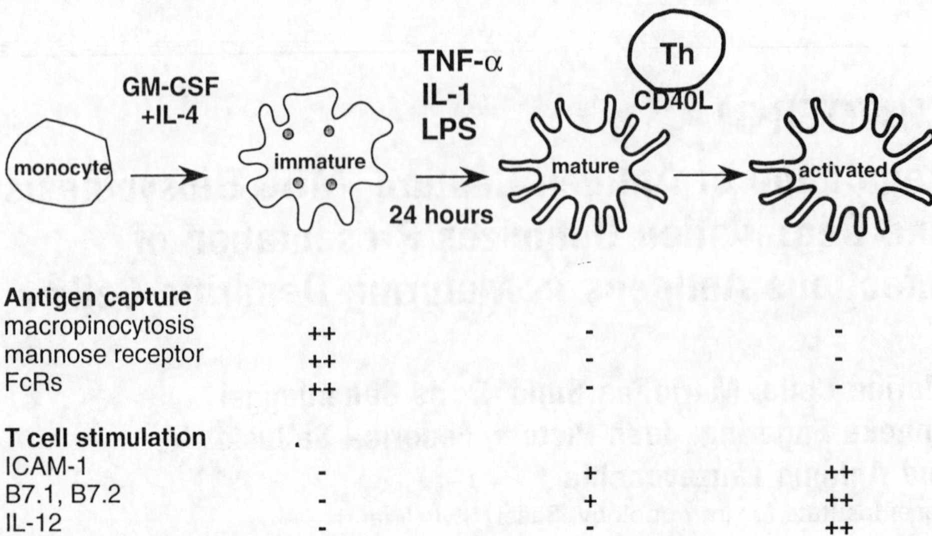

Fig. 1. Generation, maturation, and activation of dendritic cells. Human peripheral blood monocytes cultured in medium supplemented with GM-CSF and IL-4 develop into typical veiled cells characterized by high endocytic activity, but low T cell stimulatory capacity. Inflammatory cytokines (TNF-α and IL-1 or LPS) rapidly convert these cells into mature DC. This involves the downregulation of endocytic activity and the upregulation of adhesion, costimulatory, and MHC molecules. Stimulation by T cells via CD40 ligand may further upregulate costimulatory and adhesion molecules and selectively trigger IL-12 production. The whole process from monocytes to immature, mature, and activated DC is highly efficient (up to 80–90% of initial input) and does not involve cell proliferation as demonstrated by BrdU incorporation.

address the mechanisms that optimize presentation of infectious antigens on class I and class II molecules in maturing DC and discuss the relevance of these findings for immunotherapy.

IMMATURE DC EFFICIENTLY PRESENT SOLUBLE ANTIGENS TAKEN UP BY FLUID-PHASE OR RECEPTOR-MEDIATED ENDOCYTOSIS

Immature DC have extraordinarily high levels of endocytic activity (Sallusto *et al.*, 1995). They have a high constitutive level of macropinocytosis that allows them to take up large volumes of fluid (as much as the cell's own volume every 2 hours) and concentrate the macrosolutes in the endocytic compartment. In addition, they possess the mannose receptor, a pattern-recognition molecule that allows efficient uptake of mannosylated and fucosylated antigens, as well as the Fc receptor, CD32, which allows capture of immune complexes. As shown in Fig. 2a, immature DC are extremely efficient APC. They can present tetanus toxoid (TT), which is taken up by fluid phase at concentrations of $\sim 10^{-10}$ M, and are therefore as efficient as TT-specific B cells that take up this antigen via specific mIg (Fig. 2b). Presentation of soluble antigen by DC can be further boosted ~100-fold by targeting the antigen to CD32 or to the mannose receptor (Engering *et al.*, 1997; Sallusto and Lanzavecchia, 1994). When mannosylated TT or TT complexed with specific IgG antibodies was used, presentation was observed at tetanus toxoid (TT) concentrations lower than 10^{-12} M,

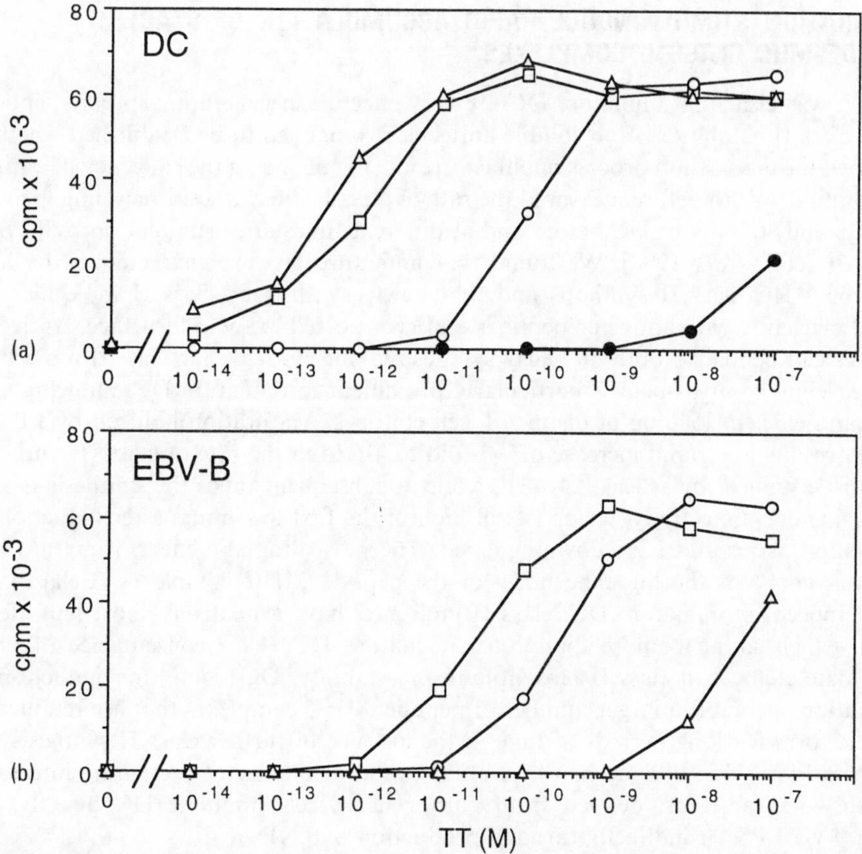

Fig. 2. Immature DC are the most efficient APC for presentation of soluble antigens. Proliferative response of a tetanus toxoid (TT)-specific class II-restricted T cell clone to increasing concentrations of TT in the presence of different APC. (a) Presentation by immature DC (open symbols) or by mature DC (solid symbols). The antigen was soluble TT (circles), mannosylated TT (triangles), or TT complexed to IgG antibodies (squares). (b) Presentation of soluble TT by nonspecific (triangles) or TT-specific (squares and circles) EBV-transformed B cell clones.

definitively demonstrating that immature DC are the most efficient APC for capture and presentation of soluble antigen. As originally reported by Schuler and coworkers (Kampgen *et al.*, 1991), mature DC, although highly stimulatory for allogeneic T cells, are unable to take up and present soluble antigens (Fig. 2a), a fact that is explained by the rapid downregulation of both endocytic activity and MHC class II biosynthesis upon maturation. One should note that these experiments were performed with T cell clones which did not require high levels of costimulatory molecules. Thus the dose–response curves reflect the generation of specific peptide–MHC complexes and are minimally affected by T cell stimulatory capacity. In fact, the capacity to stimulate a primary mixed leukocyte response (MLR) from naive cord blood T cells is far superior in mature than in immature DC (Cella *et al.*, 1996; Sallusto and Lanzavecchia, 1994).

MATURATION STIMULI INDUCE RAPID ACCUMULATION OF STABLE PEPTIDE–MHC CLASS II COMPLEXES

While it was clear that immature DC are very effective in generating specific peptide–MHC class II complexes from soluble antigens, it remained to be established whether, and how, the maturation process might contribute to enhancing the efficiency of antigen presentation. We therefore measured the rate of class II biosynthesis, recycling, peptide loading, and stability in DC before and at different times after stimulation by LPS or TNF-α (Cella *et al.*, 1997). We found that immature DC are characterized by high levels of MHC class II synthesis and that newly synthesized class II molecules are loaded efficiently with antigenic peptides and transported to the cell surface. Antigenic peptides can be loaded both on newly synthesized and on recycling class II molecules. The recycling compartment is particularly prominent in immature DC, allowing very rapid and efficient loading of distinct T cell epitopes. Maturation induced by LPS or TNF-α results in a rapid increase of ~3-fold to 4-fold in the rate of class II synthesis, which is sustained for at least 24–48 h, while at subsequent times the synthesis is shut off. The endocytic activity, which is still high in the first few hours after induction of maturation, is progressively downregulated. The most dramatic effect of maturation, however, concerns the life expectancy of the peptide–MHC complexes (Cella *et al.*, 1997). Indeed, in immature DC, class II molecules have a relatively short half-life of ~10 h, which shifts to more than 100 h in mature DC. As a consequence of these coordinate changes in class II biosynthesis and stability, DC, soon after induction of maturation, assemble a larger number of peptide–MHC complexes that are retained in a stable form for long periods of time in the absence of further class II synthesis. As shown in Plate 34.3, this mechanism optimizes the possibility of presenting infectious antigens—i.e., antigens, derived from pathogens, which stimulate DC directly, for instance via LPS, or indirectly through production of TNF-α.

ENHANCED AND SUSTAINED SYNTHESIS OF CLASS I MOLECULES IN MATURE DC FAVORS PRESENTATION OF VIRAL ANTIGENS

When biosynthesis and stability of class I molecules were measured in maturing DC, a different picture emerged (Cella *et al.*, 1997). As shown in Plate 34.4, maturation stimuli such as TNF-α and LPS induce a very dramatic upregulation of class I biosynthesis (up to 10-fold). In contrast to what is observed for class II molecules, the biosynthesis of class I molecules is sustained for several days. In addition, the half-life of class I molecules does not change significantly after maturation, remaining relatively short (~10–20 h) even at late times. This relatively short half-life may reflect an intrinsically greater instability of class I as compared to class II molecules in living cells.

The difference in stability between class I and class II molecules makes good sense if we consider the different functions of these two systems of peptide presentation (Germain, 1994). Class II molecules should present antigens which are transiently encountered in the surrounding environment of a DC present in a peripheral tissue, so it is important that DC make a maximum effort to load antigenic peptides over a short period of exposure to the antigen and then retain them as stable complexes. On the other hand, class I molecules should present endogeneously synthesized antigens, so that it is instrumental that these complexes be continuously generated inside the cell to allow expression of all possible viral proteins for the time that the cell remains infected.

IMPLICATIONS FOR THE THERAPEUTIC EXPLOITATION OF DENDRITIC CELLS

With the increased understanding of the mechanism of DC maturation, new avenues for the potential exploitation of these cells can be considered.

A first possiblity would be to enhance or modify the antigen-presenting capacity of DC *in vivo*. This could be achieved by improved adjuvants that may include cytokines or drugs to enhance or modulate DC maturation. Targeting of antigen or bioactive compounds could be carried out by exploiting the high endocytic activity and the presence of the mannose receptor.

A second possibility is to use DC themselves as adjuvants for vaccination (Young and Inaba, 1996; Schuler and Steinman, 1997). There are two critical steps to be considered: antigen loading and T cell stimulatory capacity. As to the first, we know how to load antigens efficiently on the class II pathways by pulsing with soluble antigen during maturation or with peptide after maturation is induced. In both cases the stability of peptide–MHC complexes will ensure efficient and protracted presentation *in vivo*. Class I molecules can also be loaded with exogenous peptides. However, this approach may suffer from the limitation that the complexes generated have a short half-life. Thus this approach may be effective only when using high concentrations of particularly good binders that may be sufficient for enough complexes to remain displayed after some days. In principle, a better method for loading class I molecules could be the transfection of DC, since this approach will exploit the sustained increase of class I synthesis. Efficient methods for transfection of nondividing monocyte-derived DC are absolutely required to pursue this approach. Approaches alternative to transfection for loading class I molecules endogenously, such as loading of DC with macropinocytosed antigen (Norbury *et al.*, 1997) or apoptotic bodies (Albert *et al.*, 1998), might be particularly successful.

As to the stimulatory capacity of DC, it remains to be established how the functional properties of DC could be modulated to obtain the desired stimulatory effect. As we suggested earlier (Cella *et al.*, 1996), the mechanism of T to T cell help via APC activation may be exploited therapeutically. This may be feasible by providing on the DC, in addition to the CTL epitope, a recall antigen such as TT, which could be recognized by memory T cells. This will allow stimulation of DC by T helper cells via CD40L–CD40 interaction to occur at the appropriate sites in the lymph nodes, thus increasing the stimulatory capacity of the DC and inducing IL-12 production at sites where it can most effectively stimulate a CTL response.

ACKNOWLEDGMENTS

We thank Klaus Karjalainen and Marco Colonna for critical reading and comments. The Basel Institute for Immunology was founded and is supported by F. Hoffmann La Roche Ltd, Basel, Switzerland.

REFERENCES

Albert, M.L., Sauter, B. and Bhardwaj, N. (1998). Dendritic cells acquire antigen from apoptotic cells and induce class I-restricted CTLs. *Nature* **392**, 86–89.

Cella, M., Scheidegger, D., Palmer Lehmann, K., Lane, P., Lanzavecchia, A. and Alber, G. (1996). Ligation of CD40 on dendritic cells triggers production of high levels of interleukin-12 and enhances T cell stimulatory capacity: T–T help via APC activation. *J. Exp. Med.* **184**, 747–752.

Cella, M., Engering, A., Pinet, V., Pieters, J. and Lanzavecchia, A. (1997). Inflammatory stimuli induce accumulation of MHC class II complexes on dendritic cells [In Process Citation]. *Nature* **388**, 782–787.

Engering, A.J., Cella, M., Fluitsma, D., Brockhaus, M., Hoefsmit, E.C.M., Lanzavecchia, A. and Pieters, J. (1997). The mannose receptor functions as a high capacity and broad specificity antigen receptor in human dendritic cells. *Eur. J. Immunol.* **27**, 2417–2425.

Germain, R.N. (1994). MHC-dependent antigen processing and peptide presentation: providing ligands for T lymphocyte activation. *Cell* **76**, 287–299.

Heufler, C., Koch, F., Stanzl, U., Topar, G., Wysocka, M., Trinchieri, G., Enk, A., Steinman, R.M., Romani, N. and Schuler, G. (1996). Interleukin-12 is produced by dendritic cells and mediates T helper 1 development as well as interferon-gamma production by T helper 1 cells. *Eur. J. Immunol.* **26**, 659–668.

Kampgen, E., Koch, N., Koch, F., Stoger, P., Heufler, C., Schuler, G. and Romani, N. (1991). Class II major histocompatibility complex molecules of murine dendritic cells: synthesis, sialylation of invariant chain, and antigen processing capacity are downregulated upon culture. *Proc. Natl Acad. Sci. USA* **88**, 3014–3018.

Norbury, C.C., Chambers, B.J., Prescott, A.R., Ljunggren, H.G. and Watts, C. (1997). Constitutive macropinocytosis allows TAP-dependent major histocompatibility complex class I presentation of exogenous soluble antigen by bone marrow-derived dendritic cells. *Eur. J. Immunol.* **27**, 280–288.

Pure, E., Inaba, K., Crowley, M.T., Tardelli, L., Witmer Pack, M.D., Ruberti, G., Fathman, G. and Steinman, R.M. (1990). Antigen processing by epidermal Langerhans cells correlates with the level of biosynthesis of major histocompatibility complex class II molecules and expression of invariant chain. *J. Exp. Med.* **172**, 1459–1469.

Romani, N., Koide, S., Crowley, M., Witmer-Pack, M., Livingstone, A.M., Fathman, C.G., Inaba, K. and Steinman, R.M. (1989). Presentation of exogenous protein antigens by dendritic cells to T cell clones. Intact protein is presented best by immature, epidermal Langerhans cells. *J. Exp. Med.* **169**, 1169–1178.

Sallusto, F. and Lanzavecchia, A. (1994). Efficient presentation of soluble antigen by cultured human dendritic cells is maintained by granulocyte/macrophage colony-stimulating factor plus interleukin 4 and downregulated by tumor necrosis factor alpha. *J. Exp. Med.* **179**, 1109–1118.

Sallusto, F., Cella, M., Danieli, C. and Lanzavecchia, A. (1995). Dendritic cells use macropinocytosis and the mannose receptor to concentrate macromolecules in the major histocompatibility complex class II compartment: downregulation by cytokines and bacterial products. *J. Exp. Med.* **182**, 389–400.

Schuler, G. and Steinman, R.M. (1985). Murine epidermal Langerhans cells mature into potent immunostimulatory dendritic cells in vitro. *J. Exp. Med.* **161**, 526–546.

Schuler, G. and Steinman, R.M. (1997). Dendritic cells as adjuvants for immune-mediated resistance to tumors. *J. Exp. Med.* **186**, 1183–1187.

Steinman, R.M. (1991). The dendritic cell system and its role in immunogenicity. *Annu. Rev. Immunol.* **9**, 271–296.

Watts, C. (1997). Inside the gearbox of the dendritic cells. *Nature* **388**, 724–725.

Young, J.W. and Inaba, K. (1996). Dendritic cells as adjuvants for class I major histocompatibility complex-restricted antitumor immunity. *J. Exp. Med.* **183**, 7–11.

CHAPTER 35
Development and Testing of Dendritic Cell Lines

Giampiero Girolomoni[1], Maria Rescigno[2] and Paola Ricciardi-Castagnoli[2]
[1]Laboratory of Immunology, Istituto Dermopatico dell'Immacolata, IRCCS, Rome, Italy; [2]CNR Center of Cellular and Molecular Pharmacology, Milan, Italy

Time is what you make of it.

Elisabeth M. Swatch

INTRODUCTION

Dendritic cells (DC) are now recognized as major players in the orchestration of immune responses against a variety of antigens, including allergens, infectious agents, and tumors (Schuler *et al.*, 1997). DC direct both the quality and the quantity of the immune response, and thus they can represent a very appropriate means for the manipulation of harmful or protective immunity, for example, against cancer (Girolomoni and Ricciardi-Castagnoli, 1997; Schuler and Steinman, 1997). However, the difficulties in preparing cells in sufficient numbers and in a reasonably pure form, and the short life-span of DC in culture have greatly hindered the progress of knowledge of DC biology. In particular, the molecular basis of the unique immunostimulatory properties of DC, the fine mechanisms of antigen handling, and the biochemical pathways of signal transduction have been only marginally investigated. On the other hand, a more complete characterization of DC physiology and the identification of DC-specific genes appear necessary prerequisites for an optimal use of DC in immunotherapy and for selective targeting of DC functions. In the last few years, several laboratories have successfully approached these issues by establishing DC lines from animal tissues. Both the availability of these DC lines and the methodologies used for their growth have enhanced our understanding of DC biology, and have provided important information that can be more easily confirmed in DC derived from humans. In general, two types of DC lines have been generated: (a) immortalized DC lines, which do not require continuous stimulation with growth factors for their propagation, and (b) growth factor-dependent DC lines.

Dendritic Cells: Biology and Clinical Applications
ISBN 0-12-455860-7

IMMORTALIZED DC LINES

Several immortal DC lines have been prepared, mainly by introducing immortalizing oncogens into DC primary cultures (Table 1). Retroviral vectors are among the most efficient means of transferring genes into cells. A major advance in their use has been the construction of packaging cell lines containing a helper-retrovirus defective in the RNA packaging signal (ψ sequence), but with intact structural genes. When these cells are infected with a replication-defective retrovirus bearing the gene(s) of interest and with an intact ψ sequence, they produce pure stocks of the engineered viruses without the recipient cell becoming a retrovirus producer (Mann *et al.*, 1983). Avian retroviruses with the v-*myc* oncogene can transform hematopoietic cells with a monocytic phenotype and recombinant retrovirus carrying the v-myc^{MH2} gene inserted in the mouse AKRv viral genome were shown to immortalize *in vitro* mouse macrophages and microglial cells (Lutz *et al.*, 1994; Pirami *et al.*, 1991). Using the helper-free retroviral vector MIBψ2-N11, immortalized DC lines were generated from spleen (Granucci *et al.*, 1994; Paglia *et al.*, 1993) and fetal skin (Girolomoni *et al.*, 1995) that did not require additional exogenous factors for their growth. These DC lines exhibited many phenotypical and functional features of DC, including the capacity to induce primary T cell response when injected *in vivo*. The FSDC line, generated from mouse fetal skin, exhibited characteristics common to macrophages, and thus could be representative of early DC progenitors. Accordingly, the FSDC lines showed a different sensitivity to cytokine activation signals compared to DC isolated from adult mice (Girolomoni *et al.*, 1995; Riva *et al.*, 1996). The mechanism that drives indefinite proliferation of these cells is not completely clarified. Analysis of the molecularly cloned proviral genome sequence showed a possible env^{AKR}–myc^{MH2} fusion and several point mutations within the *myc* region, compared with the original avian v-myc^{MH2} sequence (Sassano *et al.*, 1994). This fusion gene containing an altered *myc* oncogene may encode for a particular DNA-binding protein with enhanced transforming potential.

More recently, Shen *et al.* (1997) have successfully established immortalized DC lines by transducing GM-CSF into bone marrow cultures followed by supertransfection with *myc* and *raf* oncogenes. In this system, GM-CSF probably acts in a paracrine fashion by expanding infectable DC, because indefinite proliferation was maintained without the DC producing detectable levels of the growth factor. DC clones derived by limiting dilution showed some differences in the surface phenotype and were very efficient in presenting exogenous protein antigens on both MHC class II and class I molecules.

Table 1. Immortalized mouse DC lines

Name	Source	Mouse strain	Immortalizing agent	Reference
CB1	Spleen	DBA/2	env^{AKR}–myc^{MH2} fusion gene	Paglia *et al.* (1993)
D2SC/1	Spleen	BALB/c	env^{AKR}–myc^{MH2} fusion gene	Granucci *et al.* (1994)
FSDC	Fetal skin	(DBA/2 × C57BL/6)F_1	env^{AKR}–myc^{MH2} fusion gene	Girolomoni *et al.* (1995)
tsDC	Bone marrow	(CBA/Ca ×C57BL/10)F_1-tsA58	Thermolabile SV40 large T antigen	Volkmann *et al.* (1996)
DC1.2, DC2.4, DC2.5.1, DC4.1	Bone marrow	C57BL/6	GM-CSF + *myc* and *raf*	Shen *et al.* (1997)
JAWS II	Bone marrow	C57BL/6	Not reported	Brossart *et al.* (1997)

An alternative approach to generating immortal DC was described by Volkmann *et al.* (1996). They took advantage of transgenic mice carrying a temperature-sensitive mutant of the Simian virus 40 large T antigen under the control of the MHC class I K^b promoter, which allows the conditional immortalization of cells at the permissive temperature of 33–37°C. When the cells were transferred to 39°C, the transgene product was rapidly degraded, and cells stopped dividing. DC isolated from bone marrow in the presence of GM-CSF showed continuous growth when cultured at 33°C; upon exposure to 39°C, DC (tsDC) underwent differentiation and functional maturation similarly to primary DC, a process that was enhanced when tsDC were cultured in the presence of T cells, skin cells, or supernatants from activated T cells.

An interesting property of some immortalized DC lines is that they can be loaded with exogenous protein antigens *in vitro* and initiate protective MHC class I-restricted cytotoxic T cell responses *in vivo*, a function that can be augmented when the antigen is administered in a particulate form or associated with cell debris (Bachmann *et al.*, 1996; Brossart *et al.*, 1997; Paglia *et al.*, 1996). Furthermore, recent studies on the skin-derived DC line, FSDC, allowed the identification of an intracellular compartment where exogenous antigens are stored. In this way, antigens can be accumulated without massive degradation until DC have migrated from the peripheral tissue (e.g., the skin) to the draining lymph nodes (Lutz *et al.*, 1997). Information derived from such experiments may ultimately prove to be very important for optimal use of DC in the immunotherapy of tumors or viral diseases.

Finally, it has been reported that infection with an estrogen-inducible v-*rel*, the oncogenic version of c-*rel* contained within the avian retrovirus complex REV-T/REV-A, induced an estrogen-dependent transformation *in vitro* of chicken bone marrow cells. These cells exhibited B cell determinants, but when the v-Rel estrogen receptor fusion protein (v-RelER) was inactivated by an estrogen antagonist, cells differentiated into DC as assessed by several morphological and functional criteria (Boehmelt *et al.*, 1995). However, changing the culture medium gave rise to cells with the characteristics of polymorphonuclear neutrophils, suggesting that a hormone-activated v-RelER can transform a DC/neutrophil progenitor, and that members of the NF-κB transcription factor family are involved in DC development. In agreement with this hypothesis, mice with a defective expression of the *relB* gene have impaired differentiation of DC in lymphoid organs (Burkly *et al.*, 1995). An important limitation of most immortalized DC lines is that they retain an immature phenotype and cannot be stimulated to acquire a fully mature status, probably because the immortalization itself inhibits the complete differentiation of DC. In contrast, growth factor-dependent DC lines can be more easily induced to mature *in vitro*, and thus they can more closely mimick the *in vivo* behavior of DC.

GROWTH FACTOR-DEPENDENT DC LINES

Several DC lines have been obtained from mouse skin, especially from fetuses and newborns (Table 2). Elbe *et al.* (1994) first reported the generation of long-term DC lines from mouse fetal skin. These lines (80/1, 18, 86/2) were established by stimulating skin cells with IL-2 and Con-A or with GM-CSF, and required the continuous presence of these factors for their protracted growth. The surface phenotype was similar to that of fetal Langerhans cells with high MHC class I expression and no class II, thus

Table 2. Growth-factor dependent mouse DC lines

Name	Source	Mouse strain	Growth factor requirements	Reference
80/1, 18, 86/2	Fetal skin	C3H/He/Han	GM-CSF or IL-2 and Con-A	Elbe *et al.* (1994)
XS series	Newborn epidermis	BALB/c	GM-CSF, CSF-1, skin fibroblast supernatant, keratinocyte supernatant	Xu *et al.* (1995a)
D1	Spleen	C57BL/6	Supernatant from GM-CSF-treated fibroblasts	Winzler *et al.* (1997)
FSDDC	Fetal skin	C57BL/6	GM-CSF and CSF-1	Jakob *et al.* (1997)

allowing a detailed analysis of the capacity of DC to induce $CD8^+$ T cell responses. 80/1 and 18 DC were indeed strong activators of naive allogeneic $CD8^+$ T lymphocytes, a property that was critically dependent on physical contact between stimulator and responder cells and on the expression of B7-1 costimulatory molecule. In addition, MHC class I^+ DC line 18 pulsed *in vitro* with particulate hepatitis B surface antigen (HBsAg) could efficiently prime class I-restricted, HBsAg-specific cytotoxic T cells when injected into a naive host (Böhm *et al.*, 1995), and were sufficient to sensitize naive animals for transplantation immunity, leading to accelerated skin allograft rejection (Lenz *et al.*, 1996). This line was phenotypically stable, and attempts to induce MHC class II expression failed.

Takashima and coworkers have been successful in generating long-term DC lines from the epidermis of newborn mice by culturing epidermal cell suspensions with recombinant GM-CSF and culture supernatant from the Pam 212 keratinocyte cell line (Xu *et al.*, 1995a, c). These cells (XS series) have been maintained by feeding with GM-CSF and culture supernatants from Pam 212 keratinocytes and skin-derived nurse cells (NS series), and in phenotype and function resembled immature Langerhans cells. Further characterization of the growth factor requirements indicated that both GM-CSF and CSF-1 promoted cell proliferation. In contrast, IL-1–12, G-CSF, and stem cell factor had no effect, and TNF-α and IFN-γ were inhibitory when used in combination with GM-CSF (Xu *et al.*, 1995b). In following experiments, nurse cells turned out to be fibroblasts with the capacity to produce high amounts of CSF-1 (Schuhmachers *et al.*, 1995; Takashima *et al.*, 1995). The capacity of CSF-1 to sustain the growth of immature DC has recently been confirmed by Jakob *et al.* (1997), who propagated DC lines from mouse fetal skin by culturing cells in GM-CSF and CSF-1-supplemented medium.

Regarding growth factor-dependent DC lines generated from organs other than the skin, a spleen DC line (D1) was obtained by culturing cell suspensions in medium supplemented with fibroblast (NIH/3T3) supernatant and GM-CSF (Winzler *et al.*, 1997). Studies on these DC cell lines provided very important information about the maturation stages of DC and the reciprocal interactions between DC and T cells (Kitajima *et al.*, 1995; Kitajima *et al.*, 1996; Winzler *et al.*, 1997).

Two distinct maturation stages of DC have been identified: an immature stage, called 'processing phenotype', in which DC are highly phagocytic and have low levels of MHC and costimulatory molecules on the cell surface, and a mature stage, called 'presenting phenotype', in which DC have lost the capacity to take up particles and have acquired high T cell activating functions (Winzler *et al.*, 1997). A T cell-dependent maturation of DC has also been described and appears to be mediated by T cell-derived cytokines such as IFN-γ (Kitajima *et al.*, 1996), as well as by interactions between surface molecules (e.g., CD40L–CD40) (Cella *et al.*, 1996). These findings have important implications for the design of more effective DC-based immunotherapeutic strategies. For example, from such observations it has been suggested that to facilitate cytotoxic T cell responses against tumor antigens, DC should be pulsed simultaneously with the tumor antigen and a recall antigen (e.g., tetanus toxoid). DC emigrated from the lymphoid organs will rapidly recruit recall antigen-specific T cells that in turn will foster DC maturation and ultimately enhance their capacity to trigger tumor antigen-specific T cell responses (Cella *et al.*, 1996).

In conclusion, the possibility of having large numbers of DC in different stages of differentiation can be very useful for understanding at the molecular level the mechanisms of DC maturation. In particular, the identification of DC-specific genes should be greatly facilitated, thus opening the possibility of targeting selective DC functions.

REFERENCES

Bachmann, M.F., Lutz, M.B., Layton, G.T., Harris, S.J., Fehr, T., Rescigno, M. and Ricciardi-Castagnoli, P. (1996). Dendritic cells process exogenous viral proteins and virus-like particles for class I presentation to $CD8^+$ cytotoxic T lymphocytes. *Eur. J. Immunol.* **26**, 2595–2600.

Boehmelt, G., Madruga, J., Dörfler, P., Briegel, K., Schwarz, H., Enrietto, P.J. and Zenke, M. (1995). Dendritic cell progenitor is transformed by a conditional v-Rel estrogen receptor fusion protein vRelER. *Cell* **80**, 341–352.

Böhm, W., Schirmbeck, R., Elbe, A., Melber, K., Diminky, D., Kraal, G., van Rooijen, N., Barenholz, Y. and Reimann, J. (1995). Exogenous hepatitis B surface antigen particles processed by dendritic cells or macrophages prime murine MHC class I-restricted cytotoxic T lymphocytes *in vivo. J. Immunol.* **155**, 3313–3321.

Brossart, P., Goldrath, A.W., Butz, E.A., Martin, S. and Bevan, M.J. (1997). Virus-mediated delivery of antigenic epitopes into dendritic cells as means to induce CTL. *J. Immunol.* **158**, 3270–3276.

Burkly, L., Hession, C., Ogata, L., Reilly, C., Marconi, L.A., Olson, D., Tizard, R., Cate, R. and Lo, D. (1995). Expression of relB is required for the development of thymic medulla and dendritic cells. *Nature* **373**, 531–536.

Cella, M., Scheidegger, D., Palmer-Lehmann, K., Lane, P., Lanzavecchia, A. and Alber, G. (1996). Ligation of CD40 on dendritic cells triggers production of high levels of interleukin-12 and enhances T cell stimulatory capacity: T–T help via APC activation. *J. Exp. Med.* **184**, 747–752.

Elbe, A., Schleischitz, S., Strunk, D. and Stingl, G. (1994). Fetal skin-derived MHC class I^+, MHC class II^- dendritic cells stimulate MHC class I-restricted responses of unprimed $CD8^+$ T cells. *J. Immunol.* **153**, 2878–2889.

Girolomoni, G., Lutz, M.B., Pastore, S., Assmann, C.U., Cavani, A. and Ricciardi-Castagnoli, P. (1995). Establishment of a cell line with features of early dendritic cell precursors from mouse fetal skin. *Eur. J. Immunol.* **25**, 2163–2169.

Girolomoni, G. and Ricciardi-Castagnoli, P. (1997). Dendritic cells hold promise for immunotherapy. *Immunol. Today* **18**, 102–104.

Granucci, F., Girolomoni, G., Lutz, M.B., Foti, M., Marconi, G., Gnocchi, P., Nolli, L. and Ricciardi-Castagnoli, P. (1994). Modulation of cytokine expression in mouse dendritic cell clones. *Eur. J. Immunol.* **24**, 2522–2526.

Jakob, T., Saitoh, A. and Udey, M.C. (1997). E-cadherin-mediated adhesion involving Langerhans cell-like dendritic cells expanded from murine fetal skin. *J. Immunol.* **159**, 2693–2701.

Kitajima, T., Ariizumi, K., Mohamadzadeh, M., Edelbaum, D., Bergstresser, P.R. and Takashima, A. (1995). T cell-dependent secretion of IL-1β by a dendritic cell line (XS52) derived from human epidermis. *J. Immunol.* **155**, 3794–3800.

Kitajima, T., Caceres-Dittmar, G., Tapia, F.J., Jester, J., Bergstresser, P.R. and Takashima, A. (1996). T cell-mediated terminal maturation of dendritic cells. Loss of adhesive and phagocytotic capacities. *J. Immunol.* **157**, 2340–2347.

Lenz, P., Elbe, A., Stingl, G. and Bergstresser, P.R. (1996). MHC class I expression on dendritic cells is sufficient to sensitize for transplantation immunity. *J. Invest. Dermatol.* **107**, 844–848.

Lutz, M.B., Granucci, F., Winzler, C., Marconi, G., Paglia, P., Foti, M., Assmann, C.U., Cairns, L., Rescigno, M. and Ricciardi-Castagnoli, P. (1994). Retroviral immortalization of phagocytic and dendritic cells clones as a tool to investigate functional heterogeneity. *J. Immunol. Methods* **174**, 269–279.

Lutz, M.B., Assmann, C.U., Girolomoni, G. and Ricciardi-Castagnoli, P. (1996). Different cytokines regulate antigen uptake and presentation of a precursor dendritic cell line. *Eur. J. Immunol.* **26**, 586–594.

Lutz, M.B., Rovere, P., Kleijmeer, M.J., Rescigno, M., Assmann, C.U., Oorschot, V.M., Geuze, H.J., Trucy, J., Demandolx, D., Davoust, J. and Ricciardi-Castagnoli, P. (1997). Intracellular routes and selective retention of antigens in mildly acidic cathepsin D/lysosome-associated membrane protein-1/MHC class II-positive vesicles in immature dendritic cells. *J. Immunol.* **159**, 3707–3716.

Mann, R., Mulligan, R.C. and Baltimore, D. (1983). Construction of a retrovirus packaging mutant and its use to produce helper-free defective retrovirus. *Cell* **33**, 153–159.

Paglia, P., Girolomoni, G., Robbiati, F., Granucci, F. and Ricciardi-Castagnoli, P. (1993). Immortalized dendritic cell line fully competent in antigen presentation initiates primary T cell responses *in vivo*. *J. Exp. Med.* **178**, 1893–1901.

Paglia, P., Chiodoni, C., Rodolfo, M. and Colombo, M.P. (1996). Murine dendritic cells loaded *in vitro* with soluble protein prime cytotoxic T lymphocytes against tumor antigen *in vivo*. *J. Exp. Med.* **183**, 317–322.

Pirami, L., Stockinger, B., Betz-Corradin, S., Sironi, M., Sassano, M., Valsasnini, P., Righi, M. and Ricciardi-Castagnoli, P. (1991). Mouse macrophage clones immortalized by retroviruses are functionally heterogenous. *Proc. Natl Acad. Sci. USA* **88**, 7543–7547.

Riva, S., Nolli, M.L., Lutz, M.B., Citterio, S., Girolomoni, G., Winzler, C. and Ricciardi-Castagnoli, P. (1996). Bacteria and bacterial cell wall constituents induce the production of regulatory cytokines in dendritic cell clones. *J. Inflamm.* **46**, 98–105.

Sassano, M., Granucci, F., Seveso, M., Marconi, G., Foti, M. and Ricciardi-Castagnoli, P. (1994). Molecular cloning of a recombinant retrovirus carrying a mutated env^{AKR}–myc^{MH2} fusion gene immortalizing cells of the monocytic-macrophage lineage. *Oncogene* **9**, 1473–1477.

Schuhmachers, G., Xu, S., Bergstresser, P.R. and Takashima, A. (1995). Identity and functional properties of novel skin-derived fibroblast lines (NS series) that support the growth of epidermal-derived dendritic cell lines. *J. Invest. Dermatol.* **105**, 225–230.

Schuler, G. and Steinman, R.M. (1997). Dendritic cells as adjuvants for immune-mediated resistance to tumors. *J. Exp. Med.* **186**, 1183–1187.

Schuler, G., Thurner, B. and Romani, N. (1997). Dendritic cells: from ignored cells to major players in T-cell-mediated immunity. *Int. Arch. Allergy Immunol.* **112**, 317–333.

Shen, Z., Reznikoff, G., Dranoff, G. and Rock, K.L. (1997). Cloned dendritic cells can present exogenous antigens on both MHC class I and class II molecules. *J. Immunol.* **158**, 2723–2730.

Takashima, A., Edelbaum, D., Kitajima, T., Shadduck, R.K., Gilmore, G.L., Xu, S., Taylor, R.S., Bergstresser, P.R. and Ariizumi, K. (1995). Colony-stimulating factor-1 secreted by fibroblasts promotes the growth of dendritic cells (XS series) derived from murine epidermis. *J. Immunol.* **154**, 5128–5135.

Volkmann, A., Neefjes, J. and Stockinger, B. (1996). A conditionally immortalized dendritic cell line which differentiates in contact with T cells or T cell-derived cytokines. *Eur. J. Immunol.* **26**, 2565–2572.

Winzler, C., Rovere, P., Rescigno, M., Granucci, F., Penna, G., Adorini, L., Zimmermann, V.S., Davoust, J. and Ricciardi-Castagnoli, P. (1997). Maturation stages of mouse dendritic cells in growth factor-dependent long-term cultures. *J. Exp. Med.* **185**, 317–328.

Xu, S., Ariizumi, K., Caceres-Dittmar, G., Edelbaum, D., Hashimoto, K., Bergstresser, P.R. and Takashima, A. (1995a). Successive generation of antigen-presenting, dendritic cell lines from murine epidermis. *J. Immunol.* **154**, 2697–2705.

Xu, S., Ariizumi, K., Edelbaum, D., Bergstresser, P.R. and Takashima, A. (1995b). Cytokine-dependent regulation of growth and maturation in murine epidermal dendritic cell lines. *Eur. J. Immunol.* **25**, 1018–1024.

Xu, S., Bergstresser, P.R. and Takashima, A. (1995c). Phenotypic and functional heterogeneity among murine epidermal-derived dendritic cell clones. *J. Invest. Dermatol.* **105**, 831–836.

CHAPTER 36
Dendritic Cell-derived Exosomes: Potent Immunogenic Cell-free Vaccines

Laurence Zitvogel[1], Armelle Regnault[2], Anne Lozier[1], Graça Raposo[3] and Sebastian Amigorena[2]
[1]Laboratoire d'Immunologie Cellulaire, Département de Biologie Clinique, Institut Gustave Roussy, Villejuif, France; [2]CJF 95-01 INSERM; [3]UMR144 CNRS, Institut Curie, Paris, France

INTRODUCTION

Antigen-presenting cells (APC) contain a specialized late endocytic compartment, MIIC (MHC class II-enriched compartment), that harbors newly synthesized MHC class II molecules in transit to the plasma membrane (Nijman, 1995; Kleijmeer, 1995). MIIC have lysosomal characteristics (they are acidic and bear lysosomal marker molecules, i.e., LAMP, tetraspanins) and are involved in antigen processing and peptide binding to class II molecules. However, functionally different subclasses of MIIC exist, encompassing membrane sheet and/or internal vesicle (multivesicular bodies, MVB) containing compartments. Ultrastructural studies of EBV-transformed B cells demonstrate that multivesicular bodies are exocytic compartments in that their limiting external membrane can fuse with the plasma membrane resulting in the release, into the extracellular milieu, of their internal vesicular content. The externalized vesicles, termed exosomes, carry in their membrane MHC class II molecules with their peptide-binding domain oriented toward the extracellular milieu. During their formation, internal vesicles arise from the budding of a portion of the outer endosomal membrane toward the endosomal lumen (Raposo *et al.*, 1997; Fig. 1). These MHC class II molecules are functional and induce antigen-specific MHC class II-restricted T cell responses *in vitro* (Raposo *et al.*, 1996). Interestingly, Kleijmeer *et al.* (1998) reported that MHC class I molecules colocalize with MHC class II and tetraspanin molecules in the external membrane and internal vesicles of these MVB.

We now show that dendritic cells (DC) secrete antigen-presenting vesicles in a regulated manner. Importantly, tumor peptide pulsed DC-derived exosomes mediate potent MHC-dependent anti-tumor immune responses that induce tumor rejection in mice (Zitvogel *et al.*, 1998).

Dendritic Cells: Biology and Clinical Applications
ISBN 0-12-455860-7

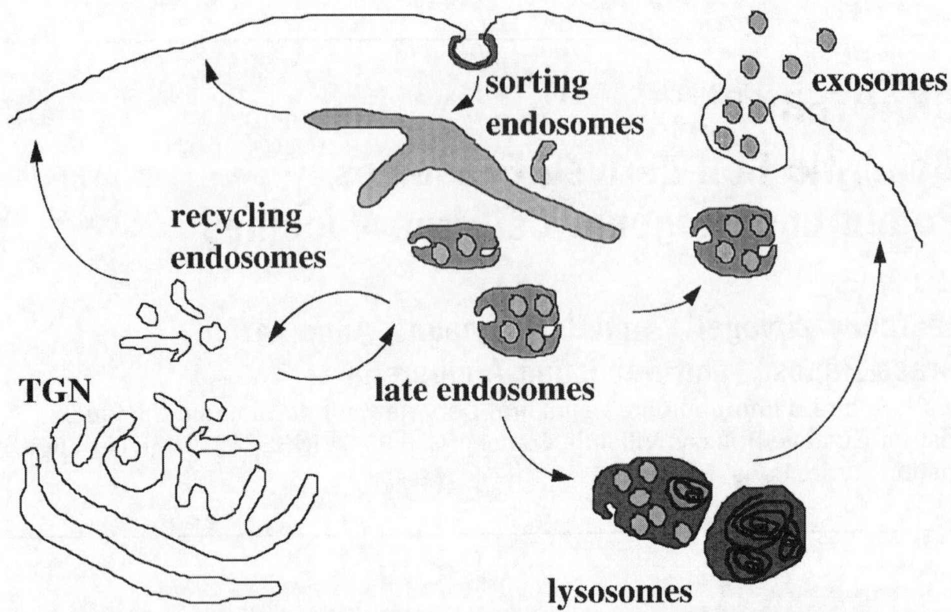

Fig. 1. Schematic representation of the endocytic and exocytic system of antigen-presenting cells. Ultrastructural studies have revealed that the vast majority of MHC class II molecules reside in lysosome-related late endocytic compartments, the MIIC. MIIC encompass both multilamellar-containing compartments and/or multivesicular bodies (MVB). MVB represent a meeting point between the endocytic and the exocytic pathways. At the electron-microscopic level, the late endosome appears as a 200–300 nm membrane compartment containing in its lumen variable amounts of small 60–90 nm vesicles. The internal vesicles of the MVB are thought to arise from budding of a portion of the limiting membrane into the endosomal lumen. During the invagination toward the intraluminal milieu, some membrane proteins are sequestered in the internal vesicles, whereas others remain in the limiting membrane of the MVB. The external membrane of MVB fuses with the plasma membrane, resulting in the exocytosis of the internal vesicular content, the exosomes, into the extracellular milieu. TGN, trans-Gdgi network.

HUMAN AND MOUSE DC SECRETE THE INTERNAL VESICLES OF MULTIVESICULAR LATE ENDOSOMES

We first examined secretory lysosomes from immature human monocyte-derived DC cultured in IL-4 + GM-CSF. Ultrastructural studies revealed that these cells contain numerous internal vesicles (multivesicular MIIC) as well as MIIC displaying electron-dense concentrically arranged membrane sheets (multilamellar MIIC). As described by Kleijmeer *et al.* (1998) in EBV-transformed B cells, we also found that in human monocyte-derived (MD)-DC generated in IL-4 + GM-CSF for 7–10 days, multivesicular MIIC express MHC class I molecules (Zitvogel *et al.*, 1998). Both markers were found in the external membrane of the endosomes and the intraluminal 60–90 nm vesicles (not shown). Multilaminar compartments were not labeled with anti-MHC class I antibodies (not shown). In contrast to CD63 (Metzelaar, 1991) or CD82, MHC class I molecules were also detected at the cell surface (Zitvogel *et al.*, 1998). Multivesicular MHC class I- and class II-containing compartments were often observed in close apposition to the cell surface, suggesting their direct fusion with the plasma membrane (Zitvogel *et al.*, 1998). Consistent with this possibility, 60–90 nm vesicles were often observed close to the outer side of the plasma membrane. These vesicles were abundantly labeled with anti-MHC class I and II, CD63, and CD82 specific antibodies. Therefore, 60–90 nm vesicles, bearing the same markers as the internal vesicles of multivesicular MIIC (class I, class II, CD63, CD82) are released by human DC.

These vesicles were isolated from DC culture supernatants following differential ultracentrifugation (Raposo *et al.*, 1996) and analyzed by whole-mount immuno-electron microscopy. A homogeneous population of vesicles of 60–90 nm diameter was observed (Fig. 2, lower panel). Like the vesicles from the exocytic profiles, over 95% of these vesicles were labeled with the anti-CD63 and anti-CD82 antibodies, as well as with anti-MHC class I and class II antibodies (not shown).

Similar vesicles were observed in the supernatants of mouse DC. We used the well-characterized growth factor-dependent D1 DC line (Winzler *et al.*, 1997) and bone marrow-derived DC (BM-DC) to analyze the exosomal production by mouse DC. As in the case of human DC, immature murine DC exhibit abundant multivesicular endosomal compartments (Fig. 2, upper panel), which were occasionally observed in close apposition to the plasma membrane. This Lamp-1 positive endosomal population stained for MHC class I and II molecules by confocal immunofluorescence (data not shown). Exosomes, harvested from D1 (Fig. 2, lower panel) or BM-DC supernatants, expressed MHC class I, class II (Fig. 2, upper panel) and costimulatory signal molecules as detected by whole-mount electron microscopy and Western blot (not shown). MHC class I and class II as well as CD86 and transferrin receptors (TfRs) were found on exosomes; the three latter markers were enriched in exosomes as compared with the cell lysates. In contrast, although detected in the cell lysates, H2-M, Ii chain, and calnexin (an endoplasmic reticulum-specific marker) were undetectable in the exosomal preparations. The size and morphology of immature mouse DC-derived exosomes were similar to the size and morphology of those derived from human DC.

EXOSOMES HAVE ALLOSTIMULATORY CAPACITIES AND ARE MHC CLASS I-RESTRICTED ANTIGEN PRESENTING VESICLES *IN VITRO*

Allogeneic lymphocytes were capable of proliferating when cocultured with DC-derived exosomes in a day 5 *in vitro* thymidine incorporation assay. Their proliferation rate was 50 times greater when whole irradiated DC were used as stimulators (not shown).

To determine whether exosomes may directly stimulate a $CD8^+$ cytotoxic, HLA-A2-restricted T cell clone (Duffour *et al.*, 1997), HLA-A2-positive human monocyte-derived DC were pulsed with MART-1/$MelanA_{(27-35)}$ peptides and exosomes were isolated from the cell culture supernatants.

The MART-1/MelanA-pulsed DC-derived exosomes were capable of stimulating IFN-γ production of a MART-1/MelanA-specific HLA-A2-restricted CTL clone LTl2 in a dose-dependent manner. Exosomes produced by DC pulsed with a control peptide ($gp100_{(280-288)}$) had no stimulatory effect on this clone. Thus, MHC class I molecules displayed at the surface of DC-derived exosomes are functional but to a lesser extent than the cells from which they are secreted (Zitvogel *et al.*, 1998).

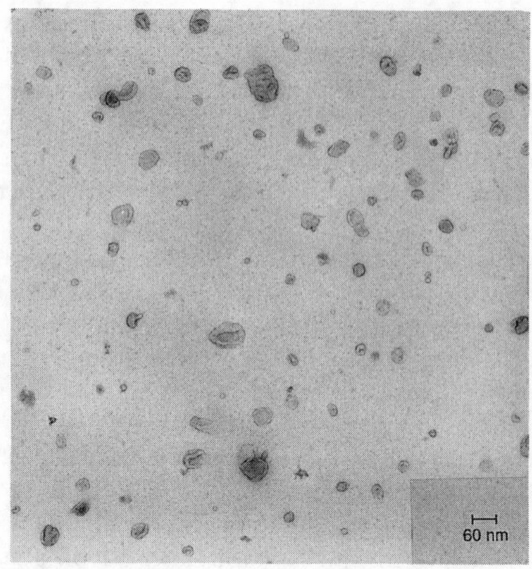

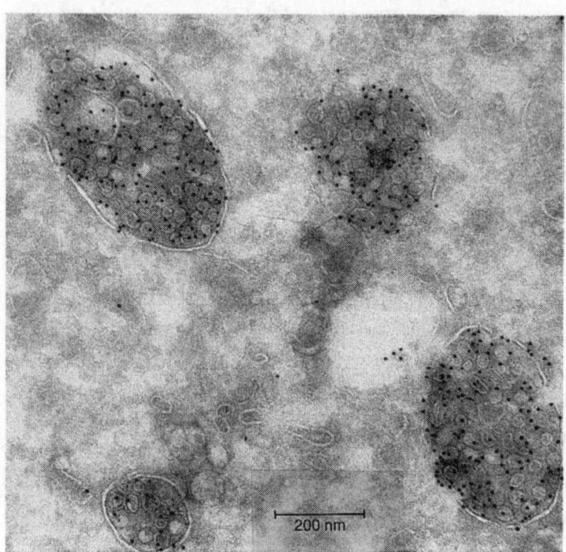

Fig. 2. MHC class II compartments of mouse D1 DC. Upper panel: Ultrathin cryosections of D1 cells were immunogold labeled for MHC class II (protein A–10 nm gold). MHC class II are localized in compartments displaying internal membrane vesicles (MVB). Lower panel: Whole-mount electron microscopy of D1-derived exosomes. The 100 000*g* pellets obtained after differential ultracentrifugation of D1 supernatants are composed of small vesicles with diameter varying from 50 to 90 nm. Bars: 250 nm.

TUMOR PEPTIDE-PULSED DC-DERIVED EXOSOMES INDUCE TUMOR GROWTH SUPPRESSION IN TUMOR-BEARING MICE

We tested the capacity of these vesicles to induce T cell-mediated immune responses *in vivo*. Bone marrow-derived DC cultured in IL-4 + GM-CSF (BM-DC) (Mayordomo *et al.*, 1995; Zitvogel *et al.*, 1996), loaded with acid-eluted tumor peptides, were previously shown to mediate specific anti-tumor immune responses. P815 is an immunogenic but aggressive mastocytoma, syngeneic for DBA/2 (H-2^d), for which very few effective immunotherapies on day-10 established tumors have been reported. Acid-eluted tumor (P815) peptides were pulsed onto syngeneic mouse BM-DC as previously described (Zitvogel *et al.*, 1996). Exosomes were prepared from the DC supernatants by differential ultracentrifugation and utilized for *in vivo* immunization.

As shown in Fig. 3A, therapy of day-10 established P815 tumors (50–90 mm^2 in size) was carried out using a single intradermal (i.d.) administration of 3–5 μg of exosomes per mouse. Within a week, tumor growth stopped in the groups receiving exosomes derived from autologous tumor peptide-pulsed DC and 40–60% mice were tumor free at day 60 (Fig. 3A). These animals had a long-lasting immune response and rejected a lethal tumor challenge with P815 but not with the syngeneic leukemia L1210 (not shown). Groups of mice immunized with exosomes derived from self splenic peptide-pulsed DC showed no effect on tumor growth as compared with control mice groups (Fig. 3A). Thus, P815 peptide-pulsed DC-derived exosomes promoted tumor regression.

Similar anti-tumor effects were achieved in the day 3–4 established TS/A tumor model. These anti-tumor effects were not found in athymic Nu/Nu counterparts, indicating that T cells are required for the exosome-induced anti-tumor immune responses. In addition, exosomes directly prime tumor-specific CTL responses in P815-bearing hosts. Splenocytes from mice that rejected P815 tumors following immunization with exosomes were harvested at day 90 and cultured for 5 days in the presence of irradiated B7.1-expressing P815 cells to enhance specific precursor frequency. These effector cells were tested in a 4 h ^{51}Cr-release assay against the autologous tumor cells P815 (H-2^d), against the irrelevant leukemia (H-2^d) L1210, and against YAC cells. Significant specific lytic activity on P815 was achieved in splenocytes from exosome-immunized mice (not shown). Interestingly, none of the spleens from littermates spontaneously rejecting P815 or bearing growing P815 tumors displayed cytolytic activity against P815 under the same conditions (not shown). Therefore, a single injection of exosomes derived from DC pulsed with the relevant peptides efficiently primed specific antitumor CTL responses *in vivo*.

Exosomes Induce MHC-Restricted Response

To determine whether exosome-induced immune responses are MHC restricted and not simply due to any direct effect of acid-eluted tumor peptides, day-5 BM-DC derived from H-2^d (DBA/2) or H-2^b (C57BL/6) mice were pulsed in parallel with acid-eluted P815 tumor peptides. Exosomes were then isolated and separately utilized for direct i.d. injection of DBA/2 mice bearing 6–10-day established P815 tumors. Only the syngeneic tumor peptide-bearing exosomes were potent tumor vaccines (with up to 60% tumor-free mice), whereas the allogeneic counterparts did not promote significant anti-tumor effects. These results suggest that these antigen-presenting vesicles induce MHC-restricted anti-tumor effects *in vivo* (Fig. 3A). When the exosomes derived from BM-DCs (DBA/2) pulsed with the tumor-specific subdominant epitope P1A were injected i.d. to protect mice against subsequent challenge with P815, up to 75% of mice were efficiently capable of preventing the onset of the tumor, whereas control peptide

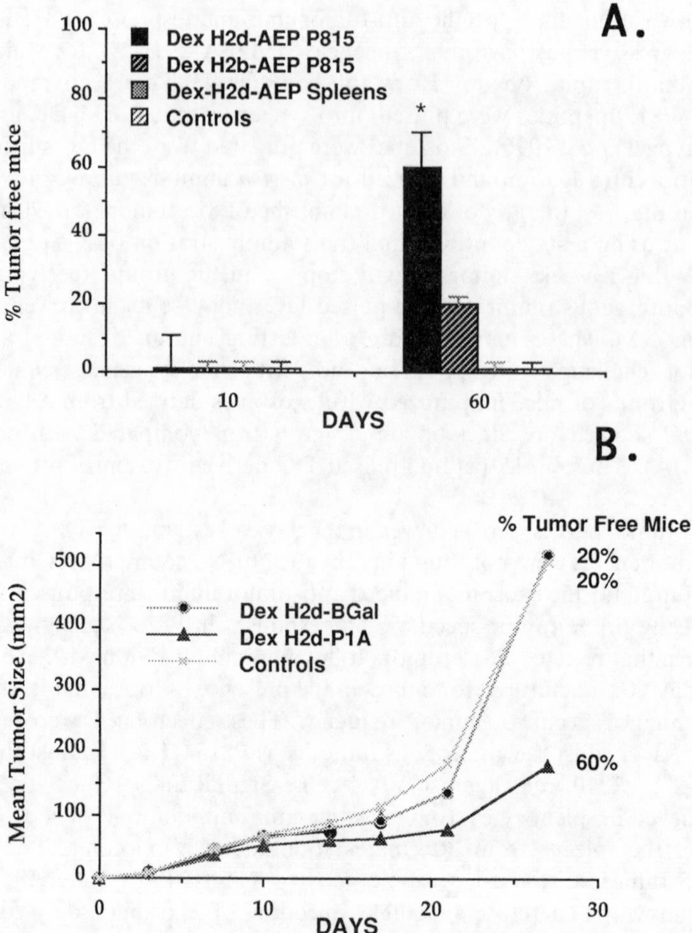

Fig. 3. Anti-tumor effects following administration of exosomes derived from tumor peptide-pulsed BM-DC. (A) DBA/2 animals bearing 50–80 mm^2 tumors were immunized intradermally in the lower part of ipsilateral flank with exosomes (3–5 μg/mouse) from BM-DC H2^d pulsed with acid-eluted P815 tumor peptides (DexH2^d-AEP P815) or with acid-eluted DBA/2 spleen peptides (DexH2^d-AEP Spleens) or with acid-eluted P815 tumor peptides (DexH2^b-AEP P815). Tumor sizes were monitored twice a week. The percentages of tumor-free mice at days 10 and 60 are represented. Five DBA/2 mice per group were vaccinated and two subsequent experiments were performed with similar results. (B) Exosomes derived from BM-DC DBA/2 pulsed with the subdominant P1A tumor epitope were injected i.d. 15 days prior to tumor challenge with a lethal dose of P815 tumor cells. Control groups were protected either with saline or with exosomes derived from BM-DC DBA/2 pulsed with the H2d-BGal epitope TPHPARIGL. The percentage of tumor-free mice at day 60 is represented as well as the tumor growth over time.

(BGal, H2d)-bearing exosomes were not efficient (Fig. 3B). Importantly, intravenous or i.d. adoptive therapy using 5–10 × 10^5 immature BM-DC pulsed with acid-eluted tumor peptides was not as efficient as i.d. administration of exosomes derived from the same cells (Fig. 4) in curing mice. Similar results were achieved on established TS/A tumors in BALB/c animals and on prophylaxis studies using the P1A tumor peptide (not shown).

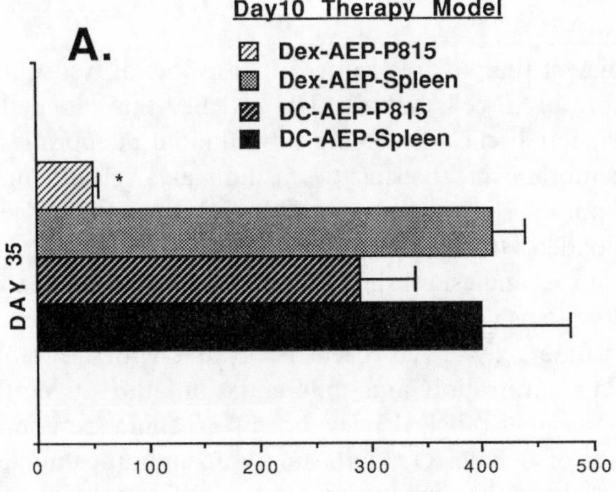

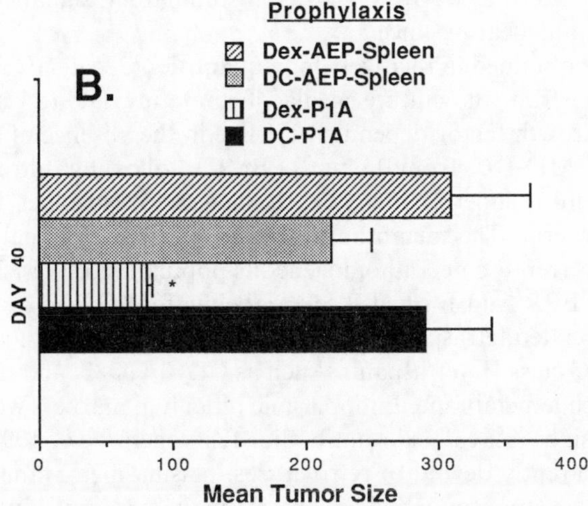

Fig. 4. Exosomes are more potent than immature dendritic cells, from which they derive, in eradicating established tumors *in vivo*. (A) DC (5×10^6) pulsed with either acid-eluted splenic peptides (AEP) or P815 tumor peptides were administered i.v. or i.d. at days 8–10 following P815 i.d. establishment in 5 mice. In parallel, the supernatants of these cells were harvested following 18 h incubation with splenic peptides or P815 relevant peptides, ultracentrifuged, and characterized for exosome production (DC exosomes, Dex). Up to 5 μg/5×10^6 DC allow i.d. immunization of 5 mice in the ipsilateral flank. A single administration of exosome was performed at day 8–10. The mean tumor size at day 35 is depicted. * represents significant results at 95% using Fisher's exact method compared with injection of saline or peptide-pulsed DC. Representative data are shown among additional similar experiments. (B) Similar experiments but DC or Dex were injected as prophylaxis, 15 days prior to tumor challenge with P815. P1A is used instead of acid-eluted tumor peptide in this setting. The mean tumor size at day 40 is depicted. * represents significant results at 95% using Fisher's exact method compared with injection of peptide-pulsed DC.

DISCUSSION

Ultrastructural studies of the possible routes of transport of lysosomal constituents to the cell surface in not only B cells but also DC revealed that late endosomal compartments, i.e., multivesicular bodies displaying intraluminal membrane vesicles, can fuse with the plasma membrane in an exocytic fashion and release, in the extracellular environment, 60–90 nm exosomes (Raposo, 1996; Raposo, 1997; Kleijmeer,1998). We report that antigen-loaded DC-derived exosomes bear functional class I molecules that allow CTL priming *in vivo* and established tumor growth suppression in various murine experimental model systems (Zitvogel *et al.*, 1998).

Even though exosome release has been associated with clearance of transferrin receptors, reticulocyte maturation and differentiation into an erythrocyte pathway (Bockxmeer, 1979), the physiological relevance of exosome secretion and function *in vivo* are still a matter of debate. Our data imply an immunostimulatory role of this exosome release and show that immature mouse and human dendritic cells secrete exosomes in a regulated manner (unpublished data) that bear not only MHC class II molecules but also MHC class I as well as costimulatory signal molecules and are immunogenic in tumor-bearing mice.

Exosomes can be obtained in relatively high quantities (2–5 μg/10^6 DC per 18 h using the Bradford assay) from the culture media of immature DC (d5 mouse BM-DC in GM-CSF + IL-4, growth factor-dependent D1 line in the absence of activating stimuli, or CD83-negative MD-DC from human PBMC) following ultracentrifugation at 100 000*g* of the culture supernatants. We characterized exosomes by morphological and biochemical criteria. The membranes pelleted at 100 000*g*, analyzed by immunoelectron microscopy, represented a homogeneous population of vesicles that resembled those described for EBV-transformed B cells, labeling for MHC class I, class II, CD86, and lysosomal-associated tetraspan molecules (Metzelaar, 1991). Exosomes abundantly overexpressed MHC class II, tetraspanins such as CD63/CD82, and CD86 molecules as compared with plasma membrane. Endoplasmic reticulum markers were not detected in western blotting using anti-calnexin antibodies (Zitvogel *et al.*, 1998). Exosome preparations were apparently devoid of retroviruses, plasma membrane shedding, microsome constituents or apoptotic bodies. Interestingly, we reproducibly reduced the amounts of vesicles secreted by inducing maturation of the mouse DC D1 line or BM-DC, as assessed by Bradford assay, western blotting with MHC class I antibodies, and immuno-electron microscopy (unpublished data). The basal secretion can be further and significantly enhanced by lowering the culture pH or incubating with defined cytokines, strongly suggesting that exocytosis of antigen-presenting vesicles by DC is regulated.

The striking observation is that immature DC, purportedly considered to be poor antigen-presenting cells (Cella, 1997), are actually capable of secreting antigen-presenting exosomes that account for efficient T cell priming *in vivo*. Indeed, intradermal injection of a single dose of exosome derived from 5×10^5 tumor peptide-pulsed DC was associated with tumor growth suppression in established mammary or mastocytoma tumor models. DC-derived exosomes are more effective in prophylaxis and therapy of mouse tumors than whole DC-based vaccines. Indeed, 2–5 μg of exosomes secreted from 10^6 DC pulsed with tumor peptides were more protective or curative than the DC themselves. Although not yet biochemically defined, exosomes bear high amounts of MHC class II, tetraspanins, and costimulatory molecules compared with DC lysates. The lipid composition of these compartments may be different from that of the plasma membrane and facilitates their *in vivo* uptake and/or transport to T cell-enriched areas. *Ex vivo* expanded DC represent valuable immunotherapeutic options for cancer-bearing patients (Steinman, 1991, 1996; Girolomoni, 1997) but phenotypic changes (surface markers, migration pathways, etc.) can be anticipated following withdrawal from the culture medium (Bender, 1996). In addition, MHC class I molecules on mature DC seem to have a relatively short half-life compared with MHC class II molecules (Cella, 1997). However, further molecular characterization of their composition and further investigation of their mechanisms are needed to better understand their *in vivo* efficacy.

The physiological role of DC-derived exosomes remains unclear. It is conceivable that T-helper cytokines are delivered to the DC upon arrival in the lymph node T cell-enriched areas. Antigen-presenting vesicles would then be released to amplify specific T cell clonal expansion. Alternatively, other host APC could take up these exosomes to transport these antigenic vesicles to specific sites where priming of naive T cells and/or B cell cross-talk could be elicited.

These data support the implementation of DC-derived exosomes for cancer immunotherapy as a novel dendritic cell-free therapeutic cancer vaccine and suggest that exosomes may represent a physiological means of communication between DC and T-lymphocytes.

SUMMARY

Dendritic cells (DC) are professional antigen-presenting cells having a unique ability to induce primary immune responses *in vitro* and *in vivo* (Inaba *et al.*, 1990; Caux *et al.*, 1992; Hart, 1997). Here, we show that antigen-presenting vesicles from endosomal MHC class II-enriched compartments can be secreted by DC and induce potent T cell-mediated anti-tumor immune responses *in vivo*. These vesicles, called 'exosomes', represent the internal vesicles of multivesicular endosomes, which are secreted following fusion of the external membrane of endosomes with the plasma membrane (Raposo *et al.*, 1996). Exosomes harvested from immature DC culture supernatants by ultracentrifugation were characterized by immuno-electron microscopy and western blotting. These vesicles harbor not only endosomal markers absent from the cell surface, but also express high levels of major histocompatibility complex (MHC) class I, class II, and costimulatory molecules. MHC class I molecule-bearing exosomes stimulate antigen-specific $CD8^+$ T cell clones *in vitro*. Importantly, intradermal injection of tumor peptide-pulsed DC-derived exosomes is capable of priming specific cytotoxic T-lymphocytes *in vivo* and suppressing growth of day 3–10 established murine tumors in a T cell-dependent and MHC-restricted manner. Cell-free-based exosome vaccines may be superior to dendritic cell adoptive therapy for controlling tumor growth. The anti-tumor effects of DC-derived exosomes support their implementation for cancer immunotherapy and suggest that exosomes represent a novel 'liposome-like' means of communication between cells of the immune system.

REFERENCES

Bender, A., Sapp, M., Schuler, G. *et al.*, (1996). Improved methods for the generation of dendritic cells from nonproliferating progenitors in human blood. *J. Immunol. Methods* **196**, 121–135.

Bockxmeer, F.V. and Morgan, E. (1979). Transferrin receptors during rabbit reticulocyte maturation. *Biochim. Biophys. Acta* **584**, 76–83.

Cella, M., Engering, A., Pinet, V. *et al.* (1997). Inflammatory stimuli induce accumulation of MHC class II complexes on dendritic cells. *Nature* (*London*) **388**, 782–786.

Dufour, E., Carcelain, G., Gaudin, C. *et al.* (1997). Diversity of the cytotoxic melanoma-specific immune response. *J. Immunol.* **158**, 3787–3795.

Girolomoni, G., Ricciardi-Castagnoli, P. (1997). Dendritic cells hold promise for immunotherapy. *Immunol. Today* **18**, 102–104.

Kleijmeer, M., Ossevoort, M., Veen, C.V. *et al.* (1995). MHC class II compartments and the kinetics of antigen presentation in activated mouse spleen dendritic cells. *J.Immunol.* **154**, 5715–5724.

Kleijmeer, N., Escola, J.M., Griffith, J., Geuze, H. (1998). MHC class I molecules are present in MHC class II compartments from dendritic cells and B lymphocytes. In: *Cellular and Molecular Biology of Dendritic Cells*, Keystone Symposia. Abstr. 220, p. 64.

Mayordomo, J.I., Zorina, T., Storkus, W.J. *et al.* (1995). Bone marrow-derived dendritic cells pulsed with synthetic tumour peptides elicit protective and therapeutic antitumour immunity. *Nature Medicine* **1**, 1297–1302.

Metzelaar, M., Wijngaard, P., Peters, P. *et al.* (1991). CD63 antigen: a novel lysosomal membrane glycoprotein, cloned by a screening procedure for intracellular antigens in eukaryotic cells. *J. Biol. Chem.* **266**, 3239–3245.

Nijman, H., Kleijmeer, M., Ossevoort, M. *et al.* (1995). Antigen capture and MHC class II compartments in freshly isolated and cultured blood dendritic cells. *J. Exp. Med.* **182**, 163–174.

Raposo, G., Kleijmeer, M., Posthuma, J. *et al.* (1997). Immunogold labeling of ultrathin cryosections: application in immunology. *Exp. Immunol.* **4**, 1–10.

Raposo, G., Nijman, H., Stoorvogel, W. *et al.* (1996). B lymphocytes secrete antigen presenting vesicles. *J. Exp. Med.* **183**, 1161–1172.

Raposo, G., Vidal, M. and Geuze, H. (1997). Secretory lysosomes and the production of exosomes. In: *Unusal Secretory Pathways: From Bacteria to Man* (ed. Karl Kuchler), Landes, pp. 161–184.

Steinman, R.M. (1991). The dendritic cell system and its role in immunogenicity. *Annu. Rev. Immunol.* **9**, 271–296.

Steinman, R. (1996). Dendritic cells and immune-based therapies. *Exp. Hematol.* **24**, 859–862.

Winzler, C., Rovere, P., Rescigno, M. *et al.* (1997). Maturation stages of mouse dendritic cells in growth factor-dependent long term cultures. *J. Exp. Med.* **185**, 317-328.

Zitvogel, L., Mayordomo, J.I., Tjandrawan, T. *et al.* (1996). Therapy of murine tumors with tumor peptide-pulsed dendritic cells: dependence on T cells, B7 costimulation, and T helper cell 1-associated cytokines. *J. Exp. Med.* **183**, 87–97.

Zitvogel, L., Regnault, A., Lozier, A., Wolfers, J., Flament, C., Tenza, D., Ricciardi-Castagnoli, P., Raposo, G. and Amigorena, S. (1998). Eradication of established murine tumors using a novel cell-free vaccine: dendritic cell-derived exosomes. *Nature Medicine* **4**, 594–600.

CHAPTER 37
Dendritic Cells as Donors and Recipients of Cytokine Signals

Nikolaus Romani[1], Franz Koch[1], Christine Heufler[1], Eckhart Kämpgen[2] and [3]Gerold Schuler

Departments of Dermatology, Universities of [1]Innsbruck, Austria, [2]Würzburg, Germany and [3]Erlangen-Nürnberg, Germany

INTRODUCTION

With the recent boom in dendritic cell (DC) research our knowledge about these cells as producers of or responders to cytokines is expanding rapidly. This was made possible by the refinement of methods for isolating and enriching dendritic cells from the tissues or blood and—even more so—by the development of techniques for growing large numbers of dendritic cells from blood (mainly in the human system) or bone marrow (mainly in rodent systems) (see Chapter 27). Previously, it was difficult to obtain sufficient numbers of DC in sufficient purity for detailed cytokine analyses. In a 1994 review article on cytokines and dendritic cells, particularly Langerhans cells (Romani *et al.*, 1994b), we wrote that 'a few years from now it will be easier to write a conclusive review about Langerhans cells and cytokines. We are looking forward to that day.' That day has come and certainly there is now a wealth of data on this topic. We doubt, however, whether it has become 'easier' to compose this review. Rather than trying to give a complete account of presently available cytokine data, it is the aim of this chapter to outline some important (and currently busy) areas of research about dendritic cells as donors and recipients of cytokine signals.

TECHNIQUES FOR ANALYZING CYTOKINE EXPRESSION BY DENDRITIC CELLS

Not only have the methods for obtaining DC been improved, but also the technology for analyzing cytokine production as well as responsiveness to cytokines has advanced (reviewed in Carter and Swain, 1997). Some examples will be given. Methods will be grouped by the levels of detection, i.e., mRNA, protein, bioactivity.

Analyses at the mRNA Level

Polymerase Chain Reaction (PCR)

This very sensitive technique has advanced in terms of quantification of the amplification product. Methods are now available that allow the quantitative comparison of

Dendritic Cells: Biology and Clinical Applications
ISBN 0-12-455860-7

PCR data. The great advantage of PCR is its high sensitivity; very low levels of message can be detected. If PCR is applied for the analysis of DC it is mandatory to monitor rigorously the purity of DC populations because even minute contamination with nondendritic cells may give 'false positives.' The disadvantage of PCR (as well as of northern blotting) is that bulk populations are examined. A possible heterogeneity of populations remains undiscovered.

Single-cell PCR

An interesting variant of the PCR was recently reported. Neumann and colleagues. (Neumann *et al.*, 1997) used the tools of patch clamp electrophysiology to extract RNA from single cells (neurons) in culture. They amplified the RNA by reverse transcription PCR and were able to detect the expression of cytokine genes (interferon-γ and TNF-α). Although difficult to perform, this method holds promise of help in answering important questions. Whether it is feasible to extract mRNA from single cells *in situ* (in sections) has not been tested. Alternatively, it is possible to perform the amplification step itself *in situ*, e.g., on cytospin preparations. The amplified mRNA is subsequently visualized by in-situ hybridization ('in-situ PCR') (Bagasra *et al.*, 1993).

In-situ Hybridization

A better established method for the detection of mRNA *in situ* (but without amplification) is in-situ hybridization (Hoefakker *et al.*, 1995). It was originally done with radioactively labeled probes and autoradiography. This is increasingly being displaced by techniques of nonradioactive in-situ hybridization. The most widely distributed protocol uses digoxigenin-conjugated probes that—after hybridization—are visualized by means of anti-digoxigenin antibodies that are tagged either with a fluorochrome or with an enzyme (peroxidase or alkaline phosphatase). Nonradioactive in-situ hybridization holds the potential to be combined with immunohistochemistry, thus allowing the simultaneous visualization of cytokine mRNA expression and a desired cell marker molecule. An example was the localization of IL-12 mRNA in mature murine spleen dendritic cells identified immunohistochemically by a monoclonal antibody (mAb) (Heufler *et al.*, 1996).

Analyses at the Protein Level

Enzyme-linked Immunosorbent Assays (ELISA)

Sandwich ELISAs have become the method of choice for the determination of cytokine production of cells in culture or of cytokine levels in body fluids. Cell homogenates can also be subjected to ELISA analyses (Holliday *et al.*, 1996). The sandwich consists of a *capture antibody* that is coupled to the bottom of microtiter wells and that 'pulls out' the cytokine molecules from the samples, and a *detection antibody* that is conjugated to peroxidase or biotin and serves to visualize the plate-bound (captured) cytokine. Capture and detection antibodies must not interfere with each other and therefore must be selected such that they recognize different epitopes on the cytokine molecule. A typical example for a cytokine ELISA has been described recently for IL-12 (Wilkinson *et al.*, 1996). When absolute values for cytokine concentration are discussed, one should not neglect the possibility that data obtained from ELISA and cytokine standards from different manufacturers may vary (Ledur *et al.*, 1995).

Flow Cytometry

The staining and subsequent analysis in the flow cytometer of permeabilized, isolated cells in suspension with antibodies to cytokines is an emerging and very promising method (Carter and Swain, 1997). An important advantage of this approach is the possibility of combining cell lineage markers with the anti-cytokine antibodies and thus to identify the cytokine-producing cells. Production of different cytokines in one cell can also be assessed. This methodology has even been taken further in that live T cells were sorted according to the cytokines they secreted (Manz *et al.*, 1995). It should be noted, though, that generally it is required to stimulate cells in order to be able to detect the cytokines. Moreover, a trick has to be applied: cells to be analyzed must be treated with Brefeldin A or monensin to prevent the cytokine from being secreted and thus to promote its accumulation within the cell. This results in a higher intracellular cytokine concentration and, as a consequence, a better detectability (Carter and Swain, 1997). The full potential of this method for the analysis of DC is starting to be exploited.

Immunohistochemistry

This is the traditional technique for localizing cytokines *in situ* (reviewed in Hoefakker *et al.*, 1995). The advantage is that the cytokine *proteins* are visualized. A disadvantage is that it cannot be ruled out that cytokine protein has been taken up rather than synthesized by the cell proper. Owing to the soluble nature of cytokines (as opposed to more robust membrane-anchored molecules), immunohistochemistry is not easy. Fixation and permeabilization protocols have to be worked out carefully and tested. Yet there are examples where this technique has been successfully applied to detect cytokines in DC (e.g., Gruschwitz and Hornstein, 1992; Macatonia *et al.*, 1995; Cella *et al.*, 1996)

Analyses at the Level of Bioactivity

Bioassays in Vitro

The ultimate proof that a given cytokine is functional can only be derived from bioassays. A large number of such assays for different cytokines is available (Mire-Sluis *et al.*, 1995). They are often based on the proliferation-promoting properties of cytokines (e.g., CTLL assay for IL-2) or on their cytotoxic properties (e.g., L929 assay for TNF-α). The bioactivity of chemokines is measured by their capacity to induce chemotactic or chemoattractive migration of cells. A recent example is the observation that a DC-derived chemokine (DC-CK1) attracts naive T lymphocytes in migration assays (Adema *et al.*, 1997).

Some General Considerations

When analyzing or judging experimental data on cytokines and DC, it is important to keep in mind some general principles. These points may seem trivial, yet, we feel that they are worth being mentioned and emphasized.

In Vivo–in Situ–in Vitro

In vitro assays of cytokine production measure a DC's ability to make a given cytokine. Moreover, we can learn how the production of cytokines can be augmented or inhibited. Such data do not necessarily reflect the true situation in the living human or mouse. *In vivo* assays have to be applied to approach these questions. This often means measuring cytokine levels in body fluids such as blood, or in culture supernatants of organ cultures. Again, these values may not always accurately describe the cytokine milieu in a particular, biologically relevant organ or tissue (e.g., lymph node, skin). The closest that one can get to this is by immunohistochemistry and/or in-situ hybridization of organ or tissue sections. Immunohistochemistry for cytokines is difficult and often tricky. In-situ hybridization is widely used but it has certainly not yet reached the degree of 'foolproofness' of immunohistochemistry. Both methods yield qualitative or at most semiquantitative data. It is important to be aware of the fact that actual concentrations of cytokines *in situ* cannot be determined with the tools that we have presently at hand. For example, it would be interesting to know the actual concentration of TNF-α that induces the emigration of Langerhans cell from the epidermis after the application of contact sensitizers or in organ culture. It would also be exciting to learn about the actual concentrations of IL-4, IL-10, IL-12, etc. within the microenvironment of the T cell area of the lymph node, where the T_H1/T_H2 decision takes place. Such questions await the development of appropriate methods with which one could tackle them.

Mature versus Immature Dendritic Cells

It has already been shown in the first reports on DC cytokine production that these cells express different cytokine patterns at different stages of differentiation: for example, the IL-1β mRNA expression is upregulated upon maturation in culture (Heufler *et al.*, 1992). It is therefore important to consider the maturational status of DC whenever comparing data from different sources. It should also be kept in mind that populations of immature or mature DC may not always be 100% of the one or the other type! For example, populations of freshly isolated Langerhans cells (i.e., immature DC) contain a small percentage of strongly MHC class II-expressing cells. These Langerhans cells appear to have started maturation already *in situ*. Conversely, populations of cultured Langerhans cells (i.e., mature dendritic cells) contain a minority of invariant chain-expressing cells. These Langerhans cells appear to lag behind in their maturation process (Koch *et al.*, 1995b). Cytokine production by such minority fractions will certainly be detected by sensitive methods like the PCR and can lead to incorrect conclusions.

Source of Dendritic Cells

Much of the work that is presently undertaken utilizes DC derived from blood monocytes or from $CD34^+$ progenitor cells. Caux and colleagues (Caux *et al.*, 1997) have recently differentiated subsets of DC by phenotype and function. Most likely, these variants of DC also express different cytokine/cytokine-receptor profiles. Another example that should alert us to consider this point is TNF-α: Langerhans cells do not make this cytokine (Enk and Katz, 1992; Heufler *et al.*, 1992); dendritic cells from the blood do, however, express mRNA for TNF-α (Zhou and Tedder, 1995).

TECHNIQUES FOR ANALYZING CYTOKINE EFFECTS ON DENDRITIC CELLS

These techniques comprise all those protocols where purified cytokines are administered experimentally *in vitro* or *in vivo*, or where neutralizing anti-cytokine reagents (antibodies, antagonists) are given. A major advance has been the development of mice that either overexpress genes encoding given cytokines (transgenic mice) or mice that lack given cytokine genes, because they have been experimentally disrupted (*knockout mice*). Both technologies have evolved to the point where genes can be specifically expressed or knocked out (Cre/loxP technique; Fässler *et al.*, 1995) in selected cells or tissues of the body. This renders these methods very powerful for studying the complex effects of cytokines. For example, the transgene encoding the chemokine MCP-1 was specifically expressed in the basal layer of the murine epidermis and this led to a recruitment of DC (Langerhans cells) into the skin (Nakamura *et al.*, 1995). Another dimension of these approaches is the possibility of cross-breeding different knockout or transgenic animals. A recent example is a TNF-α/lymphotoxin-α double knockout mouse that has already yielded interesting insights into the biology of TNF-α (Eugster *et al.*, 1996).

In spite of researchers' enthusiasm about the new technologies, a word of caution is warranted. It has been observed repeatedly that animals that lack seemingly vital genes can survive for significant periods—at least in the protected environment of germ-free animal facilities. This should alert us that there are backup mechanisms operative in the living organism. It is difficult to determine whether such backup mechanisms function in the normal animal or whether they are activated specifically when the default mechanism of action is rendered nonfunctional by the experimentor. This concern should not invalidate the usefulness of genetically modified mice for cytokine research with dendritic cells.

DENDRITIC CELLS AS PRODUCERS OF CYTOKINES

Many studies dealing with the cytokine production of dendritic cells are currently ongoing. Different types of DC at different stages of development and maturation are being investigated with different methods. We have not yet arrived at a clear picture. Therefore, we do not attempt to cover the current knowledge comprehensively. Rather, we will mention some interesting foci of DC-related cytokine research.

Inflammatory Cytokines

Dendritic cells fulfill a sentinel function in the different tissues where they reside. In response to many antigens or to danger they respond by elaborating inflammatory cytokines. Most notably, mRNA for IL-1β is expressed by DC as they mature both *in vitro* (Heufler *et al.*, 1992) and *in vivo* (Enk and Katz, 1992). Only few reports show secretion of IL-1β protein (Ragg *et al.*, 1997). IL-6 was shown repeatedly to be made by DC (Romani *et al.*, 1994b; Cumberbatch *et al.*, 1996). Like IL-1β it is also upregulated upon maturation. TNF-α was not found in mature and immature DC from skin

(Heufler *et al.*, 1992). Immature DC derived from human blood monocytes (Thurnher *et al.*, 1997; Verhasselt *et al.*, 1997) or mature DC obtained by CD40 triggering (Caux *et al.*, 1994), however, produce this cytokine.

In addition to these classical pro-inflammatory cytokines it is also conceivable that the extraordinarily large amounts of IL-12 (nanogram quantities) that are made by immature DC upon phagocytosis of bacteria or CD40 ligation (Cella *et al.*, 1996, and our own unpublished observations) may contribute to the inflammatory process.

T Cell-regulating Cytokines

Several reports have shown that DC can make the cytokine IL-12. Production of IL-12 can be boosted from low constitutive levels (Heufler *et al.*, 1996) to very high levels via two pathways of stimulation, namely microbes/microbial products and T cells (via ligation of CD40 and/or MHC class II on DC) (Koch *et al.*, 1996; Cella *et al.*, 1996). Inflammatory stimuli such as a combination of TNF-α and prostaglandin E_2 have the same effect (Rieser *et al.*, 1997). IL-10 can inhibit both pathways; IL-4 appears to inhibit only the microbial pathway of IL-12 induction, though under certain conditions it enhances the CD40-mediated induction of IL-12 (Takenaka *et al.*, 1997). Preliminary reports indicate that another T cell-regulating cytokine, namely IL-18 (interferon-γ-inducing factor) is produced in functional form by DC (Stoll *et al.*, 1998; Scheicher *et al.*, 1998).

Chemokines

It has been known for some time that DC can elaborate MIP-1α and MIP-2 (Heufler *et al.*, 1992; Zhou and Tedder, 1995). A number of very recent publications has made it clear that DC are important producers of a whole array of chemokines (Godiska *et al.*, 1997; Mohamadzadeh *et al.*, 1996). In contrast to other cytokines, whose expression is normally shared by DC and various other cell types, some chemokines appear to be exclusively made by DC, examples being a T cell-attracting C-C chemokine named DC-CK1 (Adema *et al.*, 1997) and a C-C chemokine that is made specifically by thymic DC named TECK (thymus-expressed chemokine) (Vicari *et al.*, 1997). This field is presently evolving at a very fast pace.

DENDRITIC CELLS AS RESPONDERS TO CYTOKINES

Expression of Cytokine Receptors on Dendritic Cells

By definition, any cytokine that acts directly on DC must do so via a receptor on the surface of the DC. Owing to the large numbers of cells required, the classical radioligand binding assays (Scatchard analyses) were hard to perform and therefore rarely done. Now, DC can be obtained in large numbers and, in addition, more and better (monoclonal) antibodies have become available that allow the detection of receptors by flow cytometry (Larregina *et al.*, 1997). A recent review by Kämpgen *et al.*, 1995) sums up much of our current knowledge on this point. As expected, DC express on their surfaces receptors for the various cytokines that exert known effects on these cells, e.g.,

GM-CSF, IL-1, TNF-α. Still enigmatic is the presence of the low-affinity IL-2 receptor (CD25) on mature DC.

Chemokine Receptors

This particular family of cytokine receptors has attracted much interest because some of its members serve as coreceptors, together with CD4, for the entry of HIV-1 into target cells (Baggiolini *et al.*, 1997). Human DC express the chemokine receptors CCR5 (for RANTES and for macrophage-tropic HIV strains) and CXCR4 (for SDF-1 and for T cell-tropic HIV strains) and, accordingly, HIV-1 can enter the cells although this does not lead to replication of the virus (Granelli-Piperno *et al.*, 1996; Rubbert *et al.*, 1998). In addition, CCR1, -2, and -3 and CXCR-1 and -2 were detected on the surface of human DC (Sozzani *et al.*, 1997; Ayehunie *et al.*, 1997). A novel receptor (CCR6) for the C-C chemokine MIP-3α was recently identified on CD34-derived human blood DC (Greaves *et al.*, 1997) and on lung DC (Power *et al.* 1997). The presence of as yet undefined CCRs on DC can be postulated from their chemotactic responses to the corresponding chemokines, e.g., DC-CK1 (Adema *et al.*, 1997) or macrophage-derived chemokine/MDC (Godiska *et al.*, 1997). The expression of several chemokine receptors on DC emphasizes the importance of chemokines in the regulation of DC function, particularly migration.

Cytokines Regulate Dendritic Cell Ontogeny

GM-CSF

Myeloid DC, macrophages and granulocytes arise from a common precursor cell in the bone marrow (Inaba *et al.*, 1993; and Chapter 5 by Caux *et al.*). Therefore, it is not surprising that GM-CSF is an essential cytokine for the generation of DC by culture from multipotent ($CD34^+$) precursors in the marrow (Inaba *et al.* 1992a; Young *et al.*, 1995), in cord blood (Caux *et al.*, 1992), peripheral blood (Inaba *et al.*, 1992b), spleen (Lu *et al.*, 1995a), or liver (Lu *et al.*, 1994). In cultures of murine bone marrow it suffices to add GM-CSF in order to obtain populations containing a large percentage of mature DC (Inaba *et al.*, 1992a; Yamaguchi *et al.*, 1997; Lutz *et al.*, 1998). The cocktail of 'self-made' cytokines that is operative in cultures of developing bone marrow DC, in addition to experimentally added GM-CSF, has not yet been determined. Experiments with transgenic mice producing excessive levels of GM-CSF showed an increase of dendritic cells that could be isolated from lymphoid organs (Vremec *et al.*, 1997). This underscores the importance of GM-CSF. Conversely, however, the examination of mice that have a targeted disruption of their genes for GM-CSF or for the GM-CSF receptor β-chain (CDw131; shared with IL-3 and IL-5 receptors) did not reveal dramatic deficits in the numbers of DC in lymphoid organs (Vremec *et al.*, 1997). This suggests that the development of most DC in lymphoid tissues is dependent on more cytokines than GM-CSF.

An additional pathway of DC ontogeny has recently been described in thymus (Chapter 6 by Maraskovsky *et al.*). These DC stem from a progenitor that they share with T cells. They are therefore referred to as 'lymphoid dendritic cells.' They can be grown from thymic precursors in the absence of exogenously added GM-CSF as well as from precursors of GM-CSF knockout mice (Saunders *et al.*, 1996). They were also found in the above-mentioned GM-CSF receptor knockout mice (Vremec *et al.*, 1997). Thus, their development appears to be independent of GM-CSF.

TNF-α

This cytokine is essential when DC are generated from CD34$^+$ progenitors in bone marrow or umbilical cord blood. TNF-α cooperates with GM-CSF (Reid *et al.*, 1992; Caux *et al.*, 1992). How TNF-α is involved in the ontogeny of DC *in vivo* is not known. Preliminary data from our laboratory show that in TNF-α/lymphotoxin-α double knockout mice (Eugster *et al.*, 1996) the development of dendritic cells is not abrogated (unpublished data). Certainly, TNF-α ensures that DC procured in this way are mature at the end of the culture (Caux *et al.*, 1992).

Flt3 Ligand

Another ontogenetically important cytokine is the Flt3 ligand. Mice that were injected with this cytokine possessed markedly elevated numbers of dendritic cells in lymphoid and nonlymphoid tissues (Maraskovsky *et al.*, 1996). *In vitro*, Flt3 ligand enhanced the development of DC from both murine (Saunders *et al.*, 1996) and human (Siena *et al.*, 1995) precursors. This was reflected *in vivo* by the fact that Flt3 ligand-treated mice were effectively protected against a malignant experimental tumor (Lynch *et al.*, 1997).

Stem Cell Factor/c-kit Ligand

A similar but less pronounced effect was observed with stem cell factor. In cultures of developing human DC from CD34$^+$ progenitors in marrow and umbilical cord blood, the addition of stem cell factor enhanced both size and numbers of dendritic cell colonies as well as the final DC progeny (Young *et al.*, 1995; Saraya and Reid, 1996; Siena *et al.*, 1995). This effect occurred only in a synergistic combination with GM-CSF and TNF-α.

IL-4

The observation in murine bone marrow cultures that, in the hands of some investigators, the addition of IL-4 (together with GM-CSF) leads to better yields of more potent DC (Lu *et al.*, 1995b; Mayordomo *et al.*, 1997; Dillon *et al.*, 1997) suggests that IL-4 modulates the developmental pathway, probably by suppressing the monocyte/macrophage lineage (Jansen *et al.*, 1989). A hint for a role of IL-4 *in vivo* comes from studies with IL-4 transgenic mice: IL-4-overexpressing mice have a higher density of epidermal Langerhans cells (Elbe *et al.*, unpublished observations). At a later stage in ontogeny, however, IL-4 does play an important role, at least *in vitro*. Those methods that attempt to generate DC from monocytes in the human blood depend critically on IL-4 (Sallusto and Lanzavecchia, 1994; Romani *et al.*, 1994a). IL-4 serves to suppress the differentiation along the macrophage pathway (Jansen *et al.*, 1989). The importance of this pathway, which was entirely defined *in vitro*, for the *in vivo* situation is unknown.

TGF-β1

The effect of this cytokine is primarily qualitative rather than quantitative. TGF-β_1 seems to direct the differentiation of $CD34^+$ DC progenitors toward the subset of dendritic cells with epidermal destiny, namely Langerhans cells. The most direct *in vivo* evidence for this stems from experiments with TGF-β_1 knock-out mice. These animals specifically lack Langerhans cells; other types of DC are present (Borkowski *et al.*, 1996). *In vitro*, Strobl *et al.*, (1997) noted that $CD34^+$ progenitor cells cultured in the presence of TGF-β_1 (together with GM-CSF and TNF-α and under serum-free conditions) gave rise to Birbeck granule-containing DC. Similar findings were reported for monocyte-derived DC from human blood (Geissmann *et al.*, 1998). Moreover, a substantial part of human $CD34^+$ progenitors that coexpress the cutaneous lymphocyte antigen (CLA/mAb HECA-452) (Strunk *et al.*, 1997) or E-cadherin (Caux *et al.*, 1996) develop into Birbeck granule-containing Langerhans cells upon culture in the presence of GM-CSF and TNF-α; progenitors that do not express either of these molecules never become Langerhans cells. These data, together with the observation that TGF-β_1 induces the cutaneous lymphocyte antigen on T cells (Picker *et al.*, 1993) and DC (Geissmann *et al.*, 1998), lead to a hypothesis whereby TGF-β_1 causes the upregulation of CLA on developing DC and, as a consequence, their selective homing to the skin.

Cytokines Regulate Dendritic Cell Maturation

Dendritic cell maturation was first described with epidermal Langerhans cells as a model (Schuler and Steinman, 1985; Romani *et al.*, 1989). It has since been observed with other types of DC as well. After having developed from progenitors in the bone marrow or in the thymus, DC populate lymphoid and nonlymphoid tissues and reside there as *immature* (or *early stage*) DC. In response to appropriate stimuli, a process is triggered whereby DC quickly develop a strong capacity for processing native protein antigens (efficient antigen uptake, massive MHC biosynthesis; abundance of processing organelles such as class II-containing vesicles (MIICs); Pierre *et al.*, 1997). They are now still *immature* but functionally highly active (*intermediate stage*). Freshly isolated (i.e., trypsinized) epidermal Langerhans cells are the prototype for this stage. The differentiation process continues and leads to mature (*late stage*) DC. They are characterized by a very poor capacity for antigen uptake and processing but by a strong T cell sensitizing function. Inflammatory stimuli, including the cytokines TNF-α and IL-1β were identified as inducers of the previously described (Kämpgen *et al.*, 1991; Puré *et al.*, 1990) transient boost in MHC class II biosynthesis that occurs at the onset of maturation (Cella *et al.*, 1997). These cytokines are also responsible for the shutdown of macropinocytosis (Sallusto *et al.*, 1995) and TNF-α was shown to enhance the upregulation of MHC class II and CD86 in cultures of murine bone marrow DC (Yamaguchi *et al.*, 1997).

In vivo, the cellular sources of maturation-inducing inflammatory cytokines can be different cell types in the vicinity of DC. In the skin, for example, keratinocytes have been shown to elaborate TNF-α and IL-1α in response to danger such as the experimental application of contact sensitizers. IL-1β on the other hand, is made by DC themselves in response to the same stimuli (Enk and Katz, 1992). Also, the phagocytosis of bacterial particles or soluble bacterial products (LPS) elicits the production of inflammatory cytokines in DC: IL-1β (Henderson *et al.*, 1997; Granuccia *et al.*, 1994; Kanangat *et al.*, 1995), TNF-α (Henderson *et al.*, 1997; Thurnher *et al.*, 1997), and IL-6 (Riva *et al.*, 1996). This would enable DC that become infected or that are located in a microbially infested environment to set off the maturation process in an autocrine way and thus induce immunity.

Two molecules were recently described that appear to be critically involved in dendritic cell survival and maturation. TRANCE (TNF-related activation-induced cytokine) is made by T cells and was shown to rescue DC from apoptosis (Wong *et al.*, 1997). RANK (receptor activator of NF-κB), a homolog of the TNF receptor, is expressed on DC and binding of the ligand molecule (RANKL) enhances the immunstimulatory capacity of DC for naive T cells (Anderson *et al.*, 1997).

An important counterregulator of DC maturation is the cytokine IL-10 (De Smedt *et al.*, 1997). This cytokine prevents the upregulation of costimulatory molecules on DC. DC treated in this way induce not proliferation but anergy in $CD4^{+}T$ cells and T_H1 clones (Steinbrink *et al.*, 1997; Enk *et al.*, 1993a; Takenaka *et al.*, 1997). IL-10 thus acts in a tolerogenic way. When administered *in vivo*, IL-10 impairs the development of contact hypersensitivity (Enk *et al.*, 1994), a process that is critically dependent on the maturation and migration of cutaneous DC. It is important to note that once DC are fully mature they are no longer susceptible to the effects of IL-10 (Steinbrink *et al.*, 1997). Another maturation-inhibiting cytokine appears to be TGF-β (Yamaguchi *et al.*, 1997).

As mentioned above, it is now well established that TNF-α is a main inducer of DC maturation. This conclusion is derived from many experiments in which TNF-α is added to cultures containing other cytokines as well. There may, however, be circumstances where TNF-α leads to a disturbed maturation. We were also to show previously that highly enriched Langerhans cells that were cultured with TNF-α in the absence of any other cytokines (except possible undetermined 'self-made' cytokines) did not acquire high T cell stimulatory capacity like their counterparts cultured in the presence of GM-CSF, or keratinocyte-conditioned media (Koch *et al.*, 1990). We identified a loss of immunogenic peptides from the MHC class II molecules as well as a diminished capacity to cluster resting T cells as reasons for these phenomena (Koch *et al.*, 1995a). These data should remind us of the manifold and crucial interactions between different cytokines. The data also suggest that TNF-α by itself is not sufficient for complete maturation.

Cytokines Regulate Dendritic Cell Migration

Migration from Nonlymphoid to Lymphoid Tissues—Induction

Maturation and migration are tightly linked processes. They appear to be initiated by inflammatory cytokines. This was shown directly in experiments in which LPS was injected into mice. This led to both a loss or numerical reduction of DC from nonlymphoid tissues such as hearts, kidney, and skin (Roake *et al.*, 1995a) and a concomitant recruitment of MHC class II-negative precursor DC into these tissues (Roake *et al.*, 1995b). The depletion of DC could also be achieved by systemic administration of TNF-α and—to a lesser degree—IL-1 (Roake *et al.*, 1995a). LPS treatment also causes a translocation of DC within lymphoid tissues: in the spleen, DC migrate from the marginal zone between red and white pulp to the T cell areas (De Smedt *et al.*, 1996). In an *in vivo* model it was shown that the intradermal application of TNF-α induces both the reduction of Langerhans cell densities within the epidermis (Cumberbatch *et al.*, 1994), indicating emigration, and the accumulation of DC in the draining lymph nodes (Cumberbatch and Kimber, 1992). Similarly, in both murine and human skin organ cultures (Ortner *et al.*, 1996) TNF-α enhances and anti-TNF-α inhibits the migration of Langerhans cells and dermal DC out of their cutaneous environment into the culture medium (unpublished observations). Finally, when the accumulation of hapten (FITC)-bearing cutaneous DC in the draining lymph nodes was studied, an effect of TNF-α on the migration was observed: blocking of TNF-R2 (p75) with a mAb significantly inhibited the influx of DC into the node (Wang *et al.*, 1996). In the classical model of contact hypersensitivity, the production of cytokines was studied in detail at the level of mRNA. Upon application of contact allergens, i.e., under circumstances where Langerhans cells had been shown to emigrate from the epidermis (Bergstresser *et al.*, 1980; Weinlich *et al.*, 1998), keratinocytes were induced to express mRNA for TNF-α and IL-1α, whereas Langerhans cells expressed IL-1β message (Enk and Katz, 1992). TNF-α was also induced by chemically related, nonsensitizing compounds (that also did not cause migration); IL-1 expression, in contrast, appeared to be triggered specifically by contact allergens that also led to the emigration of Langerhans cells (Enk and Katz, 1992). When IL-1β was injected into murine skin it mimicked all those phenomena that were seen upon application of contact allergens, i.e., upregulation of message for TNF-α, IL-1α, IL-10, IP-10 and MIP-2 in keratinocytes and of IL-1β and MHC class II in Langerhans cells (Enk *et al.*, 1993b). Like contact allergens, intradermal IL-1β also caused emigration of Langerhans cells from the epidermis (Enk *et al.*, 1993b; Nylander-Lundqvist and Bäck, 1990). The blocking of IL-1 by administration of IL-1 receptor antagonist resulted in clearly impaired contact hypersensitivity reactions (Kondo *et al.*, 1995a). Thus, it is obvious that TNF-α and IL-1β are central to the migration of DC (Cumberbatch *et al.*, 1997).

How these two cytokines cooperate with each other may be elucidated in knockout models. Contact hypersensitivity can be induced in TNF-R1 knockout mice (also in combination with antibody blocking of TNF-R2 (Kondo *et al.*, 1995b). In contrast, contact hypersensitivity was found to be defective in IL-1β (Shornick *et al.*, 1996) knockout mice. Dendritic cell/Langerhans cell migration was not directly monitored in these experiments. Yet the data could mean that the two cytokines work in a cascade-like fashion, IL-1β being the 'master cytokine' (Knop and Enk, 1995): TNF-α induces IL-1β and IL-1β, in turn, induces downregulation of E-cadherin (see below).

Migration from Nonlymphoid to Lymphoid Tissues—Adhesion Molecules and Chemotactic Cytokines

Langerhans cells are anchored between the surrounding epidermal keratinocytes by homophilic adhesion mediated by E-cadherin molecules (Udey, 1997). TNF-α, IL-1β, short-term culture, and epicutaneous application of contact sensitizers can downregulate E-cadherin expression on Langerhans cells (Schwarzenberger and Udey, 1996), thus loosening their contacts with keratinocytes and making them ready to migrate.

Once unleashed by the downregulation of E-cadherin, Langerhans cells migrate through the basement membrane. Thereby, cytokine-regulated adhesive interactions with basement membrane components such as laminin are critical (Price *et al.*, 1997). Dendritic cells move further through the collagen network until they reach afferent dermal lymphatic vessels where they get carried to the lymph nodes. It is not known to what degree this process is regulated by cytokines. It is likely that the cells follow chemotactic signals. Fibroblasts were reported to be a source of as yet undefined chemoattractants (Kobayashi *et al.*, 1994). Endothelial cells make a chemotactic factor that promotes the migration of human DC across vessel walls (Rahdon *et al.*, 1997). *In vitro*, human DC respond to a number of chemotactic stimuli: C5a (Sozzani *et al.*, 1995; Xu *et al.*, 1996), MCP-3, MIP-1α, RANTES (Sozzani *et al.*, 1995; Xu *et al.*, 1996), and a novel C-C chemokine, MDC (macrophage-derived chemokine) (Godiska *et al.*, 1997). Which of these chemoattractants are operative *in vivo* is not known.

Migration from Bone Marrow to Nonlymphoid Tissues

The first event in the life of DC is to leave the bone marrow and to enter a nonlymphoid tissue, for example, the epidermis. This aspect of DC migration is less well studied. Observations in knockout mice point to TGF-β_1 as an important regulator of this process. In TGF-β_1 knockout mice there are no Langerhans cells in the epidermis; lymph nodes, however, do contain DC (Borkowski *et al.*, 1996) and DC can be grown from the bone marrow (Borkowski *et al.*, 1997). Another important cytokine was revealed in a transgenic model. Mice were 'constructed' in which the gene for the chemokine MCP-1 was expressed under the control of the promoter for keratin of the basal layers. MCP-1 was produced abundantly by the basal keratinocytes. These mice showed increased numbers of MHC class II-positive cells in the skin, presumably Langerhans cells (Nakamura *et al.*, 1995). The novel C-C chemokine MIP-3α appears to be critically involved in the recruitment of DC to the tissues since receptors for it were selectively detected on human DC (Greaves *et al.*, 1997; Power *et al.*, 1997).

Cytokines Regulate T Cell Sensitization by Dendritic Cells

Migrating dendritic cells from various nonlymphoid tissues arrive—antigen-laden—in the lymph nodes or in the spleen. There, they are strategically well positioned to meet as many lymphocytes as possible and to find and bind antigen-specific T cells. This random event can be improved by a recently discovered chemokine. Human DC are the exclusive producers of a C-C chemokine, termed DC-CK1, that selectively attracts naive T lymphocytes (Adema *et al.*, 1997). In-situ hybridization revealed that mRNA for DC-CK1 is indeed expressed by DC within lymphoid organs. Similar, though less specific, T cell-attracting cytokines are IL-15 and MIP-1γ which were recently shown to be secreted in functional form by human blood DC (Blauvelt *et al.*, 1996; Jonuleit *et al.*, 1997) and mouse spleen DC (Mohamadzadeh *et al.*, 1996), respectively.

Once a DC has bound ('clustered') many antigen-specific T cells, another DC-derived cytokine plays a decisive role. IL-12, which is constitutively produced by DC in small amounts (Heufler *et al.*, 1996), is dramatically upregulated when MHC class II molecules engage with the T cell receptor and—later in time—when CD40 on the surface of the mature dendritic cell engages with the CD40 ligand (CD154) on the surface of an activated T cell (Koch *et al.*, 1996). Very high levels of IL-12 can be measured under these conditions (Cella *et al.*, 1996). Unless IL-4 is present, this ensures the development of a T_H1 response, i.e., the clonal expansion of T-helper cells that produce interferon-γ. This is particularly important when DC present nonmicrobial antigens, e.g., tumor peptides in the case of immunotherapy. In contrast to bacteria or bacterial products (LPS) such antigens do not induce IL-12 production in DC. That DC-derived IL-12 can indeed drive T cell responses toward a T_H1 pattern has been shown both in the mouse (Macatonia *et al.*, 1995; Heufler *et al.*, 1996) and in man (Ohshima and Delespesse, 1997).

CONCLUDING REMARKS

Data on the expression of many different cytokines at different levels (mRNA, protein, bioactivity) in different types of DC and at different stages of maturation have been corroborated over the past few years. From this heterogeneous accumulation of valuable data some common features can be extracted and some important questions formulated.

- In the ontogeny of DC, TGF-β appears to be a crucial cytokine that directs the development toward epidermal Langerhans cells. The mechanism by which this occurs is not yet known.
- Inflammatory cytokines (TNF-α, IL-1β) are critical inducers of DC maturation. The interactions of these cytokines with each other and with other cytokines are still incompletely understood.
- Dendritic cells express several chemokine receptors and are chemotactically responsive to various chemokines. It is not known where, *in vivo*, this chemotaxis takes place.
- Dendritic cells make chemokines themselves and use them, for example, for the attraction of T-lymphocytes. This contributes to their high immunostimulatory potential. This field of research is only in its beginnings.
- IL-12 has proved to be an important DC product. It promotes the development of T_H1 responses. Its production can be induced either by a mechanism of 'natural immunity', i.e., uptake of bacteria or by a mechanism of 'adaptive immunity', i.e., interaction with T cells, the latter mechanism being more efficient.

We are now in a period where all sorts of cytokine knockout mice are being tested with regard to their influence on the development and on the maturation of DC (see Table 1). Data from each knockout as well as transgene models will add important stones to the mosaic of our knowledge. This will lead to a better understanding of how the different cytokines are orchestrated *in vivo*. This in turn will render more efficient all those approaches that aim at improving DC-based immunotherapies with adjuvant cytokine treatment. To sum it all up, there is still 'lots to do in the field of DC and cytokines'.

Table 1. Investigations *in vivo* of dendritic cells in cytokine/cytokine receptor knockout mice or in mice overexpressing certain cytokine genes (transgenic mice)

Cytokine	Genetic manipulation	Findings/References
GM-CSF	Transgenic	50–150% increase of DC in lymphoid organs (Vremec *et al.*, 1997)
GM-CSF	Knockout	Almost normal numbers of DC in lymphoid organs (Vremec *et al.*, 1997) Development of DC from thymic precursors not impaired (Saunders *et al.*, 1996)
GM-CSF-R β-chain CDw131	Knockout	Almost normal numbers of DC in lymphoid organs (Vremec *et al*,, 1997)
IL-2-R CD25	Knockout	No effect on T cell stimulatory capacity (Kronin *et al.*, 1998)
IL-4	Transgenic	Increased density of epidermal Langerhans cells (Elbe *et al.*, in preparation)
TGF-β_1	Knockout	Langerhans cells absent; CD11c$^+$ lymph node DC present (Borkowski *et al.*, 1996; Borkowski *et al.*, 1997)
MCP-1	Transgenic (in basal keratinocytes)	Recruitment of Langerhans cells to the epidermis (Nakamura *et al.*, 1995)
Interferon-γ	Transgenic (in suprabasal keratinocytes)	Reduced density of epidermal Langerhans cells (Carroll *et al.*, 1997)
TNF-α-R1 (p55)	Knockout	No effect on migration of DC during the induction phase of contact hypersensitivity to FITC (Wang *et al.*, 1996)

ACKNOWLEDGMENTS

The support and encouragment of P. Fritsch, Chairman of the Department of Dermatology, Innsbruck is greatly appreciated. Our research over the years was financed by the Austrian Science Fund (FWF grants P-8549-Med, P-9967-Med, P-12163-Med, SFB/F002/7 to N.R. and G.S.), the Austrian National Bank (Jubiläumsfonds 4370, 4889, 5481, and 6575) and the German Science Foundation (DFG grants Ka753l1-1 to E.K. and SFB263 to G.S.). We apologize to all colleagues whose work could not be cited here owing to space constraints.

REFERENCES

Adema, G.J., Hartgers, F., Verstraten, R., de Vries, E., Marland, G., Menon, S., Foster, J., Xu, Y.M., Nooyen, P., McClanahan, T., Bacon, K.B. and Figdor, C.G. (1997). A dendritic-cell-derived C-C chemokine that preferentially attracts naive T cells. *Nature* **387**, 713-717.

Anderson, D.M., Maraskovsky, E., Billingsley, W.L., Dougall, W.C., Tometsko, M.E., Roux, E.R., Teepe, M.C., DuBose, R.F., Cosman, D. and Galibert, L. (1997). A homologue of the TNF receptor and its ligand enhance T-cell growth and dendritic-cell function. *Nature* **390**, 175–179.

Ayehunie, S., Garcia-Zepeda, E.A., Hoxie, J.A., Horuk, R., Kupper, T.S., Luster, A.D. and Ruprecht, R.M. (1997). Human immunodeficiency virus-1 entry into purified blood dendritic cells through CC and CXC chemokine coreceptors. *Blood* **90**, 1378–1386.

Bagasra, O., Seshamma, T. and Pomerantz, R.J. (1993). Polymerase chain reaction *in situ*: intracellular amplification and detection of HIV-1 proviral DNA and other specific genes. *J. Immunol. Methods* **158**, 131–145.

Baggiolini, M., Dewald, B. and Moser, B. (1997). Human chemokines: an update. *Annu. Rev. Immunol.* **15**, 675–705.

Bergstresser, P.R., Toews, G.B. and Streilein, J.W. (1980). Natural and perturbed distributions of Langerhans cells: Responses to ultraviolet light, heterotopic skin grafting, and dinitrofluorobenzene sensitization. *J. Invest. Dermatol.* **75**, 73–77.

Blauvelt, A., Asada, H., Klaus-Kovtun, V., Altman, D.J., Lucey, D.R. and Katz, S.I. (1996). Interleukin-15 mRNA is expressed by human keratinocytes, Langerhans cells, and blood-derived dendritic cells and is downregulated by ultraviolet B radiation. *J. Invest. Dermatol.* **106**, 1047–1052.

Borkowski, T.A., Letterio, J.J., Farr, A.G. and Udey, M.C. (1996). A role for endogenous transforming growth factor $\beta 1$ in Langerhans cell biology: The skin of transforming growth factor β null mice is devoid of epidermal Langerhans cells. *J. Exp. Med.* **184**, 2417–2422.

Borkowski, T.A., Letterio, J.J., Mackall, C.L., Saitoh, A., Wang, X.J., Roop, D.R., Gress, R.E. and Udey, M.C. (1997). A role for TGFβ_1 in Langerhans cell biology—further characterization of the epidermal Langerhans cell defect in TGFβ_1 null mice. *J. Clin. Invest.* **100**, 575–581.

Carroll, J.M., Crompton, T., Seery, J.P. and Watt, F.M. (1997). Transgenic mice expressing IFN-gamma in the epidermis have eczema, hair hypopigmentation, and hair loss. *J. Invest. Dermatol.* **108**, 412–422.

Carter, L.L. and Swain, S.L. (1997). Single cell analyses of cytokine production. *Curr. Opin. Immunol.* **9**, 177–182.

Caux, C., Dezutter-Dambuyant, C., Schmitt, D. and Banchereau, J. (1992). GM-CSF and TNF-α cooperate in the generation of dendritic Langerhans cells. *Nature* **360**, 258–261.

Caux, C., Massacrier, C., Vanbervliet, B., Dubois, B., Van Kooten, C., Durand, I. and Banchereau, J. (1994). Activation of human dendritic cells through CD40 cross-linking. *J. Exp. Med.* **180**, 1263–1272.

Caux, C., Vanbervliet, B., Massacrier, C., Dezutter-Dambuyant, C., De Saint-Vis, B., Jacquet, C., Yoneda, K., Imamura, S., Schmitt, D. and Banchereau, J. (1996). CD34$^+$ hematopoietic progenitors from human cord blood differentiate along two independent dendritic cell pathways in response to GM-CSF+TNFα. *J. Exp. Med.* **184**, 695–706.

Caux, C., Massacrier, C., Vanbervliet, B., Dubois, B., Durand, I., Cella, M., Lanzavecchia, A. and Banchereau, J. (1997). CD34$^+$ hematopoietic progenitors from human cord blood differentiate along two independent dendritic cell pathways in response to granulocyte-macrophage colony-stimulating factor plus tumor necrosis factor α. 2. Functional analysis. *Blood* **90**, 1458–1470.

Cella, M., Scheidegger, D., Palmer-Lehmann, K., Lane, P., Lanzavecchia, A. and Alber, G. (1996). Ligation of CD40 on dendritic cells triggers production of high levels of interleukin-12 and enhances T cell stimulatory capacity: T–T help via APC activation. *J. Exp. Med.* **184**, 747–752.

Cella, M., Engering, A., Pinet, V., Pieters, J. and Lanzavecchia, A. (1997). Inflammatory stimuli induce accumulation of MHC class II complexes on dendritic cells. *Nature* **388**, 782–787.

Cumberbatch, M. and Kimber, I. (1992). Dermal tumour necrosis factor-α induces dendritic cell migration to draining lymph nodes, and possibly provides one stimulus for Langerhans' cell migration. *Immunology* **75**, 257–263.

Cumberbatch, M., Fielding, I. and Kimber, I. (1994). Modulation of epidermal Langerhans' cell frequency by tumour necrosis factor-α. *Immunology* **81**, 395–401.

Cumberbatch, M., Dearman, R.J. and Kimber, I. (1996). Constitutive and inducible expression of interleukin-6 by Langerhans cells and lymph node dendritic cells. *Immunology* **87**, 513–518.

Cumberbatch, M., Dearman, R.J. and Kimber, I. (1997). Langerhans cells require signals from both tumor necrosis factor α and interleukin-1β for migration. *Immunology* **92**, 388–395.

De Smedt, T., Pajak, B., Muraille, E., Lespagnard, L., Heinen, E., De Baetselier, P., Urbain, J., Leo, O. and Moser, M. (1996). Regulation of dendritic cell numbers and maturation by lipopolysaccharide *in vivo*. *J. Exp. Med.* **84**, 1413–1424.

De Smedt, T., Van Mechelen, M., De Becker, G., Urbain, J., Leo, O. and Moser, M. (1997). Effect of interleukin-10 on dendritic cell maturation and function. *Eur. J. Immunol.* **27**, 1229–1235.

Dillon, S.M., Hart, D.N.J., Abernethy, N., Watson, J.D. and Baird, M.A. (1997). Priming to mycobacterial antigen *in vivo* using antigen-pulsed antigen presenting cells generated *in vitro* is influenced by the dose and presence of IL-4 in APC cultures. *Scand. J. Immunol.* **46**, 1–9.

Enk, A.H. and Katz, S.I. (1992). Early molecular events in the induction phase of contact sensitivity. *Proc. Natl Acad. Sci. USA* **89**, 1398–1402.

Enk, A.H., Angeloni, V.L., Udey, M.C. and Katz, S.I. (1993a). Inhibition of Langerhans cell antigen-presenting function by IL-10: a role for IL-10 in induction of tolerance. *J. Immunol.* **151**, 2390–2398.

Enk, A.H., Angeloni, V.L., Udey, M.C. and Katz, S.I. (1993b). An essential role for Langerhans cell-derived IL-1b in the initiation of primary immune responses in skin. *J. Immunol.* **150**, 3698–3704.

Enk, A.H., Saloga, J., Becker, D., Mohamadzadeh, M. and Knop, J. (1994). Induction of hapten-specific tolerance by interleukin 10 in vivo. *J. Exp. Med.* **179**, 1397–1402.

Eugster, H.P., Müller, M., Karrer, U., Car, B.D., Schnyder, B., Eng, V.M., Woerly, G., Le Hir, M., Di Padova, F., Aguet, M., Zinkernagel, R., Bluethmann, H. and Ryffel, B. (1996). Multiple immune abnormalities in tumor necrosis factor and lymphotoxin-α double-deficient mice. *Int. Immunol.* **8**, 23–36.

Fässler, R., Martin, K., Forsberg, E., Litzenburger, T. and Iglesias, A. (1995). Knockout mice: how to make them and why. The immunological approach. *Int. Arch. Allergy Immunol.* **106**, 323–334.

Geissmann, F., Prost, C., Monnet, J.P., Dy, M., Brousse, N. and Hermine, O. (1998). Transforming growth factor β1 in the presence of granulocyte/macrophage colony-stimulating factor and interleukin 4, induces differentiation of human peripheral blood monocytes into dendritic Langerhans cells. *J. Exp. Med.* **187**, 961–966.

Godiska, R., Chantry, D., Raport, C.J., Sozzani, S., Allavena, P., Leviten, D., Mantovani, A. and Gray, P.W. (1997). Human macrophage-derived chemokine (MDC), a novel chemoattractant for monocytes, monocyte-derived dendritic cells, and natural killer cells. *J. Exp. Med.* **185**, 1595–1604.

Granelli-Piperno, A., Moser, B., Pope, M., Chen, D.L., Wei, Y., Isdell, F., O'Doherty, U., Paxton, W., Koup, R., Mojsov, S., Bhardwaj, N., Clark-Lewis, I., Baggiolini, M. and Steinman, R.M. (1996). Efficient interaction of HIV-1 with purified dendritic cells via multiple chemokine coreceptors. *J. Exp. Med.* **184**, 2433–2438.

Granucci, F., Girolomoni, G., Lutz, M.B., Foti, M., Marconi, G., Gnocchi, P., Nolli, L. and Ricciardi-Castagnoli, P. (1994). Modulation of cytokine expression in mouse dendritic cell clones. *Eur. J. Immunol.* **24**, 2522–2526.

Greaves, D.R., Wang, W., Dairaghi, D.J., Dieu, M.C., De Saint-Vis, B., Franz-Bacon, K., Rossi, D., Caux, C., McClanahan, T., Gordon, S., Zlotnik, A. and Schall, T.J. (1997). CCR6, a CC chemokine receptor that interacts with macrophage inflammatory protein 3α and is highly expressed in human dendritic cells. *J. Exp. Med.* **186**, 837–844.

Gruschwitz, M.S. and Hornstein, O.P. (1992). Expression of transforming growth factor type beta on human epidermal dendritic cells. *J. Invest. Dermatol.* **99**, 114–116.

Henderson, R.A., Watkins, S.C. and Flynn, J.A.L. (1997). Activation of human dendritic cells following infection with *Mycobacterium tuberculosis*. *J. Immunol.* **159**, 635–643.

Heufler, C., Topar, G., Koch, F., Trockenbacher, B., Kämpgen, E., Romani, N. and Schuler, G. (1992). Cytokine gene expression in murine epidermal cell suspensions: interleukin 1β and macrophage inflammatory protein 1α are selectively expressed in Langerhans cells but are differentially regulated in culture. *J. Exp. Med.* **176**, 1221–1226.

Heufler, C., Koch, F., Stanzl, U., Topar, G., Wysocka, M., Trinchieri, G., Enk, A., Steinman, R.M., Romani, N. and Schuler, G. (1996). Interleukin-12 is produced by dendritic cells and mediates T helper 1 development as well as interferon-gamma production by T helper 1 cells. *Eur. J. Immunol.* **26**, 659–668.

Hoefakker, S., Boersma, W.J.A. and Claassen, E. (1995). Detection of human cytokines *in situ* using antibody and probe based methods. *J. Immunol. Methods* **185**, 149–175.

Holliday, M.R., Dearman, R.J., Basketter, D.A. and Kimber, I. (1996). Stimulation by oxazolone of increased IL-6, but not IL-10, in the skin of mice. *Toxicology* **106**, 237–242.

Inaba, K., Inaba, M., Romani, N., Aya, H., Deguchi, M., Ikehara, S., Muramatsu, S. and Steinman, R.M. (1992a). Generation of large numbers of dendritic cells from mouse bone marrow cultures supplemented with granulocyte/macrophage colony-stimulating factor. *J. Exp. Med.* **176**, 1693–1702.

Inaba, K. Steinman, R.M., Pack, M.W., Aya, H., Inaba, M., Sudo, T., Wolpe, S. and Schuler, G. (1992b). Identification of proliferating dendritic cell precursors in mouse blood. *J. Exp. Med.* **175**, 1157–1167.

Inaba, K., Inaba, M., Deguchi, M., Hagi, K., Yasumizu, R., Ikehara, S., Muramatsu, S. and Steinman, R.M. (1993). Granulocytes, macrophages, and dendritic cells arise from a common major histocompatibility complex class II-negative progenitor in mouse bone marrow. *Proc. Natl Acad. Sci. USA* **90**, 3038–3042.

Jansen, J.H., Wientjens, G.-J.H.M., Fibbe, W.E., Willemze, R. and Kluin-Nelemans, H.C. (1989). Inhibition of human macrophage colony formation by interleukin 4. *J. Exp. Med.* **170**, 577–582.

Jonuleit, H., Wiedemann, K., Muller, G., Degwert, J., Hoppe, U., Knop, J. and Enk, A.H. (1997). Induction of IL-15 messenger RNA and protein in human blood-derived dendritic cells—a role for IL-15 in attraction of T cells. *J. Immunol.* **158**, 2610–2615.

Kanangat, S., Nair, S., Babu, J.S. and Rouse, B.T. (1995). Expression of cytokine mRNA in murine splenic dendritic cells and better induction of T cell-derived cytokines by dendritic cells than by macrophages during *in vitro* costimulation assay using specific antigens. *J. Leukocyte Biol.* **57**, 310–316.

Kämpgen, E., Koch, N., Koch, F., Stöger, P., Heufler, C., Schuler, G. and Romani, N. (1991). Class II major histocompatibility complex molecules of murine dendritic cells: Synthesis, sialylation of invariant chain, and antigen processing capacity are down-regulated upon cuiture. *Proc. Natl Acad. Sci. USA* **88**, 3014–3018.

Kämpgen, E., Romani, N., Koch, F., Eggert, A. and Schuler, G. (1995). Cytokine receptors on epidermal Langerhans cells. In: *The Immune Functions of Epidermal Langerhans Cells* (ed. H. Moll). Springer-Verlag, Austin, New York, Berlin, pp. 37–56.

Knop, J. and Enk, A.H. (1995). Cellular and molecular mechanisms in the induction phase of contact sensitivity. *Int. Arch. Allergy Immunol.* **107**, 231–232.

Kobayashi, Y., Staquet, M.-J., Dezutter-Dambuyant, C. and Schmitt, D. (1994). Development of motility of Langerhans cell through extracellular matrix by *in vitro* hapten contact. *Eur. J. Immunol.* **24**, 2254–2257.

Koch, F., Heufler, C., Kämpgen, E., Schneeweiss, D., Böck, G. and Schuler, G. (1990). Tumor necrosis factor alpha maintains the viability of murine epidermal Langerhans cells in culture but in contrast to granulocyte/macrophage colony-stimulating factor without inducing their functional maturation. *J. Exp. Med.* **171**, 159–171.

Koch, F., Kämpgen, E. and Trockenbacher, B. (1995a). TNFα interrupts antigen-presenting function of Langerhans cells by two mechanisms: loss of immunogenic peptides and impairment of antigen-independent T cell clustering. *Adv. Exp. Med. Biol.* **378**, 207–209.

Koch, F., Trockenbacher, B., Kämpgen, E., Grauer, O., Stössel, H., Livingstone, A.M., Schuler, G. and Romani, N. (1995b). Antigen processing in populations of mature murine dendritic cells is caused by subsets of incompletely matured cells. *J. Immunol.* **155**, 93–100.

Koch, F., Stanzl, U., Jennewein, P., Janke, K., Heufler, C., Kämpgen, E., Romani, N. and Schuler, G. (1996). High level IL-12 production by murine dendritic cells: upregulation via MHC class II and CD40 molecules and downregulation by IL-4 and IL-10. *J. Exp. Med.* **184**, 741–746.

Kondo, S., Pastore, S., Fujisawa, H., Shivji, G.M., McKenzie, R.C., Dinarello, C.A. and Sauder, D.N. (1995a). Interleukin-1 receptor antagonist suppresses contact hypersensitivity. *J. Invest. Dermatol.* **105**, 334–338.

Kondo, S., Wang, B.H., Fujisawa, H., Shivji, G.M., Echtenacher, B., Mak, T.W. and Sauder, D.N. (1995b). Effect of gene-targeted mutation in TNF receptor (p55) on contact hypersensitivity and ultraviolet B-induced immunosuppression. *J. Immunol.* **155**, 3801–3805.

Kronin, V., Vremec, D. and Shortman, K. (1998). Does the IL-2 receptor α chain induced on dendritic cells have a biological function? *Int. Immunol.* **10**, 237–240.

Larregina, A.T., Morelli, A.E., Kolkowski, E., Sanjuan, N., Barboza, M.E. and Fainboim, L. (1997). Pattern of cytokine receptors expressed by human dendritic cells migrated from dermal explants. *Immunology* **91**, 303–313.

Ledur, A., Fitting, C., David, B., Hamberger, C. and Cavaillon, J.M. (1995). Variable estimates of cytokine levels produced by commercial ELISA kits: results using international cytokine standards. *J. Immunol. Methods* **186**, 171–179.

Lu, L., Woo, J., Rao, A.S., Li, Y., Watkins, S.C., Qian, S., Starzl, T.E., Demetris, A.J. and Thomson, A.W. (1994). Propagation of dendritic cell progenitors from normal mouse liver using granulocyte/macrophage colony-stimulating factor and their maturational development in the presence of type-1 collagen. *J. Exp. Med.* **179**, 1823–1834.

Lu, L., Hsieh, M., Oriss, T.B., Morel, P.A., Starzl, T.E., Rao, A.S. and Thomson, A.W. (1995a). Generation of DC from mouse spleen cell cultures in response to GM-CSF: immunophenotypic and functional analyses. *Immunology* **84**, 127–134.

Lu, L., McCaslin, D., Starzl, T.E. and Thomson, A.W. (1995b). Bone marrow-derived dendritic cell progenitors (NLDC 145^+, MHC class II^+, B7-1^{dim}, B7-2^-) induce alloantiger-specific hyporesponsiveness in murine T lymphocytes. *Transplantation* **60**, 1539–1545.

Lutz, M.B., Kukutsch, N., Ogilvie, A.L.J., Rossner, S., Koch, F., Romani, N. and Schuler, G. (1998). An advanced culture method for generating large quantities of highly pure dendritic cells from mouse bone marrow. *J. Immunol. Methods*, in press.

Lynch, D.H., Andreasen, A., Maraskovsky, E., Whitmore, J., Miller, R.E. and Schuh, J.C.L. (1997). Flt3 ligand induces tumor regression and antitumor immune responses *in vivo*. *Nature Medicine* **3**, 625–631.

Macatonia, S.E., Hosken, N.A., Litton, M., Vieira, P., Hsieh, C.-S., Culpepper, J.A., Wysocka, M., Trinchieri, G., Murphy, K.M. and O'Garra, A. (1995). Dendritic cells produce IL-12 and direct the development of Th1 cells from naive CD4+ T cells. *J. Immunol.* **154**, 5071–5079.

Manz, R., Assenmacher, M., Pflüger, E., Miltenyi, S. and Radbruch, A. (1995). Analysis and sorting of live cells according to secreted molecules, relocated to a cell-surface affinity matrix. *Proc. Natl Acad. Sci. USA* **92**, 1921–1925.

Maraskovsky, E., Brasel, K., Teepe, M., Roux, E.R., Lyman, S.D., Shortman, K. and McKenna, H.J. (1996). Dramatic increase in the numbers of functionally mature dendritic cells in Flt3 ligand-treated mice: multiple dendritic cell subpopulations identified. *J. Exp. Med.* **184**, 1953–1962.

Mayordomo, J.I., Zorina, T., Storkus, W.J., Zitvogel, L., Garcia-Prats, M.D., Deleo, A.B. and Lotze, M.T. (1997). Bone marrow-derived dendritic cells serve as potent adjuvants for peptide-based antitumor vaccines. *Stem Cells* **15**, 94–103.

Mire-Sluis, A.R., Page, L. and Thorpe, R. (1995). Quantitative cell line based bioassays for human cytokines. *J. Immunol. Methods* **187**, 191–199.

Mohamadzadeh, M., Poltorak, A.N., Bergstresser, P.R., Beutler, B. and Takashima, A. (1996). Dendritic cells produce macrophage inflammatory protein-1gamma, a new member of the CC chemokine family. *J. Immunol.* **156**, 3102–3106.

Nakamura, K., Williams, I.R. and Kupper, T.S. (1995). Keratinocyte-derived monocyte chemoattractant protein 1 (MCP-1): analysis in a transgenic model demonstrates MCP-1 can recruit dendritic and Langerhans cells to skin. *J. Invest. Dermatol.* **105**, 635–643.

Neumann, H., Schmidt, H., Cavalie, A., Jenne, D. and Wekerle, H. (1997). Major histocompatibility complex (MHC) class I gene expression in single neurons of the central nervous system: Differential regulation by interferon (IFN)-gamma and tumor necrosis factor (TNF)-α. *J. Exp. Med.* **185**, 305–316.

Nylander-Lundqvist, E. and Bäck, O. (1990). Interleukin-1 decreases the number of Ia+ epidermal dendritic cells but increases their expression of Ia antigen. *Acta Dermatol. Venereol.* **70**, 391–394.

Ohshima, Y. and Delespesse, G. (1997). T cell-derived IL-4 and dendritic cell-derived IL-12 regulate the lymphokine-producing phenotype of alloantigen-primed naive human CD4 T cells. *J. Immunol.* **158**, 629–636.

Ortner, U., Inaba, K., Koch, F., Heine, M., Miwa, M., Schuler, G. and Romani, N. (1996). An improved isolation method for murine migratory cutaneous dendritic cells. *J. Immunol. Methods* **193**, 71–79.

Picker, L.J., Treer, J.R., Ferguson-Darnell, B., Collins, P.A., Bergstresser, P.R. and Terstappen, L.W.M.M. (1993). Control of lymphocyte recirculation in man: II. Differential regulation of the cutaneous lymphocyte-associated antigen, a tissue-selective homing receptor for skin-homing T cells. *J. Immunol.* **150**, 1122–1136.

Pierre, P., Turley, S.J., Gatti, E., Hull, M., Meltzer, J., Mirza, A., Inaba, K., Steinman, R.M. and Mellman, I. (1997). Developmental regulation of MHC class II transport in mouse dendritic cells. *Nature* **388**, 787–792.

Power, C.A., Church, D.J., Meyer, A., Alouani, S., Proudfoot, A.E.I., Clark-Lewis, I., Sozzani, S., Mantovani, A. and Wells, T.N.C. (1997). Cloning and characterization of a specific receptor for the novel CC chemokine MIP-3α from lung dendritic cells. *J. Exp. Med.* **186**, 825–835.

Price, A.A., Cumberbatch, M., Kimber, I. and Ager, A. (1997). Alpha 6 integrins are required for Langerhans cell migration from the epidermis. *J. Exp. Med.* **186**, 1725–1735.

Puré, E., Inaba, K., Crowley, M.T., Tardelli, L., Witmer-Pack, M.D., Ruberti, G., Fathman, G. and Steinman, R.M. (1990). Antigen processing by epidermal Langerhans cells correlates with the level of biosynthesis of major histocompatibility complex class II molecules and expression of invariant chain. *J. Exp. Med.* **172**, 1459–1469.

Ragg, S.J., Woods, G.M., Egan, P.J., Dandie, G.W. and Muller, H.K. (1997). Failure of carcinogen-altered dendritic cells to initiate T cell proliferation is associated with reduced IL-1b secretion. *Cell. Immunol.* **178**, 17–23.

Rahdon, R.A., Lin, C.L., Suri, R.M., Morris, P.J., Austyn, J.M. and Roake, J.A. (1997). An endothelial cell-derived chemotactic factor promotes transendothelial migration of human dendritic cells. *Transplant. Proc.* **29**, 1121–1122.

Reid, C.D.L., Stackpoole, A., Meager, A. and Tikerpae, J. (1992). Interactions of tumor necrosis factor with granulocyte-macrophage colony-stimulating factor and other cytokines in the regulation of dendritic cell growth *in vitro* from early bipotent CD34+ progenitors in human bone marrow. *J. Immunol.* **149**, 2681–2688.

Rieser, C., Böck, G., Klocker, H., Bartsch, G. and Thurnher, M. (1997). Prostaglandin E2 and tumor necrosis factor α cooperate to activate human dendritic cells: synergistic activation of interleukin-12 production. *J. Exp. Med.* **186**, 1603–1608.

Riva, S., Nolli, M.L., Lutz, M.B., Citterio, S., Girolomoni, G., Winzler, C. and Ricciardi-Castagnoli, P. (1996). Bacteria and bacterial cell wall constituents induce the production of regulatory cytokines in dendritic cell clones. *J. Inflamm.* **46**, 98–105.

Roake, J.A., Rao, A.S., Morris, P.J., Larsen, C.P., Hankins, D.F. and Austyn, J.M. (1995a). Dendritic cell loss from nonlymphoid tissues after systemic administration of lipopolysaccharide, tumor necrosis factor, and interleukin 1. *J. Exp. Med.* **181**, 2237–2248.

Roake, J.A., Rao, A.S., Morris, P.J., Larsen, C.P., Hankins, D.F. and Austyn, J.M. (1995b). Systemic lipopolysaccharide recruits dendritic cell progenitors to nonlymphoid tissues. *Transplantation* **59**, 1319–1324.

Romani, N., Koide, S., Crowley, M., Witmer-Pack, M., Livingstone, A.M., Fathman, C.G., Inaba, K. and Steinman, R.M. (1989). Presentation of exogenous protein antigens by dendritic cells to T cell clones: intact protein is presented best by immature epidermal Langerhans cells. *J. Exp. Med.* **169**, 1169–1178.

Romani, N., Gruner, S., Brang, D., Kämpgen, E., Lenz, A., Trockenbacher, B., Konwalinka, G., Fritsch, P.O., Steinman, R.M. and Schuler, G. (1994a). Proliferating dendritic cell progenitors in human blood. *J. Exp. Med.* **180**, 83-93.

Romani, N., Heufler, C., Koch, F., Topar, G., Kämpgen, E. and Schuler, G. (1994b). Cytokines and Langerhans cells, In: *Epidermal Growth Factors and Cytokines* (ed T.A. Luger and T. Schwarz). Marcel Dekker, New York, pp. 345–363.

Rubbert, A., Combadiere, C., Ostrowski, M., Arthos, J., Dybul, M., Machado, E., Cohn, M.A., Hoxie, J.A., Murphy, P.M., Fauci, A.S. and Weissmann, D. (1998). Dendritic cells express multiple chemokine receptors used as coreceptors for HIV entry. *J. Immunol.* **160**, 3933–3941.

Sallusto, F. and Lanzavecchia, A. (1994). Efficient presentation of soluble antigen by cultured human dendritic cells is maintained by granulocyte/macrophage colony-stimulating factor plus interleukin 4 and downregulated by tumor necrosis factor α. *J Exp. Med.* **179**, 1109–1118.

Sallusto, F., Cella, M., Danieli, C. and Lanzavecchia, A. (1995). Dendritic cells use macropinocytosis and the mannose receptor to concentrate macromolecules in the major histocompatibility complex class II compartment: downregulation by cytokines and bacterial products. *J. Exp. Med.* **182**, 389–400.

Saraya, K. and Reid, C.D.L. (1996). Stem cell factor and the regulation of dendritic cell production from $CD34^+$ progenitors in bone marrow and cord blood. *Br. J. Haematol.* **93**, 258–264.

Saunders, D., Lucas, K., Ismaili, J., Wu, L., Maraskovsky, E., Dunn, A. and Shortman, K. (1996). Dendritic cell development in culture from thymic precursor cells in the absence of granulocyte/macrophage colony-stimulating factor. *J. Exp. Med.* **184**, 2185–2196.

Schuler, G. and Steinman, R.M. (1985). Murine epidermal Langerhans cells mature into potent immunostimulatory dendritic cells *in vitro*. *J. Exp. Med.* **161**, 526–546.

Scheicher, C., Kuppner, M., Keikavoussi, P., Brocker, E-B., Giegerich, G. and Kämpgen, E. (1998). Interferon-gamma-inducing factor (IL-18) and IL-12 are differentially regulated in dendritic cells. *Arch. Dermatol. Res.* **290**, 92 (abstract).

Schwarzenberger, K. and Udey, M.C. (1996). Contact allergens and epidermal proinflammatory cytokines modulate Langerhans cell E-cadherin expression *in situ*. *J. Invest. Dermatol.* **106**, 553–558.

Shornick, L.P., De Togni, P., Mariathasan, S., Goellner, J., Strauss-Schoenberger, J., Karr, R.W., Ferguson, T.A. and Chaplin, D.D. (1996). Mice deficient in IL-β manifest impaired contact hypersensitivity to trinitrochlorobenzene. *J. Exp. Med.* **183**, 1427–1436.

Siena, S., Di Nicola, M., Bregni, M., Mortarini, R., Anichini, A., Lombardi, L., Ravagnani, F., Parmiani, G. and Gianni, A.M. (1995). Massive *ex vivo* generation of functional dendritic cells from mobilized $CD34^+$ blood progenitors for anticancer therapy. *Exp. Hematol.* **23**, 1463–1471.

Sozzani, S., Sallusto, F., Luini, W., Zhou, D., Piemonti, L., Allavena, P., van Damme, J., Valitutti, S., Lanzavecchia, A. and Mantovani, A. (1995). Migration of dendritic cells in response to formyl peptides, C5a, and a distinct set of chemokines. *J. Immunol.* **155**, 3292–3295.

Sozzani, S., Luini, W., Borsatti, A., Polentarutti, N., Zhou, D., Piemonti, L., D'Amico, G., Power, C.A., Wells, T.N.C., Gobbi, M., Allavena, P. and Mantovani, A. (1997). Receptor expression and responsiveness of human dendritic cells to a defined set of CC and CXC chemokines. *J. Immunol.* **159**, 1993–2000.

Steinbrink, K., Wölfl, M., Jonuleit, H., Knop, J. and Enk, A.H. (1997). Induction of tolerance by IL-10-treated dendritic cells. *J. Immunol.* **159**, 4772–4780.

Stoll, S., Jonuleit, H., Schmitt, E., Müller, G., Yamauchi, H., Kurimoto, M., Knop, J. and Enk, A. (1998). Production of functional IL-18 by different subtypes of murine dendritic cells. Dendritic cell-derived IL-18 enhances IL-12-dependent Th1 development. *Arch. Dermatol. Res.* **290**, 41 (abstract).

Strobl, H., Bello-Fernandez, C., Riedl, E., Pickl, W.F., Majdic, O., Lyman, S.D. and Knapp, W. (1997). flt3 ligand in cooperation with transforming growth factor-β1 potentiates *in vitro* development of Langerhans-type dendritic cells and allows single-cell dendritic cell cluster formation under serum-free conditions. *Blood* **90**, 1425–1434.

Strunk, D., Egger, C., Leitner, G., Hanau, D. and Stingl, G. (1997). A skin homing molecule defines the Langerhans cell progenitor in human peripheral blood. *J. Exp Med.* **185**, 1131–1136.

Takenaka, H., Maruo, S., Yamamoto, N., Wysocka, M., Ono, S., Kobayashi, M., Yagita, H., Okumura, K., Hamaoka, T., Trinchieri, G. and Fujiwara, H. (1997). Regulation of T cell-dependent and -independent IL-12 production by the three Th2-type cytokines IL-10, IL-6, and IL-4. *J. Leukocyte Biol.* **61**, 80–87.

Thurnher, M., Ramoner, R., Gastl, G., Radmayr, C., Böck, G., Herold, M., Klocker, H. and Bartsch, G. (1997). Bacillus Calmette-Guerin mycobacteria stimulate human blood dendritic cells. *Int. J. Cancer* **70**, 128–134.

Udey, M.C. (1997). Cadherins and Langerhans cell immunobiology. *Clin. Exp. Immunol.* **107** (Suppl. 1), 6–8.

Verhasselt, V., Buelens, C., Willems, F., De Groote, D., Haeffner-Cavaillon, N. and Goldman, M. (1997). Bacterial lipopolysaccharide stimulates the production of cytokines and the expression of costimulatory molecules by human peripheral blood dendritic cells—evidence for a soluble CD14-dependent pathway. *J. Immunol.* **158**, 2919–2925.

Vicari, A.P., Figueroa, D.J., Hedrick, J.A., Foster, J.S., Singh, K.P., Menon, S., Copeland, N.G., Gilbert, D.J., Jenkins, N.A., Bacon, K.B. and Zlotnik, A. (1997). TECK: A novel CC chemokine specifically expressed by thymic dendritic cells and potentially involved in T cell development. *Immunity* **7**, 291–301.

Vremec, D., Lieschke, G.J., Dunn, A.R., Robb, L. and Shortman, K. (1997). The influence of granulocyte/macrophage colony-stimulating factor on dendritic cell levels in mouse lymphoid organs. *Eur. J. Immunol.* **27**, 40–44.

Wang, B., Kondo, S., Shivji, G.M., Fujisawa, H., Mak, T.W. and Sauder, D.N. (1996). Tumour necrosis factor receptor II (p75) signalling is required for the migration of Langerhans' cells. *Immunology* **88**, 284–288.

Weinlich, G., Heine, M., Stössel, H., Zanella, M., Stoitzner, P., Ortner, U., Smolle, J., Koch, F., Sepp, N.T., Schuler, G. and Romani, N. (1998). Entry into afferent lymphatics and maturation in situ of migrating cutaneous dendritic cells. *J. Invest. Dermatol.* **110**, 441–448.

Wilkinson, V.L., Warrier, R.R., Truitt, T.P., Nunes, P., Gately, M.K. and Presky, D.H. (1996). Characterization of anti-mouse IL-12 monoclonal antibodies and measurement of mouse IL-12 by ELISA. *J. Immunol. Methods* **189**, 15–24.

Xu, L.L., Warren, M.K., Rose, W.L., Gong, W.H. and Wang, J.M. (1996). Human recombinant monocyte chemotactic protein and other C-C chemokines bind and induce directional migration of dendritic cells *in vitro*. *J. Leukocyte Biol.* **60**, 365–371.

Yamaguchi, Y., Tsumura, H., Miwa, M. and Inaba, K. (1997). Contrasting effects of TGF-β1 and TNF-α on the development of dendritic cells from progenitors in mouse bone marrow. *Stem Cells* **15**, 144–153.

Young, J.W., Szabolcs, P. and Moore, M.A.S. (1995). Identification of dendritic cell colony-forming units among normal human CD34$^+$ bone marrow progenitors that are expanded by c-*kit*-ligand and yield pure dendritic cell colonies in the presence of granulocyte macrophage colony-stimulating factor and tumor necrosis factor α. *J. Exp. Med.* **182**, 1111–1119.

Wong, B.R., Josien, R., Lee, S.Y., Sauter, B., Li, H.L., Steinman, R.M. and Choi, Y. (1997). TRANCE (tumor necrosis factor [TNF]-related activation-induced cytokine), a new TNF family member predominantly expressed in T cells, is a dendritic cell-specific survival factor. *J. Exp. Med.* **186**, 2075–2080.

Zhou, L.J. and Tedder, T.F. (1995). A distinct pattern of cytokine gene expression by human CD83$^+$ blood dendritic cells. *Blood* **86**, 3295–3301.

CHAPTER 38
Apoptosis in Dendritic Cells

Michael R. Shurin, Clemens Esche, Anna Lokshin and Michael T. Lotze
Biological Therapeutics Program, University of Pittsburgh Cancer Institute, Pittsburgh, Pennsylvania, USA

INTRODUCTION

Apoptosis, together with differentiation, proliferation, and survival, is a highly regulated fundamental biological process that is involved in development, responsiveness, and homeostasis. After its discovery by Carl Vogt in 1842 (see Peter *et al.*, 1997), studies of apoptosis were dormant for more than a century. 'Apoptosis' is a name that was chosen in 1972 for a particular morphology of cell death that was easily distinguished from necrosis (Kerr *et al.*, 1972). The initial description of apoptosis was based on cellular morphology and is characterized by condensation of chromatin and DNA, blebbing and shrinkage of cytoplasm, and eventual disintegration of dead cells into membrane-bound apoptotic bodies that are rapidly engulfed by neighboring cells. The biochemical characterization of apoptosis includes internucleosomal cleavage of DNA into oligonucleosomal fragments ('ladders') of 180–200 bp multiples, activation of intracellular cysteine proteases (caspases), and control of cell death by negative regulatory elements such as Bcl-2 family proteins or the inhibitors of apoptosis (IAP) family of proteins.

The cell death machinery comprises effectors, activators, and negative regulators. Apoptosis can be induced by a variety of intracellular and extracellular stimuli, such as growth factor deprivation, hyperthermia, glucocorticoids, radiation, viruses, chemotherapy, and active killing by cytotoxic T cells. Certain cytokines of the TNF family and their cognate receptors, including TNF/TNF-R 1 and 2, FasL/Fas (CD95/APO/T), and TRAIL/TRAIL-R1 and 2 (DR4 and DR5), are classic triggers of the suicide response (Nagata, 1997). There is growing evidence that mitochondrial function is disturbed early in the apoptotic response and may be important in mediating apoptosis. Following exposure of cells to stimuli that trigger apoptosis, cytochrome *c* is rapidly released from mitochondria into the cytoplasm where it activates caspases. Apoptosis induced by TNF-related receptors appears to directly activate caspases independently of cytochrome *c* release. In the case of Fas-induced apoptosis, FADD, an adapter molecule, binds to the receptor and physically engages caspase-8, which represents the most upstream protease involved in the generation of the death signal. Following activation of caspases, biochemical events occur that lead to DNA degradation and the

Dendritic Cells: Biology and Clinical Applications
ISBN 0-12-455860-7

characteristic morphological changes associated with apoptosis. At least ten different members of the caspase family have been identified in mammals (Cohen, 1997).

The transduction of multiple apoptotic stimuli into caspase activation is regulated by a large family of proteins, including the Bcl-2 family. Products of the *bcl-2* gene family were originally identified as cell death receptors and later the existence of both pro-apoptotic and anti-apoptotic Bcl-2 homologues was demonstrated. Mcl-1 and Bcl-x_L are Bcl-2 homologues that can protect from apoptosis, while other homologues, such as Bax, Bak, and Bad, all inhibit the ability of Bcl-2 to block cell death (Uren and Vaux, 1996).

Despite increasing interest in the field of physiological and pathological cell death, the mechanisms of regulated induction and protection of different cell populations from death signals are poorly understood. Unregulated excessive apoptosis may be the reason for various degenerative and infectious diseases that are characterized by an abnormal loss of normal or protective cells. Conversely, an inappropriately low rate of apoptosis may promote survival of abnormal cells. It seems likely that identification of pro- and anti-apoptotic factors holds great promise for elucidating the pathogenesis of a variety of diseases and for developing more specific and effective treatments. Here, we focus on apoptosis in dendritic cells (DC), since the understanding of all aspects of DC immunobiology, including regulation of their death, is crucial for further development of effective DC-based immunotherapies.

DENDRITIC CELL LIFE CYCLE

The origin and ontogeny of DC have been reviewed in detail (Thomas and Lipsky, 1996; Hart, 1997; Banchereau and Steinman, 1998). DC originate from $CD34^+$ progenitor cells in the bone marrow. Within nonlymphoid tissues, they apparently develop into immature DC with the capacity to take up and process antigen. These DC can then migrate into secondary lymphoid tissues and mature into activated DC with the ability to present antigen to T cells and stimulate their proliferation. Thus, four sequential stages of DC development and maturation—pro-(pre-)DC, immature DC, mature (activated) DC, and apoptotic DC—could be defined and characterized.

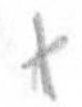

There is evidence that the maturation of DC is crucial for the initiation and development of immune responses. Following their egress from the bone marrow, DC-progenitor cells, or pro-DC, enter the blood and migrate to the tissues. In most tissues, DC are present in an immature stage, characterized by the unique capability to acquire antigen. Once the DC have captured an antigen, they leave nonlymphoid tissue and travel to lymphoid tissue such as the spleen and lymph nodes. While migrating toward regional lymph nodes, DC undergo maturational events involving reduction of antigen-processing capacity and enhancement of antigen-presenting function. Furthermore, the maturational changes in DC are associated with alteration in expression of surface molecules involved in DC function. This includes a decrease or loss of molecules important for antigen uptake, such as FcR and mannose receptor, and increase in the expression levels of MHC class I and II and costimulatory molecules. In addition, during this process, actin-based cytoskeleton and surface adhesion molecules are also rearranged, and cell motility is increased. This is likely to allow DC migration to lymphoid organs (Winzler *et al.*, 1997). The functional maturation of DC ends by

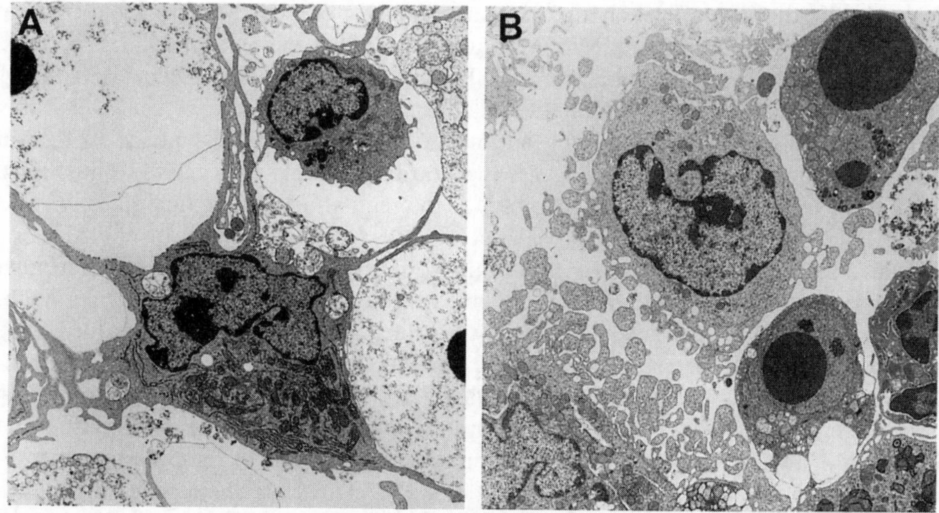

Fig. 1. Live and apoptotic DC. Electron micrographs of murine bone marrow-derived normal (A) and apoptotic DC (B). Ultrastructural changes are associated with dilatation of endoplasmic reticulum, swelling and condensation of mitochondria, and cytoplasmic and chromatin condensation (original magnification ×7250).

apoptotic cell death, and reversion to the immature phenotype cannot be detected (Fig. 1).

Little is known about the fate of DC after they have delivered antigen and presented it to T-lymphocytes in the lymph node. Few DC are found in the efferent lymph. It is possible that central migration of antigen-loaded DC and subsequent activation of T cells triggers terminal differentiation of DC, resulting in DC death (Hart, 1997). No direct data of DC death within lymph nodes have been reported. Early reports suggested that after encountering antigen, DC could become targets for NK cell-mediated killing (Shah *et al.*, 1986). It is feasible that, in order to reduce multiple antigen processing and presentation, DC, following effective interaction with T cells, should receive negative stimuli that render them ineffective antigen-presenting cells (APC). The role of apoptosis in elimination of DC has been addressed recently.

DC have been shown to undergo apoptosis during antigen-specific interaction with T cells (Matsue *et al.*, 1998). When splenic DC were cultured with both KLH-specific $CD4^+$ T_H1 clone and KLH, less than 13% of DC were viable by propidium iodide (PI) uptake after 20 h. By contrast, more than 50% of DC remained alive when cocultured with either T-lymphocytes or antigen alone. These data suggest that DC die following antigen-specific interaction with $CD4^+$ T cells. It is likely that Fas/FasL interaction plays an important role in this process (see below).

Estimated DC life span *in vivo* depends on the method, tissue, and species used. It varies from 3 days to 4 weeks, although the duration of homing of Langerhans cells (LC) in the epidermis might be longer (Steinman and Cohn, 1973; Thomas and Lipsky, 1996). Mature DC have been demonstrated to express high levels of protein from the NF-κ family such as p65, c-Rel, RelB, p50/p105, and p52/p100 (Granelli-Piperno *et al.*,

1995; Feuillard *et al.*, 1996). Mice with a disruption of *relB* gene lacked a thymic medulla, and had impaired splenic APC activity, higher susceptibility to infections, and reduced number of thymic but not skin DC (Burkly *et al.*, 1995; Weih *et al.*, 1997). It is possible that RelB might regulate expression of certain genes, possibly MHC class II, related to DC differentiation (Carrasco *et al.*, 1993). In fact, expression of RelB was strongly induced during DC maturation (Kikuchi *et al.*, 1998). Thus, RelB seems to be one of the factors responsible for the regulation of DC differentiation and maturation.

Finally, it is important to note that apoptotic events, occurring before terminal maturation, play a role in supporting DC lineage selection and homeostasis. Santiago-Schwarz *et al.* (1997) outlined functionally distinct apoptotic schedules, which were associated with different phases of DC development from multipotent $CD34^+$ progenitor cells. During early phases of growth, unselected progenitors underwent apoptosis. At the level of progenitors/precursors, apoptosis appeared to ensure the selection and expansion of $DR^+CD33^+CD13^+$ DC precursors. Late phases of apoptosis were associated with the death of terminally differentiated DC. Thus, regulated programmed cell death during DC generation from progenitors likely represents a biological mechanism, which maintains hematological homeostasis by preventing uncontrolled proliferation and renewal of progenitor/stem cells. Interestingly, TGF-β_1 promotes the generation of DC *in vitro* by protecting progenitor cells from apoptosis, which correlates with significantly reduced Fas expression on cultured cells (Riedl *et al.*, 1997). These results indicate that, although suppression of apoptosis may prolong the survival of late DC elements, an earlier apoptotic program appears to be required for the selective expansion of DC elements from multipotent progenitor cells (Santiago-Schwarz *et al.*, 1997).

INFECTION AND DEATH OF DENDRITIC CELLS

Both viral and bacterial infection of DC can cause their death. For instance, using different variants of a lymphocytic choriomeningitis virus (LCMV), Borrow *et al.* (1995) observed that LCMV clone 13 caused a high level of infection in APC in the white pulp of spleen, including periarterial interdigitating DC. This infection was associated with a CD8-dependent loss of DC from periarteriolar lymphoid sheaths and, functionally, with an impairment of splenocytes from infected animals to stimulate activation of naive T cells in a primary mixed leukocyte response (MLR).

Infection of human CD34-derived DC by measles virus caused 25% of DC to undergo apoptosis after 4 days of infection, as detected using Annexin V and PI staining (Grosjean *et al.*, 1997). Another group, using TUNEL techniques, has demonstrated that in measles virus-infected monocyte-derived human DC cultures, $\sim$45% of cells undergo apoptosis by the conclusion of the culture (Fugier-Vivier *et al.*, 1997). In contrast, UV-inactivated measles virus does not induce apoptosis of DC, suggesting that this death is largely due to viral replication. It is possible that members of the TNF family are upregulated on DC after viral infection, which may induce paracrine-killing of T cells and autocrine-killing of DC cultures (Fugier-Vivier *et al.*, 1997). Virus, both infectious and UV-inactivated, was able to inhibit IL-12 production by CD40-activated DC (Fugier-Vivier *et al.*, 1997). This represents an important factor contributing to the T_H2 polarization observed in virus-infected patients. HIV infection could also induce functional polarization to T_H2 responses. Similarly, stimulation of type-2 cytokine production and suppression of type-1 cytokine synthesis has been described in tumor-bearing hosts (Ghosh *et al.*, 1995).

Several reports raise the possibility that HIV-1 may induce DC killing. LC in the skin and mucous membranes are productively infected with HIV *in vivo* (Braathen *et al.*, 1987; Weissman *et al.*, 1995). Evaluation of LC in patients with AIDC revealed a significant reduction of LC number per square millimeter of body surface area (Belsito *et al.*, 1984). In another early study, Daniels *et al.* (1987) demonstrated that epithelial LC were absent or greatly reduced in the lesions of oral hairy leukoplakia, a described manifestation of HIV infection in which EBV has been shown to replicate. In non-lesional oral mucosa from the same patients, LC were detected in approximately normal numbers. Furthermore, the exposure of DC in culture to HIV-1 was shown to promote severe DC morphological alterations and killing (Beaulieu *et al.*, 1996). Progressive destruction of follicular DC has been reported to be associated with the later stage of HIV infection (Petrasch *et al.*, 1994) and LP-BM5 murine leukemia virus infection (murine acquired immunodeficiency syndrome) (Masuda *et al.*, 1993). Knight (1995) summarized clinical and experimental evidence and proposed that a major mechanism producing immunological abnormalities in HIV-1 infection was the infection and subsequent dysfunction of DC. Thus, these results illustrate an additional mechanism for virus-induced immunosuppression, which might contribute to the clinically important inhibition of immunity which accompanies many virus infections, including HIV type 1.

Infection of murine spleen DC line or bone marrow-derived DC by *Listeria monocytogenes* was also found to induce apoptotic death of DC (Guzman *et al.*, 1996). Using several isogenic mutants deficient in the production of individual listerial virulence factors, authors were able to identify a protein, so-called listeriolysin, responsible for the induction of DC death. Apoptosis in DC was also induced by purified listeriolysin, suggesting that this protein directly induces death of DC. Thus, invasion of DC by *Listeria monocytogenes* causes cell death, which may play an important role in the pathogenesis of listerial infections by inhibiting development of immune responses, hindering bacterial clearance, and promoting spread of the infection.

On the other hand, it is well documented that infection of DC stimulates their maturation and activation (Henderson *et al.*, 1997). Thus, it is possible that both processes, activation and apoptosis, induced in DC upon infection with virus or bacteria, play an important syngeneic role in the initiation of specific immune responses. In fact, Young *et al.* (1985) noted that some LC were associated with epithelial cells that appeared to be undergoing apoptosis, and they first suggested that these LC might be involved in phagocytosis of apoptotic cells. Parr *et al.* (1991) confirmed these data, presenting the ultrastructural details of phagocytosis of apoptotic vaginal epithelial cells by LC. Rubartelli *et al.* (1997) demonstrated that DC, unlike macrophages, failed to take up opsonized particles or necrotic cells, while apoptotic bodies were efficiently engulfed by DC. Interestingly, DC and macrophages required different surface receptors involved in recognition of apoptotic bodies, such as vitronectin receptor, CD36, and phosphatidylserine receptor. An important role of CD14 in recognition and phagocytosis of apoptotic cells has just been revealed (Devitt *et al.*, 1998). An elegant study underlying the functional significance of DC phagocytosis was recently reported by Albert *et al.* (1998). They showed that human DC, but not macrophages, present antigen derived from influenza-infected apoptotic cells and stimulate class I-restricted

CTL. However, it has also been observed that exogenous HIV-1 Tat was able in a time- and dose-dependent manner to inhibit the engulfment of apoptotic bodies by DC (Zocchi *et al.*, 1997). All these findings suggest a mechanism by which DC acquire antigen from infected and apoptotic cells (possibly DC) for further presentation to T cells. Thus, these and other studies are leading to a new appreciation of the role of DC in both protective and pathogenic aspects of viral infection (Bhardwaj, 1997).

TUMOR-INDUCED APOPTOSIS OF DENDRITIC CELLS

O'Mahony *et al.* (1993) first demonstrated that immunosuppressive factors derived from human esophageal squamous carcinoma induced apoptosis in normal and transformed JURKAT T cells. Tumor-induced immunosuppression can also be mediated by elimination of immune cells within the tumor microenvironment. Tumor-induced apoptosis of T-lymphocytes has now been demonstrated in colorectal cancer (O'Connell *et al.*, 1996), melanoma (Hahne *et al.*, 1996), hepatocellular carcinoma (Strand *et al.*, 1996), breast cancer (Gimmi *et al.*, 1996), lung carcinoma (Niehans *et al.*, 1997), astrocytoma (Saas *et al.*, 1997), multiple myeloma (Villunger *et al.*, 1997), and virtually every tumor type which has been examined carefully. In addition, the total number of NK cells is also decreased substantially in cancer patients (Vujanovic *et al.*, 1996), which allows one to hypothesize that tumor-induced apoptosis of NK cells may also contribute to the impairment of anti-tumor immune response observed in cancer patients and tumor-bearing animals. Recent findings of Kolde *et al.* (1998) suggest

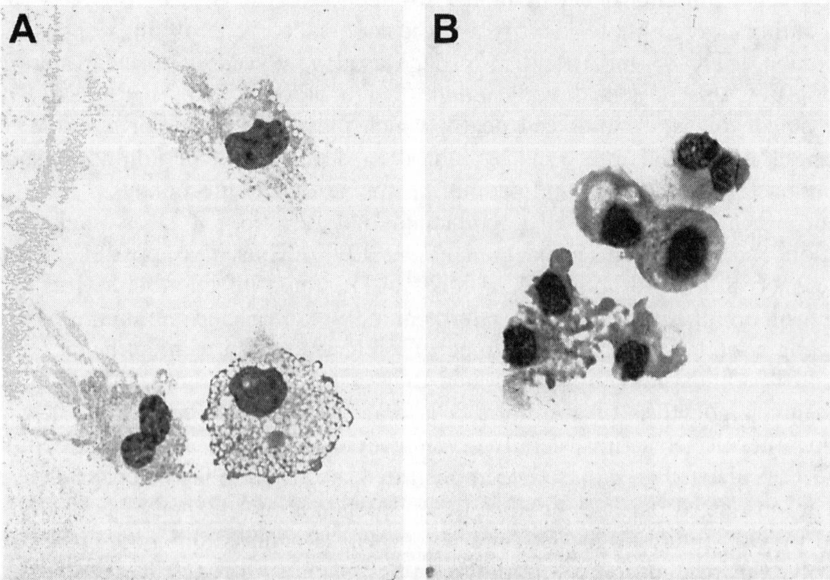

Fig. 2. Tumor-induced apoptosis in murine DC. Morphological evaluation of DC apoptosis after pre-incubation with B16 melanoma cells (B) in comparison with control DC (A). Cytospin slides were fixed in methanol and stained with eosin Y, methylene blue, and azure A. The typical features of apoptosis include condensation of cytoplasm and shrinkage of the cell, membrane blebbing, chromatin condensation, and nuclear fragmentation.

that FasL-expressing tumors are capable of inducing apoptotic elimination of not only lymphocytes but eosinophils as well.

We have demonstrated that both murine and human DC undergo apoptosis to varying degrees *in vitro* and *in vivo* after contact with tumors (Shurin *et al.*, submitted). Death of DC by apoptosis was detected based on the distinctive morphology which allowed them to be relatively easily distinguished from healthy cells and from those dying by necrosis. As shown in Fig. 2, mouse bone marrow-derived DC underwent apoptosis after preincubation with the highly lethal and very poorly immunogenic B16 melanoma cells. The typical features of apoptosis, including condensation of cytoplasm and shrinkage of the cell, membrane blebbing, chromatin condensation, and nuclear fragmentation, were observed. These data were confirmed by analysis of DNA fragmentation in DC cultures preincubated with different tumor or control cells. DNA laddering was a typical feature in DC samples obtained from tumor-conditioned cocultures (Fig. 3). Furthermore, using [^{3}H]DNA release assay to assess DNA fragmentation, we found that coincubation of both murine and human DC with a variety of tumor cell lines resulted in significant time- and dose-dependent apoptosis of DC. In contrast, incubation of DC with splenocytes, PBMC, or PHA-activated blasts was not associated with significant death of DC. As an example, Fig. 4 shows the results of a representative experiment. Results suggesting that tumor causes apoptosis in DC were

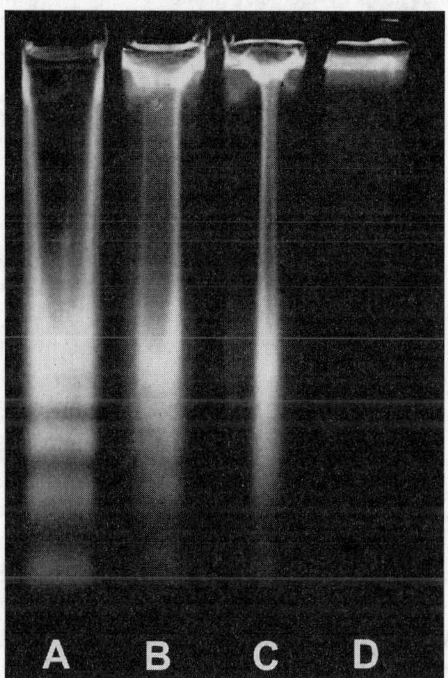

Fig. 3. Tumor-induced DNA fragmentation in murine DC. Agarose gel electrophoresis of DNA extracted from murine DC after coincubation with B16 melanoma cells or splenocytes. 10 μg DNA/lane was run on a 2% agarose gel stained with ethidium bromide. Analysis of these data shows the characteristic 'laddering of DC DNA after coculture with B16 melanoma for 48 h (A) or 24 h (B). No DNA fragmentation was detected when DC were coincubated with splenocytes for 24 h (D) or 48 h (C).

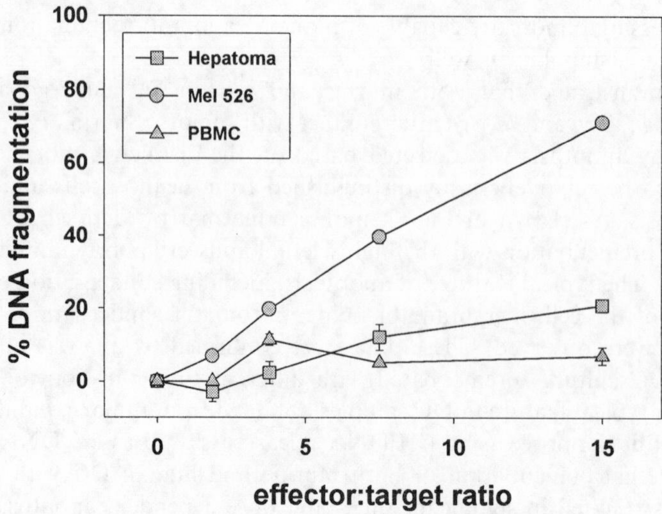

Fig. 4. Tumor-induced apoptosis in human DC. Determination of DNA fragmentation in human CD34-derived DC by a JAM assay. DC were labeled with [^{3}H]thymidine (3 μCi/ml) for 24 h, washed, purified by density centrifugation, and coincubated with different tumor cells or control cells at tumor : DC ratios up to 15 : 1 in 96-well round-bottom plates. Eight hours later, cells were harvested onto glass-fiber filter and the intact [^{3}H]DNA was measured by liquid scintillation counting. A significant tumor-specific and dose-dependent killing of DC by tumor cells was reproducibly detected.

confirmed by live microscopy, which allowed us to directly visualize alterations of DC morphology and the development of apoptotic bodies following contact between DC and the tumor cell (Fig. 5).

Although these and other data clearly demonstrate induction of DC apoptosis by tumor-derived factors, exact mechanisms of this effect are not clear. Since direct contact between DC and tumor cell resulted in a faster appearance of apoptotic figures, it is likely that both soluble and membrane-bound molecules are involved. Different tumor cells may release and express on the surface different pro-apoptotic factors, such as NO, TGF-β, IL-10, gangliosides, FasL, TRAIL, and others. The roles of these factors, as well as the intracellular signal transduction pathways responsible for tumor-induced apoptosis in DC, remain to be determined. These studies are in progress in our laboratory.

DC play an important role in the initiation and regulation of the anti-tumor immune response (Shurin, 1996). Thus, impairment of APC number or activity could result in deficient expansion or activation of specific T-lymphocytes. There are numerous clinical observations suggesting a positive correlation between the number of tumor-infiltrating dendritic cells (TIDC) and improved tumor prognosis (Becker, 1993; Lotze, 1997). The infiltration of DC into primary tumor lesions has been associated with significantly prolonged patient survival and a reduced incidence of metastatic disease in patients with oral, head and neck tumors, nasopharyngeal tumors, lung, bladder, esophageal, and gastric carcinomas (Lotze, 1997). Furthermore, regression of primary cutaneous melanomas was associated with Langerhans cell infiltration (Bröcker *et al.*, 1982; Poppema *et al.*, 1983; Nestor and Cochran, 1987). Using FLT3 ligand, a pluripotent

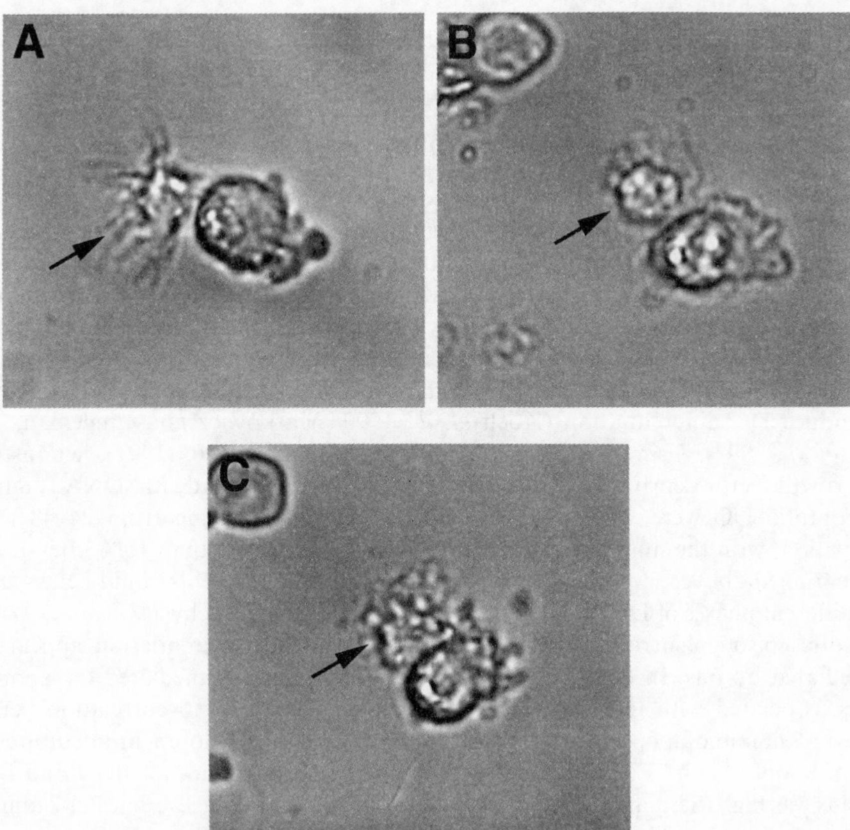

Fig. 5. Kinetic study of tumor-induced apoptosis in DC. Direct contact between MC38 colon adenocarcinoma cell and DC (arrow) results in a rapid DC apoptosis as demonstrated on time-lapse images obtained by live microscopy. (A), (B), and (C) correspond to 5, 30, and 60 min of cell–cell contact on a microscope cover slip (37°C). Similar results were obtained for B16 melanoma cells, suggesting that various tumor cells cause contact-induced apoptotic death of DC.

hematopoietic growth factor (Shurin *et al.*, 1998), we have recently demonstrated that its anti-tumor effect was accompanied by the accumulation of DC at the tumor site (Esche *et al.*, 1998). Interestingly, FLT3-ligand not only stimulates the generation of DC *in vivo* (Shurin *et al.*, 1997), but also causes redistrubution of mature and immature DC in the skin (Esche *et al.*, 1998).

It was shown in early studies that the number of epidermal LC was decreased in malignant tumors. For instance, Gatter *et al.* (1984), using an immunohistochemical approach, demonstrated that in benign skin lesions LC were increased, whereas in malignant tumors they were not only markedly depleted or absent but also grossly stunted and deformed in outline. Similar data were reported by Facchetti *et al.* (1984), who observed that epidermal LC were rare in the central part of tumor biopsies which showed a primary malignant melanoma in the vertical growth. LC are often depleted above 'deeply invasive' melanomas and they decline in number as melanoma progresses (Stene *et al.*, 1988). These results were recently confirmed by

Toriyama *et al.* (1993), who reported a substantial reduction in LC in the epidermis over melanoma.

MECHANISMS OF APOPTOSIS IN DENDRITIC CELLS

The spontaneous death of DC in cultures and its regulation by cytokines and growth factors has been evaluated intensively. For instance, it has been shown that the spontaneous decrease of human LC viability during culture is due to apoptosis (Ludewig *et al.*, 1995). This was shown by the rapid onset of internucleosomal DNA fragmentation, appearance of morphological characteristics of apoptosis (dilation of the endoplasmic reticulum, chromatin condensation and membrane blebbing) and susceptibility to phagocytosis. GM-CSF, TNF-α, and CD40L have been reported to promote DC survival and induce DC differentiation (Koch *et al.*, 1990; Markowicz and Engleman, 1990; Caux *et al.*, 1994). Using long-term DC cultures, Winzler *et al.* (1997) demonstrated that growth factor deprivation led to DC growth arrest and cell death. DNA fragments in apoptotic DC were visualized by TUNEL staining, starting from 24–48 h after deprivation, with the number of viable cells decreasing to less than 10% after 1 week. As mentioned above, several functionally distinct apoptotic events could be associated with different phases of DC development in cultures (Santiago-Schwarz *et al.*, 1997). The apoptotic episodes surrounding the earlier stage of DC differentiation appeared to be mediated by Fas. In contrast, a Fas-independent pathway mediated the apoptotic events associated with terminally differentiated DC, because no correlation between Fas expression and apoptosis was observed. By peak DC development in cultures, the level of apoptosis and Fas expression was low and the expression of Bcl-2 and Bcl-x_L proteins was high (Santiago-Schwarz *et al.*, 1997). These data suggest that Bcl-2 family of anti-apoptotic proteins may protect DC against cell death at the peak of DC development and that Fas and Bcl-2 inversely regulate apoptotic events during DC generation.

In spite of the growing evidence for the role of Fas/FasL interaction in the developmental selection and functions of T lymphocytes and NK cells, less attention has been paid to the function of Fas in APC, including DC. Immature DC have been shown to express low levels of both Fas and FasL (Winzler *et al.*, 1997). We and others demonstrated expression of both Fas and FasL in murine bone marrow-derived dendritic cells (Lu *et al.*, 1997a,b; Fig. 6). The role of Fas/FasL interaction in DC apoptosis during antigen-specific interaction with T cells has been demonstrated recently by Matsue *et al.* (1998) using a long-term DC line XS52 and a KLH-specific T_H1 clone. DC remained >87% viable when cultured with either T cells or antigen alone, whereas >66% of them were dead by PI uptake after 16 h of incubation with both the T cell clone and KLH. Anti-CD95L antibody significantly inhibited T cell-mediated apoptosis of XS52 cells, and ligation of CD95 with specific antibody triggered XS52 death in a T cell-independent manner. Thus, ligation of Fas on the DC cell line with FasL expressed on T cells was required and sufficient to trigger DC death (Matsue *et al.*, 1998). Interestingly, addition of anti-Ia antibody to DC/T-cell/antigen cocultures prevented DC apoptosis. Similar data were also reported earlier, suggesting that activated $CD8^+$ T cells were able to kill APC by both perforin and Fas-mediated mechanisms (Sad *et al.*, 1996). Thus, antigen-specific interaction of DC with T cells may induce Fas-mediated apoptosis of DC and might serve as a unique regulatory mechanism to prevent the continual activation of T cells (Fig. 7).

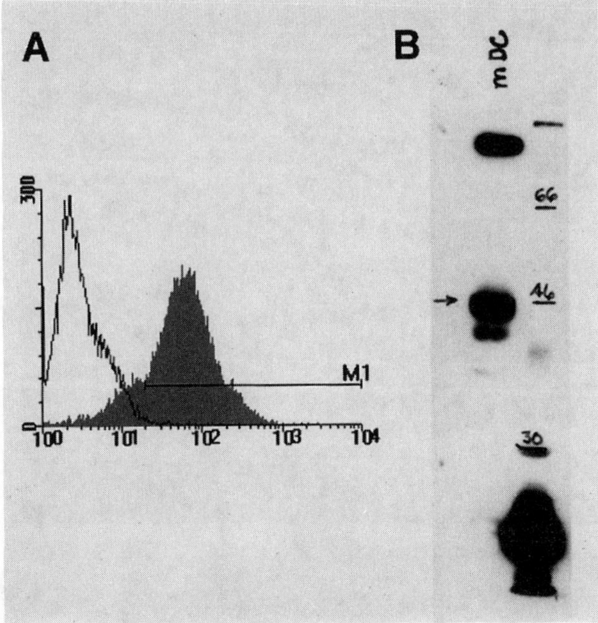

Fig. 6. Detection of Fas expression in murine cultured bone marrow-derived DC by FACScan analysis (A) and western blotting (B). These data demonstrate that cultured murine DC produce and express a high level of Fas molecules.

Interestingly, using human LC, von Stebut *et al.* (1997) demonstrated LC apoptosis in cultures which engaged Fas signaling pathways. Expression of Fas (CD95) was revealed in approximately 40% of isolated LC and addition of anti-CD95 IgM induced an accelerated but not enhanced decrease of LC viability within the next 72 h. After 2 days of culture without cytokines, CD95 expression was completely downregulated and anti-CD95-IgM failed to induce apoptosis in these cells. Caux *et al.* (1994) and Ludewig *et al.* (1995) demonstrated that spontaneous apoptosis of human DC and LC was efficiently inhibited by CD40 ligation. Using human peripheral blood DC, Koppi *et al.* (1997) reported that the addition of recombinant soluble CD40L strongly inhibited CD95-mediated apoptosis in these cells. Furthermore, Björck *et al.* (1997) proposed a mechanism by which CD40 ligation inhibits Fas-mediated apoptosis of DC. This study indicates that when DC are partially mature they may have a propensity to undergo apoptosis either spontaneously or in response to Fas triggering. In contrast, fully mature DC that have received CD40-mediated stimulation following T cell encounter are apparently resistant to cell death after Fas ligation. The different responses of these two DC populations correlated with differences in the levels of Bcl-2 protein. This was further strengthened by finding that CD40 triggering stimulated expression of Bcl-2 protein, which was associated with the observed resistance to Fas-induced apoptosis. These findings suggest that the interaction between DC and T cells may have implications for both the activation of naive T lymphocytes and, subsequently, the fate of DC (Björck *et al.*, 1997). It is possible that the regulation of DC apoptosis by CD95L and

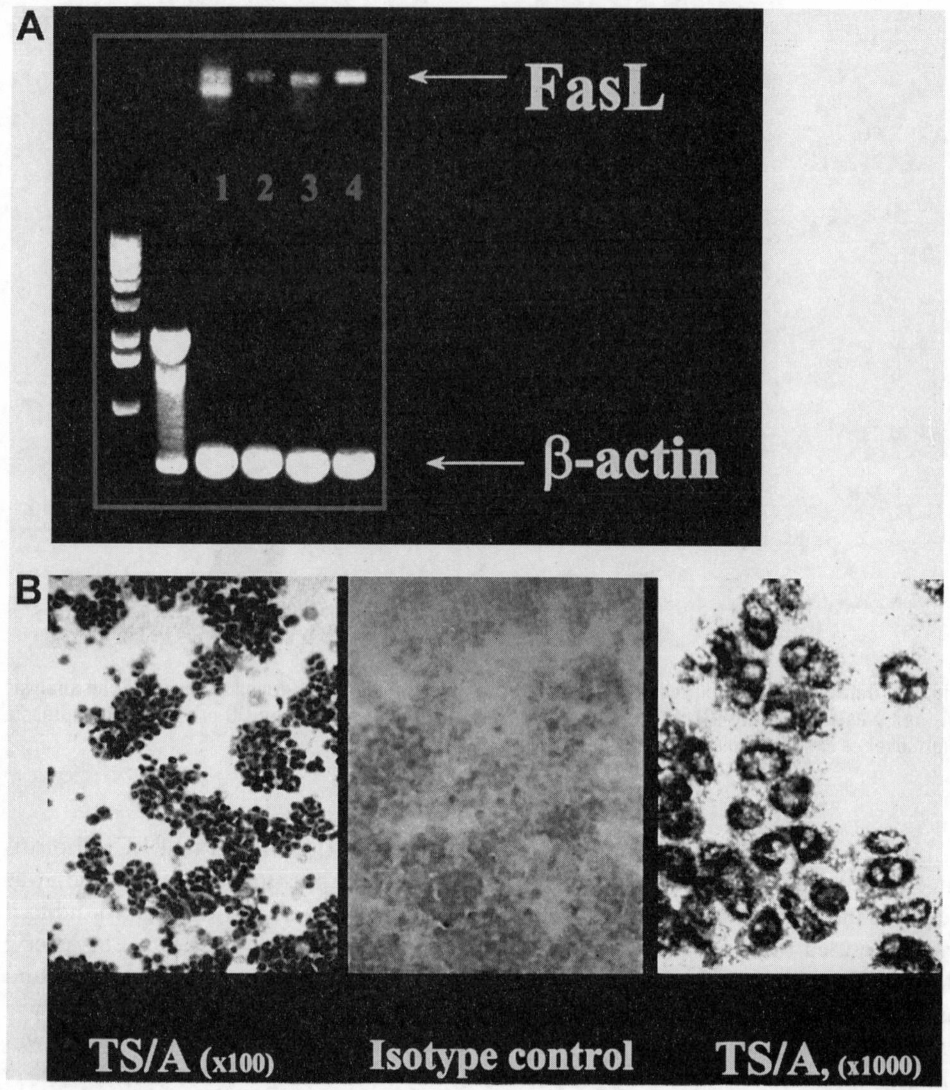

Fig. 7. Expression of FasL (CD95L) on tumor cells. Detection of FasL on murine tumor cell lines using RT-PCR (A) and immunohistochemistry (B). (A) Amplification products were visualized in 2% agarose gels after staining with ethidium bromide. 1-TS/A carcinoma, 2-C3 sarcoma, 3-B16 melanoma, and 4-MC38 adenocarcinoma. (B) TS/A mammary adenocarcinoma cells were immunocytochemically stained using anti-FasL antibody NOK-1. Left and right panels demonstrate two magnifications (originally ×100, ×1000) of FasL$^+$ tumor cells, whereas the central panel shows negative isotype control staining. These data suggest that murine tumor cells express high levels of both FasL mRNA and protein.

CD40L may represent an important mechanism responsible for the feedback control of DC activity by activated T cells.

Recently, TRANCE (TNF-related activation-induced cytokine), a novel ligand of the TNF family, was cloned and characterized. Remarkably, TRANCE receptors were only detected on DC, suggesting that a major function of TRANCE is to modulate

DC activity (Wong *et al.*, 1997). In fact, it was shown that TRANCE inhibits apoptosis of mouse bone marrow-derived DC and human monocyte-derived DC *in vitro* and can be considered as a DC-specific survival factor. Similar to CD40L, TRANCE promotes the survival of mature DC by regulating the expression of Bcl-x_L. Signaling by TRANCE receptor appeared to be dependent on TNF-receptor-associated factor 2 (TRAF-2) (Wong *et al.*, 1997). Finally, it would be of interest to test the role of IL-12, a potent anti-tumor cytokine (Shurin *et al.*, 1997b), in the regulation of DC sensitivity to apoptotic signals, since it was shown that CD40 ligation stimulates IL-12 production via activation of NF-κB (Yoshimoto *et al.*, 1997) and TRAF-2 activates NF-κB as well (Rothe *et al.*, 1995).

Thus, DC express both Fas and FasL, but the involvement of this pathway in apoptotic death could be effector-specific. An important observation was described recently by Um *et al.* (1996) suggesting that human monocytes express Fas irrespective of their activation status, and that engagement of Fas by its agonistic antibody could induce apoptosis. The lethal effect of Fas was most pronounced when monocytes were activated by TNF-α and IL-1β, whereas LPS-treated monocytes were resistant to the apoptotic action of Fas. LPS rescued monocytes from Fas-mediated death, at least in part, by inhibiting the Fas-dependent elevation of reactive oxygen intermediates (Um *et al.*, 1996). It is possible that DC may also have a protective mechanism that directly interferes with the Fas/FasL-induced transduction pathway and controls their destiny. Thus, it appears that Fas signaling might be different depending upon the cell populations involved as well as their stage of maturation and activation.

Both murine and human DC can be activated following infection with different bacteria or viruses (Johnston *et al.*, 1996; Henderson *et al.*, 1997; Winzler *et al.*, 1997). Paracrine induction of TNF-α expression in DC infected with Gram-positive and Gram-negative bacteria has been also detected (Riva *et al.*, 1996). Thus, maturation of DC, as well as their sensitivity to the induction of apoptosis, requires stimulation with living bacteria, LPS, or cytokines such as TNF-α or, likely, IL-1β. This may suggest that the sensitivity of DC to pro-apoptotic stimuli may depend on the maturational stage of DC development. In fact, it was demonstrated that human peripheral blood monocytes undergo apoptosis when cultured in the absence of growth factors or activation stimuli; addition of inflammatory mediators, such as TNF-α, IL-1β, or LPS effectively inhibited this apoptotic process (Mangan *et al.*, 1991). Kämpgen *et al.* (1994b) reported that both GM-CSF and TNF-α significantly inhibited the levels of spontaneous apoptosis of both cultured murine LC and splenic DC. Similar data were obtained using cultured human LC (Ludewig *et al.*, 1995). Apoptosis in cultured human monocytes could also be efficiently prevented by GM-CSF and IFN-γ (Mangan and Wahl, 1991). These findings are consistent with the hypothesis that cells are programmed to die unless they receive a survival signal.

On the other hand, high levels of DC infiltration were found in different tissues during chronic inflammation. It is likely that greater DC attraction, reduced emigration and decreased rates of apoptosis of DC are all involved in this phenomenon. The production of factors such as GM-CSF and TNF-α at the site of inflammation implies that a number of mechanisms, including local proliferation and apoptosis, may play a role in the maintenance of large numbers of DC locally (Thomas and Lipsky, 1996). Furthermore, as inflammation wanes, the number of DC in the lesion declines owing to emigration and programmed cell death of DC.

Nitric oxide (NO) could also be considered a tumor-derived or macrophage-derived factor able to cause DC apoptosis. In fact, Lu *et al.* (1996) demonstrated that exposure of DC to the NO donor SNAP (*S*-nitroso-*N*-acetylpenicillamine) caused apoptosis of DC. In addition, they showed that endogenous NO production by DC, stimulated by IFN-γ and LPS, resulted in DC apoptosis. Thus, these data suggest that increased concentration of NO in the local microenvironment and/or hyperactivation of DC may cause apoptosis of DC and, in turn, failure in antigen recognition and presentation to T-lymphocytes. For instance, utilizing UV radiation as an apoptotic signal, Kitajima *et al.* (1996b) suggested that DC undergoing apoptosis deliver unusual activation signals to T cells during antigen presentation, signals that lead to cellular unresponsiveness rather than to effective immunity.

It has also been shown that UV radiation substantially reduced the viability of DC cell lines (Tang and Udey, 1992; Schuhmachers *et al.*, 1996). Furthermore, Kitajima *et al.* (1996) demonstrated that radiation doses that cause only minimal direct cytotoxicity sensitized the DC cell line to become highly susceptible to apoptosis when subsequently confronted either with LPS or with antigen plus antigen-specific T-cells. The mechanism of this effect is unknown, but the authors hypothesized that irradiation might stimulate the expression of Fas on DC. Another possible factor responsible for DC apoptosis is IL-10, a factor produced by tumor cells, T cells, B cells, and macrophages (Howard and O'Garra, 1992; Gastl *et al.*, 1993). Ludewig *et al.* (1995) demonstrated that IL-10 induced apoptosis of human DC *in vitro* and reversed the effect of TNF-α and TRAP (CD40L), which inhibited spontaneous DC apoptosis in cultures. It is possible that IL-10 is involved in a negative feedback mechanism during initiation of adaptive immune responses, as even low doses of IL-10 induce apoptosis and reverse the effect of TNF-α (Ludewig *et al.*, 1995).

Both topical and systemic administration of various glucocorticoids cause a marked decrease in LC density in animals and humans (Belsito *et al.*, 1982; Shaieb *et al.*, 1987; Bernateck *et al.*, 1996). Ultrastructural examination of the skin from animals treated topically with glucocorticoids revealed alterations in the LC including clumping of nuclear chromatin, dilation of endoplasmic reticulum, and swelling and condensation of mitochondria. These observations suggest that cell injury and induction of cell death may be one of the mechanisms mediating LC depletion induced by glucocorticoids. Effect of dexamethasone on LC was also evaluated using both freshly isolated and cultured murine LC (Furue and Katz, 1989). It was found that dexamethasone directly decreased the number of LC in a dose- and time-dependent manner. This early suggestion was recently confirmed by Kämpgen *et al.* (1994a), who demonstrated that steroids are potent inducers of programmed cell death in LC. Stimulation of apoptosis in LC by steroids in that study was demonstrated *in vitro* by the appearance of typical DNA ladders after steroid exposure of purified LC and was also visible *in situ* using TUNEL staining. Using murine splenic DC, Moser *et al.* (1995) reported that DC yield in cultures in the presence of dexamethasone was reduced by up to 50% as compared to the control population. Interestingly, a single injection of dexamethasone results in a dose-dependent loss of splenic DC (Moser *et al.*, 1995). Our data with cultured bone marrow-derived DC also suggested that corticosterone dose-dependently inhibited DC viability after 24 h treatment *in vitro*. Additionally, we found that the acute surgical stress resulted in suppression of the ability of splenic cells to stimulate proliferation of naive T-lymphocytes in a primary MLR in mice (Shurin *et al.*, in preparation). The mechanisms of this effect remain to be determined and could be result of DC emigration out of the spleen, loss of expression of MHC or costimulatory molecules on DC, or, alternatively, the induction of DC apoptosis by released corticosterone or other stress hormones and neuromediators. Finally, a new mechanism of glucocorticoid-induced immune suppression has recently been suggested. Working with the murine epidermal-derived DC line XS52, Kitajima *et al.* (1996a) demonstrated that dexamethasone directly inhibited T cell-mediated terminal maturation of DC. Thus, additional experiments will be required to clarify the effect of corticosteroids on murine and human DC maturation, survival, and function *in vitro* and *in vivo*.

Aiba *et al.* (1998) have demonstrated that various haptens induce maturation and/or apoptosis in cultured monocyte-derived DC in a dose-dependent fashion. For instance, DNCB, $NiCl_2$, and $MnCl_2$ stimulate DC maturation as determined by downregulation of c-Fms/CSF-1R expression and enhancement of CD86 (B7-2) expression. At a higher dose, $NiCl_2$, $MnCl_2$, and $CoCl_2$, but not DNCB, induce apoptosis in DC measured by Annexin V binding. These data suggest that haptens could stimulate maturation and apoptosis of DC through different signal transduction pathways. Treatment with zinc sulfate, which directly inhibits endonuclease activity, drastically diminished spontaneous DNA fragmentation in 12–24 h cultures of murine LC or splenic DC (Kämpgen *et al.*, 1994b). Interestingly, the inhibition of protein synthesis by cycloheximide markedly increased spontaneous apoptosis of murine LC and splenic DC, as was determined by TUNEL staining (Kämpgen *et al.*, 1994b).

Thus, studies aimed at determining mechanisms of apoptosis in DC and factors involved in pro- and anti-apoptotic signaling in DC are incomplete. Further investigations are required to characterize the mechanisms of DC apoptosis and the role of this phenomenon in the etiology and pathogenesis of different diseases.

CONCLUSIONS

Of significant clinical interest is the existence of a relationship between DC infiltration of tumor mass and prognosis in malignancy. The infiltration of DC into primary tumor lesions has been associated with significantly prolonged patient survival and reduced incidence of metastatic disease in patients with oral, head and neck tumors, nasopharyngeal tumors, and lung, bladder, esophageal, and gastric carcinomas (Lotze, 1997). Our finding of tumor-induced apoptotic death of DC may explain these clinical observations. More 'aggressive' tumors may cause higher levels of DC apoptosis at the tumor site and, in turn, stronger inhibition of antigen recognition, processing and presentation by DC, which are necessary for the initiation and maintenance of an effective anti-tumor immune response. In fact, Stene *et al.* (1988) reported that melanoma-associated Langerhans cells declined in number as melanoma progressed. Similarly, examination of the frequency of epidermal Langerhans cells in the epidermis overlying primary melanoma revealed a substantial reduction in these cells (Toriyama *et al.*, 1993). Subsequent investigation of the mechanisms involved in tumor-induced apoptosis of DC will allow us to determine effective means to protect DC from premature death and thus improve tumor-specific immune responses.

Investigation of factors responsible for DC apoptosis is important for the development of effective strategies designed to protect DC from tumor-induced cell death. It is important to remember that such studies should involve not only tumor-related compounds but also infection-derived factors. As discussed above, several virus infections may be associated with viral-induced death of infected DC, including HIV-1 and measles virus infections. As an example, AIDS has caused almost 2 million deaths in the last decade, and measles virus infection results in the death of more than 1 million children per year (Borrow *et al.*, 1995). These infections in humans are often accompanied by clinically important immune suppression. The pathogenesis of this phenomenon is still poorly understood, but it is possible that loss of DC and defects in antigen presentation and stimulation of T-lymphocytes play an important role.

In summary, understanding the primary signals and intracellular pathways involved in regulation of apoptosis in DC will bring new means to control both initiation and termination of the immune response. Thus, such studies will have both theoretical and practical significance.

ACKNOWLEGMENTS

This study was supported in part by the Competitive Medical Research Fund (M.R.S), 97-007-1RNI from the AUHS (A.L.), Es 132/1-1 from the Deutsche Forschungsgemeinschaft (C.E.) and NIH RO1 CA 73816-01 (M.T.L.). The authors thank Drs G. Shurin, P. Hershberger and S. Watkins for their invaluable help in our studies and for helpful comments on the manuscript.

REFERENCES

Aiba, S., Manome, H. and Tagami, H. (1998). The induction of maturation and apoptosis of CD1a+ dendritic cells by haptens. *J. Invest. Dermatol.* **110**, 563a.

Albert, M.L., Sauter, B. and Bhardwaj, N. (1998). Dendritic cells acquire antigen from apoptotic cells and induce class I-restricted CTLs. *Nature* **392**, 86–89.

Banchereau, J. and Steinman, R.M. (1998). Dendritic cells and the control of immunity. *Nature* **392**, 245–252.

Beaulieu, S., Kessous, A., Landry, D., Montplaisir, S., Bergeron, D. and Cohen, E.A. (1996). In vitro characterization of purified human dendritic cells infected with human immunodeficiency virus type 1. *Virology* **222**, 214–226.

Becker, Y. (1993). Dendritic cell activity against primary tumors: an overview. *In Vivo* **7**, 187–191.

Bernateck, M., Jonas, L. and Diezel, W. (1996). Histochemical, immunohistochemical and ultrastructural studies on the action of glucocorticoids on epidermal Langerhans cells (ELC) of murine skin. *Acta Histochem.* **98**, 101–106.

Belsito, D.V., Flotte, T.J., Lim, H.W., Baer, R.L., Thorbecke, G.J. and Gigli, I. (1982). Effect of glucocorticosteroids on epidermal Langerhans cells. *J. Exp. Med.* **155**, 291–302.

Belsito, D.V., Sanchez, M.R., Baer, R.L., Valentine, F. and Thorbecke, G.J. (1984). Reduced Langerhans cell 1a antigen and ATPase activity in patients with the acquired immunodeficiency syndrome. *N. Engl. J. Med.* **310**, 1279–1282.

Bhardwaj, N. (1997). Interactions of viruses with dendritic cells: a double-edged sword. *J. Exp. Med.* **186**, 795–799.

Björck, P., Banchereau, J. and Flores-Romo, L. (1997). CD40 ligation counteracts Fas-induced apoptosis of human dendritic cells. *Int. Immunol.* **9**, 365–372.

Borrow, P., Evans, C.F. and Oldstone, M.B. (1995). Virus-induced immunosuppression: immune system-mediated destruction of virus-infected dendritic cells results in generalized immune suppression. *J. Virol.* **69**, 1059–1070.

Braathen, L.R., Ramirez, G., Kunze, R.O.F. and Gelderblom, H. (1987). Langerhans cells as primary target cells for HIV infection. *Lancet* **2**, 1094 (letter).

Bröcker, E., Poppema, S., Terbrack, D., De Leij, L., Macher, E. and Sorg, C. (1982). Analysis of mononuclear cell infiltrates in human malignant melanoma—an immunohistological study. *Immunobiology* **162**, 333–334.

Burkly, L., Hession, C., Ogata, L., Reilly, C., Marconi, L.A., Olson, D., Tizard, R., Cate, R. and Lo, D. (1995). Expression of *relB* is required for the development of thymic medulla and dendritic cells. *Nature* **373**, 531–536.

Carrasco, D., Ryseck, R.P. and Bravo, R. (1993). Expression of *relB* transcripts during lymphoid organ development: specific expression in dendritic antigen-presenting cells. *Development* **118**, 1221–1231.

Caux, C., Massacrier, C., Vanbervliet, B., Dubois, B., van Kooten, C., Durand, I. and Banchereau, J. (1994). Activation of human dendritic cells through CD40 cross-linking. *J. Exp. Med.* **180**, 1263–1272.

Cohen, G.M. (1997). Caspases: the executioners of apoptosis. *Biochem. J.* **326**, 1–16.

Daniels, T.E., Greenspan, D., Greenspan, J.S., Lennette, E., Schiodt, M., Petersen, V. and de Souza, Y. (1987). Absence of Langerhans cells in oral hairy leukoplakia, an AIDS-associated lesion. *J. Invest. Dermatol.* **89**, 178–182.

Devitt, A., Moffatt, O.D., Raykundalia, C., Capra, J.D., Simmons, D.L. and Gregory, C.D. (1998). Human CD14 mediates recognition and phagocytosis of apoptotic cells. *Nature* **392**, 505–509.

Esche, C., Subbotin, V.M., Maliszewski, C., Lotze, M.T. and Shurin, M.R. (1998). FLT3 Ligand administration inhibits tumor growth in murine melanoma and lymphoma. *Cancer Res.* **58**, 380–383.

Esche, C., Subbotin, V.M., Hunter, O., Lotze, M.T. and Shurin, M.R. (1998). FLT3 Ligand and interleukin-12 regulate accumulation of dendritic cells and mast cells in murine skin. *Arch. Dermatol. Res.* **290**, 87a.

Facchetti, F., de Wolf-Peeters, C., de Greef, H. and Desmet, V.J. (1984). Langerhans cells in various benign and malignant pigment-cell lesions of the skin. *Arch. Dermatol. Res.* **276**, 283–287.

Feuillard, J., Körner, M., Israel, A., Vassy, J. and Raphael, M. (1996). Differential nuclear localization of p50, p52 and RelB proteins in human accessory cells of the immune response *in situ*. *Eur. J. Immunol.* **26**, 2547–2551.

Fugier-Vivier, I., Servet-Delprat, C., Rivailler, P., Rissoan, M.C., Liu, Y.J. and Rabourdin-Combe C. (1997). Measles virus suppresses cell-mediated immunity by interfering with the survival and functions of dendritic and T cells. *J. Exp. Med.* **186**, 813–823.

Furue, M. and Katz, S.I. (1989). Direct effects of glucocorticosteroids on epidermal Langerhans cells. *J. Invest. Dermatol.* **92**, 342–347.

Gastl, G.A., Abrams, J.S., Nanus, D.M., Oosterkamp, R., Silver, J., Liu, F., Chen, M., Albino, A.P. and Bander, N.H. (1993). Interleukin-10 production by human carcinoma cell lines and its relationship to interleukin-6 expression. *Int. J. Cancer* **55**, 96–101.

Gatter, K.C., Morris, H.B., Roach, B., Mortimer, P., Fleming, K.A. and Mason, D.Y. (1984). Langerhans cells and T cells in human skin tumours: an immunohistological study. *Histopathology* **8**, 229–244.

Ghosh, P., Komschlies, K.L., Cippitelli, M., Longo, D.L., Subleski, J., Ye, J., Sica, A., Young, H.A., Wiltrout, R.H. and Ochoa, A.C. (1995). Gradual loss of T-helper 1 populations in spleen of mice during progressive tumor growth. *J. Natl Cancer Inst.* **87**, 1478–1483.

Gimmi, C.D., Morrison, B.W., Mainprice, B.A., Gribben, J.G., Boussiotis, V.A., Freeman, G.J., Park, S.Y.L., Watanabe, M., Gong, J.L., Hayes, D.F., Kufe, D.W. and Nadler, L.M. (1996). Breast cancer-associated antigen, DF3/MUC1, induces apoptosis of activated human T cells. *Nature Medicine* **2**, 1367–1370.

Granelli-Piperno, A., Pope, M., Inaba, K. and Steinman, R.M. (1995). Coexpression of NF-κB/REL and Sp1 transcription factors in human immunodeficiency virus-1 induced, dendritic cell-T cell syncytia. *Proc. Natl Acad. Sci. USA* **92**, 10944–10948.

Grosjean, I., Caux, C., Bella, C., Berger, I., Wild, F., Banchereau, J. and Kaiserlian, D. (1997). Measles virus infects human dendritic cells and blocks their allostimulatory properties for CD^+ T cells. *J. Exp. Med.* **186**, 801–812.

Guzman, C.A., Domann, E., Rohde, M., Bruder, D., Darji, A., Weiss, S., Wehland, J., Chakraborty, T. and Timmis, K.N. (1996). Apoptosis of mouse dendritic cells is triggered by listeriolysin, the major virulence determinant of *Listeria monocytogenes*. *Mol. Microbiol.* **20**, 119–126.

Hahne, M., Rimoldi, D., Schröter, M., Romero, P., Schreier, M., French, L.E., Schneider, P., Bornand, T., Fontana, A., Lienard, D., Cerottini, J.C. and Tschopp, J. (1996). Melanoma cell expression of Fas (Apo-1/CD95) ligand: implications for tumor immune escape. *Science* **274**, 1363–1366.

Hart, D.N.J. (1997). Dendritic cells: unique leukocyte populations which control the primary immune response. *Blood* **90**, 3245–3287.

Henderson, R.A., Watkins, S.C. and Flynn, J.L. (1997). Activation of human dendritic cells following infection with *Mycobacterium tuberculosis. J. Immunol.* **159**, 635–643.

Howard, M. and O'Garra, A. (1992). Biological properties of interleukin 10. *Immunol. Today* **13**, 198–200.

Johnston, L.J., Halliday, G.M. and King, N.J.C. (1996). Phenotypic changes in Langerhans cells after infection with arboviruses: a role in the immune response to epidermally acquired viral infection? *J. Virol.* **70**, 4761–4766.

Kämpgen, E., Gold, R., Eggert, A., Kleudgen, S., Toyka, K.V. and Bröcker, E. (1994a). Evidence for apoptotic cell death within the dendritic cell system and its modulation by GM-CSF and TNF alpha. *Arch. Dermatol. Res.* **286**, 230a.

Kämpgen, E., Gold, R., Eggert, A., Keikavoussi, P., Grauer, O., Toyka, K. and Bröcker, E. (1994b). Steroids and UV-B are potent inducers of programmed cell death in immature and mature dendritic cells. *J. Cell. Biochem.* **18B**, 12a (suppl.).

Kerr, J.F.R., Wyllie, A.H. and Currie, A.R. (1972). Apoptosis: a basic biological phenomenon with wide-ranging implications in tissue kinetics. *Br. J. Cancer* **26**, 239–257.

Kikuchi, A., Franzoso, G., Siebenlist, U. and Udey, M.C. (1998). NFκB/Rel protein expression and activity in a model of dendritic cell (DC) activation and maturation. *J. Invest. Dermatol.* **110**, 487a.

Kitajima, T., Ariizumi, K., Bergstresser, P.R. and Takashima, A. (1996a). A novel mechanism of glucocorticoid-induced immune suppression: the inhibition of T cell-mediated terminal maturation of a murine dendritic cell line. *J. Clin. Invest.* **98**, 142–147.

Kitajima, T., Ariizumi, K., Bergstresser, P.R. and Takashima, A. (1996b). Ultraviolet B radiation sensitizes a murine epidermal dendritic cell line (XS52) to undergo apoptosis upon antigen presentation to T cells. *J. Immunol.* **157**, 3312–3316.

Knight, S.C. (1995). Mechanisms of retrovirally induced immunosuppression acting via dendritic cells. *Adv. Exp. Med. Biol.* **378**, 423–427.

Koch, F., Heufler, C., Kämpgen, E., Schneeweiss, D., Böck, G. and Schuler, G. (1990). Tumor necrosis factor α maintains the viability of murine epidermal Langerhans cells in culture, but in contrast to granulocyte/macrophage colony-stimulating factor, without inducing their functional maturation. *J. Exp. Med.* **171**, 159–171.

Kolde, G., Wesendahl, C. and Ringling, M. (1998). Fas ligand expression in Langerhans cell histiocytosis: evidence for an immune privileged disorder. *Arch. Dermatol. Res.* **290**, 47a.

Koppi, T.A., Tough-Bement, T., Lewinsohn, D.M., Lynch, D.H. and Alderson, M.R. (1997). CD40 ligand inhibits Fas/CD95-mediated apoptosis of human blood-derived dendritic cells. *Eur. J. Immunol.* **27**, 3161–3165.

Lotze, M.T. (1997). Getting to the source: dendritic cells as therapeutic reagents for the treatment of patients with cancer. *Ann. Surg.* **226**, 1–5.

Lu, L., Bonham, C.A., Chambers, F.G., Watkins, S.C., Hoffman, R.A., Simmons, R.L. and Thomson, A.W. (1996). Induction of nitric oxide synthase in mouse dendritic cells by IFN-gamma endotoxin and interaction with allogeneic T cells: nitric oxide production is associated with dendritic cell apoptosis. *J. Immunol.* **157**, 3577–3586.

Lu, L., Qian, S., Hershberger, P., Rudert, W.A., Li, Y., Chambers, F.G., Starzl, T.E., Lynch, D.H. and Thomson, A.W. (1997a). Blocking of the B7-CD28 pathway increases apoptosis induced in activated T cells by in vitro-generated CD95L (FasL) positive dendritic cells. *Transplant. Proc.* **29**, 1094–1095.

Lu, L., Qian, S., Hershberger, P.A., Rudert, W.A., Lynch, D.H. and Thomson, A.W. (1997). Fas ligand (CD95L) and B7 expression on dendritic cells provide counter-regulatory signals for T cell survival and proliferation. *J. Immunol.* **158**, 5676–5684.

Ludewig, B., Graf, D., Gelderblom, H.R., Becker, Y., Kroczek, R.A. and Pauli, G. (1995). Spontaneous apoptosis of dendritic cells is efficiently inhibited by TRAP (CD40-ligand) and TNF-α, but strongly enhanced by interleukin-10. *Eur. J. Immunol.* **25**, 1943–1950.

Mangan, D.F. and Wahl, S.M. (1991). Differential regulation of human monocyte programmed cell death (apoptosis) by chemotactic factors and pro-inflammatory cytokines. *J. Immunol.* **147**, 3408–3412.

Mangan, D.F., Welch, G.R. and Wahl, S.M. (1991). Lipopolysaccharide, tumor necrosis factor-α, and IL-1β prevent programmed cell death (apoptosis) in human peripheral blood monocytes. *J. Immunol.* **146**, 1541–1546.

Markowicz, S. and Engleman, E.G. (1990). Granulocyte-macrophage colony-stimulating factor promotes differentiation and survival of human peripheral blood dendritic cells in vitro. *J. Clin. Invest.* **85**, 955–961.

Marland, G., Bakker, A.B., Adema, G.J. and Figdor, C.G. (1996). Dendritic cells in immune response induction. *Stem Cells* **14**, 501–507.

Masuda, A., Burton, G.F., Fuchs, B.A., Szakal, A.K. and Tew, J.G. (1993). Destruction of follicular dendritic cells in murine acquired immunodeficiency syndrome (MAIDS). *Adv. Exp. Med. Biol.* **329**, 411–416.

Matsue, H., Edelbaum, D., Hartmann, A.C., Morita, A., Bergstresser, P.R., Okumura, K., Yagita, H. and Takashima, A. (1998). Dendritic cell apoptosis during antigen-specific interaction with $CD4^+$ T cells. *J. Invest. Dermatol.* **110**, 488a.

Moser, M., de Smedt, T., Sornasse, T., Tielemans, F., Chentoufi, A.A., Muraille, E., van Mechelen, M., Urbain, J. and Leo, O. (1995). Glucocorticoids down-regulate dendritic cell function *in vitro* and *in vivo*. *Eur. J. Immunol.* **25**, 2818–2824.

Nagata, S. (1997). Apoptosis by death factor. *Cell* **88**, 355–365.

Nestor, M.S. and Cochran, A.J. (1987). Identification and quantification of subsets of mononuclear inflammatory cells in melanocytic and other human tumors. *Pigment Cell Res.* **1**, 22–27.

Niehans, G.A., Brunner, T., Frizelle, S.P., Liston, J.C., Salerno, C.T., Knapp, D.J., Green, D.R. and Kratzke, R.A. (1997). Human lung carcinomas express Fas ligand. *Cancer Res.* **57**, 1007–1012.

O'Connell, J., O'Sullivan, G.C., Collins, J.K. and Shanahan, F. (1996). The Fas counterattack: Fas-mediated T cell killing by colon cancer cells expressing Fas ligand. *J. Exp. Med.* **184**, 1075–1082.

O'Mahony, A.M., O'Sullivan, G.C., O'Connell, J., Cotter, T.G. and Cillins, J.K. (1993). An immune suppressive factor derived from esophageal squamous carcinoma induces apoptosis in normal and transformed cells of lymphoid lineage. *J. Immunol.* **151**, 4847–4856.

Parr, M.B., Kepple, L. and Parr, L. (1991). Langerhans cells phagocytose vaginal epithelial cells undergoing apoptosis during the murine estrous cycle. *Biol. Reprod.* **45**, 252–260.

Peter, M.E., Heufelder, A.E. and Hengartner, M.O. (1997). Advances in apoptosis research. *Proc. Natl Acad. Sci. USA* **94**, 12736–12737.

Petrasch, S., Brittinger, G., Wacker, H.H., Schmitz, J. and Kosco-Vilbois, M. (1994). Follicular dendritic cells in non-Hodgkin's lymphomas. *Leukemia Lymphoma* **15**, 33–43.

Poppema, S., Bröcker, E., De Leij, L., Terbrack, D., Visscher, T., Terhaar, A., Macher, E., The, T.H. and Sorg, C. (1983). In situ analysis of the mononuclear cell infiltrate in primary malignant melanoma of the skin. *Clin. Exp. Immunol.* **51**, 77–82.

Riedl, E., Strobl, H., Majdic, O. and Knapp, W. (1997). TGF-β1 promotes in vitro generation of dendritic cells by protecting progenitor cells from apoptosis. *J. Immunol.* **158**, 1591–1597.

Riva, S., Nolli, M.L., Lutz, M.B., Citterio, S., Girolomoni, G., Winzler, C. and Ricciardi-Castagnoli, P. (1996). Bacteria and bacterial cell wall constituents induce the production of regulatory cytokines in dendritic cell clones. *J. Inflamm.* **46**, 98–105.

Rothe, M., Sarma, V., Dixit, V.M. and Goeddel, D.V. (1995). TRAF2-mediated activation of NF-κB by TNF receptor 2 and CD40. *Science* **269**, 1424–1427.

Rubartelli, A., Poggi, A. and Zocchi, M.R. (1997). The selective engulfment of apoptotic bodies by dendritic cells is mediated by the alpha(v)beta3 integrin and requires intracellular and extracellular calcium. *Eur. J. Immunol.* **27**, 1893–1900.

Saas, P., Walker, P.R., Hahne, M., Quiquerez, A.L., Schnuriger, V., Perrin, G., French, L., van Meir, E.G., de Tribolet, N., Tschopp, J. and Dietrich, P.Y. (1997). Fas ligand expression by astrocytoma in vivo: maintaining immune privilege in the brain? *J. Clin. Invest.* **99**, 1173–1178.

Sad, S., Kägi, D. and Mosmann, T.R. (1996). Perforin and Fas killing by $CD8^+$ T cells limits their cytokine synthesis and proliferation. *J. Exp. Med.* **184**, 1543–1547.

Santiago-Schwarz, F., Borrero, M., Tucci, J., Palaia, T. and Carsons, S.E. (1997). In vitro expansion of $CD13^+CD33^+$ dendritic cell precursors from multipotent progenitors is regulated by a discrete fas-mediated apoptotic schedule. *J. Leukocyte Biol.* **62**, 493–502.

Schuhmachers, G., Ariizumi, K., Kitajima, T., Edelbaum, D., Xu, S., Shadduck, R.K., Gilmore, G.L., Taylor, R.S., Bergstresser, P.R. and Takashima, A. (1996). UVB radiation interrupts cytokine-mediated support of an epidermal-derived dendritic cell line (XS52) by a dual mechanism. *J. Invest. Dermatol.* **106**, 1023–1029.

Shah, P.D., Keji, J., Gilbertson, S.M. and Rowley, D.A. (1986). $Thy\text{-}1^+$ and $Thy\text{-}1^-$ natural killer cells. Only $Thy\text{-}1^-$ natural killer cells suppress dendritic cells. *J. Exp. Med.* **163**, 1012–1017.

Shaieb, A.M., Berman, B., Smith, B. and Krumpe, P. (1987). Epidermal Langerhans cell density in patients with pulmonary malignancies and chronic obstructive pulmonary disease. *J. Dermatol. Surg. Oncol.* **13**, 991–996.

Shurin, MR. (1996). Dendritic cells presenting tumor antigen. *Cancer Immunol. Immunother.* **43**, 158–164.

Shurin, M.R., Pandharipande, P.P., Zorina, T.D., Haluszczak, C., Subbotin, V.M., Hunter, O., Brumfield, A., Storkus, W.J., Maraskovsky, E. and Lotze, M.T. (1997a). FLT3 ligand induces the generation of functionally active dendritic cells in mice. *Cell. Immunol.* **179**, 174–184.

Shurin, M.R., Esche, C., Peron, J.M. and Lotze, M.T. (1997b). Antitumor activities of interleukin-12 and mechanisms of action. *Chem. Immunol.* **68**, 153–174.

Shurin, M.R., Esche, C. and Lotze, M.T. (1998). FLT3: receptor and ligand. Biology and potential clinical application. *Cytokine Growth Factor Rev.*, in press.

Shurin, M.R., Lokshin, A., Esche, C. and Lotze, M.T. (1998). Tumors induce apoptosis of dendritic cells: role of Flt3-ligand and IL-1α in tumour-associated dendritic cell function. *Proc. AACR* **39**, 550–551.

Steinman, R.M. and Cohn, Z.A. (1973). Identification of a novel cell type in peripheral lymphoid organs of mice. I. Morphology, quantitation, tissue distribution. *J. Exp. Med.* **137**, 1142–1162.

Stene, M.A., Babajanians, M., Bhuta, S. and Cochran, A., J. (1988). Quantitative alterations in cutaneous Langerhans cells during the evolution of malignant melanoma of the skin. *J. Invest. Dermatol.* **91**, 125–128.

Strand, S., Hofmann, W.J., Hug, H., Mller, M., Otto, G., Strand, D., Mariani, S.M., Stremmel, W., Krammer, P.H. and Galle, P.R. (1996). Lymphocyte apoptosis induced by CD95 (APO-1/Fas) ligand-expressing tumor cells—a mechanism of immune evasion? *Nature Medicine* **2**, 1361–1366.

Tang, A. and Udey, M.C. (1992). Effects of ultraviolet radiation on murine epidermal Langerhans cells: doses of ultraviolet radiation that modulate ICAM-1 (CD54) expression and inhibit Langerhans cell function cause delayed cytotoxicity in vitro. *J. Invest. Dermatol.* **99**, 83–89.

Thomas, R. and Lipsky, P.E. (1996). Dendritic cells: origin and differentiation. *Stem Cells* **14**, 196–206.

Toriyama, K., Wen, D.R., Paul, E. and Cochran, A.J. (1993). Variations in the distribution, frequency, and phenotype of Langerhans cells during the evolution of malignant melanoma of the skin. *J. Invest. Dermatol.* **100**, 269S–273S.

Um, H.D., Orenstein, J.M. and Wahl, S.M. (1996). Fas mediates apoptosis in human monocytes by a reactive oxygen intermediate dependent pathway. *J. Immunol.* **156**, 3469–3477.

Uren, A.G. and Vaux, D.L. (1996). Molecular and clinical aspects of apoptosis. *Pharmacol. Ther.* **72**, 37–50.

Villunger, A., Egle, A., Marschitz, I., Kos, M., Böck, G., Ludwig, H., Geley, S., Kofler, R. and Greil, R. (1997). Constitutive expression of Fas (Apo-1/CD95) ligand on multiple myeloma cells: a potential mechanism of tumor-induced suppression of immune surveillance. *Blood* **90**, 12–20.

von Stebut, E., Philipp, S., Würz, C., Ringling, M. and Kolde, G. (1997). Apoptosis of cultured Langerhans cells is mediated by the CD95 (APO-1/Fas)/ CD95L-system. *J. Invest. Dermatol.* **109**, 406a.

Vujanovic, N.L., Basse, P., Herberman, R.B. and Whiteside, T.L. (1996). Antitumor functions of natural killer cells and control of metastases. *METHODS: A Companion to Methods in Enzymology* **9**, 394–408.

Weih, F., Warr, G., Yang, H. and Bravo, R. (1997). Multifocal defects in immune responses in *RelB*-deficient mice. *J. Immunol.* **158**, 5211–5218.

Weissman, D., Li, Y., Orenstein, J.M. and Fauci, A.S. (1995). Both a precursor and a mature population of dendritic cells can bind HIV. *J. Immunol.* **155**, 4111–4117.

Winzler, C., Rovere, P., Rescigo, M., Granucci, F., Penna, G., Adorini, L., Zimmermann, V.S., Davoust, J. and Ricciardi-Castagnoli, P. (1997). Maturation stages of mouse dendritic cells in growth factor-dependent long-term cultures. *J. Exp. Med.* **185**, 317–328.

Wong, B.R., Josien, R., Lee, S.Y., Sauter, B., Li, H.L., Steinman, R.M. and Choi, Y. (1997). TRANCE (tumor necrosis factor [TNF]-related activation-induced cytokine), a new TNF family member predominantly expressed in T cells, is a dendritic cell-specific survival factor. *J. Exp. Med.* **186**, 2075–2080.

Yoshimoto, T., Nagase, H., Ishida, T., Inoue, J. and Nariuchi, H. (1997). Induction of interleukin-12 p40 transcript by CD40 ligation via activation of nuclear factor-kappaB. *Eur. J. Immunol.* **27**, 3461–3470.

Young, W.G., Newcomb, G.M. and Hosking, A.R. (1985). The effect of atrophy, hyperplasia and keratinization accompanying the estrous cycle on Langerhans cells in mouse vaginal epithelium. *Am. J. Anat.* **174**, 173–186.

Zocchi, R., Poggi, A. and Rubartelli, A. (1997). The RGD-containing domain of exogenous HIV-1 tat inhibits the engulfment of apoptotic bodies by dendritic cells. *AIDS* **11**, 1227–1235.

CHAPTER 39
Studies of Endocytosis

Wendy S. Garrett and Ira Mellman
Department of Cell Biology and Section of Immunobiology, Yale University School of Medicine, New Haven, Connecticut, USA

INTRODUCTION

Dendritic cells (DC) are the preeminent antigen-presenting cells (APC) of the immune system. They are sentinel cells capable of a variety of antigen capture mechanisms including receptor-mediated endocytosis, macropinocytosis, and phagocytosis. DC possess several specializations relevant to antigen uptake. Both the features and distribution of their endocytic compartments, MHC class II (cII) compartments and Langerhans cell granules (LCG), and their modes and levels of endocytic uptake are modulated upon maturation. A consideration of the endocytic machinery of dendritic cells should provide information for a variety of questions in dendritic cell biology. The goal of this chapter is to provide a brief summary of the literature on DC endocytosis, a review of the current methods used to study endocytosis, and a discussion of the developmental regulation of the endocytic pathway in DC.

PHAGOCYTOSIS

Phagocytosis is a receptor-mediated, actin- and ATP-dependent phenomenon that is triggered by the binding of particles or organisms to specific plasma membrane receptors (Silverstein *et al.*, 1979). Actin assembles around the particle when ligands expressed by the particle ligate cell surface receptors. F-actin-driven pseudopods engulf the particle, which is internalized in a cytoplasmic phagosome. Members of the rho family of GTPases have been implicated in a number of actin-mediated cytoskeletal rearrangements. Recent studies have demonstrated a role for cdc42 and rac-1 in the recruitment of F-actin to the phagocytic cup (Cox *et al.*, 1997) Mannose, β-glucan, Fc, scavenger, and complement receptors can transduce the signals essential for phagocytic internalization (Brown, 1995). Fc receptor-mediated phagocytosis involves a tyrosine kinase-dependent pathway. Several cytoskeletal proteins, including paxillin, that associate with early phagosomes are tyrosine kinase substrates that are phosphorylated in response to Fc receptor ligation (Greenberg *et al.*, 1994). The signals and the pathways involved in triggering phagocytic internalization are still not fully understood and are active areas of investigation.

Dendritic Cells: Biology and Clinical Applications
ISBN 0-12-455860-7

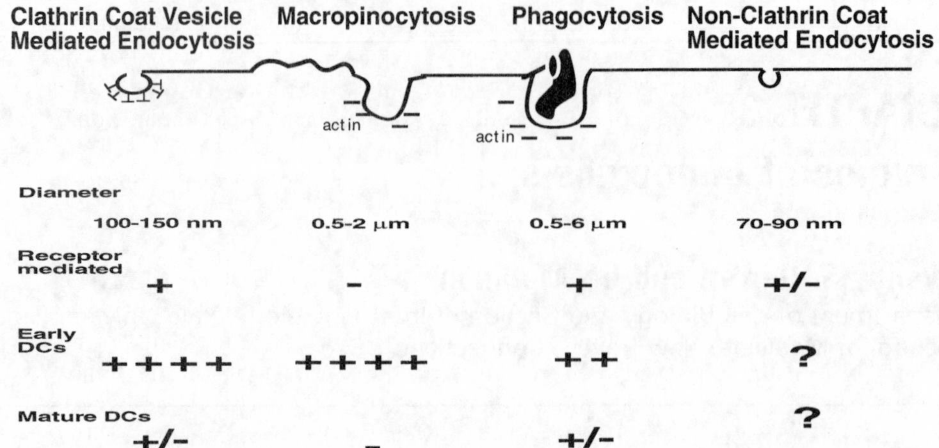

Fig. 1. Mechanisms of endocytic uptake.

Phagocytosis provides a means for the internalization of both a selective and a broad range of receptor-bound antigenic ligands. Dendritic cells seem specially engineered for the internalization and presentation of phagocytic ligands, as evidenced by the observation that the antigen-presenting capacity of DC was much higher for bead-adsorbed antigen than for the soluble form of the antigen (Scheicher *et al.*, 1995).

PINOCYTOSIS

Pinocytosis encompasses both fluid-phase uptake and receptor-mediated endocytosis. Fluid-phase uptake includes micropinocytosis and macropinocytosis: two distinct forms of solute uptake. Micropinocytosis involves internalization of macromolecules less than 0.2 μm in diameter via both clathrin-coated and uncoated vesicles (Robinson *et al.*, 1996).

Clathrin Coat-Mediated Endocytosis

Most receptor-bound ligands are internalized via a clathrin coat-mediated process. Certain membrane receptors, e.g., FcγR, are efficiently clustered in clathrin-coated vesicles. These receptors usually have an internalization signal in their cytoplasmic domain. Such signals work by binding to adaptor proteins to which the clathrin coat attaches. Coats consist of a clathrin cage, a trimer of heterodimers (clathrin heavy and light chain) and a heterotetrameric adaptor complex (Schmid, 1997; Robinson, 1994). An important component of the clathrin-coated vesicle machinery is dynamin, a GTPase, which is required for coated pits to pinch off as coated vesicles. After internalization in a clathrin-coated pit, receptor–ligand complexes have two possible fates (Mellman, 1996). The complexes can traffic through the endosomal–lysosomal pathway, encountering lower and lower pH and increasing concentrations of proteases and hydrolytic enzymes (Mellman, 1996). Alternatively, the receptor–ligand complexes can dissociate within the endosomal network where they can be sorted. Upon sorting to the recycling arm of the endocytic pathway, receptors can return to the cell surface, where they can initiate multiple rounds of ligand internalization (Mellman, 1996). Clathrin coat receptor-mediated endocytosis provides a selective means for efficiently concentrating the internalization of specific ligands. It is necessary for the uptake of nutrients and other components essential for the maintenance of cellular homeostasis (Mellman, 1996).

Macropinocytosis

Macropinocytosis is mediated by the actin cytoskeleton and is independent of clathrin and membrane receptors. Macropinosomes are heterogeneous in size, ranging from 0.2 to 5 μm in diameter. Three differentially regulated processes are essential for macropinocytosis: actin cytoskeleton-driven ruffle formation, closure of the ruffle into a vesicle, and dissociation of actin filaments from the vesicle so that it can participate in intracellular trafficking and fusion with other vesicles (Swanson and Watts, 1995).

In contrast to micropinocytosis, macropinocytosis is most prevalent in a select number of cells. Several agonists are capable of inducing macropinocytosis. EGF induces macropinocytosis in fibroblasts, while PMA stimulates the process in macrophages (Swanson and Watts, 1995). Studies examining *Salmonella*-induced macropinocytosis have demonstrated that cdc42 is essential for macropinocytosis and that dominant negative cdc42 expressed in the host cell can block macropinocytosis of *Salmonella* (Chen *et al.*, 1996). Bacterial products of the *Salmonella* type III secretion system appear to activate cdc42 in the host cell, resulting in membrane ruffling (Hardt *et al.*, 1998). Cells usually require inductive signals to macropinocytose and downregulate macropinocytosis in the absence of these stimulating factors. However, immature dendritic cells constitutively macropinocytose (Sallusto *et al.*, 1995).

Macropinocytosis is a nonselective form of endocytosis. It has been unclear how internalized ligands are concentrated in macropinosomes. However, preliminary experiments suggest that aquaporins, water channels, may play a role by mediating water egress from macropinosomes (A. Lanzavecchia, personal communication).

The fate of macropinosomes is cell-type-dependent. In EGF-stimulated A431 cells, a human epithelioid cell line, macropinosomes may fuse with each other but fail to deliver their contents to early or late endosomes (Hewlett *et al.*, 1994). In macrophages, macropinosomes gradually acquire lysosomal markers, progressing through three stages—a transferrin receptor positive phase (TfnR); a TfnR^- rab 7^+ mannose 6-phosphate receptor $(\text{M6PR})^+$ phase; and a TfnR^-, rab 7^-, M6PR^-, cathepsin L^+, lgpA^+, and lgpB^+ phase—before fusing with the tubular lysosomal compartment (Racoosin and Swanson, 1993). In the fetal skin-derived dendritic cell line (FSDC) (Girolomoni *et al.*, 1995), macropinosomes acquire proteases and decrease pH but do not possess all lysosomal markers (Lutz *et al.*, 1997), suggesting that a macropinosome-derived compartment may function as an antigen-retention compartment.

Macropinocytosis is a nonselective form of uptake by which a relatively large of volume of antigen-rich solute can be internalized. It is an appealing concept that sentinel DC in the periphery may be able to internalize vast quantities of a variety of antigens and eventually prime naive T cells to mount an immune response. A recent study of macropinocytosis in the mouse GM-CSF BM DC system focused on the cross-priming phenomenon (Brossart and Bevan, 1997) Cross-priming involves the presentation of exogenous antigens by the class I molecules in addition to the presentation of the antigen by the class II molecules (Carbone and Bevan, 1990). Ovalbumin internalized by immature DC by macropinocytosis was presented by class I molecules to $CD8^+$ ovalbumin-specific T cell clones. Potentially, macropinocytosis may provide a unique pathway in DC for efficient channeling of antigenic peptide to both the class I and class II pathways.

However, there is scant evidence that macropinocytosis actually serves a purpose *in situ*. The epidermis is a tight meshlike network of keratinocytes in which Langerhans cells interdigitate. It seems unlikely that Langerhans cells are capable of generating large membrane ruffles while in the skin. Similarly, macropinocytosis presents a conceptual problem for the sentinel DC of the tissues. Perhaps macropinocytosis is an *in vitro* activity that simply reflects an inherent capability to generate the pseudopod extensions that engulf phagocytic ligands. There are several similarities between phagocytosis and macropinocytosis. Both are dependent on remodeling of the actin cytoskeleton and cdc42 is an important effector in regulating these changes (Cox, 1997; Chen *et al.*, 1996). There are also morphological similarities between the generation of macropinocytic ruffles and phagocytic cups. However, the receptor dependence of phagocytosis and ligand/receptor-mediated zippering of the phagocytic pseudopods around the particle may suggest that the two are distinctive processes that share several mechanistic similarities. Alternatively, macropinocytosis results from culturing effects and has little *in vivo* relevance. Perhaps macropinocytosis is the moral equivalent of phagocytosis.

Endocytic Receptors

Below is a brief summary of the numerous receptors that are expressed by dendritic cells during their development and that are capable of mediating receptor-mediated endocytosis and in several cases phagocytosis as well.

Mannose/β-Glucan Receptor

The mannose receptor (MR) is expressed on immature DC (Engering *et al.*, 1996; Sallusto *et al.*, 1995; Reis e Sousa *et al.*, 1993). MR contains multiple carbohydrate-binding domains and internalizes a variety of glycoproteins. The receptor binds a range of oligosaccharides with different affinities: D-mannose = L-fucose ≫ D-*N*-acetylglucosamine ⩾ D-glucose ≫ D-xylose ≫ galactose (Pontow *et al.*, 1992). Unlike FcR, MR recycles and can mediate multiple rounds of ligand internalization (Pontow *et al.*, 1992). MR plays an important role in host defense, mediating phagocytosis of unopsonized targets, and internalizes a variety of microorganisms that have exposed mannosylated glycoproteins: *Candida albicans*, *Leishmania* promastigotes, and *Pneumocystis carinii* (Ezekowitz and Hoffmann, 1996). In antigen presentation experiments, MR enhanced the ability of DC to present low concentrations (10^{-9}–10^{-12} ng/ml) of soluble mannosylated ligands (Engering *et al.*, 1997). The maturation factor LPS (40-hour treatment) reduced the capacity of DC to present both mannosylated and nonmannosylated ligands by 10–100-fold (Engering *et al.*, 1997).

DEC-205R

DEC-205R, a member of the C-type lectin receptor family, is an orphan receptor. Initial experiments using rabbit polyclonal antibodies directed against the ectodomain of the receptor demonstrated that the receptor is internalized by receptor-mediated endocytosis and was delivered to class II-positive multivesicular structures (Jiang *et al.*, 1995). Rabbit antibodies specific for the DEC-205R ectodomain were presented to reactive T cell hybridomas with 100-fold more efficiency that nonspecific rabbit antibodies (Jiang *et al.*, 1995). Although total DEC-205R expression increases with maturation, cell surface expression decreases during development (M. Nussenzweig, personal communication). Downmodulation during development and preliminary data on its antigen-presenting function suggest that it may serve as an antigen receptor. The increasing levels of expression with development and intracellular localization suggest an additional role.

FcR

Both murine and human epidermal Langerhans cells express high-affinity receptors for IgE molecules (Wang *et al.*, 1992; Bieber *et al.*, 1992; Maurer *et al.*, 1996; Stingl and Maurer, 1997) and low-affinity receptors for IgG molecules (Schmitt *et al.*, 1990; Esposito-Farese *et al.*, 1995). The high-affinity receptor for IgE (FcεRI) is expressed on Langerhans cells, dermal DC (Wang *et al.*, 1992), and peripheral blood (PB) DC (Maurer *et al.*, 1996). On DC, FcεRI functions to augment allergen presentation in an IgE-dependent manner. Peripheral blood human DC, Langerhans cells, and dermal DC lack FcεR1β and express FcεRI as a multimer of FcεR1α and FcεRIγ chains (Maurer *et al.*, 1996). Immature murine Langerhans cells (LC) express two membrane-anchored isoforms of FcγR, FcγRIIb2 (CD32b2) and FcγRIII (CD16). LC are capable of internalizing IgG–Ag complexes via receptor-mediated endocytosis by their cell surface FcγRs. The FcRs expressed by LC and DC may not be internalized for the destruction of opsonized particles in phagolysosomes but rather internalized for antigen-processing and presentation.

Complement Receptor

The complement system plays a role in enhancing a number of immune phenomena: phagocytosis of pathogens, inflammation, antigen focusing, and cell lysis (Burke and Gigli, 1980). There are several receptors for components of the complement system: C3b, C3bi, C3d, and C4b receptors. Many cells express C3b receptor (C3bR) and some subsets of these cells express a form of C3bR that cross-reacts with C4b. Receptors specific for C4b are more limited in expression (eosinophils, peripheral B-lymphocytes, neutrophils). Langerhans cells express C3bR but do not express C4bR (Stingl *et al.*, 1977). LC also express C3biR and downregulate expression after 1–3 days in culture (Schuler and Steinman, 1985). The significance of complement receptors on DC is an issue of speculation. Some have proposed that C3R my allow for antigen bridges between DC and naive T cells expressing C3 (Burke and Gigli, 1980).

Scavenger Receptor

There are three known classes of scavenger receptors: A, B, and C. Initial studies on the scavenger receptors focused on their binding of oxidized and acetylated low-density lipoprotein. However, they are capable of binding a variety of negatively charged molecules (Rigotti, 1997). The first scavenger receptors identified were the class A type I and II receptors which are expressed on macrophages. Class A receptors are also expressed on dendritic cells (S. Gordon, personal communication). Recently, scavenger type A receptors have been implicated in the clearance of apoptotic cells in the thymus (Platt *et al.*, 1996). Class B scavenger receptors (SR-B) are members of the CD36 protein family and bind negatively charged liposomes, HDL (Rigotti, 1997), acetylated and oxidized LDL, and apoptotic cells (Fukasawa, 1996). Class C receptors have been cloned from *Drosophila* and are expressed by *Drosophila* embryonic hemocytes and macrophages and the Schneider L2 cell line. Preliminary characterization of this receptor demonstrates affinity for acetylated LDL and polyanionic ligands (Pearson *et al.*, 1995). The expression of scavenger receptors has not been characterized for all the different dendritic cell populations.

ASSAYS

Experimental Approaches

Endocytosis assays are conceptually simple: cells are incubated in the presence of a ligand and then the uptake of the ligand is measured. The complexity of these assays using DC is introduced in four basic ways: the preparation of the cell population, the choice of the ligand, the conditions under which the cells are exposed to the ligand, and how ligand uptake is assessed. The techniques used to assess ligand uptake can be qualitative and/or quantitative. Fluorescently conjugated ligands in conjunction with flow cytometry and immunofluorescence microscopy can be used to examine uptake in viable and fixed populations of cells. Antibodies or enzymatic reactions can be employed to follow the uptake of a ligand using immunohistochemical techniques at the light- and electron-microscopic level. In addition, fluorometric substrates can be used to quantitate enzymatic ligands. The quantity of internalized versus exocytosed ligands and the rates of internalization and exocytosis are easily deduced from data analysis of these techniques.

Subcellular fractionation and free-flow electrophoresis are standard cell biological techniques utilized in studying the intracellular trafficking of ligands through the endocytic pathway when the ligand can be assessed by an enzymatic activity or antibody-mediated detection system. Alternatively, antigen presentation assays have demonstrated the uptake and processing of a ligand when appropriate T cell clones or hybridomas are available.

Endocytic Ligands

FM3-25

FM3-25 (*N*-(3-triethylammoniumpropyl)-4-(4-(dioctadecylamino)styryl)pyridinium di-4-chlorobenzenesulfonate) and FM4-64 (*N*-(3-triethylammoniumpropyl)-4-(6-(4-(diethylamino)phenyl)hexatrienyl)pyridinium dibromide) are vital lipophilic styryl dyes that have been used to assay for endocytosis (Ziv and Smith, 1996; Melikyan *et al.*, 1995). The dye molecules insert into the outer leaflet of the plasma membrane, where they fluoresce when excited (Vida and Emr, 1995). FM3-25 and FM4-64 are tracers for membrane turnover and plasma membrane dynamics. These dyes may be quite helpful in understanding the maturation of macropinosomes in DC.

Lucifer Yellow

The potassium salt of Lucifer Yellow CH (LY) is a hydrophilic tracer for fluid-phase pinocytosis with a peak absorbance at 425 nm and peak fluorescence emission at 528 nm. At A488 nm, the excitation wavelength of an argon laser, the emission is rather low, $\sim 700\,cm^{-1}\,M^{-1}$. Lucifer yellow CH bears a carbohydrazide group allowing for aldehyde fixation which allows for immunocytochemical analysis. In macrophages, LY is not degraded and is nontoxic at concentrations up to 6 mg/ml (Swanson *et al.*, 1985). Although LY has been used successfully in labeling the endocytic pathway of macrophages and PBMC GM-CSF + IL-4 DC, LY membrane impermeance should be evaluated by examining for cytosolic leakage in different cell types (Swanson, 1989). Intense light excitation of lysosomes loaded with LY occasionally results in lysosomal explosion and leaking of LY into the cytoplasmic space (Swanson, 1989).

Dextrans

Dextrans are electroneutral, hydrophilic branched polymers of poly-D-glucose that do not cross biological membranes (Thorbol, 1981). Fluoresceinated dextrans (F-DXs) are commercially available from Pharmacia, Sigma, and Molecular Probes. Molecular Probes provides a range of fluorescein-dextrans (moleular mass 3000–2 000 000 Da) with a high degree of dye substitution (2–4 dye molecules 40 000 Da: 3–6 dye molecules 70 000 Da). Commercially available F-DXs may contain free fluorescein, which is highly adsorptive and potentially cytotoxic. Gel exclusion chromatography or dialysis should be used to reduce the levels of unconjugated fluorescein.

Seminal studies using FITC-DXs demonstrated their usefulness in studies of fluid-phase pinocytosis (Berlin and Oliver, 1980). DC have been pulsed with 0.1 to 10 mg/ml F-DX and typically assayed for uptake using three basic methods. Cell detergent lysates have been analyzed in fluorometers, live or fixed DC have been assayed by flow cytometry, or cells have been examined using fluorescence or confocal microscopy. Quantitative measurement of intracellular F-DX are often inaccurate because fluorecein fluorescence varies as an inverse function of pH (Mellman *et al.*, 1986). Thus, visualization of F-DX in the acidic milieu of endosomes and lysosomes often reflects a fluorescence overshoot. Fluorescence overshoot with acidic pH values is less of a problem with Texas red- and rhodamine-conjugated dextrans and proteins. However, these fluors are more adsorptive (Swanson, 1989).

Horseradish Peroxidase

Horseradish peroxidase (HRP) is a glycoprotein that is absent from most mammalian cells. It can be employed as both a fluid-phase and a receptor-mediated probe (Steinman *et al.*, 1974b). HRP was demonstrated to be a ligand for MR (Stahl *et al.*, 1978). It is a convenient tracer for immunocytochemistry; *in situ*, HRP can be detected by reaction with diaminobenzidine. Its concentration can be measured by colorimetric assay using *o*-phenylenediamine (OPD) and hydrogen peroxide (Straus, 1964). Polyclonal sera directed against HRP are commercially available and are useful for fluorescence microscopy imaging. HRP has been a standard tracer for the endocytic pathway for almost four decades. It is relatively nontoxic and has only been demonstrated to perturb the endocytic pathway in thioglycolate-stimulated macrophages (Swanson *et al.*, 1985).

Nonfluorescent, Nonenzymatic Ligands

A number of ligands that have been used in endocytic assays have not been mentioned explicitly. These ligands have been used in conventional light microscopy and ultrastructural studies. Colloidal carbon, latex microspheres/beads, paramagnetic latex, and iron-containing beads have been valuable tools in a variety of uptake assays. Paramagnetic latex and iron-containing beads can be used in conjunction with magnets to isolate different cell populations or to separate subcellular organelles. Pathogens, including bacteria, mycobacteria, and yeast, have been used to ask questions about host–pathogen interactions as well as endocytosis. Such organisms can easily be labeled directly with FITC, TRITC, or biotin, or indirectly with appropriate antibodies.

ENDOCYTIC CAPACITIES OF DENDRITIC CELLS

Initially, endocytosis was of interest to those studying DC because it provided a means to functionally characterize and differentiate DC from other splenic or epidermal cells. Three basic techniques dominated studies of dendritic cell endocytosis: electron microscopy, flow cytometry, and antigen presentation assays. Until 1992, bulk culturing methods for the generation of developmentally homogeneous DC did not exist, and previous to that time endocytosis assays were performed on LC or DC *in situ*, or from short term culture of tissue explants/isolates (for reviews see Steinman and Swanson, 1995; Austyn, 1996; Cella *et al.*, 1997).

Electron Microscopy Studies

Early analysis of the endocytic capacities of LC were performed at the ultrastructural level using ferritin or horseradish peroxidase (HRP) as an uptake tracer. These studies demonstrated that LC could use endocytosis to internalize exogenous protein, but that LC were weakly endocytic as compared to keratinocytes (Nordquist *et al.*, 1966; Wolff and Schreiner, 1970; Sagbiel, 1972). Initial studies of the endocytosis of soluble HRP, colloidal carbon, and thorium dioxide by splenic DC *in vitro* and *in vivo* demonstrated poor DC uptake of soluble endocytic markers as compared to macrophages (Steinman and Cohn, 1974; Steinman, 1974a). The LC and DC that these groups examined would be characterized as mature by the morphological phenotyping that is employed today. Thus, these experiments demonstrated that mature/late DC have low endocytic capacity.

Phagocytosis by sentinel DC, such as LC and organ DC, have been studied in detail. DC isolated from mouse spleen, lymph nodes, thymus, liver (Steinman and Cohn, 1974; Steinman *et al.*, 1980), and rat solid organs and tissue (Hart and Fabre, 1981) demonstrated low levels of phagocytosis. As observed in a transmission electron microscopy (EM) study, LC isolated from epidermal suspensions phagocytose zymosan and latex microspheres (Reis e Sousa *et al.*, 1993). *In vivo* antigen uptake studies in rats and sheep have contributed to the understanding of DC antigen uptake and migration in an intact immune system. Following subcutaneous injection of HRP in complete Freund's adjuvant (CFA) and boosting, HRP immune complexes were visualized within veiled DC (Hall and Robertson 1984). EM studies demonstrated that dendritic cells can internalize *Borrelia burgdorferi* by coiling phagocytosis (Filgueira *et al.*, 1996).

In freshly isolated and cultured human peripheral blood DC, the trafficking of pulse-chased BSA-gold was compared. The antigen trafficked through the endocytic pathway and accumulated in class II^{+} endosomal/lysosomal compartments similar to those observed in B cells (Nijman *et al.*, 1995).

Ultrastructural studies have been important in demonstrating that, in DC, phagocytosis is required not only for the uptake of immune complexes, bacteria, fungi, and yeast but also for the clearance of dead cells. Several EM studies have demonstrated that IDC phagocytose necrotic and apoptotic cells. Allogeneic lymphocytes have been visualized within IDC in lymph node and spleen (Fossum and Rolstad, 1986; Fossum *et al.*, 1984) and irradiated necrotic thymocytes have also been identified within IDC (Duijvestijn *et al.*, 1982). In murine vaginal epithelia during late metestrus and early diestrus, LC phagocytosis apoptotic vaginal epithelial cells (Parr *et al.*, 1991).

Flow Cytometry

Flow cytometry, which can assay bulk populations at the level of a single cell, is an amenable system for analysis of heterogeneous dendritic cell preparations. Bulk populations of homogeneous cells are required for the subcellular fractionation and spectrophotometry/fluorometry traditionally used to accurately determine the localization of ligands in different compartments of the endosomal–lysosomal system. DC isolated from mouse spleen and incubated for 24 h had heterogeneous endocytic activities in flow cytometric assays (Levine and Chain, 1992). The uptake of *Staphylococcus aureus*, latex microspheres, and zymosan was investigated in freshly isolated Langerhans cells and splenic DC using flow cytometry (Reis e Sousa *et al.*, 1993). Flow cytometry was also used to follow the internalization of FITC by sentinel DC isolated from heart and kidney (Austyn *et al.*, 1994).

Macropinocytosis and mannose receptor-mediated endocytosis are extremely efficient means for internalizing macromolecules in immature DC from the GM-CSF, IL-4 PBMC culture system (Sallusto *et al.*, 1995). Mannose receptor mediated the saturable uptake of F-DX as judged by competition studies using anti-mannose receptor antibody, mannan, mannosylated-BSA, and EDTA. LY uptake was nonsaturable in the flow cytometric assays and was inhibited by cytochalasin D (actin cytoskeleton inhibitor) and amiloride ($Na\text{-}H^{+}$ pump inhibitor), suggesting that its uptake is mediated by macropinocytosis.

Cord blood $CD34^{+}$ hematopoietic progenitor cells treated with GM-CSF and TNF-α differentiate into two distinct DC lineages in culture: a LC type DC and a $CD14^{+}$-derived DC (Caux *et al.*, 1997). The two lineages have similar functional capacities in T cell activation assays but have differences in their endocytic capacities (Caux *et al.*, 1997). The $CD14^{+}$ DC bound immune complexes, while the LC-type lineage DC demonstrated greatly reduced immune complex binding in a FACS-based assay (Caux *et al.*, 1997). The endocytic activity of CD14-derived DC was approximately

10-fold higher than that of the LC-type DC. Mannose receptor mediated the uptake of F-DX and HRP in both lineages (Caux *et al.*, 1997).

Antigen Presentation Assays

In the past decade, several groups have explored the antigen capture function of DC by assaying for antigen presentation. The majority of these studies do not directly address the mechanisms by which DC take up antigen but are instructive for a number of reasons. Freshly purified splenic DC could internalize, process, and present keyhole limpet hemocyanin (KLH). The processing of KLH was chloroquine-sensitive, suggesting that an acidified intracellular compartment, an endosome or lysosome, was necessary for processing (Chain *et al.*, 1986). Freshly isolated epidermal LC present soluble, intact myoglobin (Romani *et al.*, 1989). In LC, antigen processing of myoglobin and conalbumin was inhibited by both chloroquine and cycloheximide. This observation suggests that both an acidified compartment and newly synthesized proteins were required for processing. Antigen could be retained in cultured, antigen-pulsed LC for up to 2 days in an immunogenic form (Romani *et al.*, 1989; Puré *et al.*, 1990). Splenic DC efficiently generated and presented immunogenic fragments of intact hen egg lysozyme (HEL) to an I-A^k-restricted T cell hybridoma-specific HEL. When splenic DC and LPS blasts were used as APC in presentation assays, DC required 100-fold less HEL to induce the same level of T cell proliferation as with LPS blasts (DeBruijn *et al.*, 1992). LC process and present phagocytic ligands to antigen-specific T cells, e.g., *Leishmania major* (Moll *et al.*, 1995). Mouse bone marrow-derived GM-CSF-cultured dendritic cells phagocytose particulate antigen and can process and present Bacillus Calmette-Guerin (BCG) to antigen-specific T cells (Inaba *et al.*, 1993). In addition to phagocytosing a variety of particles and pathogens, DC phagocytose apoptotic cells. Human PBMC internalize flu-infected apoptotic macrophages and present derived antigens via both the class I and class II pathways (Albert *et al.*, 1998).

DEVELOPMENT REGULATION

Recent studies have confirmed a concept inferred from earlier studies, namely, that endocytosis is a developmentally regulated process in dendritic cells. Immature dendritic cells constitutively macropinocytose, endocytose, and phagocytose. In response to stress and 'danger', in the form of explantation, pathogen, and inflammatory stimuli (Matzinger 1994), DC mature and undergo striking morphological and functional changes (Banchereau and Steinman, 1998). One functional alteration is the downregulation of endocytosis. A shutdown of endocytosis is consistent with DC changing their metier from antigen sentinels to T cell primers. A sentinel DC with its high endocytic capacity and with an additional T cell stimulatory capacity trafficking through or located in a lymph node might result in autoimmunity. Studies examining the internalization and presentation of myoglobin in fresh versus cultured LC and splenic DC demonstrated that processing and presentation of exogenous protein was lost during culture, suggesting that endocytosis was developmentally regulated (Romani *et al.*, 1989). Particulate uptake and presentation studies in mouse bone marrow DC clearly indicated that progenitor/early DC pulsed and chased with BCG were much more efficient in presentation assays compared to pulsed and chased mature DC (Inaba *et al.*, 1993). Studies of DC in the peripheral hepatic lymph established that DC go through a transitory phagocytic stage and that they downregulate their phagocytic activity when they enter their migratory stage (Matsuno *et al.*, 1996). Investigations of CD34$^+$-derived LC-lineage DC and CD14$^+$-lineage DC suggested that LC endocytic activity is temporally restricted to an early stage of their development, 'day 6', while CD14$^+$ lineage DC vigorously endocytose for a longer duration, 'days 8–13'.

Maturational stimuli downregulate macropinocytosis and receptor-mediated endocytosis. Treatment of PBMC-derived dendritic cells with TNF-α, CD40L, IL-1β, and LPS, inflammatory stimuli, resulted in a marked reduction of endocytosis (Sallusto *et al.*, 1995). Ceramide has emerged as a down stream effector and intracellular signal common to pathways mediated by the above inflammatory stimuli (Sallusto *et al.*, 1996). Ceramide inhibited the uptake of F-DX and LY in PBMC-derived DC (Sallusto *et al.*, 1996). Treatment with TNF-α, IL-1β, and CD40L decreased endocytosis and increased intracellular levels of ceramide. However, ceramide did not upregulate cII and costimulatory molecules. This finding is inconsistent with the observation that upregulation of cell surface cII molecules in mature DC results at least in part from a shutdown of endocytic recycling (Cella *et al.*, 1997). Thus ceramide cannot be the only intracellular signaling molecule responsible for downregulating endocytosis.

Using the mouse bone marrow DC culturing system, we have obtained data suggesting that there is precipitous, stage-specific control of endocytic activity. Preliminary results suggest that the endocytic activity of mature cells remains intact and that cdc42 is involved at an endocytosis control point.

SPECIALIZATIONS OF THE DC ENDOCYTIC PATHWAY

Antigen-processing compartments have been a subject of intensive research and much debate in recent years (Pierre and Mellman, 1998; Amigorena *et al.*, 1994; Qiu *et al.*, 1994; Tulp *et al.*, 1994; West *et al.*, 1994; Peters *et al.*, 1991; Neefjes *et al.*, 1990; Harding, 1990). The discovery of novel endocytic compartments enriched in cII molecules proved a major conceptual advance in the cell biological basis of antigen processing (Mellman *et al.*, 1996). Examinations of class II compartments in DC have been carried out at the level of fluorescence (Sallusto and Lanzavecchia, 1994) and immunoelectron microscopy (Nijman *et al.*, 1995). Two recent studies have examined the organization of class II pathways during the *in vitro* development of DC (Cella *et al.*, 1997; Pierre *et al.*, 1997). These studies provided insight into how the antigen-processing machinery of DC is a dynamic device reconfiguring itself in response to environmental stimuli (Watts, 1997).

In the human PBMC GM-CSF IL-4 DC system, cII molecules in immature DC are rapidly internalized and recycled ($t_{1/2} = 10$ h), however, cII molecules in DC exposed to maturational factors have a cII $t_{1/2}$ (> 100 h) and increase their synthesis of cII (Cella *et al.*, 1997). As the DC mature, the cII half-life appears to increase as a result of a general shutdown of the recycling of cII. Previous studies have observed a downregulation in DC endocytosis in response to inflammatory stimuli (Sallusto *et al.*, 1995). The increased cII synthesis and $t_{1/2}$ result in a large pool of long-lived peptide-loaded cII molecules on the cell surface awaiting recognition by the appropriate T cell.

In the mouse BM GM-CSF DC system, three distinct developmental stages differentiated by their cII compartmentalization were identified (Pierre *et al.*, 1997). cII in immature DC accumulates in lysosomes instead of trafficking to the cell surface. As maturation progresses, cII redistributes to peripherally located vesicles that resemble CIIV (reviewed in Pierre and Mellman, 1998; described in Amigorena *et al.*, 1994). Finally, in fully mature DC, peptide loaded cII traffics to the cell surface ready to stimulate relevant T cells. In addition to endocytic structures specialized for the loading of cII molecules with immunogenic peptides, other unique endocytic structures exist in Langerhans cells.

There has been a long-standing interest in the function of LCG, or Birbeck granules. Their origin and purpose remain elusive. The two most commonly debated origins are secretory and endocytic. In the secretory model, the granules bud from the Golgi stacks and fuse with the plasma membrane, exocytosing their putative contents; while in the endocytic model, the granules invaginate from the plasma membrane, bringing antigens and/or nutrients into the cell (Bucana *et al.*, 1992; Bartosik, 1992; Hashimoto and Tarnowski, 1968). The evidence supporting an endocytic function for LCG has at times seemed contradictory. While some groups found that HRP did not accumulate in LC (Wolff and Schreiner, 1970) others demonstrated the accumulation of HRP in LCG (Bartosik, 1992). LCG appeared to concentrate lectins and lectin conjugates, such as conalbumin and ferritin-conjugated conalbumin, but did not accumulate ferritin (Takigawa *et al.*, 1985). Ferritin immune complexes were also internalized and accessed LCG (Takigawa *et al.*, 1985). Using immunogold histochemistry and electron microscopy, the trafficking of CD1 and HLA-DR antibodies was followed in the endocytic pathway of LC. At successive time points, the antibodies localized to coated vesicles, Birbeck granules, endosomes, and lysosomes, providing evidence that LCG are part of the endocytic pathway (Hanau *et al.*, 1987). Although LCG do not appear to be essential for the normal function of human LC (Mommaas *et al.*, 1994), many have speculated that LCG play a role in antigen sequestration, accounting for the ability of LC to retain antigen in an immunogenic form for several days.

CONCLUSIONS

Over the past twenty five years, numerous studies have contributed to an emerging understanding of endocytosis in dendritic cells. While initial studies suggested that dendritic cells were weakly endocytic, the development of bulk culturing methods has helped to establish that early/immature dendritic cells are endocytically active and that endocytosis is developmentally downregulated in dendritic cells. Bulk culturing methods have facilitated careful studies of dendritic cell developmental and cell biology in recent years. Endocytic internalization and recycling assays and subcellular fractionation have been instrumental in elucidating the nature of the endocytic specializations that make DC the preeminent APC of the immune system. Many questions remain regarding the characteristics of the novel endocytic organelles present in DC. In addition, the nature of the signals involved in the downregulation of endocytosis and in the developmental remodeling of its cII trafficking pathway are an active area of inquiry.

REFERENCES

Albert, M.L., Sauter, B. and Bhardwaj, N. (1998). Dendritic cells acquire antigen from apoptotic cells and induce class I-restricted CTLs. *Nature* **392**(6671), 86–89.

Amigorena, S., Drake, J., Webster, P. and Mellman, I. (1994). Transient accumulation of new class II MHC molecules in a novel endocytic compartment in B lymphocytes. *Nature* **369**, 113–120.

Austyn, J.M. (1996). New insights into the mobilization and phagocytic activity of dendritic cells. *J. Exp. Med.* **183**, 1287–1292.

Austyn, J.M., Hankins, D.F., Larsen, C.P., Morris, P.J., Rao, A.S. and Roake, J.A. (1994). Isolation and characterization of dendritic cells from mouse heart and kidney. *J. Immunol.* **152**, 2401–2410.

Banchereau, J., and Steinman, R.M. (1998). Dendritic cells and the control of immunity. *Nature* **392**(6673), 245–252.

Bartosik, J. (1992). Cytomembrane-derived Birbeck granules transport horsedash peroxidase to the endosomal compartment in the human Langerhans cells. *J. Invest. Dermatol.* **99**, 53–58.

Berlin, R.D. and Oliver, J.M. (1980). Surface functions during endocytosis II. Quantification of pinocytosis and kinetic characterization of mitotic cycle with a new fluorescence technique. *J. Cell Biol.* **85**, 660–671.

Bieber, T., de la Salle, H., de la Salle, C., Hanau, D. and Wollenberg, A. (1992). Expression of high-affinity receptor for IgE (Fc epsilon R1) on human Langerhans cells: the end of a dogma. *J. Invest. Dermatol.* **99**, 105–115.

Brown, E. (1995). Phagocytosis. *Bioessays* **17**(2), 109–117.

Brossart, P. and Bevan, M. (1997). Presentation of exogenous protein antigens on major histocompatability complex class I molecules by dendritic cells: pathway of presentation and regulation of cytokine. *Blood* **90**, 1594–1599.

Bucana, C.D., Munn, C.G., Song, M.J., Dunner, K. and Kripke, M.L. (1992). Internalization of Ia molecules into Birbeck granule-like structures in murine dendritic cell. *J. Invest. Dermatol.* **99**(4), 365–373.

Burke, K. and Gigli, I. (1980). Receptors for complement on Langerhans cells. *J. Invest. Dermatol.* **75**, 46–51.

Carbone, B.F. and Bevan, M. (1990). Class I-restricted processing and presentation of exogeneous cell-associated antigen in vivo. *J. Exp. Med.* **171**(2), 377–387.

Caux, C., Massacrier, C., Vanbervliet, B., Dubois, Durand, Cella, M., Lanzavecchia, A., and Banchereau, J. (1997). $CD34^+$ hempatopoietic progenitors from human cord blood differentiate along two independent dendritic cell pathways in response to GM-CSF plus TNFα: II. Fcn analysis. *Blood* **90**, 1458–1470.

Cella, M., Engering, A., Pinet, V., Pieter, J. and Lanzavecchia, A. (1997). Inflammatory stimuli induce the accumulation of MHC class II complexes on dendritic cells. *Nature* **388**, 782–786.

Cella, M., Sallusto, F. and Lanzavecchia, A. (1997). Origin, maturation, and antigen presenting function of dendritic cells. *Curr. Opin. Immunol.* **9**, 10–16.

Chain, B.M., Kay, P.M., and Feldman, M. (1986). The cellular pathway of antigen presentation: biochemical and functional analysis of antigen processing in dendritic cells and macrophages. *Immunology* **58**, 271–276.

Chen, L.M., Hobbes, S. and Galan, J.E. (1996). Requirement of CDC42 for *Salmonella*-induced cytoskeletal and responses. *Science* **274**(5295), 2115–2118.

Cox, D., Chang, P., Zhang, Q., Reddy, P.G., Bokoch, G.M., and Greenberg, S. (1997). Requirements for both Rac1 and Cdc42 in membrane ruffling and phagocytosis in leukocytes. *J. Exp. Med.* **186**(9), 1487–1494.

De Bruijn, M.L.H., Nieland, J.D., Harding, C.V., and Melief, C.J. (1992). Processing and presentation of intact hen egg-white lysozyme by dendritic cells. *Eur. J. Immunol.* **22**, 2347–2352.

Duijvestijn, A.M., Kohler, Y.G., and Hoefsmit, E.C.M. (1982). Interdigitating cells and macrophages in the acute involuting rat thymus. *Cell Tissue Res.* **224**, 291-301.

Engering, A.J., Cella, M., Fluitsma, D.M., Hoejsmit, E.C., Lanzavecchia, A. and Pieter, J. (1997). The mannose receptor functions as a high capacity and broad specificity antigen receptor in human dendritic cells. *Eur. J. Immunol.* **27**, 2417–2425.

Esposito-Farese, M.E., Sautes, de la Salle, Latour, Bieber, de La Salle, Ohlmann, Fridman, Cazenave, Teilaud, Daeron, Bonnerot and Hanau. (1995). Membrane and soluble FcγRII/III modulate the antigen presenting capacity of murine dendritic epidermal Langerhans cells for IgG-complexed antigens. *J. Immunol.* **154**, 1725–1735.

Ezekowitz, R.A.B. and Hoffmann, J.A. (1996). Innate immunity *Curr. Opin. Immunol.* **8**(1), 1–2.

Filgueira, L., Nestle, F., Rittig, M., Joller, H. and Groscurth, F. (1996). Human dendritic cells phagocytose and process *Borrelia burgdoferi*. *J. Immunol.* **158**, 2998–3005.

Fossum, S. and Rolstad, B., (1986). The role of interdigitating cells and NK cells in the rapid rejection of allogeneic lymphocytes. *Eur. J. Immunol.* **15**, 440–449.

Fossum, S., Rolstad, B. and Ford, W.L. (1984). Thymus independence, kinetics, and phagocytic ability of interdigitating cells. *Immunobiology* **168**, 403–413.

Fukasawa, M., Adachi, H., Hirota, K., Tsujimoto, M., Arai, H. and Inoue, K. (1996). SRB1, a class B scavenger receptor, recognizes both negatively charged liposomes and apoptotic cells. *Exp. Cell Res.* **221**, 246–250.

Girolomoni, F., Lutz, M.B., Pastore, S.S., Abmann, C.U., Cavani A. and Ricciardi-Castagnoli, R. (1995). Establishment of a cell line with features of early dendritic cell precursors from fetal mouse skin. *Eur. J. Immunol.* **25** , 2163.

Greenberg, S., Chang, P. and Silverstein, S.C. (1994). Tyrosine phosphorylation of the gamma subunit of Fc gamma receptors, p72syk, and paxillin during Fc receptor-mediated phagocytosis in macrophages. *J. Biol. Chem.* **269**(5), 3897–3902.

Hall, S.G. and Robertson, D. (1984). Phagocytosis, in vivo, of immune complexes by dendritic cells in the lymph of sheep. *Int. Arch. Allergy Appl. Immunol.* **73**, 155–161.

Hanau, D., Fabre, M., Schmitt, D.A., Garaud, J., Pauly, G., Tongio, M., Mayer S. and Cazanave, J. (1987). Human epidermal Langerhans cells cointernalize by receptor mediated endocytosis 'nonclassical' major histocompatibility complex class I molecules (T6 antigens) and class II molecules (HLA-DR antigens) *Proc. Natl Acad. Sci. USA* **84**, 2901–2905.

Harding, C.V., Unanue, E.R., Slot, J.W., Schwartz, A.L. and Geuze, H.J. (1991). Functional and ultrastructural evidence for intracellular formation of major histocompatibility complex classII–peptide complexes during antigen processing. *Proc. Natl Acad. Sci, USA* **87**, 5553–5357.

Hardt, W., Chen, L., Schuebel, K., Bustelo, X., and Galán, J. (1998). *S. typhimurium* encodes an activator of rho GTPases that induces membrane ruffling and nuclear responses in host cells. *Cell* **93**, 815–826.

Hart, D. and Fabre, J. (1981). Demonstration and characterization of Ia-positive dendritic cells in the interstitial connective tissues of rat hearts and other tissues but not in brain. *J. Exp. Med.* **153**, 347.

Hashimoto, K. and Tarnowski, W.M. (1968). Some new aspects of the Langerhans cell. *Arch. Dermatol.* **97**, 450–464.

Hewlett, L.J., Prescott, A.R., and Watts, C. (1994). The coated pit and macropinocytic pathways serve distinct endosome populations. *J. Cell Biol.* **124**, 689–703.

Inaba, K., Inaba, M., Naito, M. and Steinman, R.M. (1993). Dendritic cell progenitors phagocytose particulates, including Bacillus Calmette-Guerin organisms, and sensitize mice to mycobacterial antigens in vivo. *J. Exp. Med.* **178**, 479–488.

Jiang, W., Swiggard, Heufler, Peng, Mirza, Steinman, and Nussensweig (1995). The receptor DEC-205 expressed by dendritic cells and thymic epithelial cells is involved in antigen processing. *Nature* **375**, 151–154.

Levine, T.P. and Chain, B.H. (1992). Endocytosis by antigen presenting cells: dendritic cells are as endocytically active as other antigen presenting cells. *Proc. Natl Acad. Sci. USA* **89**, 8342–8346.

Lutz, M.N., Rovere, P., Kleijmeer, M., Recigno, M., Abmann, C.U., Oorschot, V.M.J., Geuze, H.J., Trucy, J., Demandolx, D., Davoust, J. and Ricciardi-Castagnoli, P. (1997). Intracellular routes and selective retention of antigens in mildly acidic cathepsin D/lysosome-associated membrane protein-1/MHC class II-positive vesicles in immature dendritic cells. *J. Immunol.* **159**, 3707–3716.

Matsuno, K., Ezaki, T. Kudo, S. and Uehara (1996). A life stage of particle-laden rat dendritic cells in vivo: their terminal division, active phagocytosis, and translocation from the liver to hepatic lymph. *J. Exp. Med.* **183**, 1865–1878.

Matzinger, P. (1994). Tolerance, danger, and the extended family. *Annu. Rev. Immunol.* **12**, 991–1045.

Maurer, D., Fiebiger, S., Ebner, C., Reininger, B., Fischer, G.F., Wichlas, S., Jouvin, M.H., Schmitt-Egenolf, M., Kraft, D., Kinet, J.P. and Stingl, G. (1996). Peripheral blood dendritic cells express Fc epsilon RI as a complex composed of Fc epsilon RI alpha- and Fc epsilon RI gamma-chains and can use this receptor for IgE-mediated allergen presentation. *J. Immunol.* **157**(2), 607–616.

Melikyan, G., White, J., and Cohen, F. (1995). GPI-anchored influenza hemagglutinin induces hemifusion to both red blood cell and planar bilayer membranes. *J. Cell Biol.* **131**, 679–691.

Mellman, I. (1996). Endocytosis and molecular sorting. *Annu. Rev. Cell Dev. Biol.* **12**, 575–625.

Mellman, I., Fuchs, R. and Helenius, A. (1986). Acidification of the endocytic and exocytic pathways. *Annu. Rev. Biochem.* **55**, 663–700.

Mellman, I., Pierre, P. and Amigorena, S. (1996). Lonely MHC molecules seeking immunogenic peptides for meaningful relationships. *Curr. Biol.* **7**, 564–572.

Moll, H. Flohe, S. and Rollinghoff (1995). Dendritic cells in *Leishmania major*-immune mice harbor persistent parasites and mediate an antigen-specific T cell immune response. *Eur. J . Immunol.* **25**, 693–699.

Mommaas, M., Mulder, A., Vermeer, B.J. and Koning, F. (1994). Functional human epidermal Langerhans cells that lack Birbeck granules. *J. Invest. Dermatol.* **103**, 807–810.

Neefjes, J.J., Stollorz, V., Peters, P.J., Geuze, H.J. and Ploegh, H.L. (1990). The biosynthetic pathway of MHC class II but not class I molecules intersects the endocytic route. *Cell* **61**, 171–183.

Nijman, H.W., Kleijmeer, M., Ossevoort, M., Oorschot, V., Vierboo, M., van der Keur, M., Kenemans, P., Kast, W., Geuze, H.J. and Melief, S.J. (1995). Antigen capture and major histocompatibility class II compartments of freshly isolated and cultured human blood dendritic cells. *J. Exp. Med.* **182**, 163–174.

Nordquist, R.E., Olson, R.L. and Everett, M.A. (1966). The transport, uptake, and storage of ferritin in human epidermis. *Arch. Dermatol.* **94**, 482–490.

Parr, M.B., Kepple, L. and Parr, E.L. (1991). Langerhans cells phagocytose vaginal epithelial cells undergoing apoptosis during the murine estrous cycle. *Biol. Reprod.* **45**, 252–260.

Pearson, A., Lux and Kieger (1995). Expression cloning of dSR-c1, a class C macrophage-specific scavenger receptor from *Drosophila melangaster. Proc. Natl Acad. Sci. USA* **92**, 4056–4060.

Peters, P.J., Neefjes, J.J., Oorschot, V., Ploegh, H.L. and Geuze, H.J. (1991). Segregation of MHC class II molecules from MHC class I molecules in the Golgi complex for transport to lysosomal compartments. *Nature* **349**, 669–676.

Pierre, P. and Mellman, I. (1998). Exploring the mechanisms of antigen processing by cell fractionation. *Curr. Opin. Immunol.* **10**, 145–153.

Pierre, P., Turley, S., Gatti, E., Hull, M., Meltzer, J., Mirza, A., Inaba, K., Steinman, R.M. and Mellman, I. (1997). Developmental regulation of MHC class II transport in mouse dendritic cells. *Nature* **388**, 787–792.

Platt, N., Suzuki, H., Kurihara, T., Kodama, T. and Gordon, S. (1996). Role for the class A macrophage scavenger receptor in the phagocytosis of apoptotic thymocytes in vitro. *Proc. Natl Acad. Sci. USA* **93**, 12456–12490.

Pontow, S.E., Kery, V. and Stahl, P.D. (1992). Mannose receptor. *Int. Rev. Cytol.* **137b**, 221–244.

Puré, E., Inaba, K., Crowley, M., Tardelli, L., Witmer-Pack, M.D., Ruberti, G., Fathman, G. and Steinman, R.M. (1990). Antigen processing by epidermal Langerhans cells correlates with the level of biosynthesis of major histocompatibility complex class II molecules and expression of invariant chain. *J. Exp. Med.* **172**, 1459–1469.

Qiu, Y., Xu, X., Wandinger-Ness, A., Dalke, D.P. and Pierce, S.K. (1994). Separation of subcellular compartments containing distinct functional forms of MHC class II. *J. Cell Biol.* **125**, 595–605.

Racoosin, E.L. and Swanson, J.A. (1993). Macropinosome maturation and fusion with tubular lysosomes in macrophages. *J. Cell Biol.* **121**, 1011–1020.

Reis e Sousa, C., Stahl, P.D. and Austyn, J.M. (1993). Phagocytosis of antigens by Langerhans cells in vitro. *J. Exp. Med.* **178**, 509–519.

Rigotti, A., Trigutti, B., Babitt, J., Penman, M., Xu, S. and Krieger, M. (1997). Scavenger receptor B1 – a cell surface receptor for high density lipoprotein. *Curr. Opin. Lipidol.* **8**, 181–188.

Robinson, M.S., Watts, C. and Zerial, M. (1996). Membrane dynamics in endocytosis. *Cell* **84**, 13–21.

Robinson, M.S. (1994). The role of clathrin, adaptors, and dynamin in endocytosis. *Curr. Opin. Cell Biol.* **6**, 538–544.

Romani, N., Koide, S., Crowley, M., Witmer-Pack, M., Livingstone, A.M., Fathman, C.G., Inaba, K. and Steinman, R.M. (1989). Presentation of exogenous protein antigens by dendritic cells to T cell clones. *J. Exp. Med.* **169**, 1169–1178.

Sagbeil, R.W. (1972). *In vivo* and *in vitro* uptake of ferritin by Langerhans cells in the epidermis. *J. Invest. Dermatol.* **58**, 47–54.

Sallusto, F. and Lanzavecchia, A. (1994). Efficient presentation of soluble antigen by cultured human dendritic cells in maintained by GM-CSF plus IL-4 and downregulated by TNFα. *J. Exp. Med.* **179**, 1109–1118.

Sallusto, F., Cella, M., Danieli and Lanzavecchia, A. (1995). Dendritic cells use macropinocytosis and the mannose receptor to concentrate macromolecules in the major histocompatibility complex class II compartment: downregulation by cytokines and bacterial products. *J. Exp. Med.* **182**, 389–400.

Sallusto, F., Nicolo, De Marai, Corinti and Testi (1996). Ceramide inhibits antigen uptake and presentation by dendritic cells. *J. Exp. Med.* **184**(6), 2411–2416.

Scheicher, C., Mehlig, M., Dienes, H. and Reske, K. (1995). Uptake of microparticle-adsorbed dendritic cells results in up-regulation of interleukin-1a and interleukin-12 p40/p35 and triggers prolonged, efficient antigen presentation. *Eur. J. Immunol.* **25**, 1566–1572.

Schmid, S.L. (1997). Clathrin-coated vesicle formation and protein sorting: an integrated process. *Annu. Rev. Biochem.* **66**, 511–548.

Schmitt, D.A., Bieber, T., Cazenave, J.P. and Hanau, D. (1990). Fc receptors of human Langerhans cells. *J. Invest. Dermatol.* **94**, 155–215.

Schuler, G. and Steinman, R.M. (1985). Murine epidermal Langerhans cells mature into potent immunostimulatory dendritic cells in vitro. *J. Exp. Med.* **161**, 526–546.

Silverstein, S.C., Steinman, R.M. and Lohn, Z.A. (1977). Endocytosis. *Annu. Rev. Biochem.* **46**, 669–722.

Stahl, P.D., Rodman, J.S., Miller, M.J. and Schlesinger, P.H. (1978). Evidence for receptor mediated binding of glycoprotein, glycoconjugates, and lysosomal glycosidases by alveolar macrophages. *Proc. Natl Acad. Sci USA* **75**, 1399-1403.

Steinman, R.M. and Swanson, J. (1995). The endocytic activity of dendritic cells. *J. Exp. Med.* **182**, 283–288.

Steinman, R.M. and Cohn, Z.A. (1974). Identification of a novel cell type in peripheral lymphoid organs of mice II. Functional properties in vitro. *J. Exp. Med.* **139**(2), 380–397.

Steinman, R.M., Lustig, D.S. and Cohn, Z.A. (1974a). Identification of a novel cell type in peripheral lymphoid organs of mice 3. Functional properties in vivo. *J. Exp. Med.* **139**(6), 1431–1445.

Steinman, R.M., Silver, J.M. and Cohn, Z.A. (1974b). Pinocytosis in fibroblasts. Quantitative studies in vitro. *J. Cell Biol.* **63**(3), 949–969.

Steinman, R., Witmer, M.D., Nussenzweig, M.C., Chen, L.I., Schlesinger, S. and Cohn, Z.A. (1980). Dendritic cells of the mouse: identification and characterization. *J. Invest. Dermatol.* **75**, 14–16.

Stingl, G. and Maurer, D. (1977). IgE-mediated allergen presentation via Fc epsilon R1 on antigen-presenting cells. *Int. Arch. Allergy Immunol.* **113**, 24–29.

Stingl, G., Wolff-Schreiner, E.C., Pichler, W.J., Gschnait, F., Knapp, W. and Wolff, K. (1977). Epidermal Langerhans cells bear Fc and C3 receptors. *Nature* **268**, 245–246.

Straus, W. (1964). Cytochemical observations on the relationship between lyosomes and phagosomes in kidney and liver by combined staining for acid phosphatase and intravenously injected HRP. *J. Cell Biol.* **20**.

Swanson, J.A. (1989). Endocytic Compartment Fluorescent Labeling. In: *Fluorescence Microscopy of Living Cells in Culture. Part A. Methods in Cell Biology*, Vol. 29 (eds. Y.L. Wang and D. Taylor). Academic Press, London.

Swanson, J.A. and Watts, C. (1995). Macropinocytosis. *Trends Cell Biol.* **5**, 424–428.

Swanson, J.A., Yirinec, B.D. and Silverstein, S.C. (1985). Phorbol esters and horseradish peroxidase stimulate pinocytosis and redirect the flow of pinocytosed fluid in macrophages. *J. Cell Biol.* **100**, 851–859.

Takigawa, M., Iwatsuki, K., Yamada, M., Okamoto, H. and Imamura, S. (1985). The Langerhans cell granule is an adsorptive endocytic organelle. *J. Invest. Dermatol.* **85**, 12-15.

Tulp, A., Verwoerd, D., Dobbertein, B., Ploegh, H.L., and Pieters, J. (1994). Isolation and characterization of the intracellular MHC class II compartment. *Nature* **368**, 120–126.

Vida, T.A. and Emr, S.D. (1995). A new vital stain for visualizing membrane dynamics and endocytosis in yeast. *J. Cell Biol.* **128**(5), 779–792.

Wang, B., Rieger, A., Kilgus, O., Ochai, K., Maurer, D., Fodenger, D., Kinet, J.P. and Stingl, G. (1992). Epidermal Langerhans cells from normal human skin bind monomeric IgE via Fc epsilon R1. *J. Exp. Med.* **175**, 1353–1365.

Watts, C. (1997). Inside the gearbox of the dendritic cell. *Nature* **388**, 724–725.

West, M.A., Lucocq, J.M. and Watts, C. (1994). Antigen processing and class II MHC peptide-loading compartments in human B-lymphoblastoid cell. *Nature* **369**, 147–151.

Wolff, K. and Schreiner, E. (1970). Uptake, intracellular transport and degradation of exogenous protein by Langerhans cells. An electron microscopic-cytochemical study using peroxidase as tracer substance. *J. Invest. Dermatol.* **54**(1), 37–47.

Ziv, N.E. and Smith, S.J. (1996). Evidence for a role of dendritic filopodia in synaptogenesis and spine formation. *Neuron* **17**(1), 91-102.

Index

63 def. 75! 80! 93! 100 (phag)

67 VEILED C! 104!
PL. 7-2 284 325 296

STELLATE C. (PHOTO) 17 327
69 403

FIG. p69 DEF. 63

(72)

See yellow sheet

MICROENVIRONM. 112

DENDRIPHAGES 467

691! Appt

417

(R) 293 (Cal) 418 (4)

419 (2)

336 Marshall (Ag)

690

510, 509, 506

PHOTOS: 410! 411! L